Complications
in
Anesthesiology

J. B. LIPPINCOTT COMPANY
PHILADELPHIA • TORONTO

Complications in Anesthesiology

EDITED BY

Fredrick K. Orkin, M.D., M.B.A.

Associate Professor of Anesthesiology
Hahnemann Medical College and Hospital
Philadelphia, Pennsylvania

AND

Lee H. Cooperman, M.D.

Professor of Anesthesia
University of Pennsylvania School of Medicine
Philadelphia, Pennsylvania

With 60 Contributors

Sponsoring Editor: Richard Winters
Manuscript Editor: Helen Ewan
Indexer: Deana Fowler
Production Supervisor: N. Carol Kerr
Production Assistant: J. Corey Gray
Compositor: Black Dot Computer Typesetting Corp.
Printer/Binder: Halliday Lithographic

1 3 5 6 4 2

Library of Congress Cataloging in Publication Data
Main entry under title:

Complications in anesthesiology.

Includes index.
   1. Anesthesia—Complications and sequelae.
I. Orkin, Fredrick K. II. Cooperman, Lee H.
[DNLM: 1. Postoperative complications.
2. Anesthesia—Adverse effects. WO 245 C737]
RD82.5.C64   617′.96   82-15242
ISBN 0-397-50409-8

The authors and publisher have exerted every effort to ensure that drug
selection and dosage set forth in this text are in accord with current
recommendations and practice at the time of publication. However, in
view of ongoing research, changes in government regulations, and the
constant flow of information relating to drug therapy and drug reactions,
the reader is urged to check the package insert for each drug for any
change in indications and dosage and for added warnings and
precautions. This is particularly important when the recommended
agent is a new or infrequently employed drug.

Contents

Part Nine

The Blood

Part Ten

Obstetrics, Gynecology, and Neonatology

Part Eleven

Special Techniques

Part Twelve

Iatrogenesis

Part Thirteen

Hazards to the Anesthesiologist

Contributors

Jeffrey M. Baden, M.D.
Associate Professor of Anesthesia
Stanford University School of Medicine
Stanford, California
Staff Anesthesiologist
Veterans Administration Medical Center
Palo Alto, California

Lawrence S. Berman, M.D.
Assistant Professor of Anesthesiology and Pediatrics
University of Florida College of Medicine
Gainesville, Florida

Richard L. Bitner, M.D.
Anesthesiologist
Community General Hospital
Reading, Pennsylvania

Burton A. Briggs, M.D.
Assistant Professor of Anesthesia and Surgery
Loma Linda University School of Medicine
Director of Surgical Intensive Care
Loma Linda University Medical Center
Loma Linda, California

Beverley A. Britt, M.D.
Associate Professor of Anaesthesia
Associate Professor of Pharmacology
University of Toronto
Senior Staff Anaesthetist
Toronto General Hospital
Toronto, Ontario

Burnell R. Brown, Jr., M.D., Ph.D.
Professor and Head, Department of Anesthesiology
Professor of Pharmacology
Arizona Health Sciences Center
University of Arizona
Tucson, Arizona

David L. Bruce, M.D.
Professor of Anesthesiology
New York University School of Medicine
New York, New York

Marion A. Carnes, M.D.
Professor of Anesthesiology
School of Medicine
University of California, Davis
Davis, California

Lee H. Cooperman, M.D.
Professor of Anesthesia
University of Pennsylvania School of Medicine
Philadelphia, Pennsylvania

David J. Cullen, M.D.
Associate Professor of Anaesthesia
Harvard Medical School
Anesthetist
Massachusetts General Hospital
Boston, Massachusetts

J. Kenneth Denlinger, M.D.
Anesthesiologist
Lancaster General Hospital
Lancaster, Pennsylvania

Jay S. DeVore, M.D.
Assistant Professor of Clinical Anesthesia
University of Wisconsin School of Medicine
Madison, Wisconsin
Chairman, Department of Anesthesiology
Mercy Hospital
Janesville, Wisconsin

Jules L. Dienstag, M.D.
Associate Professor of Medicine
Massachusetts General Hospital
Harvard Medical School
Boston, Massachusetts

Hillary Don, M.D. F.R.C.P.(C)
Associate Professor of Anesthesia
University of California, San Francisco
Director, Intensive Care Unit
Moffitt Hospital
San Francisco, California

James R. Dooley, M.D.
Attending Anesthesiologist
St. Vincent's Hospital and Medical Center
New York, New York

Christopher W. Dueker, M.D.
Clinical Assistant Professor of Anesthesia
Stanford University School of Medicine
Stanford, California
Anesthesiologist
Palo Alto Medical Clinic
Palo Alto, California

McIver W. Edwards, Jr., M.D.
Associate Professor of Anesthesiology
University of Pennsylvania School of Medicine
Chief of Anesthesia
The Veterans Administration Hospital
Philadelphia, Pennsylvania

Lorne G. Eltherington, M.D., Ph.D.
Associate Professor of Anesthesia
Director, Stanford Pain Service
Stanford University Medical Center
Stanford, California

B. Raymond Fink, M.D., F.F.A.R.C.S.
Professor of Anesthesiology
University of Washington School of Medicine
Seattle, Washington

Joan W. Flacke, M.D.
Professor of Anesthesia
School of Medicine
Center for Health Sciences
University of California, Los Angeles
Los Angeles, California

Werner E. Flacke, M.D.
Professor of Anesthesiology and Pharmacology
School of Medicine

Center for Health Services
University of California, Los Angeles
Los Angeles, California

David C. Flemming, M.B., F.F.A.R.C.S.
Director of Anesthesia
Freeport Memorial Hospital
Freeport, Illinois

Jeffrey G. Garber, D.M.D.
Assistant Professor of Anesthesia
University of Pennsylvania School of Medicine
Assistant Professor of Pharmacology and Dental Surgery
University of Pennsylvania School of Dental Medicine
Chairman, Department of Dental Medicine
The Graduate Hospital
Philadelphia, Pennsylvania

Dwight C. Geha, M.D.
Assistant Professor of Anesthesiology
Arizona Health Sciences Center
University of Arizona
Tucson, Arizona

John P. Gilbert, Ph.D.†
Staff Statistician
Office of Information Technology
Harvard University
Cambridge, Massachusetts
Associate in Biostatistics
Department of Anaesthesia
Massachusetts General Hospital
Boston, Massachusetts

James R. Harp M.D.
Professor and Chairman, Department of Anesthesiology
Temple University School of Medicine
Philadelphia, Pennsylvania

Lawrence K. Harris, M.D., F.R.C.P. (C)
Chief of Cardiology
Community General Hospital
Reading, Pennsylvania

†*Deceased*

Andrew Herlich, D.M.D.
Formerly Instructor of Anesthesia
University of Pennsylvania School of Medicine
Philadelphia, Pennsylvania

Robert E. Johnstone, M.D.
Director of Anesthesia
Southeast Alabama Medical Center
Dothan, Alabama
Clinical Associate Professor of Anesthesiology
University of Alabama School of Medicine
Birmingham, Alabama

Nancy Joy, A.O.C.A.
Professor and Chairman, Art as Applied to
Medicine
Faculty of Medicine
University of Toronto
Toronto, Ontario

Tamas Kallos, M.D.
Clinical Associate Professor of Anesthesiology
University of Miami School of Medicine
Anesthesiologist
South Miami Hospital
Miami, Florida

Leah E. Katz, C.R.N.A., Ed.D.
Adjunct Associate Professor of Anesthesiology
School of Medicine
Center for Health Sciences
University of California, Los Angeles
Los Angeles, California

Ronald L. Katz, M.D.
Professor and Chairman, Department of
Anesthesiology
School of Medicine
Center for Health Sciences
University of California, Los Angeles
Los Angeles, California

Arthur S. Keats, M.D.
Clinical Professor of Anesthesiology
University of Texas Medical School at Houston
Division of Cardiovascular Anesthesia
Texas Heart Institute
Houston, Texas

Jonathan M. Kelley, M.D.
Anesthesiologist
El Camino Hospital
Mountain View, California

Kenneth F. Lampe, Ph.D.
Division of Drugs
American Medical Association
Chicago, Illinois

John H. Lecky, M.D.
Associate Professor of Anesthesia
University of Pennsylvania School of Medicine
Philadelphia, Pennsylvania

Jerry D. Levitt, M.D.
Associate Professor of Anesthesiology
Hahnemann Medical College and Hospital
Philadelphia, Pennsylvania

David E. Longnecker, M.D.
Professor of Anesthesiology
University of Virginia School of Medicine
Charlottesville, Virginia

Margot B. Mackay, B.Sc. A.A.M.
Associate Professor of Art as Applied to Medicine
University of Toronto
Toronto, Ontario

Alix Mathieu, M.D.
Professor of Anesthesia
University of Cincinnati School of Medicine
Cincinnati, Ohio

Richard I. Mazze, M.D.
Professor of Anesthesia
Stanford University School of Medicine
Stanford, California
Chief, Anesthesiology Service
Veterans Administration Medical Center
Palo Alto, California

Bucknam McPeek, M.D.
Associate Professor of Anaesthesia
Harvard Medical School
Anesthetist
Massachusetts General Hospital
Boston, Massachusetts

John D. Michenfelder, M.D.
Professor of Anesthesiology
Mayo Clinic and Mayo Medical School
Rochester, Minnesota

Ronald D. Miller, M.D.
Professor of Anesthesia and Pharmacology
Department of Anesthesia
University of California, San Francisco
San Francisco, California

Emerson A. Moffitt, M.D.
Professor of Anaesthesia
Dalhousie University
Halifax, Nova Scotia

Sharon B. Murphy, M.D.
Associate Member, Division of
Hematology–Oncology
St. Jude Children's Research Hospital
Memphis, Tennessee

Terence M. Murphy, M.B., Ch.B., F.F.A.R.C.S.
Professor of Anesthesiology
Director, Clinical Pain Service
School of Medicine
University of Washington
Seattle, Washington

Gordon R. Neufeld, M.D.
Associate Professor of Anesthesia and
Bioengineering
University of Pennsylvania School of Medicine
Philadelphia, Pennsylvania

Fredrick K. Orkin, M.D., M.B.A.
Associate Professor of Anesthesiology
Hahnemann Medical College and Hospital
Philadelphia, Pennsylvania

Otto C. Phillips, M.D.†
Clinical Professor of Anesthesiology
University of Pittsburgh
Chairman, Division of Anesthesiology
The Western Pennsylvania Hospital
Pittsburgh, Pennsylvania

†*Deceased*

P. Prithvi Raj, M.D.
Professor of Anesthesia
Director, Pain Control Center
College of Medicine
University of Cincinnati
Cincinnati, Ohio

Russell C. Raphaely, M.D.
Associate Professor of Anesthesiology and
Pediatrics
University of Pennsylvania School of Medicine
Medical Director, Pediatric Intensive Care Unit
Children's Hospital of Philadelphia
Philadelphia, Pennsylvania

Henrietta Rosenberg, M.D.
Clinical Assistant Professor of Radiology and
Pediatrics
University of Pennsylvania School of Medicine
Senior Radiologist
Director, Subdivision of Ultrasound
Children's Hospital of Philadelphia
Philadelphia, Pennsylvania

Henry Rosenberg, M.D.
Professor and Chairman, Department of
Anesthesiology
Hahnemann Medical College and Hospital
Philadelphia, Pennsylvania

John F. Ryan, M.D.
Associate Professor of Anaesthesia
Harvard Medical School
Anesthetist
Director of Pediatric Anesthesia
Massachusetts General Hospital
Boston, Massachusetts

Bradley E. Smith, M.D.
Professor and Chairman, Department of Anesthesia
Vanderbilt University School of Medicine
Nashville, Tennessee

Eldon J. Swenson, M.D.
Anesthetist
St. Mary's Hospital
Milwaukee, Wisconsin

Leroy D. Vandam, Ph.B, M.D.
Anesthesiologist
Brigham and Womens Hospital
Hospital at Parker Hill, Boston
Professor of Anaesthesia, Emeritus
Harvard Medical School
Boston, Massachusetts

Robert S. Wharton, M.D.
Assistant Professor of Anesthesia
Stanford University School of Medicine
Stanford, California

Alon P. Winnie, M.D.
Professor and Head, Department of Anesthesiology
University of Illinois Medical Center
Chicago, Illinois

Harry Wollman, M.D.
Robert Dunning Dripps Professor
Chairman, Department of Anesthesia
Professor of Pharmacology
University of Pennsylvania School of Medicine
Philadelphia, Pennsylvania

Preface

Rarely are the services of the anesthesiologist an end in themselves. Rather, our principal effort is to enable another therapy, surgery, to be undertaken. This fact is so obvious that it is seldom even acknowledged, but because of it anesthesiology compels considerable attention. With an aging population and advances in surgical care and technology, we find ourselves treating increasingly sicker patients who are undergoing increasingly more complex procedures. It should not be forgotten that our anesthetic agents and adjuvants are among the most potent and rapidly acting drugs used in medicine. The anesthetics and technics that we have recourse to have the power to impair or abolish a variety of essential bodily functions, in addition to bearing potentially serious risks to the major organ systems. Thus, these medications and practices leave the patient open to the risk of anesthetic-related complications before the successful completion of surgery can be contemplated.

Complications noted after surgery and anesthesia may be categorized epidemiologically into those related to the surgical procedure, to the patient's medical condition, and to the anesthetic. Texts dealing with surgical complications abound. A number of excellent articles and books in the genre of medical management of the surgical patient have appeared in the past 5 years. Unfortunately, there has not been an equivalent comprehensive work covering anesthetic-related complications.

To fill this void, we, with acknowledged authorities, have put together a sourcebook of anesthetic-related complications that both the practitioner and academician should find helpful. Although it is often difficult to ascribe a given complication to anesthetic administration, as opposed to the surgical procedure, the patient's disease, or other factors, we have tried to include any topic that may be related to the anesthetic.

We have been fortunate to have enlisted the enthusiastic assistance of some five dozen colleagues from throughout North America who share our interest. Without their commitment, this book could not exist. Each has presented a specific complication or a set of related problems in his own way. Yet, each has written with three objectives in mind: to present a foundation of information accounting for the development of the complications; to provide the practicing anesthesiologist with guidance for the clinical management; and to set forth what is known about the prevention of the complications. Finally, each chapter includes an extensive reference list and suggestions for further reading.

In addition to our contributors, we are indebted to several persons whose efforts enabled publication of this volume: Lewis Reines, former Editor-in-Chief of Medical Books at J. B. Lippincott Company, launched this project; his successor, Stuart Freeman, spurred us to completion with unfailing vigor. Richard Winters, Lisa A. Biello, Kenneth Cotton, and Helen Ewan spared us much editorial detail. Joan Meranze, Librarian of the Dripps Memorial Library at the University of Pennsylvania, provided bibliographic assistance for a number of chapters. Drs. Harry Wollman and Henry Rosenberg provided advice. Lastly, we are grateful for the understanding and support of our families.

Novices in the practice of anesthesia encounter many complications. Experience enables them to recognize and treat complications and, later, to avoid them altogether. We hope that this sourcebook will aid all anesthesiologists in reaching the third and final stage sooner.

Fredrick K. Orkin, M.D.
Lee H. Cooperman, M.D.

Part One

General Considerations

1 Role of Anesthesia in Surgical Mortality

Arthur S. Keats, M.D.

On two previous occasions I wrote about mortality resulting from anesthesia from the perspective of "anesthetic risk."[1,2] To do this required not only a review of studies specifically directed to anesthetic and surgical mortality; collateral data sources were necessary to document the tenuous basis for risk estimates. The following conclusions were drawn:[2]

The poor predictability of anesthetic mortality should be expected, since a significant portion of this mortality is due to human error which cannot be predicted and to other factors which never have been quantified. To a small degree physical status and the operation contemplated provide some predictive basis. To a large degree, unknown factors related to the skill of the personnel and the environment of therapy contribute to anesthetic risk. Estimates of anesthetic risk for individual patients remain, therefore, almost entirely intuitive and one cannot deny an anesthetic to any patient who urgently requires operation.

Since 1969, little has happened to alter this general conclusion, which applied to risk, a concept whose essential element is ability to predict. In contrast, the subject of this chapter ignores predictability and asks instead, What do we in fact know about deaths caused by anesthesia? The data previously reviewed apply equally here; some new data are now available. Assuming that few patients who urgently require surgery are denied an anesthetic today (a reasonable assumption), to what degree can the role of anesthesia in surgical mortality be quantified?

EARLY STUDIES OF THE ROLE OF ANESTHESIA IN SURGICAL MORTALITY

Basic to the answer of the foregoing question is the definition of the term *anesthetic death*. Today this term is still largely undefined, except in guidelines put forth by individual reporters (or their select committees) who rendered opinions as to the role of anesthesia in a surgical death. Unfortunately, the bias of those who made these judgments tainted all published estimates of death rates from anesthesia and probably stifled alternate approaches to this same question.

When anesthesiology emerged from its status as a subspecialty of surgery, it maintained much of the format of training for general surgery, including the systematic review of all postoperative deaths, a practice that continues to the present in all anesthesia training programs. In conferences on morbidity and mortality, the relative roles of the patient's disease, errors in surgical management, and errors in anesthetic management in mortality were discussed and assigned. It is probably fair to say that in the earliest of these conferences surgeons tended to ascribe complications that were not clearly surgical or disease-related to the anesthetic. Anesthesiologists tended to be defensive and denying. It was not surprising, then, that the first systematic study of the death rate from anesthesia in the post-World War II era utilized the approach of the surgical death review to approximate the role of anesthesia in overall surgical mortality.

The study of death rate by Beecher and Todd is a landmark of clinical investigation: Ten institutions participated; the study was prospective, reflecting current anesthesia practice (records of surgical deaths were reviewed shortly after the event); the investigation was multidisciplinary (in each institution both surgeon and anesthesiologist examined all surgical death records); and it included large numbers of patients (almost 600,000 anesthetic administrations during 1948–1952).[3] Anesthesia deaths were not defined for the institutional committees that made the judgments. Instead, a series of examples was provided as a guide to the types of situations to be included. The data from this study, published in 1954, provided estimates of the incidence of primary anesthesia deaths and incidence of deaths in which anesthesia was secondary or contributory, based on a total of 384 "anesthesia deaths." Unfortunately, neither a description of the circumstances surrounding these deaths nor a tabulation by cause was ever made available. The investigators chose to interpret their data in terms of death rates for specific anesthetic agents and concluded that the death rate associated with the use of muscle relaxants was several times that of any other agent. Although they attributed this high death rate to the "inherent toxicity of curare," they classified 79 per cent of the "curare deaths" as caused by errors of anesthetic technique, choice, or management. Charges of bias in interpretation of the "curare deaths" and in data presentation promptly followed, as did a rebuttal.[4] The impact of these data on the clinical use of muscle relaxants was profound but was rapidly diminished over the next few years by the wide acceptance of succinylcholine. Compared to older muscle relaxants, the ability of succinylcholine to facilitate tracheal intubation was so dramatic and obvious that the stigma of "curare deaths" was ignored but not forgotten. No prospective study of anesthesia deaths of this magnitude has since been undertaken, although the same study design was employed subsequently in the National Halothane Study.

In response to the general unhappiness with the Beecher-Todd report, Dripps, Lamont, and Eckenhoff reviewed deaths of patients who received 33,000 administrations of anesthetics over a 10-year period in the investigators' own institution.[5] However, the study included only patients who received a spinal anesthetic or a general anesthetic, plus a muscle relaxant during the procedure. Regarding their own bias in reviewing death records, they wrote the following in 1961:

There is nothing to be gained in a mortality study by omitting a particular death merely to lower a statistical death rate. Avoiding responsibility or taking refuge in the fact that a patient was desperately ill prior to anesthesia and operation may improve one's mortality figures, but it will not advance general knowledge or change one's own practices. On the other hand, one should not resort to self-flagellation, assuming responsibility for a fatality merely because an anesthetic was administered and death occurred.

The last sentence above is a moderate expression of the bias then prevailing in the review of postoperative death records. It was thought that improvement in anesthesia practices would follow if anesthesiologists would substitute for denial a generous acceptance of responsibility for the unfavorable outcomes of surgical procedures. Dripps and colleagues also noted the most serious defect common to every study of anesthesia mortality: "We cannot provide individual protocols because of lack of space. This we realize is a serious omission, because it prevents others from gauging our material by their own standards."[2] Instead of individual protocols, they tabulated the contribution of anesthesia to surgical mortality under broad categories such as inadequate preoperative preparation, hypotension, inexperience in anesthetic management, and inadequate postoperative ventilation. In only 10 of their 80 patients in whom anesthesia definitely or probably contributed to death did they find "no anesthetic or surgical error in light of present knowledge." From records of the remaining 70 patients, they tallied 160 errors. With regard to the Beecher-Todd report, they concluded, "When deaths were related to the use of muscle relaxants, errors of omission or commission were always apparent. A plea is made for the preparation of detailed written death reports."

To some degree, written death reports had, in fact, been implemented as early as 1945 by Ruth with the establishment of a community-wide anesthesia study commission.[6] During the next two decades, many community- or state-wide commissions were established. These usually relied on voluntary submission of surgical death reports from a group of participating hospitals. Alternately, some commissions, such as the well known Baltimore Anesthesia Study Committee,[7] reviewed all death certificates filed with the Department of Health in order to collect all deaths within 36 hours of anesthetic administration. Detailed reports of these deaths were solicited from the hospitals and were reviewed by the Committee. A similar voluntary reporting system with committee review existed in Great Britain.[8] Study of anesthesia deaths by retrospective review of death records was of course the classical approach to the study of all disease. The expectation was that careful analysis of a large number of deaths would identify patterns or common denominators that would then clarify the role of anesthesia in surgical deaths and, as a consequence, improve anesthetic care. None of these studies could arrive at an incidence or rate, because the population from which the voluntarily submitted sample was drawn was never known.

An operative death was considered to be related to anesthesia by the opinion of a committee or, in some institutional studies, by the opinion of one reviewer. In view of the previously described bias, review of a death record actually consisted of a search for errors in surgical or anesthetic management and, finding neither, death was usually ascribed to the inexorable course of disease. With regard to anesthetic errors, there were always more errors than patients. "Errors" were departures from whatever was considered optimal anesthetic management at the time of review, and a causal relationship between "error" and death was not required to label a death as anesthetic-related. For example, the Baltimore Anesthesia Study Committee asked the following questions of each submitted death report: Did the anesthetic management contribute to the death of this patient? If yes, was it primary or contributory? Which phase of the anesthetic management was principally *at fault?* Five choices were given for classifying the fault or error, and all anesthetic deaths were included in some error category. Without an error, anesthesia management did not contribute to death. Details of these judgments were unrecorded, and no allowance was made for a subsequent review based on changing concepts or knowledge. In their study of operating and recovery room deaths, Boba and Landmesser did not include deaths unless "anesthetic error contributed to or caused the collapse."[9] With this bias in review of death records, it is not surprising that all published studies of anesthetic mortality report a predominance of "errors" and classify most anesthetic deaths as preventable. For example, regarding the almost 1,600 anesthetic-related deaths collected on a voluntary basis in Great Britain over a 15-year period,[8,10] the investigators noted that "in the great majority of the reports there were departures from accepted practices." In a survey of anesthetic-contributory death in Groote Schuur Hospital, Harrison considered 54 to 93 per cent as probably to possibly preventable.[11] Memery classified all anesthetic deaths collected from a large private practice as "errors."[12]

In these studies, the patient population from whom these anesthetic "errors" were collected showed some annoying inconsistencies. Most studies recognized patients in whom surgical therapy was undertaken in desperation, and a fatal outcome was expected. Dripps and associates included patients with an ASA physical status of Class 5 (moribund patient not expected to survive 24 hours with or without operation) in their anesthetic-related mortality,[5] whereas others excluded "inevitable deaths."[11,13] Deaths considered fortuitous, such as those due to pulmonary embolism and coronary thrombosis, were inconsistently included[10] or excluded.[11] Finally, some studies identified a group of deaths "which cannot at present be fully explained and for which countermeasures are either lacking or largely empirical" but were still considered anesthetic-contributory deaths.[5,11] In view of the bias in all these studies, their most serious defect is the failure to describe even briefly the circumstances of the deaths leading to the judgments so meticulously tabulated. Considering the vast changes in surgical practice, concepts of surgical care and diseases, and the rapid growth of knowledge of anesthetics even in the past decade, these tediously collected data are largely uninterpretable today.

RECENT STUDIES OF THE ROLE OF ANESTHESIA IN SURGICAL MORTALITY

Since 1969, data of several additional studies directly relating to the epidemiology of anesthetic deaths have become available.[2] Although improved in some aspects of design and reporting compared to earlier studies, none have answered any critical questions, and none are immune to the general criticism expressed above.

In 1970, a special committee that investigated anesthetic deaths in New South Wales during the period of 1960 to 1968 published its accumulated findings.[14] Relying on voluntary reporting of deaths and coroners' reports, the committee classified deaths by three degrees of relationship to the anesthetic: "reasonably certain," "some elements of doubt," and "caused by both the anesthetic and the surgical techniques." These three categories were considered "true" anesthetic deaths, and 286 were collected. Five other categories included surgical deaths, inevitable deaths, fortuitous deaths, deaths that could not be assessed despite considerable data, and deaths not assessed because of inadequate data. The number of "Committee-defined" deaths (all eight categories) was 745, of which 151 were attributable entirely to the surgical technique and 234 were considered to be inevitable deaths. Of their bias, they state the following:

In those cases classified in categories 1, 2, and 3, the Committee held that the anesthetic was in part or wholly responsible for the patient's death. This implies that there has been some error of judgement, management or technique on the part of the anesthetist and these cases have been analyzed according to error thought to have been involved.

They then identified 1,215 errors in the 286 deaths and classified them in 12 categories, such as inadequate preoperative preparation, inade-quate resuscitation, incorrect choice of anesthetic technique, hypoxic gas mixture, overdose, or inadequate ventilation. The remainder of the report discusses each of these types of errors in a tutorial manner without further analysis of the specific event in each category. Of special interest is that the Committee's opinion with regard to errors in each death report was made available to the reporting anesthetist. In 141 (49%) of the 286 deaths, the responsible anesthetist disagreed with the Committee's judgment of error. Of additional special interest is one conclusion of this report which states, "anesthetic agents themselves are not lethal except when they are misused."

Marx, Mateo, and Orkin reviewed all postanesthetic deaths in their institution over the 5-year period of 1965 to 1969.[15] The review was facilitated by computer storage of anesthetic records. Of all deaths, 83 per cent were attributed to the patient's preexisting disease, 10 per cent to the operation, 4 per cent to anesthesia, and 3 per cent to the postoperative management. Their report was unique in providing reasonably descriptive, although brief, details of the deaths related to anesthesia. Of the 27 deaths primarily related to the anesthetic, 20 (74%) were considered preventable. The single most common cause was aspiration of vomitus, which occurred in six patients. The seven unpreventable deaths "primarily related to anesthetic management" included three patients with obstruction of a Carlen's tube by blood clot or tumor, one premature infant with hypothermia during laparotomy despite vigorous warming efforts, and three deaths in elderly patients on the 5th or 6th postoperative day from "bilateral bronchopneumonia following endotracheal intubation." These events are not further detailed, and the basis for judging those primarily related to the anesthetic was not recorded. Of additional interest, five of the 20 deaths attributed to errors in postoperative management were the result of pulmonary aspiration in nonanesthetized patients.

Bodlander[16] continued for a second decade the study of postanesthetic deaths first reported by Clifton and Hotten[13] from the same institution. Despite a large increase in the incidence of all postoperative deaths in their institution, deaths ascribed solely to anesthesia decreased from 29.9 to 3.7 per cent, an enviable statistic, which they ascribed to improvement in numbers of senior anesthetic staff and the use of regional anesthesia for obstetrics. Primary anesthetic deaths are not described but are classified by cause in broad categories.

In a retrospective study of cardiac arrests in infants and children, Salem and colleagues collected 73 instances in which anesthesia was primarily responsible or importantly contributory to the arrest.[17] Unfortunately, cardiac arrests not attributable to the anesthetic were not similarly collected, and no incidence was obtainable. They classified causes of arrest according to cardiovascular and respiratory factors responsible and described some well known patterns leading to cardiac arrest. One-third of these patients died following arrest, and they considered "most of these accidents preventable."

In a unique study, Taylor, Larson, and Prestwich reviewed 41 instances of cardiac arrest during operation from records supplied by a professional liability insurance company.[18] Presumably, all instances were the subject of litigation and represented a highly selective sample. More than half of the patients were healthy and had an ASA physical status of Class 1; none were categorized in Class 4 or 5. Sixteen of the operations were minor, and 32 were elective. The probable causes of cardiac arrest, according to a single reviewer who judged them, were anesthetic mismanagement in nine, cardiovascular abnormality in nine, hypoxia owing to hypoventilation in 18, and miscellaneous causes in five patients. Judgments as to causes of arrest are only very briefly listed, and no details of events leading to cardiac arrest in this group of healthy patients were given. The most surprising conclusion was the apparent failure to recognize arrest and institute resuscitation, since only three of the 41 patients survived without neurological deficit.

The pattern of these recent studies is not greatly different from earlier studies. Analyses of death continue to focus on "errors" that are barely described and that are the consequence of a judgment that the investigators do not believe requires documentation. In all early and recent studies, no reporter believed it necessary to assure the reader that the cause ("error") led to the death.

ERROR AS A CAUSE OF ANESTHETIC DEATH

In 1948, Macintosh wrote, "I hold there should be no deaths due to anesthesia."[19] He is also claimed to have said, "The causes of anesthetic death are all too often mundane and obvious and rarely require much, if any, scientific investigation to establish them, provided a truthful account of the facts can be obtained."[20] Considering Macintosh's stature during the many decades encompassing the modern anesthetic era, it is likely that the statement above represented the prevailing and enlightened view of anesthetic deaths during this period. It is not surprising, then, that studies devised to discover the role of anesthesia in surgical mortality were actually designed to discover errors only. They were indeed successful in discovering an extraordinary number of "errors," most of which remain undescribed. What is surprising is the persistence and pervasiveness of this "error" bias to the present time.

Obviously human errors play a role in the contribution of anesthesia to surgical mortality. Admitting that any error would constitute too large a role, it is of special importance in today's litigious medical climate to know if the term *large* represents 10 or 90 per cent of anesthetic deaths. High estimates of error have resulted from the deliberate seeking out of errors, failure to seek out anesthetic causes other than error, lack of knowledge, until recently, of mechanisms of anesthetic death other than by error, and particularly the loose equating of "departure from current practice" with death. The failure to publish sufficient details of death, so that the quality of judgments could be reviewed by others, is a serious limitation to any reasonable estimate of error frequency. From the brief details of some judgments included in published reports, the relationship of an identified error with a death strains one's cause-effect imagination.

Despite this general criticism, the generous

reporting of errors clearly pointed to some patterns of anesthetic-associated deaths. When these patterns were sufficiently specific, such as aspiration of vomitus, circulatory collapse on change of position, or failure of oxygen supply, attention was called to clinical situations that merit precaution, prevention, or special attention. When patterns were identified as inadequate preparation for anesthesia, incorrect choice of anesthetic technique, hypoventilation, or hypotension, little of educational value and nothing of value in identifying mechanisms or methods of prevention were gained.

Two categories of anesthetic death by error, overdose and aspiration of vomitus, merit special comment. In almost every study reviewed, "overdose" is prominent as a cause of anesthesia mortality. Most reports identify overdose specifically with thiopental, while others do not specify, and still others include overdose with inhalation agents as well. Amazingly, *in no report is there a definition of what constituted the toxic dose or "overdose" of thiopental* or any other agent. Regarding thiopental, Edwards states, "as little as 0.15 or 0.2 g. caused sudden death."[8] If this is indeed so, the hemodynamic effects of thiopental urgently need reappraisal, considering its wide use even in seriously ill patients. Either the toxicity of thiopental is unappreciated, or "overdose" was not the cause of death. One can only speculate why this presumably common cause of anesthetic death was never investigated by experimentation.

Aspiration of vomitus continues to lead as a cause of mortality, even in the most recently published retrospective survey.[15] Although anesthesiologists now generally agree that no method will prevent aspiration of vomitus with absolute certainty in a patient with a full stomach, whether he is awake or anesthetized, this event continues to be considered as a cause of death solely related to the anesthetic and always preventable. A reappraisal of this position is certainly necessary. In patients with a full stomach who urgently require surgery, for whom there is no choice other than general anesthesia, and who then aspirate despite all proper precautions, death cannot be considered an error and preventable. The proper alternative is that of a known risk of anesthesia in such patients, a risk accepted by the patient as part of his informed consent.

Other patterns of anesthetic death clearly pointed to errors that are preventable and do not strain the cause-effect relationship. Among these are death from high spinal or epidural anesthesia in patients given conventional doses, death from excessive doses of local anesthetics or of neostigmine, death from obstructed endotracheal tubes, death from intubation of the esophagus, death from failure of oxygen supply, death from a disconnected ventilator, death from air embolism as a result of infusion, death from bilateral pneumothorax unrelated to the operation, and death from administration of the wrong drug. This list serves only to provide examples of clearly preventable errors that can lead to death and that require little judgment to establish a mechanism of death. Fortunately, knowledge of these errors has led to the invention or provision of devices or methods to decrease the likelihood of error and death. For example, wide availability of resuscitation drugs and equipment, improved non-kinking endotracheal tubes with improved cuffs, fail-safe oxygen delivery systems, alarms to indicate disconnected ventilators, plastic infusion containers, and the improved labeling of drug containers, still to be achieved. The recent study of cardiac arrests suggests the need for a sturdy monitor of inspired oxygen concentration, with an alarm system.[18] Identification of such error patterns can promptly lead to remedial measures or may at least stimulate a search for them.

An even more promising approach to the detection of error patterns and direction of preventive measures was described by Cooper and associates.[21] Their approach does not require a death to identify an error. Using a nonspecific interview technique, recorders asked anesthesiologists and trainees to describe "near misses" experienced or observed at any time in the past during conduct of anesthesia. These critical incidents were categorized as attributable to human error (82%) or equipment failure (14%). The study is ongoing and hopefully will describe specific error patterns, which can then be eliminated. Certainly this is a fruitful approach to identifying the *potential* role of errors in anesthesia mortality. Although it will not define the actual role of errors, these data can significantly strengthen any cause-effect relationships between error and postanesthetic death. For example, how long can a ventilator be disconnected without death? How often was X milliliters of drug Y mistakenly injected for drug Z without ill effects? How often did air embolism not lead to mortality? With such data supporting or not supporting cause-effect relationships, the true role of error in anesthesia mortality may one day be approximated.

ANESTHETIC DEATHS THAT ARE NOT THE RESULT OF ERROR

The pervasive bias of error in all considerations of anesthetic death probably impeded progress in discovery of causes of anesthetic death by other means, because the implications of this bias are so profound.

First, such bias leads to the assumption that drugs used during anesthesia are different from all other drugs, that they exhibit no idiosyncrasies, that patients do not show hypersensitivity, and that interactions with other drugs and disease do not occur. Adverse responses to these drugs are thought to result only when they are misused. Perhaps this view is derived secondarily from the concepts, once widely held as fundamental, that inhalation agents were inert and were not metabolized, and that blood and brain levels of anesthetics could be controlled at will. The naiveté of assuming anesthetics are innocuous is equivalent to believing that antibiotic toxicity is always caused by an overdose error and is unrelated to the severity of infection; or, that digitalis toxicity is caused by an error unrelated to the degree of heart failure. The same naiveté characterizes drug surveillance studies that ascribe all untoward events in patients with disease treated by medication to adverse drug reactions, regardless of whether a cause-effect relationship can be demonstrated and is independent of the stage of disease treated. These attitudes completely ignore well established concepts of clinical pharmacology, such as the variations in response to average doses, influence of specific diseases on drug responses, drug interactions, enzyme induction, active drug metabolites, and pharmacogenetics.

Until recently, pharmacologic events were not even conceived as applying to anesthetic drugs in man. The recurrent opinion has been that anesthetic agents themselves are not lethal except when misused. Drugs used in clinical anesthesia are potent and potentially lethal, and, like all drugs, anesthetics have primary desired actions and unwanted side effects. At times side effects become unintentionally severe and noxious, such as an adverse drug reaction, which may be fatal. Fatalities from drug administration, anesthetic or otherwise, *even when cause and effect can be demonstrated*, are not tantamount to error. For example, suppose atropine in a dose of 0.2 mg. is given to treat sudden bradycardia and hypotension secondary to traction reflex in a digitalized patient with mitral stenosis, during vaginal hysterectomy with spinal anesthesia. Instead of the anticipated result of this logical action, severe tachycardia and pulmonary edema develop, resulting in death. Clearly this is an adverse drug reaction during anesthesia. It is not an error, but it is related to the hazard of administration of atropine to patients with mitral stenosis. Similar examples include the consequences of excessive hypertension from an average dose of vasopressor or profound respiratory depression from a conventional dose of narcotic. Drugs, like all therapeutic modalities, are prescribed in anticipation of benefits and at the risk of adverse responses. There has never been any justification for excluding drugs used during anesthesia from this basic therapeutic principle. This also applies equally to anesthetic techniques, as in the following example. Profound muscle relaxation is required to permit a surgeon to accomplish a therapeutic operation to relieve severe intestinal obstruction in a seriously ill patient. This relaxation is best achieved by large but conventional doses of muscle relaxants. Failure to breathe after operation is an accepted risk, and its consequence is prolongation of tracheal intubation and the need for mechanical ventilation. When such a patient develops bilateral bronchopneumonia and dies several days later, prior use of large doses of muscle relaxants does not constitute an error or adverse drug reaction; it is simply a risk necessarily taken to effect a life-saving therapy.

A second implication of the bias of ever present errors in anesthesia mortality is that it explicitly precludes any new knowledge concerning mechanisms of death attributable to anesthesia. I indicated the few instances in which deaths that are not obviously due to any error are even mentioned. Precisely in this group, one should explore for undescribed and subtle mechanisms by which anesthetics contribute to mortality. Here it is relevant to note that discovery of major new mechanisms of anesthetic death during the past 15 years did not follow from any study directed to anesthesia mortality by review of death reports. Succinylcholine-induced hyperkalemia, malignant hyperpyrexia, genetic variants in plasma cholinesterase, post-halothane hepatitis, and methoxyflurane nephrotoxicity were discovered by alert clinicians investigating adverse effects not attributable to error. Current studies of the immunosuppressant properties of general anesthetics may yet reveal even more subtle mechanisms. One can properly wonder how deaths from these causes were classified by omniscient committees before these new mechanisms were described.

Delineation of the role of anesthesia in surgical mortality still requires a definition of those anesthetic deaths that are not the result of error. Elements of this definition are described in this book. Difficulties in identifying other elements have been considered.[2] The most obvious difficulty is that, with rare exception, anesthesia is not therapeutic and is administered only to facilitate some other therapy. No control study of the hazards of operation without anesthesia will ever be performed. The hazards of anesthesia can therefore never be considered independent of a second procedure. Both risks and benefits of anesthesia are confounded with a disease state, with an operation or manipulation by a second set of persons who act largely independently, and, finally, with a third set of persons who care for patients during a period when they are still vulnerable to the adverse effects of anesthesia. In this complex interaction of procedures and personnel, it is difficult to differentiate adverse effects of anesthetics from surgically induced effects, nonanesthetic drug-induced effects, and adverse responses induced by nursing procedures. This complexity applies particularly to patients with serious systemic disease undergoing hazardous operations and requiring maximum postoperative care. In such patients an anesthetic may contribute importantly to overall surgical mortality, but complexity and ignorance of what to look for impede progress.

The challenge seems almost overwhelming in view of the difficulties now recognized in attempting to identify factors contributing to overall surgical mortality, of which anesthesia mortality is only a part. A by-product of the National Halothane Study was the discovery of the large differences in surgical mortality for specific operations among the participating hospitals.[22] These could not be explained by any readily identifiable differences in patient populations and led to a larger study undertaken by the Stanford Center for Health Care Research.[23,24] The outcomes following 15 categories of surgical operations in 17 hospitals were adjusted for physical status, stage of surgical disease, age, sex, stress level, and insurance coverage. When so standardized, substantial and significant differences in mortality and severe morbidity measures still existed among hospitals. These differences were poorly correlated with qualifications of medical and nursing staffs. At the moment, these investigators postulate that postoperative adjusted mortality and morbidity rates are most likely to correlate with hospital features related to organizational and sociological structure rather then measurable characteristics of the patient mix. Anesthesia mortality as a subset of surgical mortality incorporates most of these same variables. Identification of its role in overall surgical mortality is not readily forthcoming.

Discovery of other mechanisms in anesthesia mortality may be more feasible in a less complex milieu. For example, a study of anesthesia limited to patients not expected to die might reveal new mechanisms, although they would not be subtle or applicable to the critically ill. In a study including patients of ASA physical status of Classes 1 and 2 (healthy or with mild systemic disease), undergoing operations that are not life-threatening, adverse effects of anesthesia might become more visible in relation to the smaller distortions secondary to operation. Unfortunately, detailed reports of deaths in this type of patient have been rarely published and have never been collected.[18] However, in such a group at least the frequency of error as a cause of death could be more easily identified. Among the rest, a search for new mechanisms could realistically begin. Those of us who have participated regularly in mortality conferences for a sufficiently long period remember at least one reasonably healthy patient who underwent a non-life-threatening operation and who died unexpectedly during or shortly after operation. As a hypothetical example, suppose a 50-year-old man undergoing subtotal gastrectomy for peptic ulcer disease can not be resuscitated after cardiac arrest during operation. According to the death record, a summary prepared by the anesthesiologist, preoperative anesthetic and surgical management are impeccable. Autopsy reveals diffuse mild coronary disease without occlusion, lung changes consistent with chronic bronchitis, and duodenal ulcer. None of these changes can account for death. How can such an event be explained? There are only three possibilities: Death was fortuitous and part of the obligitory mortality of hospitalized patients (see below); death was caused by a mechanism as yet undiscovered; or, the final alternative (if Macintosh's view is accepted), the anesthesiologist who prepared the death report lied, and no further investigation is necessary. This last possibility is no longer tenable intellectually in view of increasing knowledge of clinical pharmacology of anesthetic drugs. The image of the guilt-laden anesthesiologist accepting all unanticipated and unexplained outcomes of surgical therapy as a consequence of his error has become counterproductive. Further progress requires that reports be accepted as true accounts, that they be collected in a repository or registry, that cause-effect relationships be sought according to rigorous scientific standards, and that admission of ignorance is acceptable when no causes can be found.

Study of the suggested healthy population may also quantify the role of the obligatory death rate of hospitalization in surgical mortality described originally in the author's earlier publication.[2] It has been estimated that 350,000 Americans die annually of *sudden death syndrome*, defined as unexpected natural death occurring within 1 hour after collapse of an individual in apparent good health.[25] Assuming that 16 million operations are performed annually, with a mean hospitalization of 5 days per patient, there are 80 million person-days during which any death would be part of surgical mortality. If the day of and day after operation is assumed to be the vulnerable period for anesthetic-associated mortality, there are 32 million person-days during which any of the 350,000 occurrences of sudden death syndrome could be considered anesthetic mortality. Although almost all of these deaths are assumed to be the result of a fatal arrhythmia secondary to coronary artery disease, increasing recent interest in sudden death reveals a disconcerting number that cannot be accounted for by autopsy findings. Not surprisingly, many patients with occult or even clinically identified coronary artery disease do not show anatomical cause for the fatal event at autopsy. Mitral valve prolapse syndrome, coronary artery spasm (Prinzmetal's angina), and prolonged Q-T interval syndromes lead to sudden death without evidence at autopsy. Sudden deaths that are not the result of heat stroke occur every fall among football players and among other college students. Autopsies often show cardiovascular abnormalities, but they are usually insufficient to account for death. Unexplained sudden death is well known among healthy soldiers. Crib death (sudden infant death syndrome) is a similar enigma in infants; cardiovascular abnormalities may be present at autopsy, but they are not severe enough to have been diagnosed ante mortem or to cause death. Since these events occur in apparently healthy individuals and presumably result from ventricular fibrillation, psychological factors have been suggested as one precipitating cause. By no reasonable approximation can sudden death syndrome account for a large portion of deaths associated with anesthesia. Of great significance, however, is its existence and its potential to cause death during anesthesia. A diagnosis of anesthetic death should never be made by exclusion. The possibility of sudden death syndrome requires that anesthetic causes be reasonably related to death before a judgment of anesthetic death is accepted.

WHAT IS KNOWN ABOUT THE ROLE OF ANESTHESIA IN SURGICAL MORTALITY?

Precious little is known about the role of anesthesia in surgical mortality. Thirty years of self-flagellation in the form of anesthesia mortality studies have generated an abundance of anesthetic "errors." Some of these "errors" survive the test of the cause-effect relationship. Some anesthetic deaths have been caused by human error or equipment failure. We have no idea of their frequency. All other generated "errors" now exist only in the vague memory of omniscient committees that equated deviation from accepted practice, as perceived during the particular year of review, with "error," and "error," with anesthetic death. The need for evidence of a casual relationship was waived in the belief that inclusion of even the most remote relationships would improve standards of practice. Knowing the bias that generated the data, all published estimates of the incidence of anesthetic deaths are unacceptable; for all practical purposes such estimates are unknown. Some potential mechanisms of anesthetic death are the subject of this book. Their frequency as a contribution to overall surgical mortality is yet to be determined.

A fresh approach is needed in this new determination. The practice of anesthesiology consists of the administration of a variety of potent drugs, employs a number of maneuvers requiring technical skill and utilization of mechanical equipment, and necessitates knowledge of equipment function and malfunction. In every aspect of this activity, something is actively done to a patient. At any phase of this activity, any untoward event may be attributed to an immediately preceding reaction by simple post-hoc reasoning. Whereas untoward patient events in less activist specialties of medicine are readily ascribed to the patient's disease or an unrelated fortuitous event, the almost continuous ministrations of the anes-

thesiologist leave him vulnerable to the easy post-hoc hypothesis. Demonstration of cause-effect relationship is absolutely essential if any secure knowledge of mechanisms of anesthetic death is to be achieved. In consideration of deaths during anesthesia, it is time to substitute a presumption of innocence for one of guilt until cause and effect are demonstrated.

Further, the anesthesiologist's application of drugs, maneuvers, techniques, and machines to patients must be viewed on the same risk-benefit scale as all forms of medical therapy, as well as non-therapy. Each is designed to benefit total surgical care of a patient. However, each also has its risk in terms of adverse drug reactions, unwanted outcomes of technical manuevers, and malfunction of machines, including the risk of receiving and acting on erroneous information from monitors designed to increase safety. Risks exist because they are not completely preventable by the most skilled and knowledgeable human. Patients react to drugs individually, with a spectrum of responses not usually predictable, and at times adverse. All humans are not anatomically the same, and all technical maneuvers cannot be consistently successful. Machines do not perform optimally at all times. These are risks that may occur in the hands of the most competent anesthesiologist, using drugs and techniques faultlessly and conscientiously caring for the patient. Such risks, alone or in combination may lead to anesthetic death. Death during anesthesia is possible without error or toxicity. It is precisely these risks that need to be quantified to determine the role of anesthesia in surgical mortality. With respect to prevention, if no actions are taken, no risks are assumed, and all untoward events are prevented.

Finally, more attention needs to be given to the sudden death syndrome in the hospital population, both in adults and children. Activist specialties of medical practice, such as anesthesiology and surgery, are absorbing these deaths as related to their therapy. Not only do these deaths confound estimates of risk and mortality, but they lead to malpractice litigation and costly defensive anesthesia practices that do not represent optimal anesthetic patient care.

REFERENCES

1. Keats, A. S.: The estimate of the anesthetic risk in medical evaluations. Am. J. Cardiol. *12*:330, 1963.
2. Goldstein, A., Jr., and Keats, A. S.: The risk of anesthesia. Anesthesiology, *33*:130, 1970.
3. Beecher, H. K., and Todd, D. P.: A study of the deaths associated with anesthesia and surgery. Ann. Surg., *140*:2, 1954.
4. Abajian, J., Jr., Arrowwood, J. G., Barrett, R. H., et al.: Critique of "A study of the deaths associated with anesthesia and surgery." Ann. Surg., *142*:138, 1955.
5. Dripps, R. D., Lamont, A., and Eckenhoff, J. E.: The role of anesthesia in surgical mortality. J.A.M.A., *178*:261, 1961.
6. Ruth, H. S.: Anesthesia study commissions. J.A.M.A., *127*:514, 1945.
7. Phillips, O. C., Frazier, T. M., Graff, T. D., et al.: The Baltimore anesthesia study committee: Review of 1024 postoperative deaths. J.A.M.A., *174*:2015, 1960.
8. Edwards, G., Morton, H. J. V., Pask, E. A., et al.: Deaths associated with anaesthesia: Report on 1000 cases. Anaesthesia, *11*:194, 1956.
9. Boba, A., and Landmesser, C. M.: Total cardiorespiratory collapse (cardiac arrest). N. Y. State J. Med., *61*:2928, 1961.
10. Dinnick, O. P.: Deaths associated with anaesthesia. Anaesthesia, *19*:536, 1964.
11. Harrison, G. G.: Anesthetic contributory death—its incidence and causes. Part I: Incidence; Part II: Causes. S. Afr. Med. J., *42*:514, 1968.
12. Memery, H. N.: Anesthesia mortality in private practice. A ten year study. J.A.M.A., *194*:1185, 1965.
13. Clifton, B. S., and Hotten, W. I. T.: Deaths associated with anaesthesia. Br. J. Anaesth., *35*:250, 1963.
14. Special Committee Investigating Deaths Under Anaesthesia: Report on 745 classified cases, 1960–1968. Med. J. Aust., *1*:573, 1970.
15. Marx, G. F., Mateo, C. V., and Orkin, L. R.: Computer analysis of postanesthetic deaths. Anesthesiology, *39*:54, 1973.
16. Bodlander, F. M.: Deaths associated with anaesthesia. Br. J. Anaesth., *47*:36, 1975.
17. Salem, M. R., Bennett, E. J., Schweiss, J. F., et al.: Cardiac arrest related to anesthesia. Contributing factors in infants and children. J.A.M.A., *233*:238, 1975.
18. Gordon, T., Larson, C. P., Jr., and Prestwich, R.: Unexpected cardiac arrest during anesthesia and surgery: an environmental study. J.A.M.A., *236*:2758, 1976.
19. Macintosh, R.: Deaths under anaesthetics. Br. J. Anaesth., *21*:107, 1948.
20. Wylie, W. D.: "There, but for the grace of God . . .". Ann. R. Coll. Surg. Engl., *56*:171, 1975.
21. Cooper, J. B., Newbower, R. S., Long, C. B., et al.: Preventable anesthesia mishaps: a human factors study. Anesthesiology, *49*:399, 1978.
22. Moses, L. E., and Mosteller, F.: Institutional differences in postoperative death rates. J.A.M.A., *203*:492, 1968.
23. Scott, W. R., Forrest, W. H., Jr., and Brown, B. W., Jr.: Hospital structure and postoperative mortality and morbidity. In Shortell, S. M., and Brown, M. (eds.): Organizational Research in Hospitals. pp. 72–89. Chicago, Blue Cross Association, 1976.
24. Stanford Center for Health Care Research: Comparison of hospitals with regard to outcomes of surgery. Health Serv. Res., *11*:112, 1976.
25. Doyle, J. T.: Mechanisms and prevention of sudden death. Mod. Concepts of Cardiovasc. Dis., *45*:111, 1976.

FURTHER READING

Keats, A. S.: What do we know about anesthesia mortality? Anesthesiology, *50*:387, 1979.

2 Epidemiologic Methods in Anesthesia

Bucknam McPeek, M.D., and John P. Gilbert, Ph.D.

Epidemiology is the branch of medicine that deals with the study of the distribution and cause of disease or injury in human populations. It differs from clinical medicine because it is concerned with the health of groups or populations of people rather than of a single patient.

ISOLATED CASE REPORTS

A clinical case report is the anesthesiologist's first signal of an anesthetic complication. A physician, observing one or more unexpected events after exposure to an anesthetic agent, may write and publish a clinical case report. Anesthesiology is constantly challenged with individual clinical case histories that suggest anesthetic problems. Such case reports are important. They alert the anesthesiologist to the possibility of undesirable therapy, thus forming the first line of defense against the continued use of such therapy. As anesthesiologists, we are absolutely dependent upon the sensitivity of individual physicians to detect unexpected events and record them accurately for publication.

A clinical case report details the disease-related experiences of a single patient. A hospital record room contains shelf upon shelf of such individual clinical case histories. A magnificent array of medical information may be available on each patient.

Despite a possible wealth of carefully documented detail, an individual clinical case report has a major defect. It is usually not possible to determine the number of cases in the group from which a single case is drawn. Thus, the probability of similar cases occurring in the future cannot be estimated. If there were a case of jaundice after an exposure to an anesthetic drug or a case of paraplegia after administration of a spinal anesthetic, it would be desirable to determine the incidence of these complications. There is a significant difference between one case of jaundice that occurs after ten exposures to anesthetics and one case that occurs after 10,000 exposures. Three cases of paraplegia drawn from an experience of 300 spinal anesthetic administrations carries a greater impact than a single case from a hospital's experience of 300,000 administrations.

Regardless of the care and energy with which an individual clinical case history is investigated and reported, it tells us nothing about the incidence of similar cases in a population. In other words, the numerator (observed case) is always "1," and the denominator (population) is unknown. Even if a relatively large number of individual clinical cases of a specific complication following exposure to a drug are reported in the literature, it is impossible to say anything about the incidence of the complication without some knowledge of the size of the population at risk. A statement about incidence or the probability of occurrence requires both a numerator and a denominator. The appearance of increasing numbers of clinical case histories of a specific complication may suggest that it is a more common occurrence than if only one such report had been made. Yet, it is impossible to predict exactly how much more likely is the occurrence as new reports come to our attention; nor can the probability of occurrence of a specific event be estimated, to say nothing of whether it is causally related to a particular treatment or practice.

POPULATION STUDIES

Epidemiologists have developed specialized methods in order to study the extent and cause of disease. As practicing physicians, anesthesiologists use these methods and benefit from their results, often without much understanding of the methods themselves. Nonetheless, if one wishes to use or interpret epidemiological studies, it is necessary to have a working knowledge of the underlying concepts, potentials, and limitations of the various methods involved. As one might expect, there is a large and growing literature on epidemiologic methods and experimental design. Although we explore some of the major issues here, the reader should consult the references at the end of the chapter for a more detailed treatment of specific areas.

The ability to identify a particular complication or diagnose a specific disease with reasonable reliability is vital to its epidemiologic study. If it cannot be identified it cannot be included in cases that comprise a numerator. This problem has been largely responsible for the inability to study adequately the halothane-hepatitis question.

Epidemiologists are interested in population studies because such studies enable them to discuss the incidence rate, or probability of an observed event. These studies require a denominator, which is a defined population serving as a comparison group for the individuals who are experiencing the event or undergoing the treatment under investigation. Individual case histories are important because they alert us to unsuspected events. Epidemiologic or population studies are frequently triggered by knowledge gained through individual case reports. It is the presence of a denominator that really distinguishes the two, bringing forth an epidemiological study from a collection of case histories.

Many individual details are often available from a clinical case report. Yet in a population study, if the denominator is very large, it is not uncommon to have available only a few details about each case. Ordinarily, financial considerations preclude using both a great many cases and a large number of facts per case. In the National Halothane Study, an elaborate design allowed reference to a denominator of 856,000 patients.[1] Yet the analysis was based on some 8 to 10 individual items of information about each of the surveyed patients. The epidemiologic study currently underway at the Massachusetts General Hospital has a population of some 80,000 patients, and 40 or 50 items of information are recorded for each patient.[2] Thus, there is usually an inverse relationship to be found between the size of a study's population and the number of facts available for each single case.

SAMPLING

Of course, an investigator ordinarily has available for study a specific population of patients, such as the patients treated in a particular hospital or practice. Frequently, it is not practical to study all the individuals available. A sample may be drawn of representatives from the larger population. This process is called sampling, and the extent to which information obtained may be extrapolated to the total population depends in large measure on the skill with which the sampling was done. Sometimes a process called *stratification* is used. Stratified samples are drawn to insure that specified proportions of selected groups are included. For example, it may be required that a sample consist of two groups of pregnant women: one group of those pregnant for the first time, and a second group of an equal number of those who have been pregnant before. Within specified subgroups selection may be either random or according to some system. A *random sample* is one that is drawn so that every subject in the total population has an equal chance of being represented in the sample. A *systematic sample* is one in which individuals are selected by some system; for example, every 10th person or every 100th person may be included in a sample. If the order of the population prior to drawing the sample is random, or at least not highly structured with respect to some confounding variable, systematic sampling will work. Sometimes it is disastrous. A number of years ago, the popularity of non-commissioned officers in the Army was studied using a systematic sample of every 30th man from the post list. Imagine the investigator's surprise when he found that sergeants were almost universally respected. Further investigation revealed that the post list consisted of hundreds of barracks lists, with each barrack housing 27 privates, two corporals, and a sergeant. The sergeant was the 30th name on each list.

DESCRIPTIVE AND ANALYTIC EPIDEMIOLOGIC STUDIES

It is customary to separate epidemiologic studies into two broad categories. The first, *descriptive epidemiology*, concerns the amount and range of disease within a population. The second, *analytic epidemiology*, focuses on the causes of disease or the factors influencing its extent. Descriptive studies are important because they take a first step toward uncovering the causes of disease or injury by identifying groups with a high or low rate of specific illness.

Once such an identification has been made, the next step is an attempt to understand why the rate is high or low in a particular population. The results of observational studies aid the formulation of hypotheses that can be tested by analytic studies in order to determine the underlying causes of the disease and explain its distribution.

In their purest form, analytic studies are executed to test a hypothesis that a specific factor or cause is related to a particular effect. This is accomplished by measuring both exposure to the cause and the presence or absence of the effect for each individual in the study. That is, the study is designed to test the following general hypothesis: If the frequency of illness or injury within two groups is dependent on the presence of an identified factor, then that particular factor should appear more frequently in the group with the illness or injury than in the other.

The majority of analytic epidemiologic studies survey the individual members of each group. There are, of course, some studies that examine the experience of the group as a whole, but these will not be dealt with here, since they are not very common.

Analytic studies of individual members of the group are of three general kinds: cross-sectional, case-control, and cohort. In a *cross-sectional study*, the cause and effect are measured at the same time. A study of the relationship between body build and difficulty in passing an endotracheal tube might be an example. A *case-control study* is retrospective; it starts with the effect and determines the frequency of the hypothesized cause. Persons with the illness or injury are compared to a control group free of the illness, and an attempt is made to determine whether the two groups differ in their previous exposure to the causative factor. A *cohort study*, on the other hand, is prospective. The investigator starts with the cause and looks for the development of the effect. Individuals who are exposed to the hypothesized causal factor are followed and compared with a control group composed of those individuals not exposed to the causal factor. Both groups are carefully observed through time to determine the incidence of the subsequent development of the effect.

Note that each of these methods attempts to relate cause and effect. The cross-sectional study examines cause and effect by a single measurement in time. The case-control study involves two groups that differ in the presence of the effect; the investigator looks backward in time to compare their exposure to a hypothesized cause. The cohort study involves two groups, or cohorts, which differ in their exposure to a suspected cause and follows them forward in time to determine the rates at which they may develop the effect.

OBSERVATIONAL AND EXPERIMENTAL STUDIES

There are two basic approaches to investigating hypotheses about causation: observational and experimental. In the observational approach, the investigator observes the occurrence of the disease in individuals who are already separated into groups on the basis of exposure to a factor such as a particular anesthetic agent. An example of this is the National Halothane Study. In this study, the allocation of individuals into groups on the basis of exposure to specific anesthetic agents was not done by the investigators, but instead depended on the person's previous anesthetic experience. Often this mode of classification may raise questions about the comparability of the groups.

In the experimental approach, which is always a cohort study, the investigator examines the effect of deliberately varying some causative factor under his control. This is the essential difference between observational and experimental studies. In an observational study, the differences between study groups are only observed and are not experimentally manipulated by the investigator. As mentioned, a major problem with observational studies is the comparability of the observed group. Since these groups are not created experimentally, they must be taken as the investigator finds them. They will ordinarily differ in other ways, in addition to the specific causal factor under study. One group may be older and another may have more men than women; or, the participants may show different states of general health. Thus, the role of the factor under investigation may be obscrued by a great many variables. Observational studies continue to provide much useful knowledge for medical research. Yet physicians, particularly in the last 50 years, have come to rely more and more on the experimental approach.

Experimental studies can establish causation with more surety than observational studies. This is primarily due to the increased control with which experimental studies may be conducted. The degree of control can usually be determined by examining the fundamental structure of a study. Three basic study types were found by Gilbert, McPeek, and Mosteller in a recent study of evaluations of different treatments given to patients undergoing surgery and anesthesia.[3,4] Using the National Library of Medicine medical literature analysis and retrieval system (MEDLARS), they drew a sample of 107 papers from the medical literature in surgery and anesthesia, covering the period between 1964 and 1972. Their sample papers reported on the following three kinds of studies: randomized controlled trials, nonrandomized controlled trials, and series. The term *randomized controlled trial* indicated that the investigator compared two or more treatment groups and that patients were assigned to the groups by a formal randomization process. The *nonrandomized controlled trials* were not formally randomized; patients treated concurrently in the same institution were compared, and patients treated previously by one method were compared with patients treated currently by another. A *series* consisted of reports of patients treated in a particular manner, but with no specific referent for comparison, aside from other reports in the literature dealing with similar patients.

Series

Series ordinarily tell the anesthesiologist little about causation, although much can be learned about the results of a particular treatment or the effects of a disease. The strength of an epidemiologic study, and, thus, the surety with which we can accept its results, depends on a variety of factors, but mostly upon the degree of control. Sometimes a series is just a collection of selected case reports. We have more confidence in a series if it is a census, consisting of *all* cases of complication X seen over a time period, or if an unbiased sample of *all* observed cases of complication X is drawn to form the reported series. Since a series is not a controlled trial, the results cannot be used with much certainty to form conclusions about causation. However, there are exceptions to this. For example, in some cases the causal link is short and direct, such as the appearance of tissue damage after prolonged tracheal intubation with a cuffed tube; it seems reasonable to conclude that the cuff has caused the damage. In addition, when a well verified theory can be applied or when the effect is immediate and substantial and there is no other reasonable explanation (e.g., when tissue damage follows the intra-arterial injection of thiopental), the cause is evident. Another variation of this principle is illustrated when an unusually rare event is frequently observed after a certain treatment (e.g., the defects observed in infants whose mothers took thalidomide during pregnancy).

Therefore, a series can sometimes supply information about causation, as well as information about levels of performance, outcome, and the natural history of disease. Nonetheless, the controlled study still provides the primary support for theories of cause, and its credibility rests mainly on the strength of the control. Only to the extent that the control group is truly similar to the exposed group will differences in outcome illustrate the role of the causal factor.

On very rare occasions, natural groups may be found that seem to be similar in all respects except for the degree of exposure to a hypothesized causal factor. This is called a *natural experiment*, and in these most unusual circumstances an observational study may establish causal association.

Controlled Studies

In a controlled study, assignment of patients to the exposed group or to the control group is an important issue. The principal aim is to achieve similarity between the groups. A number of considerations must be dealt with in the pursuit of this goal. For instance, the known information about the disease or complication under study should be examined. It is also necessary to identify any potentially confounding variables that might have a large effect. In a study of anesthetic drugs, it is certainly important to insure that the exposed and control groups are similar with respect to age, physical status, and the operation performed. In a study of heart disease, the groups might be matched with respect to risk factors, such as hypertension, smoking, diabetes, and previous cardiac history. Unfortunately, it is unlikely that the investigator knows enough about the specific disease or complication to guarantee that even the most careful matching has eliminated all possible confusing factors. Afterward it is difficult to eliminate the effect of previously unknown factors. To a very limited extent, this problem may be dealt with by assuring general similarity between the exposed and control groups. Thus, the groups may be drawn from the same general population, from patients seen at the same clinic or hospital, or from the same general ethnic or socioeconomic group.

Finally, it is necessary to be sure that information required in the study can be obtained from both groups in the same fashion. In other words, it is desirable to acquire the same information from the same kinds of people. Any difference in response rates between the control group and the exposed group raises serious problems.

ALLOCATION TO GROUPS IN CONTROLLED TRIALS

There are two basic methods of allocation: random and systematic. A *random allocation* is one that is drawn in such a fashion that every subject of the population to be studied has an equal chance of being represented in each group. Random allocation has great theoretical and practical advantages.

A *systematic allocation* is one in which individuals are selected systematically to form the groups. For example, every second person may be assigned to the experimental group. If the order of the study population prior to the allocation to groups is random, or at least not highly structured with respect to some confounding variable, systematic allocation will produce satisfactory results.

The method of allocation is important. It deserves careful thought, and once the procedure is selected it must be followed exactly. Little confidence can be placed in data acquired from treatment groups that have been selected in a haphazard fashion. In their survey of controlled studies in anesthesia, Gilbert and colleagues found a substantial and potentially troublesome range, both in the methods of allocating treatments in clinical trials and in the care in reporting their methods.[3] Often investigators report so briefly upon their method of allocation that the reader cannot determine how it was done. In other papers, investigators use methods that readily lead to bias. For example, when someone associated with the trial personally chooses which patients are to receive a specific treatment, the allocation is no longer unbiased.[5]

Knowing who is to receive treatment A next may influence decisions about eligibility and thus create bias. All schemes designed to balance allocation have this weakness. Eligibility must always be decided separately and prior to allocation to treatment. Furthermore, when investigators use the method of alternate cases to assign patients to two treatments, they encounter two or more candidates appearing almost simultaneously. In this case, some preference or prejudice of the person who assigns the treatment will affect the trial. If that person prefers that treatment A be administered to women or young people, then more women and young people will receive treatment A. Sometimes patients present themselves in a nearly random order and, if there were no picking and choosing, this method of assigning treatments would suffice. Yet, bunching usually occurs, which means that someone will probably influence the assignments, either consciously or unconsciously. For example, one recent study that used alternate assignments resulted in two groups of about 150 and 250, respectively, instead of groups that differed by, at most, one or two members.

Another method predisposed to nonrandom allocation involves the assignment of treatment by birthdate, depending, for example, on whether the date is odd or even. An investigator who knows the subject's birthdate and the associated treatment can decide that the subject is not eligible for the study and thereby introduce selection effect. The same objection applies to use of patients' hospital numbers in prospective studies, although not in retrospective studies. Note that the objection here is not to rules that disallow entrance into the study. Rules for exclusion are often essential, but these rules must be strictly insulated from the choice of treatment once the patient's elibility has been established. Although informal methods of random allocation can be used rather effectively, they are subject to abuse: "Let's flip the coin again since we've already had four heads in a row." Informal methods, such as coin tossing, are usually difficult to document, and therefore they cannot be checked later if questions arise, as they do with great regularity.

The use of a published table of random digits makes it easy to keep a written record of which numbers were chosen and how the numbers were used to make the assignments. Tables of random numbers are widely available and inexpensive to use. Still, the application of any randomization technique must be examined for possible bias. As randomizing devices, slips of paper marked with a treatment in a sealed envelope appear to be efficient. However, sometimes the envelopes are not opaque, especially when held against bright light, as they often are, and the assigner can shuffle envelopes, knowing the characteristics of the participant and the possible treatments. Even the use of a random number table may introduce bias, depending on the method by which numbers are assigned. If an investigator is responsible for entering each patient in the order of arrival on a list of random numbers, nonrandom assignment could occur when two patients appear at the same time, and the investigator must choose in which order to place them. As a protection against this, the investigator should not be told how the numbers correspond to the treatments.

Although these precautions may seem elaborate, it is wise to assume that if something can go wrong in an investigation, it usually will. When the quality of randomization is questionable, the guarantee of lack of bias disappears, which adds to the uncertainty of the conclusions. Of course, randomization alone does not insure that a proper experiment has been carried out or that correct results will be obtained. Therefore, when expensive and delicate studies such as randomized clinical trials are carried out, their component parts, like the steps of randomization and the degree of blindness, must be thoroughly inspected and secured. When quality control measures have been applied in a study, they should be reported in detail. The amount of care taken in the design and execution of an investigation is a major indicator of its quality. When such care is not reported, some readers may uncharitably assume that these steps have not been taken.

Blindness

One of the methodological lessons that researchers learned from early medical trials at the beginning of this century was the extreme difficulty of obtaining objective and reproducible data from human subjects. Because few people view their own death with equanimity, it is only with the greatest difficulty that a patient can admit to himself and to his physician that a long desired cure has failed. In less dramatic circumstances, the patient's respect for the physician-researcher, as well as his own personal hopes, may exert a similar inhibiting effect. Humans communicate with each other in many different ways, some completely unconscious, and so the hopes of the research team can often be communicated to the patient without either being aware of it, much like a form of infection.

Double-blind evaluation, in which neither the physician nor the patient knows which treatment he has received, is a way of preventing contamination of this sort. The requirement of a double-blind design, when it is possible, is no more an aspersion on the honesty and integrity of the investigator than is the use of rubber gloves an aspersion on the personal hygiene of a surgeon. In both cases, experience has taught us that failure to follow the best possible practices often leads to disastrous consequences. Since it is often impossible to tell, without another trial, whether bias has affected the results observed, a randomized double-blind trial carries weight because it provides the researcher with the maximum protection against these subtle sources of error. When, owing to the type of therapy being investigated, it is not possible to devise a double-blind study, it may still be possible to avoid some sources of bias by using an unbiased or blind evaluator. This does not mean that unblinded studies are always wrong, or that blind studies are always right; rather, it means that unblinded studies are more likely to be biased, and it is virtually impossible to document the absence of such effects. Thus, it is the possibility of bias that cannot be dismissed, that weakens our confidence in these studies, and that makes them less useful for decision making, even when their findings are correct.

Power and Generalization

In generalizing from the results of a clinical trial, there are two dangers. One of these is that a true difference will be overlooked. The other is that a difference will be reported erroneously. As the sizes of experimental groups are limited, there is always some risk that the data will suggest a false conclusion because of sampling fluctuation. Large differences tend to be more easily detected than small ones, and in any particular study larger samples are more likely to lead to the correct conclusions than smaller ones. Because the level of significance is affected by the degree of the true but unknown difference in effectiveness of the treatments, as well as by the strength of the evidence as determined by the sample size, it is easier to obtain significant results when the true differences are large than when they are small. The capability of a trial to detect small effects is called its *power* and depends primarily on the unknown difference between the treatment effects, the design of the trial, and the sizes of the groups. For example, consider a 5-per-cent change in a death rate. (Five per cent is about four times the average surgical death rate from all operations over the country as a whole.) Reducing a death rate from 35 to 30 per cent may be an important improvement in patient care, but this does not mean that it will be easily identified in the everyday setting of clinical practice. Indeed, statistical theory shows that a well run, randomized, controlled trial must have 1000 patients in each group to be 80-per-cent confident in detecting such a difference. Without a large formal study, uncontrolled effects of patient selection, concurrent treatments, and other factors make the reliable detection of such differences almost impossible.

The results of a carefully designed study may represent the true situation for the particular institution involved. But, how do these results apply to anesthesia as a whole? Essentially, they relate to a sample of patients having anesthesia in one institution. Thus, applicability elsewhere requires considerable argument beyond the empirical facts. The patient population in a large city charity hospital differs from that of an affluent suburban practice. Patients seen in a Veterans Administration hospital differ from those of an obstetrical or a pediatric hospital. Edinburgh is not Boston. Each physician must consider such differences and evaluate for himself how reports of studies performed by others in other settings can be applied to his own practice. This is one reason that physicians prefer more than one clinical trial and multi-institutional studies; they want to broaden the base of the inference.

FUTURE PROGRESS IN ANESTHESIA

Experience with research on different treatments in anesthesia indicates that relatively small gains or losses are to be expected from most studies.[3] Clinical trials must be routinely designed to detect these small differences accurately and reliably. When a systematic study of a new anesthetic treatment is first being considered, it is frequently viewed with great optimism. The investigators may believe that the new procedure will prove to be greatly superior, and preliminary and informal experience may seem to support their position. However, this initial optimism is frequently unwarranted. Careful trials generally seem to show only modest gains, and sometimes the new treatment is demonstrated to be inferior to the standard. A necessary part of the design of any clinical study is to insure sufficient power to detect effects of clinical importance. Just as individual innovations are likely to produce relatively small gains, much of the progress made in any area of anesthesia or any large scale research program will consist of a number of modest gains, each adding to previous results rather than providing one or two revolutionary breakthroughs. Since small gains can easily be negated by small losses if new treatments or modified practices are adopted uncritically, careful unbiased evaluation plays an important role, both in guiding research programs and in documenting their progress. An appreciation of this gradual developmental process will give physicians more realistic expectations for both the time and effort required for progress in anesthesia.

REFERENCES

1. Bunker, J. P., Forrest, W. H., Jr., Mosteller, F., et al.: The National Halothane Study. Bethesda, National Institute of General Medical Sciences, 1969.
2. Owens, W. D., Dykes, M. H. M., Gilbert, J. P., et al.: Development of two indices of postoperative morbidity. Surgery, 77:586, 1975.
3. Gilbert, J. P., McPeek, B., and Mosteller, F.: Progress in surgery and anesthesia—benefits and risks of innovative therapy. *In* Bunker, J. P., Barnes, B. A., Mosteller, F. (eds.): Costs, Risks and Benefits of Surgery. pp. 124-169. New York, Oxford University Press, 1977.
4. McPeek, B., Gilbert, J. P., and Mosteller, F.: The end result: quality of life. *In* Bunker, J. P., Barnes, B. A., and Mosteller, F. (eds.): Costs, Risks and Benefits of Surgery. pp. 170-175. New York, Oxford University Press, 1977.
5. Student: The Lanarkshire milk experiment. Biometrika, 23:398, 1931.

FURTHER READING

Friedman, G. D.: Primer of Epidemiology. New York, McGraw-Hill, 1974.
Gilbert, J. P., McPeek, B., and Mosteller, F.: Statistics and ethics in surgery and anesthesia. Science, *198*:684, 1977.
Gilbert, J. P., McPeek, B., and Mosteller, F.: The clinician's responsibility for helping to improve the treatment of tomorrow's patients. N. Engl. J. Med., *302*:630, 1980.
Hill, A. B.: Principles of Medical Statistics. ed. 9. New York, Oxford University Press, 1971.
Lowrance, W. W.: Of Acceptable Risk. Science and the Determination of Safety. Los Altos, William Kaufmann, 1976.
MacMahon, B., and Pugh, T. F.: Epidemiology Principles and Methods. Boston, Little, Brown & Co., 1970.

Part Two

Preoperative Considerations

3 Complications of Prior Drug Therapy

Lorne G. Eltherington, M.D., Ph.D.

The multiplicity of prescription and over-the-counter drugs consumed by our "pill-oriented" society leads to a high probability of adverse drug reactions and interactions occurring in surgical patients. Most surgical patients receive several drugs during their hospitalization, and it is unusual to find a patient who, during preoperative evaluation, denies taking any drugs. We should not be surprised by the report that approximately 5 per cent of hospitalized patients have an adverse drug reaction, but rather by the fact that it does not occur in *every* surgical patient.[1] Moreover, current anesthetic practice relies upon a combination of drugs, each chosen for a specific purpose, such as anesthesia, muscle relaxation, analgesia, sedation, and possibly amnesia. The probability of a drug interaction occurring varies directly with the number of drugs to which a patient is exposed.

When evaluating a patient's prior drug therapy in terms of anesthetic risk, it is not only the drugs that must be considered but perhaps more importantly, the reason, or reasons, for which the drugs are being taken. For example, the pharmacological considerations for a patient taking nitroglycerin and alpha-methyldopa are not nearly as important as the severity of the coronary artery disease and hypertension for which the medications are taken and how these diseases will alter the response to anesthesia and surgery.

MECHANISMS AND SITES OF DRUG INTERACTION

There are nine commonly accepted mechanisms of drug interaction. For each of the mechanisms, an example follows that relates particularly to anesthetic practice.

Direct Physical or Chemical Interaction

If allowed to contact thiopental in the intravenous tubing, both succinylcholine and meperidine react chemically to form a dense, white precipitate. Also, a physical interaction commonly occurs in the intravenous tubing when whole blood mixes with dextrose solutions; clumping of the red blood cells results.

Interference at Absorption Sites

Drug interactions at absorption sites provide prolonged action and diminish the toxicity of local anesthetics. The small blood vessel vasoconstriction produced by epinephrine retards absorption of local anesthetic into the blood.

Competition at the Plasma Protein Binding Site

Since many drugs bind to plasma proteins, especially the albumin fraction, competition at the plasma protein binding site presents an excellent focus for interaction. If drug A and drug B compete for the same binding site and are given simultaneously, it is obvious that more free drug (unbound A and B) than usual will be present, and toxicity will be more likely to develop. For example, 70 per cent of thiopental is bound to plasma albumin. Patients taking tolbutamide, diazoxide, phenylbutazone, or one of the coumadin anticoagulants that also bind to albumin may show increased sensitivity to thiopental induction, because more thiopental is free in the plasma to produce anesthesia and cardiovascular depression.

Competition at the Receptor Site

Drug competition at receptor sites is best exemplified clinically when atropine and neostigmine are administered to antagonize a nondepolarizing muscle relaxant. The cholinesterase inhibitor allows buildup of acetylcholine at all cholinergic synapses (*i.e.*, muscarinic sites, such as the heart, smooth muscle, and exocrine glands, and nicotinic sites, such as the autonomic ganglia and skeletal neuromuscular junctions). At skeletal muscle receptors, acetylcholine competitively antagonizes the muscle relaxant, while atropine is added to competitively antagonize the acetylcholine buildup at receptors; this buildup would otherwise potentially cause bradycardia, salivary secretions, and increased gastrointestinal motility.

Altered Drug Excretion

Altered drug excretion becomes a possible source of drug interaction in anesthesia when, for example, gallamine, a nondepolarizing muscle relaxant, is administered to patients with reduced renal function. A single dose of the drug, which is almost entirely excreted unchanged in the urine, has been reported to cause markedly prolonged respiratory paralysis in anephric patients.

Altered Acid-Base Balance That Changes the Proportion of Ionized versus Non-ionized Moiety

Altered acid-base balance can, at least theoretically, cause important changes in drug action and toxicity during anesthesia. An interesting example of this problem may occur when a woman in labor receives intramuscular narcotics for pain.

These drugs are weak bases; only the unbound, non-ionized, lipid-soluble moiety can cross the blood-brain barrier to provide analgesia and produce respiratory depression; and it is only this form that can also pass a maternal-placental barrier to cause fetal depression. The weak narcotic base in maternal plasma is exposed to an increasing *p*H (due to alkalosis induced by hyperventilation) and becomes more non-ionized (lipid soluble). Thus, hyperventilation by the mother can increase both analgesic and toxic actions of the drug. (See Fig. 43-1.)

Accelerated and Inhibited Drug Metabolism

Both acceleration and inhibition of drug metabolism by previously administered agents can lead to an altered activity of anesthetic drugs. Patients chronically receiving an enzyme-inducer, such as phenobarbital, may be better able to metabolize halothane and thus produce a greater quantity of metabolites that some researchers have speculated can cause hepatic toxicity. Likewise, patients taking liver-enzyme inhibitors, such as monoamine oxidase or cholinesterase inhibitors may develop increased sensitivity to meperidine and succinycholine.

Physiologic Changes and Homeostatic Alterations

Drugs that produce physiologic changes, such as reduced renal blood flow, and homeostatic alterations, such as blockade of reflex cardiovascular pathways, may result in increased anesthetic morbidity and mortality. Propranolol, a competitive beta-adrenergic-receptor-blocking drug may predispose patients to develop heart failure by decreasing reflex sympathetic stimulation of heart rate and contractility. However, this same action may be beneficial for patients in borderline heart failure.

DOSE-RESPONSE AND TIME-ACTION

Prior drug therapy may alter a patient's response to anesthesia in three major ways: *depression of homeostatic reflex responses; prolongation and/or intensification of anesthetic drug action; shortening and/or diminution of anes-*

thetic drug action. The latter may occur, for example, in patients who are receiving chronic anti-anxiety therapy. The patients are likely to obtain less sleep and anxiety relief from pheno-barbital premedication because of increased activity of drug-metabolizing enzymes in the liver. The consequences of shortening and/or diminishing the effect of drugs used in the perioperative period may be viewed simply as a shift to the right of a dose-response curve (Fig. 3-1, Curve 2) and a decrease in area under the time-action curve (Fig. 3-2, Curve 2). This occurrence is not likely to be harmful to the patient. However, depression of homeostatic reflex responses and prolongation or intensification of anesthetic drug action may theoretically lead to serious morbidity and even

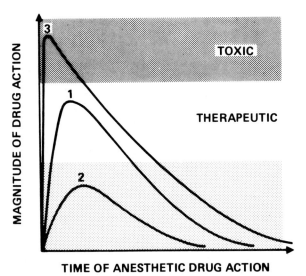

TIME OF ANESTHETIC DRUG ACTION

Fig. 3-2. These schematic time-action curves illustrate the influence that prior drug therapy may have on anesthetic drug effects. Curve 1 might represent a single bolus of morphine injected during induction of balanced anesthesia. A shift to Curve 3 is elicited in a patient who is receiving a monoamine oxidase inhibitor, whereas Curve 2 might represent a patient who chronically uses narcotics.

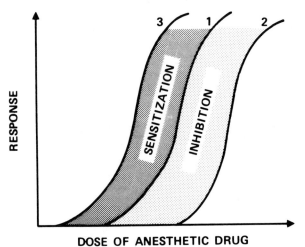

DOSE OF ANESTHETIC DRUG

Fig. 3-1. These schematic dose-response curves illustrate the influence of prior drug therapy on anesthetic drug action. Curve 1 represents the normal relationship between a drug used during surgery and the response to that drug. A shift to Curve 3 occurs when, for example, a patient using anticholinesterase eye drops for glaucoma receives succinylcholine. The inhibition of cholinesterase markedly sensitizes the patient to the muscle-relaxing action of succinylcholine. Prolonged apnea may occur in this circumstance. Curve 2 shows a shift to the right or inhibited drug response that occurs in a patient receiving propranolol who also is given isoproterenol or dopamine to increase cardiac output during anesthesia. The patient requires higher than normal rates of inotropic drug infusion, certainly not a problem as long as the competitive nature of the propranolol-isoproterenol interaction is understood.

mortality. Fortunately, the problems that arise from these responses usually lead to serious complications only when they are unsuspected or poorly treated.

Curve 3 in Figures 3-1 and 3-2 represents the response of a patient whose preanesthetic history includes drug therapy causing increased susceptibility to anesthetic drugs. That is, a displacement of the dose-response curve to the left and increased area under the time-action curve are observed. The mechanism of this sensitization might be represented by one of the drug interactions discussed on page 26. For example, prior therapy of glaucoma with echothiophate (Phospholine) eye drops, combined with muscle relaxation produced by succinylcholine, may result in prolonged apnea. Echothiophate, an anticholinesterase, blocks plasma pseudocholinesterase, the enzyme responsible for rapid breakdown of succinylcholine. This is an example of a drug interaction that results from inhibition of drug metabolism.

Prior drug therapy may also influence a patient's anesthetic course and management by drug depression of a homeostatic reflex defense mechanism that the patient would normally use as a protection against anesthetic and surgical "stress." For example, chronic use of adrenocortical steroids suppresses the response of the adrenal cortex to stress and, although very rare, the anesthetized patient can develop profound hypotension correctable only by pharmacological doses of intravenous steroids.

SELECTED DRUG INTERACTIONS

The Boston Collaborative Comprehensive Drug Surveillance Study indicated that each patient receives, on the average, nine different drugs during a hospitalization.[1] A study by May in 1977 supports this conclusion and suggests further that antihypertensive and anticoagulant drugs are responsible for the highest incidence of adverse drug reactions.[2] Thus, each patient is subjected to a considerable risk of drug interactions, as well as adverse drug effects. Although most adverse responses to drugs are transient and of minor consequence, about 3 per cent of patients experience life-threatening reactions.[3] Among the most common reactions are arrhythmia, central nervous system (CNS) depression, fluid overload, and hemorrhage. Table 3-1 lists some of the drugs administered to or taken by patients who undergo surgery, grouped according to major pharmacological classification. These drugs may elicit a broad range of adverse responses, ranging from those of doubtful clinical significance to life-threatening reactions. Several potentially serious drug interactions are discussed in more detail in the remainder of this chapter.

CARDIAC GLYCOSIDES

A constantly increasing proportion of elderly people in the population engenders an increasing prevalence of heart disease. Many patients who undergo surgery take cardiac glycosides (digitalis) for the management of atrial tachyarrhythmias and congestive heart failure (CHF). Changes in the patient's sensitivity to digitalis brought about by anesthesia and surgery are prime considera-

tions. Various factors are known to modify digitalis tolerance,[4] and anesthetic management should avoid as many of these as possible. However, patients may be over- or under-digitalized, taking diuretics that compound the potassium loss produced by digitalis, and, worst of all, their surgery may be so urgent that there is insufficient time to assess and remedy these abnormalities.

More important than the pharmacological considerations in a patient taking digitalis are the problems of managing a patient with heart disease who takes digitalis for *symptomatic relief* of CHF. Two recent papers by Goldberg,[5] and Stevens,[6] plus a thought-provoking editorial by Hamilton,[7] have greatly helped to clarify the important anesthetic considerations for patients with "sick hearts." These investigators stress that reducing myocardial work and, consequently, myocardial oxygen demand during anesthesia are of utmost importance. Since oxygen delivery to the heart is flow-limited, it makes more sense to reduce the oxygen demand, afterload, heart rate, and contractility than to attempt to increase the supply. Thus, careful blood pressure reduction and myocardial depression by agents like halothane may be very practical for patients with heart disease, especially that due to coronary artery insufficiency.

Deutsch and Dalen have recommended that all surgical patients with clinical, electrocardiographic (ECG), or radiologic evidence of organic heart disease receive prophylactic digitalis, even in the absence of heart failure.[8] This stand is strongly disputed by Selzer, who suggests that the classical concept of "digitalization" in patients who are not in CHF or do not show digitalis-sensitive arrhythmias is virtually meaningless, for no therapeutic end points are available.[9] A recent attempt by Joubert to compare serum digoxin concentrations with ECG variables revealed that correlation of serum digoxin with either clinical effect or toxicity is poor and, further, that quantitation of digitalis effect, even in the presence of CHF, is difficult, to say nothing of quantitation when failure is not present.[10] Also, Nies has warned that digitalis, more than most drugs, must be used in doses necessary to reach a predetermined goal or end point.[11] Using conven-

(Text continues on page 38.)

Table 3-1. Selected Drug Interactions

Prior Drug Therapy	Complications	Prevention, Treatment or Significance	References
Autonomic and Cardiovascular Drugs			
Anticholinesterases			
Ecothiophate eye drops (Phospholine)	Prolonged apnea with succinylcholine due to plasma pseudocholinesterase inhibition	Change to pilocrapine eye drops 4 weeks prior to surgery, or avoid succinylcholine.	52
Organophosphate insecticide exposure (e.g., Parathion)	Same as above	Avoid succinylcholine in patients with potential exposure (e.g., farm workers).	53
Alkylating anticancer drugs (Cytoxan)	Same as above	Avoid succinylcholine.	54 55
Oral contraceptives	Serum cholinesterase deficiency, reported during pregnancy, might occur with chronic oral contraceptive use.	Of doubtful clinical significance	56
Antihypertensive Drugs			
Postganglionic, presynpatic blockade Clondine (Catapres) Guanethidine (Ismelin) Methyldopa (Aldomet) Reserpine (Serpasil and other rauwolfia alkaloids)	All cause release and/or replacement of norepinephrine by a false neurotransmitter. Complete blockade does not occur with reserpine or the other drugs of this class, probably due to incomplete "sympathectomy." The minimal alveolar concentration (MAC) for halothane, and by implication other general anesthetics, may be lowered by these drugs.	Continue antihypertensive therapy up to the time of surgery. Intraoperative hypotension is treated as usual by decreasing the anesthetic dose and increasing fluid administration. Untreated hypertensives or those taken off medication before anesthesia may show very labile swings in blood pressure during anesthesia due to depleted plasma volume. All anesthetics should be carefully titrated in these patients, and hypertension vigorously treated with nitroprusside, nitroglycerin, or phentolamine and increased anesthetic dosage.	16 17 18 57
Alpha-adrenergic receptor blackade Phenoxybenzamine (Dibenzyine) Prazosin (Minipress)	May accentuate the cardiovascular depression of anesthetic agents due to blunting of the sympathetic nervous system (SNS) and might be	Low dose competitive and high dose noncompetitive blocking action (nonequilibrium block). Prazosin, unlike other alpha blockers, acts only on post-	53

(Continued)

Table 3-1. Selected Drug Interactions *(Continued)*

Prior Drug Therapy	Complications	Prevention, Treatment or Significance	References
Autonomic and Cardiovascular Drugs *Antihypertensive Drugs* (Continued)	desirable in some diseases (e.g., pheochromocytoma, thyroid storm, and cardiac disease).	synaptic receptors, diminishing the incidence of accompanying tachycardia.	
Phentolamine (Regitine)	Short-acting, expensive, and causes persistent tachycardia. Immediate blood pressure effect is due to a direct vasodilator action on vascular muscle and not adrenergic blockade.	A competitive block that may be antagonized by norephinephrine and other alpha-receptor agonists.	
Beta-adrenergic receptor blockade Propranolol (Inderal) Nadolol (Corgard) Timolol (Timoptic) Metoprolol (Lopressor)	Chronic therapy diminishes cardiac reserve due to blunted SNS activity. The drug produces direct, quinidine-like myocardial depression *only* in doses much greater than those needed for beta-receptor blockade. If the SNS is essential as a secondary compensation for congestive heart failure, propranolol will worsen the failure. Acute administration can cause bronchospasm and/or severe bradycardia and will intensify congestive heart failure.	Continue administration of the drug until just prior to anesthesia. Reduction of SNS activity, except when it is required to support a failing heart, is an excellent therapy for a "sick" heart. Isoproterenol or dopamine infusion should easily counteract any residual beta-receptor blockade during or after anesthesia.	18 24 25 26 33
Beta-adrenergic receptor facilitation Hydralazine (Apresoline) Chlorpromazine (Thorazine)	May exaggerate intraoperative hypotension due to anesthetic agents, but of doubtful clinical significance, except in the case of high doses of chlorpromazine.	Continue these drugs until surgery. Propranolol will block the cardiovascular actions of both drugs. Consequently, they have been called beta-mimetics.	53
Diuretics Hydrochlorothiazide (e.g., Esidrix) Furosemide (Lasix) Ethacrynic acid (Edecrin)	May cause hypovolemia with reduced total body potassium, even in the face of normo- or hyperkalemia, metabolic alkalosis, cardiac arrhythmias, and hypotension; may enhance nondepolarizing neuromuscular block; and, may	Low serum K+ and postural hypotension require KCl and volume replacement prior to anesthesia. KCl may be given at 40–60 mmol.(mEq.)/L./hr. with ECG and central venous pressure monitoring. In an emergency, give a 2-mmol.	58 59 60 61 62

Table 3-1. Selected Drug Interactions *(Continued)*

Prior Drug Therapy	Complications	Prevention, Treatment or Significance	References
Autonomic and Cardiovascular Drugs			
Antihypertensive Drugs (Continued)	produce coma in patients taking lithium, which competes with potassium intracellularly, increasing lithium toxity.	(mEq.) intravenous bolus of KC1 every 5 minutes to treat cardiac arrhythmias.	
Other drugs Pargyline (Eutonyl)	Introduced as an antihypertensive but used more as antidepressant (see *CNS Drugs*).	Should be discontinued at least 2 weeks prior to surgery.	57
Vasoconstrictor Drugs Ergotamine (Ergotrate)	Chronic therapy for migraine may lead to hypovolemia by virtue of systemic vasoconstriction.	Examine for signs of hypovolemia, such as postural hypotension and altered Valsalva response.	
Sympathomimetic amines (amphetamine)	Drugs used for weight reduction or abused for other reasons may cause hypovolemia (as above). Also shown to increase the MAC for halothane (see *Abused Drugs*).	Use all anesthetic drugs in carefully titrated doses.	
Cardiac Glycosides Digoxin	Causes hypokalemia alone, which is intensified by diuretics and intraoperative fluid shifts. Severe cardiac arrhythmias may occur. Preoperative, prophylactic use is dangerous, for no endpoints of "digitalization" are available.	Continue administration to fasting time prior to anesthesia. Do not give prophylactically prior to surgery. Serum K^+ below 3 mmol. (mEq.)/L. should be treated with 40-60 mmol. (mEq.)/L. of I.V. fluid per hour of anesthesia, with ECG monitoring, depending upon deficit. Any patient on chronic diuretic therapy, even though he is normokalemic or hyperkalemic, should be suspected of having reduced intracellular potassium and therefore may be more sensitive to digitalis arrhythmias. Cardiac arrhythmias during anesthesia may be treated by a 2-mmol.(mEq.) bolus injection of KCl as required or propranolol, 0.5 mg., I.V., every 2 minutes, up to 5 mg. total dose.	5 12 60 63

(Continued)

Table 3-1. Selected Drug Interactions *(Continued)*

PRIOR DRUG THERAPY	COMPLICATIONS	PREVENTION, TREATMENT OR SIGNIFICANCE	REFERENCES
Autonomic and Cardiovascular Drugs			
Antiarrhythmic Drugs			
Quinidine	All increase the duration of experimental nonpolarizing neuromuscular block. Quinidine also may poteniate succinylcholine.	Probably not clinically significant. Anticholinesterases may not antagonize the block.	64
Procaineamide (Pronestyl)			
Disopyramide (Norpace)			65
Phentoin (Dilantin)			
Propranolol (Inderal)	(See *Adrenergic Receptor Blockade.*)		
Nadolol (Corgard)			
Lidocaine (Xylocaine)			
Anticoagulants			
Heparin	Avoid regional anesthesia and reverse for surgery of brain and eye and surgery involving large raw surfaces. Reversal may cause a hypercoagulable state.	A protamine titration should be used to reverse heparin, since excess protamine may cause bleeding, and rapid injection may cause hypotension.	66 67
Oral agents	As above. Acute administration of barbiturates may theoretically displace coumarins from plasma albumin binding sites and cause bleeding. This possibility has not been documented. Likewise, chronic phenobarbital use elicits induction of coumarin-metabolizing enzymes in the liver. Stopping barbiturate use around the time of surgery would not cause increased blood levels of coumarins (and thus increased risk of bleeding), since it takes 1–2 weeks before dissipation of the inducing effect.	May be reversed in hours by intravenous vitamin K_1, the dose varying with the degree of reversal desired and the degree of anticoagulation present. Old banked blood will cause immediate coumarin reversal, for it contains the four stable factors of the prothrombin complex.	
Warfarin (Coumadin)			
Dicoumarol			
CNS Drugs			
Sedative Hypnotics			
Long-acting barbiturates (phenobarbital)	Chronic barbiturate use causes induction of hepatic drug-metabolizing enzymes that may cause an increase in metabolites of halogenated anesthetics. This may increase the risk of liver damage if the metabolites prove to be hepatic toxins or sensitizers. The benzodiazepines and sedative antihistaminics have been	Clinical significance is uncertain	68
Benzodiazepines			
Diazepam (Valium)			
Antihistaminics			
Hydroxyzine (Visteril)			

Table 3-1. Selected Drug Interactions *(Continued)*

Prior Drug Therapy	Complications	Prevention, Treatment or Significance	References
CNS Drugs			
Sedative Hypnotics (Continued)	reported to cause sensitization to coumarin anticoagulants by an unknown mechanism and may theoretically cause bleeding in anticoagulated patients. Premedication for anxiety may require higher than usual doses of sedative hypnotics. High dose, chronic use-abuse of this group may lead to withdrawal problems.		
Alcohol	The acute alcoholic usually has a full stomach from alcohol-induced gastric secretions and food. The chronic alcoholic may be hyponatremic, malnourished, and hypovolemic; depressed liver function may cause hypoalbuminemia and reduced plasma binding and metabolism of drugs. Decreased binding and hypovolemia-induced lowered volume of distribution may sensitize the patient to anesthetic drugs, but alcoholics are usually resistant.	Administer 30 ml. of antacid, preoxygenate, and use a rapid sequence induction with cricoid pressure. Awake intubation is usually difficult because the patients are uncooperative. Titrate all drugs carefully in the chronic alcoholic because of multiple factors that tend to both increase and decrease drug effects. Using a technique that allows at least 50% inspired oxygen will provide some compensation for the probable decreased tissue oxygen delivery from anemia, reduced blood volume, and shunting by way of AV malformations (spiders).	69 70 71 72
Antipsychotics Phenothiazine tranquilizers Chlorpromazine (Thorazine) Butyrophenone tranquilizers Haloperidol (Haldol)	May cause postural hypotension through alpha-adrenergic receptor blockade. The agents also cause beta-adrenergic receptor stimulation. Use of epinephrine or isoproterenol during anesthesia is expected to cause increased cardiac stimulation and peripheral vasodilatation. Institutionalized patients receiving large doses may show marked hypotension during general anesthesia.	Continue administration up to time of surgery. Beta-adrenergic stimulation, hypotension, and tachycardia are blocked by propranolol. Hypotension may be effectively treated by alpha-adrenergic agonists.	73

(Continued)

Table 3-1. Selected Drug Interactions *(Continued)*

Prior Drug Therapy	Complications	Prevention, Treatment or Significance	References
CNS Drugs			
Antipsychotics			
Lithium (Lithane)	Causes sodium retention and thus an increased intravascular volume, threatening congestive heart failure in those with limited reserve. T wave depression is seen without evidence of cardiac dysfunction.	Heart failure may be treated with digitalis or other inotropes without discontinuing lithium. Lithium potentiates the actions of pancuronium, succinylcholine, and decamethonium in dogs, but not curare or gallamine. Therefore, a nerve stimulator should be used in order to rationally give muscle relaxants to patients taking lithium. Also, since it has been demonstrated that the drug enhances morphine analgesia and barbiturate or diazepam sleeping times in mice, more care than usual should be taken when giving *any drug* to patients receiving lithium.	62
Antidepressants			
Tricyclics			
Amitriptyline (Elavil)	Problems similar to phenothiazine tranquilizers. They also block norepinephrine re-uptake into nerve endings, thus sensitizing the myocardium. Chronic use may reduce cardiac reserve.	Patients on chronic therapy usually have little problem with anesthesia. Continue administration of the drug to the fasting time prior to surgery. Therapeutic effects of the drugs (2–3 weeks) far outlast its presence in serum. (Half-life of nortryptyline is 15–90 hours.)	76
Monoamine oxidase inhibitors

Hydrazine type phenelzine (Nardil)

Non-hydrazine type tranylcypromine (Parnate) | Besides inhibiting monoamine oxidase (MAO), they inhibit enzymes which metabolize sedative-hypnotics, narcotics, and tranquillizers. Death or coma has followed the use of meperidine in patients using MAO drugs. The potentially lethal sensitization is probably due to a central action of MAO inhibition to increasing serotonin levels. Sympathomimetic amines, especially ephedrine and metaraminol, are markedly potentiated. | If possible, switch to tricyclics at least 3 weeks prior to surgery. If not possible, give much smaller doses of all CNS depressants and consider regional techniques. Avoid all indirectly acting sympathomimetics, and use norepinephrine or phenylephrine. Probably, it is best to avoid narcotics, especially meperidine and morphine. | 76
77
78
79 |

Table 3-1. Selected Drug Interactions *(Continued)*

Prior Drug Therapy	Complications	Prevention, Treatment or Significance	References
CNS Drugs			
Anticonvulsant Drugs			
Phenytoin (Dilantin)	(See *Antiarrhythmic Drugs*.)	Continue administration up to the fasting time before surgery to minimize the possibility of withdrawal seizures. It is wise to use phenobarbital for sleep and premedication, since it is a very good anticonvulsant drug, and to avoid use of enflurane.	80
Phenobarbital	(See *Sedative-hypnotic Drugs*.)		
Other anticonvulsants	No known interaction with anesthetic drugs		
Anti-Parkinsonism Drugs			
Levodopa	Cardiac contractility is increased for 2 hours following a 1–2 g. oral maintenance dose. Patients may have postural hypotension during early therapy, may be more sensitive to the hypotensive effects of anesthesia and blood loss, and may be more sensitive to myocardial sensitization resulting from halothane or cyclopropane. Both phenothiazines and butyrophenones, even as premedicants, may antagonize dopamine and aggravate the disease. Many patients taking L-dopa have arteriosclerotic vascular disease and vital organ compromise that are of far greater importance with regard to anesthetic risk than the possibility of the drug itself causing problems.	Propranolol will block arrhythmias should they occur. Avoid phenothiazines and butyrophenones, which may cause extrapyramidal symptons. Continue use of the drug up to time of surgery. Chronic clinical doses of 1–2 g. usually do not affect blood pressure or heart rate. If patients receiving L-dopa also take a decarboxylase inhibitor, such as carbidopa which does not cross the blood-brain barrier, L-dopa will be converted to its active form, dopamine, only in the brain where it acts and not in the periphery where it elicits toxicity.	76 81
Endocrines			
Adrenocortical Steroids	Traditional belief is that chronic steroid therapy, even for only a week during the year prior to surgery, will cause depression of the adrenal cortex and predispose the patient to "stress-induced" (caused by anesthesia and surgery) hypotension, shock, and even death. Sudden increase in steroid dosage may lead to delayed wound healing, in-	Suggested premedication consists of cortisone acetate, 100 mg, I.M., at bedtime, and hydrocortisone, 100 mg. parenterally, 1 hour before anesthesia, and every 6 hours thereafter for 12–24 hours. There is *no* relationship between prior steroid therapy, plasma cortisol levels during surgery, and response of the adrenal cortex to ACTH. *No* pre-	42 43 48 82

(Continued)

Table 3-1. Selected Drug Interactions *(Continued)*

Prior Drug Therapy	Complications	Prevention, Treatment or Significance	References
Endocrines			
Adrenocortical Steroids (Continued)	fection, exacerbation of hypertension, and extension of venous thrombosis.	operative steroids are recommended, but I.V. hydrocortisone is used to treat *unexplained* intraoperative hypotension unresponsive to fluid administration and anesthesia dose-reduction.	
Drugs for Diabetes Insulin	Anesthetic risk relates to coronary and cerebral vascular disease primarily. Very high blood sugar may result in an osmotic diuresis with resultant hypovolemia, hyponatremia, and hypokalemia. On the other hand, the CNS manifestations of hypoglycemia are masked by general anesthesia.	Ketosis-prone diabetics should be admitted to the hospital at least 2 days prior to surgery. Mature onset, ketosis-resistant diabetics may be treated much like any other patient in terms of admission and premedication, except for blood sugar testing 1 hour prior to surgery. Striving for exact blood sugar control in these patients over the short perioperative period is not rational and may predispose to hypoglycemia, much more dangerous than mild hyperglycemia.	49
Oral hypoglycemic drugs Chlorpropamide (Diabinase) Tolbutamide (Orinase)	Hypoglycemia may occur up to 60 hours following the last dose. Predisposing factors include starvation, and renal and hepatic failure. The hypoglycemia may mimic a cerebrovascular accident in the elderly.	Patients should be followed with frequent blood sugar measurements, and if insulin is required only short-acting preparations should be used.	83
Oral Contraceptives	(See *Anticholinesterases*.) Metabolism of meperidine and promazine is impaired, and other drug metabolism may be similarly affected.	CNS depressants may have prolonged action.	84 85 86
Chemotherapeutic Agents *Antimicrobial Drugs* Polymyxins, colistins, lincomycin, tetracycline and clindamycin	Cause neuromuscular block by themselves. Both depolarizing and nondepolarizing blocks may be prolonged and intensified.	Not antagonized by calcium; neostigmine will worsen the block, except perhaps with lincomycin.	87 88

Table 3-1. Selected Drug Interactions *(Continued)*

Prior Drug Therapy	Complications	Prevention, Treatment or Significance	References
Chemotheraprutic Agents			
Antimicrobial Drugs			
Streptomycin, neomycin, viomycin, kanamycin, gentamicin	As above	Both neostigmine and calcium may antagonize the block; sodium bicarbonate will antagonize a neomycin block.	89 90
Penicillins, chloramphenicol, erythromcin, cephalosporins, bacitracin, rifampin, ristocetin, vancomycin	Not shown to cause or increase neuromuscular block		
Penicillins and carbenicillin	Cause hypokalemic alkalosis by acting as nonreabsorbable anions	Same problems and precautions as with the diuretics	91
Gentamycin, kanamycin, tetracycline	Severe nephrotoxicity when patients receive methoxyflurane	Avoid methoxyflurane in these patients	92
Anticancer Drugs			
Alkalating agents (Cytoxan)	(See *Anticholinesterases*.)	Monitor the effect of neuromuscular agents with a nerve stimulator.	93
Nitrogen mustards (thio-TEPA)	May cause or potentiate nondepolarizing neuromuscular blockade		
Abused Drugs			
Alcohol	(See *CNS Drugs*.)	(See *CNS Drugs*.)	
Narcotics	These patients have a high prevalence of hepatitis and diminished hepato-renal function; therefore drugs that depend upon hepatic metabolism and renal excretion may have prolonged effect. Heroin users who have recently had a dose and who require emergency surgery are an especially difficult problem. They often have large ventilation-perfusion mismatch and increased pulmonary extravascular water due to capillary leak and adult respiratory distress syndrome.	Use general anesthesia, preferably a balanced technique to prevent withdrawal during surgery. Halogenated agents may confuse the etiology of postoperative hepatitis. Potent inhalation agents may be used when pulmonary dysfunction demands high inspired oxygen. It is very important to establish a timed dosage schedule for these patients postoperatively and not to attempt tapering or withdrawal. These patients fully monitored and have several large intravenous lines, using internal and external jugular placement and/or peripheral cutdowns. All drugs should be carefully titrated, as there are no "usual doses" for this group of patients.	95 72

(Continued)

Table 3-1. Selected Drug Interactions *(Continued)*

Prior Drug Therapy	Complications	Prevention, Treatment or Significance	References
Abused Drugs			
CNS Stimulants			
Cocaine	Increases halothane MAC in dogs and sensitizes the heart to halothane and endogenous catecholamines. Nasal application results in detectable plasma levels for 6 hours. Sympathetic stimulation from chronic use may be associated with diminished plasma volume and resultant hypotension during anesthesia.	Avoid "light" anesthesia to reduce the possibility of cardiac arrhythmias.	95 96
Amphetamines	MAC is increased, probably due to catecholamine depletion in the CNS. The same process occurring in the periphery with chronic use may result in blunted SNS activity, thus accentuating the effects of hypovolmeia.	Carefully evaluate the patient's volume status, and aggressively replace fluid losses. As with other drug abuse, a high hepatitis incidence makes halothane a secondary choice (see *Narcotics*).	97
Cannabinoids	Reduction in halothane MAC, cholinesterase inhibition, and liver enzyme induction occur in animals. Excessive smoking eventually causes obstructive airway disease. A dose-related increase in heart rate is blocked by propranolol, suggesting a sympathomimetic action on the heart.	Acute episodic use is probably without clinical significance. Chronic abusers *may be* more susceptible to anesthetic agents, since cannabinoids have several pharmacological properties of sedative-hypnotic drugs.	98

tional "digitalizing doses" has resulted in a 20-per-cent incidence of toxicity in hospitalized patients.[11]

A primary concern regarding digitalized patients is their total body potassium, especially the intracellular–extracellular ratio. Many patients receiving digitalis for CHF also take diuretics, even though Nies has cautioned that diuretics should be used only when maximum effect has been achieved from digitalis alone, and signs and symptoms of volume overload, such as *severe* peripheral edema, ascites, dyspnea on exertion, or paroxysmal nocturnal dyspnea, are still present.[11]

Digitalis itself causes depletion of intracellular potassium by inhibition of the sodium pump, increase in intracellular sodium, and movement of potassium out of the cell to maintain a normal electrical gradient across the cardiac cell membrane. The potassium loss produced by a diuretic may greatly contribute to the loss of cardiac cell potassium caused by digitalis. This loss may be 1 to 10 mmol. (10 mEq.) per kg., even in the face of normal or elevated serum potassium.[12] This depletion makes patients very susceptible to digitalis toxicity, manifested by cardiac arrhythmias and, infrequently, increasing CHF.

A digitalized patient scheduled for emergency surgery and showing signs and symptoms of CHF should be evaluated carefully to be reasonably sure that the failure is not due to digitalis toxicity, a poorly appreciated aspect of digitalis overdose. Administration of additional cardiac glycoside to the patient who is receiving digitalis and who is still in mild CHF preoperatively is somewhat controversial. It is the author's belief that before he is given digitalis, the patient should be visited by an empathetic anesthesiologist who explains the details of the proposed anesthetic, surgery, and postoperative course, after which a reasonable dose of anti-anxiety drug (e.g., pentobarbital, 1.5–2 mg./kg., or diazepam, 10–20 mg.) may be administered. This preoperative sequence will often calm the patient sufficiently to reduce sympathoadrenal activity, so that myocardial work is decreased and additional digitalis becomes unnecessary.

The widely held notion that anesthesia is a "stress," especially to the heart, is open to some question. Hamilton suggests that anesthesia is a relatively non-stressful event and, in fact, actually protects a patient from the stress of surgery.[7] For example, Theye showed that halothane anesthesia decreases the oxygen consumption of the heart and other organs.[13] These organs then require less blood flow and therefore less cardiac output to maintain a normal state of cellular metabolism. Recently, Bland and Lowenstein showed that halothane, in the absence of CHF, favorably influences the relationship between myocardial oxygen need and supply in dogs.[14] These results point out that *perhaps* lowered blood pressure and myocardial depression, as produced by halothane, *may* be desirable. That is, halothane should improve CHF by reducing myocardial work and thereby lowering cardiac demand for oxygen. The data also suggest that the common use of morphine-oxygen relaxant techniques for coronary artery bypass grafting and the use of a balanced anesthetic for very sick patients are less desirable than halothane and enflurane which are associated with more hypotension. For very sick patients, especially those with coronary artery disease, the most rational anesthetic management may be one that produces a controllable degree of cardiac depression.

Overt CHF in the operating room is sometimes treated with a small dose of intravenous digoxin, which has an onset within 30 minutes and a peak effect in 2 hours. A more rational therapy for acute failure developing during anesthesia is the infusion of a short-acting inotropic agent such as dopamine and dobutamine or, as a second choice, isoproterenol. Glucagon is also useful when failure is present together with cardiac arrhythmias that may be due to digitalis toxicity.[4] The second-to-second control provided by a dopamine infusion alone or with an isoproterenol infusion (providing venous constriction and increased preload, decreased total peripheral resistance and decreased afterload, maintenance of renal perfusion and increased contractility) allows excellent regulation of failure during the unstable surgical and postoperative period. Once the patient receives adequate pain control and achieves hemodynamic and respiratory stability postoperatively, digitalis can be slowly and carefully administered as needed. In this relatively stable situation, fluctuations in serum potassium levels will be minimized and much more controllable than, for example, during cardiopulmonary bypass; however, potassium should certainly be administered intraoperatively if required.

It is the author's contention that prophylactic digitalis is *not* indicated prior to anesthesia unless the patient is in CHF. Should signs of CHF appear during anesthesia, the failure is rationally treated with short-acting, titratable, cardiotonic drugs. In the postoperative period, should failure continue or return, digitalis may be started slowly and carefully, with dose and frequency determined by the patient's individual response to well-defined treatment goals.

ANTIHYPERTENSIVE DRUGS

The 1963 review by Alper, Flacke, and Krayer concludes that chronic reserpine medication for the control of hypertension need not be discontinued prior to anesthesia, since there is only a slight danger that hemodynamic depression will be caused by the drug; and, this hypotension may be treated easily, should it occur during anesthesia.[15] This conclusion has been confirmed and extended by Katz[16] and Ominsky and Wollman[17] to include other antihypertensive agents, except for mono-amine oxidase inhibitors (MAOI), which are seldom used, and perhaps beta-adrenergic blocking drugs.

Föex and Prys-Roberts performed elegant studies on the effects of anesthetic agents on the hypertensive patient. The studies culminated in a 1974 review.[18] They conclude that pharmacological considerations of prior antihypertensive therapy, except for MAOI and propranolol-like drugs, should not present a problem during anesthesia. Also, ischemic heart disease and depressed myocardial performance often associated with hypertension should be major considerations. Geer and Greenhow stress that untreated or poorly controlled hypertensive patients experience large and potentially dangerous blood pressure variations during and after anesthesia.[19] Unfortunately, some physicians (usually not anesthesiologists) still recommend discontinuation of antihypertensive treatment several days prior to surgery.[20]

Intraoperative hypotension occurring in patients on antihypertensive therapy who show diminished myocardial work, such as that which occurs during halothane anesthesia, should be well tolerated as long as lowered diastolic pressure does not seriously compromise coronary blood flow. What level of hypotension is tolerable? Certainly ECG monitoring is essential, and ischemia-induced changes of S-T segments should not be permitted. Cerebral perfusion is another problem, because many hypertensive patients have generalized occlusive vascular disease. Again, an anesthetic agent such as halothane, which lowers brain oxygen consumption (CMR_{O_2}), will allow considerable lowering of cerebral blood flow (CBF) without brain damage. As a practical matter, the intraoperative blood pressure of hypertensive patients with signs and symptoms of cerebral vascular disease should probably be maintained at a level no lower than 80 per cent of the usual value. Patients with ischemic heart disease should be treated as described above.

If therapy becomes necessary for the control of intraoperative hypotension in a chronically hypertensive patient, it should be based upon the usual differential diagnoses, such as anesthetic overdose, blood loss, volume depletion, reflexes, position, and surgical manipulation. As a last resort, or in an acute situation as other corrective steps are being taken, a pressor drug should be given. Ephedrine is an excellent choice, since it has both vasoconstrictor and inotropic properties.

Hypertensive episodes during anesthesia may be treated with drugs, after excluding hypoxia, hypercardia, hyperthermia, and light anesthesia as likely causes. Sodium nitroprusside has become very popular as a potent, finely controllable agent used to decrease blood pressure. The author feels that it is the drug of choice for treating hypertensive episodes during anesthesia (see Chap. 48). A recent report on intravenous nitroglycerin suggests that it causes more reduction in left ventricular filling pressure (preload) for a given blood pressure decrease (afterload) than does sodium nitroprusside.[21] Phentolamine and chlorpromazine are also used to treat hypertension, but they cannot be regulated as precisely as sodium nitroprusside or, perhaps, nitroglycerin, which show a rapid onset and ultrashort action. Ganglionic blocking drugs such as trimethaphan and pentolinium have fallen into disuse since the rediscovery of sodium nitroprusside, but they are still practical drugs for intraoperative control of hypertension as well as procedures requiring deliberate hypotension (See Chap. 48).

BETA-ADRENERGIC RECEPTOR ANTAGONISTS

Propranolol, the most widely administered beta-adrenergic receptor antagonist in the United States, is used to treat a wide variety of diseases and syndromes, including ischemic heart disease, hypertension, cardiac arrhythmias, thyrotoxicosis, pheochromocytoma, obstructive cardiomyopathy, and simple anxiety, among many others.[22] The primary mechanism of drug action is competitive antagonism at beta-adrenergic receptors of endogenous sympathomimetic amines, especially those mediating increases in heart rate and myocardial contractility. It is not established that all therapeutic effects of propranolol are a consequence of beta-receptor blockade, but the effects on the heart most likely are a result of this. The nonspecific "quinidine-like" myocardial depression of propranolol requires concentrations two or three times higher than those needed for beta-receptor blockade.[23] When endogenous sympathetic tone of dogs is eliminated by epidural block, propranolol has no depressant effect on cardiac function in doses that cause profound beta-receptor blockade.[24] Prys-Roberts has confirmed this finding in humans: ". . . propranolol may impair the contractile state of the heart when the comparison is made with the enhanced state of the innervated heart . . . but the final contractile state is no more depressed than that of the denervated heart."[25]

An understanding of the pharmacological action and pharmacokinetic properties of propranolol allows continuation of therapy with this drug up to the time of surgery. A report from the Cleveland Clinic suggests that the duration of the effect of propranolol may persist for several days after discontinuing administration of the drug, and that it compromises the cardiac reserve of patients undergoing routine cardiac surgery.[26] This has made many anesthesiologists somewhat apprehensive when patients undergo surgery only 24 to 48 hours after discontinuing propanolol use, as suggested by Coltant.[27] Data from Kaplan suggest that the apprehension is unnecessary and perhaps irrational.[28] In fact, continuing propranolol up to the time of surgery may be excellent premedication for patients with "sick hearts." Of major importance in this context is that the drug is a competitive antagonist. This means that, should evidence of unexpected myocardial depression occur during anesthesia or in the postoperative period, isoproterenol or other beta-receptor agonists will reverse the depression.[29] Further, beta-receptor blockade has been reported to provide excellent myocardial protection from the sympathetic stimulation induced by preoperative fear and anxiety.[30] This same protective effect will occur when sympathetic stimulation is elicited by anesthesia induction, intubation, surgical manipulation, and postoperative pain. Coltant recommended that propranolol be discontinued prior to surgery because it attenuates sympathetic responses of the heart;[27] perhaps this actually constitutes a rationale to *continue* use of the drug.

The relatively new and frequent use of propranolol for treatment of acute myocardial infarction supports the contention that it has beneficial effects in cardiac patients. Examination of the pharmacological action of propranolol provides a logical explanation for this use. Blockade of sympathetic stimulation results in less myocardial work, decreased oxygen consumption, and, hence, reduction in the size of infarcted cardiac muscle, as well as protection against arrhythmias. Maroko and Braunwald have shown this in dogs.[31] The recent use of vasodilators in acute myocardial infarction is also based upon reduction of myocardial work by a decrease in aortic pressure afterload, thus allowing a reduction in infarct size.[32]

Patients in CHF tolerate propranolol poorly because they depend upon sympathetic stimulation of the hypertrophied and dilated heart as secondary compensation for pump failure, and they require treatment with inotropic drugs such as digitalis. This does not mean that beta-adrenergic blocking drugs should not be used *following digitalization.* Adverse reactions to propranolol are *not* dose-related but appear early in treatment and usually follow administration of small doses.[23] Patients coming to surgery with chronic beta-receptor blockade are stabilized, therefore, and sudden drug toxicity should not occur unless an overdose is given.

Discontinuation of beta-blockade in patients with angina has been associated with sudden exacerbation of ischemic symptoms[33]; this is another reason for continuing propranolol administration until the time of surgery. Also, it is commonly accepted that the sudden discontinuation of anithypertensive drugs may lead to serious rebound hypertension. Beta-adrenergic receptor blockade should be considered an excellent "stress attenuator," and administration should be continued up until surgery.

A rather intriguing idea, based upon pharmacological considerations, is premedication of cardiac patients not in CHF with both beta- and alpha-adrenergic antagonists! A rational choice would be propranolol and phentolamine, both competitive blocking agents. This *partial* pharmacological, sympathetic "denervation" renders the cardiovascular system somewhat passive to anesthetic or surgical "stress." Vlachakis and Mendlowitz have used just such a combination: a high dose of dibenzyline, a noncompetitive alpha blocker (unlike phentolamine), plus propranolol, to treat ambulatory hypertensive patients. Using isolated kidney perfusion, McCombs and Berkowitz have shown that phentolamine reduces renal vascular resistance and increases cortical blood flow.[35] In the same experiment, propranolol increased sodium reabsorption and decreased cortical perfusion by way of afferent glomerular arteriolar vasoconstriction. A combination of both drugs may provide normal renal vascular resistance and help maintain intravascular volume by enhancing sodium (and water) reabsorption.

The anesthetized patient undergoing surgery is probably not exposed to the degree of stress encountered by the ambulatory hypertensive patient. In fact, activation of the sympathetic nervous system (SNS) during anesthesia is a liability for the heart because it leads to increased cardiac work and the oxygen demand. During the surgical procedure, complete functional integrity of the SNS may be required in cases of severe blood and third-space fluid losses that produce hypovolemia. The responses of the SNS to hypovolemia are peripheral vasoconstriction, tachycardia, and increased contractility. These are potentially unfavorable events for a patient with cardiac disease. With drug-induced, attenuated SNS activity, hypovolemia causes hypotension in proportion to the depletion of vascular volume. The obvious treatment for this is transfusion. Even if a sudden large drop in blood pressure occurs (an unlikely event according to the above discussion), the competitive nature of the "dual adrenergic block" would allow the temporizing use of vasoconstrictors and/or myocardial stimulants.

Other benefits of premedication with beta- and alpha-adrenergic antagonists are protection against arrhythmias, the safer use of anesthetic agents that stimulate the SNS, such as ketamine and cyclopropane, and markedly reduced swings in cardiac "stress." Obviously, patients in overt CHF are not candidates for this scheme. Ideally, the "premedication" should begin several days prior to surgery. This unusual treatment to reduce SNS activity may not appear practical now.

It is, perhaps, in the same stage of development as was the use of mild hypotension with halothane for patients with heart disease several years ago.

ADRENOCORTICOSTEROIDS

Cope stated the following in 1965: "We still eagerly await evidence that adrenal failure of stress response is a significant risk after steroid therapy."[36] However, preoperative and intraoperative steroid supplementation in patients who have received oral corticosteroids during the prior year is commonly advocated and assumes that they may be relatively "Addisonian" in their response to anesthesia and surgery. In fact, the schedule of steroid replacement is usually the same used for patients who are to have their pituitary or both adrenal glands removed and appears excessive for someone who might show relative adrenal insufficiency during anesthesia. It is important to examine carefully the evidence regarding whether anesthesia is a "stress" that activates the pituitary-adrenal system.

Stress as described by Cannon and Selye refers to a situation whereby an animal reacts to external stimuli by activation of the pituitary-adrenal axis in an attempt to maintain homeostasis.[37,38] Behaviorally, the animal "fights or takes flight." This activation is manifested biochemically by elevation of plasma levels of 17-hydroxycorticosteroids and catecholamines. For example, pain caused by surgery with inadequate anesthesia is a marked stress. Selye further refines the stress concept by defining death as *complete freedom from stress.*

There is considerable evidence that anesthesia does not cause stress but does, in fact, protect our patients from the stress of surgery. Virtue and Helmrich showed that thiopental, cyclopropane, and nitrous oxide do not elevate plasma corticosteroid levels.[39] Carnes showed that halothane and regional anesthesia depress the adrenocortical response to surgery,[40] and other studies have demonstrated that adequate blood replacement will abort the adrenocortical response to surgical stimulation.

The second biochemical indicator of "stress" is elevated plasma catecholamines. Deep surgical anesthesia with halothane causes no change in plasma catecholamines compared to preanesthetic levels, whereas deep ether and cyclopropane anesthesia cause elevations.[41] Light general anesthesia with halothane, diethyl ether, cyclopropane, and thiopental-nitrous oxide, as well as spinal anesthesia, prevents a significant rise in catecholamines during surgery.

These results suggest that "light" anesthesia blocks surgical "stress" and that "deep" cyclopropane and ether anesthesia produces or allows "stress," as evidenced by elevated catecholamines. However, this suggestion makes no sense at all. It is well known and widely accepted that general anesthesia produced by any agent blocks surgical stimulation in a linear, dose-related manner. It is also true that ether and cyclopropane, well known activators of the SNS, produce elevations in plasma catecholamines in a linear, dose-related manner. The separation of two pharmacological properties, anesthesia and plasma catecholamine elevation, is quite reasonable and explains why some anesthetic agents and, thus, anesthesia in general may be erroneously regarded as stressful to patients when, in fact, they function to prevent the pituitary-adrenal stimulation of surgery. That is, true stressors such as pain produce elevation of plasma catecholamines by way of the following sequence: noxious stimuli, afferent sensory nerve stimulation, CNS processing of the information, pain perception, pain affect, cortical activation of the SNS, and subsequent catecholamine and adrenocortical steroid release. Drugs such as cyclopropane and ether also happen to increase plasma catecholamines. However, this evidence is not proof that anesthesia in general is a true stress. Anesthesia must be examined separately from the drugs that produce anesthesia. All drugs have multiple pharmacological actions; thus, it seems fair to conclude that the state of anesthesia protects the patient from stress, although other pharmacological properties of the many diverse anesthetic drugs used (e.g., ketamine) may produce biochemical signs of stress, such as catecholamine elevation.

Wylie and Churchill-Davidson conclude that, "Anesthesia itself can be regarded, at the most, as no more than a minor form of stress."[42] Conse-quently, general anesthesia, especially combined with anxiety-relieving premedication and a preoperative visit, rather than causing stress, should be particularly beneficial in the critically ill surgical patient. The idea that a patient is too ill to stand the "stress of general anesthesia" and thus should have surgery under local anesthesia is outmoded and dangerous. This view is supported by the above argument and by the skill with which new agents such as halothane and enflurane are administered.

It is doubtful that patients who have received steroids over the year prior to surgery need prophylactic steroid administration before anesthesia and surgery. Kehlet and Binder studied 104 glucocorticoid-treated patients who underwent surgery without supplementary steroid coverage.[43] Of eight patients who developed unexplained hypotension during anesthesia, only one patient showed concomitantly low plasma cortisol levels. Other surgical patients showed minimal adrenal cortical activity preoperatively and yet no signs of adrenal insufficiency during anesthesia. The investigators concluded that acute "stress-induced" adrenal insufficiency during surgery in steroid-treated patients must be infrequent. Furthermore, when hypotension did occur during anesthesia, blood pressure returned to normal either spontaneously or with volume correction.

A study in 1974 from the same laboratory investigated the possibility that patients receiving steroids can develop deficits in plasma volume.[44] The results suggest that hypotension occurring during surgery in steroid-treated patients is not due to plasma volume insufficiency, since postoperative plasma volumes were the same as those in patients who had not received steroids prior to surgery.

The traditional steroid premedication for patients who have received corticosteroids during the year prior to surgery has little or no scientific foundation. However, the most important consideration regarding continued use of this practice is the benefit versus risk to the patient. A false sense of security may develop when the anesthesiologist accepts the contention that intraoperative hypotension is automatically due to adrenal insufficiency. This belief can delay and confuse the diagnosis and treatment of hypotension, which only rarely will be due to adrenal failure. Vandam stressed that all possible causes of intraoperative hypotension should be investigated before steroids are given.[45] In those rare situations in which steroid injection reverses hypotension, isotonic sodium chloride and glucose should be administered, and other causes, such as unrecognized hypovolemia, should be sought.

In support of steroid premedication, however, Hayes and Larner state quite unequivocally, "Short courses of systemic corticosteroid therapy in large doses may be properly given for diseases [and presumably conditions] that do not threaten life, in the absence of specific contraindications."[46] This permissive attitude developed from experience with medical patients and the short-term therapy of diseases such as asthma. There is no question that chronic steroid treatment will alter collagen restructuring and that this, in turn, will delay wound healing. Also, the incidence and severity of infection is much greater in patients receiving long-term corticosteroids. Do these considerations apply, to a lesser degree, to the short-term steroid "umbrella" given the surgical patient? This question has not been well answered, but a report by Winstone and Brooke suggests that it is true.[47] Another study reports that a sudden increase in steroid dosage may exacerbate hypertension and venous thrombosis, and this also suggests caution.[48] Until these reports are refuted by careful studies, rational therapeutic principles suggest that surgical patients who have received or are receiving steroids preoperatively *do not need* supplemental cortisol as part of their premedication and that our present policy of supplemental steroid coverage is based not on data but on tradition. If steroids are needed in the operating room to treat unexplained hypotension, then an intravenous dose of 100 mg. of hydrocortisone should be more than sufficient to reverse the hypotension if it is the result of adrenal insufficiency.

HYPOGLYCEMIC AGENTS

Over 90 per cent of the approximately 4 million diabetic patients in the United States have maturity-onset diabetes and are ketosis-resistant. Consequently, the preoperative and intraoperative control of their blood sugar is of minor importance compared to the necessity for awareness and expectant treatment of their probable cardiovascular and neurologic pathology. Approximately 70 per cent of diabetic patients die from vascular disease, most commonly due to involvement of the coronary arteries and resultant myocardial infarction. Also, they may have blunting of reactivity of the autonomic nervous system and thus be less able to respond to the cardiovascular challenges that occur during anesthesia and surgery.

Intraoperative hypoglycemia may be masked by anesthesia and yet may result in severe, permanent heart and brain damage. For example, the signs and symptoms of hypoglycemia in the awake patient are anxiety, confusion, hyperactivity, hallucinations, convulsions, and coma. These warning signals are not obvious during general anesthesia. However, the anesthesiologist should consider hypoglycemia in a patient showing evidence of unexplained catecholamine activity, such as tachycardia, sweating, pallor, and elevated blood pressure. Twenty to 30 ml. of 50-percent dextrose given intravenously should rapidly reverse these symptoms if they are due to hypoglycemia. Since even overnight fasting can deplete the normal liver of its glycogen stores, thus making the liver more prone to hypoxic and drug-induced damage, perhaps *all patients* having anesthesia should receive 5-per-cent dextrose and water as their first intravenous fluid. This rule can be altered if the diabetic patient's blood sugar is elevated 1 hour prior to induction.

Should it occur in the maturity-onset diabetic patient during the relatively short preoperative fast and operative period, hyperglycemia will produce only minor physiological changes. Since it is well known that even optimum blood sugar control over many years may not prevent the cardio-vascular and neurological sequelae of diabetes, it makes little sense to strive for exact control during the relatively short perioperative period. This traditional concept of treatment is pharmacologically unsound because the *risk* of insulin-induced hypoglycemia is considerably greater than the *benefit* of exact blood sugar control or even mild hyperglycemia (< 300 mg/dl) of short duration. Thus, the most rational and simple treatment for this large group of diabetic patients is to withhold insulin and hypoglycemic drugs the night before surgery and during the immediate postoperative period. A blood sugar determination performed 1 hour prior to surgery (when possible, this should be the first morning case) will alert the anesthesiologist to hypoglycemia due to long-acting insulin or oral hypoglycemics (*e.g.*, chloropropamide) given the day before. Should hypoglycemia occur, it can be easily treated by intravenous dextrose administration.

A common method of managing the preoperative insulin requirements of ketone-resistant diabetic patients is to give one-half their NPH dose the morning of surgery and to start intravenous dextrose (5%) in water.[49] However, this practice makes little therapeutic sense. It will indeed provide lower blood sugar over the 6 to 12 hours of peak activity and last up to 28 hours following injection, but it will be of little or no value during the actual anesthetic period. Moreover, the immediate postoperative period is usually unstable in terms of pain control, bleeding, and anxiety. This is the time when there should be more exact control of the patient based upon serial blood sugar measurements.

Justification for preoperative insulin administration is given by Rossini in two papers from the Joslin Research Laboratory.[50,51] These are based upon the contention that *short-term, uncontrolled* diabetes mellitus can result in ketoacidosis and hyperosmolar coma, lipid abnormalities, electrolyte imbalance, intracellular dehydration, impairment of wound healing, and decreased immunologic, lymphocytic, and phagocytic function. The two major problems are the terms *short-term* and *uncontrolled*. Certainly, brittle diabetic patients who are prone to ketoacidosis should be carefully and skillfully managed. However, for 90 per cent or more of the patients with diabetes (insulin-dependent or not) who are not subject to develop ketoacidosis, hyperglycemia during the *very short-term* period of anesthesia will not be harmful and is much preferred to the risks of hypoglycemia. An obvious compromise is to measure the blood sugar of all diabetic patients 1 hour before anesthesia and base therapy upon

these results and not upon any set formula of management.

Juvenile diabetics and those few maturity-onset, brittle patients subject to ketoacidosis must be carefully managed with respect to probable underlying cardiovascular and neurologic disorders, as well as the propensity for developing ketoacidosis, electrolyte abnormalities, and volume deficits. This group of high-risk patients should be admitted to the hospital at least 2 days before an elective operation, so that blood sugar, ketone, and electrolyte status can be adequately evaluated and adjusted using regular (crystalline) insulin. The anesthesiologist should be informed of the proposed surgery well in advance of the operation and should confer with the patient's internist regarding proper preanesthetic, intraoperative, and postoperative insulin management.

The physical status of the brittle, juvenile diabetic having emergency surgery should be designated as ASA Class 4E and handled accordingly. It is imperative that serial blood sugars and acetone be monitored and treated with glucose and regular insulin before and during surgery. The internist who will be involved in the postoperative management should be nearby for rapid consultation.

REFERENCES

1. Jick, H., Miettinen, O. S., Shapiro, S., et al.: Comprehensive drug surveillance. J.A.M.A., 213:1455, 1970.
2. May, F. E., Stewart, R. B., and Cluff L. E.: Drug interactions and multiple drug administration. Clin. Pharmacol. Ther., 22:322, 1977.
3. Boston Collaborative Drug Surveillance Program, Drug Surveillance Utilizing Epidemiologic Methods. Am. J. Hosp. Pharm., 30:584, 1973.
4. Ivankovic, A. D.: Anesthetic management problems posed by therapeutic advances. II. Digitalis and glucagon. Anesth. Analg., 51:607, 1972.
5. Goldberg, A. H.: The patient with heart disease: preoperative evaluation and preparation. Anesth. Analg., 55:618, 1976.
6. Stevens, W. C.: Anesthetic management. Anesth. Analg., 55:622, 1976.
7. Hamilton, W. K.: Do let blood pressure drop and do use myocardial depressants. Anesthesiology, 45:273, 1976.
8. Deutsch, S., and Dalen, J. E.: Indications for prophylactic digitalization. Anesthesiology, 30:648, 1969.
9. Selzer, A., Kelly, J., Jr., Gerbode F., et al.: Case against routine use of digitalis in patients undergoing cardiac surgery. J.A.M.A., 195:549, 1966.
10. Joubert, P., Kroening, B., Weintraub, M.: Serial serum digoxin concentrations and quantitative electrocardiographic changes. Clin. Pharmacol. Ther., 18:757, 1975.

11. Nies, A., Melmon, K. L., and Morrelli, H. (eds.): Clinical Pharmacology: Basic Principles in Therapeutics. pp. 189–189. New York, Macmillan, 1972.
12. Braden, D. C., and Morrelli, H. G.: Digoxin toxicity in patients with normokalemic potassium depletion. Clin. Pharmacol. Ther., 22:21, 1977.
13. Theye, R. A.: The contributions of individual organ systems to the decrease in whole-body VO2 with halothane. Anesthesiology, 33:367, 1972.
14. Bland, J. H. L., and Lowenstein, E.: Halothane-induced decrease in experimental myocardial ischemia in the non-failing canine heart. Anesthesiology, 45:287, 1976.
15. Alper, M. H., Flacke, W., and Krayer, O.: Pharmacology of reserpine and its implications for anesthesia. Anesthesiology, 24:524, 1963.
16. Katz, R. L., Weintraub, H. D., and Papper, E. M.: Anesthesia, surgery and rauwolfia. Anesthesiology, 25:142, 1964.
17. Ominsky, A. J., and Wollman, H.: Hazards of general anesthesia in the reserpinized patients. Anesthesiology, 30:443, 1969.
18. Föex, P., and Prys-Roberts, C.: Anaesthesia and the hypertensive patient. Br. J. Anaesth., 46:575, 1974.
19. Geer, R. T., and Greenhow, D. E.: Antihypertensive medication and surgery. J.A.M.A., 234:1221, 1975.
20. Perlroth, M. G., and Hultgren, H. N.: The cardiac patient and general surgery. J.A.M.A., 232:1279, 1975.
21. Lappas, D. G., Powell, W. M., Jr., and Daggett, W. M.: Cardiac dysfunction in the perioperative period: pathosphsiology, diagnosis and treatment. Anesthesiology, 47:117, 1977.
22. Morrelli, H. F.: Propranolol. Ann. Intern. Med., 78:913, 1973.
23. Nies, A. S., and Shand, D. G.: Clinical pharmacology of propranolol. Circulation, 52:6, 1975.
24. Flacke, J. W., Osgood, P. F., and Bendixen, H. H.: Propranolol and isoproterenol in dogs deprived of sympathetic nerve activity. J. Pharmacol. Exper. Therap., 158:519, 1967.
25. Prys-Roberts, C., Föex, P., Biro, G. P., et al.: Studies of anaesthesia in relation to hypertension. V: Adrenergic beta-receptor blockade. Br. J. Anaesth., 45:671, 1973.
26. Viljoen, J. F., Estafanous, G., and Kellner, G. A.: Propranolol and cardiac surgery. J. Thorac. Cardiovasc. Surg., 64:826, 1972.
27. Coltant, D. J., Cayen, M. N., Stinson, E. B., et al.: Investigation of the safe withdrawal period for propranolol in patients scheduled for open heart surgery. Br. Heart J., 37:1228, 1975.
28. Kaplan, J. A., Dunbar, R. W., Bland, J. W., et al.: Propranolol and cardiac surgery: a problem for the anesthetist? Anesth. Analg., 54:571, 1975.
29. Bodem, G., Brammell, H. L., Weil, J. V., et al.: Pharmacodynamic studies of beat-adrenergic antagonism induced in man by propranolol and practolol. J. Clin. Invest., 52:747, 1973.
30. Taggart, P., and Carruthers, M.: Supression by oxprenolol of adrenergic response to stress. Lancet, 2:256, 1972.
31. Maroko, P. R., and Braunwald, E.: Modification of myocardial infarction size after coronary occlusion. Ann. Intern. Med., 79:720, 1973.
32. Cohn, J. N.: Vasodilator therapy of myocardial infarction. N. Engl. J. Med., 290:1433, 1974.
33. Harrison, D. C., and Alderman, E. L.: Discontinuation of propranolol therapy: cause of rebound angina pectoris and acute coronary events. Chest, 69:1, 1976.
34. Vlachakis, N. D., and Mendlowitz, M.: Alpha- and beta-adrenergic receptor blocking agents combined with a diuretic in the treatment of essential hypertension. J. Clin. Pharmacol., 16:352, 1976.
35. McCombs, P. R., and Berkowitz, H. D.: Adrenergic blockade and renal hemodynamics. Surgery, 80:246, 1976.
36. Cope, C. L.: Some adrenal facts and fancies. Proc. R. Soc. Med., 58:55, 1965.
37. Cannon, W. B.: The Wisdom of the Body. pp. 286–304. New York, W. W. Norton, 1932.
38. Selye, H.: Stress Without Distress. pp. 25–32. Philadelphia, J. B. Lippincott, 1974.
39. Virtue, R. W., and Helmrich, M. L.: Adrenal response to stress before operation, during anaesthesia and during surgery. Proc. R. Soc. Med., 49:492, 1956.
40. Carnes, M. A.: Anesthetic considerations in adrenocortical disease. Clin. Anesth., 1:141, 1963.
41. Hamelberg, W., Sprouse, J. H., Mahaffey, J. E., et al.: Catecholamine levels during light and deep anesthesia. Anesthesiology, 21:297, 1960.
42. Wylie, W. D., and Churchill-Davidson, H. C.: A Practice of Anaesthesia. ed. 2 pp. 1201–1212. Chicago, Year Book Medical Publishers, 1966.
43. Kehlet, H., and Binder C.: Adrenocortical function and clinical course during and after surgery in unsupplemented glucocorticoid-treated patients. Br. J. Anaesth., 45:1043, 1973.
44. Kehlet, H., Engquist, A., and Greibe, J.: Plasma volume during surgery in unsupplemented glucocorticoid-treated patients. Br. J. Anaesth., 46:452, 1974.
45. Vandam, L. D., and Moore, F. D.: Adrenocortical mechanisms related to anesthesia. Anesthesiology, 21:531, 1961.
46. Hayes, R. C., Jr., and Larner, J.: Andrenocorticotropic hormone: adrenocortical steroids and their synthetic analogs; inhibitors of adrneocortical steroid biosynthesis. *In* Goodman, L. S., and Gillman, A. (eds.): The Pharmacological Basis of Therapeutics. ed 5. pp. 1472–1506. New York, MacMillan, 1975.
47. Winstone, N. E., and Brooke, B. N.: Effects of steroid treatment on patients undergoing operation. Lancet, 1:973, 1961.
48. Pooler, H. E.: A planned approach to the surgical patient with iatrogenic adrenocortical insufficiency. Br. J. Anaesth., 40:539, 1968.
49. Stehling, L.: Hypoglycemic drugs. Clin. Anesth., 10:233, 1973.
50. Rossini, A. A.: Why control blood glucose levels? Arch. Surg., 111:229, 1976.
51. Rossini, A. A., and Hare, J. E.: How to control the blood glucose in the surgical diabetic patients. Arch. Surg., 111:945, 1976.
52. Pantuck, E. J.: Ecothiopate iodine eye drops and prolonged response to suxamethonium. Br. J. Anaesth., 38:406, 1966.
53. Meyers, F. H., Jawetz, E., and Goldfein, A.: Review of Medical Pharmacology. ed 4. p. 61. Los Altos, Lange Medical Publications
54. Gurman, G. M.: Prolonged apnea after succinycholine in a case treated with cytostatics for cancer. Anesth. Analg., 51:761, 1972.
55. Zsigmond, E. K., and Robins, G.: The effect of a series of anti-cancer drugs on plasma cholinesterase activity. Can. Anaesth. Soc. J., 19:75, 1972.
56. Robertson, G. S.: Serum cholinesterase deficiency. II Pregnancy. Br. J. Anaesth., 38:361, 1966.
57. Miller, R. D., Way, W. L., and Eger, E.I., II. The effects of

alpha-methyldopa, reserpine, guanethidine and iproniazid on minimum alveolar anesthetic requirement (MAC). Anesthesiology, *29*:1153, 1968.

58. Potassium formulations and therapy. Med. Lett. Drugs Ther. *11*:77, 1969.

59. Miller, R. D., Yung, J. S., and Matteo, R. S.: Enhancement of d-tubocurarine neuromuscular blockade by diuretics in man. Anesthesiology, *45*:442, 1976.

60. Clemetsen, H. J.: Potassium therapy. A break with tradition. Lancet, *2*:175, 1962.

61. Katz, R. L., and Bigger, J. R., Jr.: Cardiac arrhythmias during anesthesia and operation. Anesthesiology, *33*:193, 1970.

62. Oh, T. E.: Frusemide and lithium toxicity. Anaesth. Intens. Care, *5*:60, 1977.

63. Cohn, K. E., Aginon, F., and Gamble, O. W.: The effect of glucagon on arrhythmias due to digitalis toxicity. Am. J. Cardiol., *25*:683, 1970.

64. Harrah, M., Way, W. L., and Katzung, B.: The interaction of d-tubocurarine with antiarrhythmic drugs. Anesthesiology, *33*:406, 1970.

65. Miller, R. D., Way, W. L., and Katzung, B. G.: The potentiation of neuromuscular blocking agents by quinidine. Anesthesiology, *28*:1036, 1967.

66. Ellison, N., and Ominsky, A. J.: Clinical considerations for the anesthesiologist whose patient is on anticoagulant therapy. Anesthesiology, *39*:328, 1973.

67. DeAngelis, J.: Hazards of subdural and epidural anesthesia during anticoagulant therapy. A case report and review. Anesth. Analg., *51*:676, 1972.

68. Martin, E. W.: Hazards of Medication. pp. 421–832. Philadelphia, J. B. Lippincott, 1971.

69. Orkin, L. R.: Anesthetic management of the drug abuse patient. Avoiding the pitfalls. Clinical Trends in Anesthesiology, *6*:1, 1976.

70. Johnstone, R. E., Kulp, R. A., and Smith, T. C.: Effects of acute and chronic ethanol administration on isoflurane requirement of mice. Anesth. Analg., *54*:277, 1975.

71. Keilty, S. R.: Anesthesia for the alcoholic patient. Anesth. Analg., *48*:659, 1969.

72. Rubin, E., Gang, H., Misra, P. S., et al.: Inhibition of drug metabolism by acute ethanol intoxication. Am. J. Med., *49*:801, 1970.

73. Gold, M. I.: Profound hypotension associated with preoperative use of phenothiazines. Anesth. Analg., *53*:844, 1974.

74. Hill, G. E., Wong, K. C., and Hodges, M. R.: Lithium carbonate and neuromuscular blocking agents. Anesthesiology, *46*:122, 1977.

75. Mannisto, P. T., and Saarnivaara, L.: Effect of lithium and rubidium on the sleeping time caused by various intravenous anaesthetics in the mouse. Br. J. Anaesth., *48*:185, 1976.

76. Schwartz, A. J., and Wollman, H.: Anesthesia considerations for patients on chronic therapy: L-dopa, monoamine oxidase inhibitors, tri-cyclic and antidepressants and propranolol. Refresher Courses in Anesthesiology, *4*:99, 1976.

77. Perks, E. R.: Monoamine oxidase inhibitors. Anaesthesia, *19*:376, 1964.

78. Evans-Prosser, C. D.: The use of pethidine and morphine in the presence of monoamine oxidase inhibitors. Br. J. Anaesth., *40*:279, 1968.

79. Vigran, I. M.: Dangerous potentiation of meperidine hydrochloride by pargyline hydrochloride. J.A.M.A., *187*: 953, 1964.

80. Greer, J.: Anesthesia and seizures. Int. Anesth. Clin., *6*:351, 1968.

81. Goldberg, K. I.: Anesthetic management of patients treated with antihypertensive agents or levodopa. Anesth. Analg., *51*:625, 1972.

82. Bass, B. F.: Steroids. Clin. Anesth., *10*:249, 1973.

83. Schen, R. J., and Khazzam, A. S.: Postoperative hypoglycemic coma associated with chlorpropamide. Br. J. Anaesth., *47*:899, 1975.

84. Hansten, P. D.: Meperidine and combination oral contraceptives. J. Clin. Pharmacol., *15*:640, 1975.

85. Crawford, J. J., and Rudofsky, S.: Some alterations in the pattern of drug metabolism associated with pregnancy oral contraceptives and the newly born. Br. J. Anaesth., *38*:446, 1966.

86. Jaclau, M. R., and Fouts, J. R.: Effect of norethynodrel and progesterone on hepatic microsonal drug-metabolizing enzyme systems. Biochem. Pharmacol., *15*:891, 1966.

87. Miller, R. D.: Factors affecting the action of muscle relaxants. *In* Katz, R. (ed.): Muscle Relaxants. pp. 163–192. Exerpta Medica, (Amsterdam), 1975.

88. Fogdall, R. P., and Miller, R. D.: Prolongation of a pancuronium-induced neuromuscular blockade by clindamycin. Anesthesiology, *41*:407, 1974.

89. Stanley, V. F., Giesecke, A. H., Jr., and Jenkins, M. T.: Neomycin-curare neuromuscular block and reversal in cats. Anesthesiology, *31*:228, 1969.

90. Pittinger, C., and Adamson, R.: Antibiotic blockade of neuromuscular function. Ann. Rev. Pharmacol., *12*:169, 1972.

91. Cabizuca, S. V., and Desser, K. B.: Carbencillin-associated hypokalemic alkalosis. J.A.M.A., *236*:956, 1976.

92. Barr, G. A., Mazze, R. I., Cousins, M. J., et al.: An animal model for combined methoxyflurane and gentamycin nephrotoxicity. Br. J. Anaesth., *45*:306, 1973.

93. Bennett, E. J., Schmidt, G. B., Patel, K. P., et al.: Muscle relaxants, myasthenia and mustards? Anesthesiology, *46*:220, 1977.

94. New York State Society of Anesthesiologists, Anesthesia Study Committee, Clinical Anesthesia Conference. Hypotension during anesthesia in narcotic addicts. N. Y. State J. Med., *66*:2685, 1966.

95. Van Dyke, C., Barash, P. G., Jatlow, P., et al.: Cocaine: plasma concentrations after intranasal application in man. Science, *191*:859, 1976.

96. Stoelting, R. K., Creasser, C. W., and Martz, R. C.: Effect of cocaine administration on halothane MAC in dogs. Anesth. Analg., *54*:422, 1975.

97. Johnston, R. R., Way, W. L., and Miller, R. D.: Alteration of anesthetic requirement by amphetamine. Anesthesiology, *36*:357, 1972.

98. Stoelting, R. K., Mantz, R. C., GArtner, J., et al.: Effects of delta-9-tetrahydrocannabinol on halothane MAC in dogs. Anesthesiology, *38*:521, 1973.

FURTHER READING

Smith, N. T., Miller, R. D., and Corbascio, A. N. (eds.): Drug Interactions in Anesthesia. Philadelphia, Lea & Febiger, 1981.

Part Three

Regional Anesthesia

4 Immediate Reactions to Local Anesthetics

P. Prithvi Raj, M.D., and Alon P. Winnie, M.D.

The complications of regional anesthesia are primarily caused by either the untoward effects of local anesthetic drugs and their adjuvants or trauma associated with the injection technique. The complications may be immediate (e.g., within 2 hours) or delayed. Immediate reactions are usually reversible, provided immediate and correct treatment is administered. The trauma to the tissues, on the other hand, produces slowly developing pathological changes that may result in serious sequelae (see Chaps. 5, 6, and 7). Each practitioner of regional anesthesia should be fully aware of the inherent dangers of immediate and delayed reactions and should have facilities to institute remedial treatment for these complications. This chapter deals mainly with complications owing to the immediate reactions and their management.

Immediate reactions occurring at the time at which a regional block is performed may be classified as psychogenic; systemic and related to local anesthetic drugs; systemic and related to adjuvant vasoconstrictor drugs; and allergic.

PSYCHOGENIC REACTION TO LOCAL ANESTHETICS

Psychogenic reaction to local anesthetics is very often seen in people who tend to faint at the mere sight of a needle or a drop of blood; who agree reluctantly to the regional procedure, but still prefer another technique (e.g., general anesthesia); and who hyperreact in the presence of their immediate relatives (e.g., children).

The reaction can take the form of fainting, agitation, or frank hostility. In patients who pretend to faint, the vital signs remain stable and lid reflexes remain intact. Conversely, agitated patients do increase their blood pressure, pulse, and respiratory rate and may sweat profusely. The vocal reaction of the agitated patient to the touch of the needle tip is highly exaggerated, and some patients may sob.

A psychogenic reaction to regional anesthesia can be prevented by correctly selecting and preparing the patient,[1] beginning with the preoperative visit. During this visit, the nature of the technique should be explained to the patient in layman's terms with calmness and assurance. The efficacy of the procedure should be emphasized and the alternatives discussed. The discomfort and pain, if any, caused by the technique itself should be explained realistically, along with the common complications and their sequelae. After informed consent has been obtained, suitable preoperative medication should be prescribed. In the operating room, each step of the block procedure should be explained to the patient prior to its execution. In our experience, psychogenic reactions are extremely rare and occur only in patients who are ill prepared.

51

SYSTEMIC REACTIONS TO LOCAL ANESTHETICS

Whenever a local anesthetic is injected, a portion of the drug is absorbed by the circulation. Presence of the anesthetic in blood means that the drug is carried to every cell, and it therefore has the potential to affect the function of many organs. Because of its action on excitable membrane, a local anesthetic can produce distant and widespread secondary effects on the CNS and cardiovascular system. These indirect effects often are quite different from the direct effects on the intended organ. For example, an extensive epidural anesthetic may block conduction in the white rami of the cardiac accelerator nerves and, thus, may slow the heart rate, whereas the concurrently high blood level of the anesthetic may indirectly affect the conducting and contractile mechanisms of the heart. Local anesthetics do, in fact, diffuse from vessel to nerve and can block impulse conduction when given systemically.[2,3]

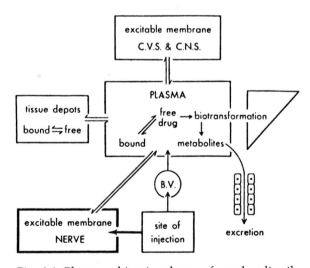

Fig. 4-1. Pharmacokinetic scheme of uptake, distribution, and elimination of local anesthetic drugs from the epidural space (site of injection). Uptake into nerve and blood vessels (*B.V.*) leads to redistribution into plasma, tissue depots, and potentially toxic sites in the cardiovascular and central nervous systems (*C.V.S., C.N.S.*). (Bromage, P. R.: Epidural Analgesia. p. 87. Philadelphia, W. B. Saunders, 1978)

CONCENTRATIONS OF LOCAL ANESTHETICS IN BLOOD

Pharmacokinetics

Once injected, the local anesthetic is absorbed by blood vessels, which carry the dose to the plasma of the central blood volume. Following pharmacokinetic principles akin to those involved in the uptake and distribution of general anesthetics, redistribution occurs in accordance with regional blood flows, concentration gradients, and solubility coefficients. The high blood flow to the CNS and cardiovascular system and the high lipid solubility of local anesthetics predispose to the delivery of concentrations potentially toxic to these systems. Counteracting this are the processes of ionization (to charged forms that cannot cross membranes), protein binding (with bound drug also unable to cross membranes), biotransformation, and renal excretion (Fig. 4-1).[4]

Factors that determine the arterial plasma concentration and, thus, the toxicity of local anesthetic agents include the site and rate of injection, concentration and total dose, use of a vasoconstrictor, rate of redistribution in various tissues, degree of ionization, degree of plasma and tissue protein binding, and rate of metabolism and excretion.[4-8] Table 4-1 summarizes some physiochemical properties of the most commonly used local anesthetics.

For example, injection of anesthetic into the relatively vascular mucous membrane results in a higher peak level than does skin infiltration using the same dose. The addition of a vasoconstrictor to the local anesthetic solution retards systemic absorption, resulting in a lower arterial concentration. A greater degree of protein binding (e.g., 95% with bupivacaine compared to 64% with lidocaine) is associated with a larger pool of drug that exists in a pharmacologically inactive state. Thus, the risk of toxicity is reduced. The rate of metabolism of local anesthetics is related principally to their chemical structure; the ester compounds (e.g., procaine, chloroprocaine, tetracaine) are hydrolyzed rapidly in the plasma by cholinesterase, and the amide compounds (e.g., lidocaine,

Table 4-1. Physiochemical Properties of Commonly Used Local Anesthetics

Drug	Struc-ture	Molecular Weight (Base)	pK$_a$ at 25°C	% Nonionized Drug			Partition Coefficient in N-Heptane, pH 7.4	Protein Binding 1 μg./ml. plasma	
				pH 7.0	pH 7.4	pH 7.6		Maternal	Fetal
Procaine	Ester	272	8.9	1.2	3.1	4.8			
Chloro-procaine	Ester	307	8.7	2.0	4.8	7.4			
Tetracaine	Ester	300	8.5	3.1	7.4	11.2			
Lidocaine	Amide	234	7.9	11.	24.	33.	2.9	64.	24.
Mepivacaine	Amide	246	7.6	20.	39.	50.	0.8	77.	
Prilocaine	Amide	257	7.9	11.	24.	33.	0.4	55.	
Bupivacaine	Amide	288	8.1	7.	17.	24.	27.5	95.	66.
Etidocaine	Amide	276	7.7	17.	33.	44.	141.	95.	

(Modified from Ralston, D.H., and Shnider, S.M.: The fetal and neonatal effects of regional anesthesia in obstetrics. Anesthesiology, *48*:34, 1978)

mepivacaine, prilocaine, bupivacaine, etidocaine) undergo much slower and more complex degradation in the liver.

Usual Plasma Concentrations

Mazze compared plasma concentrations of lidocaine in 15 patients undergoing intravenous regional, axillary, epidural, and caudal blocks and found mean peak concentrations of 1.5, 2.5, 3.1, and 1.8 μg. per ml., respectively.[9] Tucker investigated systemic absorption of a single dose of mepivacaine (500 mg.) in commonly used regional techniques in 70 patients.[10] The highest plasma concentrations (5–10 μg./ml.) occur after intercostal block. Addition of epinephrine lowers the plasma concentration to 2 to 5 μg. per ml., which is comparable to peak levels with other techniques (Figs. 4-2, 4-3). Others have found similar results with other local anesthetics.[11–13]

Toxic Plasma Concentrations

Several investigators have studied the toxicity of lidocaine administered intravenously. Foldes found that signs and symptoms of toxicity to the CNS and cardiovascular system appear after the infusion of lidocaine, 1.4 mg. per kg., at a rate of 0.5 mg. per kg. per min., into unanesthetized volunteers.[14] This infusion resulted in a plasma concentration of 5.3 μg. per ml. Bromage and Robson infused lidocaine in patients anesthetized

with thiopental and nitrous oxide and noted that signs of toxicity occur under these circumstances when the lidocaine concentration exceeds 10 μg. per ml.[15] Although there are numerous factors that determine whether toxicity occurs, signs of toxicity may be anticipated when the arterial lidocaine concentration exceeds 5μg. per ml.

Generally, however, there is a poor correlation between a given plasma concentration and a given manifestation of toxicity, even in the same patient.[16] It is very likely that the plasma anesthetic levels in these studies were not in a steady state when the signs of toxicity appeared; hence, the rate of administration, as well as the total dose, is important.[17] In the typical clinical situation, local anesthetic is administered as a single, brief injection, so that toxicity correlates more closely with the dosage standardized to body weight. With lidocaine, for example, the threshold for symptoms of toxicity to the central venous system in humans is reached with a dosage greater than 6 mg. per kg.[16,18,19]

Concentrations With Compounded Mixtures

Many anesthesiologists are compounding local anesthetic mixtures to shorten the latency, prolong the duration of the block, and prevent toxicity.[20–23] Raj measured arterial plasma concentration in patients undergoing epidural or brachial

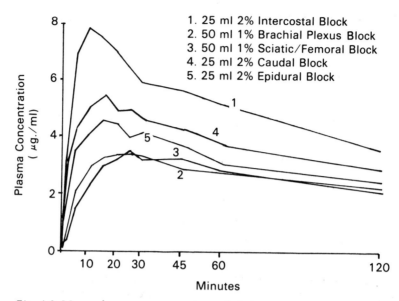

Fig. 4-2. Mean plasma concentrations of plain mepivacaine (500 mg.) after different blocks. (Modified from Tucker, G. T., Moore, D. C., Bridenbaugh, P. O., et al.: Systemic absorption of mepivacaine in commonly used regional block procedures. Anesthesiology, *37*: 277, 1972)

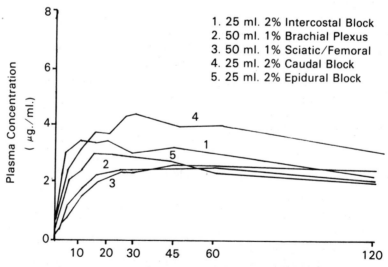

Fig. 4-3. Mean plasma concentrations of mepivacaine (500 mg.) with epinephrine (1:200,000) after different blocks. (Modified from Tucker, G. R., Moore, D. C., Bridenbaugh, P. O., et al.: Systemic absorption of mepivacaine in commonly used regional block procedures. Anesthesiology, *37*: 277, 1972)

plexus block after administering compounded mixtures of either chloroprocaine-bupivacaine or lidocaine-bupivacaine (Figs. 4-4, 4-5).[23] In these mixtures, the chloroprocaine concentration peaks and then falls earlier than that of either lidocaine or bupivacaine. Based upon these studies, the best local anesthetic mixture for rapid onset, prolonged duration, and reduced toxicity is chloroprocaine-bupivacaine with epinephrine. In patients with atypical cholinesterase, one should reduce the chloroprocaine dosage (Fig. 4-6). Whether the compounding of local anesthetics actually prevents toxicity is debatable and has become less clinically relevant since long-acting, highly protein-bound agents, such as bupivacaine, have become available.

EFFECTS ON THE CNS

The most dramatic and potentially the most hazardous complication of local anesthetic use is a generalized seizure. These seizures result when the anesthetic blood level exceeds a certain minimum (e.g., 7 μg./ml. with lidocaine). Yet, low blood levels (e.g., lidocaine, 0.5–4.0 μg./ml.) of local anesthetics have an *anti*convulsant action.[24-26]

In a variety of organisms including humans, the intravenous injection of a large but nonlethal dose of local anesthetic produces generalized seizures that resemble grand mal convulsions grossly and electroencephalographically.[18,27,28] Newborn infants, like adults, respond with tonic-clonic seizures to maternal overdosage of local anesthetics.

However, pronounced species differences exist in the susceptibility of local anesthetic seizures. In humans, mepivacaine 5mg./kg., procaine or chloroprocaine 3 mg./kg., tetracaine (0.5 mg./kg.), or lidocaine (1.5 mg./kg.) produces premonitory symptoms of an impending seizure when infused intravenously.[14,19] deJong infused lidocaine (4–10 mg./kg.) in six patients under investigation for refractory temporal lobe epilepsy, and typical temporal seizures were induced without causing grand mal seizures.[29]

Several experimental approaches suggest that local anesthetic-induced seizures arise from subcortical regions rather than from cortical or brain stem sites. A lower brain stem site of origin is excluded by demonstrating that convulsions occur when cocaine is injected into the carotid artery but not when it is injected into the vertebral artery of the vascularly isolated rabbit brain.[30] In addition, microinjection of local anesthetics into the midbrain does not elicit seizures.[31] Parenteral injection of cocaine produces EEG seizure patterns in the nuclear complex of the amygdala,[32] and the first suggestion of a disturbance appears within seconds of an intravenous injection. There is slowing and increased amplitude of the electrical activity in that region, followed by paroxysmal discharges of spike or spindle bursts.[17,31,33] When lidocaine or prilocaine is injected into one common carotid artery of the dog, focal discharges appear first in the ipsilateral amygdala.[34]

Generalized CNS depression follows this initial CNS excitation as the cerebral blood anesthetic concentration rises.[17] Among the manifestations of this CNS depression are respiratory depression and, later, respiratory arrest.

Effect of Seizures

The duration of seizures is an important determinant of their potential harm. Seizures raise the metabolic activity of the brain and muscles and, hence, increase oxygen demand. In mechanically ventilated dogs, seizures increase cerebral oxygen consumption by 60 per cent and cerebral blood flow by 264 per cent.[35] During electrically induced seizures, the cerebral venous oxygen tension falls to or below 20 torr (2.8 kPa) in spontaneously breathing psychiatric patients. These patients thus may develop cerebral hypoxia briefly, although lightly anesthetized subjects ventilated with oxygen during electroconvulsive therapy do not.[36]

Hence, a convulsion need not be, and should not be, fatal. The convulsant dose of most local anesthetics is 25 to 50 per cent of the dose lethal to laboratory animals.[37,38] The margin of safety is

(Text continues on page 59.)

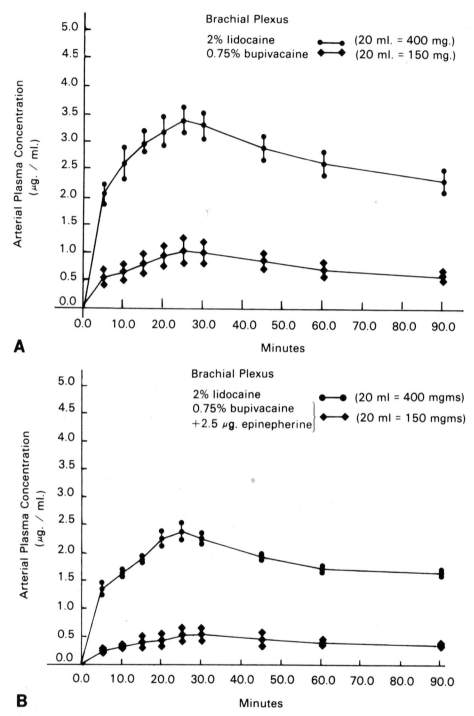

Fig. 4-4. Mean plasma concentrations after brachial plexus block with lidocaine-bupivacaine mixture (*A*) without and (*B*) with epinephrine. (Raj, P. P., Rosenblatt, R., Miller, R., et al.: Dynamics of compounded local anesthetic mixtures in regional anesthesia. Anesth. Analg., 56: 110, 1977)

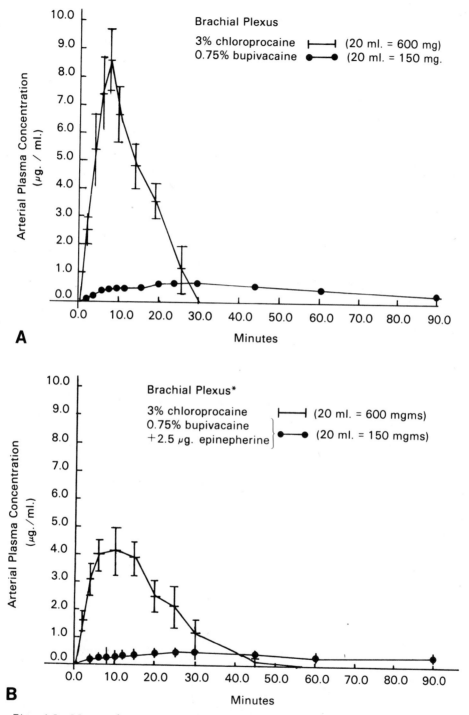

Fig. 4-5. Mean plasma concentrations after brachial plexus block with chloroprocaine-bupivacaine mixture (A) without and (B) with epinephrine. (Raj, P. P., Rosenblatt, R., Miller, R., et al.: Dynamics of compounded local anesthetic mixtures in regional anesthesia. Anesth. Analg., *56*: 100, 1977)

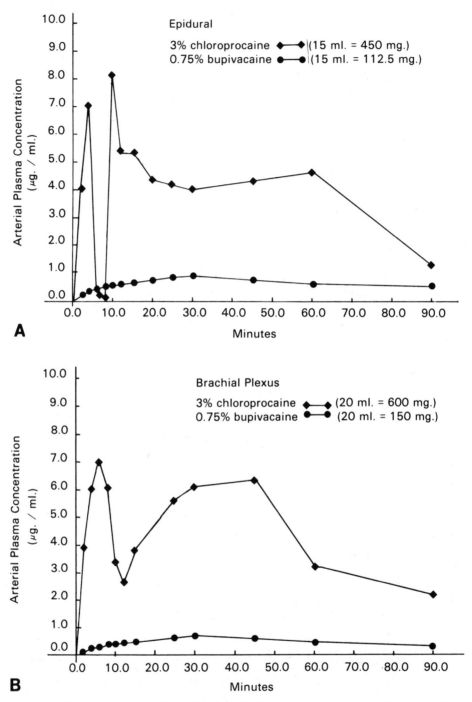

Fig. 4-6. Plasma concentrations after brachial plexus block with a chloroprocaine-bupivacaine mixture in a patient with atypical plasma cholinesterase. (Raj, P. P., Rosenblatt, R., Miller, R., et al.. Dynamics of compounded local anesthetic mixtures in regional anesthesia. Anesth. Analg., *56:* 100, 1977)

substantially greater if elementary cardiorespiratory resuscitation is instituted promptly. The rising demands of the hyperactive brain and violently contracting muscle can be met satisfactorily by proper ventilation and supplemental oxygen. Properly ventilated dogs appear normal even after extended bouts of procaine-induced seizures at weekly intervals.[35,39]

Prevention of Seizures

The abrupt onset and serious sequelae of local anesthetic-induced seizures demand that anyone who administers a local anesthetic must know how to prevent and treat them. During a convulsion, respiration is impaired because of violent and uncoordinated contraction of many muscles, superimposed upon the soft-tissue obstruction of the airway that accompanies unconsciousness. Cardiovascular function may also be impaired by the high concentration of local anesthetics in the blood (see pp. 60–62). Hence, to treat seizures, their sequelae, and other complications described in this chapter, *resuscitative equipment and drugs, as well as personnel who are competent in resuscitation and life support, should be available whenever local anesthetics are used.*

The best way to prevent a seizure is to use the smallest dose of anesthetic compatible with the desired clinical effect. Table 4-2 lists suggested maximum dosages. For some drugs this value is not known precisely; for example, bupivacaine, 400 mg. with epinephrine, has been used safely

Table 4-2. Suggested Maximum Dosages of Local Anesthetics for the Healthy 70-kg. Adult

	Plain Solutions (mg.)	Solutions Containing Epinephrine (mg.)
Cocaine	200	
Procaine		1000
Chloroprocaine	800	1000
Tetracaine	100	200
Lidocaine	300	500
Mepivacaine	300	500
Prilocaine	600	600
Bupivacaine	175	225
Etidocaine	300	400

for regional nerve blocks in healthy patients.[40] For very young or old patients and for those in poor physical condition, the dosage must be lower than usual. Patients with congestive heart failure, for example, should receive decreased dosage of amide-type local anesthetics, because heart failure is associated with diminished hepatic blood flow and, in turn, diminished hepatic extraction of these agents.[41] Whenever possible, a vasoconstrictor such as epinephrine should be added to the solution to decrease the rate of absorption of the anesthetic. However, in patients with hypertension, other cardiovascular disease, and hyperthyroidism, the use of vasoconstrictors for this purpose is relatively contraindicated. Frequent aspiration should be performed during administration of the anesthetic solution to detect inadvertent intravascular (or other aberrant) injection.

Premonitory signs usually forewarn of an impending seizure. These may include dizziness; ringing in the ears; a vague sensation of light-headedness; nystagmus; dysphoria; shivering; fine twitching and tremor of muscles of the face and digits with most local anesthetics; and, with lidocaine, somnolence. Detection of these early signs requires constant attention to and communication with the patient. If these signs occur, the anesthesiologist should stop the injection and institute treatment. Often, administering oxygen and asking the patient to breathe deeply suffices. If the patient becomes unconscious, the anesthesiologist should administer oxygen by mask, with assisted ventilation.

The prior or concomitant administration of CNS depressants, such as barbiturates, benzodiazepines, and general anesthetics, raises the convulsive threshold to local anesthetics. Unfortunately, barbiturates are of little value in clinical situations, for near-anesthetic doses are required to prevent seizures. At reasonable dosage, however, benzodiazepine derivatives such as diazepam prevent or shorten the duration of cocaine seizures in rats and cats and raise the convulsive threshold with less cardiorespiratory depression than barbiturates.[42–45] For example, the intramuscular administration of diazepam (0.25 mg./kg.)

raises the convulsive threshold to lidocaine 100 per cent in monkeys.[44] deJong recommends diazepam premedication in a dosage as small as 0.1 mg. per kg. to reduce risk of seizure.[44] Inhalation of 70-per-cent nitrous oxide raises the convulsive threshold 50 per cent, but the addition of diazepam does not result in further protection.[46] Anticonvulsants such as diphenylhydantoin are ineffective and may even increase the severity of a cocaine or procaine convulsion.[47–49] In fact, anticonvulsants prove futile in treating newborn infants who convulse subsequent to the transplacental passage of mepivacaine.[50]

Treatment of Seizures

Seizures occasionally do occur because of accidental intravascular injection or unusually rapid absorption (relative overdose), as well as excessive dosage (absolute overdose). The first step in management of the convulsing patient should be to maintain his airway and to protect him from hypoxia and self-injury. Controlled and, later, assisted respiration with 100-per-cent oxygen by mask is essential. Airway management and ventilation should not be interrupted to administer drugs, because a local anesthetic-induced seizure is usually shortlived, lasting 1 min., or 2 at most. Convulsions, being more visible, tend to obscure the insidious and potentially more threatening fall in cerebral perfusion that may occur due to hypotension as a direct result of simultaneous cardiovascular toxicity (see p. 61). Lowering the head and raising the feet will increase the brain's blood supply during this period.

In addition to basic resuscitative measures, drugs may be administered by assistants if the seizure continues. Barbiturates remain the most effective drugs to terminate a local anesthetic seizure. Remarkably small doses (e.g., thiopental, 1–2 mg./kg.) often suffice. Although ultra-short-acting barbiturates are commonly used, diazepam (0.1–0.2 mg./kg.) or long-acting barbiturates may be used. Short-acting muscle relaxants may be used if barbiturates are unsuccessful in ending seizures or if they are necessary to facilitate tracheal intubation or better control of respira-

tion. Caution is advised when barbiturates and neuromuscular blocking agents are used to treat seizures. Barbiturates per se do not lower the mortality rate.[48] On the other hand, they can depress cardiovascular function synergistically with local anesthetics.[51] Neuromuscular blocking agents stop the muscular activity of the seizure but have no effect on the electrical activity of the brain[52]; in addition, use of these agents may lead to other complications, such as aspiration owing to passive regurgitation. Therapy with neuromuscular blocking agents should be instituted only when simpler measures have failed.

EFFECTS ON THE CARDIOVASCULAR SYSTEM

Local anesthetic agents cause cardiovascular changes as a result of their indirect effects on autonomic nerves and their direct effects on cardiac or vascular smooth muscle; evoked reflexes and direct CNS actions may also be involved. Local anesthetic agents appear to depress myocardial contractility, while they may both stimulate and depress vascular smooth muscle contractility. Their action on autonomic nerves is complex. In addition to the usual effects on membranes, agents such as cocaine can alter the uptake of norepinephrine by autonomic nerves.

Indirect Effects on the Cardiovascular System

Local anesthetics may produce cardiovascular changes indirectly through the effects of the regional anesthetic technique on the autonomic nervous system. A concomitant decrease in blood pressure with spinal anesthesia is almost a universal occurrence,[53] and the magnitude of the decrease is related directly to the height of the sympathetic block produced.[54] The paralysis of preganglionic sympathetic fibers, which are responsible for maintaining vascular smooth muscle tone, results in decreased peripheral vascular resistance with secondary peripheral pooling of blood, decreased venous return, and decreased cardiac output.[55] With sympathetic block above

T5, paralysis of cardiac accelerator fibers also results, with bradycardia and secondary intensification of the hypotension. The blood pressure decrease is greater when the patient is hypovolemic, is tilted head up, or has a higher initial blood pressure level.

The hemodynamic changes produced by epidural anesthesia are qualitatively the same but usually not as great as those accompanying spinal anesthesia.[56] The lesser hemodynamic effect is due principally to the lower level of sympathetic block produced for a given sensory level; with spinal anesthesia, the sympathetic block extends two or more spinal segments above the sensory level, whereas with epidural anesthesia, there is no difference between sympathetic and sensory levels.[57] However, because relatively large doses are used in epidural anesthesia, *direct* effects on the heart and peripheral vessels may also occur (see below). The effects of epinephrine that is often added to the local anesthetic are significant in this respect. Absorption of this vasoconstrictor (which is capable of producing mixed adrenergic effects) into the systemic circulation results in an epinephrine concentration sufficient to produce beta- but not alpha-adrenergic receptor stimulation. As a result, compared to epidural anesthesia without epinephrine (or spinal anesthesia), epidural anesthesia with epinephrine results in a greater increase in heart rate, an increase in stroke volume and cardiac output, and a greater decrease in peripheral vascular resistance.[56] Overall, hypotension is *more* frequent with epidural anesthesia when epinephrine is used than with epidural anesthesia without epinephrine or spinal anesthesia (see Chap. 5).

Direct Effects on the Cardiovascular System

Cardiac Effects. Much of what is known about the cardiac effects of local anesthetics is derived from clinical experience in the use of lidocaine to treat ventricular premature contractions, although similar effects occur with other local anesthetics.

At low blood lidocaine levels (e.g., 2–5 μg./ml.) that follow intravenous doses of up to 50 μg. per kg. per min., there is prolongation or abolition of phase 4 depolarization in Purkinje fibers and a shortening of the duration of the action potential and of the effective refractory period.[58,59] These electrophysiological changes characterize the antiarrhythmic effect of lidocaine (see Chap. 14). There are no consistent accompanying cardiac (or peripheral vascular) hemodynamic effects.[60–62]

When the lidocaine blood level rises to 5 to 10 μg. per ml., conduction velocity and action potential amplitude decrease with resultant prolongation of the P-R interval and QRS duration, as well as sinus bradycardia, apparent in the ECG. Associated with these electrophysiological changes is a dose-related negative inotropic effect in animals[63,64] and humans,[65,66] which is manifested by decreased intraventricular pressure, increased end-diastolic volume, and decreased cardiac output. This cardiodepression correlates with the relative anesthetic potency of the agent; thus, tetracaine is considerably more cardiodepressant than lidocaine and chloroprocaine, which, in turn, are more depressant than procaine. Generally, however, myocardial depression following regional anesthesia occurs only when inadvertent intravascular injection occurs or when the dosage is excessive.

Should the blood lidocaine level rise above 10 μg. per ml., the aforementioned electrophysiological changes deteriorate further, with the appearance of AV block and, then, asystole.

Peripheral Vascular Effects. Local anesthetics have a biphasic effect on vascular smooth muscle. At low concentrations of lidocaine (e.g., 2–5 μg./ml.), stimulation of myogenic contractures occurs in selected peripheral vascular beds, with decreased limb blood flow secondary to an increased vascular resistance.[67,68] This stimulatory effect, which is not correlated with relative anesthetic potency, causes a redistribution of blood among peripheral vascular beds. This would account for the *increase* in mean arterial pressure noted often after the administration of local anesthetics, even in the presence of unchanged or slightly decreased peripheral resistance.

When the lidocaine blood level rises about 5 μg. per ml., vasodilation results from a direct depressant effect on peripheral smooth muscle, leading to hypotension.[67,68] Coupled with decreased myocardial contractility, peripheral dilatation may progress to circulatory collapse, particularly when the blood lidocaine level rises above 10 μg. per ml.

Treatment of Direct Effects. Clinically important hemodynamic changes resulting from *direct* effects of the local anesthetic generally do not occur until the local anesthetic blood level is sufficiently high to have caused CNS toxicity. Hence, treatment of hypotension is added to the therapy already undertaken for a seizure (see pp. 59–60). Such treatment may range from raising the legs (to promote venous return), to the administration of vasopressors (see pp. 82–84), to cardiopulmonary resuscitation (see Chap. 16), as the gravity of the patient's condition dictates what is required to restore organ perfusion.

EFFECTS ON THE UTERUS AND THE FETUS

Regional anesthesia administered to a parturient may affect the fetus indirectly through changes in maternal homeostasis and directly through fetal uptake of local anesthetics.[69]

Indirect Effects on the Uterus and the Fetus

Regional anesthesia may adversely affect uterine blood flow by producing maternal hypotension, uterine vasoconstriction, adrenergic stimulation, or uterine hyperactivity.

Maternal hypotension is a common complication of regional anesthesia and, in turn, has profound effects on uterine blood flow. The reported incidence of hypotension varies depending on the definition of hypotension, method of monitoring, height of the block, and use of prophylactic measures (see Chap. 41).[70–76]

Nearly a sixth of maternal blood volume is contained in the uterus at term.[70] Partial or complete inferior vena caval compression by the gravid uterus impedes venous return to the heart and may cause hypotension.[70,72,77,78] In most parturients, an increase in resting sympathetic tone compensates for the effects of vena caval compression.[79] However, when sympathetic tone is impaired by conduction anesthesia, marked reduction in blood pressure may result. Hypotension is further accentuated by blood loss or dehydration.

Prophylactic use of ephedrine, left uterine displacement, and infusion of lactated Ringer's solution can decrease the incidence of maternal hypotension during cesarean section from 82 to 14 per cent.* The effects of adding epinephrine to local anesthetics, however, are controversial. Some investigators[80] have found a greater decrease in blood pressure with epinephrine than without it when performing epidural anesthesia for cesarean section, whereas others[81] have observed no change.

Uterine Vasoconstriction. Uterine blood flow may decrease as a result of uterine vasoconstriction owing to high concentration of local anesthetics.[82,83] Procaine, lidocaine, mepivacaine, and bupivacaine produce a dose-related decrease in uterine blood flow in nonpregnant ewes[84]; however, uterine vasoconstriction does not occur with blood levels (2–4 μg./ml.) associated with lidocaine epidural analgesia during labor.[85] Blood levels of local anesthetics sufficiently high to cause uterine vasoconstriction may be found following routine paracervical blocks.[69]

Adrenergic Stimulation. The peripheral alpha-adrenergic effect of high blood epinephrine levels owing to inadvertent intravascular injection produces uterine vasoconstriction and resultant decreased uterine blood flow. In ewes given epinephrine (0.1–1.0 μg./kg./min.), maternal blood pressure rises 50 to 65 per cent, and uterine blood flow decreases by 55 to 75 per cent.[86] Metaraminol, with mixed alpha- and beta-adrenergic activity, restores uterine flow without any improvement in fetal acidosis.[87,88] Mephentermine and ephedrine have minimal effects on uterine blood flow and increase maternal blood pressure primarily by central inotropic and chronotropic activity. Hence, these vasopressors are preferred for treatment of maternal hypotention.

---

*Personal communication, S. H. Shnider

Uterine Hyperactivity. Local anesthetics and vasopressor drugs administered during conduction anesthesia can alter uterine tone[89,90] through stimulation of alpha- and beta-adrenergic receptors in uterine muscle. Epinephrine, commonly used with local anesthetics, has both alpha- and beta-adrenergic activity. Alpha-adrenergic stimulation causes uterine vasoconstriction and increases muscle tone, whereas beta-adrenergic stimulation results in decreased uterine tone, as well as vasodilatation. The beta-adrenergic effect predominates with low blood levels of epinephrine that follow absorption from the epidural space.[91,92] Inadvertent vascular injection, however, may produce high blood levels of epinephrine, which, in turn, produce alpha-adrenergic effects. Studies of uterine muscle strips demonstrate that local anesthetics increase tone but decrease the rate and strength of contraction.[93] In common clinical situations, the blood levels of local anesthetics have little effect on uterine muscle. The impairment of uterine contractility commonly associated with regional anesthesia is due most probably to interruption of uterine innervation rather than blood-borne anesthetic, because epidural saline injection and clinical spinal anesthesia both produce such impairment.[94,95]

Fetal Consequences. The hazard to the fetus of decreased uterine blood flow is dependent on its severity and duration. When uterine perfusion is impaired severely, fetal asphyxia results.[96–102] Fetal asphyxia is deleterious principally to the CNS, heart, and lungs.[101,103,104]

In halothane-anesthetized monkeys, the fetus tolerates a reduction in maternal pressure to 50 torr for as long as 2 hours, but pressures of 40 torr or lower regularly produce fetal asphyxia. Fetal P_{O_2} is decreased from 29 to 34 torr (3.9–4.5 kPa), to 3 to 16 torr (0.4–2.1 kPa), and fetal heart rate deceleration occurs.[101,105,106] Fetal death occurs from myocardial failure with severe asphyxia (*p*H 7.0) lasting several hours. Permanent brain injury occurs with asphyxia of intermediate severity.[101,103,104] Idiopathic respiratory distress syndrome may also follow intrauterine fetal asphyxia.[69]

During epidural anesthesia, late deceleration fetal heart rate changes can develop when maternal systolic blood pressure is less than 100 torr for 5 to 7 min.[107] The fetal heart rate returns to normal with oxygen administration and correction of hypotension. When systolic blood pressure remains below 100 torr longer than 15 min., fetal depression (as measured by low Apgar scores) results.[108,109] However, more severe hypotension often has no apparent deleterious effect if treated promptly.[108–111]

Thus, prompt therapy is indicated when maternal blood pressure falls below 100 torr or below 70 per cent of normal. This is particularly important when placental function is already impaired, as in preeclampsia. Therapy includes left uterine displacement, volume expansion, and oxygen administration.[70] If further measures are needed, a vasopressor with predominantly beta-adrenergic effect is used (e.g., ephedrine, 5–10 mg., I.V.).

Direct Effects on the Uterus and Fetus

That local anesthetics traverse the placenta is well known.[112–120] They do so by passive diffusion.[118,119] The amount transferred per unit time varies directly with the maternal–fetal concentration gradient and surface area available.[118] Transfer is also dependent upon characteristics of individual local anesthetics, such as lipid solubility, protein binding, and fraction of unionized drug (see Table 4-1).

Dosage. Increasing dosage of local anesthetics administered by epidural, paracervical, or pudendal block results in higher peak blood level.[121–124] Blood levels of lidocaine[121,125–127] and mepivacaine[122–124] are decreased 20 to 50 per cent by the addition of epinephrine. However, the blood levels of prilocaine, bupivacaine, and etidocaine do not change significantly with the use of epinephrine.[125,128,129] The high lipid solubility of bupivacaine and etidocaine—which may facilitate adipose tissue uptake—and their greater vasodilating effect may counteract vasoconstriction by epinephrine.[129]

Maternal protein binding decreases placental transfer of local anesthetics by decreasing the free base fraction available for diffusion.[115,130–132] Protein binding of lidocaine is concentration-dependent: At 12 μg. per ml., only 30 per cent is

Table 4-3. Local Anesthetic Concentrations After Maternal Local Analgesia

DRUG	TECHNIQUE	MEAN MATERNAL DOSE (MG.)	MEAN DURATION OF ANALGESIA PREPARTUM (MIN.)	MEAN MATERNAL BLOOD CONCENTRATION (μG./ML.)	MEAN FETAL OR NEONATAL BLOOD CONCENTRATION (μG./ML.)	MEAN FETAL–MATERNAL CONCENTRATION RATIO
Bupivacaine	Epidural	95	259	0.36	0.11	0.31
	Paracervical	52	51	0.58	0.08	0.31
	Pudendal	50	50	0.22	0.05	0.25
Etidocaine	Epidural	188	25	0.70	0.23	0.33
Lidocaine	Epidural	446	151	2.1	1.2	0.57
	Paracervical	200	166	1.2	0.6	0.58
	Pudendal	200	53	0.9	0.4	0.44
Mepivacaine	Epidural	572	164	3.3	2.1	0.69
	Paracervical	275	113	2.9	2.3	0.79
Prilocaine	Epidural	484	120	1.3	1.5	1.20

(Modified from Ralston, D.H., and Shnider, S.M.: The fetal and neonatal effects of regional anesthesia in obstetrics. Anesthesiology, 48:34, 1978)

bound, while at 2 μg. per ml., nearly all the drug is bound.[138] These findings imply saturation of binding sites and, thus, much greater placental transfer with higher concentrations. Of the local anesthetics studied, bupivacaine and etidocaine are bound to the greatest extent, followed in decreasing order by mepivacaine, lidocaine, and prilocaine (Table 4-1). Recently, differential binding of local anesthetics by maternal and fetal blood has been proposed to explain the fetal–maternal concentration gradient.[112,114,133–135] Maternal plasma protein binding capacities are much higher than fetal capacities.[131,136,137] A direct relationship also exists between the maternal protein binding and fetal–maternal drug ratios. Bupivacaine has the lowest fetal–maternal ratio, while prilocaine the highest (Table 4-3).

Placental Transfer. Lidocaine appears in the umbilical vein 2 to 3 min. after intravenous injection and remains there in measurable quantities for 30 to 45 min.[137] Absorption of the anesthetic from the mother's epidural space begins within 3 to 5 min. after injection. Peak blood levels are reached in 25 to 40 min. in the maternal blood and in 30 to 45 min. in the fetal blood.[138] The lidocaine or mepivacaine concentration of the fetal circulation is approximately 50 to 70 per cent of that in the maternal circulation. The placenta evidently presents a type of barrier to the passage of lidocaine and mepivacaine.[137] Procaine and chloroprocaine cross the placenta, too, but their rapid hydrolysis in the maternal and fetal blood precludes accurate measurement. Procaine concentration in fetal blood at birth is about one-half of that in maternal circulation.[139] Less than 4 mg. per kg. of procaine injected into the maternal vein cannot be detected in fetal or maternal blood.

Fetal Toxicity. Regional anesthesia in obstetrics is associated on the whole with a lower incidence of neonatal depression than is general anesthesia. Local anesthetics do cross the placenta soon after maternal injection and enter the fetal circulation; however, small amounts of these drugs evidently are harmless. In utero, fetal mepivacaine levels below 7 μg. per ml. are never associated with bradycardia or other prepartum signs of fetal distress. When the fetal scalp blood has a plasma concentration of about 14 μg. per ml., fetal distress is always present.

Newborn infants tolerate as much as 3 to 4 μg. per ml. of lidocaine or mepivacaine in the cord blood without difficulty.[138,140] Higher blood levels have been incriminated in contributing to neonatal depression. Even so, the majority of infants are resuscitated readily and have high Apgar scores 5 min. after birth. One might conclude, then, that either the anesthetic is redistributed, metabolized, or excreted exceedingly rapidly after delivery, or that the drug contributes little to neonatal depression.

Occasionally large amounts of a local anesthetic reach the fetal circulation. When mepivacaine is injected inadvertently into the fetal scalp instead of the maternal sacral canal, the infant is apneic at birth or soon thereafter, has refractory bradycardia, and convulses periodically.[141] If vital functions can be maintained, the mepivacaine level in the blood drops from 75 μg. per ml. at 4 hours to 8 μg. per ml. at 30 hours, at which time the infant finally stops convulsing and the EEG reverts to normal.

While well managed lumbar or caudal epidural block is seldom associated with unduly high fetal anesthetic levels, this does not seem to be true with paracervical injection, which is associated with fetal bradycardia in 20 to 30 per cent of cases.[69] Fetal bradycardia occurs following intravenous administration of local anesthetic in the mother, even without maternal hypotension. This suggests that the local anesthetic is responsible for the bradycardia.[142] As fetal scalp blood levels oftentimes exceed those in maternal arterial blood, local anesthetic may reach the fetus by a more direct route than the maternal systemic one. It has been suggested that the anesthetic either finds its way into nearby paracervical blood vessels or migrates along fascial planes and so reaches the placental intervillous space.

Newborns who experience local anesthetic toxicity have a high death rate. Of four infants inadvertently injected with mepivacaine into the scalp, only two survived and developed normally.[141] Other investigators reported one stillbirth and one infant who survived less than 2 days with

the syndrome of intrauterine bradycardia, followed at birth by apnea and convulsions.[50]

Even when neonates are not depressed at birth as indicated by low Apgar scores, more subtle neurobehavioral changes in the subsequent neonatal period have been noted. Scanlon[143,144] has developed a neurobehavioral examination that combines standard neurologic testing[145-147] and evaluation of the newborn's response to external stimuli. He found decreased attentiveness, muscular hypotonia, less vigorous Moro and rooting responses, and altered decremental response to pin prick in neonates 2 to 8 hours old following uncomplicated vaginal delivery with mepivacaine or lidocaine epidural anesthesia.[144] However, no neurobehavioral changes are apparent in neonates after maternal epidural anesthesia with bupivacaine (Fig. 4-7) or chloroprocaine for vaginal delivery,[148] or with bupivacaine for cesarean section.[149] Tronick evaluated neonatal neurobehavioral performance for as long as 10 days following maternal regional anesthesia with lidocaine and mepivacaine.[150] Although there were changes in muscle tone, they were transient and of minimal consequence.

Therefore, although subtle neurobehavioral changes can be demonstrated in neonates shortly after birth following maternal epidural anesthesia with lidocaine or mepivacaine, there is no evidence that these changes are detrimental. Of course, the long-term significance of these findings, if any, is unknown. Nevertheless, it seems prudent to minimize fetal exposure to local anesthetics that alter neurobehavioral states by using the lowest dosage that produces the desired maternal analgesia, and by choosing agents such as bupivacaine or chloroprocaine, which do not alter neonatal neurobehavioral status.[69]

SYSTEMIC REACTION TO VASOCONSTRICTOR DRUGS

Vasoconstrictors are used in regional anesthesia for three purposes: to prolong the anesthetic effect; to decrease the rate of absorption into systemic circulation; and to correct (or prevent) hypotension. The addition of vasoconstrictors to

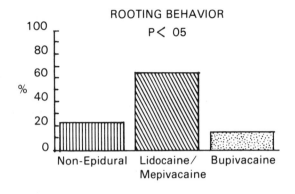
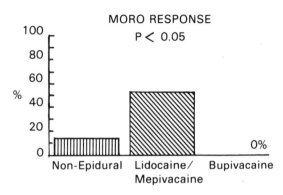
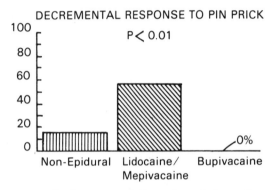
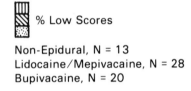

Fig. 4-7. Performance of 61 newborn infants, 2 to 4 hours of age, on several neurologic and behavioral tests that characterize adaptive capacity. Compared are the percentages of low scores among infants delivered with epidural analgesia with lidocaine or mepivacaine (*Lidocaine/Mepivacaine*) or bupivacaine (*Bupivacaine*), and those delivered without epidural analgesia (*Non-Epidural*). (Scanlon, J. W.: Effects of local anesthetics administered to parturient women on the neurological and behavioral performance of newborn children. Bull. N.Y. Acad. Med., *52:* 231, 1976)

the local anesthetic solution achieves the first two.

Systemic toxic reactions to vasoconstrictor drugs may be the result of an allergy or a high blood concentration. Halle observed spasmodic sneezing in a number of cases following the use of epinephrine in the nasal passages.[151] Gordonoff and Steube have suggested that death or severe reactions after procaine-epinephrine injection in two of their patients might have been due to allergic reactions.[152] This interpretation is open to question. While allergic reaction to vasoconstrictor drugs is certainly rare, reactions to a high blood level of a vasoconstrictor is not infrequent and may be confused with an anaphylactic reaction. Patients may complain of shortness of breath, fear, anxiety, headache, palpitation, nausea, and faintness. Of these, palpitation and headache are perhaps the most frequent symptoms of high blood levels of vasoconstrictors. The physician may note tachypnea, tachycardia, hypertension, pallor, tremor, and/or vomiting. Thus, the reaction to vasoconstrictor drugs may also resemble the early stages of a toxic reaction to a local anesthetic—that is, stimulation of the CNS.

Moore[153] and Adriani[154] believe that vasoconstrictor drugs should be employed only for a specific purpose: prolonging the anesthetic effect and/or reducing the rate of absorption of the local anesthetic solution. They feel that if the dosage of vasoconstrictors is not excessive, then even intravascular injection of the drugs produces only transient side effects that are likely to be of no particular significance in normal persons. However, in patients with hypertension, coronary artery disease, and hyperthyroidism, the use of vasoconstrictors is relatively contraindicated.

The anesthesiologist should avoid vasoconstrictor drugs when blocking the digits, the nose, and the penis. In these areas, the volume of the solution that may be accomodated without causing mechanical pressure on the blood vessel is small. The chance of completely occluding the blood supply to the area by mechanical compression and vasoconstriction is enhanced. The anesthesiologist must not add vasoconstrictors to cocaine, which possesses vasoconstrictive properties, for such a practice can result in tissue slough.

Though many vasoconstrictor drugs are available, those commonly used are epinephrine and phenylephrine. The optimum concentration of epinephrine is 1:200,000 (5 μg./ml.): that is, 0.1 ml. of 1:1000 epinephrine in 20 ml. of local anesthetic solution. The corresponding concentration of phenylephrine is 1:20,000. Exceeding the total dose of 0.25 mg. of epinephrine or 2 mg. of phenylephrine increases the incidence of reactions.

ALLERGY TO LOCAL ANESTHETICS

The incidence of true allergic reactions to local anesthetics is unknown but is probably exceedingly low compared to their widespread use. In fact, in most reports it is impossible to determine the etiology of a given reaction or even to differentiate a true allergic reaction from rapid absorption owing to a highly vascular site or intravascular injection (relative overdose), or a toxic dose (absolute overdose), and from psychogenic reaction or idiosyncrasy. Moreover, an allergic reaction may be caused by another drug (e.g., preanesthetic medication) administered at about the same time and may be confused with the systemic response to a vasoconstrictor in the local anesthetic solution. Too often a patient is labeled as "allergic to local anesthetics" without adequate justification.

Allergy to local anesthetics may be manifested as dermatitis,[155] urticaria,[156] or anaphylaxis[157]; pruritis and bronchospasm frequently accompany allergic drug reactions. Eighty-three per cent of dermatitis-like reactions to procaine occur in health professionals, mostly dentists.[158] Virtually all reports of allergy involve the *p*-aminobenzoic ester groups rather than the amide group of local anesthetics. There is also cross-sensitivity between these *p*-aminobenzoic acid derivatives and the preservative methylparaben,[158–160] which is structurally similar and is used in many multiple-dose preparations of local anesthetics and other drugs, including many nonprescription agents. In contrast, allergic reactions to local anesthetics of the amide group are exceedingly rare; upon subsequent testing almost all alleged reactions are found to be due to methylparaben sensitivity.[158] There have been only a few well documented cases of allergy to amide-type agents.[157,161,162] Hence, amide-type local anesthetics, especially without preservative (e.g., in single-dose preparations), are preferred to avoid allergic reactions.

Diagnosis of Allergy to Local Anesthetics

At special risk to allergic reactions are atopic persons who have a genetic tendency to respond three to ten times more frequently[163] to antigens by producing reaginic antibodies (IgE). These patients usually have a history of periodic eczema, rhinitis, bronchial asthma, or chronic urticaria. Patients with a history of allergy to local anesthetics should be tested for allergy to the agent, preservative, placebo, and other chemically related agents.

Skin Tests. The suspected allergen is administered intradermally, scratched or pricked into the skin, or applied to the skin as a patch. The vehicle in which the drug is dissolved and any preservatives in the local anesthetic solution must be tested separately. Since severe reactions may occur in sensitized persons, these tests should be conducted with utmost caution, with all treatment modalities available. An immediate reaction, or one occurring within 2 hours, usually indicates histamine and serotonin release mediated by reaginic antibody (IgE), which attaches to mast cells and basophils. A reaction occurring 24 to 48 hours later indicates delayed hypersensitivity or contact sensitization caused by sensitized thymus-derived lymphocytes. Since both IgE antibody and lymphocytes require the complete antigen for response, a negative reaction may occur owing to the use of the hapten (the drug) without its carrier macromolecule.[164] In addition, Adriani feels that the skin test may give a false negative result because the protein of skin is different from protein elsewhere in body, and the hapten may be a metabolite and not a drug itself.[165] Thus, these tests are helpful only when positive.

Arora and Aldrete suggest the following intradermal procedure:[166] First, explain the procedure and obtain written consent from the patient, whose vital signs are monitored closely. Then, without applying antiseptic over the area of skin to be tested, inject intracutaneously 0.01 ml. of the following local anesthetics, without epinephrine (which might mask a positive reaction): 0.5-per-cent lidocaine with and without methylparaben; 0.25-per-cent bupivacaine with and without methylparaben; 0.25-per-cent tetracaine; 1-per-cent procaine; 0.5-per-cent mepivacaine; and sterile saline with and without methylparaben. Grade the reaction at 30 min. with the following criteria: negative—no visible change at the injection site; positive— + (1 cm.), ++ (2 cm.), or +++ (3 cm.) wheal with erythema. A + reaction is probably due to localized histamine release rather than an antigen-antibody reaction. In patients with a negative response, inject 50 mg. of 1-per-cent lidocaine, 1-per-cent mepivacaine, 0.1-per-cent tetracaine, or 0.125-per-cent bupivacaine. There should be a 25-min. interval between the injections. They are assessed as follows: A

negative response indicates that the local anesthetic in question can be administered safely in larger doses; patients with positive reactions require more precise immunological testing.

Prausnitz-Kustner Test. Serum from the suspected allergic patient is injected intradermally at several sites in either another normal human or a monkey; the latter is preferable to eliminate the risk of transmission of viral hepatitis. Twenty-four hours later, the presumed allergen is injected at the same sites. A wheal and flare within 2 hours denote a positive test. The test avoids the risk of anaphylaxis in the suspected patient and is very sensitive in detecting an IgE-mediated immediate reaction.[164]

In vitro tests have the obvious advantage of not risking the occurrence of a potentially serious reaction. The lymphocyte transformation test (LTT) reflects the delayed type of hypersensitivity reaction. In this test, peripheral lymphocytes are cultured with different amounts of suspected antigen. Lymphocytes from unsensitized persons do not divide. Cells from sensitized persons, however, are stimulated to undergo cell transformation in preparation for cell division, which is detected by uptake of radioactive RNA and DNA precursors. The efficacy of this test in the detection of drug allergy has been attested to by many investigators.[164,167,168] The macrophage inhibition test,[169] another correlate of delayed hypersensitivity, seems to be less specific than the LTT.[164]

Immediate hypersensitivity (histamine release) can be measured by the basophil degranulation test. The patient's basophils or leukocytes, or rabbit basophils, are incubated sequentially with the patient's serum and the drug. Histamine release is measured fluorometrically or by radioimmunoassay. The sensitivity of this test is poor.[164]

Treatment of Allergic Reactions

Prevention is always more desirable than treatment. However, allergic reactions cannot always be predicted and averted. Should such a reaction occur, oxygenation and ventilation must be supported, as needed. The following drugs should be considered for sequential intravenous administration to help maintain cardiac output and peripheral perfusion, as well as to counteract the effects of the released mediators (histamine, serotonin, slow-reacting substance of anaphylaxis):[164]

Epinephrine. In addition to stimulating alpha- and beta-adrenergic receptors, epinephrine potentiates adenyl cyclase activity, thus effectively increasing the tissue concentration of 3',5'-cyclic adenosine monophosphate (cAMP), which inhibits release of mediators and relaxes bronchial smooth muscle. Typically, epinephrine is administered as a dilute intravenous infusion. Epinephrine may cause arrhythmias when used with halothane, particularly in the presence of hypercarbia. Hence, it must be used cautiously with this agent.

Isoproterenol, a sympathomimetic amine, stimulates beta-adrenergic receptors almost exclusively, and its action is of shorter duration than epinephrine. Until a beta-adrenergic stimulator specific for the lung is widely available, isoproterenol may be used to treat bronchospasm without hypotension. During general anesthesia, the aerosol route is preferable, since it permits rapid bronchodilatation.

Ephedrine, a sympathomimetic amine, stimulates alpha-adrenergic receptors, causing vasoconstriction, and central beta-adrenergic receptors, increasing both myocardial contractility and bronchodilatation. Although its use for bronchospasm is limited, it is extremely effective for eliminating hypotension secondary to extreme vasodilatation and other causes. During general anesthesia, it may be administered intravenously or intramuscularly, depending on the rapidity and duration of action desired. Intravenously, it is given in doses of 0.15 mg. per kg. and acts for 30 to 45 minutes; intramuscularly, larger doses of 0.3 mg. per kg. may be administered, and the effect lasts 1.5 to 2 hours.

Antihistamines compete with histamine for tissue receptor sites in bronchial or intestinal smooth muscle. The intravenous route is preferred. Diphenhydramine in doses of 10 to 20 mg.,

intravenously may be repeated every 2 to 3 hours if symptoms persist.

Methylxanthines inhibit phosphodiesterase, resulting in an increased level of 3',5'-cAMP intracellularly and thus inhibiting further release of mediators. Efficacious in the treatment of bronchospasm, methylxanthines may cause arrhythmias and hypotension. A recommended dose of aminophylline is 250 to 500 mg. to be administered intravenously over 20 to 30 min.

Steroids are believed to enhance the effect of epinephrine on adenyl cyclase, and they seem to interfere with histamine release. Hydrocortisone in bolus intravenous doses of 100 mg., followed by intravenous infusions at a rate of 100 mg. every 6 to 8 hours, is recommended.

Atropine. By blocking cholinergic receptors, atropine effectively decreases intracellular cyclic 3',5'-guanosine monophosphate, in turn diminishing histamine and slow-reacting substance release. Also, inhibitory parasympathetic effects on the cardiovascular system are eliminated. Atropine may be given in small intravenous increments of 0.5 mg.

When the allergen has been given intramuscularly or subcutaneously, the injection of 0.1 to 0.2 mg. of epinephrine subcutaneously in the area of injection may delay absorption of the offending drug; ice packs placed on the area and a tourniquet on the limb have a similar effect.

REFERENCES

1. Bonica, J. J.: Management of Pain. Philadelphia, Lea & Febiger, 1953.
2. Cotev, S., and Robin, G. C.: Experimental studies on intravenous regional anaesthesia using radioactive lignocaine. Br. J. Anaesth., 38:936, 1966.
3. deJong, R. H., and Nace, R. A.: Nerve impulse conduction during intravenous lidocaine injection. Anesthesiology, 29:22, 1968.
4. Covino, B. G., and Vassallo, H. G.: Local Anesthetics: Mechanisms of Action and Clinical Use. pp. 95–121. New York, Grune & Stratton, 1976.
5. Englesson, S., Paymaster, N. J., and Hill, T. R.: Electrical seizure activity produced by Xylocaine and Citanest. Acta Anaesthesiol. Scand. 16[Suppl.]:47, 1965.
6. Bromage, P. R., and Gertel, M.: Improved brachial plexus blockade with bupivacaine hydrochloride and carbonated lidocaine. Anesthesiology, 36:479, 1972.

7. Boullin, D. J., and Sullivan, T. J.: Relationship between the uptake, binding and pharmacological action of procaine in the isolated heart. Br. J. Pharmacol., 35:322, 1969.

8. Stewart, D. M., Rogers, W. P., Mahaffey, J. E., et al.: Effect of local anesthetics on the cardiovascular system of the dog. Anesthesiology, 24:620, 1963.

9. Mazze, R. I., and Dunbar, R. W.: Plasma lidocaine concentrations after caudal, lumbar epidural, axillary block, and intravenous regional anesthesia. Anesthesiology, 27:574, 1966.

10. Tucker, G. T., Moore, D. C., Bridenbaugh, P. O., et al: Systemic absorption of mepivacaine in commonly used regional block procedures. Anesthesiology, 37:277, 1972.

11. Scott, D. B., Jebson, P. J. R., Braid, D. P., et al.: Factors affecting plasma levels of lignocaine and prilocaine. Br. J. Anaesth., 44:1040, 1972.

12. Braid, D. P., and Scott, D. B.: The systemic absorption of local analgesic drugs. Br. J. Anaesth., 37:394, 1965.

13. Lund, P. C., Bush, D. F., and Covino, B. G.: Determinants of etidocaine concentration in the blood. Anesthesiology, 42:497, 1975.

14. Foldes, F. F., Molly, R., McNall, P. G., et al.: Comparison of toxicity of intravenously given local anesthetic agents in man. J.A.M.A., 172:1493, 1960.

15. Bromage, P. R., and Robson, J. G.: Concentrations of lignocaine in the blood after intravenous, intramuscular, epidural, and endotracheal administration. Anaesthesia, 16:461, 1961.

16. Scott, D. B.: Evaluation of the toxicity of local anaesthetic agents in man. Br. J. Anaesth., 47:56, 1975.

17. Wagman, I. H., deJong, R. H., and Prince, D. A.: Effects of lidocaine on the central nervous system. Anesthesiology, 28:155, 1967.

18. Usubiaga, J. E., Wikinski, J., Ferrero, R., et al.: Local anesthetic-induced convulsions in man. An electroencephalographic study. Anesth. Analg., 45:611, 1966.

19. Foldes, F. F., Davidson, G. M., Duncalf, D., et al.: The intravenous toxicity of local anesthetic agents in man. Clin. Pharmacol. Ther., 6:328, 1965.

20. Bromage, P. R., and Gertel, M.: Improved brachial plexus blockade with bupivacaine, hydrochloride and carbonated lidocaine. Anesthesiology, 36:479, 1972.

21. Moore, D. C., Bridenbaugh, L. D., Bridenbaugh, P. O., et al.: Does compounding of local anesthetic agents increase their toxicity in humans? Anesth. Analg., 51:579, 1972.

22. Cunningham, N. L., and Kaplan, J. A.: A rapid onset long-acting regional anesthetic technique. Anesthesiology, 41:509., 1974.

23. Raj, P. P., Rosenblatt, R., Miller, J., et al.: Dynamics of compounded local anesthetic mixtures in regional anesthesia. Anesth. Analg., 56:110, 1977.

24. Julien, R. M.: Lidocaine in experimental epilepsy: correlation of anticonvulsant effect with blood concentrations. Electroencephalogr. Clin. Neurophysiol., 34:639, 1973.

25. deJong, R. H.: Local Anesthetics. ed. 2. pp. 86–88. Springfield, Charles C Thomas, 1977.

26. Lemmen, L. J., Klassen, M., and Duiser, B.: Intravenous lidocaine in the treatment of convulsions. J.A.M.A., 239:2025, 1978.

27. Acheson, F., Bull, A. B., and Glees, P.: Electroencephalogram of the cat after intravenous injection of lidocaine and succinylcholine. Anesthesiology, 17:802, 1956.

28. Sorel, L., and LeJeune, R.: Modifications de l'EEG du lapin sous l'action de divers succedanes de la cocaine injectes par voie intraveineuse. Arch. Int. Pharmacodyn., 102:314, 1955.

29. deJong, R. H., and Walts, L. F.: Lidocaine-induced psychomotor seizures in man. Acta Anaesthesiol. Scand., 23[Suppl.]598, 1966.

30. Jolly, E. R., and Steinhaus, J. E.: The effect of drugs injected into limited portions of the cerebral circulation. J. Pharmacol. Exp. Ther., 116:273, 1956.

31. Tuttle, W. W., and Elliott, H. W.: Electrographic and behavioral study of convulsants in the cat. Anesthesiology, 30:48, 1969.

32. Eidelberg, E., Lesse, H., and Gault, F. P.: An experimental mode of temporal lobe epilepsy. Studies of the convulsant properties of cocaine. In Glaser, G. H. (ed.): EEG and Behavior. Chap. 10. New York, Basic Books, 1963.

33. Prince, D. A., and Wagman, I. H.: Activation of limbic system epileptogenic foci with intravenous lidocaine. Electroencephalogr. Clin. Neurophysiol., 21:416, 1966.

34. Englesson, S., Paymaster, N. J., and Hill, T. R.: Electrical seizure activity produced by Xylocaine and Citanest. Acta Anaesthesiol. Scand., 16[Suppl.]47, 1965.

35. Plum, F., Posner, J. B., and Troy, B.: Cerebral metabolic and circulatory responses to induced convulsions in animals. Arch. Neurol., 18:1, 1968.

36. Posner, J. B., Plum, F., and Van Poznak, A.: Cerebral metabolism during electrically induced seizures in man. Arch. Neurol., 20:388, 1969.

37. Beutner, R., and Calesnick, B.: The essential characteristics of local anesthetics. Anesthesiology, 3:673, 1942.

38. Steinhaus, J. E.: Local anesthetic toxicity: a pharmacological reevaluation. Anesthesiology, 18:275, 1957.

39. Mark, L. C., Brank, L., and Goldensohn, E. S.: Recovery after procaine-induced seizures in dogs. Electroencephalogr. Clin. Neurophysiol., 16:280, 1964.

40. Moore, D. C., Bridenbaugh, L. D., and Thompson, G. E., et al.: Bupivacaine: a review in 11,080 cases. Anesth. Analg., 57:42, 1978.

41. Zito, R. A., and Reid, P. R.: Lidocaine kinetics predicted by indocyanine green clearance. N. Engl. J. Med., 298:1160, 1978.

42. deJong, R. H., and Heavner, J. E.: Local anesthetic seizure prevention: diazepam versus pentobarbital. Anesthesiology, 36:449, 1972.

43. deJong, R. H., and Heavner, J. E.: Diazepam prevents local anesthetic seizures. Anesthesiology, 34:523, 1971.

44. deJong, R. H., and Heavner, J. E.: Diazepam prevents and aborts lidocaine convulsions in monkeys. Anesthesiology, 41:226, 1974.

45. deJong, R. H.: Local Anesthetics. ed. 2. pp. 108–109. Springfield, Charles C. Thomas, 1977.

46. deJong, R. H., Heavner, J. E., and deOliverira, L. F.: Effects of nitrous oxide on the lidocaine seizure threshold and diazepam protection. Anesthesiology, 37:299, 1972.

47. Eidelberg, E., Neer, H. M., and Miller, M. K.: Anticonvulsant properties of some benzodiazepine derivatives. Neurology, *15*:223, 1965.
48. Sanders, H. D.: A comparison of the convulsant activity of procaine and pentylenetetrazol. Arch. Int. Pharmacodyn. Ther., *170*:165, 1967.
49. Feinstein, M. B., Lenard, W., and Mathias, J.: The antagonism of local anesthetic induced convulsions by the benzodiazepine derivative diazepam. Arch. Int. Pharmacodyn. Ther., *187*:144, 1970.
50. Rosefsky, J. B., and Petersiel, M. E.: Perinatal deaths associated with mepivacaine paracervical-block anesthesia in labor. N. Engl. J. Med., *278*:530, 1968.
51. Richards, R. K., Smith, N. T., and Katz, J.: The effects of interaction between lidocaine and pentobarbital on toxicity in mice and guinea pig atria. Anesthesiology, *29*:493, 1968.
52. Wagman, I. H., deJong, R. H., and Prince, D. A.: Effects of lidocaine on spontaneous cortical and subcortical electrical activity: production of seizure discharges. Arch. Neurol., *18*:277, 1968.
53. Dripps, R. D., and Deming, M. V. N.: An evaluation of certain drugs used to maintain blood pressure during spinal anesthesia: comparison of ephedrine, paredrine, pitressin-ephedrine and methedrine in 2,500 cases. Surg. Gynecol. Obstet., *83*:312, 1946.
54. Defalque, R. J.: Compared effects of spinal and extradural anesthesia upon the blood pressure. Anesthesiology, *23*:627, 1962.
55. Greene, N. M.: Physiology of Spinal Anesthesia. ed. 2. pp. 43–117. Baltimore, Williams & Wilkins, 1969.
56. Ward, R. J., Bonica, J. J., Freund, F. G., et al.: Epidural and spinal anesthesia: cardiovascular and respiratory effects. J.A.M.A., *191*:275, 1965.
57. Greene, N. M.: Physiology of Spinal Anesthesia. ed. 2. pp. 227–234. Baltimore, Williams & Wilkins, 1969.
58. Bigger, J. T., and Mandel, W. J.: Effect of lidocaine on the electrophysiological properties of ventricular muscle and Purkinje fibers. J. Clin. Invest., *49*:63, 1970.
59. Bigger, J. T., and Mandel, W. J.: Effect of lidocaine on conduction in canine Purkinje fibers and at the ventricular muscle-Purkinje fiber junction. J. Pharmacol. Exp. Ther., *172*:239, 1970.
60. Austen, W. G., and Moran, J. M.: Cardiac and peripheral vascular effects of lidocaine and procaineamide. Am. J. Cardiol., *16*:701, 1965.
61. Kao, F. F., and Jalar, U. H.: The central action of lignocaine and its effects on cardiac output. Br. J. Pharmacol., *14*:522, 1959.
62. Vyden, J. K., Mandel, W., Hayakawa, H., et al.: The effect of lidocaine on peripheral hemodynamics. J. Clin. Pharmacol., *15*:506, 1975.
63. Stewart, D. M., Rogers, W. P., Mahaffey, J. E., et al.: Effect of local anesthetics on the cardiovascular system in the dog. Anesthesiology, *24*:620, 1963.
64. Nayler, W. G., McInnes, I., Carson, V., et al.: The effect of lignocaine on myocardial function, high energy phosphate stores, and oxygen consumption: a comparison with propranolol. Am. Heart J., *78*:338, 1969.
65. Harrison, D. C., Sprouse, J. H., and Morrow, A. G.: The antiarrhythmic properties of lidocaine and procaine amide: clinical and physiologic studies of their cardiovascular effects in man. Circulation, *28*:486, 1963.
66. Klein, S. W., Sutherland, R. I. L., and Morch, J. E.: Hemodynamic effects of intravenous lidocaine in man. Can. Med. Assoc. J., *99*:472, 1968.
67. Nishimura, N., Morioka, T., Sato, S., et al.: Effects of local anesthetic agents on the peripheral vascular system. Anesth. Analg., *44*:135, 1965.
68. Blair, M. R.: Cardiovascular pharmacology of local anaesthetics. Br. J. Anaesth., *47*:247, 1975.
69. Ralston, D. H., and Shnider, S. M.: The fetal and neonatal effects of regional anesthesia in obstetrics. Anesthesiology, *48*:34,1978.
70. Asling, J. H.: Hypotension after regional anesthesia. *In* Shnider, S. M. (ed.): Obstetrical Anesthesia, Current Concepts and Practice. pp. 158–163. Baltimore, Williams & Wilkins, 1970.
71. Kennedy, R. L.: An instrument to relieve inferior vena cava occlusion. Am. J. Obstet. Gynecol., *107*:331, 1970.
72. Kennedy, R. L., Friedman, D. L., Katchka, D. M., et al.: Hypotension during obstetrical anesthesia. Anesthesiology, *20*:153, 1959.
73. Marx, G. F.: Anesthesia for elective cesarean section. Clin. Anesthesiol., *10*:198, 1973.
74. Marx, G. F.: Shock in the obstetrical patient. Anesthesiology, *25*:423, 1965.
75. Shnider, S. M.: Anesthesia for elective cesarean section. *In* Shnider, S. M. (ed.): Obstetrical Anesthesia, Current Concepts and Practice. pp. 94–106. Baltimore, Williams & Wilkins, 1970.
76. Wollman, S. B., and Marx, G. F.: Acute hydration for prevention of hypotension of spinal anesthesia in parturients. Anesthesiology, *29*:374, 1968.
77. Eckstein, K. L., and Marx, G. F.: Aortocaval compression and uterine displacement. Anesthesiology, *40*:92, 1974.
78. Scott, D. B.: Inferior vena caval occlusion in late pregnancy. Clin. Anesthesiol., *10*:37, 1973.
79. Bonica, J. J.: Maternal physiologic changes during pregnancy and anesthesia. *In* Shnider, S. M., and Moya, F. (eds.): The Anesthesiologist, Mother and Newborn. pp. 3–19. Baltimore, Williams & Wilkins, 1974.
80. Akamatsu, T. J.: Cesarean section under epidural anesthesia with epinephrine. Anesthesiol. Rev., *1*:28, 1974.
81. Levinson, G., Shnider, S. M., Krames, E., et al.: Epidural anesthesia for cesarean section: effects of epinephrine in the local anesthetic solution (abstr). p. 285. American Society of Anesthesiologists Annual Meeting, 1976.
82. Gibbs, C. P., and Noel, S. C.: Human uterine artery response to lidocaine. Am. J. Obstet. Gynecol., *126*:313, 1976.
83. Gibbs, C. P., and Noel, S. C.: Response of arterial segments from gravid human uterus to multiple concentrations of lignocaine. Br. J. Anaesth., *49*:409, 1977.
84. Greiss, F. C., Jr., Still, J. G., and Anderson, S. G.: Effects of local anesthetic agents on the uterine vasculature and myometrium. Am. J. Obstet. Gynecol., *124*:889, 1976.
85. Biehl, D., Shnider, S. M., Levinson, G., et al.: The direct effects of circulating lidocaine on uterine blood flow and foetal well-being in the pregnant ewe. Can. Anaesth. Soc. J., *24*:445, 1977.

86. Greiss, F. C., Jr.: The uterine vascular bed: effect of adrenergic stimulation. Obstet. Gynecol., *21*:295, 1963.

87. Asling, J. H., Shnider, S. M., Wilkinson, G. R., et al.: Gas chromatographic determination of mepivacaine in capillary blood. Anesthesiology, *31*:458, 1969.

88. Shnider, S. M., deLorimier, A. A., and Steffenson, J. L.: Vasopressors in obstetrics. III. Fetal effects of metaraminol infusion during obstetric spinal hypotension. Am. J. Obstet. Gynecol., *108*:1017, 1970.

89. Belitzky, R., Delard, L. G., and Novick, L. M.: Oxytoxic effects of intramyometrial injection of procaine in a pregnant woman. Am. J. Obstet. Gynecol., *107*:973, 1970.

90. Vasicka, A., Hutchinson, H. E., Eng., M., et al.: Spinal and epidural anesthesia, fetal and uterine response to acute hypo- and hypertension. Am. J. Obstet. Gynecol., *90*:800, 1964.

91. Kennedy, W. F., Jr., Bonica, J. J., Ward, R. J., et al.: Cardiorespiratory effects of epinephrine when used in regional anaesthesia. Acta Anaesthesiol. Scand., *23*[Suppl.]:320, 1966.

92. Smith, N. T., and Corbascio, A. N.: The use and misuse of pressor agents. Anesthesiology, *33*:58, 1970.

93. McGaughey, H. S., Jr., Corey, E. L., Eastwood, D., et al.: Effect of synthetic anesthetics on the spontaneous mobility of human uterine muscle *in vitro*. Obstet. Gynecol., *19*:233, 1962.

94. Poppers, P. J.: Evaluation of local anaesthetic agents for regional anaesthesia in obstetrics. Br. J. Anaesth., *47*:322, 1975.

95. Bonica, J. J.: Principles and Practice of Obstetric Analgesia and Anesthesia. pp. 190–215. Philadelphia, F. A. Davis, 1967.

96. Adams, F. H., Assali, N., Cushman, M., et al.: Interrelationships of maternal and fetal circulations. Pediatrics, *27*:627, 1961.

97. Adamsons, K., and Myers, R. E.: Circulation in the intervillous space: obstetrical considerations in fetal deprivation. *In* Gruenwald, P. (ed.): The Placenta. pp.158–177. Baltimore, University Park Press, 1975.

98. Ebner, H., Barcohana, J., and Bartoshok, A. K.: Influence of post-spinal hypotension on the fetal electrocardiogram. Am. J. Obstet. Gynecol., *80*:569, 1960.

99. Lucas, W. E., Kirschbaum, T., and Assali, N. S.: Spinal shock and fetal oxygenation. Am. J. Obstet. Gynecol., *93*:583, 1965.

100. Moya, F., and Thorndike, V.: Maternal hypotension and the newborn. Proceedings of the Third World Congress of Anesthesiology, *2*:11, 1964.

101. Myers, R. E.: Two patterns of perinatal brain damage and their condition of ocurrence. Am. J. Obstet. Gynecol., *112*:246, 1972.

102. Prystowsky, H.: Fetomaternal gas exchange. Clin. Obstet. Gynecol., *3*:286, 1960.

103. Brann, A. W., and Dykes, F. D.: The effects of intrauterine asphyxia on the full-term neonate. Clin. Perinatol., *4*:149, 1977.

104. Brann, A. W., and Myers, R. E.: Central nervous system findings in the newborn monkey following severe *in utero* partial asphyxia. Neurology, *25*:327, 1975.

105. Cibils, L. A.: Clinical significance of fetal heart rate patterns during labor. II. Late decelerations. Am. J. Obstet. Gynecol., *123*:473, 1975.

106. Myers, R. E., Mueller-Heubach, E., and Adamsons, K.: Predictability of the state of fetal oxygenation from a quantitative analysis of the components of late deceleration. Am. J. Obstet. Gynecol., *115*:1083, 1973.

107. Hon, E. H., Reid, B. L., and Hehre, F. W.: The electronic evaluation of the fetal heart rate. II. Changes with maternal hypotension. Am. J. Obstet. Gynecol., *79*:209, 1960.

108. Moya, F., and Smith, B.: Spinal anesthesia for cesarean section: clinical and biochemical studies of effects on maternal physiology. J.A.M.A., *179*:609, 1962.

109. Moya, F.: Spinal anesthesia for cesarean section. Int. Anesthesiol. Clin., *1*;849, 1963.

110. Stenger, V., Eitzman, D., Anderson, T., et al.: A study of the oxygenation of the fetus and newborn and its relation to that of the mother. Am. J. Obstet. Gynecol., *93*:376, 1965.

111. Stenger, V., Eitzman, D., Gessner, I., et al.: A study of the acid-base balance of the fetus and newborn and its relation to that of the mother. Am. J. Obstet. Gynecol., *90*:625, 1964.

112. Burt, R. A.: The foetal and maternal pharmacology of some of the drugs used for the relif of pain in labour. Br. J. Anaesth., *43*:824, 1971.

113. Finster, M., and Mark, L. C.: Placental transfer of drugs and their distribution in fetal tissues. Handbook Exp. Pharmacol., *28*:276, 1972.

114. Ginsburg, J.: Placental drug transfer. Ann. Rev. Pharmacol., *11*:387, 1971.

115. Goldstein, A., Aronow, L., and Kelman, S. M.: Principles of Drug Action. The Basis of Pharamcology. ed. 2. pp. 198–210. New York, John Wiley & Sons, 1973.

116. Heymann, M. A.: Interrelations of fetal circulation and the placental transfer of drugs. Fed. Proc., *31*:44, 1972.

117. Long, R. F., and Marks, J.: The transfer of drugs across the placenta. Proc. Soc. Med., *62*:318, 1969.

118. Mirkin, B. L.: Perinatal pharmacology: placental transfer, fetal localization, and neonatal disposition of drugs. Anesthesiology, *43*:156, 1975.

119. Moya, F., and Smith, B. E.: Uptake, distribution and placental transport of drugs and anesthetics. Anesthesiology, *26*:465, 1965.

120. Villee, C. A.: Placental transfer of drugs. Ann. N.Y. Acad. Sci., *123*:237, 1965.

121. Braid, D. P., and Scott, D. B.: The systemic absorption of local analgesic drugs. Br. J. Anaesth., *37*:394, 1965.

122. Shuner, K. G., Harthon, J. G. L., Herbring, B. G., et al.: Blood levels of mepivacaine after regional anaesthesia. Br. J. Anaesth., *37*:746, 1965.

123. Shnider, S. M., and Way, E. L.: Plasma levels of lidocaine (Xylocaine) in mother and newborn following obstetrical conduction anesthesia: clinical applications. Anesthesiology, *29*:951, 1968.

124. Tucker, G. T., Moore, D. C., Bridenbaugh, P. O., et al.: Systemic absorption of mepivacaine in commonly used regional block procedures. Anesthesiology, *37*:277, 1972.

125. Mather, L. E., Tucker, G. T., Murphy, T. M., et al.: The effects of adding adrenaline to etidocaine and lignocaine

in extradural anaesthesia. II. Pharmacokinetics. Br. J. Anaesth., 48:989, 1976.

126. Thomas, J., Climie, C. R., and Mather, L. E.: The influence of adrenaline on plasma levels and placental transfer of lignocaine following lumbar epidural administration. Br. J. Anaesth., 41:1029, 1969.

127. Tucker, G. T., and Mather, L. E.: Pharmacokinetics of local anaesthetic agents. Br. J. Anaesth., 47:213, 1975.

128. Covino, B. G., and Vassallo, H. G.: Local Anesthetics: Mechanisms of Action and Clinical Use. p. 104. New York, Grune & Stratton, 1976.

129. Lund, P. C., Cwik, J. C., and Gannon, R. T.: Extradural anaesthesia: choice of local anaesthetic agents. Br. J. Anaesth., 47:313, 1975.

130. Lant, A. F.: The factors affecting the action of drugs. In Scurr, C., and Feldman, S. (eds.): Scientific Foundations of Anaesthesia. ed. 2. pp. 405–428. London, William Heinemann, 1974.

131. Tucker, G. T., Boyes, R. N., Bridenbaugh, P. O., et al.: Binding of anilide-type local anesthetics in human plasma. II. Implications in vivo, with special reference to transplacental distribution. Anesthesiology, 33:304, 1970.

132. Tucker, G. T.: Plasma binding and distribution of local anesthetics. Int. Anesthesiol. Clin., 13:33, 1975.

133. Shnider, S. M., and Way, E. L.: The kinetics of transfer of lidocaine (Xylocaine) across the human placenta. Anesthesiology, 29:944, 1968.

134. Covino, B. G.: Comparative clinical pharmacology of local anesthetic agents. Anesthesiology, 35:158, 1971.

135. Mather, L. E., Long, G. J., and Thomas, J.: The binding of bupivacaine to maternal and foetal plasma proteins. J. Pharm. Pharmacol., 23:359, 1971.

136. Ehrnebo, M., Agurell, S., Jalling, S., et al.: Age of differences in drug binding by plasma proteins: studies on human foetuses, neonates and adults. Eur. J. Clin. Pharmacol., 3:189, 1971.

137. deJong, R. H.: Arterial carbon dioxide and oxygen tensions during spinal block. J.A.M.A., 191:698, 1965.

138. Clark, R. B., Jones, G. L., Barclay, D. L., et al.: Maternal and neonatal effects of 1% and 2% mepivacaine for lumbar extradural analgesia. Br. J. Anaesth., 47:1283, 1975.

139. Usubiaga, J. E., La Iuppa, M., Moya, F., et al.: Passage of procaine hydrochloride and para-aminobenzoic acid across the human placenta. Am. J. Obstet. Gynecol., 100:918, 1968.

140. deJong, R. H.: Anesthetic complications during continuous caudal analgesia for obstetrics. Anesth. Analg., 40:384, 1961.

141. Sinclair, J. C., Fox, H. A., Lentz, J. F., et al.: Intoxication of the fetus by a local anesthetic. A newly recognized complication of maternal caudal anesthesia. N. Engl. J. Med., 273:1173, 1965.

142. Teramo, K., and Rajamaki, A.: Foetal and maternal plasma levels of mepivacaine and fetal acid-base balance and heart rate after paracervical block during labour. Br. J. Anaesth., 43:300, 1971.

143. Scanlon, J. W., and Alper, M. H.: Perinatal pharmacology and evaluation of the newborn. Int. Anesthesiol. Clin., 11:163, 1973.

144. Scanlon, J. W., Brown, W. U., Jr., Weiss, J. B., et al.: Neurobehavioral responses of newborn infants after maternal epidural anesthesia. Anesthesiology, 40:121, 1974.

145. Brazelton, T. B.: Neonatal Behavioral Assessment Scale. pp. 1–61. Philadelphia, J. B. Lippincott, 1973.

146. Hogan, G. R., and Ryan, N. J.: Neurological evaluation of the newborn. Clin. Perinatol., 4:31, 1977.

147. Prechtl, H., and Beintema, D.: The Neurological Examination of Full-term Newborn Infants. London, William Heinemann, 1964.

148. Scanlon, J. W., Ostheimer, G. W., Lurie, A. O., et al.: Neurobehavioral responses and drug concentrations in newborns after maternal epidural anesthesia with bupivacaine. Anesthesiology, 45:400, 1976.

149. McGuinness, G. A., Merkow, A. J., Kennedy, R. L., et al.: Epidural anesthesia with bupivacaine for cesarean section: neonatal blood levels and neurobehavioral responses. Anesthesiology, 49:270, 1978.

150. Tronick, E., Wise, S., Als, H., et al.: Regional obstetric anesthesia and newborn behavior: effect over the first ten days of life. Pediatrics, 58:94, 1976.

151. Halle, Idiosynkrasie gegen Nebennierenpraparate. Ztschr Laryng Rhin., 19:445, 1930.

152. Gordonoff, T., and Steube, P.: Lokalanasthesie und ihre Gefahren. Schweiz Monatsschr Zahn-Heilkunde, 56:1, 1946.

153. Moore, D. C.: Complications of Regional Anesthesia: Etiology, Signs and Symptoms, Treatment. Springfield, Charles C. Thomas, 1955.

154. Adriani, J.: Some practical aspects of the chemistry and pharmacology of local anesthetic drugs. South. Med. J. 39:143, 1946.

155. Lang, C. G., and Luikart, R.: Dermatitis from local anesthetics with a review of one hundred and seven cases from the literature. J.A.M.A., 146:717, 1951.

156. Hart, G. L.: Generalized urticaria following third molar extraction. Oral Surg., 30:325, 1970.

157. Holti, G., and Hood, F. J. C.: An anaphylactoid reaction to lignocaine. Dent. Prac. Dent. Res., 15:294, 1965.

158. Aldrete, J. A., and Johnson, D. A.: Allergy to local anesthetics. J.A.M.A., 207:356, 1969.

159. Schorr, W. F.: Paraben allergy. A cause of intractable dermatitis. J.A.M.A., 204:859, 1968.

160. Nagel, J. E., Fuscaldo, J. T., and Fireman, P.: Paraben allergy. J.A.M.A., 237:1594, 1977.

161. Eyre, J., and Nally, F. F.: Nasal test for hypersensitivity, including a positive reaction to lignocaine. Lancet, 1:264, 1971.

162. Rood, J. P.: A case of lignocaine hypersensitivity. Br. Dent. J., 135:411, 1973.

163. Miller, F. F.: History of drug sensitivity in atopic persons. J. Allergy, 40:46, 1967.

164. Mathieu, A., Battit, G. E., and DiPadua, D.: Anaphylactic and anaphylactoid reactions to anesthetic agents and other drugs used during anesthesia. In Mathieu, A., and Kahan, B. D. (eds.): Immunologic Aspects of Anesthetic and Surgical Practice. pp. 261–287. New York, Grune & Stratton, 1975.

165. Adriani, J.: Reactions to local anesthetics. J.A.M.A., 196:119, 1966.

166. Arora, S., and Aldrete, J. A.: Investigation of possible allergy to local anesthetic drugs: correlation of intradermal with intramuscular injections. Anesthesiol. Rev., 3:13, 1976.
167. Sarkany, I.: Clinical and laboratory aspects of drug allergy. Proc. Roy. Soc. Med., *61*:891, 1968.
168. Halpern, B., and Ky, N. T.: Diagnosis of drug allergy in vitro with the lymphocyte transformation test. J. Allergy, *40*:168, 1967.
169. Rocklin, R. E., Rosen, R. S., and David, J. R.: An in vitro assay for cellular hypersensitivity in man. J. Immunol., *104*:95, 1970.

FURTHER READING

Bromage, P. R.: Pharmacology. *In* Bromage, P. R.: Epidural Analgesia. pp. 68–118. Philadelphia, W. B. Saunders, 1978.

Covino, B. G., and Vassalo, H. G.: Local Anesthetics: Mechanisms of Action and Clinical Use. New York, Grune & Stratton, 1976.
deJong, R. H.: Local Anesthetics. ed. 2. Springfield, Charles C. Thomas, 1977.
Mathieu, A., Battit, G. E., and DiPadua, D.: Anaphylactic and anaphylactoid reactions to anesthetic agents and other drugs used during anesthesia. *In* Mathieu, A., and Kahan, B. D. (eds.): Immunologic Aspects of Anesthetic and Surical Practice. pp. 261–287. New York, Grune & Stratton, 1975.
Ralston, D. H., and Shnider, S. M.: The fetal and neonatal effects of regional anesthesia in obstetrics. Anesthesiology, *48*:34, 1978.
Scott, D. B., and Cousins, M. J.: Clinical pharmacology of local anesthetic agents. *In* Cousins, M. J., and Bridenbaugh, P. O. (eds.): Neural Blockade in Clinical Anesthesia & Management of Pain. pp. 86–121. Philadelphia, J. B. Lippincott Company, 1980.

5 Complications of Spinal and Epidural Anesthesia

Leroy D. Vandam, Ph.B., M.D.

The practice of anesthesia reflects the art as well as the knowledge of the times, and the same may be said of the complications that ensue. With experience and study, the results of a certain technique should improve; if not, the technique should be abandoned in favor of methods offering more acceptable morbidity and mortality. In this context, the popularity of both spinal and epidural anesthesia has waxed and waned over the years, but their widespread use today is an indication of better understanding and progressive improvement in their administration. As background to a presentation of the complications resulting from these kinds of regional anesthesia, a brief history may provide insight into the problems that concern us.

HISTORY OF SPINAL AND EPIDURAL ANESTHESIA

Within a year of the demonstration of the local anesthetic properties of cocaine in 1884, Leonard Corning, a surgeon of New York City, attempted to relieve the symptoms of a patient with urologic complaints by injecting a solution of cocaine into the vicinity of the spinal cord. Numbness in the lower half of the body was apparent after 20 minutes. We shall never know whether Corning succeeded in giving a spinal or epidural anesthetic, because the needle was capped with a syringe, and Corning does not comment on the escape of cerebrospinal fluid (CSF). However, Quincke, in

1891, performed subarachnoid puncture for the first time. It was but a step further to inject cocaine into the subarachnoid space, and this Bier attempted in 1898. After several administrations to patients, he, as the subject, became the first to suffer the common complication of spinal anesthesia, postural headache. Copious quantities of CSF escaped because the syringe did not fit the needle. Others followed suit—Matas in America and Tuffier in France—with anticipated success. Subsequent reports contain more than a few references to headache, nausea and vomiting (because of the practice of barbotage), and meningitis. Moreover, because it was impossible to assure the sterility of solutions of cocaine, residual neurologic deficits developed later. Furthermore, the immediate onset of arterial hypotension was noted, so it became the custom to operate on patients given spinal anesthesia using the head-down position.

In 1901 Cathelin succeeded in producing epidural anesthesia by injection by way of the sacro-coccygeal ligament into the caudal canal. In the 1st decade of the 20th century, many of the details of spinal anesthesia as we know them today were introduced: the use of dextrose to weight the anesthetic solution, thereby permitting hyperbaric control; substitution for cocaine of the more easily sterilized procaine (Novocain); and addition of epinephrine to prolong the effect of nerve block. As early as 1921, Antoni advocated the use of a small-gauge lumbar puncture needle to minimize CSF leakage and development of headache. At about the same time, Pages achieved more uniform success with lumbar epidural anesthesia, perfected and popularized a decade later by the Italian surgeon A.M. Dogliotti.

Ultimately, the clamor over the neurologic sequelae of spinal anesthesia reached a crescendo in the 1940s, culminating in Thorsen's monograph on the subject.[1] Both he and Kennedy,[2] an emminent neurologist, proclaimed that neurologic disease and paralysis were too high a price to pay for the fine muscle relaxation achieved with spinal anesthesia. Fortunately, in America, the rise of professionalism in anesthesia led to the kinds of studies that illuminated the causes and suggested preventive measures to eliminate neurologic complications. The problem of hypotension was more or less solved by the prophylactic administration of sympathomimetic amines and intravenous fluid administration to correct the disproportion between blood volume and the dilated vascular space. Finally, new anesthetics, knowledge of their mode of action and metabolism, and detailed technical studies led to a resurgence of epidural anesthesia in the 1950s and 1960s.

Having reviewed these milestones, at the same time suggesting the dilemmas, I will present the complications of spinal and epidural anesthesia side by side, for the techniques are almost identical. Such complications may be immediate, largely owing to the physiologic effect of nerve block in the spinal region, or delayed, owing to pathophysiologic changes that result from the techniques and drugs employed. The anatomic basis of these techniques provides the clues to these complications.

FUNCTIONAL ANATOMY OF SPINAL AND EPIDURAL ANESTHESIA

Subarachnoid and Epidural Tap

For the prevention of neurologic sequelae, knowledge of the anatomy of the spinal column and its contents is essential in the performance of epidural and subarachnoid puncture. Subarachnoid puncture should always be performed well below the L2–3 interspace to avoid direct injury to the spinal cord, which usually terminates at that level. This rule is less important in epidural anesthesia, in which entry is made at any point on the spinal column, depending upon the segmental area to be anesthetized. With the lumbar vertebral spines identified by their rectangular tips, usually the L4–5 space is chosen and is approximated by a line drawn between the highest points of the iliac crests. Entry by way of the lumbosacral space, the largest of all, is not easy because of the overhanging fifth lumbar spine: The approach, from below upward, starts at the level of the second sacral foramen and angles upward and medially (the so-called Taylor approach). Because repeated attempts at lumbar puncture per se may result in back pain and neurologic sequelae, the back should be maximally flexed to open up the interspaces. In the obese, in whom landmarks are not obvious, and patients with arthritis, the sitting position helps both to straighten and flex the spine through the weight of the torso.

Progressing inward, the needle passes through several structures easily recognized by sensation of touch and resistance (Fig. 5-1). Disinfection of the skin must be meticulous, while attention should be paid to epidermal abnormalities (e.g., pigmentation, alopecia, or dimpling) that might indicate spinal dysraphism or low termination of the cord, as in the Arnold-Chiari syndrome. A needle with a close-fitting stylet is essential to avoid introduction of bits of epidermis, subcutaneous tissue, or periosteum into the epidural or subarachnoid space, which can result in infection or transplantation of epidermal cells to the meninges.[3,4] The longitudinal furrow of the back results from fixation of the skin by connective tissue to the supraspinous ligament and vertebral spines but does not always represent the midline, unless the spine is erect and flexed. The supraspinous ligament spans the apices of the spinal processes and, similar to other ligaments, contains relatively few pain receptors, so that midline puncture may be pain-free. Any pain elicited is felt deep in the back or segmentally and is rarely referred to buttocks or thighs. A paresthesia, the characteristic sensation of electric

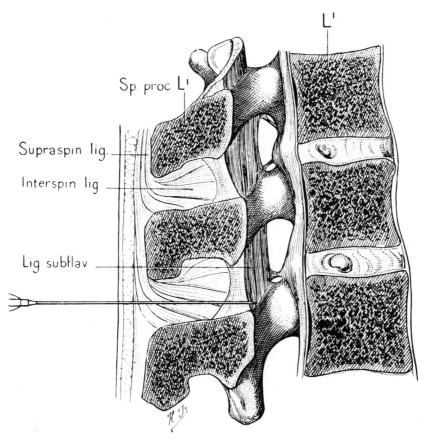

Fig. 5-1. Saggital section of the lumbar spine shows the direction of the needle perpendicular to the surface of the skin and the anatomical structures through which it passes. (Labat, G.: Regional Anesthesia. Philadelphia, W.B. Saunders, 1923)

shock referred to a component of the lumbosacral plexus, suggests that a nerve has been touched. Repeated paresthesias call for abandonment of the procedure. Once the needle is in the subarachnoid space, the local anesthetic should never be injected when a paresthesia is present, because permanent damage is very likely to occur. Introduction of catheters into the epidural or subarachnoid space results in a higher incidence of paresthesias than introduction of the needle alone.[5]

The interspinous ligament is a dense collagenous structure, a good guide to the midline, offers resistance to injection, and provides the anatomic basis for the loss of resistance test upon entering the epidural space. Just beyond the

junction of the vertebral arches is the paired ligamentum flavum, consisting of yellow elastic tissue confluent in the midline and offering less resistance as the needle is advanced. This alteration in resistance is often mistaken as entry into the subarachnoid space. However, it is just as likely to be the epidural or subdural space.

Epidural Space

The epidural space is within the spinal column surrounding the dural sac. It extends from the foramen magnum above to the sacrococcygeal ligament below and varies in capacity according to the cross-sectional area of the canal and diameter of the spinal cord, which is larger in the cervical, upper thoracic, and lumbar regions. The contents of this space include nerve roots partly ensheathed in meninges, semiliquid fat, areolar tissue, and radicals of the peridural plexus of veins. The space may be partially occluded by fibrous tissue adhesions between dura mater and vertebrae, particularly in the aged.

The perivertebral plexus of veins, a valveless system of great capacity subject to changes in pressure transmitted from the abdomen, drains the structures of the back. The veins act as accessory pathways for the caval system in returning blood from the periphery. The plexus is ladder-like, without venous radicals in the midline, where lumbar puncture is ordinarily done. Perforation of one of these veins is the usual cause of a bloody spinal tap and the source of epidural hematoma formation in individuals with clotting abnormalities. Occasionally, the tip of a catheter placed in the epidural space may enter one of the veins. If not recognized, injection of anesthetic solution may result in a generalized toxic reaction, as well as failure to obtain anesthesia. Changing pressures in this venous system affect pressure within the dural sac because dilation of the veins, both inside and outside of the dura, elevates CSF pressure. The resulting change in CSF pressure can be seen during myelography when the patient coughs or strains and the contrast medium rises several segments. This is the basis of Queckenstedt's test and is the reason that straining or coughing after injection of a local anesthetic may lead to high levels of anesthesia. In the relief of spinal headache owing to CSF hypotension, application of a tight abdominal binder may be effective through increasing intra-abdominal venous pressure and thereby raising pressure in the epidural plexus and secondarily elevating CSF pressure.

A negative pressure in the lumbar epidural space is found just after the lumbar puncture needle perforates the ligamentum flavum and is a useful sign in detecting entry into the space during administration of epidural anesthesia. The negative pressure has been ascribed to one or more of several influences: tenting of the dura as the needle is inserted, with creation of a partial vacuum; spinal flexion, which increases the ca-

pacity of the epidural space through an accordion-like effect; and transmission of negative intrathoracic pressure to the lumbar epidural space.

Dura

The dura is an avascular collagenous membrane with vertically directed fibers, recognizable by a characteristic loss of resistance as the membrane is tented and perforated by the needle. The poor vascularity of the dura leads to slow healing, with the result that the opening may persist after needle puncture and allow leakage of CSF. It has been recommended that the dura be entered with the bevel of the needle parallel to the long axis of the fibers to diminish the size of the opening, but this has not been shown to be effective in preventing headache.*

Subdural Space

The subdural space is a true space between dura and arachnoid that is observed during laminectomy, when the dura is incised and the underlying arachnoid prevents escape of CSF. The importance of this space in spinal anesthesia lies in the possibility that the local anesthetic may be injected here, rather than into the subarachnoid space, and cause failure.[6]

Arachnoid

The arachnoid is a web-like membrane that contains the CSF and acts as a framework for blood vessels supplying the spinal cord. It is not sensed as a distinct structure when lumbar puncture is performed. CSF and local anesthetics are absorbed by the spinal arachnoidal granulations by way of perineural lymphatics and in epidural anesthesia after exit through intervertebral perineural spaces.

Subarachnoid Space and Spinal Cord

In the lumbar area, the structures of importance in the subarachnoid space consist of the anterior and posterior nerve roots forming the cauda equina, which pass laterally from their

---

*Personal communication, R. D. Dripps

origins through the intervertebral foramina, where the dorsal root ganglia are found. Each nerve root, both dorsal and ventral, is comprised of many rootlets, arising in a continuous line from the lateral spinal sulcus. The individuality of the fibers, rather than conglomeration in bundles as in peripheral nerves, allows for easy penetration and rapid onset of anesthesia. The fibers are both myelinated and unmyelinated with nodes of Ranvier, where local anesthetic penetration is said to take place. In the lumbar area, the nerve roots may be traumatized during puncture, as indicated by paresthesias. Yet, because they are not under tension, the roots are usually not transfixed by the needle and, therefore, are deflected readily. They may be injured more frequently than we realize, however, particularly the motor roots, for contact does not result in paresthesia. Injection of local anesthetic into a nerve root, suggested by intensification of pares-

thesia, severe pain, and, occasionally, loss of consciousness, results in permanent neurologic damage, because the anesthetic diffuses along the nerve into the spinal cord, where pressure ischemia occurs.[7]

Above the cauda equina, the subarachnoid space is incompletely divided into anterior and posterior compartments by the dentate ligament, which arises from the cord in a continuous line between anterior and posterior nerve roots to attach by a series of digitations to the dura-arachnoid (Fig. 5-2). As such, the dentate ligament acts as a baffle that is possibly of importance in localizing anesthesia when an attempt is made to produce unilateral block.

The blood supply to the spinal cord is segmentally derived from cervical, thoracic, lumbar, and sacral arteries by passage medially along the nerve roots to anastomose on the surface with the anterior and posterior spinal arteries (Fig. 5-3).

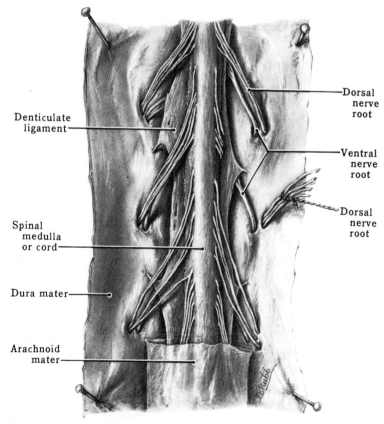

Denticulate ligament

Spinal medulla or cord

Dura mater

Arachnoid mater

Dorsal nerve root

Ventral nerve root

Dorsal nerve root

Fig. 5-2. A portion of the spinal cord and its membranes from behind are shown. The dura mater is unopened below; the arachnoid is removed above. Note the transparency of the latter, the multiple radicles of the spinal nerve roots, the dentate ligament, and the ganglia ensheathed in dura. (Reproduced by permission from J.C.B. Grant's Atlas of Anatomy, ed. 7. Copyright © 1978, Williams & Wilkins)

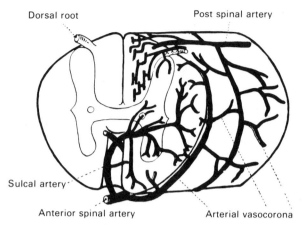

Fig. 5-3. The blood supply of the spinal cord, showing the anterior and posterior spinal arteries, the anastomoses on the surface, and the manner of penetration of the cord. (Vandam, L. D.: Spinal anesthesia. In Hale, D.E. (ed.): Anesthesiology. Philadelphia, F.A. Davis, 1963)

High in the cord, the anterior and posterior spinal arteries originate from the vertebral, basilar, and branches of the thyrocervical arteries. The cord is thus vascularized by an anastomosing network with the vessels penetrating the cord from the periphery. These vessels are usually not injured during lumbar puncture; blood-stained CSF usually comes from the peridural venous plexus. However, subarachnoid apoplexy may follow rupture of a sclerotic vessel, and ischemia of the cord may result from arteriosclerotic occlusion of one of these vessels, producing characteristic neurologic syndromes. Some observers believe that the progressive development of neurologic disease owing to arachnoiditis results from occlusion of the blood vessels by an organizing inflammatory process at the periphery of the cord.

PHYSIOLOGIC EFFECTS OF SPINAL AND EPIDURAL ANESTHESIA

Background

When an anesthetic is injected into the epidural or subarchnoid space, anesthesia begins at the point of injection. Spinal nerve roots, dorsal root ganglia, and the periphery of the cord are the sites of action. In epidural anesthesia, the local anes-thetic affects these structures by diffusion across the meninges and passage outward through the intervertebral foramina, where the spinal nerves are reached. The major effects ultimately result from anesthetization of anterior and posterior spinal nerve roots. Because of the initial high concentration gradient and lipoid solubility of the local anesthetics, absorption takes place rapidly, according to the diameter of the nerve fiber. As in all forms of local anesthesia, fibers of smallest diameter are affected first, because a lesser concentration is needed, and the surface area for penetration is larger. However, structure may be important, for sympathetic B fibers seem to be most susceptible. Thus, neurologic function disappears, more or less, in the following order: autonomic activity, sensation to pinprick, sensation of heat and cold, vibratory and position sense, motor power, and, finally, touch. From this sequence of action, it can be deduced that differential block is possible, depending upon concentration of anesthetic injected.

Respiratory Insufficiency

The excellent muscle relaxation obtained with spinal anesthesia is unrivaled by any other anesthetic technique, including use of neuromuscular blocking agents, which act only at the neuromuscular junction, and deep ether anesthesia, which acts at the sensory side of the reflex arc, internuncially in the spinal cord and at the neuromuscular junction. The muscle paralysis of spinal anesthesia results from interference with conduction in motor nerves and is aided by blockade on the sensory side of the spinal reflex arc. Skeletal muscular relaxation requires use of high concentrations of anesthetic to block the large motor fibers. Paralysis of the lower intercostal muscles is the price paid for good operating conditions in the upper abdomen. If, in addition, abdominal packs and retractors interfere with diaphragmatic action, respiration may be seriously compromised.[8] This must be detected, and, if it is marked, ventilation must be assisted. Many patients complain of subjective difficulty in breathing, probably because proprioceptive sense from intercostal and abdominal muscles is lost. High intercostal paralysis is accompanied by a feeling of suffocation and signs of motor and sensory paralysis in the arms. If phrenic nerve roots are blocked, accessory muscles of respiration may be called into action, although these too may be weakened. The patient is unable to talk owing to inability to move air, and consciousness may be lost. Paralysis of respiration is treated with positive pressure oxygen by way of a mask or tracheal intubation, until the level of anesthesia recedes.

Repiratory paralysis is rare during epidural anesthesia, because the anesthetic does not diffuse as easily in the epidural space as in the CSF. In a survey of complications of epidural anesthesia involving 30,088 administrations, Dawkins reported the onset of massive anesthesia in approximately 0.2 per cent.[9] After apparently uneventful administration and a lapse of some 20 min., respiration ceased and pupils dilated, with no fall in blood pressure. With respiratory support, recovery took place in about 1.75 hours. To account for this reaction, either intravenous injection eventually occurred, or massive transudation into CSF took place.

Circulatory Depression

The appearance of marked degrees of arterial hypotension after administration of spinal anesthesia was an early concern and still is a controversial aspect of this technique, despite prophylactic and therapeutic use of vasopressor drugs. Even a temporary major fall in blood pressure may so decrease cerebral or coronary blood flow that ischemic accidents may occur in patients with arteriosclerosis who lack the intrinsic ability to increase blood flow by vasodilation.

The arterial hypotension of spinal anesthesia results from interruption of sympathetic innervation to systemic vessels, both veins and arteries, and interference with reflexes that control the level of pressure. The consistency and magnitude of the fall in pressure are directly proportional to—and the chance for compensatory vasoconstriction in unanesthetized areas of the body is indirectly proportional to—the height of the sympathetic blockade. Blood pressure tends to fall more if the initial level of pressure is high. Postural effects are marked, as in any kind of neurogenic hypotension. The hypotension may be further aggravated by a reduced blood volume. In a study of spinal anesthetics given without prophylactic vasopressors, Dripps and Deming found that 90 per cent of individuals sustained a fall in blood pressure, and the average fall in systolic pressure was 35 per cent of control level.[10] Studies of the circulation indicate that a decrease in total peripheral vascular resistance accounts for the hypotension in some patients, while in others a decrease in cardiac output is found.[11] The latter probably results from systemic venous dilation and pooling of blood, with decreased venous return to the heart. Accessory factors include bradycardia resulting from block of accelerator impulses to the heart and, possibly, from a decrease in endogenous release of catecholamines from sympathetic nerve endings, which thereby decreases myocardial contractility. Skeletal muscle relaxation and decrease in the amplitude of respiration, with consequent diminution in negative intrathoracic pressure and venous return to the thorax, seem not to be major factors in the development of the hypotension. Vasoconstriction in unanesthetized areas of the body may compensate partially for the fall in pressure. With total autonomic blockade, the reflex response to hypotension initiated by way of the baroreceptors, comprising vasoconstriction and accleration of the pulse, is inactivated.

In treating hypotension, it is wise to concentrate less on blood pressure than on organ perfusion. For example, a modest degree of hypotension might be better for the heart, as the lesser afterload, in the presence of vasodilation, decreases the work and oxygen demand of the myocardium. Consequently, the need to perfuse the heart at normal end-diastolic pressure is lessened.

Hypotension as a consequence of epidural anesthesia occurs under the same circumstances as does hypotension during spinal anesthesia. At the same levels of anesthesia, the circulatory response to epidural block is qualitatively the same as for spinal anesthesia, but there is a difference: Absorption of local anesthetic from the epidural space into the circulation can cause depressant systemic vascular effects. All of the local anesthetics exert a quinidine-like effect on the myocardium, reducing contractility, diminishing irritability, and slowing conduction time; in addition, peripheral vasodilation occurs. In comparisons of spinal and epidural anesthesia of equal extent, the hypotension observed with the latter technique tends to be less profound. A possible reason for this difference is that, in epidural anesthesia, there is little or no gap between sensory and sympathetic levels; that is, sympathetic block does not ascend as high as in spinal anesthesia. The concomitant use of epinephrine in epidural anesthesia does not quite prevent development of hypotension. Despite an increase in heart rate and stroke volume, peripheral resistance is diminished. Pressor drugs are seldom given prophylactically before epidural anesthesia, but their use before spinal anesthesia is not uncommon. As in spinal anesthesia, many accessory factors are concerned in the circulatory depression observed with epidural anesthesia: adequacy of blood volume; height of sympathetic blockade; the amount of local anesthetic and epinephrine absorbed into the systemic circulation; and a tendency in aged patients for the level of anesthesia to ascend to greater heights.

Both cerebral and coronary blood flow may remain unchanged during the hypotension of spinal and epidural anesthesia because of vasodilation and decrease in resistance to flow, the means by which the circulation is ordinarily maintained in these vascular beds.[12] However, if arteriosclerosis is present, precluding vasodilation, or if the mean arterial blood pressure falls below 60 or 70 torr, vasodilation may be insufficient to compensate, and ischemia may result. Thus, the hypotension that can be tolerated depends upon the pressure to which the patient is accustomed and the presence of vascular disease. Since little decrease in cerebral metabolic rate occurs during spinal anesthesia, hypotension may be more of a threat to the brain than to the heart. Measurements of cerebral blood flow indicate that vasodilation compensates for the hypotension, but signs of cerebral ischemia, such as yawning, fainting, and nausea, are seen frequently in normal patients in the supine position, when systolic blood pressure falls below 70 to 80 torr.

Both hepatic and renal blood flow are maintained up to a point during spinal and epidural anesthesia, because the decline in mean arterial pressure is accompanied by vasodilation, and perfusion remains adequate. Urinary output usually ceases below systolic pressures of 60 or 70 torr, but the renal parenchyma may still be well perfused. Despite the vasodilation, if hypotension is marked, antidiuresis occurs. Changes in hepatic function following spinal anesthesia differ little from those observed after general anesthesia of various kinds.[12] The operation performed is a much more important influence. During hypotensive spinal anesthesia, estimated hepatic blood flow is markedly decreased, but there is greater degree of hepatic dysfunction postoperatively than in normotensive anesthesia. Vasodilation in liver and kidneys is considered helpful in the prevention of ischemia and avoidance of certain changes associated with irreversible shock in the experimental animal.

In the early 1930s, prophylactic injection of vasopressor drugs was first employed to counteract the fall in blood pressure encountered during spinal anesthesia. The rationale is to maintain normal tissue perfusion in heart and brain, despite vasoconstriction produced in kidneys and liver. In a study of the actions of several vasopressor drugs, Dripps and Deming found methamphetamine to be quite useful, but there was little statistical difference among the drugs studied (Fig. 5-4).[10] Practically every vasopressor drug has been utilized prophylactically in spinal anesthesia. In view of the circulatory alterations found, it would seem logical to use a drug with both myocardial and peripheral stimulating properties, so that cardiac output and peripheral vascular resistance are maintained. Some prefer ephedrine because of its predominantly central actions, while others elect methoxamine or phenylephrine, both with peripheral actions. In Table 5-1 the commonly employed pressor drugs with suggested dosage are listed. The drug should be injected intramuscularly before injection of the spinal anesthetic. If pressure falls to threatening levels after anesthesia has taken effect, the vasopressor should again be injected both intravenously to raise the pressure quickly and intramuscularly for a sustained effect. If more than one or two subsequent injections are required, a continuous infusion of vasopressor may be begun

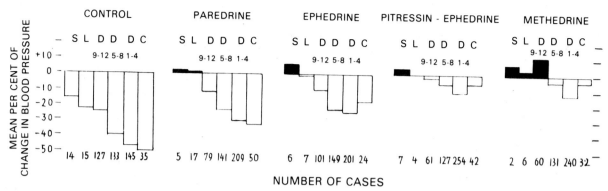

Fig. 5-4. The mean percentage of fall in blood pressure at various levels of anesthesia for the control and each pressor drug group: sacral, S; lumbar, L: dorsal 9–12, D9–12; dorsal 5–8, D5–8; dorsal 1–4, D1–4; and cervical, C. The total number of cases in each group is also given. Note the increased percentage of fall in blood pressure at higher levels of anesthesia. Also, the tendency for the blood pressure to fall is less when pressor drugs are used; this is particularly striking at the higher levels of anesthesia, when more effective pressors are used. (By permission of Dripps, R.D., and Deming, M. V. N.: An evaluation of certain drugs used to maintain blood pressure during spinal anesthesia: comparison of ephedrine, paredrine, pitressinephedrine and methedrine in 2,500 cases. Surg. Gynecol. Obstet. 83:312, 1946)

to titrate a blood pressure to an appropriate level. Some clinicians attempt to lessen the degree of hypotension by infusion of approximately 1 L. of fluids, intravenously, before giving spinal anesthesia. This helps to some degree in obstetric patients, but the incidence of postanesthetic catheterization increases, owing to diuresis and overdistention of the urinary bladder.

Bowel and Urinary Dysfunction

Interruption of sympathetic innervation to the bowel leaves the parasympathetic nerves unopposed, with resultant smooth muscle contraction, hyperactive peristalsis, and relaxation of sphincters. Along with muscle paralysis, the contracted bowel is one of the reasons that abdominal relaxation appears to be so good during spinal anesthesia; this accounts for the scaphoid appearance of the abdomen. Excessive peristalsis, however, should alert the surgeon to anticipate intestinal spillage during intestinal anastomoses. Hyperactive peristalsis is one of the reasons that spinal anesthesia is deemed dangerous in the presence of intestinal obstruction, for fear of perforation. There are no documented instances of this accident. Defecation and colostomy move-

Table 5-1. Average Doses of Common Vasopressor Drugs Used to Treat Hypotension in Spinal Anesthesia*

VASOPRESSOR	INTRAMUSCULAR† (mg.)	INTRAVENOUS† (mg.)	INTRAVENOUS INFUSION‡ (mg./500 ml.)
Ephedrine	25–50	15	§
Phenylephrine	2–5	0.2–0.5	10
Methoxamine	10–20	5–10	60

*Vandam, L. D.: Drugs for arterial hypotension and shock. *In* Modell, W. (ed.): Drugs of Choice. St. Louis, C. V. Mosby, 1974.

†I.M. or I.V. route is preferred for rapid absorption.

‡In 5% dextrose in water or 0.9% sodium chloride. The concentration of the vasopressor in solution and the rate of infusion should sustain blood pressure without overloading the circulation with fluid. Stronger solutions may be prepared as needed.

§Not given by infusion because of tachyphylaxis and central nervous stimulation.

ments often occur because of sphincter relaxation. Preanesthetic use of morphine, with its secondary depressant effect on intestinal smooth muscle, may counteract these parasympathetic stimulatory effects.

Spinal and caudal anesthesia have always been associated with a high incidence of inability to void postoperatively and the need for catheterization. In the sacral region, both sympathetic and parasympathetic nerves are blocked, with consequent detrusor and sphincter paralysis. These autonomic effects considerably outlast motor and sensory blockade. Inability to empty the bladder is exaggerated by overdistention when intravenous fluid therapy is overzealous.

Nausea and Vomiting

In 1923, Labat, commenting on spinal anesthesia, stated, "Under the best conditions nausea frequently occurs in the Trendelenburg position and in the case of operations on the organs of the upper abdominal cavity, especially the stomach. This is increased by rough manipulation and heavy packing of the bowels against the diaphragm."[13] Babcock, one of the pioneers in spinal anesthesia, found that vomiting occurred in 13 per cent and nausea in 18 per cent of his patients. He believed that nausea was a premonitory sign of hypotension, cyanosis, or respiratory depression.[14] Among other reasons suggested for the onset of nausea during spinal anesthesia are cerebral ischemia, psychic factors, presence of bile in the stomach owing to relaxation of the sphincters, increased peristalsis, a specific action of the drug on the spinal medulla, the effect of preanesthetic medication and bodily motion, and use of a vasoconstrictor drug. Nausea and vomiting occur in at least 13 per cent and perhaps as many as 42 per cent of spinal anesthetics.[15]

Vomiting is a complex coordinated motor reflex. The neural pool is in the lateral gray reticular formation of the medulla, which coordinates the several components of vomiting. Vomiting may be incited directly or reflexively by direct stimulation of the chemoreceptive trigger zone in the floor of the fourth ventricle, sensitive to drugs with central actions as morphine, apomorphine, or nicotine. On the other hand, vagal and sympa-

thetic afferent nerve fibers transmit the effects of emetics acting locally on bowel and carry other kinds of reflexes from the thorax and abdomen. Thus, the medulla is the integrative area, but vomiting may be initiated from almost any site in the body. Stretch of the wall of the stomach, esophagus, or duodenum stimulates the same nerve endings as those that carry visceral pain. Hence, pain, whether produced in viscera or parietes, may cause vomiting, which does not necessarily connote a gastrointestinal disturbance. Davis and Pollock stated that ". . . the persistance of vomiting after blocking of the pain fibers (cerebrospinal) indicates that strong visceral afferent impulses continue to reach the higher centers through the sympathetic and vagal chains" (See Chap. 31).[16]

According to these concepts, many instances of nausea and vomiting during spinal anesthesia must be initiated reflexively from the operative field, as supported by the data presented in Table 5-2.[15] Among patients with a sensory level to pinprick at the fourth thoracic segment or higher, there was an increased incidence of nausea and vomiting, even though pain was not experienced. Since few of the operations performed necessitated such high levels, it is probable that the local anesthetic had spread in the subarachnoid space without providing complete anesthesia. Table 5-3 shows that intrathecal use of epinephrine was associated with a higher incidence of vomiting. Epinephrine not only prolongs anesthesia but delays onset and the time for full attainment of a satisfactory sensory level. For these reasons, the level of anesthesia is difficult to control, and it is often the practice to reduce the dose of anesthetic drug when epinephrine is added. Under these circumstances, inadequate sensory blockade may easily ensue.

NEUROLOGIC SEQUELAE OF SPINAL AND EPIDURAL ANESTHESIA

Because of neurologic sequelae (see pp. 91–104), criticism of spinal anesthesia reached a peak in the late 1940s. To this day, neurologists, neurosurgeons, and the public fear the method, because they believe that neurologic sequelae are inevita-

Table 5-2. Frequency of Nausea and Vomiting During Spinal Anesthesia in Relation to Operative Position, Sensory Level of Anesthesia, and the Need for Supplementation with General Anesthesia

CATEGORY	NAUSEA & VOMITING (176 CASES)		NO NAUSEA & VOMITING (763 CASES)		AVERAGE P VALUE
	(NUMBER)	(%)	(NUMBER)	(%)	
Position					
Supine	82	47	400	53	
Lithotomy	29	16	139	18	
Lateral	25	14	69	9	
Trendelenburg	27	15	58	8	<0.30
Prone	8	5	69	9	
Fowler	3	2	10	1	
Other	2	1	18	2	
Sensory level					
Tenth thoracic & below	37	21	205	27	
Fourth to ninth thoracic	111	63	439	57	
Above fourth thoracic	26	15	45	6	
Not recorded	2	1	74	10	
Supplementation					
Intravenous	58	33	265	35	
Inhalation	11	6	18	2	
Intravenous-inhalation	80	46	180	24	
None	27	15	300	39	

(Crocker, J. S., and Vandam, L. D.: Concerning nausea and vomiting during spinal anesthesia. Anesthesiology, *20*:587, 1959)

ble. Many anesthesiologists avoid the technique owing to the possibility of a law suit, should postanesthetic complications develop. Yet, carefully observed series of anesthetics have demonstrated that major neurologic consequences need not occur, and that the frequency of minor neurologic sequelae is minimal with reasonable care.[17] Analysis of postanesthetic deaths places spinal anesthesia in a favorable position with regard to mortality.[18] A paradox is therefore evident: Clinical impressions have overruled careful observation, and patients may be denied a valuable anesthetic technique.

As it was believed that spinal anesthesia was the method of choice for certain operations and offered additional advantages in others, spinal anesthesia was studied prospectively and objectively during the period from 1948 to 1951 at the University of Pennsylvania. A total of 8,460 patients given 10,098 spinal anesthetics was available for study. Incidents associated with lumbar puncture, details of the local anesthetic

Table 5-3. Prevalence of Pain, Hypotension, the Need for Supplementary Vasopressor Drugs, and the Use of Intrathecal Epinephrine in Relation to Nausea and Vomiting During Spinal Anesthesia

CATEGORY	NUMBER OF CASES	NAUSEA & VOMITING		NO NAUSEA & VOMITING		AVERAGE P VALUE
		(NUMBER)	(%)	(NUMBER)	(%)	
Pain	176	72	41	80	10	<0.01
Hypotension	176	79	45	172	23	<0.01
Supplementary vasopressor drugs	176	79	45	194	26	<0.01
Intrathecal epinephrine	97	48	50	136	33	<0.01

(Crocker, J. S., and Vandam, L. D.: Concerning nausea and vomiting during spinal anesthesia. Anesthesiology, *20*:587, 1959)

employed, and immediate and postoperative effects were carefully recorded. During the hospital stay, patients were seen daily by the anesthesiologist concerned or by a trained nurse. Questions were asked that could lead to early discovery of the kinds of neurologic disease alleged to result from the anesthetic. Before leaving the hospital, patients were told to expect and were requested to reply to a questionnaire that would be mailed within 6 months. The advantage of the immediate phase of the study was that all of the facts on administration of anesthesia, details of the operation, and immediate postoperative effects could be gathered in significant numbers in one institution, where the habits of the anesthesiologists were known. This search for complications probably exaggerated the reporting of symptoms and invited extraneous complaints, but only by these means could one hope to uncover neurologic problems that might have passed undetected.

A parallel study was conducted in a group of 1,000 persons given general anesthesia for the same kinds of operation performed under spinal anesthesia, to uncover those symptoms and signs that might be common to the patient or to the operation performed. A smaller series of 100 patients was given spinal anesthesia only after the induction of general anesthesia to exclude symptoms that may arise purely on a psychologic basis.

Data were obtained for 89 per cent of the anesthetics, for periods ranging from a minimum of 6 months to 10 years.[7] No instance of adhesive arachnoiditis, transverse myelitis, or cauda equina syndrome was found. Minor neurologic deficits were noted; none were progressive and none were of any consequence. Also, 11 patients were found who had exacerbation of preexisting neurologic disease after anesthesia.

It was apparent that neurologic complications of spinal anesthesia could result from lumbar puncture per se or subsequent injection of the local anesthetic. Concerning lumbar puncture, several etiologic factors are involved. Best known are those attributable to leakage of CSF, giving rise to the syndrome of decreased intracranial pressure: headache, and ocular and auditory symptoms. Another group of complications involved trauma of lumbar puncture. Backache and infection have been reported many times as sequelae of lumbar puncture, but neurologic deficit resulting from trauma has not been emphasized.

The complications of spinal anesthesia are presented below in detail and are followed by those resulting from epidural anesthesia. To some extent, the complications are classified by a system used by Thorsen in his monograph on "Neurological Complications After Spinal Anesthesia."[1] He studied patients undergoing spinal anesthesia and patients undergoing only diagnostic lumbar puncture, and he surveyed the literature on complications.

CEREBRAL COMPLICATIONS OF SPINAL AND EPIDURAL ANESTHESIA

As with any kind of anesthesia, damage to the brain can result from arterial hypotension or respiratory inadequacy; the resultant ischemia produces transient neurologic signs and symptoms, or irreversible changes if hypoxia is severe or when cardiac arrest ensues. Cerebrovascular accidents have been reported after transient hypotension during spinal anesthesia and after excessive hypertensive responses to the injection of a vasopressor drug. Bizzarre CNS symptoms, such as coma, loss of memory, mental deterioration, confusion, and psychoses, can probably be attributed to unrecognized or untreated episodes of hypoxia in the majority of cases. It is vital, however, (and this point cannot be emphasized more) to seek other causes of neurologic disease, rather than to ascribe all neurologic changes that occur in the postanesthetic period to the spinal anesthetic.

The Syndrome of Decreased Intracranial Pressure

The overall incidence of headache, and ocular, and auditory complications reported by Vandam and Dripps is shown in Table 5-4.[19] The headaches had certain special features: They were postural, with onset upon assumption of the erect position, and were usually relieved by recumbency; the location was frontal, occipital, vertex, or

Table 5-4. The Syndrome of Decreased Intracranial Pressure Following 9277 Spinal Anesthetics

COMPLICATION	NUMBER OF PATIENTS	%
"Spinal" headache	1011	11.0
Ocular difficulties	34	0.4
Auditory difficulties	35	0.4

(Vandam, L. D., and Dripps, R. D.: Long-term follow-up of patients who received 10,098 spinal anesthetics. III. Syndrome of decreased intracranial pressure (headache and ocular and auditory difficulties). J.A.M.A., *161*:586, 1956. Copyright © 1956, American Medical Association)

nuchal, or a combination of these probably depending upon the particular intracranial pain-sensitive structure involved. Severity, duration, and time of onset of headache varied. The patients described in subjective terms how or what they felt when experiencing a headache: constricting band, heaviness, vacuumlike, dead weight, lead weight, worse on moving, makes sounds, and echo-like. Occipital headache, nuchal pain, and stiff neck were not considered as signs of meningitis, for fever and pleocytosis in CSF were not found. Rather, spasm and pain in the cervical muscles were interpreted as reactions to pain similar to those that occur in the other areas of the body. Stiff neck and tender spots in cervical muscles are common accompaniments of headache, regardless of the cause. A similar incidence of headaches was found in the control series of 1,000 patients given general anesthesia, but the headaches were nonspecific in nature.

Ocular difficulties reported were double vision, blurring, difficulty in focusing, spots before the eyes, photophobia, scintillation, and difficulty in reading. Auditory complaints included decreased hearing, obstruction, plugging, popping, tinnitus, buzzing, and roaring. Few of these symptoms were found in the patients receiving general anesthesia; if so, they could be related to preexisting medical disease. The symptoms enumerated were definitely related to lumbar puncture rather than to introduction of the spinal anesthetic. In a controlled series of lumbar puncture in our hands,[19] and in those of others,[1] the same kinds of symptoms were found.

In performing a second lumbar puncture for diagnostic or therapeutic reasons in a patient after the onset of a spinal headache, CSF pressure was observed to be very low. Although not an invariable finding, the association suggested a cause and effect relationship. This, combined with other evidence (see p. 88), has led to the belief that headache and the associated symptoms result from leakage of CSF through a dural opening left by the lumbar puncture needle. When CSF pressure is lowered, compensatory intracranial vasodilation, aggravated by assumption of the erect position, results in traction on pain-sensitive dilated blood vessels and gives rise to a vascular type of headache.[19–22] No increase in CSF pressure after spinal anesthesia was found in these studies. Thus, it should not be assumed that infection or CSF hypertension plays a role in the development of the usual postural headache.

The Nature of "Spinal" Headache. The overall incidence of headache in the Pennsylvania series was 11 per cent, while an incidence of 18 per cent was found by Thorsen in 50,000 cases collected from various sources. The occurrence of headache according to age is shown in Table 5-5. Incidence decreased after the 5th decade, and the highest frequency occurred in the 3rd and 4th decades. In part, this difference among age-groups may be attributed to elevation of pain threshold in the aged, perhaps owing to a progressive decrease in sensory neural elements. Vibratory sensibility decreases with advancing age, and there is also a decrease in elasticity of the cerebral vessels. The differences among age-groups were not subject to factors that might affect CSF pressure, such as earlier ambulation in the young or more adequate parenteral fluid replacement in one group compared to the other.

The overall incidence of headache in women was almost twice that in men (Table 5-6). The main reason for this striking difference is the inclusion of obstetric cases in the group of women studied; headache following vaginal delivery carried out under spinal anesthesia occurred in 22 per cent of the patients, twice the overall figure. This may relate to the extreme changes in intra-abdominal pressure during labor, which influence CSF pressure and leakage, to

Table 5-5. Relation of the Age to the Incidence of "Spinal" Headache

AGE (YEARS)	NUMBER OF SPINAL ANESTHETICS	NUMBER OF "SPINAL" HEADACHES	%
10–19	537	51	10
20–29	1994	321	16
30–39	1833	261	14
40–49	1759	192	11
50–59	1736	133	8
60–69	1094	45	4
70–79	297	7	2
80–89	27	1	3
Total	9277	1011	11

(Vandam, L. D., and Dripps, R. D.: Long-term follow-up of patients who received 10,098 spinal anesthetics. III. Syndrome of decreased intracranial pressure (headache and ocular and auditory difficulties). J.A.M.A., *161*:586, 1956. Copyright © 1956, American Medical Association)

rapid changes in blood volume following delivery, to dehydration during labor, and to the lesser attention paid to parenteral fluid replacement after delivery. When obstetric cases are not considered, headache is still more of a problem in women (Table 5-6). Although other investigators may disagree,[23] the role of the psyche in the development of headache in either men or women seems negligible. To prove this point, Vandam and Dripps gave spinal anesthesia to 100 persons under general anesthesia. Although none of these people knew that spinal anesthesia had been administered, the percentage of postural headache was the same as in the series at large.

The most conclusive data on development of lumbar puncture headache are shown in Table 5-7, which relates the diameter of the needle to headache. The incidence of headache decreased progressively with smaller needle diameter, as did severity and duration. Employment of a 26-gauge needle resulted in a negligible incidence. When a 16-gauge needle was employed for continuous spinal anesthesia, not only were technical difficulties greater, but the number and severity of headaches as well as ocular complaints were so prohibitive that this technique was soon restricted to the older age-groups; or, the method was reserved for those conditions in which safety and better control with the continuous technique were major considerations. For routine use and freedom from technical difficulty, a 22-gauge needle proved best. The overall incidence of

Table 5-6. Relation of the Sex to the Incidence of "Spinal" Headache

SEX	NUMBER OF SPINAL ANESTHETICS		NUMBER OF "SPINAL" HEADACHES		%	
Male	4063		302		7	
Female	5214		709		14	
Spinal anesthetic for vaginal delivery		938		220		22
Spinal anesthetic for other procedures		4276		489		12
Total	9277		1011		21	

(Vandam, L. D., and Dripps, R. D.: Long-term follow-up of patients who received 10,098 spinal anesthetics. III. Syndrome of decreased intracranial pressure (headache and ocular and auditory difficulties). J.A.M.A., *161*:586, 1956. Copyright © 1956, American Medical Association)

Table 5-7. Relation of Gauge of Needle Used for Lumbar Puncture to Incidence of "Spinal" Headache

Needle Gauge	Number of Spinal Anesthetics	Number of "Spinal" Headache	%
16	839	151	18
19	154	16	10
20	2698	377	14
22	4952	430	9
24	634	37	6

(Vandam, L. D., and Dripps, R. D.: Long-term follow-up of patients who received 10,098 spinal anesthetics. III. Syndrome of decreased intracranial pressure (headache and ocular and auditory difficulties). J.A.M.A., *161*:586, 1956. Copyright © 1956, American Medical Association)

headache with this needle was nearly 9 per cent, but the headaches were generally mild.

Early ambulation of surgical patients was encouraged, and onset of lumbar puncture headache took place soon after the assumption of a head-up position. In some cases, headache appeared when the patient first lifted his head or got out of bed for the first time. If headache was severe, patients soon learned the value of recumbency in relieving symptoms. The first occurrence of headache after several days or even weeks explains why, in some reported series, the incidence is exceptionally low (Table 5-8). Patients simply were not observed postoperatively over a long enough period. The same criticism can be directed at the reported incidence of headache after diagnostic lumbar puncture. It is ususally asserted that headaches are few in number, but when a careful follow-up is done, the true incidence is obtained. In the Pennsylvania series, onset of headache was sometimes reported long after the patient had left the hospital. Just why headache should be so delayed is not easily explained. One can postulate that slow leakage of CSF continues without causing symptoms until loss overbalances production, or until a certain pain threshold is reached.

For many years, it had been the practice to require patients to remain flat in bed after spinal anesthesia to prevent or minimize headache. We have no evidence that this is effective. Leakage of CSF probably takes place during operation and afterward, even if the patient is recumbent.[24]

Surprisingly, the duration of headache from lumbar puncture is sometimes extraordinarily long; in the Pennsylvania series, the range was from 1 day to 12 months, and 53 per cent of headaches ended within 4 days (Table 5-9). However, leakage can persist for a long time. Because of poor blood supply, the dura does not readily heal. Leakage from the needle opening has been seen at laminectomy and at postmortem examination as long as 14 days after lumbar puncture. Experimentally, Wolff produced headache consistently by drainage of 20 ml. of CSF, with the subject in the erect position.[20] The headache was relieved readily by raising CSF pressure artificially with saline solution. When headache does not follow lumbar puncture, even when a large-gauge needle is employed, it is possible that the arachnoid may have prolapsed to occlude the dural opening, thereby preventing leakage; this, too,

Table 5-8. The Time of Onset of "Spinal" Headache in the Postoperative Period

Time Of Onset After Operation	Number of "Spinal" Headaches (1,011)	%
Day of Operation	89	9
1st	302	29
2nd	216	21
3rd	123	13
4–6th	115	11
7–12th	12	1
1 month	2	0.2
5 months	2	0.2
no data	150	15

(Vandam, L. D., and Dripps, R. D.: Long-term follow-up of patients who received 10,098 spinal anesthetics. III. Syndrome of decreased intracranial pressure (headache and ocular and auditory difficulties). J.A.M.A., *161*:586, 1956. Copyright © 1956, American Medical Association)

Table 5-9. The Duration of "Spinal" Headache

DURATION	NUMBER OF "SPINAL" HEADACHES (1,011)	%
1–2 days	245	24
3–4 days	296	29
5–7 days	193	19
8–14 days	79	8
3–6 weeks	49	5
3–6 months	19	2
7–12 months	38	4
no data	92	9

(Vandam, L. D., and Dripps, R. D.: Long-term follow-up of patients who received 10,098 spinal anesthetics. III. Syndrome of decreased intracranial pressure (headache and ocular and auditory difficulties). J.A.M.A., *161*:586, 1956. Copyright © 1956, American Medical Association)

has been observed at laminectomy. Because leakage occurs so readily, a variety of lumbar puncture techniques and special needles have been devised. I do not believe that oblique insertion of the needle can be done consistently to puncture dura and arachnoid at different levels, so that prolapse of arachnoid occurs. Similarly, it has been suggested that the bevel of the needle be inserted parallel to the longitudinal fibers of the dura, so that fibers are spread rather than sectioned. Vandam and Dripps performed a series of 100 spinal anesthetics in which the bevel of the needle was inserted parallel to the fibers; headaches were slightly fewer in number, but not significantly different from the larger series.

Treatment of Spinal Headache. Headache need not follow spinal anesthesia if careful technique and small needles are employed. When headache occurs, the pain can be relieved with analgesics or by raising CSF pressure artificially. Hydration and application of a tight abdominal binder may relieve the milder headache. A second puncture with replacement of fluid alleviates headache immediately. Often, relief is permanent, despite the fact that the dura has been reentered. The mechanism of relief of headache by way of epidural placement of fluid is not clear; perhaps, the dura is buttressed, or epidural fluid passing through the opening raises CSF pressure directly. Artificial elevation of CSF pressure should be reserved for treatment of incapacitating headache when nausea, vomiting, or dizziness is protracted

and when ocular nerve palsy is imminent. Over the last few years, almost uniform success in relieving headache has been achieved by means of a "blood patch."[25] About 10 ml. of the patient's own venous blood is collected aseptically and injected into the epidural space at the leakage site. The clot thus formed stems escape of CSF.

Ocular Symptoms of Decreased Intracranial Pressure. In the spinal anesthesia study in Pennsylvania, there were 34 patients who had difficulty with vision (Table 5-4). Complaints ran the gamut of double vision, blurring, inability to read, sensitivity to light, spots before the eyes, and difficulty in focusing. In all but eight cases, visual complaints were associated with typical postural headache. There were three proven cases of lateral rectus muscle palsy, and the symptom of prolonged double vision in three others suggested that palsy might also have been present. These cases followed use of a 16-gauge needle for continuous spinal anesthesia. Five of the headaches were severe, and three of these were localized to the occiput. Thus, the palsies and the other ocular complaints seemed related to CSF leakage. Ocular nerve palsies appeared rather suddenly, about 1 week after anesthesia, and persisted from a few weeks to 6 months, with eventual restitution of functional vision. Many reports of cranial nerve palsy after spinal anesthesia have appeared and the abducens was usually involved.[26] One theory contends that, with brain displacement and traction on supporting structures, a motor nerve such as the abducens, with its long intracranial course, can be compressed against bone, or, as the nerve passes through the cavernous sinus, venous dilation might result in pressure.

Because of the possibility of development of abducens palsy, it is best to avoid use of a large-gauge needle, as in continuous spinal anesthesia, except for aged patients in whom headache is not common. When confronted with intractable severe headache, all available means of increasing CSF pressure should be tried to avoid nerve palsy.

Auditory Difficulties. Thirty-five patients in the Pennsylvania series described difficulty in hearing (Table 5-4). In many there was associated dizziness, and nausea was common. In Thorsen's series, dizziness was found in 9.1 per cent, but he could not determine if this was of vestibular or cerebellar origin.[1] Dizziness, nausea, and hearing difficulty were found in a control series receiving general anesthetics, but these could usually be ascribed to underlying medical disease; for example, an aged man with dizziness and severe headache after general anesthesia also had severe hypertension.[19] After spinal anesthesia, patients noted buzzing, popping and clogging of the ears, loss of hearing, humming, roaring, and stuffiness. With few exceptions, these complaints were also associated with postural headache. Hence, a decrease in CSF pressure was implicated. It is well known that there is an anatomic communication between subarachnoid space and cochlea. Hughson demonstrated that, with decrease in CSF pressure, there is a fall in intralabyrinthine pressure, followed by inability of the ear to transmit high tones.[27] In several patients, an audiogram was restored to normal when CSF pressure was artificially elevated.

INJURIES LOCALIZED TO THE SPINAL CORD AND ITS COVERINGS

Another group of complications results from traumatic lumbar puncture. In a comparison of single-dose and continuous spinal anesthesia, Dripps found a much higher incidence of technical difficulties, production of paresthesias, and bloody taps with continuous spinal anesthesia, but he did not mention any difference in neurologic sequelae.[5] While backache and infection have been emphasized as sequelae of lumbar puncture, neurologic deficit has not been emphasized. The following is a typical case:

Case 5-1. A 23-year-old man was to undergo excision of a fistula-in-ano. He had had no previous anesthetic nor history of systemic disease, but he did have occasional headache and backache, though not severe. Spinal anesthesia was selected, although the skin of the back was scarred and marked with keloid, the result of burns suffered in childhood. Many attempts at lumbar puncure with a 22-gauge needle were made at two interspaces, with the patient in the sitting position. Paresthesias were experienced in both legs. Although the subarachnoid space was entered and clear CSF obtained, anesthesia was abandoned because paresthesias were noted every time an attempt was made to withdraw fluid. The operation was then carried out under general anesthesia.

On the 1st postoperative day, severe postural headache developed, beginning in the nuchal region and radiating around the side of the face to the eyes. Tenderness and pain at the lumbar puncture site were noted, with radiation to the low back. There was no numbness nor difficulty in voiding or walking. A week later, the patient still had postural headache and severe back pain. He walked with the aid of a cane, in a semi-stooped position. He complained of pain in the left calf, but there were no paresthesias or numbness. After urination, there was a sensation that the bladder was incompletely emptied, and he had experienced considerable diminution in sexual drive. Neurologic examination was normal, except for tenderness over the L3–5 spines. Subsequently, his condition improved, and he resumed work as a machinist. However, 8 months after operation following exacerbation of back and leg pain, findings were suggestive of a protruded disc, either at L3–4 or L4–5. He was treated conservatively.

There can be little doubt about the relation between traumatic puncture and development of back and leg pain in Case 5-1. Since the anesthetic was not injected into the subarachnoid space, an intraneural or intraspinal injection was not the cause. The decision to abandon spinal anesthesia was correct; the deciding factor was inability to avoid paresthesias with repositioning of the needle, which alone can cause nerve injury.[28]

Case 5-2. A 32-year-old woman was scheduled for cesarean section. She had had spinal anesthesia for section 4 years previously, without complication. With the patient in the lateral decubitus position, numerous attempts at lumbar puncture with a 22-gauge needle were made, producing many paresthesias to both legs, thighs, and feet, that were more severe on the left. At one time, blood-tinged CSF was recovered. Ultimately, subarachnoid tap produced a scant quantity of clear CSF. The anesthetic was injected without additional paresthesias, but anesthesia was unsatisfactory; supplementary general anesthesia was required.

Postoperatively, this intelligent woman stated that sensation returned more slowly in the left than the right leg. Early complaints were backache at the puncture sites and a feeling of weakness in the left leg. At first, she was unable to lift the left leg because of motor weakness and loss of sense of position. On standing she tended to lose balance, and she bore her weight on the right leg. She also complained of spasmodic pain on voiding. Symptoms gradually abated, and on the 8th postoperative day, residual neurologic signs were minimal: hypalgesia over the anterior left thigh and slight motor weakness in the entire limb, but with normal reflexes.

Three months later, the patient showed marked improvement but complained of occasional loss of balance, a sensation as though the third and fourth toes were flexed, and several episodes of involuntary defecation. Neurologic examination was normal. After 5 years of observation, residual complaints were pain and numbness in the heels and toes during fatigue.

This patient had had spinal anesthesia before, the method was accepted by her, and there was no antecedent neurologic disease. Difficulty in lumbar puncture was not easily explained. Inexperience on the part of a beginner, failure to flex the spine adequately in a pregnant woman, and faulty selection of landmarks were probably responsible. Back pain at the puncture site, experience of multiple paresthesias particularly in the left leg, subsequently severely involved, and recovery of blood-stained CSF all suggest the relation to trauma.

MINOR SEQUELAE OF TRAUMATIC LUMBAR PUNCTURE

The remainder of the cases in the Pennsylvania series (Table 5-10) comprised a group of individuals with no antecedent neurologic disease, and the anesthetic tetracaine-dextrose solution was used in 13 of the 17 cases. The common denominator in all was multiple insertion of the lumbar puncture needle, with production of paresthesias in lumbar and sacral dermatomes; blood-stained fluid was seen only once. In all patients, subsequent complaints, of pain, paresthesia, or numbness, could be related to paresthesia experienced at lumbar puncture. Duration of complaints ranged from 1 day to many months, and the symptoms were never incapacitating or progressive.

Some characteristics of the pain deserve mention. Symptoms in patients 7, 10, and 14 resembled the syndrome of meralgia paresthetica.[29] Patient 10 was unusual, in that pain and paresthesias at puncture were experienced in the shoulder girdle, a symptom known as "Lhermitte's sign," ascribed to reduction in CSF pressure with traction on adhesions, or other mechanial effects on the spinal cord.[30] It is doubtful that an intraneural or intraspinal injection was made in any case, since this usually results in excruciating paresthesia with injection, often loss of consciousness, and onset of permanent sensory and motor deficit immediately postoperatively.

Some of the complaints probably resulted from damage to deep tissues of the back, with resultant painful foci. Trauma to ligaments, fascia, or bone with localized hemorrhage can give rise to low back pain and sciatic radiation, a syndrome produced experimentally upon injection of hypertonic saline into the back.[31] Infected disc as a sequel of traumatic puncture has also been reported.[32] It is also possible that injury to the cauda equina may have caused a radiculitis not extensive enough to be associated with sensory deficit. Still another possibility is the occurrence of a sterile inflammatory reaction, owing to introduction of blood into the subarachnoid space.[33]

Not all traumatic lumbar punctures are followed by neurologic complaints, and paresthesias are not preventable even in the best of hands. In a large series, paresthesias were encountered during lumbar puncture in 13 per cent of single-dose spinal anesthetics and in 30 per cent with continuous spinal anesthetics using a catheter, yet few patients subsequently suffered disability.[5]

Perhaps, the patient with marked obesity, spi-

Table 5-10. Minor Sequelae of Lumbar Puncture in 17 Patients*

Patients No.	Age	Sex	Operation	No. of Attempts	Site of Paresthesia	Complaint	Duration of Side Effects
1	24	M	Coccygeal sinus	3	R leg	Shooting pains, R leg	1 day
2†	28	F	Coccygeal sinus	1	L leg	Shooting pain and numbness, L leg	2 days
3	34	M	Appendectomy	1	L buttock, penis	Paresthesia, L buttock & penis	2 days
4	43	F	Hemorrhoidectomy	4	L thigh, buttock	Pain, L thigh to knee	1 day
5	47	F	Hysterectomy	2	R buttock, groin	Weakness & pain, R leg	8 days
6	29	F	Cesarean section	2	R leg	R leg paralyzed, pain	2 wks.
7‡	36	M	Appendectomy	2	R thigh	Numbness & tingling, R thigh	3 wks.
8‡	41	M	Varicose veins	1	R leg	Numb area, R foot	2 wks.
9	54	F	Cholecystectomy	1	L leg	Sharp pains, L leg	few wks.
10	30	F	Laparotomy	2	R leg & shoulder	Pain, R shoulder & thigh, numbness, R thigh, paresthesias	1 mo.
11	31	F	Vaginal plastic	4	None	Pain, L calf & foot, numbness	1 mo.
12	35	F	Hysterectomy	1	L leg	Pain, L leg	Months
13	38	M	Appendectomy	Many	R toes, both heels	Burning pain in heels	Months
14	29	F	Delivery	2	R leg	Numbness, R thigh	6 mos.
15	39	M	I & D rectal abscess	2	L leg	Pain, L leg	1 yr. intermittent
16	40	M	Cholecystectomy	5	R leg	Shooting pain, R foot	6 mos.
17	55	M	Cholecystectomy	1	L leg	Pain, L leg	Intermittent

*Vandam, L. D., and Dripps, R. D.: Long-term follow-up of patients who received 10,098 spinal anesthetics. IV. Neurological disease incident to traumatic lumbar puncture during spinal anesthesia. J.A.M.A., 172:1483, 1960. Copyright © 1960, American Medical Association

†Cerebrospinal fluid was bloody in this patient only.

‡A 22-gauge needle was used in all but these patients, in whom a 20-gauge needle was used.

nal curvature, or arthritis should be offered another form of anesthesia. If not, attention should be given to a position and technique that will make lumbar puncture easier. When difficulty is encountered with midline insertion, the lateral approach should be tried. Blood-stained CSF should be allowed to clear before injection of anesthetic. Injection should never be made in the presence of paresthesia, test injection be made into a nerve root or spinal cord. When paresthesia is produced, the needle should be repositioned or inserted at another interspace. Finally, the question of when to abandon lumbar puncture will always arise. It is not easy to take an objective viewpoint in the midst of a technical procedure performed just before operation, but blind persistence is unwarranted. If a technique other than spinal anesthesia can be utilized safely (and usually it can), a patient should be spared further discomfort and the complications described here.

INFECTIOUS SEQUELAE OF TRAUMATIC LUMBAR PUNCTURE

Meningitis

Chemical or bacterial meningitis may occur following diagnostic lumbar puncture or the administration of spinal or epidural anesthesia. Such complications are essentially unknown with epidural anesthesia, unless the dural sac is inadvertently entered and blood or bacteria thereby introduced. It is also possible that, in the presence of an epidural abscess following a catheter or needle insertion into the epidural space, infection can spread to the subarachnoid space. Soon after its introduction, meningism and meningitis were occasional findings following subarachnoid block. Meningism (stiff neck, headache, and fever) may merely accompany spinal headache. Bacterial meningitis, on the other hand, is accompanied by more serious signs and symptoms. Diagnostic puncture to identify the organism and appropriate antibiotic treatment are essential. Repeated lumbar puncture after spinal anesthesia occasionally yields CSF with elevated protein content and pleocytosis. At one time, these findings were interpreted as indicators of meningitis.[34] However, the raised protein content is thought to be merely a reflection of raised protein levels in the general circulation, following operation.[35] In addition, increased numbers of cells are usually seen after traumatic lumbar puncture with production of paresthesias.[35]

Chemical Meningitis. From time to time there have been epidemics of chemical meningitis occurring in several institutions.[36,37] This complication, which may also occur after paravertebral nerve block and epidural and caudal anesthesia, is characterized by fever, headache, cervical rigidity, nausea and vomiting, transient neurologic signs, prostration, and coma. The CSF is opalescent and sterile, although it contains a variety of white cells in increased number. The syndrome lasts for no more than several days and has been attributed to pyrogens in apparatus and the solutions used. Treatment is purely symptomatic, not requiring use of antibiotics. The possibility of Coxsackie viral disease must also be entertained under certain circumstances.

Bacterial Meningitis. Meningitis has ceased to be a problem in spinal anesthesia with increased attention to asepsis. Vandam and Dripps discovered no case of meningitis arising in direct association with anesthesia but reported a case of meningitis arising after 12 days.[38] The following report of coincident, acute, purulent otitis media gives rise to interesting speculation.

Case 5-3. A 12-year-old mentally retarded boy had incapacitating bilateral pes planus. A diagnostic spinal anesthesia was done to exclude an element of spasm in his orthopaedic problem. A tetracaine spinal anesthetic to the level of T12 was given by means of a 22-gauge needle, inserted at the L3–4 interspace, following recovery of clear CSF. Mild headache was present 2 days afterward. Twelve days after anesthesia, there was abrupt onset of frontal headache, neck stiffness, and fever to 39.1°C. Blood pressure was 110/70, pulse rate, 100, and respirations, 24 per min. Purulent secretion was seen in the right auditory canal, and the ear drum was injected. Marked stiffness of the anterior and posterior cervical muscle groups was elicited, with referred pain to forehead and low back. Brudzinski's and Kernig's signs were present.

The white blood cell count was 8,100. Lumbar puncture produced grossly clear CSF, with 20 red blood cells and 150 white cells, of which 60 per cent were neutrophiles, and 40 per cent, lymphocytes. Protein content was 58 mg. per dl., sugar, 56 mg. per dl., and chloride, 118 mg. per dl. The initial pressure was 20.0 torr. Culture was negative. Within 24 hours of the start of treatment with penicillin G and tetracycline, signs and symptoms disappeared. The boy had recovered completely at 6 months.

The 12-day interval between anesthesia and onset of meningitis tends to exclude anesthesia as the cause of meningitis. Meningism and meningitis are not uncommon in association with acute otitis media. Early disappearance of symptoms and paucity of CSF changes suggested a diagnosis of meningism rather than frank bacterial meningitis.

Despite these contentions, there is good reason to believe that spinal anesthesia should not be administered in the presence of infection, especially if blood stream invasion is a possiblity. Weed was able to produce meningitis repeatedly in several animal species by performing occipital or lumbar puncture within 5 hours of intravenous injection of pathogenic bacteria.[39] Meningitis began not at the puncture site but intracranially, and the injected bacteria were recovered from the subarachnoid space. Thus, the concept of lowered resistance to infection induced by spinal puncture was established. Others have reported onset of meningitis, as well as epidural abscess, in humans when spinal anesthesia was associated with acute infectious disease.[40,41] Caution should be the rule when considering spinal anesthesia for operations complicated by infection.

COMPLICATIONS RELATED TO INJECTION OF THE LOCAL ANESTHETIC

Two major complications of spinal anesthesia deserve special mention because of the resulting disabling illness: cauda equina syndrome and chronic adhesive arachnoiditis.

Cauda Equina Syndrome

The cauda equina syndrome is so called because signs and symptoms are localized to areas innervated by the lumbar and sacral nerves. In any chemical, neural injury, the small fibers are affected first, just as they are the first to be affected by local anesthetics. Thus, a patient with the syndrome presents with autonomic disability, problems in evacuation of bladder and bowel, and disturbed sweating and temperature control in lumbar and sacral dermatomes. In addition, sensation to pinprick, temperature, and position may be altered. There is a form of cauda equina syndrome that can follow traumatic lumbar puncture. The typical picture is seen when an intraneural injection of local anesthetic is made. The solution spreads along the nerve root to origins in the spinal cord, which it enters and then causes both dissolution and ischemia of cell bodies. When neither traumatic tap nor intraneural injection can be implicated and the cauda equina syndrome develops, it is assumed that a toxic substance, possibly a detergent used in cleaning apparatus or a contaminant of the local anesthetic, like an antiseptic such as phenol, must have been introduced into the subarachnoid space. At one time, when ampules were soaked in phenol solution, it was possible for the caustic substance to seep into a local anesthetic through inapparent cracks in ampules. Such an occurrence was implicated in the development of neurologic complications in a celebrated law suit in Great Britain.[42] For this reason, apparatus and ampules are sterilized today by either autoclaving or ethylene oxide treatment. Suspicious-looking ampules that have discolored solutions or seem to have less than the volume of solution listed should be discarded and not used in spinal anesthesia.

Adhesive Arachnoiditis

Adhesive arachnoiditis, a somewhat stereotyped central nervous pathologic reaction, occurred long before spinal anesthesia was employed.[43] Appearing diffusely, or in patchy distribution, this sterile organizing inflammatory process may be idiopathic or a response to trauma, chemical irritant, or infection. The subarachnoid space becomes obliterated by adhesions to the spinal cord, with dense attachment of the arachnoid to dura. At laminectomy, the dura can hardly be peeled away from the underlying arachnoidal membrane. Blood vessels are entrapped in the organizing inflammatory process, with resultant ischemia and destruction of cells and tracts within the spinal cord, which produces a variety of neurologic deficits. On pathologic examination, the blood vessels themselves are obliterated by a vasculitis or organizing endarteritis.

Adhesive arachnoiditis occuring after spinal anesthesia presents additional features of variable location and progressive involvement of the spinal cord and brain; hence, it is called *chronic progressive* adhesive arachnoiditis. Hydrocephalus, syringomyelia, and the gamut of paraplegia and tetraplegia typify the end stage of this process. The cause is unknown, and it has been attributed to contamination of the local anesthetic with a chemical irritant preservative (methylparaben) or to an allergic response to the anesthetic. The latter is suggested by the concomitant vasculitis sometimes found. The lesion has been reproduced experimentally by injection of a variety of chemical irritants, including detergents, into the subarachnoid space.[44] Figure 5-5 shows a normal-looking spinal cord at laminectomy, with the picture of adhesive arachnoiditis juxtaposed.

Arachnoiditis does not seem to occur now, although we cannot be certain that it has been eliminated, without continued surveillance of spinal and epidural techniques. If there has been improvement, credit should go to wiser choice of techniques and use of equipment and solutions meticulously prepared, sterilized, and continuously surveyed in pharmaceutical houses and hospital pharmacies. Storage times, lot numbers, and date of expiration of drug efficacy must be known.

Arachnoiditis presents typical manifestations at myelography, although many physicians would prefer not to inject an additional chemical irritant for diagnosis. To exclude other lesions, laminectomy is necessary. The best treatment for adhesive arachnoiditis is to attempt to decompress the cord and reestablish CSF communication. There are no data to show that the parenteral use of adrenocortical steroids is efficacious in treating the disease.

MINOR NEUROLOGIC SEQUELAE OF SPINAL AND EPIDURAL ANESTHESIA

Vandam and Dripps reported 71 cases in which subjective or both subjective and objective evidence of neurologic disease was found following spinal anesthesia.[45] In a control series of general anesthetics, similar complaints were not encountered. Subjective complaints consisted of numbness, tingling, heaviness, or burning; some were associated with neurologic defect. Symptoms and signs were usually present in the immediate postoperative period, lasting from a few days to more than 6 months without progression. It is significant that the majority of complaints were confined to the lumbar and sacral areas of the body. A few patients had tingling of the fingers without objective change, but this was probably of little significance. In 85 others (1.0% of the total number of patients), symptoms were reported that were called "irritative," for want of a better term. These were complaints of cramps and twisting, pulling, or drawing sensations, in the lower extremities; they arose and subsided in the first few days after operation. As 0.9 per cent of patients given general anesthesia had identical symptoms, the investigators believed that they were not peculiar to spinal anesthesia.

Many of these people were apparently symptom-free postoperatively, yet 6 months later they said that neurologic symptoms were experienced from the time of operation. There is little doubt that the investigation sensitized patients to the possibility of development of disease and that they were, therefore, prone to associate minor complaints with the anesthetic. Nevertheless, the complaints were genuine, and similar findings were not encountered in a control group of patients given general anesthesia.

Numbness usually is not found as a sequela of lumbar puncture, and few of the 71 individuals had headache. There were comparatively few instances of traumatic lumbar puncture, and on only a few occasions was blood-stained CSF obtained. When paresthesias were produced at the

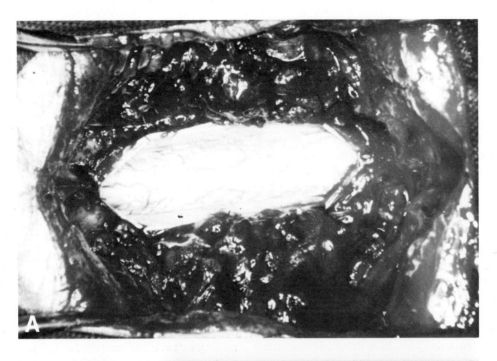

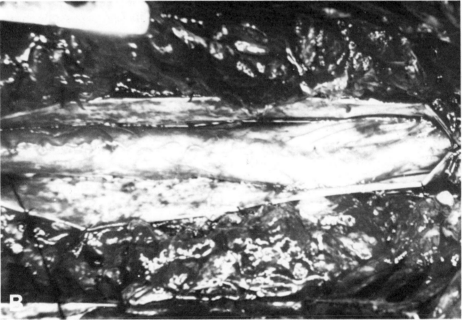

Fig. 5-5. (*A*)Normal spinal cord at laminectomy. The dura has been opened, and the arachnoid is still intact. Note the transparency of the latter and the delicate anastomosing network of blood vessels on the sùrface of the cord. (*B*)A case of adhesive arachnoiditis shown at laminectomy. In contrast to *A*, the dura has been opened and stripped, only with difficulty, from the underlying arachnoidal membrane. The latter is opaque, thickened, vascularized, and adherent to the underlying spinal cord, which cannot be seen. The subarachnoid space is obliterated. (Vandam, L.D.: Spinal anesthesia. In Hale, D.E. (ed.): Anesthesiology. Philadelphia, F.A. Davis, 1963)

time of lumbar puncture, they showed no obvious relation to the subsequent site of neurologic involvement. One must conclude, then, that the trauma of lumbar puncture played little part in the development of disease. Was trauma of another kind responsible? Can the kind of operation performed or mechanical factors associated with operation be implicated? In some instances, such complaints can be related to positioning of legs in stirrups. There might have been a direct relation in these patients, in whom varicose veins were ligated, hemorrhoidectomy was performed, or herniorrhaphy was carried out in proximity to the area of numbness. These operations did not comprise a large share of those reported. A relation to position on the operating table, to the application of restraining straps, or to subsequent intramuscular injection of antibiotics into the thigh could not be established.

Consideration of the part played by the local anesthetic remains. Complaints were confined almost entirely to the lumbar and sacral areas, the general level of the spine at which lumbar puncture is done and, consequently, where the concentration of anesthetic is highest in contact with neural tissues. No relation between the specific anesthetic injected and number of complications was found. Weighting the anesthetic with dextrose and position at the time of injection could not be related to the side on which the difficulty was experienced subsequently.

It seems likely, then, that these neurologic complaints were related in a nonspecific way to the injection of the anesthetic agent. Perhaps it is significant that the majority of injectable spinal anesthetic solutions are hypertonic, with mean values for osmolality falling outside the CSF range, 257 to 305 mOsm. per L.; the damage caused by these anesthetics is related directly to the variation from isotonicity of the solution employed.[46] Moreover, vasoconstrictor drugs injected into the subarachnoid space may cause neurologic sequelae in the rhesus monkey.[47] But the concentrations of vasoconstrictor used were far higher than those employed in clinical practice, and the Pennsylvania study failed to implicate these drugs in the development of disease. Neurologic sequelae have followed injection of various foreign substances into the subarachnoid space.[48] The delicacy of spinal structures and their peculiar vascularity almost invite trouble.

Finally, there is a similarity between the neurologic complaints described and the syndrome of meralgia paresthetica. The latter is characterized by numbness and paresthesias in the area of distribution of the lateral femoral cutaneous nerve, not an uncommon ailment.[49] The cause of the syndrome is unknown and has been attributed to arthritis of the spine, spinal trauma, excessive tobacco smoking, or lower abdominal stresses such as pregnancy, wearing of a truss, or a cartridge belt. The course of the lateral femoral cutaneous nerve in the retroperitoneal space and lower abdomen, its proximity to the anterior superior spine of the ilium, and final penetration of the fascia lata suggest that the nerve may be inordinately susceptible to trauma. Was it a coincidence that in approximately half of the patients described numbness coincided with the distribution of the lateral femoral cutaneous nerve? It hardly seems possible that specific nerve fibers comprising the lateral femoral cutaneous nerve can be selectively affected by a substance injected into the subarachnoid space.

ANTECEDENT NEUROLOGIC DISEASE AND DEVELOPMENT OF POSTANESTHETIC SEQUELAE

An important means of prevention of neurologic disease after spinal anesthesia involves proper selection of patients for the method. In general, it had been a basic tenet, hitherto undocumented, that afflictions of the CNS and spinal column contraindicate the use of the spinal anesthesia. In the Pennsylvania series, despite care in selection, spinal anesthesia was inadvertently given to 11 patients with preexisting neurologic disease.[38]

Spinal Cord Tumor

A preexisting, but symptomless spinal cord meningioma resulted in symptoms immediately postoperatively. Early lack of recognition and later preoccupation with a relation to spinal anesthesia delayed diagnosis and therapy.

Case 5-4. A 42-year-old woman underwent repair of a diaphragmatic hernia. Lumbar puncture was performed with a 22-gauge needle at the L4–5 interspace, a transient paresthesia was produced in the left leg, but CSF was clear and dripped freely. Spinal anesthesia to the level of T5 was obtained. Postoperatively, the patient complained of backache. Before leaving the hopsital, she experienced heaviness in the legs and tingling sensations in the toes. Six months later, the patient wrote that she had gradually become incapacitated with backache, falling episodes, spreading numbness, loss of strength, and paresthesias in the legs.

Neurologic findings included ataxia, positive Romberg's sign, positive Babinski's sign on the left, no abdominal reflexes, diminished or loss of sense of position in the legs, hypesthesia to pinprick to the level of T10, partial loss of motor power in the left leg, and spasm of the back muscles. Red and white blood cell counts were normal, blood serology was negative, and free hydrochloric acid was present in gastric juice. CSF pressure and dynamics were normal. The protein content of the CSF was 47 mg.%, Kolmer's test was negative, and cells were not present. A cystometrogram disclosed a hypotonic bladder. Radiographic examination of the back showed degenerative and hypertrophic changes in the thoracic spine. Myelography was avoided because of the suspicion that arachnoiditis was present. Physical therapy was prescribed. One year after spinal anesthesia, a meningioma was found at laminectomy in another hospital. Postoperatively, there was rapid improvement, and 6 months later, the patient had recovered completely.

Early onset of symptoms of spinal cord compression by tumor after lumbar puncture can be attributed to displacement of the mass or to vascular engorgement. An alteration in CSF pressure, rather than injection of the spinal anesthetic, was responsible for these changes. Michelsen[50] and Nicholson and Eversole[51] reported similar experiences with spinal cord tumors and administration of spinal anesthesia. Michelsen suggests that CSF dynamics and the protein content be tested routinely in spinal anesthesia. I believe this to be an impractical approach. A spinal anesthetic should not be injected, however, if lumbar puncture yields a suspicious-looking fluid or if flow of fluid is not free.

Viral Disease of the Nervous System

Case 5-5 represents a possible relation between acute herpes zoster, spinal anesthesia, and subsequent development of neurologic disease.

Case 5-5. A 25-year-old woman with right lower quadrant abdominal pain underwent surgery for appendicitis. Spinal anesthesia to T6 was obtained with tetracaine and glucose, injected through a 22-gauge needle at the L3–4 intervertebral space. One tap was made without paresthesia, and CSF was clear. At operation, the appendix was not inflamed. On the 2nd postoperative day, herpetic lesions appeared on the left side in the distribution of dermatomes T6 and T4. These lesions persisted for 4 weeks and were treated with ergotamine. Three weeks after operation, sensations of pins-and-needles arose in both thighs, with radiation down the backs of legs. At the same time, there was severe backache, with difficulty in straightening the trunk. The sensory disturbances lasted 12 days, and backache, 2 weeks. A month following anesthesia, diminished appreciation of pinprick was elicited over the outer surface of the right foot and anterior surface of the tibia. One week later these signs disappeared, but coldness in the right foot remained. The only complaint after 1 year was a subjective difference in the temperature in the legs.

Herpes zoster is an infectious disease caused by a virus that affects the posterior root ganglion, posterior nerve roots, and dorsal horns. Persistent sensory and motor paralysis often results. Thus, a clear relationship between neurologic deficit and spinal anesthesia or herpes zoster cannot be established in Case 5-5.

Trophic lesions of an herpetiform type may, in rare instances, be induced by spinal anesthesia, one of the explanations offered by Carter for an eruption arising after lumbar puncture.[52] Trauma may be the cause if the lumbar puncture needle injures a ganglion, for herpetiform eruptions can be produced by manipulation in the distribution of a nerve root. Arnold found herepetic eruptions in three cases following 640 spinal anesthetics.[53] He found no relation to lumbar puncture site and assumed that a toxic injury had occurred. Despite these possibilities, it would seem wise to avoid spinal anesthesia if a diagnosis of viral disease is made preoperatively. This admonition is borne out by the report of Nicholson and Eversole on spinal anesthesia followed by neurologic deficit, in a patient with varicella.[51]

Mumps Encephalitis

Case 5-6. A 36-year-old woman, 134 cm. tall, weighing 89 kg., was scheduled for cholecystectomy. She was in the 3rd month of pregnancy and gave a history of eclampsia, hypertension, and jaundice. Lumbar puncture was performed without paresthesia, using a 22-gauge needle inserted at the L3–4 interspace. CSF was clear and flowed freely. Spinal anesthesia to T5 was achieved with tetracaine, glucose, and epinephrine. Immediately postoperatively, the patient experienced weakness of the right leg and diffuse impairment of pinprick sensation. A mild, transient postural headache lasted for 2 days. Within several days, the leg seemed stronger, but it buckled under her when she attempted to stand, on the 10th postoperative day. At this time, the patient volunteered that she had had mumps followed by convulsions and encephalitis 10 years previously. Both legs were affected at that time, especially the right, which weakened with exercise. When seen 3 years later her right leg, though much stronger, continued to annoy her with intermittent pain.

In this patient, spinal anesthesia seemed to precipitate symptoms that had been dormant for years. A history of encephalitis was not elicited in the preoperative visit, despite specific inquiry for antecedent neurologic disease. For one reason or another, many patients forget important events during history taking. One can only speculate on the reasons for recrudescence of disease. It may be significant that the maximum concentration of anesthetic in the subarachnoid space came in contact with the lumbar nerve roots on the previously affected right side.

Other Diseases of the CNS

The anesthesiologist is frequently confronted with selection of an anesthetic for a patient with cerebrovascular disease and its associated disorders, or combined sclerosis, disseminated sclerosis, syphillis, and amyotrophic lateral sclerosis. With respect to these patients, Yaskin states the following:[54] "It is a well recognized fact that the first clinical manifestation of some clearly defined nervous disorder may date from a severe trauma, operation or confinement." Critchley adds, "Spinal anesthesia also may be a precipitating agent in the evolution of such afflictions as disseminated sclerosis, progressive muscular atrophy or syphilis."[55]

Case 5-7. A 59-year-old woman had a cerebrovascular accident, followed by left hemiparesis and urinary bladder "weakness" 6 years before entry. These compliants cleared considerably, but she was left with intractable right leg pain. As a diagnostic and prognostic measure for treatment of the pain, a differential spinal anesthetic by means of a continuous technique was given with 0.2-per-cent procaine. Multiple taps were made with a 16-gauge needle. A paresthesia was produced in the right foot, but CSF was clear. A No. 3 ureteral catheter was inserted 3 cm. into the subarachnoid space. Although a sensory level to T4 was obtained, pain was not relieved. After anesthesia, pain in the legs increased. A typical postural headache, bladder "weakness," and frequency followed. All eventually disappeared.

Bladder "weakness" might have represented retention and overflow incontinence, since the patient was receiving large amounts of morphine for pain. Exacerbation of leg pain may have resulted from irritation by the anesthetic. From time to time after spinal anesthesia, patients are seen with leg cramps that may be ascribed to irritation. However, similar complaints were found in a series of patients given general anesthesia.[45]

Backache and Sciatic Pain

Backache is a common complaint after both spinal and general anesthesia. When followed by sciatic pain, backache becomes a neurologic problem, since there may be protrusion of an intervertebral disc and compression of a spinal nerve root. In the Pennsylvania study several cases with a common pattern were seen: recurrence of backache and sciatica after spinal anesthesia, with symptoms and signs strongly suggesting disc protrusion. Although questioned before anesthesia, none of the individuals admitted having had back pain.

Case 5-8. A 59-year-old man was given spinal anesthesia with tetracaine and glucose for suprapubic prostatectomy. Lumbar puncture was performed after two insertions of a 22-gauge needle. There was no pain or paresthesia, and CSF was clear. On standing 2 days postoperatively, the patient experienced severe low back pain with radiation to the left foot, aggravated by straining. At this time, he said that he had had shooting pains in the left leg before anesthesia. One week after anesthesia, examination disclosed right sacroiliac tenderness and straight leg raising limited to 70 degrees. Radiographs of the back showed increased density of bone, extensive osseous degenerative disease in the lower lumbar and sacral regions, marginal lipping of the vertebrae, and narrowing of the L4–5 space. He improved with traction to the affected leg, and recovery was complete 10 months later.

There are many reasons why spinal anesthesia might be inadvisable in the presence of backache. Although backache is just as common after general anesthesia, specific reasons for its occurrence after spinal anesthesia can be offered. Traumatic lumbar puncture may injure a disc or a vertebra. Hemorrhage into a ligament can act as a focus of pain, with radiation in a sciatic distribution. Psychologic aspects can by no means be neglected, as it is natural to relate pain and

tenderness at the lumbar puncture site to existing backache. Some physicians believe that muscle relaxation and positioning on a flat operating table cause back strain. Other positions on the table (e.g., lithotomy) can surely produce strain.

The situation is even more complex when there is already a protruded disc. In some clinics, spinal anesthesia is selected for laminectomy.[56] However, the incidence of persistent pain and neurologic deficit after operation for protruded disc is sufficiently high that, for this reason, spinal anesthesia should be avoided. If diagnostic myelography has been done, onset of arachnoiditis from that source is not uncommon. Finally, arachnoiditis has been found at a second laminectomy performed because of persistent backache. In some cases the arachnoiditis probably developed as a result of trauma during the first operation.[57]

Metastatic Malignancy of the Spine. Unsuspected tumor metastases to the spine may be present when spinal anesthesia is given.

Case 5-9. A 77-year-old man was given tetracaine-glucose continuous spinal anesthesia for abdomino-perineal resection of the rectum. Lumbar puncture was performed with a 16-gauge needle after two insertions, without pain or paresthesia. CSF was clear. A sensory level to T4 was obtained. Six months later, the patient developed shooting pains in the left hip and anterior thigh, with radiation to the knee. A possibility of arachnoiditis was raised by a consulting neurologist, but radiographs of the back showed destruction of the first three lumbar vertebrae by metastatic tumor.

Nicholson and Eversole also reported a case of spinal cord compression after anesthesia, owing to metastatic tumor.[51] Aside from the possibility that lumbar puncture may heighten symptoms, the most important aspect of the relation between anesthesia and spinal column disease is the likelihood that the patient will implicate the anesthetic. A patient is usually encouraged in this belief by physicians, as the prospect of death from metastatic disease is not an easy matter to discuss. Usually the possibility of spinal anesthetic complications dominates the thinking of consultants, and more likely causes for disease are relegated to a secondary role. Mistaken diagnoses have been made again and again, to the detriment of patients.

Diabetes, Senescence, and Peripheral Neuropathy

Operations on diabetic patients are often performed under spinal anesthesia, a method that does little to upset metabolic balance. However, the diabetic patient often has complicating ailments. Old age, vascular disease, and peripheral neuropathy are accompanied by neurologic signs and symptoms that may be confusing as complications of spinal anesthesia.[58]

Case 5-10. A 68-year-old man with severe diabetes, prostatic obstruction, and hematuria underwent prostatectomy. Spinal anesthesia with tetracaine and glucose was administered by means of a 22-gauge needle at the L3–4 interspace. Three insertions of the needle were made, CSF was clear, and a sensory level to T10 was obtained. Postoperative bleeding and a transfusion reaction left him with anemia; the postoperative course was marked by tachycardia, fever, mental confusion, phlebitis, and wound sepsis. Two months later, he complained of weakness and lack of control of his legs dating from the hospital stay. Although there had been subjective improvement, examination disclosed a questionable Romberg's sign, hyperactive reflexes, and a semi-shuffling gait. One month later, weakness of the muscles of the left leg and a stocking type of hypesthesia were found. Thereafter, symptoms improved. One year after operation, the patient was working as a barber and standing most of the day, but with a sense of weakness in the legs.

A few details are lacking to make this picture more interpretable. The extent of diabetic control, adequacy of circulation to the legs, and blood and spinal fluid serologies were not known. Nonetheless, the symptoms and signs may have resulted from spinal anesthesia alone. These improved, however, and one is inclined to attribute them to a number of factors: anemia, vascular disease, poor diabetic control and nutrition, and, possibly, peripheral neuropathy.

From Case 5-10, it is evident that spinal anesthesia may be held responsible for the development of any concurrent neurologic disease. Marinacci and Courville emphasized this possibility in a study of 482 patients whose complaints were attributed to spinal anesthesia.[59] Of this group, 478 were shown to have an entirely unrelated neurologic condition, either an infectious neuritis or peripheral neuropathy in the majority of cases. The electromyogram (EMG) played an important role in evaluating the complaints and differentiating them. Differentiation was based on the following criteria: distribution of denervation, that is, the EMG changes; and the time at which denervation activity is first detected by EMG. Recently Samaha has reviewed the value of electrodiagnostic studies in neuromuscular disease.[60]

COMPLICATIONS OF EPIDURAL AND CAUDAL ANESTHESIA

Because the only difference between spinal and epidural anesthesia is the injection site, complications associated with epidural anesthesia are qualitatively the same as those of spinal anesthesia. Recent studies of the physiology of epidural anesthesia amply confirm this dictum. However, a thorough prospective study of neurologic sequelae has not been done. One does have the distinct impression that such complications are rare, indeed. If so, a lack of such problems may be ascribed to the lessons learned from administration of spinal anesthesia and to the availability of more reliable anesthestics and equipment. In general, the kinds of complications that might occur (e.g., technical, physiologic, and pathologic) are suggested by Dawkins' retrospective survey of some 350 articles on epidural and caudal block, including 4,000 nerve blocks done by the author himself over a period of 25 years (Table 5-11).[9] A discrepancy exists in the total numbers of cases quoted for any one complication, because complete figures were lacking.

Blood vessel puncture is the most common

Table 5-11. Complications Following Lumbar and Thoracic Epidural Block

	NUMBER OF CASES	NUMBER OF COMPLICATIONS
Dural puncture	43,152	1,090 (2.5%)
Accidental spinal total anesthesia	48,297	102 (0.2%)
Blood vessel puncture	6,578	189 (2.8%)
Toxic reaction	66,366	144 (0.2%)
Massive epidural	16,644	28 (0.1%)
Severe hypotension	42,900	797 (1.8%)
Backache	9,107	185 (2%)
Transient paralysis	32,718	48 (0.1%)
Permanent paralysis	32,718	7 (0.02%)

(Dawkins, C. J. M.: Analysis of the complications of extradural and caudal block. Anaesthesia, *24*:554, 1969)

complication noted. No mention is made of epidural hematoma formation,[61] an accident that can also occur spontaneously,[62] particularly following needle puncture in the presence of blood clotting abnormalities that are iatrogenically or pathologically induced. Onset of severe backache following anesthesia with progressive signs of cord compression suggests hematoma formation. Myelography reveals the site of blockage, and early evacuation of the clot must be accomplished to avoid permanent deficit. Epidural abscess formation occurring after both spinal and epidural anesthesia is somewhat more delayed in onset, but with systemic signs of infection and the same kind of neurologic picture. Treatment consists of antibiotic therapy and surgical drainage.

A second common complication entails inadvertent subarachnoid puncture. Usually the needle is withdrawn, and epidural injection is made at another spinal interspace. Total spinal anesthesia may still arise, however, if the anesthetic injected epidurally enters the dural puncture opening. With accidental puncture, severe and prolonged postural headache is common because of the large-gauge needle employed. The treatment is the same as that ordinarily suggested for headache, including use of an epidural blood patch.

Dawkins gives no details on reported cases of paralysis, but he relates two incidents of his own. In one, gross destruction of the posterolateral portion of the spinal cord from T6 to T12 was

Table 5-12. Complications Following Caudal Block

	NUMBER OF CASES	NUMBER OF COMPLICATIONS
Dural puncture	13,639	171 (1.2%)
Accidental spinal	6,334	9 (0.1%)
Blood vessel puncture	639	4 (0.6%)
Failure to find sacral hiatus	2,803	87 (3.1%)
Toxic reaction	3,332	6 (0.2%)
Sepsis	3,767	8 (0.2%)
Breakage of needle	850	12 (1.4%)
Breakage of catheter	5,379	6 (0.1%)
Severe hypotension	3,189	201 (6.3%)
Transient paralysis	22,968	5 (0.02%)
Permanent paralysis	22,968	1 (0.005%)

(Dawkins, C. J. M.: Analysis of the complications of extradural and caudal block. Anaesthesia, *24*:554, 1969.)

found at necropsy following anesthesia in a 70-year-old man with inoperable carcinoma of the pancreas. In the second instance, transient sensory and motor paralysis of the lower extremities followed epidural block given for deliberate hypotension during resection of a parotid tumor. One can surmise, therefore, that neurologic sequelae may follow epidural anesthesia for the same reasons that they may follow spinal anesthesia. Finally, Dawkins notes that the sequelae of caudal block are largely those associated with the technical aspects of that approach to the epidural space (Table 5-12).

REFERENCES

1. Thorsen, G.: Neurological complications after spinal anesthesia. Acta Chir. Scand. *95* [Suppl.]: *121*, 1947.
2. Kennedy, F., Effron, A. S., and Perry, G.: The grave spinal cord paralyses caused by spinal anesthesia. Surg. Gynecol. Obstet. *91*:385, 1950.
3. Dickson, W. E. C.: Cerebrospinal fluids in meningitis. Postgrad. Med. J. *20*:69, 1944.
4. Lumbar puncture and epidermoid tumours. Lancet, *1*:635, 1977.
5. Dripps, R. D.: A comparison of the malleable needle and catheter technics for continuous spinal anesthesia. N.Y. State J. Med., *50*:1595, 1950.
6. Sechzer, P. H.: Subdural space in spinal anesthesia. Anesthesiology, *24*:896, 1963.
7. Dripps, R. D., and Vandam, L. D.: Long term follow-up of patients who received 10,098 spinal anesthetics: 1. Failure to discover major neurological sequelae. J.A.M.A. *156*:1486, 1954.
8. Freund, F. C., Bonica, J. J., and Ward, R. J.: Ventilatory reserve and level of motor block during high spinal and epidural anesthesia. Anesthesiology, *28*:834, 1967.
9. Dawkins, C. J. M.: Analysis of the complications of extradural and caudal block. Anaesthesia, *24*:554, 1969.
10. Dripps, R. D., and Deming, M.V.N.: An evaluation of certain drugs used to maintain blood pressure during spinal anesthesia: comparison of ephedrine, paredrine, pitressin-ephedrine and methedrine in 2,500 cases. Surg. Gynecol. Obstet., *83*:312, 1946.
11. Greene, N. M.: Physiology of Spinal Anesthesia. ed. 2. pp. 43–117. Baltimore, Williams & Wilkins, 1969.
12. Greene, N. M., Bunker, J. P., Kerr, W. S., et al.: Hypotensive spinal anesthesia: repiratory, metabolic, hepatic, renal and cerebral effects. Ann. Surg., *140*:641, 1954.
13. Labat, G.: Regional Anesthesia. p. 449. Philadelphia, W. B. Saunders, 1923.
14. Babcock, W. W.: Spinal anesthesia. Am. J. Surg., *5*:571, 1928.
15. Crocker, J. S., and Vandam, L. D.: Concerning nausea and vomiting during spinal anesthesia. Anesthesiology, *20*:587, 1959.
16. Davis, L., and Pollock, L. J.: Role of autonomic nervous system in production of pain. J.A.M.A., *106*:350, 1936.
17. Phillips, O. C., Ebner, H., Nelson, A. T., et al.: Neurologic complications following spinal anesthesia with lidocaine. Anesthesiology, *30*:284, 1969.
18. Beecher, H. K., Todd, D.: A study of the deaths associated with anesthesia and surgery. Ann. Surg., *140*:2, 1954.
19. Vandam, L. D., and Dripps, R. D.: Long-term follow-up of patients who received 10,098 spinal anesthetics. III. Syndrome of decreased intracranial pressure (headache and ocular and auditory difficulties). J.A.M.A., *161*:586, 1956.
20. Wolff, H.G.: Headache. Chap. 2. New York, Oxford University Press, 1948.
21. Marshall, J.: Lumbar puncture headache. J. Neurol. Neurosurg. Psychiat., *13*:71, 1950.
22. Page, F.: Intracranial hypotension. Lancet, *1*:1, 1953.
23. Redlich, F. C., Moore, B. D., and Kimbell, I.: Lumbar puncture reactions: relative importance of physiological and psychological factors. Psychosom Med., *8*:836, 1946.
24. Jones, R. J.: The role of recumbency in the prevention and treatment of spinal headache. Anesth. Analg., *53*:788, 1974.
25. DiGiovanni, A. J., and Dunbar, B. S.: Epidural injections of autologous blood for post-lumbar puncture headache. Anesth. Analg., *49*:268, 1970.
26. Bryce-Smith, R. M., and Macintosh, R. R.: Sixth-nerve palsy after lumbar puncture and spinal analgesia. Br. Med. J., *1*:275, 1971.
27. Hughson, W.: A note on the relationship of cerebrospinal and intralabyrinthine pressures. Am. J. Physiol., *101*:396, 1932.
28. Selander, D., Dhuner, K.G., and Lundborg, G. Peripheral nerve injury due to injection needles used for regional anaesthesia. An experimental study of the acute effects of needle point trauma. Acta Anaesth. Scand., *21*:182, 1977.
29. Musser, J. A., and Sailer, J.: Meralgia paresthetica of Roth. J. Nerv. Ment. Dis., *27*:16, 1900.
30. Hogeman, O.: Lhermitte's sign due to cervical exostosis. Acta Soc. Med. Upsal., *17*:192, 1952.
31. Kellgren, J. H.: On the distribution of pain arising from deep somatic strictures with charts of segmental pain areas. Clin. Sci., *4*:35, 1939.
32. Bromley, L. L., Craig, J. D., Kessel, A. W. L.: Infected intervetebral disc after lumbar puncture. Br. Med. J., *1*:132, 1949.
33. Jackson, I. J.: Aseptic hemogenic meningitis: experimental production of aseptic meningeal reactions due to blood and its breakdown products. Arch. Neurol. Psychiat., *62*:572, 1949.
34. Black, M. G.: Spinal fluid findings in spinal anesthesia. Anesthesiology, *8*:382, 1947.
35. Marx, G. F., Saifer, A., and Orkin, L. R.: Cerebrospinal fluid cells and proteins following spinal anesthesia. Anesthesiology, *24*:305, 1963.
36. Goldman, W. W., and Sanford, J. P.: An "epidemic" of chemical meningitis. Am. J. Med., *29*:94, 1960.
37. DiGiovanni, A. J.: "Chemical meningitis" tied to cleaning fluid bacteria. J.A.M.A., *214*:2129, 1970.
38. Vandam, L. D., Dripps, R. D.: Exacerbation of pre-existing neurologic disease after spinal anesthesia. N. Engl. J. Med., *255*:843, 1956.
39. Weed, L. H., Wegefarth, P., Auer, J. B., et al.: The production of meningitis by release of cerebrospinal fluid during an experimental septicemia: preliminary note. J.A.M.A., *72*:190, 1919.

40. Berman, R. S., Eisele, J. H.: Bacteremia, spinal anesthesia, and development of meningitis. Anesthesiology, *48*:376, 1978.
41. Loarie, D. J., Fairley, H. B.: Epidural abscess following spinal anesthesia. Anesth. Analg., *57*:351, 1978.
42. Foreign Letters (London). J.A.M.A., *154*:532, 1954.
43. Mackay, R. P.: Chronic adhesive arachnoiditis. A clinical and pathological study. J.A.M.A., *112*:802, 1939.
44. Hurst, E. W.: Adhesive arachnoiditis and vascular blockage caused by detergents and other chemical irritants: an experimental study. J. Path. Bact., *70*:167, 1955.
45. Vandam, L. D., and Dripps, R. D.: A long-term follow-up of patients who received 10,098 spinal anesthetics. II. Incidence and analyses of minor sensory neurological defects. Surgery, *38*:463, 1955.
46. Sawinski, V. J., Goldberg, A. F., and Goldberg, N. B.: Osmolality of spinal anesthetic agents. Anesthesiology, *27*:86, 1966.
47. Brizzee, K. R., and Wu, J. J.: Studies on the effects of intrathecal injections of ephedrine sulphate on the spinal cord. J. Neuropath. Clin. Neurol., *1*:234, 1951.
48. Wilson, G., Rupp, C., and Wilson, W. W.: The dangers of intrathecal medication. J.A.M.A., *140*:1076, 1949.
49. Schneck, J. M.: Meralgia paresthetica. J. Nerv. Ment. Dis., *105*:77, 1947.
50. Michelsen, J. J.: Neurologic manifestations following spinal anesthesia. Neurology, *2*:255, 1952.
51. Nicholson, M. J., and Eversole, U. H.: Neurologic complications of spinal anesthesia. J.A.M.A., *132*:679, 1946.
52. Carter, H. R.: Herpes zoster. A case following lumbar puncture. Am. J. Psychiat. *94*:373, 1938.
53. Arnold, D. G.: Herpes zoster as a sequel of spinal anesthesia. Int. Coll. Surg., *4*:66, 1941.
54. Yaskin, H. A., and Alpers, B. J.: Neuropsychiatric complications following spinal anesthesia. Ann. Intern. Med., *23*:184, 1945.
55. Critchley, M.: Discussion of neurologic sequelae of spinal anesthesia. Proc R. Soc. Med., *30*:1007, 1937.
56. Hunter, A. R.: Anesthesia for operations on the vertebral canal. Anesthesiology, *11*:367, 1950.
57. Smolik, E. A., and Nash, F. P.: Lumbar spinal arachnoiditis: a complication of the intervertebral disc operation. Ann. Surg., *133*:490, 1951.
58. Jordan, W. R.: Neuritic manifestations in diabetes mellitus. Arch. Intern. Med., *57*:301, 1936.
59. Marinacci, A. A., and Courville, C. B.: Electromyogram in evaluation of neurological complications of spinal anesthesia. J.A.M.A., *168*:1337, 1958.
60. Samaha, F. J.: Current concepts: electrodiagnostic studies in neuromuscular disease. N. Engl. J. Med., *285*:1244, 1971.
61. Janis, K. M.: Epidural hematoma following postoperative epidural anesthesia. Anesth. Analg., *51*:689, 1972.
62. Spurny, O. M., Rubin, S., Wolf, J. W., et al.: Spinal epidural hematoma during anticoagulant therapy. Arch. Intern. Med., *114*:103, 1964.

FURTHER READING

Bromage, P. R.: Epidural Analgesia. Philadelphia, W. B. Saunders, 1978.
Cousins, M. J., and Bridenbaugh, P. O. (eds.): Neural Blockade in Clinical Anesthesia & Management of Pain. Philadelphia, J. B. Lippincott Company, 1980.
Greene, N. M.: Physiology of Spinal Anesthesia, ed. 3. Baltimore, Williams & Wilkins, 1981.
Kane, R. E.: Neurologic deficits following epidural or spinal anesthesia. Anesth. Analg., *60*:150, 1981.
Moore, D. C.: Complications of Regional Anesthesia. Springfield, Charles C Thomas, 1955.
Thorsen, G.: Neurological complications after spinal anesthesia and results from 2493 follow-up cases. Acta Chir. Scand. *95*:[Suppl. 121] 1, 1947.
Usubiaga, J. E.: Neurological complications following epidural anesthesia. Int. Anesthesiol. Clin., *13*:1, 1975.

6 Complications of Diagnostic and Therapeutic Nerve Blocks

Terence M. Murphy, M.B., Ch.B., F.F.A.R.C.S.

Murphy's law states that, "If things can go wrong, they will,"[1] and there is a risk attached to virtually everything we do in medicine. This is equally true for nerve blocks and all other forms of anesthesia. Unfortunate sequelae of nerve blocks are identified characteristically with damage to the nerve itself, with subsequent palsies, and with pain problems. Of course, nerve blocks can produce damage to other structures both adjacent to and remote from the nerve being blocked. Damage can be caused by the needle or the injected drug; either local toxicity or systemic central nervous effects may be produced by the drug itself. Because Chapters 4 and 5 have dealt with systemic effects of local anesthetics and with the complications of spinal and epidural anesthesia, this chapter will concern itself primarily with the complications arising from peripheral nerve blocks.

BASIC CONSIDERATIONS OF NERVE BLOCKS

A knowledge of anatomy is a prerequisite for successful performance of regional anesthesia and will also help in the anticipation, interpretation, and therefore the prevention or correction of possible complications from any block. To perform nerve blocks without knowing anatomy is like "sailing the uncharted sea." Placing reliance on surface landmarks learned by rote is not only accompanied by a high incidence of failure (as high as 80% in one series[2]) but is associated with an inability to recognize the potential for involving adjacent structures other than the intended nerve. For those inexperienced in applied anatomy, frequent recourse to standard regional anesthesia texts is necessary. In the following discussion, pertinent anatomical comments are made as they relate to the individual blocks.

Knowledge of the pharmacology of local anesthetics is also essential, especially with regard to both systemic and local toxicity. Systemic toxic responses can be minimized by the prophylactic administration of diazepam prior to performing the block.[3] This raises the convulsive threshold, and, if patient cooperation and alertness are not a priority, diazepam is a useful premedicant. Similarly, because the concentration of the drug injected appears to be related to the incidence of neuritis, some authorities limit the concentration of local anesthetic applied to peripheral nerves.[4,5] For example, with lidocaine, a maximum concentration of 1 per cent is used.

Along with the knowledge of anatomy and pharmacology, it is important to employ the proper technique and to use good equipment.

Techniques of Performing Nerve Blocks

The position of the needle during the block is significant. A more efficient block is produced if the small muscles of the hand are used to hold the needle as one would hold a pen; the anesthesiologist should employ delicate movements of the fingers and wrist, instead of "locking" the needle in the hand and moving it by motion at the elbow and shoulder joints. These joints are considerably less sensitive, because there is much less cortical representation than in the small muscles of the hand.

Needle position may be determined in different ways. In some instances, the needle point is positioned adjacent to a bony landmark, such as a vertebral transverse process in a patient undergoing a stellate ganglion block. On another occasion, it may be positioned by detecting a loss of resistance, such as by "popping" the needle through fascial planes (e.g., in the posterior triangle of the neck or in the axillary sheath for brachial plexus block). Frequently, a paresthesia is elicited when the needle actually touches the nerve, and the patient experiences sensations in the dermatomic distribution of that nerve; nerve blocks can also be produced using radiographic control or a nerve stimulator. Sometimes a combination of these methods is used to place the needle accurately.

Once a quantity of local anesthetic has been injected at the intended site, it is then dangerous to "hunt" for additional sites of paresthesia in an area that might already be partially anesthetized; inadvertently, the nerve may be traumatized repeatedly.

Blocks are always performed with resuscitative equipment immediately at hand: an oxygen source, a means of administering positive pressure ventilation, an established intravenous route for resuscitative fluids and drugs, and an assistant to help or summon aid should extra hands be needed. The postoperative recovery room is usually the optimal location in which to perform these blocks.

Equipment for Performing Nerve Blocks

In regional anesthesia, equipment of good quality will repay its investment. Attempting some of the more technically difficult blocks with poor quality, disposable syringes and needles only decreases the chances of success and probably increases the risk of complications. Stainless steel needles with shallow bevels reduce the incidence of trauma to the nerves, because they tend to displace the nerve rather than to cut through it, which may occur with very sharp disposable needles.

In order to reduce the possibility of nerve damage even further, the author believes it is a distinct advantage to use a nerve stimulator attached to the needle. With this device, one may visualize the myotomal distribution of the nerve being stimulated. It is then not necessary to rely entirely upon patient cooperation for the description of paresthesias, and therefore the patient may be sedated more adequately. Nerve stimulation just prior to contact with the needle point should reduce the incidence of nerve trauma from needles and also improve the success rate of the block.[6]

A freely sliding glass "control" syringe allows the anesthesiologist to work with much greater dexterity during the injection of the anesthetic and especially during aspiration for cerebrospinal fluid and blood. Because of the possibility (albeit remote) of needle breakage during the performance of nerve blocks and the sometimes great difficulty that results in recovering the embedded portion, needles with security beads should be used. Such beads permit ready recovery if the needle separates from the hub. The use of a marker is advised for those blocks in which depth of needle insertion is critical. The marker can then be set on the needle at the appropriate distance. Although special markers are available, the rubber stopper from the local anesthetic bottle is one that is usually at hand, and it serves admirably.

GENERAL COMPLICATIONS OF NERVE BLOCKS

Inadequate Anesthesia

With diagnostic blocks, there is usually no problem in repeating the block until the desired effect is achieved. Actually, in diagnostic work the failed block can always be used as a placebo as part of a diagnostic series of blocks!

Extensive Anesthesia

The treatment of total spinal and high epidural blocks is considered in Chapter 5 and will not be discussed here, other than to reemphasize the necessity for alert diagnosis and prompt treatment of such complications to avert what is potentially a fatal complication.

Any block performed near the neuraxis (e.g., paravertebral or stellate ganglion blocks) can involve spread of the anesthetic into either the epidural or even subarachnoid compartment. At worst, such spread may lead to total spinal anesthesia. To a vigilant anesthesiologist who is used to caring for patients with epidural and spinal anesthesia, these complications, though serious, do not necessarily pose any great difficulty.

If, of course, the specific block was intended as a diagnostic maneuver, its spread to other neurological components invalidates its diagnostic value, and the procedure must be repeated. The continuity of the paravertebral space permits free flow of local anesthetic between adjacent segmental nerves. This is seen particularly in the cervical and thoracic areas, where injection at one paravertebral site will often result in anesthesia extending over several dermatomes if large volumes are used. (An alternative explanation is, of course, peridural spread.) When used for surgical purposes, this involvement of adjacent dermatomes (e.g., spread to the cervical plexus during interscalene brachial plexus block) is usually of no great importance. However, when attempting segmental paravertebral diagnostic blocks, such spread can invalidate the diagnostic value of the procedure. In this case, therefore, very small amounts of drug (1–2 ml.), with accurate placement on the desired segmental nerve, are necessary.

Prolonged Block

The treatment of prolonged block usually consists of observation until sensation returns. It is important during the long block to ensure that the anesthetized area is protected with slings, splints, and padding to prevent trauma to the insensitive part by pressure, heat, or other stimuli. With undue prolongation of block, the advice and assistance of colleagues in other specialities, such as neurology and physical medicine, can often be of a great help in both documenting the extent of the block and in following its temporal progress by means of electromyography.[7,8] No instance of irreversible block with the long-acting agents such as bupivacaine and etidocaine has been reported, although the duration of action of these agents can vary considerably, even lasting as long as 20 hours.[9] The author recalls a 0.5-per cent bupivacaine axillary block used for hand surgery; when the patient required re-operation the next day, the anesthetic was still effective, and the patient was able to undergo two operations with the same anesthetic 24 hours apart!

LOCAL COMPLICATIONS OF NERVE BLOCK

Local Tissue Toxicity of the Anesthetic Agent

When used in conventional clinical concentrations, local anesthetics have not been shown to produce any localized nerve damage. In the experimental laboratory, it is necessary to use concentrations of local anesthetics far in excess of those used clinically to produce irreversible nerve block.[10] When chemical preservatives were used in spinal anesthetic solutions, studies were unable to demonstrate any toxic effect of these additives.[11] Local anesthetic agents can cause histological alterations in muscle, although this appears to be reversible, and recovery is complete within a matter of weeks.[12]

Local Tissue Toxicity of Epinephrine

The addition of epinephrine to local anesthetic solutions is frequently employed for both prolongation of the block and beta-adrenergic stimulation of the cardiovascular system. Provided a solution of appropriate strength is used (1:200,000 appears optimal[5]), the addition of epinephrine does not appear to be associated with any undue complications. In fact, in more than 28,000 blocks, there appeared to be no toxic effects associated with the addition of epinephrine.[13] However, most investigators advise against using epinephrine in digital blocks because of the possible ischemic sequelae, such as gangrene;[4] similar precautions also pertain to ring blocks of the penis.

Infection

Although infection has occurred subsequent to nerve block occasionally with disastrous results,[14,15] it is rarely seen if correct techniques of sterilization and asepsis are followed. One explanation for this infrequent occurrence is that local anesthetics appear to have antimicrobial activity, inhibiting the growth of pathogenic bacteria and some fungal organisms. Gram-negative bacteria are especially sensitive to these agents, as is the tubercle bacillus. Both lidocaine and procaine appear to interfere with protein production in the cell wall or cytoplasmic membrane of these organisms.[16] Rare severe infections have been reported and attributed to sequelae of peripheral nerve blocks. Pudendal block at the time of delivery has been implicated in infection with bowel organisms, especially *Escherichia coli* in deep structures; this organism produces dramatic and occasionally fatal infection in the sub-gluteal, retropsoal, and retroperitoneal areas, along with peritonitis.[14]

DIFFERENTIAL DIAGNOSIS OF NERVE DAMAGE (NEURITIS)

Nerve damage can be caused by factors other than the regional anesthetic technique (see Chap. 51.[17,18,19] Brachial plexus damage can occur as a result of either stretching or compression. Pressure on or trauma to many nerves in the body has been described during positioning. For example, the lateral popliteal nerve may be compressed between the head of the fibula and the lithotomy stirrups, resulting in a footdrop. If this occurs in a patient who has undergone regional anesthesia, it is quite likely that the footdrop may be attributed to the nerve block, unless the specific risk of pressure against the lithotomy stirrup had been considered. Similarly, if the leg is suspended lateral to the stirrup, the saphenous nerve can be damaged, resulting in sensory loss along the medial aspect of the calf and dorsum of the foot. The sciatic nerve can also be traumatized by intramuscular injections into the buttock either pre- or postoperatively; and, in thin emaciated patients lying on hard tables during hip-pinning operations, paralysis of all muscles below the knee, along with the hamstrings, may occur. The pudendal nerve is vulnerable in orthopedic operations involving a traction post, in which the nerve lying in Alcock's canal is compressed against the ischial tuberosity. The femoral nerve can be damaged by use of a self-retaining retractor during lower abdominal explorations. Nerve damage can follow the use of a tourniquet.[20]

It is very important to exclude the above causes before ascribing untoward sequelae to the anesthetic technique. Similarly, it is important to ascertain whether complications are dermatomic and therefore segmental, or peripheral in distribution, since this permits a diagnostic impression of the origin of the defect.

COMPLICATIONS RESULTING FROM INSERTION OF THE NEEDLE

Nerve Injury

Paresthesias are often elicited to locate a nerve before injecting the anesthetic agent. However, contact between a needle and nerve risks nerve injury. Following supraclavicular and axillary block techniques in which paresthesias are sought, the incidence of neurologic sequelae ranges from 0 to slightly over 5 per cent. These sequelae vary from mild paresthesias to severe sensory disturbances, pain, and paralysis, lasting from a few days to over 1 year.[20a, 20b] That transient nerve injury is related, at least in part, to needle trauma is suggested by a recent study that noted an incidence of 2.8 per cent when paresthesias were actively sought compared to 0.8 per cent when the axillary artery was used in axillary block.[20b] In addition, nerve injury occurs less frequently with short-beveled needles.[20a] When necessary, paresthesias should be elicited gently to minimize injury.

Pneumothorax

Pneumothorax is a risk associated with any block that involves insertion of a needle in the region of the thoracic cage.[4] The incidence varies indirectly with the experience of the anesthesiologist. Thoracic paravertebral blocks, somatic and especially sympathetic, are associated with the highest incidence of pneumothorax, 4 to 8 per cent, even in expert hands.[4] With a brachial plexus block, it occurs most frequently when the classical supraclavicular approach is used. In expert hands, the incidence of pneumothorax in such cases is about 1 per cent.[4,5] The incidence is probably lower with intercostal and stellate ganglion blocks, especially when the latter is performed from the anterior rather than posterior approach.[4] Yet, pneumothorax probably occurs more often than clinically suspected. For example, de Jong noted its presence on routine radiograph following supraclavicular brachial plexus block in 25 per cent of patients.[21]

The treatment of pneumothorax has been well established.[4] If the collapse is less than 20 per cent, symptomatic therapy and observation are usually all that is required until spontaneous recovery occurs. Above 25 per cent, closer observation is required, and preparations must be made to proceed with more active therapy should the lung fail to reexpand in the first 24 hours. Such therapy involves active decompression, usually by way of the second intercostal space in the midclavicular line with an underwater seal. However, not all chest pain that follows nerve blocks is caused by pneumothorax, and careful physical examination and chest radiograph are, of course, mandatory prior to diagnosis.

Prevention of pneumothorax during regional anesthesia is best achieved by meticulous adherence to technique and cooperation of the patient, who avoids sudden movements in response to the discomfort and paresthesia. If the anesthesiologist suspects that the needle has broached the integrity of the pleura and/or lung, it is advisable to have the patient remain at quiet bedrest for the next 12 to 24 hours. There can be a latent period between needle insertion into the pleura and the development of pneumothorax, which may conceivably be precipitated by exertion.[4] In those patients who require chest tubes, further observation in a hospital is necessary once the chest tube is withdrawn, because re-collapse can occur, necessitating reinsertion of the drainage catheter (see Chap. 12).

Bleeding Following Nerve Block

Bleeding can occur any time a blood vessel is damaged during needle insertion and is usually of greater significance within, rather than outside the neuraxis. Of course, it is a greater risk in patients who are taking anticoagulants. Permanent nerve damage has been attributed to the effect of hematoma on the brachial plexus nerves[22] and the spinal cord. To prevent this, nerve blocks should be avoided in patients with bleeding disorders and in patients taking anticoagulants, especially if the coagulation studies are abnormal.

COMPLICATIONS OF SPECIFIC NERVE BLOCKS

NERVE BLOCKS OF THE HEAD AND NECK

Prior to the advent of routine endotracheal anesthesia, much head and neck surgery was performed under regional anesthesia, as perusal of old anesthesia textbooks will confirm. With the use of oral or nasal tracheal intubation, the need for specific blocks about the head and neck diminished, as did routine use for surgical practice. However, there are still many occasions when optimal anesthesia is achieved by utilizing some of these blocks, either alone or in conjunction with general anesthesia. These blocks are especially useful in the diagnostic and therapeutic management of painful conditions.

With their compact and complicated anatomy, the head and neck pose a challenge to the regional anesthetist. Meticulous placement of needle and small doses of local anesthetic are required for accurate and discrete results. However, landmarks in this region tend to be constant and predictably located; for the practitioner who acquires the requisite skills, it can be a most useful and satisfactory method, for surgical anesthesia and especially for diagnostic anesthesia.

Trigeminal Nerve Block

Gasserian ganglion block is performed less frequently now that thermal gangliolysis is used to treat tic douloureux.[23] The complications of gasserian block stem primarily from the entrance of the needle and subsequent injection of drug into the subarachnoid space by way of the invagination of dura that surrounds the gasserian ganglion (Meckel's cavity). A very small quantity of local anesthetic injected into this space can produce quite profound anesthesia of the ipsilateral cranial nerves. For example, a patient in our clinic was given a test injection of 0.25 ml. of 1 per cent lidocaine, which produced anesthesia of all the ipsilateral cranial nerves and was associated with brief loss of consciousness. Thus, it is of paramount importance to be certain that there is no backflow of cerebrospinal fluid prior to injecting local anesthetics, especially neurolytic agents. Ideally, this block is performed under radiographic control, because advancement of the needle too far can result in damage to intracranial structures, particularly the cavernous sinus and its contents (cranial nerves II, VI) and the brain itself. Also, if the needle is directed too far posteriorly and misses the foramen ovale, it may enter the middle meningeal artery at the foramen spinosum or even the carotid artery itself in the foramen lacerum. To prevent the needle from entering the oral cavity en route, a finger is placed in the mouth during insertion to guide its path.

Mandibular Nerve Block

In "walking" the needle posteriorly off the lateral pterygoid plate to block the mandibular nerve, it is possible to miss the nerve completely and to enter the pharynx. Upon injection into the pharnyx, the patient complains of a bitter taste in the mouth and may even spit the local anesthetic out! Although injecting into the pharynx is of no great consequence, the needle has now been inserted into an infected area, and withdrawal through the infratemporal fossa may lead to infection. However, in dentistry numerous intraoral injections are made into branches of the cranial nerves by way of the oral cavity without a high morbidity.

Maxillary Nerve Block

The approach to the maxillary nerve block traverses the infratemporal fossa, by passing the needle through the coronoid notch of or anterior to the anterior ramus of the mandible. The object is to place the needle in the pterygopalatine fossa. The complications here are primarily those of damage to or injection into the very rich vascular plexus of both arteries and veins lying in this fossa, containing the five terminal branches of the maxillary artery and the veins draining the orbit by way of the inferior orbital fissure. Therefore, hematoma is not uncommon after this particular block, and because of the venous communications through the inferior orbital fissure with this fossa, fairly extensive orbital hematoma (black eye!) can be produced. It might also be possible to advance the needle through the inferior orbital fissure into the back of the orbit and produce local tissue damage. Therefore, depth of needle insertion is important, and a marker should be used. This is less likely to happen with an approach from the coronoid notch with the jaw closed, since then the line of the needle impinges upon the back of the maxilla. The higher elevation necessary to enter the orbit by way of the inferior orbital fissure is then unlikely to occur.

The maxillary nerve can also be approached along the inferolateral aspect of the floor of the orbit.[24] Here, there is danger of damage to orbital contents if strict adherence to instruction is not followed.

Frontal Nerve Block

Nerve blocks of the supratrochlear and supraorbital branches of the first division of the trigeminal nerve are best performed at or above the eyebrow. Attempts to block the nerve from within the orbit below the eyebrow are likely to produce a black eye because of injury to the loose vascular connective tissue in the orbit, which permits excess spread of hematoma should a blood vessel be punctured.

Facial Nerve Block

Block of the facial nerve results in ipsilateral facial weakness and occurs occasionally as a complication during the performance of both mandibular and maxillary nerve blocks by the extraoral route. It is caused by infiltration of the superficial and deep subcutaneous tissues over the ramus of the mandible, which produces anesthesia of the pes anserinus, those branches of the facial nerve that are lying in the parotid gland. Block of the facial nerve can also occur as a complication of glossopharyngeal block performed at the styloid process, where the facial nerve trunk can be involved as it emerges from the stylomastoid foramen.

Glossopharyngeal Nerve Block

The glossopharyngeal nerve may be blocked from an intraoral or extraoral approach.[24,25] With regard to the latter, the usual route is by way of a site halfway between the angle of the mandible and the mastoid process, using the styloid process as an end point. Invariably, block of the glossopharyngeal nerve produces a block of cranial nerves X and XI also, resulting in weakness of the trapezius and the sternomastoid muscles, as well as hoarseness on occasion. The glossopharyngeal block itself will interfere with gag reflex on the ipsilateral side. Of course, the proximity of the carotid arterial system and internal jugular vein calls for mandatory aspiration tests.

A recently reported series of glossopharyngeal nerve blocks from within the oral cavity reported very few complications and a high success rate.[25]

Vagus Nerve Block

The main trunk of the vagus nerve is rarely, if ever, blocked as a primary therapeutic maneuver. But the branches to the larynx are often blocked when attempting intubation without the use of muscle relaxants or deep general anesthesia. To render the laryngeal inlet analgesic, the superior laryngeal nerves (primarily the internal branches) are blocked as they pass beneath the greater cornu of the hyoid. This is a relatively simple block with a low morbidity, restricted to damage at the point of needle insertion. The recurrent laryngeal nerves are rarely blocked, except as a complication of stellate ganglion block. However, their distribution is blocked with a transtracheal spray of the region in which the needle is inserted, between the thyroid and cricoid cartilages in the sagittal plane. This is an effective means of anesthetizing this area with low morbidity.

Phrenic Nerve Block

The phrenic nerves are seldom the primary target for regional anesthesia, although attempts are occasionally made to block them to abort persistent attacks of singultus (hiccups). The phrenic nerve is adherent to the anterior surface of the anterior scalene muscle. Thus, it is probably blocked more often than we realize as a complication of other local anesthetic procedures in and around the base of the neck, particularly deep cervical plexus, interscalene, and stellate ganglion blocks. For example, during interscalene block, the nerve may be anesthetized either by direct involvement or by the paravertebral spread of the anesthetic to the cervical plexus that invariably accompanies this procedure.

Investigators have speculated on the inadvisability of performing bilateral interscalene blocks because of the possible risk of bilateral phrenic nerve block and, hence, of possible respiratory embarrassment.[26] However, unless the patient's respiratory function is severely compromised, blocking one and maybe even two phrenic nerves is unlikely to produce any detectable effects and probably can only be demonstrated by fluoroscopy. The phrenic nerve supplies only the central part of the diaphragm; the remainder is supplied by intercostal nerves. For the otherwise healthy patient at rest, phrenic nerve block appears to pose no respiratory embarrassment. In the respiratory cripple, however, it is conceivable that phrenic nerve block may be followed by respiratory embarrassment.

CERVICOTHORACIC SYMPATHETIC BLOCK

For the diagnosis and therapy of upper extremity pain, it is often necessary to perform a stellate ganglion block. *Stellate ganglion* is the name given to that group of autonomic fibers believed to be the confluence of the upper thoracic and inferior cervical ganglion on the sympathetic chain. Through this ganglion pass most, though not necessarily all, of the sympathetic efferents to the upper extremity.[27] Many approaches have been described for this block, and Moore has written a whole book on the subject.[28] However, the anterior approach is used most frequently; the local anesthetic is usually deposited at the level of C7 or C6, in the hope that caudal spread of the anesthetic solution in the prevertebral plane will block those fibers passing from the upper thoracic sympathetic chain to the extremity. Depending on the technique chosen, the needle is introduced in the paratracheal region at the base of the neck, either at the level of C7 or C6, and passes in close proximity to several very important structures. The two most serious and not infrequent complications of this technique are inadvertent intravascular injection into a vertebral or even the carotid artery and pneumothorax.

The anterior approach for this block depends, like other blocks, on locating a bony landmark, such as the transverse process of C6 (Chassaignac's tubercle) or C7. Having done so, the needle is withdrawn anteriorly until the point clears the prevertebral muscle mass and, more importantly, the prevertebral fascia. If the needle is advanced in error between the transverse processes into the paravertebral space, such that it locates the posterior tubercle, which may be erroneously interpreted as the anterior tubercle, then withdrawal of the needle can leave the needle point in the lumen of the vertebral artery. The injection of very small quantities of local anesthetic drug into this artery will result in profound effects. The author has had personal experience with three of such cases, in which quantities less than 0.25 ml. of 1-per-cent lidocaine resulted in unconsciousness and gross convulsions. Although an aspiration test should prevent such complications, in the three instances cited, aspiration tests were negative. Therefore, a small test dose, perhaps as little as 0.125 ml., injected slowly, is advisable. The treatment of such convulsions is discussed elsewhere (see Chap. 4) and involves airway support, the administration of oxygen, and the intravenous administration of diazepam or thiopental.

Pneumothorax following stellate ganglion block is due to direct puncture of the parietal pleura of the cupula in the thoracic inlet, and its likelihood varies with the vertical extent of the apical lobe of the lung. Thus, it is more frequent in subjects in whom the apical pleura is higher, such as tall, thin individuals rather than short, fat individuals, in whom the pleura does not reach quite so high. The incidence of pneumothorax is also higher with blocks done at the lower level (C7), compared with blocks performed at C6. The

treatment of pneumothorax is described above and in Chapter 12.

Other less serious complications of stellate ganglion block result from spread to adjacent nerves, the somatic nerves of the brachial plexus, and the recurrent laryngeal nerve. Involvement of the latter is quite common, since it lies in the same fascial compartment, anterior to prevertebral fascia, as the sympathetic chain. However, if the needle is advanced too far posteriorly and not withdrawn to prevertebral fascia, then spread to the nerves of the brachial plexus may well occur; with the volumes usually used (10–15 ml.), this often results in blocks of the cephalic components of the brachial plexus (determatomes and myotomes of C5, C6, and perhaps C7 and C8). With reversible agents, this is usually just a transient problem. However, spread to the recurrent laryngeal nerve is often distressing to the patient, and he should be warned about this possibility prior to the block. It usually results in hoarseness, cough, and a diminution of the voice to a whisper for the duration of the block. Thus, this unilateral cord paralysis and tracheal analgesia are often the most distressing features of a stellate ganglion block to the patient.

Subarachnoid spread due to incorrect needle positioning or by way of dural sleeves is possible, but infrequently encountered; in the event that it occurs, the patient may well need urgent resuscitative and supportive treatment for the resulting total spinal anesthesia (see Chap. 5). Horner's syndrome of ptosis, miosis, enophthalmos, and anhydrosis is not really a complication, but a result of the sympathetic block produced; although occasionally bothersome, it is usually tolerated well by most patients. Thoracic duct trauma has also been reported with this block.[5]

NERVE BLOCKS OF THE TRUNK

Lumbar Sympathetic Block

Lumbar sympathetic block is frequently performed for diagnosis and treatment of reflex sympathetic dystrophy; it has also been used for intermittent claudication[29] and relief of pain in the first stage of labor. The lumbar sympathetic chain is situated on the anterolateral border of the lumbar vertebrae. Invariably it is approached posteriorly. In the preferred approach, a needle is inserted 10 cm. from the midline, usually at the level of L2 or L3, advanced at a 45-degree angle, and "walked" along the vertebral body until it just slips off, at which time it should be adjacent to the lumbar sympathetic chain.[30,31] It will then have advanced beyond the psoas sheath, and therefore injected local anesthetic will be distributed in that retroperitoneal fascial plane, wherein lies the lumbar sympathetic chain. If the needle is not advanced far enough anteriorly, then the injected drug will be confined within the limits of the psoas sheath, involving the lumbar plexus as it is formed within the psoas muscle and producing a somatic rather than a sympathetic block. Even if the needle is correctly placed, it is still possible for the drug to diffuse back between the origins of the psoas major muscle, following the path of the lumbar arteries into the paravertebral space, and thence to the paravertebral nerves, especially if the patient is turned supine.[32] If the needle is advanced too far anteriorly, it may enter either the aorta or the inferior vena cava from the left or right side, respectively, or their tributaries. Another complication of the more lateral approach is puncture of the lower pole of the kidney. The author has demonstrated this in two of six cadavers tested with the needle at the level of L2, but not at L3. There is no mention in the literature of the clinical significance of this, but probably it is advisable to insert the needle at L3.

The lateral approach is more comfortable for the patient; pain is encountered at the skin, the lumbar fascia, and the periosteum of the vertebral body. With the classic paravertebral approach, in addition to these painful sites, the sensitive periosteum of the transverse process is encountered, and frequently paresthesia occurs upon contact with the paravertebral nerve. As with all blocks around the neuraxis, there is the complication of peridural and/or subarachnoid spread.[33] Inadvertently, the needle may be inserted through the paravertebral foramen. This can result from faulty technique or from poor landmarks, as found in an extremely obese patient. Local anesthetic can spread up the perineural sheaths that have been described to accompany the segmental nerves beyond the paravertebral foramina.[34]

Careful aspiration and the use of a test dose should markedly reduce the risk of intravascular and intradural complications. The most frequent complication of lumbar sympathetic block is that of somatic spread. This occurs despite the use of good technique in about 5 to 15 per cent of patients. Depending upon the agent used, the sequelae of somatic spread can have relatively little or no significance. That is, when the block is done for reflex sympathetic dystrophies, the sequela may be just a band of temporary numbness over the L2 and/or L3 dermatomes. However, if the concentration of local anesthetic is sufficient to produce motor blockade, spread can seriously compromise the patient's ability to walk for some time following the block. Therefore, it is advisable to use an agent such as 0.25-per-cent bupivacaine, which will give prolonged sympathetic blockade and, yet, even if it spills over into the lumbar plexus, will produce only somatic analgesia and not motor block. To prevent this spread to somatic nerves, the anesthesiologist must abstain from infiltrating the whole track with local anesthetic; instead, he should raise a skin wheal and perhaps a small amount (1–2 ml.) of local anesthetic at the sensitive lumbar fascia. Excessive infiltration, including the intrapsoas path of the needle, may well result in anesthetizing components of the lumbar plexus and produce weakness of hip flexion. Theoretically, complications may arise from a position of the needle point that is too anterior, resulting in the injection of drugs into the peritoneal cavity and/or viscera. However, the author is unaware of such an occurrence. Retroperitoneal hemorrhage may also occur.[35]

Thoracic Paravertebral Block

Both somatic and sympathetic paravertebral nerve blocks performed in the thoracic region are associated with a higher risk of pneumothorax than are other blocks performed in this region, such as brachial plexus and intercostal blocks. This is probably because of the increased depth of needle insertion, which leads to some degree of loss of control, and because of the proximity of pleura to the target nerves. As with other paravertebral blocks, there is also the risk of peridural and/or subarachnoid spread resulting from misplaced needles or spread of anesthetic by way of dural sheaths that accompany the nerves.

Celiac Plexus Block

The celiac plexus block, in combination with intercostal blockade, is used with success by skilled enthusiasts as a form of anesthesia for surgical patients. However, it is more frequently employed as a diagnostic maneuver when attempting to clarify causes of obscure abdominal pain. It is often used successfully in patients whose source of pain is an intra-abdominal malignancy. Because blockade of the celiac plexus leads to sympathetic denervation of a large area of the splanchnic bed, the patient's ability to maintain an adequate blood pressure is compromised, and postural hypotension is a frequent complication.

Another possible complication is the puncture of large vessels, such as the aorta or inferior vena cava. This complication occurs occasionally, and although it could lead to a retroperitoneal hematoma, this does not appear to be a frequent problem. Unless meticulous attention to needle direction is maintained, it is also possible to produce a pneumothorax.

INTRAVENOUS REGIONAL BLOCK

There appear to be very few complications of an intravenous regional block. This attests to its safety. In a series of 100 subjects, Kew and Lowe detected sinus bradycardia upon release of the tourniquet in 65 per cent, but with most of these, bradycardia was limited to a reduction of less than 10 beats per minute.[36] One patient had an asystole lasting 3 seconds, but no S-T depression was noted. In another series of 967 patients by Thorn-Alquist, only one patient required any resuscitative measure.[37] Prilocaine was used and some transient falls in blood pressure were noted in 10 patients after the release of the cuff. In one series of 77 patients, seven patients were noted to have arrhythmias, with one patient suffering an asystole requiring external cardiac massage following release of the tourniquet.[38] The cardiovascular complications appear to be self-limiting in most of these studies, and if it were not for close monitoring of the ECG, they would probably have gone undetected. Provided an adequate, intact tourniquet system can be assured, this form of regional anesthesia is surprisingly free from complications. Thrombophlebitis has been reported with use of chloroprocaine in this technique, but not with other agents.[39]

EPIDURAL AND SPINAL ADMINISTRATION OF NARCOTICS

Very recently, several investigators have shown that prolonged, unusually intense, segmental analgesia results from the epidural or subarachnoid administration of very small doses of narcotics (e.g., morphine 1 mg.). The site of action is believed to be the opiate receptors in the central nervous system demonstrated only a few years earlier.[40] Profound analgesia has been produced in patients having obstetric labor, and acute postoperative and chronic pain, without the autonomic or respiratory depression customary with regional analgesia (see pp. 80–84) or parenteral narcotics. However, several patients have experienced hypotension and respiratory depression or arrest 6 to 12 hours following the narcotic administration.[41-44] Curiously, naloxone immediately counteracted the adverse responses without affecting the analgesia. The delayed onset of respiratory and cardiovascular depression may reflect the diffusion of the narcotic in the cerebrospinal fluid from the site of injection, usually the lumbar area, to the fourth ventricle, where the respiratory and vasomotor nuclei are located.[42]

REFERENCES

1. Murphy, E.: "Murphy's Law," *Quoted In* Frank, E., Winelhake, W., Van deStadt, J., et al.: Formulations of natural law. Journal of Irreproducible Results, *21*:4, 1974.
2. Brechner, T., and Brechner, V.: Accuracy of needle placement during diagnostic and therapeutic nerve block. *In* Advances in Pain Research and Therapy I. pp. 679–683. New York, Raven Press, 1976.
3. de Jong, R. H., and Heavner, J. E.: Diazepam prevents local anesthetic seizures. Anesthesiology, *34*:523, 1971.
4. Moore, D. C.: Complications of regional anesthesia. Clin. Anesth., 7:217, 1969.
5. Bonica, J. J.: The Management of Pain, Philadelphia, Lea & Febiger, 1953.
6. Magora, F.: Obturator nerve block: evaluation of technique. Br. J. Anaesth., *41*:695, 1969.
7. Jebsen, R. H.: Electrodiagnosis in the nerve root syndrome. N. Z. Med. J., *65*:107, 1966.
8. Lofstrom, B., Wennberg, A, and Widen, L.: Late disturbances in nerve function after block with local anesthet-

ics: an electroneurographic study. Acta Anaesthesiol. Scand., 10:111, 1966.

9. Bromage, P. R., O'Brien, P., and Dunford, L. A.: Etidocaine: a clinical evaluation for regional analgesia in surgery. Can. Anaesth. Soc. J., 21:523, 1974.

10. Skou, J. C.: Toxicity of local anesthetics. Acta Pharmacol. Toxicol., 10:292, 1954.

11. McDonald, A. D., and Watkins, K. H.: An experimental investigation into the cause of paralysis following spinal anaesthesia. Br. J. Surg., 25:879, 1938.

12. Benoit, P. W., and Belt, W. D.: Destruction and regeneration of skeletal muscle after treatment with a local anesthetic, bupivacaine (Marcaine). J. Anat., 107:547, 1970.

13. Dhuner, K. G.: Frequency of general side reactions after regional anaesthesia with mepivacaine with and without vasoconstrictors. Acta Anaesthesiol. Scand., 48[Suppl.]:23, 1972.

14. Hibbard, L. T., Snyder, E. N., and McVann, R. M.: Subgluteal and retropsoal infection in obstetric practice. Obstet. Gynecol., 39:137, 1972.

15. Wenger, D. R., and Gitchell, R. G.: Severe infections following pudendal block in anesthesia: need for orthopaedic awareness. J. Bone Joint Surg., 55A:202, 1973.

16. Schmidt, R. M., and Rosenkranz, H. S.: Anti-microbial activity of local anesthetics: lidocaine and procaine. J. Infect. Dis. 121:597, 1970.

17. Atkinson, R. S., Rushman, G. B., Lee, J. A.: A Synopsis of Anaesthesia. ed. 8. pp. 828–831. Bristol, John Wright & Sons, 1977.

18. Lincoln, J. R., and Sawyer, H. P.: Complications related to body positions during surgical procedures. Anesthesiology, 22:800, 1961.

19. Britt, B. A., and Gordon, R. A.: Peripheral nerve injuries associated with anesthesia. Can. Anaesth. Soc. J., 11:514, 1964.

20. Moldaver, J.: Tourniquet paralysis syndrome. Arch. Surg., 68:136, 1954.

20a. Selander, D., Dhuner, K-G, and Lundborg, G.: Peripheral nerve injury due to injection needles used for regional anesthesia. An experimental study of the acute effects of needle point trauma. Acta Anaesth. Scand., 21:182, 1977.

20b. Selander, D., Edshage, S., and Wolff, T.: Paresthesiae or no paresthesiae? Nerve lesions after axillary blocks. Acta Anaesth. Scand., 23:27, 1979.

21. de Jong, R. H.: Axillary block of brachial plexus. Anesthesiology, 22:215, 1961.

22. Wooley, E. J., and Vandam, L. D.: Neurological sequelae of brachial plexus nerve block. Ann. Surg., 149:53, 1959.

23. Sweet, W. T., and Wepsic, J. G.: Controlled thermocoagulation of trigeminal ganglion and rootlets for differential destruction of pain fibres, Part I: Trigeminal neuralgia. J. Neurosurg., 39:143, 1974.

24. Adriani, J.: Labat's Regional Anesthesia: Techniques and Clinical Applications. ed. 3. Philadelphia, Saunders, 1967.

25. DeMeester, T. R.: Glossopharyngeal nerve block for endoscopy. Clinical Trends in Anesthesiology, 6:2, 1976.

26. Kumar, A., Battit, G. E., Froese, A. D., et al.: Bilateral cervical and thoracic epidural blockade complicating interscalene block: reports of two cases. Anesthesiology, 35:650, 1971.

27. Kuntz A: Autonomic Nervous System. ed 3. Philadelphia, Lea & Feiger, 1945.

28. Moore, D. C.: Stellate Ganglion Blocks. Springfield, Charles C Thomas, 1954.

29. Boas, R. A., Hatangdi, V.S., and Richards, E. G.: Lumbar sympathectomy percutaneous chemical technique. In Advances in Pain Research and Therapy I, pp. 685–689. New York, Raven Press, 1976.

30. Parks, F. W., and Chalmers, J. A.: Paravertebral sympathetic block in treatment of superficial and deep thrombosis of leg veins. J. Obstet. Gynaecol. Br. Commonw., 64:419, 1957.

31. Reid, W., Watt, J. K., and Gray, T. C.: Phenol injection of the sympathetic chain. Br. J. Surg., 57:45, 1970.

32. Bryce-Smith, R.: Injection of the lumbar sympathetic chain. Anaesthesia, 6:150, 1951.

33. Evans, J. A., Dobben, G. D., and Gay, G. R.: Peridural infusion of drugs in sympathetic blockade. J.A.M.A., 200:573, 1967.

34. Gay, G. R., Evans, J. A.: Total spinal anesthesia following lumbar paravertebral block: a potentially lethal complication. Anesth. Analg., 50:344, 1971.

35. Learned, L. O., and Calhoun, R. F.: Retroperitoneal hemorrhage as a complication of lumbar paravertebral injections: report of three cases. Anesthesiology 12:391, 1951.

36. Kew, M. C., and Lowe, J. P.: The cardiovascular complications of intravenous regional anaesthesia. Br. J. Surg., 58:179, 1971.

37. Thorn-Alquist, A. M.: Intravenous regional anaesthesia. A seven year survey. Acta Anaesthesiol. Scand., 15:23, 1971.

38. Kennedy, B. R., Duthie, A. M., Parbrooke, G. D.: Intravenous regional aneasthesia. Br. Med. J., 1:954, 1965.

39. Harris, W. H., Slater, M., and Bell, H. M.: Regional anesthesia by the intravenous route. J.A.M.A., 194:1273, 1965.

40. Stoelting, R. K.: Opiate receptors and endorphins: Their role in anesthesiology. Anesth. Analg., 59:874, 1980.

41. Scott, D. B., and McClure, J.: Selective epidural analgesia. Lancet, 1:1410, 1979.

42. Glynn, C. J., Matter, L. E., Cousins, M. J., et. al.: Spinal narcotics and respiratory depression. Lancet, 2:356, 1979.

43. Liolios, A., and Anderson, F. H.: Selective spinal analgesia. Lancet, 2:357, 1979.

44. Davies, G. K., Tolhurst-Cleaver, C. L., and James, T. L.: CNS depression from intrathecal morphine. Anesthesiology, 52:280, 1980.

FURTHER READING

Covino, B. G., and Vassallo, H. G.: Local Anesthetics: Mechanisms of Action and Clinical Use. New York, Grune and Stratton, 1976.

de Jong, R. H.: Local Anesthesia. ed 2. Springfield, Charles C Thomas, 1977.

Moore, D. C.: Complications of Regional Anesthesia. Springfield, Charles C Thomas, 1955.

Swerdlow, M.: Complications of local anesthetic neural blockade. In Cousins, M. J., and Bridenbaugh, P. O. (eds.): Neural Blockade in Clinical Anesthesia & Management of Pain. pp. 526–542. Philadelphia, J. B. Lippincott Company, 1980.

7 Complications of Neurolytic Blocks

Terence M. Murphy, M.B., Ch.B., F.F.A.R.C.S.

Neurolytic blocks are used primarily for the treatment of pain in cancer patients and also for the relief of persistent spasticity in patients with spinal cord injuries or progressive neurological diseases, such as multiple sclerosis. The main hazard of using these agents is possible spread to other adjacent and vital structures; this leads to a complication rate of approximately 10 per cent in the immediate post-block period, but recovery usually occurs, and the long-term complication rate is lower.

The incidence of complications has been reported by several investigators. Swerdlow describes a complication rate of 50 per cent, but this includes use of chlorocresol, a particularly toxic agent.[1] Using phenol for intrathecal block, Nathan described a 10-percent-cent incidence of complications.[2] Kuzucu, in a large series of 300 neurolytic subarachnoid blocks using alcohol, described a 7-per-cent incidence of complications in the immediate post-block period, but a long-term incidence of only 1 per cent.[3] In a series of 1000 patients receiving phenol lumbar sympathetic blocks, the most common complication was neuritis, which occurred in approximately 10 per cent of patients, but was usually mild, responded well to simple analgesics, and was self-limiting, lasting only a few weeks.[4]

Complications arise because it is not possible to guarantee that the agent, when it is injected by a percutaneous needle technique, will be deposited at and only produce an effect upon the intend-ed target. Even in experienced hands and with meticulous attention to technique, tissues other than the intended target will sometimes be involved.

NEUROLYTIC AGENTS AND OTHER TECHNIQUES USED IN NEUROLYTIC BLOCK

Alcohol

Absolute alcohol is used to effect somatic nerve block, either peripherally or within the subarachnoid space. For sympathetic blockade, 50-per-cent alcohol suffices.

Alcohol is very irritating to tissues and therefore very painful on injection. However, this discomfort is short-lived, as analgesia rapidly follows the burning sensation, and the temporary discomfort is usually tolerated well by most patients. Supplemental analgesia can reduce this discomfort upon injection but is not advisable, because it is important to have patient response to follow more closely the extent of analgesia. Analgesia lasts up to several months, and when pain returns, injection can be repeated. In contrast to phenol, the effect of alcohol is immediate, and thus any deficiencies noted in the extent of the blockade at the time of the procedure can be rectified promptly. When injected into the subarachnoid space, neurolytic concentrations tend to be limited to the site of injection.[5] If an extensive block is required, it is usually advisable to extend the block by using further injections at different levels, rather than attempting to inject larger volumes at one site. Being lighter than cerebrospinal fluid, alcohol floats to form a layer on the surface. Thus, during subarachnoid alcohol blocks it is important to ensure that the desired nerve is uppermost. If it is accidentally injected intravascularly, it is rapidly diluted, with little or no undesirable effects.

Phenol

Phenol is used for both peripheral somatic and subarachnoid nerve blocks, as well as sympathetic blocks. Concentrations from 1 to 10 per cent have been recommended. Usually, at least 5-per-cent phenol is needed, and often 10 per cent is necessary. When used in the subarachnoid space, phenol is usually mixed with glycerine, which effects a hyperbaric solution but delays its release into the tissues. As a result, the final extent of the block is often not evident until the following day. What may appear to be an adequate block at the time of the procedure usually diminishes significantly by the next day. Diminution occurs because phenol probably has a dual effect, acting both as a local anesthetic in weaker concentrations at the periphery of the injected bolus and as a neurolytic agent in stronger concentrations at the injection site.[6] Therefore, it is usually advisable, to produce a more extensive block than is required. Phenol is less predictable than alcohol; however, it is usually less irritating to the tissues and is better tolerated by patients. Like other neurolytic agents, the duration of analgesia of phenol is variable and may last for several weeks to months.

Systemic side effects are mild and nonspecific, since usually only small doses of 500 to 1000 mg., much less than the toxic dose of 8 to 15 g., are injected at any one time.[7]

Miscellaneous Agents and Techniques

Chlorocresol. Used as a 2-per-cent solution in glycerine, chlorocresol is very effective but has a higher incidence of toxic side effects than phenol, because it appears to diffuse and penetrate more.[1] Though more efficacious in pain relief than phenol, this agent also produces almost twice the degree of urinary and bowel sphincter paralysis, persistent numbness, and paresthesia.[1] Pain relief is sometimes delayed for as long as 24 hours.

Silver Nitrate. This agent should be avoided because its use has been associated with meningitis.[6,8]

Ammonium Compounds. These compounds have been used in different concentrations (5–20%) in an attempt to produce selective damage to pain fibers and hopefully preserve other fiber function.[9,10] However, this differentiation does not appear to be possible. The use of these compounds does not prevent the appearance of the post-neurolytic neuralgia seen with destructive blocks. The place of ammonium compounds in neurolytic block is undecided at this time.

Tetracaine. Tetracaine in concentrations in excess of those used for clinical anesthesia (e.g., 1%, with total dose restricted to 50 mg.) has been used to effect prolonged block.[11]

Osmotic Neurolysis. The instillation of normothermic or hypothermic, hypertonic saline solution into the subarachnoid space is frequently very uncomfortable for the patient and is associated with severe but transient, pain, vertigo, weakness, and vomiting.[12,13,14] Among the complications of this procedure are severe hypertension, sinus tachycardia or bradycardia, ventricular ectopic beats, and pulmonary edema.[15,16] Some of these untoward effects are avoided by performing the procedure under general anesthesia.[12,13] The place of osmotic neurolysis in our therapeutic repertoire is controversial.

Barbotage. This is a relatively new technique, and its analgesic effect is speculated to result from a partial demyelinization of the spinal cord due to the altered local pressure produced.[16] The principal complication is severe headache in 80 per cent of the patients. In that series there was one death attributed to thrombosis of the basilar vessels.

GENERAL COMPLICATIONS OF NEUROLYTIC BLOCKS

Failure of Neurolytic Block

Failure of nerve block is perhaps one of the most frustrating complications associated with all therapeutic blocks, particularly neurolytic blocks. Often after what appears to be meticulous placement of drugs in the appropriate anatomical site with confirmatory testing, the subsequent neurolytic block is short-lived, incomplete, or even absent. Knowledge of the action of these agents is incomplete and does not always permit full explanation of these enigmas. However, an incomplete block can always be repeated, if necessary. It is sometimes desirable, when working in vital areas where precision is paramount, to risk the possibility of an incomplete block by a somewhat more conservative approach and to be prepared to return later, rather than to proceed with an overly generous initial attempt and succeed in involving some vital structure.

Failure of the block can be minimized by meticulous adherence to technique and also by using ancillary aids, such as bi-plane fluoroscopy and/or a nerve stimulator, in an effort to position the needle more accurately at the target.

The pain experienced by many patients with cancer is often not due as much to the noxious afferent input as it is to other less specific, but still very real causes, such as anxiety and depression. In these patients, although it interrupts afferent input, a neurolytic block will not put an end to complaints that are generated by psychological causes. Therefore, it may be deemed to have "failed." Hence, it is of paramount importance to carry out a diagnostic evaluation prior to embarking upon a neurolytic block. Only if pain relief is obtained by repeated diagnostic procedures should a neurolytic block be considered.

Spread to Other Structures

Like conventional local anesthetics, neurolytic substances can spread to involve structures other than their intended target when injected percutaneously. The result ranges from a relatively mild focal necrosis of musculoskeletal tissue, causing some self-limiting discomfort for a day or so, to spread to vital structures such as the optic nerve or spinal cord, with consequences of blindness and myelitis.[18]

To prevent spread of hyperbaric or hypobaric neurolytic solutions with segmental neurolytic subarachnoid blocks, the patient should not be moved from the blocking position too soon. This ensures against involvement of other nerves or the spinal cord. However, concentrations of alcohol[5] and phenol[19] decrease so rapidly that within 10 to 15 minutes, it is quite safe to permit the patient to adopt a more comfortable position without risking spread of the agent by gravity or turbulence in the cerebrospinal fluid.

A test dose of local anesthetic will often confirm needle position or detect that the needle is placed in a dural sleeve or in another site that might lead to accidental intrathecal injection.[20]

Sphincter Disturbance

With neurolytic blocks involving the sacral roots or the cauda equina, disturbances of control of both bladder and bowel sphincters are often encountered. When segmental thoracic or lumbar neurolytic blocks are performed, occasional temporary disturbance of bladder or bowel function will occur and is one of the risks of the procedure that should be explained to the patient beforehand. It is usually of a limited duration, resolving within a matter of days to weeks. However, if neurolytic block of the cauda equina or sacral roots is undertaken, the possibility of long-term sphincter disturbance is very real and must be appreciated by both patient and anesthesiologist prior to the block. Thus, the patient's pelvic or lower extremity pain must be so severe that he is willing to accept the possibility of bladder or bowel incontinence, or both. Hence, neurolytic blocks involving sphincter control are usually reserved until such time that these functions are already compromised by the neoplastic disease process causing the pain.

In patients with bladder dysfunction, the most common presentation is retention of urine with overflow incontinence. This is usually caused by spillover of neurolytic agent onto sacral roots of the cauda equina, anywhere between their origins at the vertebral level of T12 to L1, to their emergence by way of the sacral foramina. In lumbar neurolytic blocks, therefore, it is advisable to deposit the neurolytic substance in the most peripheral location possible in the subarachnoid space, that is, just within the theca rather than in a central position within the cauda equina. If anesthetic effects are noted at a remote site (e.g., sacral dermatomes) and not at the intended target, the injection should be stopped immediately. This complication can often be avoided by initial use of a diagnostic dose of local anesthetic to ascertain the needle position. The likelihood of incontinence can also be reduced by tilting the table in the appropriate direction for hyperbaric and hypobaric solutions, so that the neurolytic agent tends to flow away from the sacral roots. In the treatment of bladder dysfunction, most of these difficulties are fortunately temporary; an indwelling catheter and continuous drainage will prevent urinary retention and minimize infection resulting in permanent damage. As recovery occurs and the patient can do without the catheter, he is instructed to micturate on a time-contingent basis. The anesthesiologist facing any of these complications should not hesitate to seek the assistance of a urologist.

COMPLICATIONS OF DENERVATION

Trophic Changes

Sloughing. Some investigators have described the complication of sloughing following neurolytic procedures on branches of the trigeminal nerve: areas of skin and subcutaneous tissues sloughed following alcohol injections.[18] The mechanism of this process is not entirely clear. Since the nerves are in close proximity to the corresponding arteries, injection of a neurolytic solution may involve destruction of the artery as well. It seems that the collateral circulation should be more than adequate to compensate for this vascular interruption, particularly in the head and neck. Perhaps in these patients the local conditions compromise collateral perfusion. Also, denervated tissues undergo trophic changes and become subject to undetected trauma, which may result in progression of infectious processes to tissue destruction.

Neuritis. The discomforts that follow a neurolytic block of a peripheral nerve are often referred to as post-neurolytic neuritis. This is most frequently seen when neurolytic blocks are performed on nerves distal to their emerging foramina, either in the skull or spinal cord. This neuritis can be such a problem that peripheral neurolytic block is not advised in any patient with a long life

expectancy but is reserved for the terminally ill patient. An exception is neurolytic block of the peripheral branches of the trigeminal system; this appears to be relatively free from the occurrence of a post-neurolytic neuritis.[21] However, with the success of thermogangliolysis in the treatment of tic douloureaux,[22] the need for neurolytic blocks of the trigeminal nerve seems to be decreasing.

Because of the possible occurrence of post-neurolytic neuralgia, it is preferable to produce the neurolysis centrally, at a subarachnoid level, so that the neurolytic block selectively involves the dorsal root.[21]

The appearance of a new pain after a neurolytic block is often described by the patient as a sequela of the block procedure but may, in fact, be due to other causes. Following the disappearance of the primary pain, discomforts that had previously not troubled the patient often become more evident.

The time before the appearance of post-neurolytic neuralgia is variable, but 6 months is a figure often quoted.[21] A second neurolytic block at this stage, performed proximal to the original procedure, will possibly afford a few more months of pain relief and is quite justified, again, in a terminally ill patient, but not in an individual with a long life expectancy.

Painful paresthesia is the only reported toxic effect of phenol injection of peripheral nerves for spasticity; it occurs in less than 10 per cent of cases.[23]

Anesthesia Dolorosa. Another complication of neurolytic procedures is anesthesia dolorosa, the patient's distress at the numbness produced. The denervated area itself can become a painful problem, much as an amputated extremity can be a source of phantom limb pain. The explanation for this phenomenon is poorly understood but possibly involves imbalances in the afferent neuronal input to the CNS, either at the spinal cord or at higher levels.[24] For this reason, it is important to permit the patient to experience the sequelae of a neurolytic block by initially using temporary agents, especially long-acting local anesthetic agents, such as bupivacaine and etidocaine. Some patients prefer to experience pain rather than numbness! However, even if numbness is well tolerated for the duration of a temporary diagnostic block, it may be more disturbing when present for a considerable period following neurolysis. The treatment for anesthesia dolorosa is unsatisfactory, but some patients may respond to carbamazine, in doses up to 1400 mg. per day, or to combinations of amitriptyline (75–150 mg./day) and fluphenazine (3–6 mg./day).

This long-term complication of deafferentation is one reason that the procedure is best reserved for the terminally ill. Patients whose pain is of a nonmalignant origin are not candidates for neurolytic procedures.

Corneal Damage. The sequela to neurolytic block of the gasserian ganglion, corneal damage, is often the most distressing aspect of this procedure for the patient. The cornea is rendered insensitive, and therefore the accumulation of foreign objects (e.g., dust, dirt) produces a chronic conjunctivitis that can lead to ulceration and infection. Several suggestions have been made to cope with this problem. Often a lateral tarsal fusion will reduce the conjunctival surface area at risk without impairing vision. Also, meticulous cleansing of the conjunctival sac with appropriate lubricants and antibiotics and wearing special spectacles with side screens can reduce the incidence of complications. Hemifacial numbness following gasserian ganglion block also results in analgesia of the ipsilateral half of the oral cavity and spilling of accumulated saliva from that side of the mouth. This frequently distresses the patient and is perhaps best treated with an antisialagogue (e.g., diphenhydramine, 10–25 mg., q. 6 h.) in modest doses to reduce saliva production.

COMPLICATIONS OF NEUROLYTIC EPIDURAL BLOCK

The injection of neurolytic agents in the epidural space has been used intermittently in the past. This procedure involves a relatively large volume of neurolytic agent, and therefore it is imperative to avoid accidental subarachnoid injection, a potential complication of all epidural injections. However, there appear to be relatively few other complications, except perhaps temporary sphincter impairment interfering with bladder control.[25]

Epidural alcohol is very painful unless preceded by a local anesthetic block. Epidural phenol is less painful and has been used in concentrations of 5 per cent and 10 per cent.[26,27]

Theoretically, epidural neurolytic agents offer advantages. Spread to the cranial cavity is unlikely, and meningeal irritation can be avoided.

Measures for Prevention of Complications of Neurolytic Blocks

Always perform diagnostic blocks before neurolytic blocks. A diagnostic block usually includes a short-acting agent (e.g., lidocaine), a long-acting agent (e.g., bupivacaine), and a placebo; ideally, these are administered on three separate occasions before proceeding with neurolytic blockade.

Always warn the patient beforehand regarding complications, and allow the patient to play an active part in the decision to proceed with neurolysis, once he is aware of the risks and complications. "Permanent blocks" are rarely permanent and often must be repeated in a matter of months. Obtain a signed, informed consent.

When contemplating nerve blocks in a patient with preexisting neurological deficits and/or disease of the nervous system (e.g., poliomyelitis or multiple sclerosis), it is necessary to document fully the nerve deficits prior to the block procedure, so that any preexisting defect will not be retrospectively ascribed to the anesthetic technique or agent.

Do not perform neurolytic blocks in a patient with a long life expectancy.

Avoid neurolytic blocks on peripheral nerves (with the exception of the branches of the trigeminal and glossopharyngeal), except in the terminally ill.

Segmental subarachnoid block, either unilateral or bilateral (as required), is the preferred neurolytic block for treatment of pain in the trunk.

Neurolytic blocks are best used for treatment of pain in the head, thorax, or abdomen; block of nerves of the brachial or lumbosacral plexus can compromise the function of the extremities. If neurolysis involves the cauda equina, sphincter incontinence may result.

Do not premedicate a patient undergoing neurolytic block.

Use a test dose.

Neurolytic agents should be used only by physicians experienced in regional nerve block.

A neurolytic block rarely solves a patient's pain problem. Other modalities of supportive therapy (e.g., medications, psychotherapy, or support) are frequently required, even if noxious input has been totally eliminated.

CLINICAL RECOMMENDATIONS

Neurolytic blocks used selectively have a definite role in the therapy of chronic pain and the relief of spasticity problems. Because of the meticulous technique required and the potential for complications, they probably should be undertaken only by the experienced practitioner.

Fortunately, like the pain relief achieved, which is often less than permanent, most complications are not permanent and resolve with time. Many of the reported impairments of sphincter dysfunction have lasted only a few days to a week or so.[2,9,28] Even when motor weakness complicates neurolytic block, it can resolve in a short time.[9,29,30] Because of the fact that the pain relief resulting from neurolytic nerve block is relatively finite, these blocks are eminently suitable for patients with finite pain problems, such as those that occur in terminal cancer. However, they are rarely indicated in chronic pain states due to nonmalignant causes, in which the pain may persist for years.

REFERENCES

1. Swerdlow, M.: Intrathecal chlorocresol. Anaesthesia, 28:297, 1973.
2. Nathan, P. W., and Scott, T. G.: Intrathecal phenol for intractable pain. The safety and dangers of the method. Lancet, 1:76, 1958.
3. Kuzucu, E. Y., Derrick, W. S., and Wilbur, S. A.: Control of intractable pain with subarachnoid alcohol block. J.A.M.A., 195:541, 1966.
4. Reid, W., Watt, J. K., and Gray, T. G.: Phenol injection of the sympathetic chain. Br. J. Surg., 57:45, 1970.
5. Matsuki, M., Kato, Y., and Ichiyanagi, K.: Progressive changes in the concentration of ethyl alcohol in human and canine subarachnoid spaces. Anesthesiology, 36:617, 1972.
6. Nathan, P. W., and Sears, R. A.: Effect of phenol on nervous conduction. J. Physiol., 150:565, 1960.
7. Esplin, D. W.: Antiseptics and disinfectants; fungicides; ectoparasiticides. *In* Goodman, L. S., and Gilman, A. (eds.): The Pharmaceutical Basis of Therapeutics. ed 4. p. 1036. New York, MacMillan, 1970.
8. Maher, R. M.: Intrathecal chlorocresol (parachlormetacresol) in treatment of pain of cancer. Lancet, 1:965, 1963.
9. Swerdlow, M.: Relief of Intractable Pain. pp. 148–174. New York, Excerpta Medica, 1974.
10. Wright, B. D.: Treatment of intractable coccygodynia by transsacral ammonium chloride injection. Anesth. Analg., 50:519, 1971.
11. Khalili, A. A., and Ditzler, J. W.: Neurolytic substances in relief of pain. Med. Clin. North Am., 52:163, 1968.
12. Hitchcock, E.: Hypothermic subarachnoid irrigation for intractable pain. Lancet, 1:1133, 1967.
13. Hitchcock, E.: Osmolytic neurolysis for intractable facial pain. Lancet, 1:434, 1969.
14. Robbie, D. S.: General management of intractable pain in advanced cancer of the rectum. Proc. R. Soc. Med., 62:1225, 1969.
15. Thompson, G. E.: Pulmonary edema complicating intrathecal hypertonic saline injection for intractable pain. Anesthesiology, 35:425, 1971.
16. O'Higgins, J. W., Padfield, A., and Clapp, H.: Possible complications of hypothermic-saline subarachnoid injection. Lancet, 1:567, 1970.
17. Lloyd, J. W., Hughes, J. T., Davies-Jones, G. A. B.: Relief of severe intractable pain by barbotage of cerebral spinal fluid. Lancet, 1:354, 1972.
18. Moore, D. C.: Complications of Regional Anesthesia. Springfield, Charles C Thomas, 1955.
19. Ichyanagi, K., Matsuki, M., Kinefuchi, S., et al.: Progressive changes in concentrations of phenol and glycerine in human subarachnoid space. Anesthesiology, 42:622, 1975.
20. Galizia, E. J., and Lahiri, S. K.: Paraplegia following coeliac plexus block. Br. J. Anaesth., 46:539, 1974.
21. Bonica, J. J.: The Management of Pain. Philadelphia, Lea & Febiger, 1953.
22. Sweet, W. H., Wepsic, J. G.: Controlled thermocoagulation of trigeminal ganglion and rootlets for differential destruction of pain fibers. Part I. Trigeminal Neuralgia. J. Neurosurg., 40:143, 1974.
23. Moritz, U.: Phenol block of peripheral nerves. Scand. J. Rehabil. Med. 5:160, 1973.
24. Melzack, R.: Phantom limb pain: implications for treatment of pathological pain. Anesthesiology, 35:409, 1971.
25. De Beule, F., and Schottee, A.: Nouvelle étapes daus la lutte contre la douleur. Alcoolisation paravertébrale et épidural. Alcoolisation de plexus solaire. Rev. Belge. Sci. Med., 6:357, 1934.
26. Laurie, H., and Vanasupa, R.: Comments on the use of intraspinal phenol pantopaque for relief of pain and spasticity. J. Neurosurg., 20:60, 1963.
27. Finer, B.: Epidural injection of carbolic acid in incurable cancer. Lancet, 2:1179, 1958.
28. Stovner, J., and Endresen, R.: Intrathecal phenol for cancer pain. Acta Anaesthesiol. Scand., 16:17, 1972.
29. Hughes, J. T.: Thrombosis of posterior spinal arteries. Neurology, 20:659, 1970.
30. Wilkinson, H. A., Mark, V. H., and White, J. C.: Further experiences with intrathecal phenol for relief of pain. J. Chron. Dis., 17:1055, 1964.

FURTHER READING

Swerdlow, M., Mehta, M. D., and Lipton, S.: The role of the anaesthetist in chronic pain management. Anaesthesia, 33:250, 1978.
Swerdlow, M.: Complications of neurolytic neural blockade. *In* Cousins, M. J., and Bridenbaugh, P. O. (eds.): Neural Blockade in Clinical Anesthesia and Management of Pain. pp. 543–553. Philadelphia, J. B. Lippincott Company, 1980.

Part Four

The Respiratory System

8 Airway Obstruction and Causes of Difficult Intubation

Henry Rosenberg, M.D., and Henrietta Rosenberg, M.D.

Patency of the airway is a *sine qua non* of safe anesthesia. Airway obstruction can occur at any time during administration of a general anesthetic, particularly in patients with predisposing structural abnormalities of the airway. Ideally, the anesthetist should be able to identify the patient with a potential airway disorder prior to induction of anesthesia, and he should be ready to employ special techniques to ensure easy access to the airway and adequate respiratory exchange. Such techniques may include adjustment of head position, awake intubation, fiberoptic bronchoscopy, tracheostomy, and cardiopulmonary bypass instituted prior to induction of anesthesia. However, difficulties with the airway are sometimes apparent only in retrospect. It is therefore obligatory that the anesthesiologist should always be prepared to diagnose the causes of airway obstruction and to exercise a plan for reestablishing airway patency.

This chapter discusses difficulties related to the airway and general anesthesia and intubation, and their management. Abnormalities that may cause difficult intubation are listed in Table 8–1.

CAUSES OF AIRWAY OBSTRUCTION

Partial or complete airway obstruction may occur at any time in the perioperative period.

Obstruction that occurs upon induction of anesthesia is a frightening experience, requiring rapid diagnosis and treatment. Often, airway compromise that develops upon induction of anesthesia or intraoperatively can be suspected preoperatively. However, even when such obstruction cannot be predicted, the anesthesiologist's knowledge of the patient's pathology helps to diagnose the cause and locate the site of obstruction and allows proper treatment to be selected. Preventive measures, however, are of even greater value. For example, anesthesia for a patient with a mass lesion of the pharynx can be induced more safely with a mask than with an intravenous technique; in such a patient airway obstruction may occur upon relaxation of the soft tissues, and the anesthesiologist's view of the trachea can be obstructed by the mass. In a patient with a substernal thyroid, it is often advisable to perform tracheal intubation with a tracheal tube that is smaller than is expected, since the tracheal lumen may be compromised by the mass.[6]

Compromise of the airway can occur from changes in the mouth, pharynx, trachea, or bronchi. The causes of such obstructions are discussed below, according to the regions in which they occur. In the Appendix, a more detailed discussion of some of the unusual syndromes that can

(Text continues on page 128.)

Table 8-1. Abnormalities That

Site of Abnormality	Congenital-Metabolic	Traumatic	Infectious
Head, neck, and jaws	Inability to extend the head (Klippel-Fiel syndrome[1], achondroplasia,[2] large encephalocele[3]) Inability to achieve optimal head position (craniosynostoses, encephalocele) Inability to open mouth widely (coronoid hyperplasia[4], Hurler's syndrome[5])	Maxillary or mandibular fracture, cervical fracture, burns	Trismus secondary to infection or fracture, osteomyelitis
Oral cavity	Microstomia, macroglossia (lymphangioma, muscular hypertrophy, Down's syndrome), micrognathia (hypoplasia of mandible,[5] Treacher Collins syndrome[6], Pierre Robin syndrome[5]), first arch syndrome, trisomy 18	Burns, caustic ingestion, macroglossia[9] (secondary to decreased venous return or secondary to trauma), lesions following posterior pharyngeal flap repair (surgery for cleft palate repair[10])	Ludwig's angina,[11] Vincent's angina
Nose	Choanal atresia, agenesis of the nose	Broken nose	Adenoid hyperplasia
Pharynx	Cystic hygroma,[5] lymphoid hyperplasia (Hurler's syndrome,[5] Niemann-Pick disease, Gaucher's disease)	Burns, caustic ingestion	Retropharyngeal abscess, hypertrophied tonsils with or without abscess (infectious mononucleosis,[12] bacterial infection)
Larynx and glottis	Laryngeal stenosis, cysts, laryngomalacia, laryngocele[7]	Burns, external injury, post-traumatic stenosis	
Trachea and bronchus	Stenosis, tracheomalacia, vascular rings[8] (double aortic arch, right aortic arch); may occur at any point through main bronchi		

INFLAMMATORY	NEOPLASTIC	NEUROLOGIC	OTHER
	Tumors of tongue, palate with bony extension and trismus		Casts of neck, ankylosing spondylitis,[17] scleroderma,[18] wired jaw, rheumatoid arthritis of temporomandibular joint,[19] effects of radiation, juvenile chronic polyarthritis (Still's disease)[20]
	Tumors of tongue, palate, floor of mouth; thyroglossal duct cyst; aberrant thyroid		Angioneurotic edema, radiation changes, epidermolysis bullosa,[21] pemphigus, hemorrhagic diathesis and/or surgery with dissection of blood to base of tongue
	Polyps, fibra, hemagiomas, cysts, solid tumors, encephalocele		Foreign bodies
	Carcinoma and sarcoma, fibroma (Gardner's syndrome[14]), other benign growths, hemangioma	Paralysis of pharyngeal muscles (myasthenia, Guillain-Barré syndrome, C.V.A., syringomyelia	Retropharyngeal intubation,[22] foreign body,[23] angioneurotic edema, epidermolysis bullosa, submucosal hemorrhage (hemophilia)
Epiglottitis,[13] laryngitis, arthritis and ankylosis of small joints of the larynx	Polyps and papillomas,[15] epiglottic cysts, carcinoma, hemangioma		Foreign body (cafe coronary syndrome); bilateral midline abductor paralysis: paralysis of recurrent laryngeal nerves (birth trauma, surgery)[24]; laryngeal stenosis secondary to acromegaly[25]; laryngeal spasm during anesthesia; glottic edema from allergic reactions
Laryngotracheobronchitis, retropharyngeal abscess	Papillomas, benign tumors, granuloma, hemangioma, mediastinal mass,[16] thryoid and esophageal tumors		Foreign body, hemorrhage, secondary to trauma or carcinoma

be associated with airway obstruction is presented. Although difficult intubation does not always ensue, the anesthesiologist's index of suspicion should be aroused in each of these syndromes, regardless of whether there is a past history of an episode of airway compromise.

Disorders of the Neck and Mandible

Mobility of the neck and opening of the mouth are important for the alignment of the tracheo-oral axes (Fig. 8-1) and visualization of the glottis. Often, functional impairment relating to these structures is apparent (e.g., fractures and trauma); however, sometimes such disability must be sought. Disabilities in patients with various forms of arthritis (rheumatoid[17,19] and juvenile arthritis[20]), the congenital anomalies such as Klippel-Feil syndrome,[26] and coronoid process hyperplasia[4] are examples of conditions that require testing of the patient's ability to move his neck and open his mouth. (See the section below for other means of evaluation of the airway.)

Lesions of the Oral and Nasal Cavities and the Pharynx

Many congenital abnormalities have in common micrognathia, macroglossia, and/or hypoplasia of the mandible, which can make airway maintenance and tracheal intubation difficult.[26–28] After surgical repair of these lesions, the airway may still remain narrowed, and the patient may be subject to airway obstruction.

Infants may present with large tumor masses protruding from the oral cavity that may fill the mouth and impede intubation.[5] Radiologic evaluation is often needed to assess the degree of airway compromise.[29] Since neonates are obligate nose breathers, obstruction of nasal passages owing to choanal atresia or birth trauma can be life-threatening, unless measures are taken to keep the mouth open or establish a nasal airway.[26]

Fortunately, inflammation of the submandibular space, as in Ludwig's angina, is rather uncommon today. Submandibular infection or

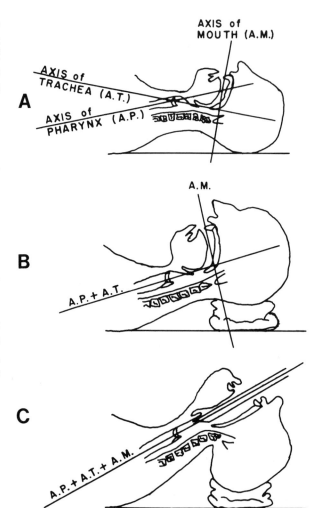

Fig. 8-1. Proper positioning for laryngoscopy and tracheal intubation. (*A*) Axes of the mouth, pharynx, and trachea are shown with head in the customary, neutral position. (*B*) Axes of the pharynx and trachea are superimposed with the head resting upon a firm pad or folded sheets. (*C*) All three axes are aligned by flexion of the cervical spine and extension at the atloidooccipital joint.

hemorrhage causes obstruction by pushing up the tongue, and dissection through tissue planes into the pharynx.[30–32] Foreign body perforation and extension of tonsillar infection, such as a retropharyngeal abscess (Fig. 8-2), are more common causes of tracheal deviation and compromise.

Airway maintenance and tracheal intubation

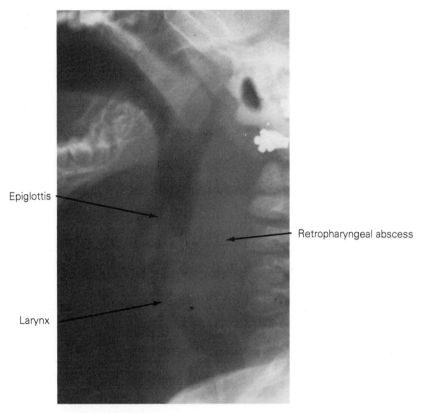

Epiglottis

Retropharyngeal abscess

Larynx

Fig. 8-2. A large retropharyngeal abscess in this infant resulted in anterolateral deviation of the trachea. Because of glottic displacement, tracheal intubation was difficult.

are often difficult under general anesthesia in patients who have undergone extensive intraoral cancer surgery. The tissues are distorted due to changes caused by radiation and surgery. Tissues may be friable, depending on the stage of healing. Furthermore, radiation can cause induration of tissues, resulting in loss of the normal elasticity of the oral and pharyngeal structures.

The pharynx is the site of partial respiratory obstruction for a variety of reasons. Cystic hygromas are frequently large and require several surgical procedures for complete removal. Each procedure carries the threat of airway compromise.[5] The forms of mucopolysaccaridosis and the lipid storage diseases may cause obstruction because of lymphoid hyperplasia.[5,33]

If care and special precautions are not taken in patients with oral and pharyngeal infection,

bleeding and rupture of abscesses can occur, with the risk of airway obstruction and aspiration.[12]

With mass lesions of the pharynx, complete airway obstruction can occur after muscle relaxation from general anesthesia or muscle relaxants. A pharyngeal mass may make it difficult to visualize the glottis or may cause airway obstruction that necessitates emergency tracheostomy. In other cases, although it may be possible to maintain the airway, intubation of the trachea may require the use of special techniques, such as fiberoptic laryngoscopy or awake intubation.

Lesions of the Glottis and Trachea

The airway is narrowest at the larynx, which is therefore a hazardous site of respiratory obstruction. This is especially true in infants. It has been calculated that edema of 1 mm. of the mucosal surface of the larynx will reduce the glottic cross-sectional area from 14 mm.[2] to 5 mm.[2 34]

Narrowing of the trachea from intrinsic or extrinsic lesions may be asymptomatic. Causes of a narrowed trachea or bronchus include substernal thyroid,[35] subglottic hemangioma,[36] and mediastinal masses.[16,30,37] Vascular rings and infectious processes of the pharynx frequently cause narrowing of the trachea or its branches.[7] Acromegalic patients may show decreased diameter of the cricoid as well.[25,38]

Use of muscle relaxants is often associated with airway problems in patients who have tracheal and glottic narrowing or with trauma to the throat. Normal muscle tone is often important in stenting the trachea and providing a clear air passage. In particular, a patient with a cut throat should not be paralyzed, since the free ends of the trachea may further separate with muscle relaxants.[39,40]

Patients with lesions that partially obstruct the glottis often refuse to lie down, since airway obstruction can occur when they are supine. The characteristic sitting position helps make more efficient use of accessory muscles of respiration. Therefore, anesthesia should be induced in the sitting position, and provision should be made for immediate tracheostomy, if necessary.

Chronic compression of the trachea owing to a tumor or a vascular structure (Fig. 8-3) may cause tracheomalacia. While the tumor and fibrotic tissue are present, the trachea may be stented. However, after reduction of the compression, tracheal collapse may occur. Tracheostomy or passage of a tube past the narrowed area is then needed.[30]

Epiglottitis is not infrequent in children of ages 2 to 7 years. It is a life-threatening condition, because the swelling may lead to narrowing of the glottis. Once treated routinely by tracheostomy, today afflicted children are treated by nasotracheal intubation, under anesthesia in the operating room with equipment for bronchoscopy and/or tracheostomy available. Intubation is maintained for 24 to 48 hours. Before extubation, laryngoscopy is performed once more, to ensure that the swelling has subsided.

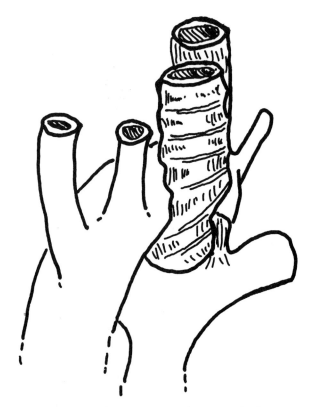

Fig. 8-3. Tracheal compression from a tight ligamentum arteriosum.

Another condition that merits special mention is papillomatosis of the larynx (Fig. 8-4).[15,41] Infants and children with papillomatosis require repeated surgery for removal of the polyps. They, too, are best anesthetized with general anesthesia without muscle relaxants, since the glottic opening may not be visible due to the multiple polyps, and ventilation with bag and mask is not always effective. Another hazard is seeding of polypoid tissue into the trachea and bronchi, which often causes polyps to develop in these structures.

ARTIFICIAL AIRWAYS AND INTUBATION OF THE TRACHEA

Endotracheal intubation is not always necessary to maintain airway patency, even in emergency situations. Oropharyngeal and nasopharyn-

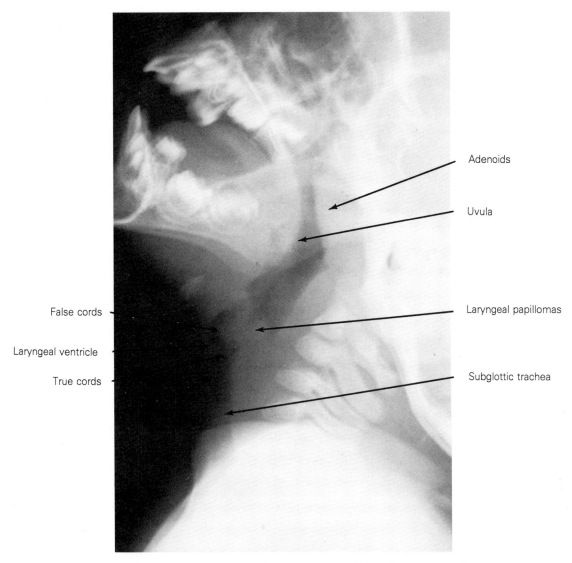

Adenoids

Uvula

False cords

Laryngeal papillomas

Laryngeal ventricle

True cords

Subglottic trachea

Fig. 8-4. Glottic narrowing shown here is due to multiple laryngeal papillomas.

geal airways will usually relieve the most common cause of airway compromise, soft tissue obstruction, and may help in other situations as well.

Although nasal airways are easier to insert, they may cause epistaxis and mucosal damage. Improper placement of an oral airway may push the tongue posteriorly and aggravate soft-tissue obstruction. Of course, neither airway protects against aspiration.

The proper position of the patient's head and neck simplifies access to the glottis and trachea.[5,42,43] Often, a difficult intubation is made easy by merely placing one or two folded sheets or firm pads under the patient's head. The main problem in visualization of the glottic opening is the proper alignment of the axes of the trachea, the mouth, and the pharynx (Fig. 8-1). Such alignment is achieved by flexing the neck, thereby straightening the cervical spine and extending the head at the atloido-occipital joint. The purpose of the laryngoscope blade is to lift the tongue and epiglottis up and away from the airway, in order to provide a view of the vocal cords, once the axes are in proper alignment.

In infants and young children, because the head is large relative to the trunk, only slight neck flexion is necessary. Flattening of the shoulders is often needed to prevent anterior displacement of the glottis beneath the mandible in this age-group.[43] Straight rather than curved blades are preferred for intubation of children, since the epiglottis is usually long and floppy and protrudes backward at an angle of 45 degrees to the anterior pharyngeal wall. In infants, the glottis is opposite the vertebral bodies of C2 to C4, while in adults it is opposite C5 and C6. It is also more anterior in children than in adults.[34]

Other routine aids to laryngoscopy are adequate jaw and soft-tissue relaxation and/or anesthetization of the airway. Patient cooperation during airway instrumentation is usually provided by adequate general anesthesia and muscle paralysis or topical anesthesia and psychologic preparation of the patient.

At least two laryngoscope blades of different sizes should be readily available before intubation, in both adults and children.

The Difficult Intubation

Even with optimal position of the head and neck in patients without obvious causes of airway pathology, it is sometimes difficult or impossible to visualize the glottis. Cass, James, and Lines discussed,[44] and more recently, White and Kander analyzed,[45] the anatomic factors that predispose patients to difficult intubation. Patients who are unable to extend their heads, flex their necks, or open their mouths widely are more difficult to intubate, as might be expected. Cass, James, and Lines also list the following factors that predispose patients to difficult intubations: a short muscular neck with a full set of teeth; a receding lower jaw with obtuse mandibular angles; protrusion of the upper incisors and reduced space between the angles of the mandible, with a high, arched palate; and increased distance from the upper incisors to the posterior border of the ramus of the mandible.

White and Kander used measurements taken from radiographs in patients with teeth (Fig. 8-5).

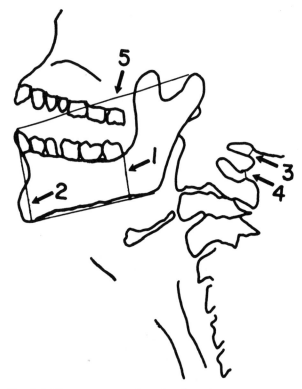

Fig. 8-5. Measurements found to be relevant in assessing the difficulty of laryngoscopy in adult:[16] *(1)* Increased posterior depth of the mandible; *(2)* Increased anterior depth of the mandible; *(3, 4)* reduction in the distances between the occiput and the spinous process of C1 and the occiput and the C1-2 interspinous gap; *(5)* effective mandibular length less than 3.6 times the posterior depth of the mandible *(1)*. However, effective mandibular length by itself is no different in those in whom laryngoscopy is difficult.

They concluded that protruding upper incisors do *not* make intubation difficult. Also, the size of the bodies of the cervical spinous processes do not differ significantly in patients in whom it is easy to perform direct laryngoscopy and in those in whom it is difficult. They found, however, that the following factors were important in making direct laryngoscopy difficult (Fig. 8-5): an increase in the posterior depth of the mandible (possibly by hindering displacement of the soft tissues by the laryngoscope); an increase in the anterior depth of the mandible; reduction in the distance between the occiput and the spinous process of C1 and, to a lesser extent, the C1–C2 interspinous gap, thus narrowing limits of head extension; and reduced mobility of the mandible because of temporomandibular joint dysfunction.[45]

Unfortunately, the distance from the chin to the thyroid cartilage was not assessed. It is an often quoted clinical observation that when this distance is below 3 to 4 cm. (two finger-breadths), difficulty in visualizing the glottis may be expected.

Miscellaneous causes of difficult intubation are listed below.

Miscellaneous Causes of Difficult Intubation

Enlarged tonsils and adenoids secondary to inflammation or tumors (lymphoma)
Retropharyngeal abscess
Cystic hygroma
Retropharyngeal tumors
  Teratoma
  Neurofibroma
  Neuroblastoma
Nasopharyngeal tumors
  Carcinoma
  Rhabdomyosarcoma
  Lymphoma
  Teratoma
Nasopharyngeal meningoencephalocele
Myxedematous thickening of retropharyngeal soft tissues
Pharyngeal tumors
  Benign polyps
  Dermoids
  Teratomas
  Thyroglossal duct cysts
  Neuroblastoma
  Neurofibromas
  Hemangiomas
Laryngeal and upper tracheal tumors
  Papillomas
  Subglottic hemangioma
Enlarged thyroid
Middle and lower tracheal compression
  Enlarged thyroid
  Mediastinal masses
    Teratoma
    Lymphoma
    Ectopic thyroid

Mechanical Problems Associated With Endotracheal Tubes

It is axiomatic that insertion of an endotracheal tube does not always guarantee that the airway is clear. In addition to malposition, a number of problems have been associated with endotracheal tube (see the following list).[22,46–60]

Obstructions of Endotracheal Tubes

Balloons
  Protrusion of the cuff past the end of the tube
  Overinflation of the balloon, with part of the balloon covering the end of the tube
  Overinflation of the balloon, leading to compression of the tube
  Asymmetric expansion of the balloon, leading to bevel compression against the tracheal wall
Tubes
  Foreign body in the tubes
  Mucous plugs
  Kinking
Amored (anode) tubes
  Kinking below the connector and above the spiral winding
  Separation of the inner wall of the tube
Miscellaneous
  Obstruction in the connectors to the tube (e.g., a manufacturer's defect or foreign body)
  Displacement of tube due to change in position of the head
  Puncture of balloon (e.g., during tracheostomy or internal jugular venipuncture)

Fortunately, herniation and slippage of the balloon past the end of the tube are less common with recent use of plastic tubes with built-in cuffs. However, compression of the tube lumen by overexpansion of the balloon still occurs, and a foreign body in the tube may still pose a problem. When airway obstruction occurs after intubation, mechanical problems with the tube should always be considered. Removing air from the balloon, passage of a suction catheter through the tube, and, finally, removal of the tube itself are steps that should be taken in such cases.

Anode (armored) tubes present a special problem. Since they consist of two coatings of latex that enclose spiral metal windings, the inner layer may peel away and cause obstruction of the lumen in the tube. Air has been reported to dissect from the balloon under the latex coating and to cause separation and obstruction during the course of anesthetic administration.[48] Kinking of an anode tube may occur between the connector and the spiral winding.

PATIENT ASSESSMENT AND GENERAL RECOMMENDATIONS

Preoperative assessment of all patients should include a history of airway problems. This in-

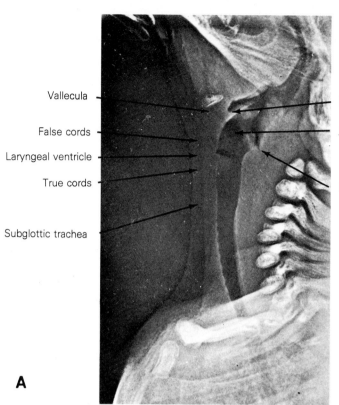

Vallecula — Epiglottis

False cords — Aryepiglottic fold

Laryngeal ventricle

True cords — Retropharyngeal space

Subglottic trachea

A

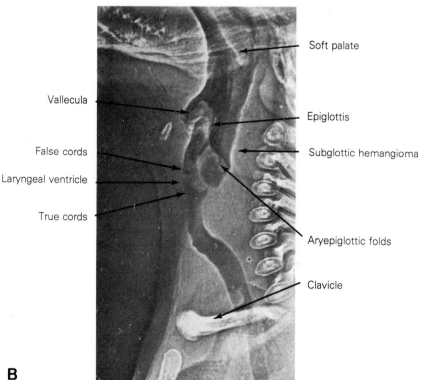

Soft palate

Vallecula — Epiglottis

False cords — Subglottic hemangioma

Laryngeal ventricle

True cords

Aryepiglottic folds

Clavicle

B

Fig. 8-6. Xeroradiograms are often helpful in evaluating the airway. (*A*) Normal examination. (*B*) Subglottic hemangioma in a child. (Xeroradiograms courtesy of Dr. John Scott, Department of Radiology, Albany Medical School)

cludes previous surgery on the airway or adjacent structures, a history of difficult intubation, hoarseness, awakening from sleep short of breath, dyspnea on exertion in the absence of heart disease, congenital heart disease, and recent infection of the mouth, pharynx, or teeth. Lesions occurring below the glottis usually do not affect the quality of the voice, whereas laryngeal lesions are associated with hoarseness and, occasionally, stridor or aphonia. Wheezing may be an indication of airway compromise.

Infants may present with a history of difficulties during feedings, occasional cyanosis, dysphonia, or use of accessory muscles of respiration and relief of respiratory difficulties when the head is extended.[8,26,34]

Lesions in the mouth or pharynx may lead to difficulties in articulation, especially when pharyngeal musculature is compromised. Sometimes, the patient's voice sounds nasal. Croupy cough is characteristic of lesions about the glottis.

Stridor is an important sign.[34] Inspiratory stridor usually indicates obstruction at or above the vocal cords, while bronchial obstruction may be associated with expiratory stridor and wheezing. Lesions that severely compromise the airway below the vocal cords may be associated with both inspiratory and expiratory stridor. A history of frequent respiratory infections, croup, or pain on swallowing are other clues to the diagnosis of airway lesions.

Preoperative examination should include inspection of the mouth and pharynx, assessment of the patient's ability to open the jaw, extend the head, and flex the neck, determination of tracheal deviation, and examination of a chest radiograph for tracheal deformity and mediastinal masses.

Limitation of movement at the temporomandibular joints may also be indicated by the inability of the patient to move his lower incisors anterior to the upper incisors. When a diagnosis is questionable, lateral neck and chest radiographs and xeroradiograms are valuable (Fig. 8-6).[29,61] Prior to anesthesia, the tracheal tube should be carefully examined for patency of the lumen. The balloon should be inflated and tested.

When difficulty is anticipated with the airway, alternatives to routine techniques of intubation are inhalation induction, awake intubation with topical anesthesia, nasotracheal intubation, use of a fiberoptic laryngoscope,[62] passage of a guide retrograde or anterograde,[63] tracheostomy, cricothyroidotomy and transtracheal ventilation, and, rarely, institution of cardiopulmonary bypass.[37]

There is no routine method of induction or maintenance of anesthesia in patients with airway compromise. Each case must be evluated in light of the existing pathology, as well as the anesthetist's skills and resources.

Muscle relaxation from general anesthesia may contribute to soft-tissue obstruction. Additionally, mucus or blood on the larynx during light planes of anesthesia can cause laryngospasm. Distortion resulting from surgery and secretions may make reintubation extremely difficult in these instances.

Patients with obstructive lesions in any area of the respiratory tract should be evaluated carefully prior to *extubation*, as well as intubation, particularly following surgical procedures.

In general, patients who require special techniques to ensure a patent airway should be extubated when their reflexes have returned completely and they are able to open their eyes and respond to commands.

REFERENCES

1. Jones, A. C. P., and Pelton, D. A.: An index of syndromes and their anaesthetic implications. Can. Anaesth. Soc. J., 23: 207, 1976.
2. Mather, J. S.: Impossible direct laryngoscopy in achondroplasia: a case report. Anaesthesia, 21:244, 1966.
3. Cordon, R. A.: Anesthetic management of patients with airway problems. Int. Anesthesiol. Clin., 10:37, 1972.
4. Shurman, J.: Bilateral hypertrophy of the coronoid processes. Anesthesiology, 42:491, 1975.
5. Bougas, T. P., and Smith, R. M.: Pathologic airway obstruction in children. Anesth. Analg. 37:137, 1958.
6. Ross, E. D. T.: Treacher-Collins syndrome: an anaesthetic hazard. Anaesthesia, 18:350, 1963.
7. Ferguson, C. F.: Treatment of airway problems in the newborn. Ann. Otol. Rhinol. Laryngol., 76:762, 1967.
8. Fearon, B.: Respiratory distress in the newborn. Otolaryngol. Clin. North Am., 1:147, 1968.
9. McAllister, R. G.: Macroglossia: a positional complication. Anesthesiology, 40:199, 1974.
10. Jackson, P., Whitaker, L. A., and Randall, P.: Airway hazards associated with paryngeal flaps in patients who have the Pierre Robin syndrome. Plast. Reconstr. Surg., 58:184, 1976.
11. Bennett, J. H.: Anesthetic management for drainage of abscess of the submandibular spade (Ludwig's angina). Anesthesiology, 4:25, 1943.
12. Meyers, E. F., and Chapin, B.: Anesthetic management of emergency tonsillectomy and adenoidectomy in infectious monomucleosis. Anesthesiology, 42:490, 1975.

13. Blanc, V. F., Weber, M. L., Levuc, C., et al.: Acute epiglottitis in children: management of 27 consecutive cases with nasotracheal intubation with emphasis on anaesthetic considerations. Can. Anaesth. Soc. J., 24:1, 1977.

14. Pappas, M. T., Katz, J., and Finestone, S. C.: Problems in anesthetic and airway management with Gardner's syndrome in report of a case. Anesth. Analg., 50:340, 1971.

15. Stein, A. A., and Volk, B. M.: Papillomatosis of trachea and lung. Arch. Pathol., 68: 468, 1959.

16. Amaranth, L., Frankmann, D. B., and Andersen, N. B.: An unusual airway obstruction secondary to congenital malformation of the thoracic inlet. Anesthesiology, 43: 106, 1975.

17. Munson, E. S., and Cullen, S. C.: Endotracheal intubation in a patient with ankylosing spondylitis of the cervical spine. Anesthesiology, 26:365, 1965.

18. Birkham, J., Heifetz, M., and Harm, S.: Diffuse cutaneous scleroderma: an anaesthetic problem. Anaesthesia, 27:89, 1972.

19. Gardner, D. L., and Holmes, F.: Anaesthetic and postoperative hazards in rheumatoid arthritis. Br. J. Anaesth., 33:258, 1961.

20. D'Arcy, E. J., Fell, R. H., Ansell, B. M., et al.: Ketamine and juvenile chronic polarthritis (Still's disease). Anesthesia, 31:624, 1976.

21. Reddy, A. R. R., and Wong, P. H. W.: Epidermolysis Bullosa: a review of anaesthetic problems and case reports. Can. Anaesth. Soc. J., 19:536, 1972.

22. Barnard, J.: An unusual accident during intubation. Anaesthesia, 3: 126, 1948.

23. Nash, P. J.: A foreign body in the larynx. Br. J. Anaesth., 48:371, 1976.

24. Butsch, J. L., Butsch, W. L., and DaRosa, J. F. T.: Bilateral vocal cord paralysis. Arch. Surg., 111:828, 1976.

25. Hassan, S. Z., Matz, G. J., Lawrence, A. M., et al.: Laryngeal stenosis in acromegaly: a possible cause of airway difficulties associated with anesthesia. Anesth. Analg., 55:57, 1976.

26. Pelton, D. A., and Whalen, J. S.: Airway obstruction in infants and children. Int. Anesthesiol. Clin., 10:123, 1972.

27. Salem, M. R., Mathrubhutham, M., and Bennett, E. J.: Difficult intubation. N. Engl. J. Med., 295:879, 1976.

28. Sklar, G. S., and King, B. D.: Endotracheal intubation and Treacher-Collins syndrome. Anesthesiology, 44:247, 1976.

29. Isdale, J. M.: The role of radiology in the assessment of the acutely ill neonate. Int. Anesthesiol. Clin., 13:49, 1975.

30. Barash, P. G., Tsai, B., and Kitahata, L. M.: Acute tracheal collapse following mediastinoscopy. Anesthesiology, 44:67, 1976.

31. Bennett, J. H.: Anesthetic management for drainage of abscess of the submandibular spade (Ludwig's angina). Anesthesiology, 4:25, 1943.

32. Gillespie, N. A.: Endotracheal Anesthesia. pp. 111–117. Madison, University of Wisconsin Press, 1963.

33. Woolley, M. M., Morgan, S., and Hays, B. R.: Heritable disorders of connective tissue in surgical and anesthetic problems. J. Ped. Surg., 2:325, 1967.

34. Holinger, P. H., and Johnston, K. C.: Factors responsible for laryngeal obstruction in infants. J.A.M.A., 143:1229, 1950.

35. Shambaugh, G. E., Seed, R., and Kurn, A.: Airway obstruction in substernal goiter: clinical and therapeutic implications. J. Chron. Dis., 26:737, 1973.

36. Lee, M. H., Ramanathan, S., Chalon, J., et al: Subglottic hemangioma. Anesthesiology, 45:459, 1976.

37. Hall, K. D., and Friedman, M.: Extracorporeal oxygenation for induction of anesthesia in a patient with an intrathoracic tumor. Anesthesiology, 42:493, 1975.

38. Kitahata, L. M.: Airway difficulties associated with anaesthesia in acromegaly, Br. J. Anaesth., 43:1187, 1971.

39. Donchin, Y., and Vered, I. Y.: Blunt trauma to the trachea. Br. J. Anaesth., 48:1113, 1976.

40. Ellis, F. R.: Management of the cut throat. Anaesthesia, 21:253, 1966.

41. Hitz, H. B., and Oesterlin, E.: A case of multiple papillomata of the larynx with aerial metastases to lungs. Am. J. Path., 8:333, 1932.

42. Bannister, F. B., and MacBeth, R. G.: Direct laryngoscopy and tracheal intubation. Lancet, 2:651, 1944.

43. Dripps, R. D., Eckenhoff, J. E., and Vandam, L. D.: Introduction to Anesthesia. pp. 186–199 and 333–335. Philadelphia, W. B. Saunders, 1972.

44. Cass, N. M., James, N. R., and Lines, V.: Intubation under direct laryngoscopy. Br. Med. J., 2:488, 1956.

45. White, A., and Kander, P. L.: Anatomical factors in difficult direct laryngoscopy. Br. J. Anaesth., 47:468, 1975.

46. Lewis, R. N., and Swerdlow, M.: Hazards of endotracheal anaesthesia. Br. J. Anaesth., 36:504, 1964.

47. Anonymous: A bizarre cause of obstruction in an oxford non-kink endotracheal tube. Anaesthesia, 7:395, 1962.

48. Bachaud, R., and Fortin, G.: Airway obstruction with cuffed flexometallic tracheal tubes. Can. Anaesth. Soc. J., 23:330, 1976.

49. Bamforth, B. J.: Complications during endotracheal anesthesia. Anesth. Analg., 42:727, 1963.

50. Blitt, C. D., and Wright, W. A.: An unusual complication of percutaneous internal jugular vein cannulation: puncture of an endotracheal tube cuff. Anesthesiology, 40:306, 1974.

51. Chiu, T. M., and Meyers, E. F.: Defective disposable endotracheal tube. Anesth. Analg., 55:437, 1976.

52. Davies, R. M.: Faulty construction of a reinforced latex endotracheal tube. Br. J. Anaesth., 35:128, 1963.

53. Dorsch, J. A., and Dorsch, S. E.: Understanding Anesthesia Equipment. pp. 249–273. Baltimore, Williams & Wilkins, 1975.

54. Ketover, A. K., and Feingold, A.: Collapse of a disposable endotracheal tube by its high-pressure cuff. Anesthesiology, 45:108, 1975.

55. Kloss, J., and Petty, C.: Obstruction of endotracheal intubation by a mobile pedunculated polyp. Anesthesiology, 43:380, 1975.

56. Pryer, D. L., Pryer, R. R. L., and Williams, A. F.: Fatal respiratory obstruction due to faulty endotracheal tubes. Lancet, 2:742, 1960.

57. Robbie, D. S., and Pearce, D. J.: Some dangers of armored tubes. Anaesthesia, 14:379, 1959.

58. Rollason, W. N.: Asphyxia due to faulty apparatus. Br. Med. J., 1:658, 1956.

59. Stark, D. C. C.: Endotracheal tube obstruction. Anesthesiology, 45:467, 1976.

60. Aro, L., Takki, S., and Aronaa, V.: Technique for difficult intubation. Br. J. Anaesth., 41:1081, 1971.

61. Moorthy, S. S., Lo Sasso, A. M., King, H., et al.: Evaluation of larynx and trachea by xeroradiography. Anesth. Analg., 55:598, 1976.

62. Tahir, A. H.: Use of fibreoptic endoscope in difficult orotracheal intubation. Anesthesiology Review, 3:16, 1976.

63. Waters, D. J.: Guided blind endotracheal intubation. Anaesthesia, 18:158, 1963.

Appendix:
Syndromes Associated with
Upper Airway Abnormalities

DISORDER OR SYNDROME	CAUSE OF DIFFICULT INTUBATION	SALIENT FEATURES
Syndromes With Features of Micrognathia (Hypoplastic Mandible)		
Aglossia-adactylia[1]	Micrognathia Intraoral bands	Agenesis of distal limb segment (digits in particular) Dental anomalies
Aminopterin-induced[2]	Micrognathia	Low birth weight Cranial dysplasia Abnormal facies Limb anomalies
Arthochalasis multiplex congenita[3]	Micrognathia	Congenital joint flaccidity with recurrent dislocation Associated anomalies include hydrocephalus and deformed feet.
Arthrogryposis[4]	Hypoplastic mandible Temporomandibular fusion	Multiple joint contracture at birth
Bird-headed dwarf[5]	Micrognathia	Bird-headed appearance Low set ears Highly arched or cleft palate Genitourinary anomalies
C syndrome of multiple congenital anomalies[6]	Micrognathia	Short stature Hypoplastic metacarpals and phalanges Soft tissue syndactyly
Cerebro-costo-mandibular[7]	Micrognathia Inadequate tracheal airway due to insufficient support from partially collapsed tracheal cartilages	Dorsal rib gaps consisting of fibrous or cartilaginous tissues, causing respiratory distress due to flail chest

DISORDER OR SYNDROME	CAUSE OF DIFFICULT INTUBATION	SALIENT FEATURES
Syndromes With Features of Micrognathia (Hypoplastic Mandible) *(Continued)*		
Cornelia de Lange[8]	Micrognathia Occasionally, choanal atresia	Microbrachycephaly Characteristic facies (low hairline, heavy confluent eyebrows) Marked mental, motor, and social retardation Limb anomalies
Cri du chat[9]	Micrognathia	Severe growth and mental retardation Cat-like cry Muscular hypotonia Various central nervous system, cardiac, genitourinary, and vertebral anomalies
Diastrophic dwarfism[10]	Micrognathia Cervical kyphosis	Micromelic dwarfism Hitchhiker's thumb Flexion contractures in peripheral joints Scoliosis Deformed ear lobes
DiGeorge's[11]	Hypoplastic mandible	Unusual facies Hypocalcemic tetany in newborns Frequent respiratory infections Absent thymus Aortic arch anomalies, esophageal atresia, tracheal and esophageal fistulas, congenital heart disease
Goldenhar's[12]	Hypoplastic mandible	Epibulbar (lipo) dermoids Hypoplastic maxilla and temporal bones Vertebral anomalies
Hemifacial microsomia[13]	Unilateral micrognathia Unilateral neck shortness	Unilateral hypoplasia with aplasia of ear, preauricular skin tag Unilateral hypoplastic maxilla Rarely, pulmonary agenesis, on affected side
Idiopathic hypercalcemia[14]	Micrognathia	In infancy: anorexia, vomiting, constipation, hypotonia, physical retardation Supravalvular aortic stenosis Mental retardation
Klippel-Feil[15]	Short or "absent" neck Decreased mobility of head in patients with atlanto-occipital fusion Micrognathia	Fused cervical or cervicothoracic vertebrae Hemivertebrae Deafness (30%) Webbed neck Torticollis

Disorder or Syndrome	Cause of Difficult Intubation	Salient Features
	Syndromes With Features of Micrognathia (Hypoplastic Mandible) *(Continued)*	
Larsen's[16]	Micrognathia Floppy epiglottis, arytenoid and tracheal cartilage secondary to diminished cartilage rigidity	Dislocated elbows, hips and knees
Mickel's[17]	Micrognathia Short neck	Occipital encephalocele Cleft lip and palate Polydactyly Polycycstic kidneys Limb, cardiovascular, and gastrointestinal anomalies
Melnick-Needles[18]	Micrognathia	Failure to thrive Sclerosis at base of skull and mastoids Tall upper cervical vertebrae Metaphyseal flaring
Noonan's (Male-Turner)[19]	Micrognathia Short neck	Short stature with delayed puberty Many patients with mild mental retardation Epicanthal folds, ptosis of eyelids (60%) Congenital heart disease
Pierre Robin[20]	Micrognathia Glossoptosis	Cleft palate Limb anomalies Congenital heart disease
Smith-Lemeli-Opitz[21]	Micrognathia Short neck	Microcephaly with moderate to severe mental retardation Hypotonia at birth with progressive spasticity Genitourinary anomalies in males Other anomalies include cleft palate, cataract, syndactyl second and third toes
Treacher Collins[22]	Hypogenesis or agenesis of mandible Occasional choanal atresia	Hypoplastic malar bones Malformed ears with conductive deafness Antimongoloid slant Congenital heart disease Underdeveloped paranasal sinuses and mastoids
Trisomy 13[23]	Micrognathia	Typical facies: microcephaly, large broad nose, cleft lip and palate, hyper- or hypo-telorism, malformed and low-set ears, anophthalmia or microphthalmia Digital anomalies "Rocker-bottom" feet Severe mental retardation

DISORDER OR SYNDROME	CAUSE OF DIFFICULT INTUBATION	SALIENT FEATURES
Syndromes With Features of Micrognathia (Hypoplastic Mandible) *(Continued)*		
Trisomy 18[24]	Micrognathia Small triangular mouth with short upper lip	Physical and mental retardation Muscular hypertonicity Shield deformity of chest Second finger overlapping third Foot deformities ("rocker-bottom") Anomalies of cardiovascular, gastrointestinal, and genitourinary systems
Trisomy 22[25]	Micrognathia	Microcephaly Preauricular skin tags Cleft palate Mental and growth retardation Congenital heart disease
Turner's[26]	Relatively small mandible Short neck	Short stature Transient lymphedema of hands and feet in infancy Shield chest, widely spaced hypoplastic nipples Cubitus nalgus Congenital heart disease (coarctation of aorta, 15%) Ovarian dysgenesis Hearing defect
Ulrich-Feichtiger[27]	Micrognathia	Mask-like facies with depressed nose Eye anomalies External ear deformations, deafness Limb anomalies Genitourinary anomalies
Wolf's[28]	Micrognathia	Mental and growth retardation Craniofacial anomalies Cleft lip and/or cleft palate
Syndromes Characterized by Macroglossia and a Small Mouth		
Beckwith-Wiedemann[29]	Macroglossia	Omphalocele or umbilical hernia Gigantism with visceromegaly Hypoglycemia Malignant neoplasms
Cowden's (multiple hamartomas)[30]	Hypoplastic mandible Microstomia	Bird-like face Gastrointestinal polyps (in 50%) Breast, mucosal, and cutaneous lesions
Down's (mongolism)[31]	Microstomia Protruding tongue	Hypotonia Epicanthal folds Mental and motor retardation Congenital heart disease

Disorder or Syndrome	Cause of Difficult Intubation	Salient Features

Syndromes With Features of Micrognathia (Hypoplastic Mandible) (Continued)

Disorder or Syndrome	Cause of Difficult Intubation	Salient Features
Hurler's[32]	Macroglossia	Grotesque facial features Severe mental retardation Coarse hair, corneal opacities Thoracolumbar gibbus, flexion contractures Hepatosplenomegaly Deficiency of α-L-iduromidase
Kocher-Debré-Sémélaigne (cretinism with muscular hypertrophy)[33]	Large tongue	Myxedema Retarded intellectual, physical, osseous and dental development Generalized increase in muscle mass
Pompe's (glycogen storage disease Type III)[34]	Macroglossia	Hypotonicity Mental retardation Cardiomegaly Deficiency of α-1,4-glucosidase

Syndromes Characterized by Small Mouth and Other Abnormalities

Disorder or Syndrome	Cause of Difficult Intubation	Salient Features
Freeman-Sheldon (whistling face)[35]	Microstomia Short, broad neck Mild pterygium colli	Ulnar deviation bands, finger contractures, non-opposable thumbs
Glossopalatine ankylosis, microglossia, hypodontia, and anomalies of the extremities[36]	Attachment of tongue to hard palate or upper alveolar ridge Ankylosis of temporomandibular joint	Anomalies of the extremities
Grieg's[37]	Macroglossia	Ocular hypertelorism Mental retardation Webbed neck Congenital heart disease
Hallerman-Streiff[38]	Microstomia Micrognathia	Dyscephaly (scapho- or brachycephaly) Small face, small pinched nose Microophthalmia, blue sclerae Hypotrichosis Proportionate dwarfism
Otopalatodigital[39]	Microstomia	Frontal bossing, prominent occiput Cleft palate Deafness Carpal, tarsal, and digital anomalies

Syndromes Characterized by Temporomandibular Joint Dysfunction

Disorder or Syndrome	Cause of Difficult Intubation	Salient Features
Ophthalmo-mandibulo-melic[40]	Jaw anomalies Temporomandibular fusion, a lack of the carotid process, obtuse mandibular angle	Limb anomalies Blindness from corneal opacities

DISORDER OR SYNDROME	CAUSE OF DIFFICULT INTUBATION	SALIENT FEATURES
Syndromes With Features of Micrognathia (Hypoplastic Mandible) *(Continued)*		
Still's[41]	Fusion of cervical spine	Arthritis Fever, weakness, weight loss Pneumonitis, pericarditis
Temporomandibular joint[42]	Limitation of motion of temporomandibular joints	Pain and limitation of motion of temporomandibular joints Muscle spasm Degenerative changes in temporomandibular joints
Syndromes That May Prohibit Nasotracheal Intubation		
Choanal atresia[43]	Nasal passage obstruction	If bilateral, severe respiratory distress occurs, especially during feeding.
Crouzon's craniofacial dysostosis[44]	Narrow nasopharynx and oropharynx	Acrocephaly with parrot-beaked nose Hypertelorism with bilateral exophthalmos Airway obstruction with cor pulmonale
Syndromes in Which Stomatitis Is a Feature		
Behçet's[45]	Aphthous stomatitis	Genital ulcers Uveitis with hypopyon Enterocolitis with ulcerations (40%) Deep vein thrombosis, pulmonary embolism, intracranial thrombophlebitis
Letterer-Siwe[46]	Stomatitis	Hepatosplenomegaly Skin rash Fever Lymphadenopathy Bleeding, anemia

APPENDIX REFERENCES

1. Harwin, S. M.: Aglossia-adacylia syndrome. Am. J. Dis. Child., *119*:255, 1970.
2. Shaw, E. G.: Fetal damage due to maternal aminopterin ingestion. Am. J. Dis. Child, *124*:93, 1972.
3. Owen, J. R.: Generalized hypermobility of joints: arthrochalasis multiplex congenita. Arch. Dis. Child., *48*:487, 1973.
4. Poznanski, A. K.: Radiographic manifestations of the arthrogryposis syndrome. Radiology, *95*:353, 1970.
5. Harper, R. G.: Bird-headed dwarfs (Seckel's syndrome). J. Pediatr., *70*:799, 1967.
6. Opitz, J. M.: The C syndrome of multiple congenital anomalies. *In* Birth Defects. Original Article Series, vol. 5, part 2. p. 161. New York, The National Foundation—March of Dimes, 1969.
7. Smith, D. W.: Rib-gap defect with micrognathai, malformed tracheal cartilages, and redundant skin: a new pattern of defective development. J. Pediatr., *69*:799, 1966.
8. Gerald, B.: The Cornelia de Lange syndrome: radiographic findings. Radiology, *88*:96, 1967.
9. James, A. E., Jr.: The cri du chat syndrome. Radiology, *92*:50, 1969.
10. Spranger, J., Longer L., and Wiedemann, H. R.: Bone Dysplasia, An Atlas on Constitutional Disorders of Skeletal Development. p. 102. Philadelphia, W. B. Saunders, 1974.
11. Kirkpatrick, J. A.: Congenital absence of the thymus. Am. J. Roentgenol. Radium Ther. Nucl. Med., *103*:32, 1968.
12. Mellor, D. H.: Goldernhar's syndrome (oculo-auriculovertebral dysplasia). Arch. Dis. Child., *48*:537, 1973.
13. Gellis, S. S.: Picture of the mouth: hemifacial microsomia. Am. J. Dis. Child., *122*:58, 1971.

14. Garcia, R. E.: Idiopathic hypercalcemia and supravalvular aortic stenosis. N. Engl. J. Med., *271*:117, 1964.

15. Morrison, S. G.:Congenital brevicollis (Klippel-Feil syndrome) and cardiovascular anomalies. Am. J. Dis. Child., *115*:614, 1968.

16. Latta, R. J.: Larsen's syndrome: a skeletal dysplasia with multiple joint dislocation and unusual facies. J. Pediatr., *78*:291, 1971.

17. Opitz, J. M.: The Mickel's syndrome (dysencephalia splanchnocystica, the Gruher syndrome). The Clinical Delineation of Birth Defects, vol. 5, Part 2. p. 167. New York, The National Foundation–March of Dimes, 1969.

18. Gorlin, R. J.: Melnick-Needles (osteodysplastia). Modern Medicine, *41*:102, 1973.

19. Riggs, W.: Roentgen findings in Noonan's syndrome. Radiology, *36*:393, 1970.

20. Farnsworth, P. B.: Glossoptotic hypoxia and micrognathia: The Pierre Robin syndrome reviewed. Clin. Pediat., (Phila.), *10*:600, 1971.

21. Smith, D. W.: A newly recognized syndrome of multiple genital anomalies. J. Pediatr., *64*:210, 1964.

22. Pavsek, E. J.: Mandibulofacial dysostosis (Treacher Collins syndrome). Am. J. Roentgenol. Radium Ther. Nucl. Med., *79*:598, 1958.

23. James, A. E., Jr.: Trisomy 13–15. Radiology, *92*:44, 1969.

24. Ozonoff, M. B.: The trisomy 18 syndrome. Am. J. Roentgenol. Radium Ther. Nucl. Med., *91*:618, 1964.

25. Hsu, L. Y. F.: Trisomy 22: Clinical entity. J. Pediatr., *79*:12, 1971.

26. Gordon, R. R.: Turner's infantile phenotype. B. Med. J., *1*:483, 1969.

27. Lowry, R. B.: Micrognathia, polydactyly, and cleft palate. J. Pediatr., *72*:859, 1968.

28. Guthrie, R. D.: The 4 p-syndrome: a clinically recognizable chromosomal deletion syndrome. Am. J. Dis. Child., *122*:421, 1971.

29. Reddy, J. K.: Beckwith Wiedemann syndrome. Arch. Pathol., *94*:523, 1972.

30. Gentry, W. C.: Multiple hamartoma syndrome (Cowden disease). Arch. Dermatol., *109*:521, 1974.

31. Austin, J. H. M.: Short hard palate in newborn: roentgen sign of mongolism. Radiology, *92*:775, 1969.

32. Leroy, J. G.: Clinical definition of the Hurler-Hunter phenotypes: a review of 50 patients. Am. J. Dis. Child., *112*:518, 1966.

33. Najjar, S. S.: The Kocher-Debré-Semelaigne syndrome. J. Pediatr., *66*:901, 1965.

34. Nahill, M. R.: Generalized glycogenosis type II (Pompe's disease). Arch. Dis. Child., *45*:122, 1970.

35. Rintala, A. E.: Freeman-Sheldon's syndrome, craniocarpo-tarsal dystrophy. Acta Paediatr. Scand., *57*:553, 1968.

36. Wilson, R. A.: Ankyloglossia superior (palato-glossal adhesion in the newborn infant). Pediatrics, *31*:1051, 1963.

37. Pendl, G.: Grieg's hypertelorism syndrome. Hdv. Paediatr. Acta, *26*:319, 1971.

38. Streiff, E. B.: Dysmorphic mandibulo-faciale (tete d'oiseau) et alteration oculaire. Ophthalmolgica, *120*:79, 1950.

39. Gorlin, R. J.: Oto-palato-digital (OPD) syndrome. Am. J. Dis. Child., *114*:215, 1967.

40. Pillay, V. K.: Ophthalmo-mandibulo-melic dysplasia: an hereditary syndrome. J. Bone Joint Surg., *46A*:858, 1964.

41. Martel, W.: Roentgenologic manifestations of juvenile rheumatoid arthritis. Am. J. Roentgenol. Radium Ther. Nucl. Med., *88*:400, 1962.

42. Sutcher, J. D.: The temporomandibular syndrome. J.A.M.A., *225*:1248, 1973.

43. Williams, H. J.: Posterior choanal atresia. Am. J. Roentgenol. Radium Ther. Nucl. Med., *112*:1, 1971.

44. Crouzon, O.: Dysostose cranio-faciale hereditaire. Bull. Soc. Med. Hop. (Paris), *33*:545, 1912.

45. O'Duffy, J. D.: Behcet's disease: Report of 10 cases, 3 with new manifestations. Ann. Intern. Med., *75*:561, 1971.

46. Sutow, W., Vietti, T., and Fernback, D.: Clinical Pediatric Oncology, p. 337. St. Louis, C. V. Mosby, 1973.

FURTHER READING

Goodman, R. M., and Gorlin, R. J.: Atlas of the Face in Genetic Disorders. ed. 2. St. Louis, C. V. Mosby Company, 1977.

9 Laryngeal Complications of General Anesthesia

B. Raymond Fink, M.D., F.F.A.R.C.S.

The complications of anesthesia affecting the larynx are of two major kinds: functional and traumatic. Functional complications are often grouped together under *laryngospasm*, a loose term applied to any unwanted muscular response that produces partial or complete obstruction of the laryngeal airway. The functional responses are usually transient and are among the least studied consequences of general anesthesia, even though they are common and sometimes potentially life-threatening. A practical approach to their diagnosis and treatment should be based on functional anatomy.[1]

DYNAMIC ANATOMY

Anatomically, the human larynx is adapted to fit an ecological niche dependent on speech and on manual labor in the bipedal erect posture. Speech involves repeated phonation with closure of the lower larynx; heavy manual labor involves repeated straining effort, with closure of both the lower and upper larynx. To achieve these closures, there has evolved a folding mechanism composed of the vocal, vestibular, and aryepiglottic folds, the preepiglottic body, and their supporting cartilages. The process of folding requires transverse apposition of the arytenoids and vertical shortening, either at the vocal folds, as in phonation, or at the vestibular and preepiglottic folds (by approximation of the thyroid cartilage and hyoid bone), as in effort. Thyroid-hyoid approximation not only forces the vestibular folds medially but also forces the preepiglottic body backward against the top of these folds. This produces a type of closure sometimes compared to a ball valve, in contrast to the shutter-like closure of the vocal folds at the glottis. Unfolding of the larynx to the all important respiratory, open configuration is partly automatic, through recoil of various springs loaded during folding; the respiratory cycle itself is marked by rhythmical partial unfolding and folding of the laryngeal folds. At laryngoscopy, the respiratory cycle is most noticeable in the vocal folds, although all other folds attached to the arytenoids necessarily also participate in the cycle. Direct laryngoscopy is likely to give a distorted view of the normal relations. Fiberscopic examination reveals that, in reality, in eupneic respiration, the transverse entrance to the laryngeal passage may be almost as narrow as the lower, anteroposterior glottic gap.

GLOTTIC OBSTRUCTION

Laryngeal obstruction at the glottis may take place upon expiration or inspiration, or both. Such obstruction is incomplete, because the air pressure throws the vocal folds into vibration, producing a stridor of definite pitch. Expiratory glottic stridor is evidence of light anesthesia and can be stopped by discontinuing the stimulus or by inducing a deeper plane of anesthesia.

144

Inspiratory glottic stridor is thought to arise when laryngeal muscle activity is depressed in the present of active ventilation. The Bernoulli effect at the glottis, added to the inspiratory fall in pressure, brings the membranous vocal cords into apposition, most readily in children and small adults. Inspiratory glottic stridor can be overcome by keeping the cords separated during inspiration; separation is achieved by applying pressure on the rebreathing bag before the onset of inspiration, thereby preventing the development of "negative" pressure, or by lightening the plane of anesthesia, which will restore the tonic laryngeal muscle activity necessary for normal glottic airflow. The possibility of rare extralaryngeal causes of stridor, such as that associated with the Arnold-Chiari malformation, must be kept in mind.[2] Laryngeal stridor may sometimes be the principal sign of residual curarization.[3]

Occasionally, inspiratory laryngeal obstruction may be supraglottic, owing to indrawing of the aryepiglottic folds or impaction of the epiglottis into the entrance.[4] In rare instances, respiratory obstruction during induction of anesthesia may be caused by a tumor of the laryngeal inlet.[5]

COMPLETE LARYNGEAL OBSTRUCTION

Spastic closure of the larynx is a sustained reflex effort closure and will last as long as the stimulus continues, even to the point of fatal hypoxia. Such a spasm cannot be broken by forcible pressure from the rebreathing bag. Forcible inflation merely distends the piriform sinuses and forces the arytenoids and aryepiglottic folds more firmly together. The upper laryngeal closure between the epiglottic cartilage anteriorly and the corniculate and cuneiform tubercles and aryepiglottic and vestibular folds behind (Fig. 9-1) can be overcome by levering the mandible forward; this produces forward displacement of not only the tongue, but also the hyoid bone and the epiglottic cartilage attached to it. Forward subluxation of the mandible through pressure behind the angles of the jaw therefore not only widens the pharynx but also opens the entrance to the larynx. This familiar mandibular maneuver is effective in "breaking" the spasm by forcibly unfolding the

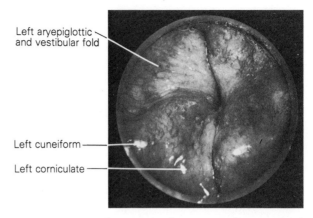

Left aryepiglottic and vestibular fold

Left cuneiform

Left corniculate

Fig. 9-1. Laryngeal spasm is shown in a photograph of the closed laryngeal entrance. The tubercle of the epiglottic cartilage has been forced up out of the picture by the laryngoscope. (Photograph by Dr. Paul Holinger. *In* Becker, W., Buckingham, R. A., Holinger, P. H., et. al.: Atlas of Otorhinolaryngology and Bronchoesophagoscopy. Stuttgart, Georg Thieme Verlag, 1969)

folds closing the upper larynx.[6] It is an excellent standby for infants, children, and patients in whom the anesthesiologist is able to overcome the force of the jaw muscles. This maneuver is always preferable to injudicious attempts to force a tube through a larynx that is tightly in spasm, which may result in pneumothorax[7] or a "burst" type of injury caused by excessive stretching of the tissue by the laryngoscope or tube.[8]

The simplest way to abolish the reflex is to discontinue the stimulation, whether it is a surgical procedure or a pharyngeal irritant, such as acid mucus or an artificial airway. Intravenous deepening of the plane of anesthesia will interrupt the reflex centrally, but peripheral block with succinylcholine is probably safer if artificial ventilation is practicable. The incidence of this complication at the end of anesthesia is best reduced by removing the endotracheal tube in a deep plane of anesthesia or after the patient has regained consciousness.

Intermittent effort closure occurs during coughing, and when an endotracheal tube is in the larynx, it is manifested as "bucking." It may progress to continuous effort closure, manifested as chest wall spasm and virtual obstruction of the bronchial passages. These responses are likely to cause damage to the laryngeal mucosa and give rise to reactive edema and airway obstruction postoperatively. It is particularly important to prevent such reactions in infants and small children, in whom a minor degree of edema may be a major encroachment of the passage.

TRAUMA

Numerous reports indicate that lesions of the larynx are not rare after endotracheal anesthesia. The larynx is open to injury at the time of insertion of the tube and remains vulnerable throughout the duration of intubation. The laryngoscope, tube, stylet, and spray nozzle are potential "weapons," but with the advent of short-acting muscular relaxants, in skilled and informed hands, these instruments no longer constitute a significant hazard to the larynx. Safe practice is based on gentleness, a knowledge of anatomy, common sense, and ever present awareness and avoidance of potential mishaps. Complete preparations include a choice of endotracheal tube sizes, preoxygenation, thorough relaxation, care in opening the mouth for orotracheal intubation, and pre-lubrication of the tube and the tip of the laryngoscope, enabling both to slide over the tissues with a minimum of friction.

The size of the tube should be at least one size smaller than the largest size possible. This is true even in children, because there is a danger of edema resulting from excessive pressure. Since the cricoid is the smallest part of an infant's airway, a tube that fits too snugly at the cords invites post-extubation subglottic edema. Use of a cuffed tube is inadvisable with a short trachea, because of the risk of pressure of the cuff in the subglottic region. It is always wise to avoid overinflation of the cuff; low pressure cuffs and relief valves have been designed. A practical, simple approach is to inflate the cuff to the point of no-leak and then to withdraw a small amount of air, which deliberately creates a slight leak around the cuff.

A stylet must never protrude from the endotracheal tube, or laceration of the vocal fold may result.[9]

The tubes used should be safety tested as recommended by Stetson: They must be supplied in a protective package and guaranteed to be sterile, nonpyrogenic, and compatible with long contact with tissues. Tubes should be marked with the designation "IT" or "Z-79"; *IT* stands for implantation tested, and *Z-79*, for Committee Z-79 (anesthesia equipment) of the U.S.A. Standards Institute. The presence of these designations indicates that the manufacturer has tested a sample from each lot manufactured, either by implantation in rabbit muscle or by a cell culture technique, and warrants the device to be free of any toxicity that can be shown by these tests. Plasticizers are added to plastics to control flexibility, stabilizers, to improve heat stability, and antioxidants, to prevent deterioration on exposure to oxygen. The additives are primary sources of tissue irritation. The physician must therefore insist that before it is sold, a polymeric or elastomeric device be tested for tissue compatibility under conditions of use.

It is now generally accepted that any object that must pass beyond the glottis should be treated as sterile." Use of equipment sterilized with ethylene oxide may be hazardous. For sterilization to be effective, there must be humidification. Ethylene oxide acts by alkylation and is absorbed by porous objects made of polymers and elastomers. An irritant film of ethylene glycol may be left on the surfaces of moist articles, including endotracheal tubes, and there may also be a surface residue of irritating detergent remaining from the cleansing operation that precedes autoclaving.

Post-extubation symptoms (Table 9-1) of hoarseness, sore throat, and even mild stridor are too often dismissed an inevitable, insignificant sequelae to intubation. Whether they resolve completely in the first 24 or 48 hours or, on the contrary, progress to more serious complications, depends on the severity of the trauma, the constitution of the patient, and the promptness and thoroughness of therapy.

Sore throat is the most common complaint after endotracheal intubation,[12] and it may be severe.[13] The incidence is increased when a cuffed tube is used and there is apparently no advantage

**Table 9-1. Post-intubation Symptoms:
Incidence in 521 Patients**

SYMPTOM	INCIDENCE (%)
Slight sore throat	16
Severe sore throat	3.3
Hoarseness	2.5
Sore throat and hoarseness	0.8
Lost voice	0.4
Incidence in females	27
Incidence in males	15

(Wolfson, B.: Minor laryngeal sequelae of endotracheal intubation. Br. J. Anaesth., *30:*326, 1958.)

to using a lubricant. The incidence of sore throat is particularly high following operations on the head and neck, although this is less true of operations in which the head is rigidly fixed. The use of a nasogastric tube is very likely to produce a sore throat.[14] Interestingly enough, Wylie noted that positive evidence of laryngeal trauma at the end of an operation does not necessarily mean that the patient will show symptoms of trauma.

The trauma of difficult intubation often occurs not at the vocal cords, but generally somewhat higher in the respiratory passages. Often, perhaps, this is not appreciated, except by anesthesiologists. In nasal intubations especially, the difficulty usually lies not in introducing the tube through the cords, but rather in placing the tube at the glottic opening.

The more common lesions are focal abrasion, hemorrhage, ulceration, and later, granuloma. Laceration of the larynx is a rare occurrence. The most serious complication is pseudomembranous laryngotracheitis, which if not immediately and appropraitely treated, may lead to sudden death of the patient. It is not necessarily a sequela to trauma; several well-documented cases have occurred following uneventful anesthesia, without known upper respiratory infection.[8]

The lowest grade injury is epithelial denudation of the vocal and vestibular folds, which is believed to occur more readily in women because of the thinness of the mucosa.[15] The thickness of the epithelium of the vestibular folds (false cords) averages 95 μm. in males and 85 μm. in females. For the vocal folds (true cords), the approximate

figures are 97 and 59 μm., respectively; and, in the subglottic area, 70 and 80 μm. There are no consistent variations with age.

Patients who succumb after surgery with endotracheal anesthesia show laryngeal lesions predominantly in the posterior subglottic region.[16,17] Hemorrhage and inflammation have been noted as early as 3.25 hours following extubation. Lateral partial or complete denudation of the epithelium and ulceration can be observed. Hyaline thrombi may be found in the neighboring blood vessels.

A fully formed pseudomembrane consists of a tubular cast conforming to the larynx and trachea. A cleavage plane appears in 48 hours and begins at the lower or tracheal end, where damage is more superficial and the membrane thinner and more easily detached. Adult post-intubation specimens were examined by Hilding after short-term intubation.[18] The most consistent evidence of trauma in the larynx was located posteriorly over the plate of the cricoid and over the arytenoids, especially the vocal processes. Desquamation was present in nearly all specimens and was greatest in patients who had undergone the longest periods of intubation. The lesions consisted of loss of part or all of the epithelium and, in some cases, included part of the submucosa. The most serious injury occurred in the posterior larynx, either from introduction of or from continued pressure by the tube during intubation or extubation. Hilding suggested that the tube commonly used in this country becomes, in effect, a curved lever when it is introduced into the trachea. Force applied at the proximal end lifts the distal end against the tracheal wall, while the posterior larynx, especially the arytenoid and cricoid cartilages, act as a fulcrum. The degree of trauma depends upon many factors: the size, shape and stiffness of the tube; the duration of intubation; the position of the head and movement between the tube and tissues; and the skill and gentleness of the anesthesiologist. Hilding showed that a cuff and swab, exerting a pressure of only 10 g. drawn once across the tracheal epithelium causes exfoliation down to and often including the basal layer of cells.

Paralysis of the vocal folds can occur as a

complication of intubation independently of operation on the neck.[19,20]

The reported cases followed operations lasting from 2 to 6 hours and were apparently sequelae of pressure from the tube or from the cuff, when paralysis was bilateral. Recently, Ellis has demonstrated anatomically how cuff pressure can produce recurrent nerve palsy.[21] Vocal paralysis is a grave complication, usually necessitating tracheostomy. Recovery of neural function takes several months.

Dislocation of the arytenoid following intubation has been reported.[22] The symptoms include hoarseness, deep voice, difficulty in swallowing, dull pain over the larynx, and inspiratory stridor, presenting on the first postoperative day. The affected cord is immobilized. The mechanism is obscure and does not necessarily represent an injury inflicted by the anesthesiologist,[22] although hooking of the arytenoid by the open end of the tube was cited by Wolfson.[23]

Johannsen claimed microtrauma was responsible for post-intubation edema observable on microlaryngoscopy.[24] Steroids are frequently administered empirically in the hope of aborting an inflammatory reaction. Hydrocortisone is given intravenously or intramuscularly, 1 hour before extubation, and cortisone acetate is given intramuscularly upon extubation and 8 and 16 hours later. Supporting experimental data have been sought. Steroids (dexamethasone) reduced the symptoms of edema in monkeys subjected to experimental intubation.[25] The anti-inflammatory effect of steroids was thought to be due to inhibition of local cellular damage and diminution of capillary dilatation and permeability.

Several techniques have been suggested to reduce the hazard of tracheal or laryngeal injury by the balloon cuff. These include the following: careful inflation of the cuff with a volume of air that is just sufficient to provide a seal with the tracheal wall; hourly deflation for 5 minutes; and alternating the site of contact by use of double cuffed tubes. The work of Bryant and colleagues suggests that careful inflation allowing an audible leak during inspiration may be the safest technique.[26] The investigators base this conclusion on a study of the condition of the mucosa and cartilage in experimental dogs.

INTUBATION GRANULOMA

The incidence of intubation granuloma, first reported by Clausen in 1932,[27] is generally estimated to be of the order of one case per 1000 endotracheal anesthesias.[28]

It must be remembered that granuloma of the vocal fold is often unrelated to intubation; even following intubation, the presence of granuloma is not of itself evidence of faulty anesthetic technique. Post-intubation laryngeal granulomas have been reported to occur in from one per 800[29] to one patient per 10,000 intubations.[30] Although laryngeal granulomas are most often found in women, they do occur in children.[31]

Contact ulcer granuloma is clearly distinguishable from post-intubation granuloma. Contact granuloma is caused by vocal fold trauma. It occurs most commonly in men and is a complication of contact ulcer. It is ascribable to misuse of the voice, which causes the cartilaginous vocal process of one arytenoid to hammer against the other. In Jackson's view, post-intubation granuloma is generally larger and broader and is found most often on the anterior third of the vocal process (Fig. 9-2).[32]

Post-intubation granulomas are thought to arise from minor or even microscopic abrasions of the delicate mucosa over the vocal process of the arytenoid cartilage that occur during intubation. The exposed surface then becomes infected. The abrasion forms an ulcer, which matures to a sessile granuloma as the denuded area becomes covered with granulation tissue in an attempt to cover the exposed cartilage. The lesion becomes an inflammatory polyp, or pyogenic granuloma, through central proliferation. It is generally 5 to 9 mm. in diameter.

Diagnosis of Intubation Granuloma

Symptoms depend on the size of the granuloma. They range from slight hoarseness and a feeling of a foreign body in the throat, to persistent sore throat, cough, and pain, to dysphonia and obstructed breathing. Occasionally, bloody sputum occurs. On the other hand, a small subglottic granuloma may be entirely symptomless. The patient's first complaint may be as early as 4 days or as late as 7 months after the anesthesia.

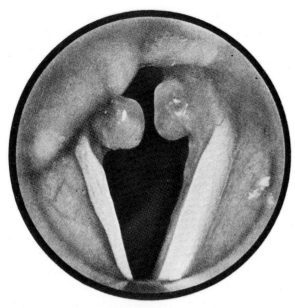

Fig. 9-2. Post-intubation granulomas of the vocal folds. Their position at the junction of the ligamentous (white) and cartilaginous portions of the folds is typical. (Becker, W., Buckingham, R. A., Holinger, P. H., et. al.: Atlas of Otorhinolaryngology and Bronchoesophagoscopy. Stuttgart, Georg Thieme Verlag, 1969)

Women are affected some five times as often as men.

Laryngoscopy reveals unilateral or bilateral tumor of the vocal fold at the vocal process of the arytneoid cartilage, near the junction of the middle and posterior third of folds.

Histological examination shows granulation tissue rich in capillaries, leukocytic infiltration. Progressive stages are edema or hematoma, fibrinous exudation and infiltration, and organization.

Etiology of Intubation Granuloma

Seven factors may contribute to the development of intubation granuloma:

Pressure exerted by the tube on the glottis leads to a lesion of the mucous membrane, at the unpadded processes vocalis, especially when the tube is of relatively big bore and remains in place a long time. The average reported duration of intubation is 2.5 hours.

Direct trauma during intubation may result in intubation granuloma.

Friction of the tube against the glottis is caused by the cyclic respiratory excursion of the carina, which may amount to several centimeters. The motion is communicated to the trachea and larynx, but not necessarily to a tube lying in the larynx, because the tube is usually immobilized by inertia, adhesive tape, or friction of the nasal passage. Frictional motion between the tube and larynx is likely to be aggravated by manipulations incident to neck operations, particularly thyroidectomy, by light narcosis, and by omission of tube lubricant.

The inherent curve of a Magill rubber tube brings the tip forward against the anterior tracheal wall. The use of plastic tubes capable of adapting to the sinuousities of the air passage minimizes this important source of pressure damage.

The position of the patient during narcosis plays a role, since over-extension of the neck tends to press the tube against the back of the glottis, again most often during thyroidectomy.[29] Often a pillow or sandbag placed under the shoulders of the patient displaces the larynx, so that the tube is forced against the posterior wall. Head and neck extension causes the infrahyoid respiratory passage to lengthen by nearly 1 cm. in adults and produces a distinct narrowing of the supraclavicular trachea. It does not prevent the inspiratory descent of the larynx, which remains observable in most subjects.[33] It is clear that extension tends to lever the tube backward against the arytenoid and increases the risk of contact pressure injury. It should be noted that the same risk does not apply to a rigid bronchoscope. The rigid tube lies more anteriorly in the glottic chink, and contact ulcer following its use is almost unknown.

Contusion of the vocal folds produced by collision during loud vocalization or coughing after removal of the tube is sometimes cited as a contributory factor.

Constitutional factors that predispose patients to intubation granuloma are related to nutrition, anemia, age, and sex. The preponderance of affected women can be attributed to the smallness of the larynx and the thinness of the mucoperichondrium. Furthermore, women are more likely to develop thyroid disorders than men.

Prophylaxis of Intubation Granuloma

Prevention of intubation granuloma is based on etiological considerations:

Antibiotic therapy should be considered following prolonged anesthesia.

The tracheal tube should be smooth and flexible, and its outer circumference should not exceed 38 mm. in men and 32 mm. in women.

The tube should be lubricated and sterile. In the event of accidental introduction into the esophagus, use of another tube is recommended.

Extension of the head after intubation should be avoided.

Surgical manipulation of the trachea should be gentle.

Relaxation should be complete. Extubation should be timed so as to avoid a paroxysm of coughing. If necessary, a small dose of succinylcholine can be administered prophylactically.

Persistent hoarseness after endotracheal anesthesia indicates that early consultation with a laryngologist is necessary.

Treatment of Intubation Granuloma

Treatment by voice conservation is difficult if the patient depends on his voice for livelihood. Voice rest after intubation is advisable if signs of laryngeal irritation are present postoperatively.[34]

Surgical removal of granuloma is curative and is necessary if danger of obstruction is to be avoided. It is easily performed by means of direct laryngoscopy during general anesthesia without intubation. The granuloma is, at first, sessile but may become pedunculated, and it may resolve itself by autoamputation. Some physicians consider strict voice rest to be the treatment of choice, as the polyp will eventually be ejected. Only when there is serious dyspnea should surgery be undertaken.

It seems that claims of negligence and lawsuits are not uncommon, even when the patient has made a complete recovery from a post-intubation granuloma, but particularly when it is unwisely managed. Close postoperative follow-up is the best protection. Barton has plausibly stated that the responsibility of the anesthesiologist ends only after the action of the drugs he has administered subsides. When complications arise from such administration, his responsibility continues until they have been obviated or properly treated.[34]

LARYNGEAL COMPLICATIONS OF GENERAL ANESTHESIA IN CHILDREN

In infants, acute lesions induced by endotracheal intubation can be classified into three types: Type I mucosal necrosis; Type II, mucosal and submucosal necrosis; and Type II, mucosal and submucosal necrosis with mild, moderate, or severe inflammation.[35] The minor lesions of Type I and those of Type II are observed in patients whose intubation lasts less than 1 hour. With longer intubations, the lesions became more severe and lead to such complications as laryngeal obstruction due to subglottic cyst, vocal cord scarring, and subglottic stenosis.

In older children, the most serious complications of endotracheal in tubation are laryngeal edema and tracheitis. The complication of subglottic edema occurs most frequently in children under 3 years of age. Onset after extubation is usually within 1 or 2 hours. As a rule, this is successfully managed by humidification, hydration, and antibiotics. Steroid therapy, though controversial, is probably helpful. Biller and associates determined experimentally that intravenous dexamethasone (4–8 mg.) prevented or hastened resolution of the edematous response to laryngeal edema.[25] (See p. 169.)

Intermittent positive pressure breathing (IPPB) combined with nebulized epinephrine may be life-saving and may change a potentially life-threatening process into a relatively benign post-anesthetic complication.[36] In children, as in adults, the incidence of all laryngeal complications can be lessened by exercising care and judgment, by the use of small sterile uncuffed tubes made of plastic, by atraumatic intubation, aseptic suction, control of infection, and by humidification with cool mist. Nebulized racemic epinephrine may be added to reduce vascular engorgement.

Spasm upon extubation is avoided by

extubating during a deep plane of anesthesia or, alternatively, as the child is waking up. A small dose of succinylcholine guarantees tranquil extubation.[37]

Long-term intubation for acute epiglottitis in children is now firmly established as a satisfactory therapy for this dangerous condition. Intubation can first be tested orally to judge the required size of tube; this should then be followed by nasal intubation, with a tube 0.5 or 1 mm. smaller. This procedure avoids all the risks and disadvantages of tracheostomy but demands skilled avoidance of laryngeal trauma.[38]

REFERENCES

1. Fink, B. R.: The Human Larynx. A Functional Study. p. 193. New York, Raven Press, 1975.
2. Fitzsimmons, J. S.: Laryngeal stridor and respiratory obstruction associated with myelomeningocele. Dev. Med. Child. Neurol., *15*:533, 1973.
3. Boliston, T. A.: Laryngeal stridor as a sign of residual curarization. Br. J. Anaesth. *43*:931, 1971.
4. Caiger, G. H., and Sichel, D. A. S.: Obstruction of the larynx during anaesthesia. Anaesthesia, *9*:177, 1954.
5. Reddy, A. R.: Unusual care of respiratory obstruction during induction of anaesthesia. Can. Anaesth. Soc. J., *19*:192, 1972.
6. Probyn-Williams, R. J.: A Practical Guide to the Administration of Anaesthetics. pp. 35–36. London, Longmans, Green & Co., 1971.
7. Kepes, E. R.: Pneumothorax complicating treatment of laryngeal spasm. N.Y. State J. Med., *72*:1848, 1972.
8. Komorn, R. M., Smith, C. P., and Erwin, J. R.: Acute laryngeal injury with shortterm endotracheal anesthesia. Laryngoscope, *83*:683, 1973.
9. Jaffe, B. F.: Postoperative hoarseness: Am. J. Surg., *123*:4 32, 1972.
10. Stetson, J. B., and Guess, W. L.: Causes of damage to tissues by polymers and elastomers used in the fabrication of tracheal devices. Anesthesiology, *33*:635, 1970.
11. Helliwell, P. J.: The sterilization and maintenance of apparatus. *In* Hewer, C. L. (ed.): Recent Advances in Anesthesia and Analgesia. ed 10. pp. 317–333. Boston, Little, Brown & Co., 1967.
12. Jones, G. O. M., Hale, D. E., Wasmuth, C. E., et al. A survey of acute complications associated with endotracheal intubation. Cleve. Clin. Q., *35*:23, 1968.
13. Wylie, W. D.: Hazards of intubation. Anaesthesia, *5*:143, 1950.
14. Brunelle, J. P., Boucher, J., Cossette, G., et al.: L'intubation orotracheale et les maux do gorge post-operatoires. Can. Anaesth. Soc. J., *8*:581, 1961.
15. Ryan, R. F., McDonald, J. R., and Devine, K. D.: Changes in laryngeal epithelium: relation to age, sex and certain other factors. Mayo Clin. Proc., *31*:47, 1956.
16. Lu. A. T., Tamura, Y., and Koobs, D. H.: The pathology of laryngotracheal complications. Arch. Otolaryngol., *74*:323, 1961.
17. Stein, A. A., Quebral, R., Boba, A., et al.: A post morten evaluation of laryngotracheal alterations associated with intubation. Ann. Surg., *151*:130, 1960.
18. Hilding, A. C.: Laryngotracheal damage during intratracheal anesthesia. Ann. Otol. Rhinol. Laryngol., *80*:565, 1971.
19. Holley, H., and Gildea, J. E.: Vocal cord paralysis after tracheal intubation. J.A.M.A., *215*:281, 1971.
20. Hahn, F. W., Martin, J. T., and Lillie, J. C.: Vocal cord paralysis with endotracheal intubation. Arch. Otolaryngol., *92*:226, 1970.
21. Ellis, P. D. M., and Pallister, W. K.: Recurrent laryngeal nerve palsy and endotracheal intubation. J. Laryngol. Otol., *89*:823, 1975.
22. Schultz-Coulon, H. J.: Luxation des arytaenoidknorpels als intubationsschaden. H. N. O., *22*:242, 1974.
23. Wolfson, B.: Minor laryngeal sequelae of endotracheal intubation. Br. J. Anaesth., *30*:326, 1958.
24. Johannsen, H. S., and Pascher, W.: Stimmstorungen durch mikrotraumen des larynx bei intubation. Arch. Otorhinolaryngol., *202*:597, 1972.
25. Biller, H. F., Harvey, J. E., Bone, R. C., et al.: Laryngeal edema. An experimental study. Ann. Otol. Rhinol. Laryngol., *79*:1084, 1970.
26. Bryant, L. R., Trinkle, J. K., and Dubilier, L.: Reappraisal of tracheal injury from cuffed tracheostomy tubes. J.A.M.A., *215*:625, 1971.
27. Clausen, R. J.: Unusual sequela of tracheal intubation. Proc. R. Soc. Med., *25*:1507, 1932.
28. Hefter, E.: Das intubationsgranulom. Anaesthetist, *8*:194, 1959.
29. Howland, W. S., and Lewis, J. S.: Mechanisms in the development of postintubation granulomas of the larynx. Ann. Otol. Rhinol. Laryngol., *65*:1006, 1956.
30. Snow, J. C., Harano, M., and Balogh, K.: Postintubation granuloma of the larynx. Anesth. Analg., *45*:425, 1966.
31. Schlorf, R. A., and Duval, A. J.: Post-intubation granuloma of the larynx. Minn. Med., *52*:717, 1969.
32. Jackson, C.: Contact ulcer granuloma and other laryngeal complications of endotracheal anesthesia. Anesthesiology, *4*:425, 1953.
33. Harris, R. S.: The effect of extension of the head and neck upon the infrahyoid respiratory passage and the supraclavicular portion of the human trachea. Thorax, *14*:176, 1959.
34. Barton, R. T.: Medicolegal aspects of intubation granuloma. J.A.M.A., *166*:1821, 1958.
35. Joshi, V. V., Mandavia, S. G., Stern, L., et al.: Acute lesions induced by endotracheal intubation. Am. J. Dis. Child., *124*:646, 1972.
36. Jordan, W. S., Graves, C. L., and Elwyn, R. A.: New therapy for postintubation laryngeal edema and tracheitis in children. J.A.M.A., *212*:585, 1970.
37. Komesaroff, D.: Extubation spasm. Anaesth. Intens. Care., *1*:443, 1973.
38. Markham, W. G., Blackwood, M. J. A., and Conn, A. W.: Prolonged intubation in infants and children. Can. Anaesth. Soc. J., *14*:11, 1967.

10 Pulmonary Aspiration of Gastric Contents

Tamas Kallos, M.D., Kenneth F. Lampe, Ph.D., and Fredrick K. Orkin, M.D.

Pulmonary aspiration of stomach contents is one of the most serious complications of the obtunded or unconscious state, which includes anesthesia. Vomiting or regurgitation with subsequent aspiration may be responsible for a considerable morbidity and mortality among obstetrical, surgical, and intensive care patients. Understanding the factors that predispose to aspiration is essential for the prevention of this complication.

PATHOPHYSIOLOGY OF PULMONARY ASPIRATION

Gastric contents may reach the pharynx as a result of active vomiting or passive regurgitation and be aspirated into the airway when the protective laryngeal reflexes are depressed. Vomiting requires coordinated muscle contraction and may occur during a stormy anesthetic induction, during maintenance of anesthesia when the anesthetic depth is insufficient, and during emergence from anesthesia (see Chap. 31). Regurgitation, more common than vomiting during anesthesia, is a passive process governed by pressure differences between the stomach and the pharynx. Silent regurgitation may occur in many patients without any clinical symptoms or signs. There are numerous factors which by themselves or in combination increase the chance of regurgitation and aspiration.[1]

Regurgitation

For regurgitation to occur, two basic and interrelated conditions must be present: increased intragastric pressure and incompetence of the gastroesophageal valvular mechanism.

Increased intragastric pressure may be present when there is delayed gastric emptying. Gastric emptying time may be prolonged by pain, anxiety, trauma, obstetrical labor, pyloric or intestinal obstruction, pressure by an intra-abdominal mass or ascites, systemic toxicity, metabolic derangements, increased intracranial pressure, and the administration of narcotic analgesics and parasympathomimetic drugs. Thus, in the pregnant patient at term, gastric emptying may be delayed by mechanical obstruction of the duodenum, endocrine depression of motility and relaxation of the gastroesophageal sphincter, anxiety, pain, and analgesic drugs (Fig. 10-1). Gastric emptying returns to normal about 8 hours postpartum. Narcotics, such as morphine and meperidine, and scopolamine, alone and in combination, double and even triple the gastric emptying time in dogs.[2,3]

Intestinal obstruction or impaired peristalsis can result in the accumulation of massive amounts of swallowed air and gastric secretions. Patients with duodenal ulcer can secrete and retain as much as 2 L. of gastric fluid overnight.[4] Similarly, 75 per cent of obese patients in the supine position have gastric fluid volumes in

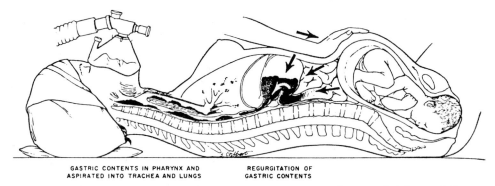

GASTRIC CONTENTS IN PHARYNX AND
ASPIRATED INTO TRACHEA AND LUNGS

REGURGITATION OF
GASTRIC CONTENTS

Fig. 10-1. Pulmonary aspiration of gastric contents during obstetrical delivery following regurgitation caused by marked increase in intraabdominal and intragastric pressure, (From Bonica, J.J.: Principles of Obstetric Analgesia and Anesthesia. Philadelphia, F.A. Davis Company, 1967)

excess of 25 ml. with a pH below 2.5,[5] a volume and level of acidity considered necessary for the development of Mendelson's syndrome (see p. 154). Fasting gastric fluid volume (and pH) varies greatly in normal persons, often being as much as 400 ml. in persons with gastrointestinal disease, particularly duodenal ulcer,[6] and in outpatients.[7] Preanesthetic doses of atropine (0.–1.0 mg.), scopolamine (0.5 mg.), and glycopyrrolate (0.2 mg.) do not decrease the proportion of adult patients whose gastric fluid contents place them at risk for Mendelson's syndrome.[8,9] Recent ingestion of food, swallowing of blood from nasal or esophageal bleeding, and aerophagia from anxiety may also distend the stomach, causing increased intragastric pressure.

Muscular fasciculation from succinylcholine given prior to tracheal intubation raises intragastric pressure sufficiently to render the gastroesophageal valve incompetent;[10–13] it may be prevented by pretreatment with a small dose of non-depolarizing neuromuscular blocking drug.[12] Succinylcholine administration in children does not raise the intragastric pressure, probably because sufficiently vigorous fasciculations do not occur.[13] (See Chap. 45.)

Gastroesophageal valve incompetence may also be present when the stomach is distended, in patients with a hiatus hernia with a short esophagus, a nasogastric tube, scleroderma or other collagen vascular diseases, those with pernicious anemia, abdominal masses including a pregnant uterus, and in patients of advanced age.[14,15] In addition, the gastroesophageal junction opens transiently during periods of respiratory obstruction in anesthetized patients.[16] Gastroesophageal sphincter tone may also decrease as anesthesia is deepened and neuromuscular block is intensified.[17] Although it had been commonly believed that atropine increases the tone of the lower esophagus,[18,19] recent studies have demonstrated that atropine in clinical doses administered intravenously *lowers* the tone at the gastroesophageal junction.[20–22] This effect can be countered by the administration of metoclopramide[22–25] and by cholinergic stimulation (e.g., bethanechol, anticholinesterase agents such as edrophonium).[26] A wide variety of other agents also produce decreased tone in the gastroesophageal valve, including ethanol, cigarette smoking, theophylline, alpha adrenergic antagonists (e.g., phentolamine), beta adrenergic agonists (e.g., isoproterenol),[14] and a fatty meal.

Laryngeal Incompetence

The lungs are generally well protected from regurgitated stomach contents by reflex closure of the glottis in response to a wide variety of noxious stimuli. However, this protective airway reflex dulls progressively with advancing age,[27] accounting for occasional aspiration in the alert person.[28] Depression of this reflex also occurs following the administration of ketamine,[29] methohexital,[30] neuroleptanalgesia,[31] and trans-laryngeal block.[32] In one study, the intravenous injection of 2 ml. of Innovar did not depress the glottic reflex; however, the authors caution that there may be considerable individual variation in response.[32] Inhalation of 50 per cent nitrous oxide from a loosely fitting nasal mask for dental analgesia may[33] or may not[34] be associated with a low incidence of aspiration. Although the effects of general anesthetics on the glottic reflex have not been studied extensively, the depression of the reflex produced lasts at least 2 and possibly as long as 8 hours following extubation, even in patients who appear alert.[35] There is evidence that the depressant effect is due also in part to tracheal intubation itself, as distinct from residual anesthesia.[36]

Types of Pulmonary Aspirate

Because the clinical consequences and treatment differ considerably, a distinction between the aspiration of particulate matter and liquid must be made.

Aspiration of particulate matter results in acute airway obstruction. Depending on the size of the particles, a main stem bronchus or smaller bronchi may become occluded. When a large area of the lung is affected, acute asphyxiation may occur. In the awake person, laryngeal or tracheal obstruction caused by a large piece of food may cause aphonia, respiratory distress, and sudden death, which in an older person may simulate an acute myocardial infarction (cafe coronary).[37,38] Following the obstruction of smaller bronchi by smaller particles, the gradual absorption of air from the affected area results in distal atelectasis, with or without mediastinal shift, and arterial oxygen desaturation from the resultant right-to-left shunt. In untreated, infection of the atelectatic area may result in pneumonia and lung abscess. If the particles aspirated are very small, airway obstruction does not occur immediately. Instead, there is a combination of edema and hemorrhage in the affected area, followed by a slowly developing granulomatous response.[39]

Aspiration of liquid gastric contents is a more common occurrence. Its consequences depend on the volume of aspirated material, its *p*H, and whether it is loaded with bacteria, as in the case of intestinal obsturction. The classic description of acid aspiration pneumonitis was first provided by Mendelson in 1946,[40] although others had reported cases earlier without making a distinction between acid and nonacid aspiration.[41–43] He observed that obstetric patients who aspirated gastric contents would present differing clinical pictures depending upon the nature and acidity of the aspirated material; he distinguished between the obstructive symptoms resulting from the aspiration of solids and the asthma-like response following the inhalation of stomach acid. The importance of *p*H was confirmed by several animal studies.[44–46] Aspiration of liquid material having a *p*H value below 2.5 results in a severe chemical burn of the tracheobronchial tree and leads to the Mendelson or acid aspiration syndrome.[44,45,47] Although the volume of gastric acid required to produce Mendelson's syndrome in humans is unknown, 1 ml./kg. of gastric juice injected into the trachea of dogs results in the syndrome, with little increase in severity following larger doses.[45] Teabeaut[44] and Roberts[48] suggest that a minimum of 25 ml. of fluid with a *p*H of less than 2.5 is required to produce Mendelson's syndrome in a healthy adult. Aspiration of materials whose *p*H is above 2.5 results in a much milder clinical course. Inhalation of feculent material almost invariably leads to death.

The pathologic changes following liquid aspiration depend on both the *p*H and the volume of the aspirated material. Aspiration of a small amount of acid material may result in a laryngotracheobronchitis manifested by hoarseness and sore throat. Larger volumes of aspirate penetrate further distally into the lung, preferentially into dependent lung areas. Chemical irritation and injury to the bronchial, bronchiolar, and alveolar lining cells results in exudation with erythrocytes and edema, with formation of hyaline membranes.[49] Animal studies suggest that thrombosis of the small pulmonary vessels may also occur.

The clinical illness of a patient who has recently aspirated acid stomach contents is characterized by the triad of tachycardia, tachypnea, and cyanosis. These are signs of arterial hypoxemia from increased ventilation-perfusion abnormalities and atelectasis, and a marked decrease in lung compliance produced by loss of surfactant. Initially, arterial hypoxemia with respiratory and metabolic acidosis is characteristic. Wheezing and coarse and fine rales in the dependent areas of the lung may be present. In severe cases, systemic arterial hypotension with pulmonary arterial hypertension and pulmonary edema can occur. Radiologically, liquid aspiration is characterized by a diffuse, patchy, pulmonary infiltrate, usually confined to the dependent areas.

INCIDENCE OF AND MORTALITY FROM PULMONARY ASPIRATION

Like other anesthetic complications, pulmonary aspiration is not a reportable event; hence, there is no registry of cases upon which to estimate incidence. The estimates from individual hospitals suffer from the relatively small numbers of cases, from differing amounts of effort expended to identify such cases, and the fact that many cases of aspiration are mild or inapparent (see next section).

"Silent" Regurgitation and Aspiration

Several investigators have introduced dye in the stomach preoperatively and inspected the patient's pharynx, larynx, and trachea at the end of surgery for the presence of the dye in an attempt to identify factors associated with aspiration during anesthesia.[50–54] Overall, they found a 14 to 26 per cent incidence of regurgitation; although no aspiration occurred in one study,[53] its incidence ranged from 7 to 20 per cent in the others. "Silent" aspiration was noted in 6 to 8 per cent of patients.[51,52]

Despite the fact that these studies were uncontrolled with respect to the presence of individual factors, some general comments may be made about the factors influencing regurgitation and aspiration in anesthetized patients. Prolonged induction or excitement is associated with inci-

dence of regurgitation and aspiration of 12 and 24 per cent, respectively, twice the rate noted during smooth inductions.[52] Swallowing, salivation, retching, and frank vomiting are particularly ominous signs.[50,52]

Anesthetic agent itself has a small effect, given the agents currently in use. The incidence of regurgitation and aspiration with halothane-nitrous oxide (8 and 3%, respectively)[54] is lower than those of nitrous oxide-thiopental (17 and 9%, respectively)[52] and of nitrous oxide-relaxant-narcotic (11% for both).[54] Considerably higher incidences were associated with diethyl ether anesthesia.[50,51] These different incidences may be reconciled by considering associated factors. For example, ether anesthesia was associated with a prolonged and often stormy induction that favors regurgitation and aspiration. Similarly, halothane is associated with a deeper level of anesthesia than nitrous oxide-relaxant techniques, which also impart periodic diaphragmatic (and, thus, gastroesophageal sphincter) relaxation.

Patient position is an important variable because gravity may enhance regurgitation. Not unexpectedly, the prone, lateral, and Trendelenburg positions are associated with higher incidences of regurgitation (as high at 50%);[51–53] aspiration in these positions was noted in 8 to 15 per cent of patients when anesthesia was administered by mask or tracheal tube without a cuff[51,52] and, in one study, never when a cuffed tracheal tube was used.[53]

Presence of a cuffed tracheal tube is a very important factor that was underemphasized in the early studies. A tracheal tube without a cuff was associated with a *higher* incidence of regurgitation and aspiration than when anesthesia was administered by mask.[51,52] Regurgitation probably occurs more often in these patients as a result of the muscle relaxation obtained to facilitate tracheal intubation. Once the cuffless tube is in place, it acts as a wick, allowing regurgitated material to flow into the trachea. Although the use of an inflatable cuff may result in laryngeal and tracheal trauma (Chaps. 9 and 11), it affords great protection against aspiration. Moreover, the use of a high-volume, low-pressure cuff is associated with a lower incidence of aspiration than the older, low-volume, high-pressure cuffs that do not conform as well to the tracheal lumen. In the intensive care unit, such low-pressure cuffs are associated with a 20 per cent incidence of aspiration.[55] However, an overly large cuff diameter relative to tracheal diameter, producing invaginations in the cuff, especially with cuff material so rigid that such invaginations do not collapse easily, may contribute to aspiration in spontaneously breathing patients.[56] In order to minimize aspiration with these newer cuffs while avoiding excessive inflation pressures that cause mucosal damage, a reservoir inflation pressure-regulating valve may be needed.[57]

Prognosis After Documented Aspiration

In contrast to those cases in which aspiration is inapparent is the grave prognosis of aspiration that is observed or documented by suctioning gastric contents from the tracheobronchial tree. Three surveys among general hospital populations indicate that the overall mortality of documented aspiration is 55 to 70 per cent.[45,57,58] One study noted that injury to only one lobe is associated with a 41 per cent mortality, whereas more extensive involvement has 86 to 100 per cent mortality.[58]

The Role of Aspiration in Maternal Mortality

Largely through the work of regional maternal mortality commissions we have some estimates of mortality due to aspiration in at least one admittedly high-risk population. Surveys conducted during the past 25 years suggest that anesthesia accounts for about 10 per cent of maternal deaths,[60] with aspiration accounting for 52 per cent of these anesthetic deaths in one large study.[61] Given a maternal death rate of 3.3 per 10,000 live births[60] and about 3.3 million live births[62] in the United States, one may estimate that aspiration results in about 100 maternal deaths per year.[63] However, recognizing that many aspiration-related deaths may be missed, others have suggested that the true number of such deaths may be twice as large.[64] Particularly alarming in British data are the *rising* maternal mortality related to anesthesia in the 1960s and the fact that anesthesia contributes to 25 per cent of maternal deaths associated with cesarean section. The rate of cesarean section is also rising.[60]

The Role of Aspiration in Surgical Mortality

Here the data are limited largely to a British survey of 1,000 deaths associated with anesthesia that noted that aspiration accounted for 10.0 per cent of surgical deaths, with 75 per cent of these deaths involving abdominal surgery.[61] Strangulated hernia was involved in 18 per cent, peritonitis in 11 per cent, and intestinal obstruction in 8 per cent, with assorted other catastrophes comprising the majority of the abdominal category. A common factor in such situations is delayed gastric emptying.

TREATMENT OF PULMONARY ASPIRATION

The overall success of treatment depends upon prompt recognition of the aspiration and the immediate institution of vigorous measures to relieve respiratory obstruction, thereby assuring adequate gas exchange and minimizing damage to the lung.

Clearing The Airway

If vomiting occurs or regurgitation is suspected, the mouth, pharynx, and trachea should be suctioned immediately to minimize the amount that can be aspirated. Tracheal suctioning also stimulates coughing and may help confirm the diagnosis of pulmonary aspiration. Patency of the airway should be assured so that high concentrations of oxygen can be administered immediately. When aspiration appears to have occurred, tracheal intubation should not be delayed. This will facilitate clearing of the airway, as well as the administration of oxygen and controlled ventilation.

Solid material aspirated into the airway requires prompt removal by bronchoscopy. In the event of aspiration of liquid stomach contents, suctioning should be performed to decrease pulmonary damage.[65] However, mucosal damage occurs within seconds, and bronchial secretions neutralize the aspirated acid within minutes. Thus, attempts to neutralize or dilute acid aspirate by lavage of the airways are useless and may result in further spreading of the damage, particularly when large volumes are used.[66,67] Small volumes (e.g., 5–10 ml.) of saline may be introduced into the airway, however, to facilitate suctioning.

Oxygenation

The main thrust of treatment after clearing the airway is directed toward maintaining adequate oxygenation and removing carbon dioxide. Arterial blood gas studies are important in following the patient's progress.

Following a minor aspiration, administration of oxygen by face mask or nasal cannula may assure an adequate arterial oxygen tension. However, in more severe cases where hypoxemia and carbon dioxide retention are present, the patient is best managed in an intensive care unit with tracheal intubation and assisted mechanical ventilation.

When large degrees of right-to-left shunt are present, positive end-expiratory pressure (PEEP) has been found helpful in improving oxygenation and allowing for lower inspired oxygen concentrations.[68] Caution is necessary with high levels of PEEP that can aggravate the pulmonary damage by causing increased transudation of fluid through injured capillary beds.[69,70] Moreover, survival may not be affected by PEEP, but rather appears related to the severity of the hypoxemia prior to the institution of PEEP.[71] Commonly associated with PEEP, pneumothorax occurs more frequently in patients with aspiration pneumonitis than in other patients receiving ventilatory support, *regardless* of whether PEEP is used.[72] In extreme cases where the lung is severely damaged and unable to maintain acceptable oxygen tensions, an extracorporeal oxygenator has been used but without improvement in survival.[73]

Bronchospasm may be treated by application of PEEP and when necessary with administration of aminophylline. A dose of 500 mg. of aminophylline may be given by slow intravenous administration.

Corticosteroids

Whether corticosteroids are efficacious in minimizing the pulmonary damage resulting from aspiration of acid gastric contents is controversial. The rationale for their use is itself controversial and rests upon the ability of steroids to decrease inflammation, stabilize lysosomal membranes,[74,75] prevent leukocyte and platelet agglutination,[76] and shift the oxyhemoglobin dissociation curve to the right (increasing oxygen release in the periphery).[77]

In one study, the intratracheal administration of hydrocortisone in cats, minutes after acid aspiration, resulted in marked improvement in the gross and microscopic appearance of the lungs.[78] However, these results could not be confirmed.[46]

Numerous studies have reported a beneficial effect of parenteral steroid administration.[65,66,79–81] Yet, these studies have important defects in experimental design that make interpretation difficult and render their conclusions tenuous at best.[68] Three recent, well-designed studies have failed to demonstrate a beneficial effect of methylprednisolone on morphologic changes or survival rates following experimental aspiration of acid.[82–84] Much less is known about the efficacy of steroids following other types of aspiration where there is less theoretical rationale for their use. In a recent study of the effect of methylprednisolone upon experimental aspiration of acid plus particulate matter, there was not only no evidence of a beneficial effect but some suggestion of interference with the healing process.[39]

Hence, no firm experimental basis exists upon which to recommend the use of steroids following aspiration. Steroids are often used in hope of lessening pulmonary inflammation and treating bronchospasm because of clinical recommendations made during the past three decades.[1,85–91] Though dosages vary, typically hydrocortisone 200 mg. is given intravenously, with 100 mg. every 6 hours intramuscularly; to avoid sodium retention, dexamethasone (10 mg. I.V., then 5 mg.

I.M. q6h) may be substituted. Most of the recommendations stress the institution of therapy immediately following aspiration if steroids are to be beneficial, and discontinuing them after 48 hours to minimize the increased risks of secondary bacterial infection and steroid-induced electrolyte imbalance. Given these risks and the lack of beneficial effect in clinical situations,[59,92] steroids should not be used indiscriminately as part of therapy. Perhaps steroid therapy will be found efficacious for some subset of patients (e.g., those with severe bronchospasm).

Antibiotics

Despite recommendations in the past[58,93–95] the administration of *prophylactic* antibiotics is now almost uniformly condemned because of the ease with which antibiotic-resistant hospital pathogens may invade the damaged lung. With the exception of aspiration of feculent gastric contents in intestinal obstruction, which contains gram-negative organisms, gastric fluid is generally sterile. Hence, not unexpectedly, there is either no demonstrable beneficial effect of prophylactic antibiotics following aspiration[59,92] or bacterial infection follows with organisms often resistant to the administered antibiotics.[47,49,95] The type of infection is influenced by host resistance and the predominant bacterial flora of the hospital environment.

Hence, with the exception of aspiration of obviously infected material (e.g., feculent aspirant, carious teeth, pus from pharyngeal abscess), antibiotics should be reserved for the treatment of the *secondary* infection that commonly develops following aspiration. Temperature elevation alone is not sufficient cause for therapy; leukocytosis, pulmonary infiltrates, and thick sputum may also be nonspecific responses to chemical pneumonitis.[68] When such signs of infection become evident, cultures for both aerobic and anaerobic organisms should be obtained before the administration of antibiotics. Whether to begin antibiotic therapy, as well as the choice of agent(s) should be based upon well collected smears. Therapy should be adjusted appropriately when culture and sensitivity reports become available.

General Supportive Measures

An absolutely essential part of therapy is frequent suctioning of the airway. Repositioning of the patient at intervals and chest physiotherapy will help reduce further complications in dependent portions of the lungs. Because intravascular volume may decrease following aspiration[46,47,49] and patients requiring prolonged mechanical ventilation tend to accumulate fluid,[97] intravenous fluid therapy should be monitored carefully with intake and output measurements, as well as daily weighings, if possible. When pulmonary edema occurs, the administration of albumin and diuretics (but not digitalis) may be beneficial.[98–100]

PREVENTION OF PULMONARY ASPIRATION

Because of the potential serious morbidity and high mortality after aspiration of gastric contents one cannot emphasize sufficiently the importance of prevention of aspiration.

General Considerations

Appreciation of the risk of aspiration in medical, surgical, and, particularly, obstetrical patients who have predisposing factors (see p. 152) is the initial first step in the prevention of aspiration. Those patients with impaired airway reflexes and especially those with depressed states of consciousness should be placed in the lateral position with, if possible, a head-down tilt to enable secretions and regurgitated or vomited gastric contents to drain from the pharynx (Fig. 10-2). Caution should be exercised with drugs having sedative properties to avoid further impairment of the protective airway reflexes. Similarly, caution is required when restarting oral intake in patients who have had tracheal intubation, because protective airway reflexes may be impaired for as long as 8 hours following extubation, even though the patient is alert.[36]

Decreasing gastric fluid volume by gentle suction applied to a nasogastric or wide bore stomach tube can remove large volumes of fluid and air from those patients predisposed to gastric retention. Because such tubes interfere with the nor-

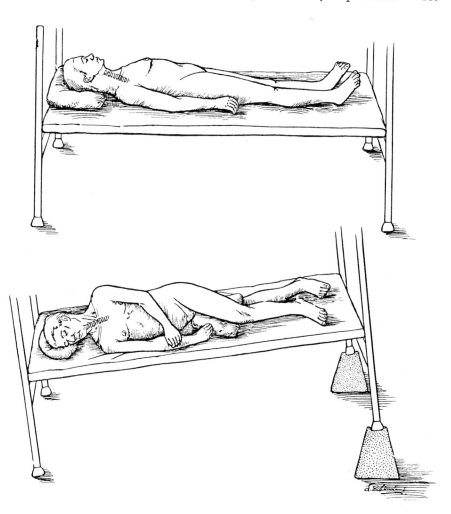

Fig. 10-2. The position of the trachea with changes in position of the unconscious patient. (A) In the supine position, in the absence of protective airway reflexes, pooling of secretions occurs and aspiration of regurgitated or vomited gastric contents is encouraged. (B) In the lateral position with head-down tilt, tracheal pooling and aspiration is less likely. (From Cameron, J.L., and Zuidema, G.D.: Aspiration pneumonia: magnitude and frequency of the problem. J.A.M.A., 219:1194, 1972)

mal valvular mechanism of the gastroesophageal junction, they should be removed just prior to the induction of anesthesia. Similarly, in those patients about to undergo anesthesia, emetics such as apomorphine[101,102] and delaying elective surgery (e.g., increasing the length of preoperative fasting)[103,104] have also been suggested as additional ways to empty the stomach prior to the administration of the anesthetic. More recently, the administration of cimetidine has been recommended to decrease gastric acid secretion (see next section). Although these measures reduce gastric volume and thereby intragastric pressure, *they do not ensure an empty stomach.*

Raising gastric pH was first suggested by Mendelson almost 35 years ago as a means of decreasing the injury following aspiration,[40] but there has been interest in this preventive approach only relatively recently following a British study of women in labor; the study demonstrated that following magnesium trisilicate no patient had a gastric-fluid pH value below 2.5, whereas 42 per cent of those patients who had not received the antacid had pH values below 2.5.[105] Similar effectiveness has been noted in patients who received 10 ml. of magnesium trisilicate within 30 minutes of elective surgery.[106,107] Although magnesium trisilicate is less commonly present in antacid preparations available in the United States, a variety of antacids have been found almost as effective in raising gastric pH in obstetrical and surgical patients.[8,108-111] Despite the introduction of antacids, except for an occasional hospital survey,[106] there is no evidence that Mendelson's syndrome occurs less frequently or with less severity.[112] Accounting in part for this apparent paradox are the problems encountered in discussing the incidence of aspiration already mentioned on page 155. Also, aspirated food particles may be irritating to the bronchial mucosa regardless of pH,[39] antacids may not mix adequately with the gastric fluid (especially if the gastric fluid volume is large and no suctioning is instituted), antacids may increase gastric fluid volume,[8] and antacids themselves may cause some degree of pneumonitis.[111,113] Overall, antacid administration represents one of the most promising preventive measures but aspiration pneumonitis may still occur.

Although anticholinergic premedication does not materially decrease gastric fluid volume,[8,9] the administration of atropine, 0.4–1.0 mg., scopolamine, 0.5 mg., or glycopyrrolate, 0.2 mg., can raise gastric pH somewhat.[9,114] The effect is small, with perhaps a third of patients who receive such premedicants having a gastric pH value below 2.5, compared to about half of those who received a placebo.

A premedicant much more effective in decreasing gastric fluid volume and pH is cimetidine.[115–117] This drug, which may be administered orally or intravenously, reduces gastric acid secretion by 90 per cent within an hour and maintains this level for 5 hours. The gastric fluid pH is increased to 5.0 or greater, with 84 to 100 per cent of patients who receive 300 mg. within 90 minutes of anesthesia having a gastric fluid pH value above 2.5.[116–118] In addition to reduced acidity, cimetidine also causes a significant reduction of total volume of gastric secretions.[119] However, it may still be too soon to know whether this new drug has undesirable effects relevant to anesthesia. In patients with delayed gastric emptying, cimetidine requires supplementation with antacids to neutralize the retained acid.

Considerations for Emergency Surgery

Any patient presenting for emergency surgery must be regarded as having a "full stomach."

Included among this group are those patients who are predisposed to regurgitation and aspiration (see p. 152) and who may be having elective surgery, as well as *all* obstetric patients in their third trimester. To the extent that time may permit, the general preventive measures just discussed should be exercised. However, when there is no time to empty the stomach (e.g., prolapsed umbilical cord, rupturing aortic aneurysm), a nasogastric tube should be passed and suction applied before the end of the anesthetic.[119a]

Consider local or regional anesthesia whenever possible to reduce the risk of aspiration. It should be remembered, however, that the danger of aspiration still exists with heavy sedation, toxic reactions to the local anesthetic (see Chap. 4), or when an unintentionally high level of spinal or epidural analgesia is produced (see Chap. 5).

Consider awake intubation in patients in whom tracheal intubation is likely to be technically difficult or especially hazardous (i.e., facial trauma, active gastrointestinal bleeding, neonate). Awake intubation may be accomplished easily in the obtunded patient without sedation. In others, judicious sedation insufficient to produce unconsciousness or depression of protective airway reflexes may be administered intravenously to relieve some of the stress of the procedure. Topical anesthesia may be applied to the tongue and pharynx, but the vocal cords and trachea are best not anesthetized.

Rapid induction with intravenous agents, followed immediately by tracheal intubation, is preferable when regional anesthesia or awake intubation are not possible. Although aspiration may occur during any part of a general anesthetic, the most dangerous periods are induction and emergence. During induction, every attempt should be made to minimize the time during which the airway is unprotected and to introduce a cuffed tracheal tube that should remain in place until the patient regains the protective airway reflexes. Although there are many variations in the technique, the typical induction and intubation proceed as follows:[120] The patient receives 3 mg. of d-tubocurarine (or 20 mg. of gallamine or 1 mg. of pancuronium) intravenously and then breathes 100 per cent oxygen at a flow rate greater than 6.1 per minute through a tight-fitting mask (a transparent one, if possible, to permit prompt recognition of regurgitation and aspiration[121]). Preoxygenation should continue at least 3 minutes without assisted or controlled ventilation (to avoid inflating the stomach). An assistant injects 250 mg. of thiopental and immediately thereafter 80 to 100 mg. of succinylcholine. In patients who are hypovolemic, ketamine in a dosage of 1 to 2 mg./kg. may be substituted for the barbiturate. In situations where succinylcholine is relatively contraindicated (i.e., lacerated globe), pancuronium (0.1 mg./kg.) may be substituted (with the omission of the defasciculating dose of curare), although the conditions for intubation are likely to be somewhat poorer.[122] When spontaneous respiration ceases, tracheal intubation is performed with a lubricated stylet within the lumen of the trachel tube. Upon passage of the tube through the vocal cords, the assistant promptly inflates the tracheal cuff.

At one time (when cyclopropane was in common use), inhalation rather than intravenous induction of general anesthesia was advocated for the patient at risk from aspiration. Once a quiet, smooth induction had been attained, the patient breathed spontaneously until an adequate depth of anesthesia for laryngoscopy and tracheal intubation had been achieved. This technique is probably no safer than an intravenous induction and requires more skill; hence the decline in its use.

Cricoid pressure (Sellick's maneuver[123]) is an effective adjunct to the safe induction of general anesthesia in these patients.[124] As soon as the patient loses consciousness, the assistant exerts firm pressure on the cricoid cartilage, occluding the esophagus between the trachea and vertebral column (Fig. 10-3). The effectiveness of this technique is impaired by the presence of a nasogastric tube, and esophageal rupture can occur if active vomiting occurs while cricoid pressure is applied.[125]

Head-up tilt of 30 to 40 degrees is another adjunct to the induction of general anesthesia that decreases the likelihood of stomach contents regurgitating into the pharynx. However, if such material reaches the pharynx, aspiration is more

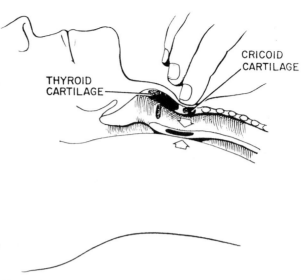

Fig. 10-3. Posterior pressure on the cricoid cartilage (Sellick's maneuver) occludes the esophagus and thereby prevents regurgitation. (From Hamelberg, W., and Bosomworth, P.P.: Aspiration Pneumonitis. p. 26. Springfield, Charles C. Thomas, 1968)

likely (if cricoid pressure is not applied). Also, patients who are hypovolemic may not tolerate this position prior to induction or may suffer further hypotension with induction; this problem can be decreased by simultaneously raising the legs about 10 degrees.

REFERENCES

1. Bannister, W. K., and Sattilaro, A. J.: Vomiting and aspiration during anesthesia. Anesthesiology, *23*:251, 1962.
2. Chase, H. F.: Role of delayed gastric emptying time in etiology of aspiration pneumonia. Am. J. Obstet. Gynecol., *56*:673, 1948.
3. Weiner, N.: Atropine, scopolamine, and related antimuscarinic drugs. In Gilman, A. G., Goodman, L. S., and Gilman, A. (eds.): The Pharmacological Basis of Therapeutics, ed. 6, pp. 120–137. New York, Macmillan, 1980.
4. Olson, W. H., and Bridgwater, A. B.: Noctural and insulin gastric secretion. J.A.M.A., *154*:977, 1954.
5. Vaughan, R. W., Bauer, S., and Wise, L.: Volume and *p*H of gastric juice in obese patients. Anesthesiology, *43*:686, 1975.
6. Brock-Utne, J. G., Moshal, M. G., Downing, J. W., *et al.*: Fasting volume and acidity of stomach contents associated with gastrointestinal symptoms. Anaesthesia, *32*:749, 1977.
7. Ong, B. Y., Palahniuk, R. J., and Cumming, M.: Gastric volume and pH in out-patients. Can. Anaesth. Soc. J., *25*:36, 1978.

8. Stoelting, R. K.: Response to atropine, glycopyrrolate, and Riopan of gastric fluid pH and volume of adult patients. Anesthesiology, 48:367, 1978.
9. Mirakhur, R. K., Reid, J., and Elliot, J.: Volume and pH of gastric contents following anticholinergic premedication. Anaesthesia, 34:453, 1979.
10. Anderson, N.: Changes in intragastric pressure following the administration of suxamethonium: preliminary report. Br. J. Anaesth., 34:363, 1962.
11. Roe, R. B.: The effect of suxamethonium on intragastric pressure. Anaesthesia, 17:179, 1962.
12. Miller, R. D., and Way, W. L.: Inhibition of succinylcholine-induced increased intragastric pressure by nondepolarizing muscle relaxants and lidocaine. Anesthesiology, 34:185, 1971.
13. Salem, M. R., Wong, A. Y., and Lin, Y. H.: The effect of suxamethonium on the intragastric pressure in infants and children. Br. J. Anaesth., 44:166, 1972.
14. Castell, D. O.: The lower esophageal sphincter: physiologic and clinical aspects. Ann. Intern. Med., 83:390, 1975.
15. Cohen, S.: Motor disorders of the esophagus. N. Engl. J. Med., 301:184, 1979.
16. Sinclair, R. N.: Oseophageal cardia and regurgitation. Br. J. Anaesth., 31:15, 1959.
17. Marchand, P.: The gastro-oesophageal 'sphincter' and the mechanism of regurgitation. Br. J. Surg., 42:504, 1955.
18. Clark, C. G., and Riddoch, M. E.: Observations on the human cardia at operation. Br. J. Anaesth., 34:875, 1962.
19. Ambache, N.: The use and limitations of atropine for pharmacological studies on autonomic effects. Pharmacol. Rev., 7:467, 1955.
20. Skinner, D. B., and Camp, T. F.: Relation of esophageal reflux to lower esophageal sphincter pressures decreased by atropine. Gastroenterology, 54:543, 1968.
21. Lind, J. F., Crispin, J. S., and McIver, D. K.: The effect of atropine on the gastroesophageal sphincter. Can. J. Physiol. Pharmacol., 46:233, 1968.
22. Brock-Utne, J. C., Rubin, J., Downing, J. W., et al.: The administration of metoclopramide with atropine. Anaesthesia, 31:1186, 1976.
23. Biancani, P., Zabinski, M. P., and Behar, J.: Pressure, tension, and force of closure of the human lower esophageal sphincter and esophagus. J. Clin. Invest., 56:476, 1975.
24. Stanciu, C., and Bennett, J. R.: Metoclopramide in gastroesophageal reflux. Gut, 14:275, 1973.
25. Dilawari, J. B., and Misiewicz, J. J.: Action of oral metaclopramide on the gastroesophageal junction in man. Gut, 14:380, 1973.
26. Roling, G. T., Farrell, R. L., and Castell, D. O.: Cholinergic response of the lower esophageal sphincter. Am. J. Physiol., 222:967, 1972.
27. Pontoppidan, H., and Beecher, H. K.: Progressive loss of protective reflexes in the airway with the advance of age. J.A.M.A., 174:2209, 1960.
28. Clark, M. M.: Aspiration of stomach contents in a conscious patient: a case report. Br. J. Anaesth., 35:133, 1963.
29. Taylor, P. A., and Towey, R. M.: Depression of laryngeal reflexes during ketamine anaesthesia. Br. Med. J., 2:688, 1971.
30. Wise, C. C., Robinson, J. S., Heath, M. J., et al.: Physiological response to intermittent methohexitone for conservative dentistry. Br. Med. J., 2:540, 1969.
31. Brock-Utne, J. G., Winning, T. J., Rubin, J., et al.: Laryngeal incompetence during neuroleptanalgesia in combination with diazepam. Br. J. Anaesth., 48:699, 1976.
32. Claeys, D. W., Lockhart, C. H., and Hinkle, J. E.: The effects of transtracheal block and Innovar on glottic competence. Anesthesiology, 38:485, 1973.
33. Rubin, J., Brock-Utne, J. G., Greenberg, M., et al.: Laryngeal incompetence during experimental "relative analgesia" using 50% nitrous oxide in oxygen. Br. J. Anaesth., 49:1005, 1977.
34. Cleaton-Jones, P.: The laryngeal-closure reflex and nitrous oxide-oxygen analgesia. Anesthesiology, 45:569, 1976.
35. Tomlin, P. J., Howarth, F. H., and Robinson, J. S.: Postoperative atelectasis and laryngeal incompetence. Lancet, 1:1402, 1968.
36. Burgess, G. E. III, Cooper, J. R., Jr., Marino, R. J., et al.: Laryngeal competence after tracheal extubation. Anesthesiology, 45:73, 1979.
37. Haugen, R. K.: The cafe coronary: sudden deaths in restaurants. J.A.M.A., 186:142, 1963.
38. Irwin, R. S., Ashba, J. K., Braman, S. S., et al.: Food asphyxiation in hospitalized patients. J.A.M.A., 231:2744, 1977.
39. Wynne, J. W., Reynolds, J. C., Hood, C. I., et al.: Steroid therapy for pneumonitis induced in rabbits by aspiration of foodstuff. Anesthesiology, 51:11, 1979.
40. Mendelson, C. L.: Aspiration of stomach contents into the lungs during obstetrical anesthesia. Am. J. Obstet. Gynecol., 52:191, 1946.
41. Hall, C. C.: Aspiration pneumonitis. An obstetric hazard. J.A.M.A., 114:728, 1940.
42. Irons, E. E., and Apfelbach, C. W.: Aspiration bronchopneumonia with special reference to aspiration of stomach contents. J.A.M.A., 115:584, 1940.
43. Gardner, A. M. N., and Pryer, D. L.: Historical and experimental study of aspiration of gastric and oesophageal contents into the lungs in anaesthesia. Br. J. Anaesth., 38:370, 1966.
44. Teabeaut, J. R. II: Aspiration of gastric contents. An experimental study. Am. J. Pathol., 28:51, 1952.
45. Awe, W. C., Fletcher, W. S., and Jacob, S. W.: The pathophysiology of aspiration pneumonitis. Surgery, 60:232, 1966.
46. Taylor, G., and Pryse-Davies, J.: Evaluation of endotracheal steroid therapy in acid pulmonary aspiration syndrome (Mendelson's syndrome). Anesthesiology, 29:17, 1968.
47. Lewis, R. T., Burgess, J. H., and Hampson, L. G.: Cardiorespiratory studies in critical illness. Arch. Surg., 103:335, 1971.
48. Roberts, R. B., and Shirley, M. A.: Reducing the risk of acid aspiration during cesarean section. Anesth. Analg., 53:859, 1974.
49. Greenfield, L. J., Singleton, R. P., McCaffree, D. R., et al.: Pulmonary effects of experimental graded aspiration of hydrochloric acid. Ann. Surg., 170:74, 1969.
50. Weiss, W. A.: Regurgitation and aspiration of gastric contents during inhalation anesthesia. Anesthesiology, 11:102, 1950.

51. Culver, G. A., Makel, H. P., and Beecher, H. K.: Frequency of aspiration of gastric contents by the lungs during anesthesia and surgery. Ann. Surg., *133*:289, 1951.

52. Berson, W., and Adriani, J.: "Silent" regurgitation and aspiration during anesthesia. Anesthesiology, *15*:644, 1954.

53. Turndorf, H., Rodis, I. D., and Clark, T. S.: "Silent" regurgitation during general anesthesia. Anesth. Analg., *53*:700, 1974.

54. Blitt, C. D., Gutman, H. L., Cohen, D. D., *et al.*: "Silent" regurgitation and aspiration during general anesthesia. Anesth. Analg., *49*:707, 1970.

55. Spray, S. B., Zuidema, G. D., and Cameron, J. L.: Aspiration pneumonia. Incidence of aspiration with endotracheal tubes. Am. J. Surg., *131*:701, 1976.

56. Pavlin, E. G., Van Nimwegan, D., and Hornbein, T. F.: Failure of high-compliance low-pressure cuff to prevent aspiration. Anesthesiology, *42*:216, 1975.

57. Bernhard, W. N., Cottrell, J. E., Sivakumaran, C., *et al.*: Adjusting of intracuff pressure to prevent aspiration. Anesthesiology, *50*:363, 1979.

58. Dines, D. E., Titus, J. L., and Sessler, A. D.: Aspiration pneumonitis. Mayo Clin. Proc., *45*:347, 1970.

59. Cameron, J. L., Mitchell, W. H., and Zuidema, G. D.: Aspiration pneumonia. Clinical outcome following documented aspiration. Arch. Surg., *106*:49, 1973.

60. Roberts, R. B.: Aspiration and its prevention in obstetrical patients. Int. Anesthesiol. Clin., *15*(1):49, 1977.

61. Edwards, G., Morton, H. J. V., Pask, E. A., *et al.*: Deaths associated with anaesthesia. A report on 1,000 cases. Anaesthesia, *11*:194, 1956.

62. Hospital Statistics. Table 1, p. 4. Chicago, American Hospital Association, 1978.

63. Merrill, R. B., and Hingson, R. A.: Studies of incidence of maternal mortality from aspiration of vomiting during anesthesia occurring in major obstetric hospitals in the U.S. Anesth. Analg., *30*:121, 1951.

64. Phillips, O. C., Frazier, T. M., Davis, G., *et al.*: The role of anesthesia in obstetric mortality. Anesth. Analg., *40*:557, 1961.

65. Hamelberg, W., and Bosomworth, P. P.: Aspiration pneumonitis: experimental studies and clinical observations. Anesth. Analg., *43*:669, 1964.

66. Bannister, W. K., Sattilaro, A. J., and Otis, R. D.: Therapeutic aspects of aspiration pneumonitis in experimental animals. Anesthesiology, *22*:440, 1961.

67. Wamberg, K., and Zeskow, B.: Experimental studies on the course and treatment of aspiration pneumonia. Anesth. Analg., *45*:230, 1966.

68. Wynne, J. W., and Modell, J. H.: Respiratory aspiration of stomach contents. Ann. Intern. Med., *87*:466, 1977.

69. Toung, T., Saharia, P., Permutt, S., *et al.*: Aspiration pneumonia: beneficial and harmful effects of positive end-expiratory pressure. Surgery, *82*:279, 1977.

70. Kudsk, K. A., Pflug, B., and Lower, B. D.: Value of positive end-expiratory pressure in aspiration pneumonia. J. Surg. Res., *24*:321, 1978.

71. Springer, R. R., and Stevens, P. M.: The influence of PEEP on survival of patients in respiratory failure: A retrospective analysis. Am. J. Med., *66*:196, 1979.

72. de Latorre, F. J., Tomasa, A., Klamburg, J., *et al.*: Incidence of pneumothorax and pneumomediastinum in patients with aspiration pneumonia requiring ventilatory support. Chest, *72*:141, 1977.

73. Workshop on Mechanisms of Acute Respiratory Insufficiency (DHEW Pub. No. (NIH) 77-981). Washington, D. C., Government Printing Office, 1976.

74. Janoff, A., Weissmann, G., Zweifach, B. W., *et al.*: Pathogenesis of experimental shock. IV. Studies on lysosomes in normal and tolerant animals subjected to lethal trauma and endotoxemia. J. Exp. Med., *116*:451, 1962.

75. Starling, J. R., Rudolf, L. E., Ferguson, W., *et al.*: Benefits of methylprednisolone in the isolated perfused organ. Ann. Surg., *177*:566, 1973.

76. Wilson, J. W.: Treatment or prevention of pulmonary cellular damage with pharmacologic doses of corticosteroid. Surg. Gynecol. Obstet., *134*:675, 1972.

77. Bryan-Brown, C. W. Baek, S., Makabali, G., *et al.*: Consumable oxygen: availability of oxygen in relation to oxyhemoglobin dissociation. Crit. Care Med., *1*:17, 1973.

78. Lewinski, A.: Evaluation of methods employed in the treatment of the chemical pneumonitis of aspiration. Anesthesiology, *26*:37, 1965.

79. Lawson, D. W., Defalco, A. J., Phelphs, J. A., *et al.*: Corticosteroids as treatment for aspiration of gastric contents: an experimental study. Surgery, *59*:845, 1966.

80. Bosomworth, P. P., and Hamelberg, W.: Etiologic and therapeutic aspects of aspiration pneumonitis. Experimental study. Surg. Forum, *13*:158, 1962.

81. Dudley, W. R., and Marshall, B. E.: Steroid treatment for acid-aspiration pneumonitis. Anesthesiology, *40*:136, 1974.

82. Downs, J. B., Chapman, R. L., Jr., Modell, J. H., *et al.*: An evaluation of steroid therapy in aspiration pneumonitis. Anesthesiology, *40*:129, 1974.

83. Chapman, R. L., Jr., Downs, J. B., Modell, J. H., *et al.*: The ineffectiveness of steroid therapy in treating aspiration of hydrochloric acid. Arch. Surg., *108*:858, 1974.

84. Chapman, R. L., Jr., Modell, J. H., Ruiz, B. C., *et al.*: Effect of continuous positive-pressure ventilation and steroid on aspiration of hydrochloric acid(pH 1.8) in dogs. Anesth. Analg., *53*:556, 1974.

85. Hausmann, W., and Lunt, R. L.: Problems of treatment of peptic aspiration pneumonia following obstetric anaesthesia (Mendelson's syndrome). J. Obstet. Gynaecol. Br. Commonw., *62*:509, 1955.

86. Marshall, B. M., and Gordon, R. A.: Vomiting, regurgitation and aspiration in anaesthesia. Can. Anaesth. Soc. J., *5*:274, 1958.

87. Dines, D. E., Baker, W. G., and Scantland, W. A.: Aspiration pneumonitis—Mendelson's syndrome. J.A.M.A., *176*:229, 1961.

88. Graham, E. C., and Choy, D.: Corticosteroids in aspiration pneumonia. J.A.M.A., *184*:976, 1963.

89. Vandam, L. D.: Aspiration of gastric contents in the operative period. N. Engl. J. Med., *273*:1206, 1965.

90. Marx, G. F.: Aspiration pneumonitis. J.A.M.A., *201*:129, 1967.

91. McCormick, P. W.: Immediate care after aspiration of vomit. Anaesthesia, *30*:658, 1975.

92. Bynum, L. J., and Pierce, A. K.: Pulmonary aspiration of gastric contents. Am. Rev. Respir. Dis., *114*:1129, 1976.

93. Ribaudo, C. A., and Grace, W. J.: Pulmonary aspiration. Am. J. Med., *50*:510, 1971.

94. Tinstman, T. C., Dines, D. E., and Arms, R. A.: Postoperative aspiration pneumonia. Surg. Clin. North Am., 53:859, 1973.

95. Arms, R. A., Dines, D. E., and Tinstman, T. C.: Aspiration pneumonia. Chest, 65:136, 1974.

96. Petersdorf, R. G., Curtin, J. A., Hoeprich, P. D., et al.: A study of antibiotic prophylaxis in unconscious patients. N. Engl. J. Med., 257:1001, 1957.

97. Sladen, A., Laver, M. B., and Pontoppidan, H.: Pulmonary complications and water retention in prolonged mechanical ventilation. N. Engl. J. Med., 279:448, 1968.

98. Skillman, J. J., Parikh, B. M., and Tanenbaum, B. J.: Pulmonary arteriovenous admixture. Improvement with albumin and diuresis. Am. J. Surg., 119:440, 1970.

99. Toung, T. J. K., Bordos, D., Benson, D. W., et al.: Aspiration pneumonia: experimental evaluation of albumin and steroid therapy. Ann. Surg., 183:179, 1976.

100. Geer, R. T., Soma, L. R., Barnes, C., et al.: Effects of albumin and/or furosemide therapy on pulmonary edema induced by hydrochloric acid aspiration in rabbits. J. Trauma, 16:788, 1976.

101. Holmes, J. A.: The prevention of inhaled vomit during anaesthesia. J. Obstet. Gynecol Br. Commonw., 63:239, 1956.

102. Crawford, J. S.: Anaesthesia for caesarean section: a proposal for evaluation with analysis of a method. Br. J. Anaesth., 34:179, 1962.

103. Stevens, J. H.: Anaesthetic problems of intestinal obstruction in adults. Br. J. Anaesth., 36:438, 1964.

104. Inkster, J. S.: The induction of anaesthesia in patients likely to vomit with special reference to intestinal obstruction. Br. J. Anaesth., 35:160, 1963.

105. Taylor, G., and Pryse-Davies, J.: The prophylactic use of antacids in the prevention of the acid aspiration syndrome. Lancet, 1:288, 1965.

106. Hutchinson, B. R., and Newson, A. J.: Pre-operative neutralization of gastric acidity. Anaesth. Intens. Care, 3:198, 1975.

107. Newson, A. J.: The effectiveness and duration of preoperative antacid therapy. Anaesth. Intens. Care, 5:214, 1977.

108. Roberts, R. B., and Shirley, M. A.: The obstetrician's role in reducing the risk of aspiration pneumonitis, with particular reference to the use of oral antacids. Am. J. Obstet. Gynecol., 124:611, 1976.

109. Hester, J. B., and Heath, M. L.: Pulmonary acid aspiration syndrome: should prophylaxis be routine? Br. J. Anaesth., 49:595, 1977.

110. White, F. A., Clark, R. B., and Thompson, D. S.: Preoperative oral antacid therapy for patients requiring emergency surgery. South. Med. J., 71:177, 1978.

111. Wheatley, R. G., Kallus, F. T., Reynolds, R. C., et al.: Milk of magnesia is an effective preinduction antacid in obstetric anesthesia. Anesthesiology, 50:514, 1979.

112. Scott, D. B.: Mendelson's syndrome. Br. J. Anaesth., 50:81, 1978.

113. Kuchling, A., Joyce, T. H., and Cooke, S.: The pulmonary lesion of antacid aspiration (abstr.). American Society of Anesthesiologists, Annual Meeting, p. 281, 1975.

114. Baraka, A., Saab, M., Salem, M. R., et al.: Control of gastric acidity by glycopyrrolate premedication in the paturient. Anesth. Analg., 56:642, 1978.

115. Henn, R. M., Isenberg, J. I., Maxwell, V., et al.: Inhibition of gastric acid secretion by cimetidine in patients with duodenal ulcer. N. Engl. J. Med., 293:371, 1977.

116. Stoelting, R. K.: Gastric fluid pH in patients receiving cimetidine. Anesth. Analg., 57:675, 1978.

117. Husemeyer, R. P., Davenport, H. T., and Rajasekaran, T.: Cimetidine as a single oral dose for prophylaxis against Mendelson's syndrome. Anaesthesia, 33:775, 1978.

118. Maliniak, K., and Vakil, A. H.: Pre-anesthetic cimetidine and gastric pH. Anesth. Analg., 58:309, 1979.

119. Coombs, D. W., Hooper, D., and Colton, T.: Pre-anesthetic cimetidine alteration of gastric fluid volume and pH. Anesth. Analg., 58:183, 1979.

119a. Arandia, H. Y., and Grogono, A. W.: Comparison of the incidence of combined "risk factors" for gastric acid aspiration: influence of two anesthetic techniques. Anesth. Analg., 59:862, 1980.

120. Stept, W. J., and Safar, P.: Rapid induction/intubation for prevention of gastric-contents aspiration. Anesth. Analg., 49:633, 1970.

121. Stetson, J. B.: Patient safety: Prevention and prompt recognition of regurgitation and aspiration. Anesth. Analg., 53:142, 1974.

122. Barr, A. M., and Thornley, B. A.: Thiopentone and pancuronium crash induction. A comparison with thiopentone and suxamethonium. Anaesthesia, 33:25, 1978.

123. Sellick, B. A.: Cricoid pressure to control regurgitation of stomach contents during induction of anaesthesia. Lancet, 2:404, 1961.

124. Fanning, G. L.: The efficacy of cricoid pressure in preventing regurgitation of gastric contents. Anesthesiology, 32:553, 1970.

125. Spence, A. A., Moir, D. D., and Finlay, W. E. I.: Observations on intragastric pressure. Anaesthesia, 22:249, 1967.

125a. Whittington, R. M., Robinson, J. S., and Thompson, J. M.: Fatal aspiration (Mendelson's) syndrome despite antacids and cricoid pressure. Lancet, 2:228, 1979.

126. Snow, R. G., and Nunn, J. F.: Induction of anaesthesia in the foot-down position for patients with a full stomach. Br. J. Anaesth., 31:493, 1959.

FURTHER READING

Hamelberg, W., and Bosomworth, P. P.: Aspiration Pneumonitis. Springfield, Charles C. Thomas, 1968.

Bonica, J. J.: Principles and Practice of Obstetrical Analgesia and Anesthesia. Chapter 39. Philadelphia, F. A. Davis Company, 1969.

Mendelson, C. L.: The aspiration of stomach contents into the lungs during obstetric anesthesia. Am. J. Obstet Gynecol., 52:191, 1946.

Roberts, R. B. (ed.): Pulmonary aspiration. Int. Anesthesiol. Clin., 15(1):1, 1977.

Wynne, J. W., and Modell, J. H.: Respiratory aspiration of stomach contents. Ann. Intern. Med., 87:466, 1977.

11 Hazards of Tracheal Intubation

David C. Flemming, M.B., F.F.A.R.C.S.

Intubation of the trachea for surgical procedures began in 1878, when MacEwen of Glasgow performed an awake orotracheal intubation prior to the administration of chloroform for a mandibular resection.[1] His reasoning included two of the basic tenets of tracheal intubation[2]:

1. Intubation allows easier access to the surgical field during head and neck surgery and,
2. Intubation "guarantees" the integrity of the airway.

Equipment and techniques for intubation did not become established clinically until the 1920s, when the troops returned for repair of their war-torn faces. Rowbotham and Magill[2-4] described equipment and techniques that enabled Sir Harold Gilles to perform his remarkable facial reconstructions. These techniques and those popularized by Waters, Guedel, and Rovenstine in America have developed into an essential part of modern anesthetic practice over the subsequent 60 years.[5,6] Originally, intubation was practiced only when essential to the conduct of surgery. Hazards were recognized, but confined to dangers surrounding the intubation process itself: however, Langton-Hewer suggested in 1924 that intubation made anesthesia easier and safer and should be used far more extensively, noting in particular the ease with which general anesthesia could be maintained during cholecystectomy in the "bucholic drayman."[7]

The proliferation of intensive care units in the 1960s allowed demonstrations that long-term intubation with crude equipment and techniques was associated with new problems. But despite the present thrust to improve intubation techniques and equipment, we are still unable to offer a guarantee that intubation of the trachea is benign.

INCIDENCE AND PREDISPOSING FACTORS

Knowledge of hazards and their incidence comes from our experience and our colleagues, morbidity conferences, and published reports. Despite numerous publications, it is difficult to state an incidence for each complication. The field is changing rapidly, with technologic improvements being introduced continually. For example, the use of high-volume, low-pressure cuffs for tracheal tubes has resulted in a reduction of tracheal injury following long-term intubation. There are numerous predisposing factors as well that vary from population to population being studied. Thus, the incidence for each complication is variable and estimates noted only a few years ago may not be valid now.

Complications are in part dependent upon the patient himself.[8] Infants, children, and adult women, all of whom have relatively small larynx and trachea, are more susceptible to airway narrowing from mucosal edema. This follows

165

from the Hagen-Poiseuille law, namely, flow in tubes varies as the fourth power of the diameter of that tube. The patient whose trachea is difficult to intubate is likely to experience more injury. Similarly, those patients with chronic or debilitating diseases are less able to tolerate the tissue trauma encountered during long-term tracheal intubation.

Other complications are influenced by the intubation process itself and the equipment used. A hurried intubation in a poorly prepared patient—improper muscle relaxation, anesthesia, or head position, or inadequate visualization—is often injurious.[8]

There are other determinants of injury associated with the tube itself. The longer a tracheal tube is in place and the larger its diameter, the greater the possibility for complications to develop.[8,9] Although early studies suggested that plastic was superior to rubber as a material for tracheal tubes, subsequent work has indicated that the various ingredients in the plastic—for example, catalysts, antioxidants, and plasticizers—are tissue irritants.[10,11] When tubes are reused, the potential exists for residual cleaning agent to remain in and on the plastic, with subsequent tissue irritation and injury. If inadequately aerated, gas-sterilized tubes may contain ethylene oxide that is released and injures airway mucosa; water and ethylene oxide form an irritant, ethylene glycol. Lindholm has pointed out that the standard endotracheal tube, because of its shape, exerts pressure on the arytenoids, posterior half of the vocal cords, and the posterior tracheal wall and he advocates tube design to minimize these pressure points.[12]

Movement of the tube in the airway with each breath is another source of injury. This happens because the tube is fixed externally yet the tracheobronchial tree moves with ventilation, especially with coughing, swallowing, and head movement.[9,13]

Much of the injury relates to the pressure exerted by the tracheal tube cuff, which in turn is influenced by cuff design.[12,14,15] Until recently, cuffs were the high-pressure, low-volume type that often inflated eccentrically, thereby exerting extreme pressure unevenly against the tracheal wall. Currently, cuffs use large inflation volumes requiring lower pressure that is distributed more evenly over a large surface area, resulting in less mucosal and submucosal injury.

CLASSIFICATION OF COMPLICATIONS

This chapter will explore briefly some hazards of intubation based on graded therapeutic urgency of which three grades are apparent:

1. Hazards requiring immediate recognition and management;
2. Chronic effects of erosion and healing; and
3. Acute trauma of lesser clinical significance.

HAZARDS REQUIRING IMMEDIATE RECOGNITION AND MANAGEMENT

Spinal Cord and Vertebral Column Injury

Ordinarily the neck is extended and the head brought anteriorly into the "sniffing position" for laryngoscopy to facilitate visualization (see Chap. 8). This position may be difficult to obtain because of jaw or neck stiffness accompanying trismus, arthritis, ankylosing spondylitis, radiation therapy, and burns; an "anterior larynx" accompanying a narrow receding mandible, heavy musculature, and a short neck; or distortion of the upper airway by tumor or trauma.[2] Cervical spine malformation, tumor, osteoporosis, or fracture all predispose to spine or cord damage with forceful hyperextension of the neck.

When one encounters a patient who has one or more of these predisposing factors, careful, gentle laryngoscopy is essential. The head should be maintained in neutral position, with the help of an assistant if necessary. Alternative intubation techniques that do not involve neck manipulation or direct laryngoscopy, such as blind nasal or fiberoptic techniques, should be considered.[8]

Autonomic Reflexes

Noxious autonomic reflexes secondary to laryngoscopy and tracheal intubation include bronchospasm, bradycardia or tachycardia, hypotension or hypertension, and cardiac arrhythmia. These are especially likely to occur in the lightly anesthetized hypoxic or hypercarbic patient. Asthmatics and poorly controlled hypertensive patients are especially at risk. Atropine can abort or prevent some of the vagal manifestations.[16] Topical anesthesia (i.e., lidocaine, 2 mg./kg.) applied to pharynx, larynx, and trachea may eliminate some of these reflexes, especially the hypertension.[17,18] Other preventive approaches include the administration of local anesthetics intravenously,[18] adrenergic blocking agents,[16,19] deep anesthesia,[20] vasodilating agents,[21] and hyperoxemia with normocarbia or hypocarbia.[22] Since these autonomic reflexes may also be present at the time of extubation, spraying lidocaine through the tracheal tube has been suggested.[23]

Airway Perforation by Mechanical Trauma or Airway Pressure

Nasal intubation frequently causes laceration of the nasal mucosa, hemorrhage, or turbinate fracture. The tube may dissect posteriorly and descend into the pharynx behind the posterior pharyngeal wall. During orotracheal intubation, pressure from the laryngoscope blade, stylet, or tube may directly perforate the airway. Raised pressure within the airway may cause rupture anywhere between the point of its application and the alveolus. Airway perforation from any cause may admit air to unusual locations and cause subcutaneous and mediastinal emphysema and pneumothorax.[24] In the awake patient, cough, hemoptysis, and cyanosis are also present and call for immediate bronchoscopy.[25] Tension pneumothorax should be included in the differential diagnosis of circulatory or respiratory instability after intubation, particularly when there is a history of thoracic or upper abdominal trauma, accidental overinflation of the lungs, obstructive airway disease with emphysema, or when positive end-expiratory pressure is in use. Nitrous oxide should be discontinued if surgical emphysema or pneumothorax is suspected, because this gas will diffuse into the trapped air and more than double its volume.[26] (see Chap. 12).

Esophageal Intubation

When visualization of the larynx is difficult, the tracheal tube is occasionally inadvertently inserted into the esophagus. Recognition of this error must be prompt to avoid the effects of hypoxia. Esophageal intubation is characterized by absence of breath sounds over the chest and a "gurgling" sound in the epigastrium, progressive abdominal distention, and signs of hypoxia, such as cyanosis, tachycardia, and dysrhythmia. Allowing the misplaced tube to remain in site while the trachea is correctly intubated may contain regurgitated gastric contents and prevent pulmonary aspiration. After correct placement of the tracheal tube, the stomach should be decompressed because a distended stomach can give rise to regurgitation, vomiting, and perforation (see Chaps. 10 and 31).

Endobronchial Intubation

Because of the acute branching of the left bronchus at the carina, an endotracheal tube, when passed beyond this point, usually goes into the right main stem bronchus. Asymmetric chest expansion, unilateral absence of breath sounds, and, with time, arterial blood gas abnormalities are diagnostic features. Clinical diagnosis is rarely difficult; occasionally a chest radiograph is required to confirm the diagnosis in the operating room. This examination is mandatory in the intensive care unit, where the margin of error is smaller than in the operating room. When endobronchial intubation is discovered, the tube should be withdrawn several centimeters and the lungs hyperinflated sufficiently to expand atelectatic segments. For longer standing atelectasis, bronchoscopy may be required to remove mucous plugs. The incidence of this complication can be minimized by measuring the endotracheal tube along the length of the airway prior to its insertion.

Tension Pneumothorax

Air filling the pleural space under pressure may enter from within or without the chest as a result of trauma and rupture of the airway, as previously mentioned. Emphysematous blebs are prone to rupture with the use of even small amounts of positive end-expiratory pressure. Continual observation of anesthetized patients draped for surgery to elicit signs of pneumothorax is clearly difficult, and the initial presentation is often abrupt circulatory collapse with distended neck veins and cardiac dysrhythmias. Hyper-resonance to percussion and distant breath sounds may also be noted. Vasopressors, understandably, are frequently administered in error as the primary treatment for some of these signs, but must be of limited value. Drainage of the pleural space is the correct treatment (see Chap. 12).

Pulmonary Aspiration

During induction of anesthesia and laryngoscopy and intubation, a variety of materials can be aspirated into the trachea. These include teeth, blood, parts of the laryngoscope, adenoidal tissue, and, most commonly, regurgitated or vomited stomach contents. See Chapter 10 for further discussion.

Airway Obstruction

After the tube has been inserted, a patent airway may still be lost. An obstruction of slow onset may present as a decrease in compliance coupled with wheezing breath sounds resembling bronchospasm, for which bronchodilators are often given in error. Acute complete obstruction is much less ambiguous in its presentation, while a problem that permits inhalation but prevents exhalation may present as circulatory collapse in the same manner as tension pneumothorax, or as rupture of the lungs with pneumothorax and surgical emphysema.

Separation of the interior latex coat of an armored tube, herniation of the endotracheal cuff, kinking, especially with the neck flexed, gradual accumulation of drying blood and secretion in the tube lumen, slow collapse of the tube by the cuff, occlusion of the bevel against the tracheal wall, even blockage of the hoses leading to the patient by foreign bodies, external pressure, or incorrectly applied one-way valves in the circle absorber system must be excluded.[8-10]

Ventilation with dry gases causes dehydration of tracheal mucus or blood, and the crusts that form may completely obstruct the endotracheal tube. This is particularly likely when using nasal tubes that are longer and of smaller diameter than oral tubes and during pediatric anesthesia or intensive care. Humidification of the inspired gas helps prevent airway obstruction and mucosal damage that could result from this.

If there is time, evaluation of the problem should include passage of a suction catheter through the endotracheal tube to confirm its patency and deflation and reinflation of the cuff. Should these measures not be successful or if there is little time, extubation and ventilation with mask or new tracheal tube should be performed.

Disconnection and Dislodgement

One of the more serious and common mechanical complications of tracheal intubation is disconnection of the tube from the rest of the breathing circuit. This problem was the most frequent "critical incident" recalled in a survey of human error and equipment failure.[27] Ordinarily such a disconnection is readily discovered by the anesthesiologist. However, when the head is not accessible to the anesthesiologist or when certain mechanical ventilators are used that continue to cycle despite the leak, the physician may be deluded in believing that the patient is being adequately ventilated. Alarms to alert personnel of an airway disconnection are recommended, as are antidisconnect devices.

Securement techniques appropriate to the nature of the surgery or accessibility of the tube are needed to prevent accidental dislodgement. Adhesive tape, benzoin, and stainless steel wire to secure the tube to the teeth are all tools that may be considered, but more important is the realization that dislodgement is a possibility. Plans to cope with dislodgement should be developed, should this occur.

Leaky Circuits

Circuit leaks cause hypoventilation and dilution of the inspired mixture by entry of air into the system. With spontaneous or manual ventilation and mechanical ventilation with the bellows above the ventilator (Air Shields), collapse of the rebreathing bellows clearly indicates that the leak exceeds the fresh gas inflow. However, ventilators having suspended bellows may give no visual warning because the bigger the leak, the easier the bellows falls to its original position and in doing so entrains more air. Continuously monitoring the thoracic stethoscope and the inspired oxygen concentration, which will be reduced by dilution with air, may reveal to the observant practitioner a developing leak, but even disconnects have been missed in this way. Frequently, cyanosis or the hypertension and tachycardia of hypercarbia has been the presenting sign of the leaking circuit. Pressure-cycled ventilators have the ability to compensate for small leaks by either increasing the flow rate or the inspiratory time. Their ability to stall in inspiration gives audible warning that the leak is too great for mechanical compensation.

Cooling by Evaporation

Evaporative water loss in children who are breathing dry gases causes loss of heat, because heat is lost in the vaporization of water. Humidification of inspired gas becomes clinically more useful for thermal conservation, particularly when anesthetizing infants and smaller children. Humidification is also useful in diminishing the incidence of sore throat and irritation of the tracheal mucosa (see below).[28]

The Difficult Extubation

On occasion, tracheal tubes are difficult to remove. Usually this is due to oversized tubes or cuffs that cannot be deflated. Rarely, a tracheal tube may be sutured inadvertently to the trachea or bronchial stump during surgery.

Laryngeal Edema

Any irritant stimulus, such as pressure from an oversized tracheal tube, dryness of inhaled gas, allergy to laryngeal sprays, or chemical irritation from rubber or ethylene oxide-sterilized tubes can initiate an inflammatory response with mucosal edema in the larynx or trachea. The edema encroaches on the laryngeal lumen, thereby increasing airway resistance. This is especially so in the young child, in whom there is a disproportionate increase in resistance with a decrease in lumen radius (Hagen-Poiseuille), resulting in

croup. The peak incidence of this occurs at 1 to 3 years of age, affecting almost 4 per cent of children who are intubated.[29,30] (See p. 150.)

Croup presents within hours of extubation with a barking, brassy cough and varying degrees of respiratory obstruction. There is also dyspnea, stridor, tachypnea, tachycardia, and suprasternal retraction. Should resolution be followed by scar formation, subglottic stenosis may then become evident but only several weeks or months after the initial insult.

Prevention of this complication begins with avoiding irritant stimuli, particularly an oversized endotracheal tube, and intubation in the presence of upper respiratory infection. There should always be a leak around the endotracheal tube in pediatric practice and the use of a face mask during anesthesia should be encouraged when possible.

Should postintubation croup occur, the beneficial role or humidification of the inspired gases, cool mist, oxygen, and administration of racemic epinephrine by aerosol is well established.[29] Steroids may also be effective. Recently, the use of helium-oxygen mixtures was suggested as a means of improving oxygen flow through edematous airways.[31]

TISSUE EROSION AND HEALING

The presence of a tracheal tube may lead to edema, desquamation, inflammation, and ulceration of the airway. The first three are generally self-limited, whereas ulceration is more serious. Typically it occurs over the posterior half of vocal cords, medial arytenoid and posterior cricoid surfaces, and the anterior portion of the trachea. The severity is related to the duration of intubation, which is why long-term laryngotracheal intubation is eventually discontinued in favor of tracheostomy. Although tracheostomy protects the larynx from further injury, trauma may still occur at the sites of the inflated cuff and, to a lesser degree, at the tip of the tube. Healing occurs by epithelial regeneration, though granuloma and polyps may develop in an ulcerated area. The fact that tissues are being damaged may be unrecognized and the sequelae may present only after prolonged intubation or months after extubation, when scarring diminishes tracheal diameter markedly.

In an attempt to prevent these injuries, tracheal tube cuffs have been redesigned to produce the lowest lateral tracheal wall pressure. The principal change has been the substitution of a large volume, low-pressure cuff for the small volume, high-pressure one of the past in order to distribute a lower pressure over a larger surface area. Other initiatives include prestretching the cuff before use,[32] periodic deflation or inflation only during inspiration, a fluted cuff, a foam-filled cuff, and pressure-regulating devices. Nonetheless, trauma still occurs.[33–35]

Tracheal Erosion

Erosion of the trachea into peritracheal tissue has been observed frequently, with the symptomatology depending upon the eroded tissue. For example, erosion into the esophagus gives rise to a tracheosophageal fistula with subsequent pulmonary aspiration. Erosion into the innominate artery results in aspiration and exsanguination. Dysphonia, hoarseness, and laryngeal incompetence may result from erosion into paratracheal nerves. Tracheomalacia, with possible tracheal collapse, results from erosion confined to the tracheal cartilage.

Tracheostomy is associated with tracheal erosion, particularly into the esophagus or innominate artery, more often than laryngotracheal intubation because tracheostomy tubes generally sit lower in the trachea and have a built-in curve. They are more rigid and do not necessarily conform to the anatomy, potentially causing pressure on tissues at the tube tip. Furthermore, hoses connected to the short tracheostomy tube are capable of exerting great leverage against the tracheal wall unless very carefully supported.

Erosion of Other Tissues

Tube pressure also damages skin at the site of insertion. Securement devices can erode the skin of the face, ears, and scalp. Salivary gland erosion can lead to suppurative parotitis. Obsessional care in tube placement may help reduce the

incidence of chronic pressure sequelae; however, the difficulty of continuous observation of all potential sites of injury makes it likely that these injuries will continue.

Healing and Granuloma Formation

Eroded tissues are ultimately replaced by scar tissue that retracts, leading to stenosis of the trachea, larynx, or nares. Granuloma occurs in 1:800[36] to 1:20,000[37] tracheal intubations, more commonly in women than men but only rarely in children. The posterior laryngeal wall is the common site of erosion and is the position of abundant overgrowth of granulation tissue. Granuloma causes cough, hoarseness, and throat discomfort. It can be prevented by minimizing the trauma associated with laryngoscopy and intubation. When it occurs, however, surgical excision is generally required.

Synechiae

Eroded vocal cords and processes may adhere together, especially when air flow through the cords is diminished by tracheostomy.[38] Surgical correction is required.

Membranes and Webs

Membranes and webs may form over sites of laryngeal and tracheal ulceration. Typically they are thick and gray. If they tear away from their site of attachment, respiratory obstruction may ensue.

Chondritis

After several days the inflammatory response to laryngeal ulceration extends to involve the laryngeal cartilages. Eventually a chondritis or chondromalacia may occur.

Stenosis and Fibrosis

This serious complication occurs several months after tracheal intubation and is the end result in a continuum beginning with erosion of the tracheal wall, weakening of the cartilages, and healing with fibrosis. Commonly associated with prolonged intubation, stenosis occurs more often in adults. The site of the stenosis is usually at the site of the cuff or, less commonly, the tip of the tube. The symptoms include a dry cough, dyspnea, and signs of respiratory obstruction. Treatment includes dilatation in the early stages and resection of the stenotic segment should the lumen size be reduced to 4–5 mm.[39,40]

Vocal Cord Paralysis

This complication can be uni- or bilateral. Symptoms of respiratory obstruction occur with bilateral paralysis, while hoarseness occurs after unilateral paralysis. It may originate from pressure exerted by the distended cuff on branches of the recurrent laryngeal nerve; hence the paralysis is usually transient.

Nerve Injury

Transient weakness, numbness, and paralysis of the tongue occurs occasionally after laryngoscopy, presumably from pressure on the laryngeal or hypoglossal nerves. The complication is short-lasting.[41]

COMPLICATIONS OF LESSER CLINICAL SIGNIFICANCE

Though the most common complication, sore throat is also one of the most benign and transient. The pain on swallowing lasts no more than 24 to 48 hours and can be alleviated to some extent by having the patient inspire humidifed air. Topical anesthesia applied to the tracheal tube may lessen this complication.

Other examples are corneal abrasion (Chap. 23), lip and tooth injury (Chap. 34), and epistasis following nasal intubation. The latter can be minimized by the prior use of a nasal decongestant (i.e., phenylephrine 0.25%) or cocaine, which shrinks the nasal mucosa.

REFERENCES

1. MacEwen, W.: Clinical observations on the introduction of tracheal tubes by the mouth instead of performing tracheotomy or laryngotomy. Br. Med. J., 2:122 and 163, 1880.
2. Atkinson, R. G., Rushman, G. B., and Lee, J. A.: A Synopsis of Anaesthesia (ed. 8). Pg. 237–259. Bristol, John Wright and Sons, Ltd., 1977.
3. Rowbotham, E. S.: Intratracheal anaesthesia by the nasal route for operations on the mouth and lips. Br. Med. J., 2:590, 1920.
4. Rowbotham, E. S., and Magill, I. W.: Anaesthetics in plastic surgery of the face and jaws. Proc. R. Soc. Med., 14:17, 1921.
5. Waters, R. M., and Guedel, A. E.: Endotracheal anesthesia: a new technique. Ann. Oto. Rhinol. Laryngol., 40:1139, 1931.
6. Waters, R. M., Rovenstine, E. A., and Guedel, A. E.: Endotracheal anesthesia and its historical development. Anesth. Analg., 12:196, 1933.
7. Langton-Hewer, C.: The endotracheal administration of nitrous oxide-ethanesol as the routine anaesthetic of choice for major surgery. Br. J. Anaesth., 1:113, 1924.
8. Applebaum, E. L., and Bruce, D. L.: Tracheal Intubation. pp. 77–94. Philadelphia, W. B. Saunders Company, 1976.
9. Blanc, V. F., and Tremblay, N. A. G.: The complications of tracheal intubation: a new classification with a review of the literature. Anesth. Analg., 53:202, 1974.
10. Dorsch, J. A., and Dorsch. S. E.: Understanding Anesthesia Equipment: Construction, Care and Complications. pg. 244–281. Baltimore, Williams and Wilkins Company, 1975.
11. Stetson, J. B., and Guess, W. L.: Causes of damage to tissues by polymers and elastomers used in the fabrication of tracheal devices. Anesthesiology, 33:635, 1970.
12. Lindholm, C. E.: Prolonged endotracheal intubation. A clinical investigation with specific reference to its consequences for the larynx and the trachea and to its place as an alternative to intubation through a tracheostomy. Acta Anaesthesiol. Scand. [Suppl.], 33, 1969.
13. Baron, S. H., and Kahlmoos, H. W.: Laryngeal sequelae of endotracheal anesthesia. Ann. Otol., 60:767, 1951.
14. Hilding, A. C.: Laryngotracheal damage during intratracheal anesthesia. Demonstration by staining the unfixed specimen with methylene blue. Ann. Otol. Rhinol. Laryngol., 80:565, 1971.
15. Cooper, J. D., and Grillo, H. C.: Analysis of problems related to cuffs on intratracheal tubes. Chest, 62:21S, 1972.
16. DeVault, M., Griefenstein, F. E., and Harris, L. C., Jr.: Circulatory responses to endotracheal intubation in light general anesthesia. The effect of atropine and phentolamine. Anesthesiology, 21:360, 1960.
17. Denlinger, J. K., Ellison, N., and Ominsky, A. J.: Effects of intratracheal lidocaine on circulatory responses to tracheal intubation. Anesthesiology, 41:409, 1974.
18. Stoelting, R. K.: Blood pressure and heart rate changes during short-duration laryngoscopy for tracheal intubation: influence of viscous or intravenous lidocaine. Anesth. Analg., 57:197, 1978.
19. Prys-Roberts, C. Foex, P., Biro, G. P., et al.: Studies of anaesthesia in relation to hypertension. V: Adrenergic beta-receptor blockade. Br. J. Anaesth., 45:671, 1973.
20. King, B. D., Harris, L. C., Jr., Greifenstein, F. E., et al.: Reflex circulatory responses to diect laryngoscopy and tracheal intubation performed during general anesthesia. Anesthesiology, 12:556, 1951.
21. Stoelting, R. K.: Attenuation of blood pressure response to

laryngoscopy and tracheal intubation with sodium nitroprusside. Anesth. Analg., *58*:116, 1979.

22. Noble, M. J., and Derricks, W. S.: Changes in the electrocardiogram during induction of anaesthesia and endotracheal intubation. Can. Anaesth. Soc. J., *6*:267, 1959.

23. Bidwai, A. V., Stanley, T. H., and Bidwai, V. A.: Blood pressure and pulse rate responses to extubation with and without prior topical tracheal anaesthesia. Can Anaesth. Soc. J., *25*:416, 1978.

24. Thompson, D. S., and Read, R. C.: Rupture of the trachea following endotracheal intubation. J.A.M.A., *204*:995, 1968.

25. Olson, R. O., and Johnson, J. F.: Diagnosis and management of intrathoracic tracheal rupture. J. Trauma, *11*:789, 1971.

26. Munson, E. S.: Transfer of nitrous oxide into body air cavities. Br. J. Anaesth., *46*:202, 1974.

27. Cooper, J. B., Newbower, R. S., Long, C. D., *et al.*: Preventable anesthesia mishaps: a study of human factors. Anesthesiology, *49*:399, 1978.

28. Chalon, J., Loew, D. A. Y., and Malebranche, J.: Effects of dry anesthetic gases on tracheobronchial ciliated expithelium. Anesthesiology, *37*:338, 1972.

29. Jordon, W. S., Graves, C. L., and Elwyn, R. A.: New therapy for postintubation laryngeal edema and tracheitis in children. J.A.M.A., *212*:585, 1970.

30. Pender, J. W.: Endotracheal anesthesia in children: advantages and disadvantages. Anesthesiology, *15*:495, 1954.

31. Duncan, P. G.: Efficacy of helium-oxygen mixtures in the management of severe viral and post-intubation croup. Can. Anaesth. Soc. J., *26*:206, 1979.

32. Geffin, B., and Pontoppidan, H.: Reduction of tracheal damage by the prestretching of inflatable cuffs. Anesthesiology, *31*:462, 1969.

33. Klainer, A. S., Turndorf, H., Wu, W., *et al*: Surface alterations due to endotracheal intubation. Am. J. Med., *58*:674, 1975.

34. Loeser, E. A., Hodges, M., Gliedman, J., *et al.*: Tracheal pathology following short-term intubation with low- and high-pressure endotracheal tube cuffs. Anesth. Analg., *57*:577, 1978.

35. Mackenzie, C. F., Shin, B., McAslan, T. C., *et al.*: Severe stridor after prolonged endotracheal intubation using high-volume cuffs. Anesthesiology, *50*:235, 1979.

36. Howland, W. S., and Lewis, J. S.: Post-intubation granulomas of the larynx. Cancer, *9*:1244, 1965.

37. Snow, J. C., Harano, M., and Balough, K.: Postintubation granuloma of the larynx. Anesth. Analg., *45*:425, 1966.

38. Kirchner, J. A., and Sasaki, C. T.: Fusion of the vocal cords following intubation and tracheostomy. Trans. Am. Acad. Ophthalmol. Otolaryngol., *77*:88, 1973.

39. Geffin, B., Bland, J., and Grillo, H. C.: Anesthetic management of tracheal resection and reconstruction. Anesth. Analg., *48*:884, 1969.

40. Webb, W. R., Ozdemir, I. A., Ikins, P. M., *et al.*: Surgical management of tracheal stenosis. Ann. Surg., *179*:819, 1974.

41. Teichner, R. L.: Lingual nerve injury: a complication of orotracheal intubation. Br. J. Anaesth., *43*:413, 1971.

FURTHER READING

Applebaum, E. L., and Bruce, D. L.: Tracheal Intubation. Philadelphia, W. B. Saunders Company, 1976.

Blanc, V. F., and Tremblay, N. A. G.: The complications of tracheal intubation: a new classification with a review of the literature. Anesth. Analg., *53*:202, 1974.

Dorsch, J. A., and Dorsch, S. E.: Understanding Anesthesia Equipment: Construction, Care and Complications. pp. 244–281. Baltimore, Williams and Wilkins Company, 1975.

Gillespie, N. A.: Endotracheal Anesthesia. Revised and edited by Bamforth, B. J., and Siebecker, K. L. (ed. 3). pp. 124–130. Madison (WI), University of Wisconsin Press, 1963.

Stauffer, J. L., Olson, D. E., and Petty, T. L.: Complications and consequences of endotracheal intubation and tracheotomy. A prospective study of 150 critically ill adult patients. Am. J. Med., *70*:65, 1981.

Sykes, W. S.: Essays on the First Hundred Years of Anaesthesia. vol. 2. pp. 95–113. Edinburgh, E. & S. Livingstone, Ltd., 1960.

12 Pneumothorax

J. Kenneth Denlinger, M.D.

Pneumothorax was recognized as a potential hazard of mechanical ventilation shortly after introduction of the technique of tracheal intubation in the 19th century.[1] As early as 1828, it was known that excessive pressure applied to the trachea by a bellows could produce lung rupture and pneumothorax. As a result, it was suggested that the handles of the bellows be equipped with a safety "stop-catch" to prevent over-distention of the lungs. Later, in 1912, several cases of pulmonary over-distention resulting in death were reported.[2] Although pneumothorax does not occur as frequently as originally feared by investigators who introduced the technique of positive pressure ventilation, case reports of intraoperative pneumothorax continue to appear. The incidence of *iatrogenic* pneumothorax has increased markedly in the past decade as a result of more frequent use of subclavian and internal jugular venipuncture, prolonged mechanical ventilation, and external cardiac massage.[3] Increased application of newer diagnostic and therapeutic procedures (e.g., laparoscopy, amniocentesis, acupuncture,) has resulted in new causes of pneumothorax.

Since tension pneumothorax may be manifested by unexplained hypotension or wheezing during anesthesia, prompt diagnosis of this complication is often difficult. Rapid cardiorespiratory failure can occur with positive pressure ventilation, and enlargement of the enclosed gas-filled space is accelerated by inward diffusion of anesthetic gases. Although pneumothorax is easily and successfully treated, it has been associated with a 16-per-cent mortality during mechanical ventilation.[3] This chapter therefore describes the pathophysiology and clinical presentation of pneumothorax, so that this potentially fatal anesthetic complication can be readily recognized.

PATHOPHYSIOLOGY

Pneumothorax can occur by way of three basic mechanisms: Type I, intrapulmonary alveolar rupture, with retrograde perivascular dissection of air, which produces mediastinal emphysema; Type II, injury to the visceral pleura, with escape of air into the pleural space; and Type III, interruption of the parietal pleura, with entry of air from adjoining structures (peritoneal cavity, mediastinum, thoracic wall). Although simple lung collapse occurring by way of any of these mechanisms may be relatively innocuous, development of *tension pneumothorax* is a life-threatening emergency.

Type I: Intrapulmonary Rupture

The mechanism by which intrapulmonary alveolar rupture leads to pneumothorax is diagrammed in Figure 12-1. Macklin and Macklin distinguished partitional alveoli, surrounded by other alveoli, from marginal alveoli, which adjoin blood vessels and bronchi.[4] Distention of parti-

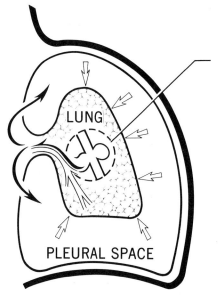

Alveolar rupture (magnified schematically) may be due to:

A. Increased airway pressure
   1. Expiratory valve dysfunction
   2. Overstretch of normal alveoli in segmental lung disease
   3. Cough, Valsalva

B. Weakened alveolar septum
   1. Infection (e.g. necrotizing pneumonia)
   2. Chronic lung disease (e.g. emphysema)
   3. Hypovolemic Shock

Fig. 12-1. A pneumothorax of Type I results from intrapulmonary rupture, perivascular dissection of air to the hilum, and rupture of the mediastinal pleura.

tional alveoli by excessive airway pressure is limited by distention of surrounding alveoli, and therefore rupture is unlikely. Distention of marginal alveoli is more likely to result in alveolar wall rupture at the interface with adjoining vascular and bronchial structures. Perivascular escape of gas then occurs from the site of alveolar rupture, toward the hilum of the lung and mediastinum, where gas ruptures and passes through the mediastinal pleura. The perivascular spread of gas can be distributed as tiny bubbles throughout the lung and in some cases produces "pulmonary interstitial emphysema." Such interstitial emphysema can cause pulmonary ventilation-perfusion abnormalities, which sometimes persist after prompt re-expansion of the collapsed lung.

Normal intrapleural pressure during quiet spontaneous respiration is slightly subatmospheric (−3 to −6 torr). However, intrapleural pressures exceeding ±100 torr may be observed during coughing, laryngospasm, and during initial expansion of the lung at birth. These pressures are physiologic extremes, required, at times, for maintenance of the structural integrity of the lung. Instantaneous airway or pleural pressures of this magnitude may be relatively unimportant in the etiology of alveolar rupture. Rather, alveolar rupture is related to distention that occurs when a pressure gradient is maintained across the alveolar wall for a given period of time.[5] The safe limits of time and pressure have not been determined in humans. A sustained intrabronchial pressure of 24 torr regularly produces interstitial emphysema in dogs.[6] In humans, it has been reported that phasic pressures less than 25 torr are relatively safe, pressures from 30 to 80 torr are potentially dangerous, and pressures above 80 torr are definitely hazardous.[7] Expiratory obstruction in anesthesia breathing systems that produces excessive positive airway pressure and tension pneumothorax has resulted from malfunction of expiratory valve mechanisms.[8] A valve disk was misplaced during reassembly of an anesthesia circle absorber system and resulted in lung rupture by way of this mechanism.[9] Lung inflation by delivery of oxygen at a pressure of 50 p.s.i., from the flush valve of an anesthesia machine to an Ayres' T-piece system, was reported to cause pneumothorax.[10] Simple inattention and failure to observe the distended breathing bag during controlled ventilation can also lead to alveolar rupture. Other mechanical

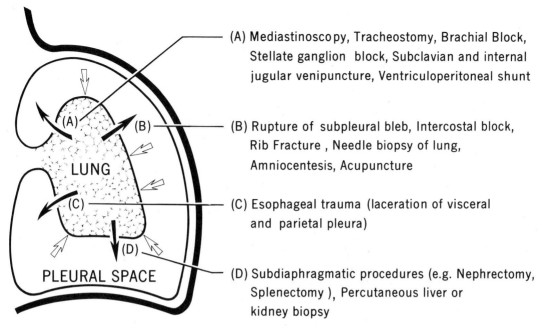

(A) Mediastinoscopy, Tracheostomy, Brachial Block, Stellate ganglion block, Subclavian and internal jugular venipuncture, Ventriculoperitoneal shunt

(B) Rupture of subpleural bleb, Intercostal block, Rib Fracture, Needle biopsy of lung, Amniocentesis, Acupuncture

(C) Esophageal trauma (laceration of visceral and parietal pleura)

(D) Subdiaphragmatic procedures (e.g. Nephrectomy, Splenectomy), Percutaneous liver or kidney biopsy

Fig. 12-2. A pneumothorax of Type II results from a break in the visceral pleura.

causes of excessively high inflation pressure include tracheal cuff overinflation, with cuff herniation over the tip of the tracheal tube, and asymmetric inflation of a tracheal cuff, causing the beveled tube orifice to rest against the tracheal wall. The flap-valve mechanism thus produced can permit lung inflation but obstruct exhalation.

Over-stretch of normal alveoli is another possible mechanism by which pneumothkrax may occur in certain lung diseases characterized by a patchy distribution of atelectasis. Meconium aspiration in the neonate and segmental airway obstruction from any cause can limit expansion of certain pulmonary segments and increase expansion of other relatively normal alveolar segments. The increased risk of pneumothorax in neonates with respiratory distress syndrome or diaphragmatic hernia may be due to pulmonary dysplasia, in addition to segmental lung distention.

Intrapulmonary rupture can also be related to weakening of the alveolar septum, such as that which accompanies pulmonary infection. The increased incidence of pneumothorax in necrotizing pneumonia, chronic lung disease, cystic fibrosis, certain collagen diseases, and hypovolemic shock may be related to structural abnormalities of the alveoli, as well as airway obstruction.

Type II: Injury to Visceral Pleura

Air can also enter the pleural space through a rent in the visceral pleura; this is shown schematically in Figure 12-2. The increased incidence of pneumothorax in parturient patients may be due to "bearing down" and rupture of a subpleural bleb during labor. Pneumothorax following laryngospasm, bronchospasm, or cough presumably results from rupture of an emphysematous bleb as well. Direct continuity is then established between the terminal bronchus and the pleural space (e.g., a bronchopleural fistula). In such cases, the ruptured emphysematous bleb can function as a valve mechanism that permits flow of gas unidirectionally from the bronchus to the pleural space. A pressure gradient from the terminal bronchus to the pleural space results in progressive accumulation of pleural gas, with tension pneumothorax.

The causes of pleural injury that may lead to

pneumothorax are many and varied. The most common are thoracic trauma with fractured ribs and iatrogenic disorders resulting from needle puncture of the pleura. Pleura laceration during internal jugular or subclavian venipuncture is not uncommon. Pneumothorax is a known complication of intercostal, thoracic, paravertebral, brachial plexus, phrenic, and stellate ganglion nerve blocks. Although it is possible for air to enter the thorax through the needle at the time of nerve block, pneumothorax following nerve block usually does not occur by way of this mechanism. Typically, pneumothorax occurs 6 to 12 hours after the block, suggesting that air entry occurs slowly and progressively through a pleural rent.[11] Pleural trauma may occur during tracheostomy (especially in children), mediastinoscopy, thoracotomy, and subdiaphragmatic procedures.[12,13] Pneumothorax secondary to pleural trauma has occurred following percutaneous liver biopsy, renal biopsy, nephrectomy, splenectomy, adrenalectomy, and insertion of a ventriculoperitoneal shunt.[5,14] Recently, pneumothorax has been reported following acupuncture.[15] Pleural laceration in utero, during amniocentesis, is known to cause neonatal pneumothorax.[16] When there is visceral pleural discontinuity, of any cause, airway pressures that ordinarily would be safe can produce tension pneumothorax.

Type III: Injury to Parietal Pleura

Air can also enter the pleural space through a break in the parietal pleura, such as that which occurs in open chest trauma (Fig. 12-3). Artificial air conduits, such as open chest tubes or cardiac pacemaker wire sheaths,[17] have also caused pneumothorax by way of this mechanism. Pneumoperitoneum induced to facilitate laparoscopy may result in retroperitoneal, para-aortic air dissection, with mediastinal pleural rupture and pneumothorax.[18] Alternatively, diaphragmatic defects may provide a pathway by which peritoneal gas enters the chest. Finally, pneumothorax may complicate thyroidectomy, tracheostomy, stellate ganglionectomy, or radial neck dissection, where exposure of the deep cervical fascia pro-

Fig. 12-3. A pneumothorax of Type III results from a break in the parietal pleura.

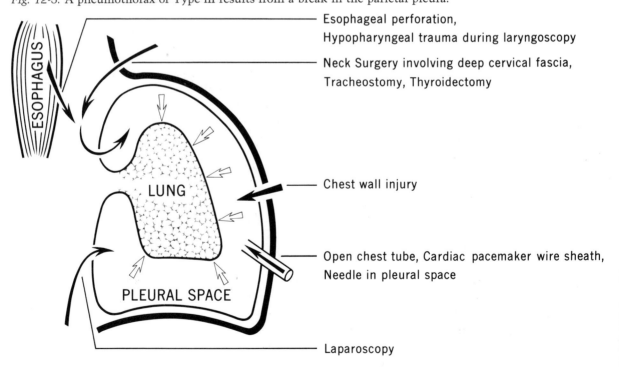

Esophageal perforation, Hypopharyngeal trauma during laryngoscopy

Neck Surgery involving deep cervical fascia, Tracheostomy, Thyroidectomy

Chest wall injury

Open chest tube, Cardiac pacemaker wire sheath, Needle in pleural space

Laparoscopy

vides a portal by which air may enter the mediastinum.[19] Anatomically, the pretracheal layer of the deep cervical fascia invests the trachea and extends directly into the mediastinum. This route of air entry was demonstrated as early as 1880, when Chapneys traced dye from tracheostomy wounds into the mediastinum during resuscitative measures in stillborn infants.[8] Simple exposure of the cervical fascia to the atmosphere is probably not sufficient to produce pneumothorax, however. Dissection of air along the cervical fascia usually is associated with excessive negative airway pressures developed during obstructed or labored respiration. Paratracheal air dissection results in pneumomediastinum, followed by pneumothorax as the mediastinal parietal pleura ruptures. Air may also enter the mediastinum by way of esophageal or hypopharyngeal perforation complicating direct laryngoscopy or esophagoscopy.[20] Positive pressure ventilation by face mask during induction of anesthesia in a patient with hypopharyngeal or esophageal perforation is reported to cause tension pneumothorax.[21]

Hemodynamic Effects of Tension Pneumothorax

Tension pneumothorax can produce hypotension and circulatory collapse by way of several different mechanisms. Mechanical obstruction to systemic venous return occurs as the mediastinal structures are displaced toward the contralateral hemithorax. A decrease in cardiac filling is associated with decreased stroke volume and arterial hypotension. In addition, hypoventilation produces hypoxia and hypercapnia, leading to circulatory depression. Studies in goats, subjected to progressive pneumothorax by pleural air injection, indicated that severe hypoxia, respiratory acidosis, tachycardia, and lowered stroke volume occurred before obstruction to venous return was significant enough to interfere with cardiac output.[22] These investigators concluded that severe hypoxia is a more likely explanation for the hemodynamic sequelae of pneumothorax than the traditional concept of mechanical venous obstruction.

It has been observed that cardiovascular depression is not always reversible, even when the chest is promptly decompressed by thoracostomy. In these rare instances, it has been postulated that pulmonary interstitial air gains entry to the pulmonary circulation, with subsequent embolization to the coronary arteries.[23] Air has been observed in the coronary circulation of patients who have expired following tension pneumothorax and cardiac arrest. Experimental lung rupture in dogs has been shown to produce coronary air embolization and reversal of pulmonary artery flow, with retrograde air entry into the right ventricle.[23] Although these data are, perhaps, not directly transferable to humans, they represent a possible explanation for the observed association of coronary air embolism and pulmonary overdistention.

The Hazard of Nitrous Oxide

Anesthetic-induced expansion of an enclosed, gas-filled space, such as a pneumothorax, can contribute to rapid development of tension pneumothorax. The solubility of nitrous oxide in blood is 34 times greater than that of nitrogen. Therefore, blood exposed to an air-filled pneumothorax discharges nitrous oxide into the space more rapidly than nitrogen is absorbed into the blood, provided that the tension gradients of the two gases are similar. Eger and Saidman quantitated the rate of increase of intrapleural gas volume in dogs breathing 68- to 78-per-cent nitrous oxide (Fig. 12-4).[24] The initial 300 ml. of air placed in the pleural space doubled in 10 minutes, tripled in 45 minutes, and, in one dog, quadrupled in 2 hours. Thus, administration of high concentrations of nitrous oxide is contraindicated in patients with closed pneumothorax or in patients who have intrapulmonary cysts or unventilated bullae.

CLINICAL PRESENTATION OF PNEUMOTHORAX

The clinical presentation of pneumothorax is dependent upon the patient's level of consciousness, associated cardiopulmonary disease, and age. In the awake adult patient, pneumothorax is first evidenced by tachycardia, cough, and chest pain that is often referred to the shoulder area and which is accentuated by deep breathing or change

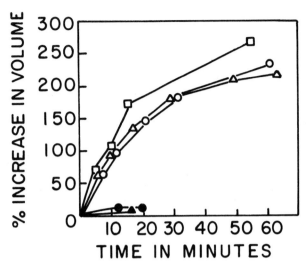

Fig. 12-4. An increase in intrapleural gas volume occurs upon administration of nitrous oxide (*open squares, circles,* and *triangles*), as opposed to a change in volume upon administration of oxygen plus halothane (*filled triangles* and *circles*). (Eger, E. I., II, and Saidman, L.J.: Hazards of nitrous oxide anesthesia in bowel obstruction and pneumothorax. Anesthesiology, 26:64, 1965)

in posture. Progressive expansion leads to tachypnea, dyspnea, and cyanosis. Severe hypoxia eventually produces loss of consciousness and cardiovascular collapse. On physical examination, breath sounds are decreased over the involved hemithorax, expiratory wheezing is frequently heard, and hyperresonance, as well as decreased vocal fremitus, may be elicited. Air in the mediastinum may be evidenced by a mediastinal "crunch," heard upon auscultation (Hamman's sign). The trachea may be deviated to the contralateral side, and subcutaneous emphysema is frequently observed. ECG changes mimicking acute myocardial infarction have been reported.[25] Left tension pneumothorax typically produces low voltage in the precordial leads.

Detection of pneumothorax in the anesthetized patient often presents a difficult diagnostic challenge. Frequently, pneumothorax under anesthesia first presents as tachycardia and hypotension. These nonspecific cardiovascular signs direct the clinician to consider more common problems,

such as anesthetic overdose or hypovolemia. As the pneumothorax expands, reduction in pulmonary compliance becomes evident. Increased airway pressure is required to maintain ventilation, and subcutaneous emphysema may appear. As in the awake patient, examination of the chest reveals decreased breath sounds, wheezing, and hyperresonance. The central venous pressure may be elevated, and the trachea may be deviated to one side. Progressive hypoxia and hypercapnia lead to obvious cyanosis, cardiac arrhythmias, and, finally, circulatory arrest. The diagnosis of unilateral tension pneumothorax is often aided by comparison of physical signs elicited over each hemithorax. However, tension pneumothorax may occur bilaterally, with decreased air entry, wheezing, and hyperresonance over the entire thorax.

In the postoperative period, pneumothorax must be considered in the differential diagnosis of either respiratory or circulatory distress. Intraoperative pleural trauma can result in a pneumothorax that develops slowly and which first presents as restlessness in the postoperative patient. In a large series of patients requiring mechanical ventilation, the most reliable signs of tension pneumothorax were subcutaneous emphysema, tachycardia, decreased breath sounds, hyperresonance, and hypotension.[3] These signs were invariably associated with rising arterial carbon dioxide tension (Pa_{CO_2}) and falling arterial oxygen tension (Pa_{O_2}).

Pneumothorax in the neonate is evidenced by tachypnea, increased irritability, grunting, retractions, and cyanosis. The chest may bulge on one side, and the apical cardiac impulse may be shifted. The sudden appearance of cyanosis and bradycardia in any neonate with pulmonary disease necessitating respiratory care should alert the physician to the immediate possibility of tension pneumothorax.

INCIDENCE OF PNEUMOTHORAX

Pneumothorax complicating anesthesia is sufficiently uncommon that precise data describing its incidence are not available, except with relation to specific high-risk procedures. Moore found a 1-per-cent incidence of pneumothorax following supraclavicular brachial plexus block.[11] Percutaneous needle biopsy of the lung is associated with pneumothorax in approximately 30 per cent of cases.[26] Etiologic classification of 544 cases of pneumothorax by Steier revealed that 209 were due to complications of hospital care, such as subclavian venipuncture and external cardiac massage.[3] Of the remaining instances, 179 were related to various types of chest trauma, 150 developed "spontaneously," and six cases were thought to be related to pulmonary infection.

The incidence of pneumothorax in patients requiring mechanical ventilation ranges from 10 to 20 per cent. It was initially thought that the use of positive end-expiratory pressure (PEEP) in the treatment of patients with respiratory failure might greatly increase the incidence of pneumothorax and pneumomediastinum. Yet, recent studies indicate that adult patients treated with PEEP plus mechanical ventilation show no greater incidence of pneumothorax than those treated with mechanical ventilation alone.[27] Only 14 per cent of patients treated with high levels of PEEP developed pneumothorax.[28]

The incidence of pneumothorax in neonates with respiratory distress syndrome (RDS) increases with the severity of the disease and with the aggressiveness of therapy used to treat it.[29] Pneumothorax occurred in 3.5 per cent (2 of 58) of infants with respiratory distress syndrome who received no assisted ventilation and in 11 per cent (14 of 124) of such infants who received continuous positive airway pressure (CPAP). Pneumothorax occurred in 24 per cent (12 of 49) of infants who were initially treated with continuous positive airway pressure but later required mechanical ventilation with positive end-expiratory pressure. In those infants with severe respiratory distress syndrome who were initially treated with mechanical ventilation plus positive end-expiratory pressure, the incidence of pneumothorax was 33 per cent (21 of 64).[29]

The incidence of spontaneous pneumothorax is higher in the neonate than in any other age-group.[30] Routine radiographic screening has revealed pneumothorax is present in 1 to 2 per cent of neonates shortly after birth. However, the incidence of symptomatic pneumothorax requiring treatment is approximately 0.05 to 0.07 per cent.

DIFFERENTIAL DIAGNOSIS OF PNEUMOTHORAX

The clinical presentation of pneumothorax may mimic that of *bronchospasm* under anesthesia. Both pneumothorax and bronchospasm are more likely to occur in patients with chronic lung disease, and both are associated with wheezing, increased airway pressure, diminished breath sounds, cyanosis, and hypotension.[31] Anesthetic-induced bronchospasm may occur following tracheal intubation in patients with bronchial asthma, especially when the tracheobronchial tree is instrumented during light planes of anesthesia. *Pulmonary embolism* and *anaphylaxis* are other causes of bronchospasm under anesthesia. The differential diagnosis must also include mechanical problems due to *overinflation of the tracheal cuff, foreign body aspiration*, and *bronchial intubation*. Deflation of the tracheal cuff and repositioning of the tracheal tube often result in improved ventilation and dissappearance of wheezing in such cases. These mechanical airway difficulties are more common than true bronchospasm during modern anesthesia practice and therefore should be excluded immediately.

Because the signs of pneumothorax are so similar to those of true bronchospasm, recognition of pneumothorax under anesthesia is sometimes delayed while bronchodilator therapy is begun. Administration of aminophylline and isoproterenol to the hypoxic, hypercapnic patient for a condition misdiagnosed as bronchospasm is dangerous and may result in fatal cardiac arrhythmias. Since the urgency of this situation does not usually permit definitive diagnosis by chest radiograph, pneumothorax must be distinguished on the basis of physical signs: hyperresonance, tracheal deviation, shifted cardiac impulse, and subcutaneous emphysema. The "scratch sign," elicited by scratching the skin over each hemithorax while listening through a stethoscope placed over the sternum, has been described as a valuable aid in the detection of unilateral tension pneumothorax.[32] A louder and more harsh sound elicited over the pneumothorax constitutes a positive sign. When pneumothorax is strongly suspected, the diagnosis is confirmed by demonstration of gas escape through a needle of large bore, inserted anteriorly into the second intercostal space.

Since hypotension and tachycardia are early signs of pneumothorax under anesthesia, congestive heart failure or *anesthetic-induced cardiac depression* must be included in the differential diagnosis. *Pulmonary edema* due to left ventricular failure also causes decreased pulmonary compliance, wheezing, and increased venous pressure, as in pneumothorax. Ischemic ECG changes may occur in both pulmonary edema and pneumothorax. However, frank pulmonary edema is associated with pink, frothy fluid on tracheal aspiration, and pneumothorax is suggested by the finding of hyperresonance, tracheal deviation, and subcutaneous emphysema. In at least one case report, tension pneumothorax was recognized only after thoracotomy was performed for direct cardiac massage, as a resuscitative measure following circulatory collapse.[33] Thoracotomy might have been avoided by simple aspiration of air from the pleural space, had the diagnosis of pneumothorax been suspected. Rapid accumulation of *pleural or mediastinal fluid* from an infiltrated or improperly positioned central venous catheter, as well as *hemothorax* complicating central venipuncture, may also produce cardiorespiratory signs simulating pneumothorax in the anesthetized patient. Pleural fluid is distinguished by dullness to percussion and is confirmed by radiographs or by thoracentesis.

Pneumothorax must be considered in the differential diagnosis of postoperative *restlessness* and *emergence delirium.* Administration of narcotics without careful evaluation of ventilation and physical examination of the chest is never justified in the presence of postoperative restlessness and tachypnea. In the awake patient, chest pain with associated tachycardia, tachypnea, and cough resulting from pneumothorax must be differentiated from that due to *pulmonary embolism* or *myocardial infarction.*

TREATMENT OF PNEUMOTHORAX

In general, a pneumothorax large enough to produce symptoms should be treated by needle aspiration and/or tube thoracostomy. A small asymptomatic pneumothorax following nerve block or minor pleural trauma frequently resolves spontaneously and requires only observation. Many cases of neonatal pneumothorax develop slowly after birth and undergo spontaneous resolution. However, neonatal pneumothorax that shows a rapid onset and is symptomatic should be treated. Repeated needle aspiration may be inadvisable because of the possibility of repeated trauma. Cardiac laceration and death has been reported following repeated needle aspiration in the neonate.[34]

Immediate treatment of tension pneumothorax is usually accomplished by insertion of a needle of large bore through the second intercostal space anteriorly. Several methods have been described for continued drainage of the pleural space. The Clagett-S needle is a blunt-tipped, S-shaped needle with multiple drainage openings, which may be inserted intrapleurally to maintain lung expansion.[8] Alternatively, a 3Fr silastic tube inserted over a rigid stylet has been advocated for the treatment of pneumothorax complicating radiologic procedures.[26] However, the most reliable method for obtaining proper pleural drainage and maintaining lung expansion in the treatment of pneumothorax is the insertion of a standard chest tube. Use of a small plastic catheter threaded through a needle is not recommended because of problems such as catheter kinking and obstruction.[35]

PREVENTION OF PNEUMOTHORAX

Since the incidence of iatrogenic pneumothorax seems to be increasing, careful consideration of the risk–benefit ratio should precede certain procedures, such as subclavian venipuncture. The mortality related to pneumothorax, however, need not be great if adequate patient surveillance is maintained. The possibility of pneumothorax should be considered whenever a central venous catheter is inserted by way of the subclavian[3] or internal jugular vein,[36] especially prior to induction of anesthesia. Positive airway pressure and the use of high concentrations of nitrous oxide may convert a small pneumothorax into a rapidly expanding tension pneumothorax. Individuals who perform intercostal nerve blocks, acupuncture, laparoscopy, percutaneous liver biopsy, or other procedures associated with pneumothorax should be prepared to treat this potential complication without delay.

Although high inflation pressures are sometimes required to re-expand atelectatic pulmonary segments, care should be exercised to avoid excessive airway pressure during administration of anesthesia. Proper functioning of each anesthesia breathing system must be checked prior to use, and new or reassembled equipment should be carefully inspected. Poorly compliant breathing bags should not be used because of higher peak pressures produced during inadvertent overdistention of the bag.[37]

Avoidance of airway obstruction or excessive negative airway pressure during neck surgery will prevent most cases of pneumothorax that are due to air dissection along the deep cervical fascia into the mediastinum. Patients with blunt chest trauma or fractured ribs should be managed by use of regional anesthesia, when possible, in order to prevent pneumothorax. When positive pressure ventilation is required in the management of chest trauma, tension pneumothkrax should be strongly suspected and treated at its earhiest hndication.

REFERENCES

1. Gillespie, N. A*: The history of endotracheal anesthesia. In Bamforth, B. J., and Siebecker, K. L. (eds.): Endotracheal Anesthesia. pp. 6–24. Madison, Ujiversity of Wisconsin Press, 1963.
2. Woolsey, W. C.: Intratracheal insufflation anesthesia. N.Y. State J. Med., 12:167, 1912.
3. Steier, M., Ching, N., Roberts, E. B., et al.: Pneumothorax complicating continuous ventilatory support. J. Thorac. Cardiovasc. Surg., 67:17, 1974.
4. Macklin, M. T., and Macklin, C. C.: Malignant interstitial emphysema of the lungs and mediastinum as an important occult complication in many respiratory diseases and other conditions. Medicine, 23:281, 1944.
5. Hamilton, W. K.: Atelectasis, pneumothorax, and aspiration as postoperative complications. Anesthesiology, 22:708, 1961.
6. Marcotte, R. J., Phillips, F. J., Adams, W. E., et al.: Differential intrabronchial pressures and mediastinal emphysema. J. Thorac. Surg., 9:346, 1940.
7. Nennhaus, H. P., Javid, H., and Julian, O.: Alveolar and pleural rupture. Arch. Surg., 94:136, 1967.
8. Martin, J. T., and Patrick, R. T.: Pneumothorax: its significance to the anesthesiologist. Anesth. Analg., 39:420, 1960.
9. Dean, H. N., Parsons, D. E., and Raphaely, R. C.: Case report: bilateral tension pneumothorax from mechanical failure of anesthesia machine due to misplaced expiratory valve. Anesth. Analg., 50:195, 1971.
10. Arens, J. F.: A hazard in the use of an Ayre T-piece. Anesth. Analg., 50:943, 1971.
11. Moore, D. C., and Bridenbaugh, L. D.: Pneumothorax, its incidence following brachial plexus block analgesia. Anesthesiology, 15:475, 1954.
12. Furgang, F. A., and Saidman, L. J.: Bilateral tension pneumothorax associated with mediastinoscopy. J. Thorac. Cardiovasc. Surg., 63:329, 1972.
13. Meade, J. W.: Tracheotomy—its complications and their management. N. Engl. J. Med., 265:519, 1961.
14. Portnoy, H. D., and Croissant, P.D.: Two unusual complications of a ventriculoperitoneal shunt. J. Neurosurg., 39:775, 1973.
15. Goldberg, I.: Pneumothorax associated with acupuncture. Med. J. Aust., 1:941, 1973.
16. Hyman, C. J., Depp, R., Pakravan, P., et al.: Pneumothorax complicating amniocentesis. Obstet. Gynecol., 41:43, 1973.
17. Linde, L. M., and Mulder, D. G.: Pneumothorax after externalization of cardiac pacemaker wires. N. Engl. J. Med., 272:682, 1965.
18. Doctor, N. H., and Hussain, Z.: Bilateral pneumothorax associated with laparoscopy. Anaesthesia, 28:75, 1973.
19. Schweizer, O.: Complications of anesthesia during radical surgery about the head and the neck. Anesthesiology, 16:927, 1955.
20. Hawkins, D. B., and House, J. W.: Postoperative pneumothorax secondary to hypopharyngeal perforation during anesthetic intubation. Ann. Otol. Rhinol. Laryngol., 83:556, 1974.
21. Dundee, J. W.: Tension pneumothorax during the induction of anaesthesia. Anaesthesia, 10:74, 1955.
22. Rutherford, R. B., Hurt, H. H., Jr., Brickman, R. D., et al.: The pathophysiology of progressive tension pneumothorax. J. Trauma, 8:212, 1968.
23. Lenaghan, R., Silva, Y. J., and Walt, A. J.: Hemodynamic alterations associated with expansion rupture of the lung. Arch. Surg., 99:339, 1969.
24. Eger, E. I., and Saidman, L. J.: Hazards of nitrous oxide anesthesia in bowel obstruction and pneumothorax. Anesthesiology, 26:61, 1965.
25. Summers, R. S.: The electrocardiogram as a diagnostic aid in pneumothorax. Chest, 63:127, 1973.
26. Sargent, E. N., and Turner, A. F.: Emergency treatment of pneumothorax, a simple catheter technique for use in the radiology department. Am. J. Roentgenol. Radium Ther. Nucl. Med., 109:531, 1970.
27. Kumar, A., Pontoppidan, J., Falke, K. J., et al.: Pulmonary baro-trauma during mechanical ventilation. Crit. Care Med., 1:181, 1973.
28. Kirby, R. R., Downs, J. B., Civetta, J. M., et al.: High level

positive and expiratory pressure (PEEP) in acute respiratory insufficiency. Chest, *67*:156, 1975.

29. Ogata, E. S., Gregory, G. A., Kitterman, J. A., et al.: Pneumothorax in the respiratory distress syndrome: incidence and effect on vital signs, blood gases and *p*H. Pediatrics, *58*:177, 1976.

30. Chernick, V., and Reed, M. H.: Pneumothorax and chylothorax in the neonatal period. J. Pediatr., *76*:624, 1970.

31. Gold, M. I., and Joseph, S. I.: Bilateral tension pneumothorax following induction of anesthesia in two patients with chronic obstructive airway disease. Anesthesiology, *38*:93, 1973.

32. Lawson, J. D.: The scratch sign—a valuable aid in the diagnosis of pneumothorax. N. Engl. J. Med., *264*:88, 1961.

33. Fitzgerald, T. B., and Johnstone, M. W.: Diaphragmatic defects and laparoscopy. Br. Med. J., *2*:604, 1970.

34. Shim, W. K. T., and Philip, A. G. S.: Danger of needle aspiration in pneumothorax in the newborn. J.A.M.A., *223*:691, 1973.

35. Withers, J. N., Fishback, M. E., Kiehl, P.V., et al.: Spontaneous pneumothorax, suggested etiology and comparison of treatment methods. Am. J. Surg., *108*:772, 1964.

36. Arnold, S., Feathers, R. S., and Gibbs, E.: Bilateral pneumothoraces and subcutaneous emphysema: a complication of internal jugular venipuncture. Br. Med. J., *1*:211, 1973.

37. Johnstone, R. E., and Smith, T. C.: Rebreathing bags as pressure-limiting devices. Anesthesiology, *38*:192, 1973.

13 Hypoxemia and Hypercapnia During and After Anesthesia

Hillary Don, M.D.

Section One: Hypoxemia During and After Anesthesia

"NORMAL" Pa_{O_2}

Hypoxemia is defined as a lower than normal partial pressure of oxygen in arterial blood (Pa_{O_2}). It does not involve, therefore, abnormalities of amount or type of hemoglobin. The interpretation of a "normal" value of Pa_{O_2} must consider the inspired oxygen fraction ($F_{I_{O_2}}$), barometric pressure, the arterial carbon dioxide tension (Pa_{CO_2}), and the age of the subject.

Breathing room air at sea level, the relationship of Pa_{O_2} to age can be approximated as follows:[1]

$$Pa_{O_2} = 100 - (0.3)(\text{age in years})$$

This presumes that there is normal alveolar and arterial carbon dioxide tension. If Pa_{CO_2} is reduced, alveolar oxygen tension ($P_{A_{O_2}}$) will increase, related by a simplified form of the alveolar gas equation:

$$P_{A_{O_2}} = P_{I_{O_2}} - \frac{P_{A_{CO_2}}}{R}$$

where $P_{I_{O_2}}$ is partial pressure of oxygen in dry inspired gas, $P_{A_{CO_2}}$ is alveolar carbon dioxide tension, and R is the respiratory quotient. Hypocapnia may therefore disguise a defect in oxygen exchange.

CAUSES OF HYPOXEMIA

Causes of hypoxemia may be divided into two categories based on the $P_{A_{O_2}}$:

Reduced $P_{A_{O_2}}$. Arterial oxygen tension will parallel any reduction in alveolar oxygen tension. A fall in $P_{A_{O_2}}$ is caused by either a reduced $F_{I_{O_2}}$ or a reduction in alveolar minute ventilation ($\dot{V}_A$).

Normal or increased $P_{A_{O_2}}$. An increase in the normally small difference between alveolar and arterial oxygen tensions may occur. This is sometimes called "venous admixture," because, conceptually, the oxygen tension in arterial blood, which "should" be the same as that of the alveolus, is reduced, as if admixture with venous blood had occurred. Traditionally, three causes of venous admixture are described: diffusion defect; abnormal distribution of ventilation–perfusion ratios, with areas of the lungs in which $\dot{V}_A$ although reduced relative to perfusion ($\dot{Q}$), is greater than zero; and complete failure of ventilation of perfused parts of the lung ($\dot{V}_A/\dot{Q} = $ zero), sometimes called a "shunt." Recognition of the latter is important, because hypoxemia resulting from complete failure of ventilation is resistant to correction by increasing $F_{I_{O_2}}$.

SIGNIFICANCE OF HYPOXEMIA

Body tissues have a critical dependence on oxygen supply. Two factors must be considered: the content of oxygen in the blood; and the actual level of Pa_{O_2}, which creates a driving pressure for movement of oxygen from the plasma to the tissues.

The content of oxygen in blood is the sum of

dissolved oxygen and that combined with hemoglobin. Dissolved oxygen ($Pa_{O_2} \times 0.003$ ml. per 100 ml. of blood or plasma) is only a small fraction of that combined with hemoglobin ([$1.37 \times$ hemoglobin] ml. oxygen at 100% saturation). The shape of the oxygen-hemoglobin dissociation curve is such that, even at a Pa_{O_2} level of 40 torr (5.3 kPa), hemoglobin is still approximately 75-per-cent saturated. Below this partial pressure, there is a rapid reduction in oxygen content. Although a level of Pa_{O_2} below 40 torr may be clinically unacceptable in terms of oxygen content, oxygen transport, which is the product of oxygen content and cardiac output, is the important consideration in terms of delivery of oxygen to the tissues. Hence, either an increase in hemoglobin or cardiac output can restore oxygen transport toward normal levels in the face of a low oxygen tension in arterial blood.

The second significant aspect in determining a satisfactory level of Pa_{O_2} is the pressure that drives oxygen from the blood to the tissue. If the head of oxygen pressure is low, it will not be corrected by changes in hemoglobin or cardiac output. It can be partially compensated by a shift of the oxygen-hemoglobin dissociation curve to the right, aiding release of oxygen at the tissues. Such a shift is found with increases in hydrogen ion concentration, P_{CO_2}, temperature, and 2,3-diphosphoglycerate (2,3-DPG).[1] In states of chronic hypoxemia, increased levels of 2,3-DPG will be found (see Chap. 16 and 35).

Determining the Pa_{O_2} that interferes with oxygen delivery at the tissues is difficult. In a study by Cullen and Eger, hypoxemia (Pa_{O_2} = 38 torr or 5.1 kPa) reduced minimum alveolar concentration (MAC) of halothane in dogs.[2] The investigators suggested that at this level of Pa_{O_2}, cerebral oxygen uptake is impaired. The fact this was not due merely to a reduction in oxygen content was supported by subsequent experiments, in which an equivalent reduction in oxygen content was produced by a decrease in hemoglobin.[3] In this situation, MAC was not reduced, suggesting that it was the "driving force" of Pa_{O_2} that was important. Therefore, a Pa_{O_2} below 40 torr (5.3kPa) is unacceptable clinically, but not principally because of a failure of oxygen transport; the lowering of oxygen-driving pressure is the significant factor.

In determining an unsatisfactory level of Pa_{O_2}, the available "safety margin" must be considered. When a patient is unstable, changes in cardiac output or a further increase in the impairment of gas exchange may drastically reduce oxygen content, if the Pa_{O_2} level approximates a value that is near the descending slope of the oxygen dissociation curve. Unless the avoidance of a high level of Pa_{O_2} is mandatory for some other reason (e.g., chronic lung disease), it is safer to maintain the Pa_{O_2} near 60 torr (8.0 kPa).

Apart from its effect on the oxygen availability to tissues, hypoxemia is also potentially harmful to pulmonary vascular resistance (PVR). In spontaneously breathing dogs anesthetized with pentobarbital, the first minute of hypoxemia (Pa_{O_2} = 28 torr or 3.7 kPa) produces a 42-per-cent rise in PVR, which then falls to control levels. This return to normal in the presence of continued hypoxemia is caused by the accompanying hyperventilation and hypocapnia. The increase in PVR is not prevented by α- and β-adrenergic blockade.[4] Although the mechanism that mediates the hypoxic pulmonary vasoconstriction is unknown, evidence suggests that local rather than nervous or humoral mechanisms are involved. Clinically, this effect of hypoxemia is significant, particularly in patients with chronic lung and cardiac disease.

Finally, patients with certain disease states are peculiarly susceptible to hypoxemia. In patients with sickle cell anemia, sickle cell trait, sickle cell hemoglobin C, and sickle cell β-thalassemia, hypoxemia is a well recognized trigger of sickle cell crisis (see Chap. 36).[5]

DIAGNOSIS OF HYPOXEMIA

Hypoxemia can be diagnosed with certainty only by measurement of Pa_{O_2}. *Cyanosis* has been defined as the presence of more than 5 g. of desaturated hemoglobin per 100 ml. of blood. However, variation in environmental lighting, the color of drapes and other surroundings, the amount of hemoglobin, and observer variation make the clinical diagnosis of cyanosis notoriously unreliable.[6] Additionally, cyanosis may be apparent without hypoxemia; common causes are the occurrence of methemoglobinemia and sulfhemoglobinemia (see Chap. 38).[7]

VENTILATORY CHANGES IN HYPOXEMIA

During anesthesia with spontaneous ventilation, the pathophysiological changes induced by hypoxemia are usually preserved. In experiments on dogs, Cullen and Eger[8] and Gray[9] reported that hypoxemia (Pa_{O_2} = 26–31 torr or 3.5–4.1 kPa) produced by lowering $F_{I_{O_2}}$ during anesthesia with halothane or methoxyflurane is associated with the following changes in respiratory function:

Increased frequency of respiration, with little change in tidal volume;

An increase in minute expired volume ($\dot{V}_E$) and alveolar minute ventilation ($\dot{V}_A$);

An increase in the fraction of dead space ventilation (V_D/V_T);

A fall in Pa_{CO_2} and rise in pH.

In studies in dogs, first awake and then anesthetized with halothane (1.1% end-tidal), Weiskopf showed that the ventilatory response to hypoxia is reduced during anesthesia.[10] In the awake dog, $\dot{V}_E$ increases markedly as Pa_{O_2} is lowered to about 40 torr (5.3 kPa). Halothane anesthesia depresses the hypoxic response by 52 per cent when the animals are normocapnic, by 65 per cent when Pa_{CO_2} is 44 torr (5.9 kPa), and by 59 per cent when Pa_{CO_2} is 48 torr (6.4 kPa). When end-tidal halothane is increased to 1.7 per cent, severe hypotension results, and the ventilatory response to hypoxemia is almost completely extinguished. Hypoxemia in the conscious state normally potentiates the effect of hypercapnia on ventilation. During anesthesia with halothane in the same experiments, hypoxemia had the reverse effect; as Pa_{O_2} was lowered, the slope of the ventilatory response to hypercapnia was reduced. Thiopental, pentobarbital, and, to a lesser extent, ketamine have also been shown to depress the hypoxemic ventilatory drive when compared to the awake state.[11]

CIRCULATORY CHANGES IN HYPOXEMIA

Cardiovascular function also changes during anesthesia in response to hypoxemia:[2,8,9,12] Cardiac output ($\dot{Q}$) increases; heart rate increases; oxygen consumption ($\dot{V}_{O_2}$) remains unchanged; delivered oxygen, Ta_{O_2} (arterial oxygen content, Ca_{O_2}, × $\dot{Q}$), decreases slightly; mean arterial pressure increases moderately; systemic vascular resistance falls; a metabolic acidosis develops as the period of hypoxemia is extended.

Cullen and Eger compared their results with further experiments on dogs in which Pa_{O_2} was reduced to 30 torr (4.0 kPa), but Pa_{CO_2} was maintained at control levels by increasing inspired carbon dioxide tension ($P_{I_{CO_2}}$).[2] The results were similar: Cardiac output and heart rate increased; systolic blood pressure also rose mildly. However, arterial pH fell, because the increasing metabolic acidosis was not compensated by hypocapnia. Calculated arterial oxygen content decreased to a greater extent during hypoxemia with normocapnia compared to those dogs in which Pa_{CO_2} was allowed to fall. This was thought due to the shift of the oxygen dissociation curve to the right, with decreased pH.

With increasing depths of anesthesia during spontaneous breathing, the cardiovascular and respiratory effects of hypoxemia are preserved. Gray showed that in dogs as end-tidal methoxyflurane is increased from 0.3 to 0.6 per cent, hypoxemia, with levels of Pa_{O_2} of 21 to 31 torr (2.8–4.1 kPa), is associated with an increase in frequency of breathing, a fall in Pa_{CO_2} and an increase in cardiac output, blood pressure, and heart rate.[9] Delivered oxygen falls, however, during the deepest level of anesthesia. Cullen studied spontaneously breathing dogs during halothane anesthesia.[8] During moderate hypoxemia (Pa_{O_2} = 40–42 torr or 5.3–5.6 kPa), frequency of respiration, heart rate, and systolic blood pressure all increase up to an alveolar concentration of 2-percent halothane. During severe hypoxemia (Pa_{O_2} = 30–32 torr or 4.0–4.3 kPa), the animals preserve the respiratory and cardiovascular response, with end-tidal halothane concentrations ranging from 0.76 to 1.25 per cent. Sudden respiratory arrest occurs at deeper levels of anesthesia.

Mechanical ventilation with intermittent positive pressure (IPPV) has been shown to alter the cardiovascular responses to hypoxemia. In studies with dogs anesthetized with pentobarbital or chloralose and urethane, with decamethonium for muscle paralysis, hypoxemia ($Pa_{O_2} = 34$ torr or 4.5 kPa) is associated with a reversal of the normal signs: Heart rate decreases, mean systolic arterial pressure and peripheral vascular resistance increase, and cardiac output is unaltered. The investigators suggest that mechanisms secondary to increased ventilation contribute significantly to the circulatory responses to hypoxemia during spontaneous breathing.[13]

This effect of IPPV is obviously significant during clinical anesthesia if it alters the cardiovascular response to hypoxemia. However, Gray[9] and Murray[14] studied dogs and found that the responses were similar to those found during spontaneous breathing. These conflicting results suggest that the effects of IPPV on the responses depend on the anesthetic agents used. This subject is not fully understood and, for obvious reasons, has not been studied in patients.

Moderate hypothermia may also alter the response to hypoxemia. Regan and Eger found in a study with anesthetized dogs that surface cooling the animal to 28°C almost completely abolishes the increase in minute ventilation seen at 37°C.[15] At 32°C, a slight increase in ventilation with hypoxemia occurs.

Beta-adrenergic blockade by propranolol in dogs does not alter the cardiovascular response to normocapnic hypoxemia (Pa_{O_2}, approximately 30 torr or 4.0 kPa) induced for 90 seconds during mechanical ventilation with halothane.[16] In these experiments, the predominant effect of hypoxemia is an increase in cardiac output (9–26%) and stroke volume, with an increase in myocardial contractility. The investigators conclude that a possible mechanism for the altered cardiac performance is as follows: Hypoxemia leads to an increase in coronary blood flow, which, in turn, decreases P_{CO_2} and increases pH in coronary sinus blood. Similar changes in these two parameters increase the contractility of isolated cardiac muscle.

In summary, hypoxemia in anesthetized dogs is associated with an increase in ventilation (mainly breathing frequency) and cardiovascular function (an increase in cardiac output, heart rate, and blood pressure; a decrease in total peripheral resistance). Oxygen transport ($\dot{Q} \times Ca_{O_2}$) is therefore preserved. Only at deep levels of methoxyflurane anesthesia (end-tidal concentrations of 0.6%) and trichloroethylene (inspired concentration of 1.5%) is oxygen transport significantly reduced. This maintenance of oxygen transport during hypoxemia may not be seen during mechanical ventilation with certain anesthetic agents or during hypothermia.

Causes of Hypoxemia During Anesthesia

Reduced $P_{A_{O_2}}$
  1. Reduced $F_{I_{O_2}}$
  2. Reduced $\dot{V}_A$
Normal $P_{A_{O_2}}$ (venous admixture)
  1. Diffusion defect
  2. $\dot{V}/\dot{Q}$ abnormal,
     where $\dot{V} >$ zero
  3. $\dot{V}/\dot{Q}$ abnormal,
     where $\dot{V} =$ zero (shunt)

CAUSES OF HYPOXEMIA DURING ANESTHESIA

Reduced $F_{I_{O_2}}$

The accidental administration of a low $F_{I_{O_2}}$, from mechanical failure of the oxygen delivery system, is a hazard during anesthesia. The contents of an oxygen cylinder, attached to an anesthesia machine, may become exhausted without being recognized. Failure to fully open a cylinder may result in cessation of flow, even though the cylinder still contains oxygen. There have also been reports of oxygen cylinders that contained a gas other than oxygen. Attachment of an oxygen cylinder to the wrong yoke should be prevented by the pin-indexing safety system, but accidental attachment of a cylinder to the incorrect yoke has occurred by use of more than one washer. Bulk oxygen systems supplying piped oxygen have reduced some of the problems associated with oxygen delivery but have introduced others.[17] The central oxygen supply may be filled with other gases (e.g., nitrogen) or may become exhausted. Infrequently, the oxygen and nitrous oxide pipelines may be accidentally switched. Finally, the central oxygen supply may be improperly attached to the anesthesia machine (see Chap. 50).

A supply of the correct gas at the correct yoke on the anesthesia machine still does not guarantee its delivery to the patient. Incorrect setting of the flowmeter or use of the wrong flowmeter, when more than one oxygen flowmeter is available, may occur. An open or cracked flowmeter has resulted in loss of oxygen. The accidental delivery of high flows of other gases has also resulted in dilution of the expected F_{IO_2}.

Once the correct gas mixture is obtained, faults in the use or assembly of the apparatus may result in failure to deliver the mixture to the patient. Within the anesthetic circuit, sticking or incorrectly assembled valves may result in rebreathing and reduction of F_{IO_2}. Many safeguards have been introduced to prevent such accidents. Colored cylinders and pin-indexing safety systems are not always preventive. "Fail-safe" systems that alarm or shut off gases other than oxygen have usually proved effective. Continuous in-line monitoring of oxygen concentration should, perhaps, be mandatory. Visual and auditory alarms must be part of the monitoring system, in the event that oxygen concentration falls below a preset limit. Failure of the oxygen monitoring system remains a hazard during anesthesia.

Reduced Alveolar Ventilation

During spontaneous ventilation, increasing depths of general anesthesia with almost any agent, except diethyl ether, result in increase of P_{ACO_2}. Therefore, P_{AO_2} will fall, and F_{IO_2}, although previously adequate, may now cause hypoxemia. Similarly, with controlled ventilation, mechanical failure of the apparatus or gas circuit may raise P_{ACO_2} and, hence, lower P_{AO_2}.

Increased Venous Admixture

The induction and maintenance of general anesthesia are usually accompanied by an alteration in gas exchange in the lung. Venous admixture increases, so that P_{AO_2} must be increased

during anesthesia to maintain Pa_{O_2} at the preanesthesia level. The exact cause of this interference with oxygen transfer is not yet clearly elucidated, but considerable data have accumulated.

In 1955 it was demonstrated that total (chest wall plus lung) compliance is reduced during general anesthesia.[18] Subsequent studies showed that this is probably due to reduction in lung compliance.[19] Since that time, many studies have shown an increase in alveolar-to-arterial oxygen gradient ($P_{(A-a)O_2}$) during anesthesia, whether breathing low (21–40%) or high (100%) oxygen concentrations. The increase in $P_{(A-a)O_2}$ has been shown to occur during either spontaneous or controlled ventilation. A comprehensive review of these data has been presented by Marshall and Wyche.[1]

Role of Functional Residual Capacity

A possible explanation for the alterations in gas exchange may be changes in functional residual capacity (FRC). During anesthesia, FRC is reduced with spontaneous[20,21] and controlled ventilation[22,23], and with controlled ventilation, FRC is reduced independently of the size of tidal volume.[24] The reduction of FRC is found to occur within, at most, 10 minutes[23] and, possibly, within 20 seconds[25] of induction of anesthesia; this reduction does not increase with duration of anesthesia.[20,21,23] The magnitude of the fall in FRC seems to be independent of inspired oxygen fraction.[20,21] A greater fall in FRC during anesthesia is found with increasing age and height–weight ratio.[20,21,23] The factors that influence the fall in FRC during anesthesia are similar to those factors that influence impairment of gas exchange. Increased $P_{(A-a)O_2}$ and shunt are found as soon as a steady state can be established after induction (within 7 minutes)[26]; these are not progressive with time[27] and, possibly, are greater with increased age.[23]

The connection between the alterations in FRC and gas exchange might be the relationship of end-expiratory lung volume to closing capacity (CC; Fig. 13-1). Closing capacity is the absolute lung volume at which the airways start to close. If FRC is near or below closing capacity, areas of the

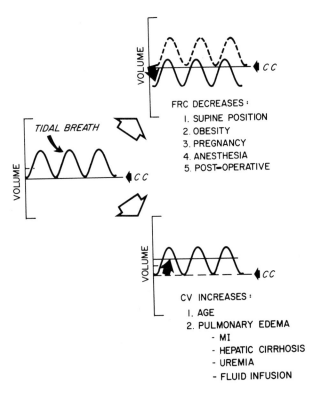

FRC DECREASES:
1. SUPINE POSITION
2. OBESITY
3. PREGNANCY
4. ANESTHESIA
5. POST-OPERATIVE

CV INCREASES:
1. AGE
2. PULMONARY EDEMA
- MI
- HEPATIC CIRRHOSIS
- UREMIA
- FLUID INFUSION

Fig. 13-1. The relationship between closing capacity (CC) and FRC can be disturbed by (*top*) decreasing FRC or (*bottom*) increasing CC.

(V_T) from 5 to 10 ml./kg.[24] This finding is unexpected, because, if the defect is associated with airway closure, less closure would be expected with high tidal volumes. In conflict with some of the data above, one study demonstrated a significant reduction in closing capacity during anesthesia. This study adapted the method for measuring closing capacity, by applying negative pressure at the airway, and makes the results more difficult to interpret.[29a]

The occurrence of airway closure during anesthesia has been demonstrated by measuring the volume of gas trapped in the lung.[30] This is achieved by manual hyperinflation of the patient's lungs following equilibration with helium in a closed circuit. A further fall in helium concentration is interpreted as representing trapped gas. When anesthesia causes FRC to fall from a value above the closing capacity, the volume of trapped gas increases from 0.12 per cent of total lung capacity (TLC) to 3.36 per cent of TLC during anesthesia.

Compared to sitting, the supine position is associated with a decrease in FRC (Fig. 13-2). Derangement of gas exchange is therefore more likely to occur in the supine position, as FRC may approximate or fall below closing capacity. One study during anesthesia with controlled ventilation in the sitting position did not demonstrate a fall in FRC.[31] Anesthesia with nitrous oxide and spontaneous breathing in seated patients, on the other hand, was associated with a decrease in FRC within 20 seconds.[25]

In summary, the induction of general anesthesia is associated with an almost immediate fall in FRC; this reduction is not progressive with time; is greater in older and more obese subjects; occurs in patients with spontaneous or controlled ventilation; is independent of inspired oxygen fraction; and may be minimized in the sitting position. General anesthesia is also associated with an increased $P_{(A-a)O_2}$ and shunt, which are influenced by factors similar to those affecting FRC. It is tempting to attribute the increase in $P_{(A-a)O_2}$ to the fall in FRC. Because of the relationship of FRC to closing capacity, gas trapping and areas of reduced (or zero) $\dot{V}_A/\dot{Q}$ may be produced in the lungs.

lung may stay closed during part or all of the tidal volume. Failure of ventilation may further lead to absorption atelectasis beyond these closed airways. The effect on gas exchange is to increase the lung regions where ventilation is low, compared to perfusion (low $\dot{V}_A/\dot{Q}$), or zero (e.g., a shunt). The fall in FRC during anesthesia, in fact, can be correlated with increase in $P_{(A-a)O_2}$.[23,28] Two studies measured closing capacity during anesthesia; investigators found that it did not change with either spontaneous or controlled ventilation as a consequence of general anesthesia.[24,29] FRC falls, and the difference between FRC and closing capacity correlates with $P_{(A-a)O_2}$, such that, as closing capacity exceeds FRC, $P_{(A-a)O_2}$ increases.[24] In one study, closing capacity, FRC, and $P_{(A-a)O_2}$ were not altered by an increase in tidal volume

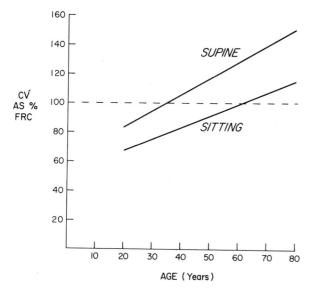

Fig. 13-2. The variations of CV (as a percentage of FRC) with age, in the sitting and supine positions. The difference is primarily due to a reduction in FRC upon assuming the supine position. (Adapted from Don, H.F., Craig, D.B., Wahba, W.M., et al.: The measurement of gas trapped in the lungs at functional residual capacity and the effects of posture. Anesthesiology, 35:582, 1971)

Although this is an attractive hypothesis, it is possible that the changes in FRC and $P_{(A-a)O_2}$ are not causally related but, instead, have a common cause.

The reason for the fall of FRC during anesthesia is not known. An intuitive explanation is that the increased tone in the abdominal muscles, observed in many patients breathing spontaneously under general anesthesia, is responsible. However, induction of total neuromuscular blockade with succinylcholine during halothane anesthesia does not alter the end-expiratory level in adults.[20] One study in children, however, showed that the end-expiratory level increased after injection of succinycholine during anesthesia.[32]

Cinefluoroscopic studies in three supine adult subjects demonstrated that the effect of either general anesthesia or muscle paralysis with succinylcholine resulted in the same degree of cepha-

lad movement of the diaphragm.[33] It has also been established that FRC falls following induction of general anesthesia with complete neuromuscular block and mechanical ventilation. The exception to this is a study that suggested that during anesthesia with Innovar, a considerable increase in end-expiratory level occurred following injection of succinycholine.[34]

Alternative explanations for the fall in FRC during anesthesia are an increase in central blood volume, alterations in lung elasticity, and a loss of inspiratory muscle tone.[21] None of the proposed explanations have so far been established.

Techniques that increase lung volume should therefore improve gas exchange during anesthesia. Results obtained with use of increased positive end-expiratory pressure (PEEP) have been variable, and only small decreases in $P_{(A-a)O_2}$ have been produced.[24,35,36] It is of interest that in one study a greater improvement of oxygenation with PEEP was found in patients anesthetized with Innovar,[37] which may have a greater effect on reducing FRC than other agents.[34]

The mean lung volume will also be a function of the size of the tidal breath and the respiratory frequency. The significance of increased tidal volume[38] and "sighs"[20,27] is disputed.

In the presence of existing abnormal venous admixture, a decrease in cardiac output will increase $P_{(A-a)O_2}$ and cause a further decline in Pa_{O_2}, due to a decrease in mixed venous oxygen content.[39] Inhibition of hypoxic pulmonary vasoconstriction might also be important in producing decreased Pa_{O_2} with constant shunt. Regional matching of perfusion to ventilation is controlled, in part, by local vasoconstriction in the presence of local alveolar hypoxia. General anesthetics (isoflurane, fluroxene, nitrous oxide, and halothane) have been shown to have variable effects on this response, but intravenous anesthetic agents do not seem to influence the response to hypoxia in isolated dog lung.[40]

A shift to the left of the oxygen-hemoglobin dissociation curve may also increase $P_{(A-a)O_2}$ in the presence of venous admixture by reducing mixed venous oxygen content. However, general anesthetic agents (e.g., halothane, enflurane, diethyl ether, nitrous oxide, and cyclopropane) have been shown to shift the curve slightly but consistently to the right.[41] Lidocaine has been shown to have no effect on the oxygen-hemoglobin relationship.[42]

Therefore, general anesthesia has an intrinsic effect of increasing $P_{(A-a)O_2}$ in some patients, and this is augmented by changes in cardiac output or hemoglobin content. Whether hypoxemia is produced, however, depends on the inspired oxygen fraction: An F_{IO_2} of at least 0.3 is recommended if hypoxemia is to be avoided during anesthesia. Epidural and spinal analgesia have no influence on $P_{(A-a)O_2}$ or shunt.[43,44]

Specific Abnormal Factors That Cause Hypoxemia

Apart from the "normal" increase in venous admixture associated with general anesthesia, hypoxemia can be caused by specific abnormal aggravating factors.

Intubation of one mainstem bronchus, either accidentally or deliberately, usually produces an increase in $P_{(A-a)}O_2$, as any shift of perfusion away from the under-ventilated lung is incomplete. Various maneuvers have been recommended to detect the presence of endobronchial intubation, but none are completely reliable, except examination of the chest radiograph.

Deliberate ventilation of one lung during anesthesia for surgery inside the thorax invariably produces an increase in $P_{(A-a)O_2}$ and, depending on the F_{IO_2}, hypoxemia. In a series of 11 patients in whom one lung was mechanically ventilated and the other allowed to collapse, mean Pa_{O_2} (F_{IO_2} = 1.0) was 160 torr (21.3 kPa), and in six of these patients arterial oxygen tension was less than 100 torr (13.3 kPa). Positive end-expiratory pressures of 5 cm.H_2O did not improve oxygenation.[45]

If the equivalent of one-lung ventilation is produced by surgical retraction, a similar increase in $P_{(A-a)O_2}$ occurs.[46] In this study of 200 patients with an F_{IO_2} of 0.5, four had a Pa_{O_2} of less than 60 torr (8.0 kPa), and two had values under 50 torr (6.7 kPa).

Endotracheal suctioning by way of catheters inserted through the endotracheal tube in pa-

tients on mechanical ventilation will reduce Pa_{O_2} for a period of time (3–4 minutes) after reinstitution of ventilation. The length of time that suction is applied affects the degree of increase of $P_{(A-a)O_2}$. Hyperinflation following suctioning reduces the severity of this effect. Boutros showed that, with a F_{IO_2} of 0.25, mean Pa_{O_2} fell from 81 to 70 torr (10.8–9.3 kPa) 60 seconds after endotracheal suctioning.[47] Unfortunately, the individual values of Pa_{O_2} were not given. In assessing the apparent hazard of a procedure, the occurrence of a life-threatening Pa_{O_2} in even one patient is of greater significance than the mean Pa_{O_2}.

A careful technique of endotracheal suctioning, with preoxygenation, utilizing a catheter of small diameter (approximately one-half the internal diameter of the endotracheal tube), and application of negative pressure only during withdrawal of the catheter will minimize this problem.

Aspiration of foreign material into the tracheobronchial tree can cause either pulmonary edema or obstruction, with consequent hypoxemia. Aspiration is common during anesthesia and can occur even in the presence of an endotracheal tube (see Chap. 10).[48]

Pulmonary edema is rare during anesthesia, even with the large volumes of intravenous fluids commonly infused. It may be associated with hypersensitivity reactions to infused blood, to its components, or to drugs.

Pulmonary embolism is associated with hypoxemia, although the exact cause is unknown. Abnormal anatomic shunts, bronchoconstriction, and atelectasis have been suggested. Possible sources of emboli are blood clots, air, blood transfusions, fat, or foreign bodies. Hypoxemia has been reported to follow the application of methyl methacrylate during total hip replacement.[49]

Bronchospasm may develop during anesthesia, with or without an antecedent history of asthma. Severe bronchospasm results in hypercapnia and hypoxemia, but milder forms may cause hypoxemia with normocapnia or hypocapnia.

Pneumothorax can occur spontaneously during anesthesia. Precipitating causes include positive airway pressures. Disruption of the lung is particularly likely to occur if high pressures are applied to limited areas of the lung (e.g., by oxygen flow through a bronchoscope (see Chap. 12).[50]

Pulmonary collapse is rare during anesthesia. Etiological factors include obstruction, hypoventilation, compression, and altered alveolar and airway surface tension.[51]

Airway obstruction may be caused by many factors. The most likely cause is soft-tissue, upper airway obstruction due to the tongue (see Chap. 8).

CAUSES OF HYPOXEMIA IN THE POSTOPERATIVE PERIOD

In normal, conscious humans, hypoxemia stimulates the cardiovascular and respiratory systems.[52,53] An increase in cardiac output, pulse rate, minute ventilation, and tidal volume occurs; however, in experiments with controlled ventilation in conscious humans, the cardiovascular response appeared to be obtunded, and pulse rate did not necessarily increase with hypoxemia.[53] Symptoms of hypoxemia include dyspnea and CNS changes, such as restlessness, confusion, and irritability. Therefore, these signs and symptoms may be found in patients who develop hypoxemia in the postoperative period. Cyanosis can be present but is often not detectable, even in the presence of significant hypoxemia. Severe hypoxemia causes both cardiovascular and respiratory depression, with hypotension, bradycardia, and decrease in minute ventilation.

Anesthesia and surgical procedures seem to be almost inevitably associated with postoperative hypoxemia, depending on the length of exposure and the site of operation. The magnitude and duration of the fall in Pa_{O_2} is directly related to the proximity of surgery to the diaphragm and the length of the procedure.

In procedures performed under general anesthesia lasting less than 22 minutes with spontaneous ventilation and without thoracic, abdominal, or oral incisions, no fall in mean Pa_{O_2} was detected postoperatively in a group of ten patients.[54] However, even in this small series, a 52-year-old woman had a postoperative Pa_{O_2} of 74 torr (9.8

kPa), compared to a preanesthesia level of 92 torr (12.2 kPa). This fall in oxygen tension was accompanied by a reduction of Pa_{CO_2} to 27 torr (3.6 kPa).

In similar types of procedures lasting longer (45–120 minutes), a decrease in Pa_{O_2} occurred up to 90 minutes after cessation of general anesthesia. Values at 3 hours had returned to preoperative levels.[54] Other studies have shown that arterial oxygen tension is significantly reduced at least 24 hours following non-abdominal surgery.[55,56]

A more significant decline in Pa_{O_2} is found following abdominal surgery. After lower abdominal surgery, the mean Pa_{O_2} while breathing air is reduced by 9.5 torr (1.3 kPa) 24 hours later.[56] After upper abdominal surgery, the decrease in arterial oxygen tension is greater[56] and may persist from 5 to 7 days.[57,58] The deficit in oxygen is greatest between the 1st and 3rd days.[57] Hypoxemia is found in patients with normal or low Pa_{CO_2} and without clinical or radiographic evidence of pulmonary disease. If a thoracic incision is involved, the fall in Pa_{O_2} may persist at least 10 to 15 days.[57]

Increased Shunt and Ventilation–Perfusion Inequality

Hypoxemia that develops in patients with a normal alveolar oxygen tension is due either to an increase in the maldistribution of ventilation and perfusion or to an increased shunt. Evidence is conflicting. One study of 18 patients showed that 24 hours after upper abdominal surgery, shunt had increased from a mean of about 1 to 5 per cent of the cardiac output.[59] The total venous admixture, however, had increased from 5.2 to 23.4 per cent of total cardiac output. Hence, the predominant effect was thought to be due to uneven distribution of ventilation–perfusion ratios. A second study also examined patients following upper abdominal surgery.[58] On the 1st, 3rd, and 6th days, $P_{(A-a)O_2}$ was significantly increased due to an increase in shunt, without change in ventilation–perfusion inequality. Finally, a third study demonstrated that both shunt and ventilation–perfusion inequality were increased 1 to 2 hours after surgery.[60] The overall conclusion is that venous admixture increases after anesthesia;

whether this is due to shunt, to ventilation–perfusion inequality, or to both cannot be stated with confidence.

The mechanism that produces the increase in shunt or ventilation–perfusion inequality can only be suggested. Changes in pulmonary function that have been documented after surgery and anesthesia include the following:

A reduction in FRC of about 20 per cent of the preoperative value persists for approximately 12 days after abdominal surgery.[61] This effect is greatest after upper abdominal surgery, is less after lower abdominal surgery, and is least after surgery outside the abdomen and thorax.[62]

A decrease in vital capacity is observed for at least 12 days after abdominal surgery. Both expiratory reserve volume and inspiratory capacity are reduced. Vital capacity after upper abdominal surgery has been reported to be 45 per cent of that preoperatively. The corresponding figure for lower abdominal surgery is 60 per cent.[63] Forced vital capacity and its component expired in one second ($FEV_{1.0}$) are also reduced.

A reduction of average tidal volume to about 80 per cent of preoperative value occurs after upper abdominal surgery, but is unchanged following inguinal herniorrhaphy. Upper abdominal surgery also markedly decreases the rate at which larger than normal tidal breaths occur. In one study, sighs (defined as 200% of preoperative mean tidal volume) were found not to occur.[64] This effect was not seen after lower abdominal surgery.

An increase in respiratory rate of 50 per cent is observed on the 2nd day following upper abdominal surgery, compared to a 10-per-cent increase after inguinal herniorrhaphy.[64]

Relationship of Functional Residual Capacity to Closing Capacity

A popular explanation of the alteration in gas exchange following anesthesia and surgery involves the relationship of functional residual capacity to closing capacity. Since closing capacity is the lung volume at which airways start to close, tidal breathing within closing capacity will result in either total failure of ventilation to parts of the lung or reduced ventilation. Measurement

of (FRC−CC) indicated an inverse relationship with $P_{(A\text{-}a)O_2}$ following upper abdominal surgery. The relationship is as follows:

$$P_{(A\text{-}a)O_2} = 28.5 - [14.6\ (FRC-CC)]\ torr,$$

where FRC and CC are measured in liters.[62] In the this study, mean values for closing capacity decreased slightly after the surgical procedures, so that the reduction in (FRC−CC) is due solely to a fall in FRC.

A study by Fibuch and colleagues demonstrated that the preoperative values of (FRC−CC) in patients undergoing upper or lower abdominal surgical procedures have an inverse relationship to postoperative changes in $P_{(A\text{-}a)O_2}$ with the patients breathing 100-per-cent oxygen.[65]

What is the cause of reduced FRC following anesthesia? The first consideration is that lung volume has been lost by atelectasis as a primary event. Immobility, depressed or absent cough reflex, altered ciliary mechanisms, small tidal volumes, and reduced inspired humidity are potent factors in producing collapse. However, radiographic evidence of atelectasis is not usually found. Failure of closing capacity to decrease significantly after anesthesia has been suggested as evidence against atelectasis.[62] Pulmonary edema is unlikely to be a primary cause of the decrease in FRC, for it should cause an increase in closing capacity due to the formation of edematous fluid around small airways.

The second consideration is that lung volume is lost by alterations in the chest wall and abdomen. Wound dressings, abdominal binders, pneumoperitoneum, or distended bowel may increase the forces tending to move the diaphragm in a cephalad direction. It is a common radiographic observation that the left diaphragm can be considerably elevated merely by air in the stomach. The supine position will exaggerate the low lung volume. Increased abdominal muscle tone due to pain or reflex stimulation tends to reduce lung volume. However, abolishing pain after abdominal surgery by epidural analgesia did not increase FRC in one study.[66] Similarly, Pa_{O_2}, $P_{(A\text{-}a)O_2}$, and Pa_{CO_2} in patients breathing either air or 100-per-cent oxygen are not altered acutely by the relief of pain following abdominal surgery.[67,68] These studies suggest that the mechanism of reduced FRC after abdominal surgery is not that of increased expiratory muscle tone induced by pain.

Factors Involved in the Occurrence of Postoperative Hypoxemia

The following items summarize the occurrence of postoperative hypoxemia:

Hypoxemia can occur after any type of surgical procedure of even the shortest duration. It occurs with greater severity and frequency following procedures near the diaphragm.

The cause of this hypoxemia is not known. A fall in FRC of approximately 20 per cent occurs following upper abdominal surgery. Whether this is a primary, causative phenomenon or is secondary to other changes in the lung or chest wall has not been demonstrated.

No alteration in anesthetic technique during surgery has been shown to influence the incidence of postoperative hypoxemia. This includes regional analgesia, the use of humidification, inspired oxygen in nitrogen, controlled ventilation, and continuous positive pressure ventilation.

Postoperative maneuvers, such as epidural analgesia and pulmonary physiotherapy, do not prevent hypoxemia but may reduce its severity.

Prolonged surgery, obesity, advanced age, an increased ratio of closing capacity to functional residual capacity preoperatively, and preexisting lung disease all tend to predispose patients to the development of hypoxemia.

It is important that hypoxemia is now recognized as an everpresent threat in the postoperative period, even if it is difficult to detect or prevent.

Disorders Associated With Hypoxemia

Factors involved in the development of hypoxemia in "routine" anesthetic practice are described in the foregoing sections. Specific disorders that are associated with hypoxemia may also occur in the postoperative period.

Pulmonary edema is uncommon in the postoperative period.[69] The combination of high left atrial or pulmonary capillary wedge pressure (>15 torr), with high or normal cardiac output producing pulmonary edema, may be seen in pulmonary congestion due to fluid overload or cardiac disease. A high pulmonary capillary wedge pressure in conjunction with a low cardiac output occurs in congestive heart failure. More commonly, pulmonary edema is associated with a low pulmonary capillary wedge pressure. In the postoperative period, this may be caused by drugs; blood, white cell, or platelet transfusions; aspiration; sepsis; pulmonary embolism (air, fat, foreign body, amniotic fluid); airway obstruction; hypoproteinemia; crystalloid fluid overload; or cerebral hypoxia.

Myocardial infarction occurs in about 0.13 per cent of patients undergoing some form of operation or diagnostic procedure.[70] Although infarction is uncommon, its occurrence is usually associated with hypoxemia. The cause of this hypoxemia is unexplained, but it may be associated with pulmonary edema and an increase in closing capacity.

Pulmonary thromboembolism also causes hypoxemia by an unexplained mechanism. Anatomic shunts, atelectasis, and bronchoconstriction have been suggested. The occurrence in the surgical population may seem to be surprisingly low, unless sensitive diagnostic techniques are used. Diagnosed pulmonary embolism occurred in 0.4 per cent of 54,183 adult patients in one survey, of whom 0.06 per cent were postoperative surgical patients.[71] However, using photoscanning on the 3rd or 4th day after surgery, slightly over half (56%) of 54 patients studied had evidence of thromboembolism. This was reduced to 19 per cent of 58 patients if prophylactic subcutaneous heparin was used.[72]

Aspiration pneumonia can occur even in the presence of a cuffed endotracheal tube. Two basic syndromes have been described. In 44,016 pregnant patients between 1932 and 1945, aspiration of stomach contents occurred in 66 patients (0.16%) during delivery. In five cases, the solid material was aspirated, and symptoms of obstruction occurred. Forty patients aspirated liquid material and showed the delayed onset of expiratory rhonchi and, in some cases, pulmonary edema (see Chap. 10).[73]

Hypoventilation is discussed more fully on page 199. Common causes of reduced alveolar ventilation are airway obstruction, sedation, or partial paralysis of the respiratory muscles. An increase in Pa_{CO_2} will inevitably cause a decrease in $P_{A_{O_2}}$, and, hence, hypoxemia, unless the inspired oxygen is increased.

Low cardiac output, in the presence of existing venous admixture, causes a decrease in Pa_{O_2}.[74] The probable mechanism is decrease of mixed venous oxygen content, which further dilutes the oxygen in pulmonary capillary blood, thereby reducing arterial oxygen tension.

Increased oxygen consumption ($\dot{V}_{O_2}$) by way of a similar mechanism tends to lower mixed venous oxygen content, producing hypoxemia, unless a compensatory increase in cardiac output occurs. Normally, this is not a significant factor postoperatively; either there is little increase in $\dot{V}_{O_2}$,[75] or there is proportionately greater increase in cardiac output, causing an increase in mixed venous oxygen content.[76] However, oxygen consumption may be increased during shivering, hyperactivity, fever, or following tissue trauma.

A decrease in oxygen-carrying capacity has a similar effect on decreasing mixed venous oxygen content if a compensatory increase in cardiac output does not occur. Hence, anemia tends to cause hypoxemia in the presence of venous admixture.

Additional causes of hypoxemia have been described. Following a period of hyperventilation, reduced body stores of carbon dioxide are replenished from the metabolic production of carbon dioxide. Hence, alveolar ventilation is reduced, and this causes a reduction in alveolar and therefore arterial oxygen tension. A normal level of ventilation is usually achieved within 1 hour. In a group of 13 patients who had been hyperventilated for an average of 2.75 hours during anesthesia and surgery, when breathing air the Pa_{O_2} fell to a mean low of 72 torr (9.6 kPa). Three patients experienced a Pa_{O_2} of less than 60 torr (8.0 kPa).[77]

Diffusion hypoxemia has also been described. The elimination of nitrous oxide in anesthetic concentrations involves excretion of large volumes of this gas due to its high solubility in blood. This movement of nitrous oxide from blood to alveolus diminishes $P_{A_{O_2}}$, and, consequently, Pa_{O_2}. In a clinical study of 20 patients during anesthesia, upon changing from a mixture of 80-per-cent nitrous oxide in oxygen to air, mean Pa_{O_2} decreased by 11 per cent. This drop was maximal within 2 minutes and had returned to control values in 4 minutes in 75 per cent of subjects. A Pa_{O_2} of less than 60 torr (8.0 kPa) was found in four patients. Spontaneous rather than controlled ventilation during the study was associated with a greater drop (18 torr) in Pa_{O_2}, which took slightly longer to return to control levels.[78]

The additive effect of diffusion hypoxemia and post-hyperventilation hypoxemia has been calculated, and results suggest that $P_{A_{O_2}}$ will fall to a low of approximately 73 torr (9.7 kPa) 5 minutes after 1 hour of controlled ventilation, with 79-percent nitrous oxide.[1]

TREATMENT OF HYPOXEMIA

Hypoxemia can usually be corrected by the enrichment of the inspired fraction of oxygen. It is impossible to predict in an individual patient whether hypoxemia is present. The mean value for Pa_{O_2}, published for a group of subjects after a particular type of procedure, can be a dangerous statistic if applied to clinical use. It is more important to examine, in any published series, the range of values of Pa_{O_2} found. If a single patient in 20 shows a Pa_{O_2} of 40 torr (5.3 kPa), it means that this life-threatening Pa_{O_2} level is possible in the presence of a mean value of 85 torr (11.3 kPa) for the group. It is reasonable practice, therefore, to provide supplemental oxygen to every patient recovering from anesthesia and surgical procedures. This is particularly true in the immediate postoperative period.

It has been claimed that a relatively low $F_{I_{O_2}}$ (up to 0.35) is adequate for reversal of hypoxemia following "routine" surgery. However, the greater decline in Pa_{O_2} in older subjects suggests that a higher $F_{I_{O_2}}$ is necessary.[79] After upper abdominal surgery, arterial oxygen tension while breathing air is calculated as follows:

$$Pa_{O_2} \simeq 81 - (0.28 \times age)$$

With an $F_{I_{O_2}}$ of 0.35 to 0.4:

$$Pa_{O_2} \simeq 166 - (1.12 \times age)$$

It is important to appreciate the difference between the actual fraction of oxygen delivered by a piece of equipment ($F_{D_{O_2}}$) and that inspired ($F_{I_{O_2}}$). For example, a flow of 5 l. per min. through nasal prongs provided an $F_{I_{O_2}}$ of 0.25 during "normal" breathing in two adult volunteers.[80] A face mask with a flow of 10 l. per min. with an $F_{D_{O_2}}$ of 1.0 provided an inspired fraction of 0.52 in the trachea during normal breathing. With a flow of 15 l. per min., the fraction of inspired oxygen rose to 0.54.[80]

Dangers of Oxygen Administration

It is not practical to measure arterial gas tensions in all patients following anesthesia. Hence, in using oxygen routinely in the recovery period, its possible dangers must be considered.

Suppression of ventilatory drive by high inspired oxygen is more likely to occur in patients who are obese; in patients who have chest wall abnormalities, chronic lung disease, metabolic alkalosis, or CNS disease; or in patients to whom narcotics have been administered.

In the newborn, retrolental fibroplasia may result from oxygen administration (see Chap. 23).

Absorption atelectasis may occur if high concentrations of oxygen are given to patients, although data on the likelihood of this occurrence are conflicting.

Pulmonary oxygen toxicity may occur if high concentrations of oxygen are administered for prolonged periods. This is not a realistic problem following short periods of administration in the immediate postoperative period.

It must also be kept in mind that the use of oxygen constitutes a fire hazard. In spite of this and the other dangers discussed above, oxygen must never be withheld from a hypoxemic patient for these reasons alone.

In patients with severe lung disease, supplementation of the inspired oxygen fraction, even with 100 per cent, may not correct the hypoxemia. In these patients, spontaneous ventilation with positive end-expiratory pressure has been used. One report has suggested that the use of raised end-expiratory pressure can avoid the need for tracheal intubation and mechanical ventilation.[81] However, in patients other than newborns, we have found this to be impractical with the equipment available. Tracheal intubation and

mechanical ventilation are usually indicated in this type of refractory hypoxemia. Although arguments have been raised that only hypoventilation requires mechanical ventilation, it is common knowledge that the greater tidal volumes delivered mechanically will usually restore Pa_{O_2} to life-supporting levels. If this, in turn, is still associated with hypoxemia, functional residual capacity can be elevated by positive end-expiratory pressure.[82]

Pain and Analgesia

Pain and its relief have been thought to modulate gas exchange. Epidural analgesia to a sensory level of the fourth thoracic dermatome has no influence on Pa_{O_2}, Pa_{CO_2}, or functional residual capacity.[83] Pain relief with epidural analgesia following upper abdominal surgery has also been shown to produce no acute change in Pa_{O_2} or $P_{(A-a)_{O_2}}$, in patients breathing air or oxygen.[67,68] Functional residual capacity also is not altered by pain relief using epidural analgesia.[66] Whether the effect of prolonged pain relief by epidural analgesics is more beneficial to gas exchange in the postoperative period is disputed. When compared to the use of morphine, epidural block with bupivacaine, following upper abdominal or hip surgery, had no influence on Pa_{O_2}, $P_{(A-a)_{O_2}}$, Pa_{CO_2}, vital capacity, or peak expiratory flow rate.[68,84]

On the other hand, Spence and Holmdahl have demonstrated a lowered $P_{(A-a)_{O_2}}$ following upper abdominal surgery in patients in whom pain relief was provided by epidural analgesia.[75,76] It is difficult to explain the differences in these results. Spence has suggested that the impaired gas exchange observed when morphine was used for pain relief was due to the comparatively large amounts of narcotic administered.[75] In no study, however, has a significant increase in Pa_{CO_2} been shown, and most patients characteristically demonstrated mild hyperventilation. The use of narcotic analgesics in excess may be associated with hypercapnia, which will cause hypoxemia, depending on the $F_{I_{O_2}}$. The use of narcotic antagonists is associated with reduction in Pa_{CO_2} and therefore improvement of Pa_{O_2}.

Even the addition of chest physiotherapy to a

program of epidural analgesia does not alter the impaired gas exchange following surgery on the upper abdomen or hip. However, the overall hospital stay is shortened by utilizing epidural analgesia.[84]

Other Considerations in the Treatment of Hypoxemia

Early mobilization and chest physiotherapy should be of value in increasing lung volume and aiding pulmonary clearance. The upright position may also be beneficial, because it is associated with an increase in FRC, compared to the supine position. In a study of obese patients following intra-abdominal surgery, Pa_{O_2} was higher, and $P_{(A-a)O_2}$, lower in the semirecumbent position than in the supine position.[85]

Prevention of pulmonary complications and hypoxemia by the use of incentive spirometry has been investigated.[86] Mean Pa_{O_2} increased in ten patients breathing either air or oxygen following surgery; changes in Pa_{CO_2} and $P_{(A-a)}O_2$ were not given, however.[86]

Treatment with intermittent positive pressure breathing (IPPB) is controversial. Used discretely in patients with reduced vital capacities, IPPB probably aids inflation of the lungs and clearance of retained secretions.

Section Two: Hypercapnia During and After Anesthesia

By definition, hypercapnia exists when Pa_{CO_2} is higher than the predicted normal level for the subject. Unlike Pa_{O_2}, Pa_{CO_2} remains remarkably constant with advancing age. With hypercapnia, the minute production of carbon dioxide may or may not be excreted from the body. Elevation of Pa_{CO_2} and, therefore, of alveolar carbon dioxide fraction is more "efficient" for removal of carbon dioxide, with a given minute ventilation of expired alveolar gas. As Pa_{CO_2} rises with the onset of hypercapnia, carbon dioxide excretion will be less than its production. However, as a steady state develops at a higher Pa_{CO_2} level, excretion must become equal to production, or Pa_{CO_2} will continue to rise.

DIAGNOSIS OF HYPERCAPNIA

Carbon dioxide activates the CNS, producing sympathoadrenal responses and resulting in increased myocardial contractility, tachycardia, and hypertension. Acting directly, carbon dioxide dilates peripheral arterioles and depresses myocardial contractility. The net effect was studied by Cullen and Eger in 41 healthy young adult male volunteers.[87] During awake spontaneous breathing and with an elevation of Pa_{CO_2} from approximately 40 to 50 torr (5.3–6.7 kPa), they observed the following changes: Heart rate increases 26 per cent; stroke volume rises 11 per cent; cardiac output increases 32 per cent; mean arterial pressure increases 10 per cent; mean right atrial pressure is unchanged; total peripheral resistance falls 14 per cent; and myocardial contractility increases.

Sechzer showed in 12 healthy, awake, spontaneously breathing male volunteers that systolic and diastolic pressures increase progressively as Pa_{CO_2} is increased to values as high as 100 torr (13.3 kPa).[88] Heart rate increases also, but cardiac arrhythmias are uncommon. The plasma levels of catecholamines (epinephrine and norepinephrine) also correlated with Pa_{CO_2}. Signs and symptoms produced by hypercapnia included headaches, hiccups, nausea, vomiting, sweating, shivering, twitching, belligerence, restlessness, excitement, and hallucinations. At Pa_{CO_2} levels above 80 torr (10.6 kPa), most subjects lose consciousness.[88]

CARDIOVASCULAR RESPONSES TO HYPERCAPNIA

General anesthesia has been shown to modify the cardiovascular responses to hypercapnia. Deliberate studies of severe hypercapnia in patients are rare, for obvious reasons. However, mild hypercapnia (up to a Pa_{CO_2} of 60 torr or 8.0 kPa) has been studied in volunteers and in patients. In these reports, $\dot{Q}$ increases with increasing Pa_{CO_2} during anesthesia with fluroxene,[89] nitrous oxide plus phenoperidine,[90] halothane,[91] enflurane,[92] isoenflurane,[93] cyclopropane,[94] and diethyl ether.[95] This increase in $\dot{Q}$ is less than that observed in the awake state. The only exception occurs during anesthesia with 1.5-per-cent halothane in 70-per-cent nitrous oxide,[91] when $\dot{Q}$ decreases as Pa_{CO_2} rises.

Heart rate rises during anesthesia in response to hypercapnia, but to a lesser extent than stroke volume. Hence, the increase in $\dot{Q}$ during anesthesia is predominantly due to an increase in stroke volume. When Pa_{CO_2} increases from 40 to 50 torr (5.3–6.7 kPa), pulse rate increases by 2 to 6 beats per minute during anesthesia with fluroxene, isoflurane, diethyl ether, or 25- to 30-per-cent cyclopropane. The mean rise in pulse rate is 10 beats per minute when 15- to 20-per-cent cyclopropane is given.

Systemic blood pressure also rises when Pa_{CO_2} is increased from 40 to 50 torr, except during anesthesia with halothane (1.5% end-tidal concentration) in oxygen or 70-per-cent nitrous oxide, when it remains unchanged, and with isoenflurane (1.8% end-tidal concentration), when it decreases. With a wide range of anesthetic agents, the increase in mean systemic pressure ranges from 1 to 8 torr for an increase in Pa_{CO_2} of 40 to 50 torr.

Therefore, the two cardiovascular parameters that are the most easily measured during anesthesia, systemic blood pressure and pulse rate, increase during mild hypercapnia (Pa_{CO_2} = 50 torr or 6.7 kPa), but these increases are too small to be useful in detecting a 10-torr increase in Pa_{CO_2}. These cardiovascular responses to hypercapnia during anesthesia are independent of whether breathing is controlled or spontaneous.

Right atrial filling pressure consistently rises with hypercapnia during anesthesia, in contrast to the conscious state. In studies of awake and anesthetized humans, total systemic vascular resistance declines, except during anesthesia with 4.5-per-cent diethyl ether.[95]

Higher levels of Pa_{CO_2} have been described during "apneic" oxygenation. Frumin studied eight patients made apeic with succinylcholine or

d-tubocurarine during or after surgical procedures.[96] Anesthesia was maintained with intermittent intravenous injections of thiopental. Pa_{CO_2} rose at the rate of 3.0 torr per minute, with a range of 2.7 to 4.9 torr per minute. The mean value for the highest Pa_{CO_2} achieved was 166 torr (22.1 kPa), with a range of 130 to 250 torr (17.3–33.3 kPa). Mean systemic blood pressure rose by 26 per cent of pre-apneic values. Systolic pressure increased by 45 torr (6.0 kPa), from a mean value of 115 torr (15.3 kPa) prior to apnea. In one subject in whom Pa_{CO_2} rose to 250 torr, systolic blood pressure increased from 120 to 150 torr. The rise in blood pressure seems to be independent of surgical stimulation, because in half of the subjects, the test apneic period was produced after the completion of surgery. Plasma epinephrine and norepinephrine values were elevated in three subjects. Values for heart rate were not presented in this study, but an "essentially constant rate" in at least one subject was noted.

More profound hypercapnia has been reported in cases in which an error in equipment assembly has led to an elevated Pa_{CO_2}. An 18-year-old patient, spontaneously breathing and anesthetized with closed circuit diethyl ether, was noted to have a Pa_{CO_2} of 234 torr (31.1 kPa) due to the absence of one-way valves in the circuit. At that time, systolic pressure was 120 torr, with a regular pulse rate of 130 beats each minute. Tachypnea, dilated, pupils, perspiration, and flushing of the face were noted. Inspired anesthetic concentration was increased, as the signs were thought to represent a light level of anesthesia. After Pa_{CO_2} had been returned slowly to 40 torr (5.3 kPa), systolic blood pressure was 130 torr, with a pulse rate of 125 beats per minute.[97]

A second report involved a 60-year-old man who was mechanically ventilated during anesthesia using nitrous oxide, oxygen, and *d*-tubocurarine. A flow of carbon dioxide that was unrecognized at the time produced an inspired concentration of approximately 35 per cent. During the initial 10 minutes of anesthetic administration, cyanosis was noted. This cyanosis disappeared, and the patient was said to be "damp." An arterial sample showed that the Pa_{CO_2} was 248 torr (33.0 kPa). At that time, systolic blood pressure was 115 torr, with a pulse rate of 100 beats per minute. The inspired carbon dioxide flow was then stopped, and Pa_{CO_2} was measured at 40 torr (5.3 kPa). Systolic blood pressure was approximately 90 torr, and the pulse rate, 70 beats per minute when Pa_{CO_2} was normal.[98]

Thus, if Pa_{CO_2} is increased in anesthetized subjects by adding carbon dioxide to the inspired gas, arterial blood pressure and pulse rate will rise, but the extent of the rise is modest. Exceedingly high values of Pa_{CO_2} may be found with little change in blood pressure or heart rate.

In patients who develop hypercapnia due to chronic lung disease, high Pa_{CO_2} can be present while the patient is awake, with little or no change in vital signs, even in the presence of considerable acidemia. We have observed one patient who experienced an increase in Pa_{CO_2} from 60 to 105 torr (8.0–14.0 kPa), which decreased the arterial *p*H to 7.0, with no change in vital signs or mental state.

Cardiac arrhythmia has been suggested as the most reliable circulatory indicator of hypercapnia.[99] However, cardiac arrhythmias are by no means universally found. In a series of 18 patients anesthetized with thiopental and succinylcholine, no arrhythmias were found when Pa_{CO_2} was about 70 torr (9.3 kPa).[100] Similarly, in nine patients anesthetized with fluroxene, a Pa_{CO_2} of 55 torr (7.3 kPa) was not associated with cardiac arrhythmias.[89] Even during severe hypercapnia (Pa_{CO_2} = 234 torr or 31.1 kPa), no alteration in cardiac rhythm was found during diethyl ether anesthesia.[97] Whether cardiac arrhythmias occur seems to depend on the surgical stimulation, the age and physical fitness of the patient, and the type of anesthetic agent. Therefore, the occurrence of cardiac arrhythmia is an unreliable indicator of hypercapnia.

VENTILATORY RESPONSES TO HYPERCAPNIA

The ventilatory response to inhaled carbon dioxide in conscious humans is increased minute ventilation. This response is blunted, but not usually eliminated, during anesthesia. For example, during halothane anesthesia tidal volume and minute ventilation, though not respiratory rate, increase with Pa_{CO_2} up to 70 torr (9.3 kPa). In the case of severe hypercapnia reported by Shultz, tachypnea was a prominent sign during anesthesia with diethyl ether.[97]

Hypercapnia may result in hypoxemia by way of two mechanisms. First, carbon dioxide may displace oxygen in the alveolar gas. For example, when patients breathe air, it is impossible for them to achieve a Pa_{CO_2} greater than 90 torr (12.0 kPa), because the displacement of alveolar oxygen will produce a Pa_{O_2} of approximately 20 torr (2.7 kPa), which would be incompatible with survival. Even enriched inspired oxygen mixtures may not protect against low $P_{A_{O_2}}$ if high levels of inspired carbon dioxide are inspired.[98]

The second mechanism is a shift of the oxygen dissociation curve to the right. The significance of this factor can be judged by the calculations of Prys-Roberts.[98] At a Pa_{O_2} level of 104 torr (13.8 kPa), and with a Pa_{CO_2} of 250 torr (33.3 kPa), the arterial saturation would be 90 per cent, whereas at normal Pa_{CO_2}, the oxygen saturation would be very close to 100 per cent.

The increase in cardiac output associated with hypercapnia, on the other hand, tends to improve arterial oxygenation. $P_{(A-a)_{O_2}}$ will decrease because of an increase in mixed venous oxygen content. Pulmonary venous admixture is not altered by hypercapnia.[92]

In summary, the signs of hypercapnia during anesthesia may not be striking, even with high levels of Pa_{CO_2}. Tachypnea, sweating, and flushed skin may occur, although they have been consistently reported only at very high levels.[96,97,98,100] A mild increase in blood pressure and pulse rate may be found.

CAUSES OF HYPERCAPNIA DURING ANESTHESIA

Increased Carbon Dioxide Production

Measurement of carbon dioxide production ($\dot{V}_{CO_2}$) during anesthesia is complicated by the size of the body stores of carbon dioxide, which affect the rate at which a new steady state will be achieved after an alteration in alveolar ventilation. Normally, it is estimated that V_{CO_2} is reduced to approximately 80 per cent of the basal state during anesthesia. An increased $\dot{V}_{CO_2}$ is found with increased body temperature. This is particularly marked in the syndrome of malignant hyperthermia during anesthesia (see Chap. 19). An artifactual increase in carbon dioxide "production" will be created when carbon dioxide is injected into a body cavity (e.g., during laparoscopy).

Altered Carbon Dioxide Transport in the Blood

Inhibition of carbonic anhydrase (CA) slows the hydration of carbon dioxide to form carbonic acid within the red cell. In this situation, the blood carries carbon dioxide almost entirely in solution. Hence, the transport from tissues to lung can be achieved only at high levels of Pa_{CO_2}. General anesthesia with ether or nitrous oxide has been shown to cause a small (approximately 6%) decrease in carbonic anhydrase activity.[101] This small decrease is probably of no consequence in the transport of carbon dioxide in the blood, for normally more than a 90-per-cent suppression of carbonic anyhdrose is needed to affect the transport of carbon dioxide.

Intrinsic Lung Disease

Disturbance of the distribution of ventilation–perfusion ratios has been shown in lung models to impair carbon dioxide output as much as oxygen uptake.[102] Uncompensated, this disturbance will cause an elevation of Pa_{CO_2}. However, this rise in Pa_{CO_2} will usually provoke an increase in minute ventilation and a return toward a normal Pa_{CO_2}, with persisting hypoxemia.

General anesthesia is associated with an increase in shunt, as yet unexplained. Without compensatory hyperventilation, this will itself cause a rise in Pa_{CO_2}. An increase in the alveolar dead space also occurs during general anesthesia and has yet to be explained. For example, a fall in pulmonary artery pressure is associated with an increase in dead space ventilation, but studies in humans have not indicated that a decrease in pulmonary artery pressure is a consequence of general anesthesia.

In summary, changes in the gas-exchanging properties of the lungs usually occur as a consequence of general anesthesia. Both shunt and alveolar dead space increase. The cause is not clear. Uncompensated, a rise in Pa_{CO_2} will occur. However, an increase in minute ventilation will usually correct the hypercapnia.

Additional pathologic changes may occur during anesthesia. The development of atelectasis causes an increase in shunt and dead space and a rise in Pa_{CO_2} when patients are mechanically ventilated at a set minute ventilation. This rise is usually easily overcome by increasing the minute ventilation. Pulmonary edema, with its multitude of causes, may develop and produce similar changes. Hypovolemia that is due to blood loss or extravasation of extracellular fluid into the so-called third space will decrease systemic and pulmonary artery perfusion pressures and increase alveolar dead space.

Central Depression of Ventilation

The carbon dioxide level in blood and extracellular fluid usually is preserved at a constant level because of its involvement on acid-base balance and cellular function. The potential effect on Pa_{CO_2} of alterations in dead space due to lung disease will be offset by the respiratory centers, which tend toward establishment of normocapnia. Failure of the centers to appropriately control ventilation will result in hypercapnia. Whereas failure of oxygenation is usually a consequence on intrinsic lung disease, a rise in Pa_{CO_2} is most often the result of failure of the control of ventilation. Although this statement bears the drawbacks of any generalization, it is made to emphasize this point. Obvious overlap occurs; for example, severe lung disease will cause elevation of Pa_{CO_2}.

In studies in anesthetized human volunteers, it has been shown that resting Pa_{CO_2} rises with increasing inspired concentrations of inhaled anesthetic agents. At the same level of MAC, halothane, methoxyflurane, cyclopropane, and fluroxene are associated with an increase in Pa_{CO_2} in a decreasing order of intensity. At 2 MAC, for example, Pa_{CO_2} is approximately 70 torr (9.3 kPa) with halothane, and 42 torr (5.6 kPa) with fluroxene.[103] The predominant effect of these agents is to cause rapid, shallow breathing. Again at 2 MAC, halothane is associated with a decrease in tidal volume from a mean of approximately 400 to 150 ml. Respiratory frequency increases from approximately 15 to 30 breaths per minute. At this same MAC, tidal volume during fluroxene anesthesia declines from approximately 450 to 200 ml., with a slightly greater increase in breathing frequency than with halothane. Tidal volumes of 100 ml. are common with halothane concentrations of 2.5 MAC. Although this tidal volume seems less than that of anatomic dead space, physiologic dead space decreases with decreasing tidal volumes, such that the ratio of dead space to tidal volume (V_D/V_T) remains constant throughout a wide range of tidal volumes.

The exception among the inhalation agents is diethyl ether, which maintains Pa_{CO_2} from light to deep planes of anesthesia (2 MAC). Above 2.9 MAC, there is an abrupt, marked rise in Pa_{CO_2}. With ether, tidal volume decreases with anesthetic depth less than with other agents. The increase in respiratory rate is approximately equal with all agents.[103] Maintenance of the arterial carbon dioxide level with ether seems to originate in CNS stimulation.[104]

The ventilatory response to increased inspired carbon dioxide is reduced with all agents, including ether. For example, with halothane (2 MAC) the response is only one-fifth of that of the conscious state. At a similar anesthetic depth with cyclopropane, the slope of the ventilatory response is maintained at 0.7 of the response during consciousness.[103]

Except with the use of diethyl ether, therefore, spontaneous breathing is usually associated with an increase in Pa_{CO_2} during inhalational anesthesia. This effect is modified by factors that increase ventilation (e.g., surgical stimulation, metabolic acidosis) and factors that further decrease Pa_{CO_2} (e.g., high inspired oxygen concentrations, metabolic alkalosis, obesity, kyphoscoliosis, drugs, CNS disease, chronic lung disease).

Narcotics depress ventilation and increase Pa_{CO_2} primarily by decreasing the rate of breathing, with less effect on tidal volume.[105]

Decrease in the Work Capacity of the Ventilatory Mechanism

An impairment of the ability of the respiratory pump may result in hypercapnia. For example, patients with neuromuscular disease, such as myasthenia gravis, or patients given muscle relaxants may develop an increase in Pa_{CO_2}. However, in awake volunteers given incremental intravenous doses of *d*-tubocurarine, the slope of the carbon dioxide response curve is not altered significantly.[106] Multiple fractured ribs or trauma to the diaphragm may result in a reduction in the effectiveness of the ventilatory pump, with consequent hypercapnia.

An Increase in the Work of Breathing

Increases in airway resistance or a decrease in compliance may result in hypercapnia.

An Increase in Inhaled Carbon Dioxide

Addition of carbon dioxide to the inspired gas may occur if carbon dioxide is turned on accidentally.[98] A fault in the valve system of the anesthetic circuit may allow rebreathing of expired gas, and failure of the soda lime abosrbing system may also result in high inspired carbon dioxide concentrations.

CAUSES OF HYPERCAPNIA IN THE POSTOPERATIVE PERIOD

The characteristic disorders of gas exchange following anesthesia and surgery are an increase in shunt and mild hyperventilation. Two factors commonly suggested as causes of elevation of Pa_{CO_2} are abdominal distension and pain. However, neither has been demonstrated to cause hypercapnia. Elevated Pa_{CO_2} levels in the postoperative period cannot be attributed to "atelectasis" or "abdominal pain"; but some other factor, usually not related to intrinsic lung disease, must be sought.

Central Depression of Ventilation

The clinical picture of the patient with elevated Pa_{CO_2} levels and without dyspnea or tachypnea is a clue to the presence of central depression of ventilation. This may, however, be complicated by the concomitant occurrence of intrinsic lung disease, and some degree of dyspnea and tachypnea may be found.

The effect of narcotics on the respiratory centers is probably the most common precipating factor. The narcotic may have been used for the induction or maintenance of anesthesia and may have an exceptionally prolonged effect. We have seen patients with depressed mental status and elevated Pa_{CO_2} 10 days after intravenous morphine; these were reversed by intravenous naloxone. This prolonged effect seems particularly evident in patients with renal failure.[107] However, one patient with apparently normal renal and hepatic function developed a slow respiratory rate (which was reversed with naloxone) 10 days after the use of methadone (30 mg.) for maintenance of anesthesia.[108] It is possible that the pain relief and respiratory depressant effect may become dissociated; and that a patient may continue to receive narcotic for pain and yet develop an increasing depression of ventilation.

Metabolic Alkalosis

The development of metabolic alkalosis may cause an elevation of Pa_{CO_2}. Although there is controversy over the occurrence of this compensatory rise in Pa_{CO_2}, there is no doubt that it does occur in some patients. It is commonly related to removal of gastric contents and the resultant hypochloremic alkalosis. Failure to find compensatory changes in Pa_{CO_2} may be due to the duration and rate of onset of the alkalosis. It is difficult to believe that these patients need to be treated for elevated Pa_{CO_2}, for it provides a more normal *pH*. The disadvantage of an elevated level of Pa_{CO_2} might be that, by causing a reduction in minute ventilation, atelectasis is more likely to occur. Otherwise, it is probably best treated by slow correction of the metabolic alkalosis.

High Levels of Inspired Oxygen and Chronic Pulmonary Lung Disease

The administration of high levels of inspired oxygen may depress ventilation. This may be a prominent feature in a patient with chronic pulmonary disease. In 26 patients with emphysema, breathing 100-per-cent oxygen caused a mean rise in Pa_{CO_2} from 49 to 62 torr (6.5–8.2 kPa). In nine of these patients with a normal Pa_{CO_2} (34–44 torr or 4.5–5.9 kPa) breathing air, arterial carbon dioxide levels rose to a mean of 53 torr (7.0 kPa).[109] High inspired oxygen may be given to a patient in whom chronic lung disease is not recognized. The cause of hypercapnia in chronic lung disease is not clearly understood. Patients with similar abnormalities of pulmonary function may have a normal or high Pa_{CO_2}. In patients who develop hypercapnia, it may be that the work of breathing is greater; or, these patients may represent those individuals who, in a normal distribution, would have a flattened carbon dioxide response, even without existing lung disease. Hence, a portion of patients without lung disease may respond to high oxygen concentrations by developing an elevated Pa_{CO_2}.

It is important to identify hypercapnia preoperatively by arterial blood gas analysis in patients with chronic lung disease.

Surgery in the Cervical Region

The name Ondine's curse was coined by Severinghaus and Mitchell to describe failure of automaticity of ventilation following cervical cordotomy for chronic pain.[110] This can occur after unilateral or bilateral cordotomy. It has also been described to follow anterior surgery at the third to fourth cervical interspace without cordotomy.[111] We have seen an elderly patient in whom methyl methacrylate cement was placed in the region of the third cervical vertebral body; this patient was discovered to be lethargic with a slow respiratory rate and a Pa_{CO_2} of 200 torr (26.6 kPa) 24 hours postoperatively. Her respiratory control returned to normal within 36 hours. There was no evidence for other causes of hypercapnia, such as narcotic effect, in this patient.

Increased Work of Breathing

It is well known that upper airway obstruction may cause hypercapnia. In obese, hypoventilating subjects, tracheostomy has been shown to restore normal Pa_{CO_2}.[112] Similarly, in children adenoidectomy has been associated with the relief of hypercapnia, hypoxemia, and pulmonary hypertension. In the postoperative period, upper airway obstruction can lead to an elevated Pa_{CO_2}. The insertion of a nasopharyngeal airway, in this case, may reverse the hypercapnia.

Decreased Work Capacity

Failure to reverse the effect of neuromuscular blocking agents will result in partial paralysis. Patients that are partially paralyzed will hypoventilate, even when there is a vital capacity that is greater than the tidal volume. It is as if the respiratory centers leave a small margin of reserve available in the ventilatory pump. The effect of the neuromuscular-junction-blocking agents pancuronium, *d*-tubocurarine, and gallamine is prolonged in patients with renal disease.

Other Causes of Hypercapnia in the Postoperative Period

Finally, two or more factors may combine to produce hypercapnia. For example, an obese patient, with mild upper airway obstruction, who is breathing high inspired oxygen and has developed a slight metabolic alkalosis from vomiting, can develop severe hypercapnia if given a small dose of narcotic.

TREATMENT OF HYPERCAPNIA DURING ANESTHESIA

The diagnosis of hypercapnia can be made only by the measurement of the carbon dioxide tension in arterial blood. Measurement of the partial pressure of carbon dioxide in a mixed venous sample ($P\bar{v}_{CO_2}$) can give some indication; this value will be about 5 torr (0.7 kPa) higher than Pa_{CO_2}.

Once hypercapnia is diagnosed, when and how should it be treated? It is obvious that high levels of Pa_{CO_2} can apparently be tolerated safely. In a study of 44 patients during anesthesia for thoracic and non-thoracic surgery, hypercapnia occurred in all patients. In the majority, maximal Pa_{CO_2} was 100 torr (13.3 kPa), and in many cases a peak of 175 to 200 torr (23.3–26.6 kPa) was found.[113] In a series of 22 patients undergoing major abdominal surgery, with spontaneous ventilation, using a face mask and "closed-circuit" halothane, most values for Pa_{CO_2} were in the range 50 to 90 torr (6.7–12.0 kPa), but in the latter half of each operation, some patients had Pa_{CO_2} levels as high as 160 torr (21.3 kPa).[114]

In spite of these case reports, it seems reasonable that a Pa_{CO_2} of over 50 torr (6.7 kPa) should be avoided during anesthesia. The treatment, obviously, is assisted or controlled ventilation. Attention to equipment, flowmeters, valves, soda lime, and unnecessary dead space are essential to prevent the development of hypercapnia.

There are a number of reported hazards of lowering an elevated Pa_{CO_2} too rapidly. It has been suggested that cardiac arrhythmias can be precipitated by rapid reduction in Pa_{CO_2}. This is not supported by most investigators, however.[96,97] Hypotension has also been reported, but again this does not occur consistently and is usually only found if Pa_{CO_2} is sufficiently elevated for a prolonged period of time.[99] Long-standing hypercapnia usually produces metabolic alkalosis due to renal compensation. Reduction to a normal Pa_{CO_2} will then produce severe alkalosis of cerebral interstitial fluid. This has been reported to result in convulsions and coma.[115]

TREATMENT OF HYPERCAPNIA FOLLOWING SURGERY

Following surgery, the same considerations apply to hypercapnia as in the intraoperative period: What is the danger of hypercapnia, and what level of Pa_{CO_2} should be treated? In a patient who has received morphine, who is sleeping but rousable, and who has a Pa_{CO_2} of 50 torr (6.7 kPa) and a *p*H of 7.32, it does not seem necessary to reverse the narcotic effect simply to improve these values. Guidelines for the treatment of hypercapnia are listed here.

Considerations in the Treatment of Hypercapnia

Is the *p*H at a dangerous level (below 7.25)?
Is the condition likely to progress, or is it stable?
Is it associated with any other harmful effect, such as hypoxemia due to hypercapnia or atelectasis due to hypoventilation?

What is the mental state of the patient?

What are the comparative dangers of the necessary treatments of hypercapnia?

The initial treatment is reversal of the cause of hypercapnia. Narcotic analgesic effects can be reversed with naloxone, which has the advantage of not causing respiratory depression, so it is relatively safe. Its disadvantages are transient nausea and vomiting and occasional hypertension. Its duration of action is short, so administration may have to be repeated at intervals.[107] Obviously, it will also reverse the analgesic effects of the narcotic. When the necessity for tracheal intubation is being considered in an obtunded patient with hypercapnia, we frequently give a trial of naloxone, particularly when the patient's drug history is not clear.

The second treatment is general stimulation and arousal, which is one of the benefits of postoperative IPPB and chest physiotherapy.

Metabolic alkalosis can be reversed slowly with acetazolamide, hydrochloric acid, or arginine hydrochloride. These agents are usually indicated in patients with a severe primary metabolic alkalosis (base excess greater than 15). If possible, it is preferable to permit renal correction.

Correction of upper airway obstruction may be helpful. Simple insertion of a nasopharyngeal airway may be curative.

Reduction of Pa_{CO_2}

Lowering the inspired oxygen can reduce the Pa_{CO_2} and will certainly lower Pa_{O_2}. Care must be taken not to produce a life-threatenning level of Pa_{O_2} when treating a relatively benign hypercapnia. This is particularly true in the postoperative period, when oxygen demands may be greater and the patient's status is likely to undergo sudden fluctuations. Employing this technique of controlled inspired oxygen requires expert nursing and medical attention.

Treatment of any underlying lung disease is also important. Intermittent positive pressure breathing, incentive spirometry, bronchodilators, chest physiotherapy, nasotracheal suctioning, mobilization, and humidification of the inspired gas all have a role when wisely and discretely used.

Finally, a reduction in Pa_{CO_2} may be brought about by the following:

Respiratory Stimulants. These agents have a controversial role in the management of hypercapnia. Opponents claim that the use of stimulants is analogous to "whipping a failing horse." If hypercapnia is of a sufficient degree to require treatment, then the use of stimulants may not be ideal.

IPPB. It is inappropriate to treat hypercapnia by giving IPPB for 15 minutes every 2 hours. However, if it appears that hypercapnia will be transient (4–6 hours), IPPB can be administered for 15 minutes every 30 to 45 minutes, and, although Pa_{CO_2} will "saw-tooth," it is a useful expedient.

Tracheal Intubation and Mechanical Ventilation. In an intensive care environment, tracheal intubation and mechanical ventilation are relatively benign procedures. In a series of 88 adult cardiac patients, we could not detect a complication attributable to 24 hours of mechanical ventilation postoperatively. However, in a series of 50 pediatric patients following cardiac surgery, there was an approximate 30-per-cent incidence of complications due to endotracheal intubation and mechanical ventilation. These included airway obstruction, accidental extubation, post-extubation airway obstruction, and accidental disconnection of the mechanical ventilator. Therefore, examination of the environment in which the patient will be treated is important in determining the possible hazards.

Guidelines for Selection of Patients Who Need Tracheal Intubation and Mechanical Ventilation

The patient's mental state should be monitored closely when mechanical ventilation is being considered. An awake, alert patient is a less likely candidate for mechanical ventilation. Not infrequently, we have decided against mechanical ventilation in patients with Pa_{CO_2} levels greater than 80 torr (10.6 kPa) on the basis of mental status.

The rate of change of Pa_{CO_2} is also an important factor. For example, two measures of 55 torr, taken at a 1-hour interval, suggest that the patient's status is stable. An increase in Pa_{CO_2} after 1 hour suggests continuing deterioration.

If the patient is distressed, has tachypnea or dyspnea, or is working hard to breathe, with intercostal muscle retraction and a tracheal "tug," intubation and mechanical ventilation are indicated.

If there is hypoxemia ($Pa_{O_2} < 55$ torr or 7.3 kPa) with an $F_{I_{O_2}}$ that is as high as can be justified by the combination of low Pa_{O_2} and high Pa_{CO_2}, then intubation should be established.

We have not found that measurement of $P_{(A-a)O_2}$, tidal volume, vital capacity, or dead space ventilation are valuable in making the decision to institute tracheal intubation and mechanical ventilation, although other investigators rely on some of these.[116,117,118,119]

When it is known that hypercapnia will be transient, intubation should be avoided if other techniques can be used to maintain the patient for the necessary period of time.

If personnel are available to determine the need for and perform tracheal intubation on short notice, the decision to intubate may be delayed.

Sometimes, the decision to intubate is based on the clinical impression that the patient "looks bad" or "will go sour," and not upon measurable quantities.

In general, it is probably better to institute tracheal intubation and mechanical ventilation if there is any doubt.

REFERENCES

1. Marshall, B. E., Wyche, M. Q., Jr.: Hypoxemia during and after anesthesia. Anesthesiology, 37:178, 1972.
2. Cullen, D. J., and Eger, E. I., II: The effects of hypoxia and isovolemic anemia on the halothane requirement (MAC) of dogs. I. The effect of hypoxia. Anesthesiology, 32:28, 1970.
3. Cullen, D. J., and Eger, E. I., II: The effects of hypoxia and isovolemic anemia on the halothane requirement (MAC) of dogs. III. The effects of acute isovolemic anemia. Anesthesiology, 32:46, 1970.
4. Malik, A. B., and Kidd, B. S. L.: Time course of pulmonary vascular response to hypoxia in dogs. Am. J. Physiol., 224:1, 1973.
5. Searle, J. F.: Anaesthesia in sickle cell states. A review. Anaesthesia, 28:48, 1973.
6. Comroe, J. H., and Botelho, S.: The unreliability of cyanosis in the recognition of arterial anoxemia. Am. J. Med. Sci., 214:1, 1947.
7. Schmitter, C. R., Jr.: Sulfhemoglobinemia and methemoglobinemia—uncommon causes of cyanosis. Anesthesiology, 43:586, 1975.
8. Cullen, D. J., and Eger, E. I., II: The effects of halothane on respiratory and cardiovascular responses to hypoxia in dogs: a dose-response study. Anesthesiology, 33:487, 1970.
9. Gray, I. G., Nisbet, H. I. A., Olley, P. M., et al.: Cardiovascular and respiratory responses to severe hypoxaemia under anaesthesia. II. Spontaneous and controlled ventilation during methoxyflurane anaesthesia. Can. Anaesth. Soc. J., 20:637, 1973.
10. Weiskopf, R. B., Raymond, L. W., and Severinghaus, J. W.: Effects of halothane on canine respiratory responses to hypoxia with and without hypercarbia. Anesthesiology, 41:350, 1974.
11. Hirshman, C. A., McCullough, R. E., Cohen, P. J., et al.: Hypoxic ventilatory drive in dogs during thiopental, ketamine, or pentobarbital anesthesia. Anesthesiology, 43:628, 1975.
12. Nisbet, H. I. A., Gray, I. G., Olley, P. M., et al.: Cardiovascular and respiratory responses to severe hypoxaemia during anaesthesia. I. The effect of various concentrations of three anaesthetic agents upon the cardiovascular response and oxygen transport. Can. Anaesth. Soc. J., 19:339, 1972.
13. Kontos, H. A., Mauck, H. P., Jr., Richardson, D. W., et al.: Mechanism of circulatory responses to systemic hypoxia in the anesthetized dog. Am. J. Physiol., 209:397, 1965.
14. Murray, J. F., and Young, I. M.: Regional blood flow and cardiac output during acute hypoxia in the anesthetized dog. Am. J. Physiol., 204:963, 1963.
15. Regan, M. J., and Eger, E. I., II: Ventilatory responses to hypercapnia and hypoxia at normothermia and moderate hypothermia during constant-depth halothane anesthesia. Anesthesiology, 27:624, 1966.
16. Roberts, J. G., Föex, P., Clarke, T. N. S., et al.: Haemodynamic interactions of high-dose propranolol pretreatment and anaesthesia in the dog. II. The effects of acute arterial hypoxaemia at increasing depths of halothane anaesthesia. Br. J. Anaesth., 48:403, 1976.
17. Feeley, T. W., and Hedley-Whyte, J.: Bulk oxygen and nitrous oxide delivery systems: design and dangers. Anesthesiology, 44:301, 1976.
18. Nims, R. G., Conner, E. H., Comroe, J. H.: The compliance of the human thorax in anesthetized patients. J. Clin. Invest., 34:744, 1955.
19. Howell, J. B. L., and Peckett, B. W.: Studies of the elastic properties of the thorax of supine anaesthetized paralyzed human subjects. J. Physiol., 136:1, 1957.
20. Don, H. F., Wahba, M., Cuadrado, L., et al.: The effects of anesthesia and 100 percent oxygen on the functional residual capacity of the lungs. Anesthesiology, 32:521, 1970.
21. Hewlett, A. M., Hulands, G. H., Nunn, J. F., et al.: Functional residual capacity during anaesthesia. II. Spontaneous respiration. Br. J. Anaesth., 46:486, 1974.
22. Laws, A. K.: Effects of induction of anaesthesia and muscle paralysis on functional residual capacity of the lungs. Can. Anaesth. Soc. J., 15:325, 1968.
23. Hewlett, A. M., Hulands, G. H., Nunn, J. F., et al.:

Functional residual capacity during anaesthesia. III. Artificial ventilation. Br. J. Anaesth., 46:495, 1974.

24. Hedenstierna, G., McCarthy, G., and Bergstrom, M.: Airway closure during mechanical ventilation. Anesthesiology, 44:114, 1976.

25. Shah, J., Jones, J. G., Galvin, J., et al.: Pulmonary gas exchange during induction of anaesthesia with nitrous oxide in seated subjects. Br. J. Anaesth., 43:1013, 1971.

26. Nunn, J. F.: Factors influencing the arterial oxygen tension during halothane anaesthesia with spontaneous respiration. Br. J. Anaesth., 36:327, 1964.

27. Panday, J., and Nunn, J. F.: Failure to demonstrate progressive falls in arterial P_{O_2} during anaesthesia. Anaesthesia, 23:38, 1968.

28. Hickey, R. F., Visick, W. D., Fairley, H. B., et al.: Effects of halothane anesthesia on functional residual capacity and alveolar-arterial oxygen tension difference. Anesthesiology, 38:20, 1973.

29. Gilmour, I., Burnham, M., and Craig, D. B.: Closing capacity measurement during general anesthesia. Anesthesiology, 45:477, 1976.

29a. Juno, P., Marsh, H. M., Knopp, T. J., et al.: Closing capacity in awake and anesthetized paralyzed man. J. Appl. Physiol., 44:238, 1978.

30. Don, H. F., Wahba, W. M., and Craig, D. B.: Airway closure, gas trapping, and the functional residual capacity during anesthesia. Anesthesiology, 36:533, 1972.

31. Rehder, K., Sittipong, R., and Sessler, A. D.: The effects of thiopental-meperidine anesthesia with succinylcholine paralysis on functional residual capacity and dynamic lung compliance in normal sitting man. Anesthesiology, 37:395, 1972.

32. Hatch, D. J., and Kerr, A. A.: Change in end-tidal position in children after suxamethonium. Br. J. Anaesth., 47:66, 1975.

33. Froese, A. B., and Bryan, A. C.: Effects of anesthesia and paralysis on diaphragmatic mechanics in man. Anesthesiology, 41:242, 1974.

34. Kallos, T., Wyche, M. Q., and Garman, J. K.: The effects of Innovar on functional residual capacity and total chest compliance in man. Anesthesiology, 39:558, 1973.

35. Wyche, M. Q., Teichner, R. L., Kallos, T., et al.: Effects of continuous positive-pressure breathing on functional residual capacity and arterial oxygenation during intraabdominal operations: studies in man during nitrous oxide and d-tubocurarine anesthesia. Anesthesiology, 38:68, 1973.

36. Frumin, M. J., Bergman, N. A., Holaday, D. A., et al.: Alveolar-arterial O_2 differences during artificial respiration in man. J. Appl. Physiol., 14:694, 1959.

37. Patton, C. M., Jr., Dannemiller, F. J., and Broennle, A. M.: CPPB during surgical anesthesia: effect on oxygenation and blood pressure. Anesth. Analg., 53:309, 1974.

38. Stone, J. G., and Sullivan, S. F.: Pulmonary shunting during alveolar hypoventilation in the dog. Anesthesiology, 42:443, 1975.

39. Sullivan, S. F.: Oxygen transport. Anesthesiology, 37:140, 1972.

40. Benumof, J. L., and Wahrenbrock, E. A.: Local effects of anesthetics on regional hypoxic pulmonary vasoconstriction. Anesthesiology, 43:525, 1975.

41. Smith, T. C., Colton, E. T. III, and Behar, M. G.: Does anesthesia alter hemoglobin dissociation? Anesthesiology, 32:5, 1970.

42. Carden, W. D., and Petty, W. C.: The lack of effect of lidocaine on oxyhemoglobin dissociation. Anesthesiology, 38:177, 1973.

43. Wahba, W. M., Craig, D. B., Don, H. F., et al.: The cardio-respiratory effects of thoracic epidural anaesthesia. Can. Anaesth. Soc. J., 19:8, 1972.

44. Askrog, V. F., Smith, T. C., and Eckenhoff, J. E.: Changes in pulmonary ventilation during spinal anesthesia. Surg. Gynecol. Obstet., 119:563, 1964.

45. Aalto-Setälä, M., Heionen, J., and Salorinne, Y.: Cardiorespiratory function during thoracic anaesthesia: a comparison of two-lung ventilation and one-lung ventilation with and without $PEEP_5$. Acta Anaesthesiol. Scand., 19:287, 1975.

46. Thomas, D. F., and Campbell, D.: Changes in arterial oxygen tension during one-lung anaesthesia. Br. J. Anaesth., 45:611, 1973.

47. Boutros, A. R.: Arterial blood oxygenation during and after endotracheal suctioning in the apneic patient. Anesthesiology, 32:114, 1970.

48. Carson, I. W., Moore, J., Balmer, J. P., et al.: Laryngeal competence with ketamine and other drugs. Anesthesiology, 38:128, 1973.

49. Park, W. Y., Balingit, P., Kenmore, P. I., et al.: Changes in arterial oxygen tension during total hip replacement. Anesthesiology, 39:642, 1973.

50. Britton, R. M., and Nelson, K. G.: Improper oxygenation during bronchofiberscopy. Anesthesiology, 40:87, 1974.

51. Amaranath, L., Dwyer, C. B., DeBoer, G., et al.: Massive pulmonary collapse during anesthesia: A case report. Anesth. Analg., 51:324, 1972.

52. Dripps, R. D., and Comroe, J. H.: The effect of the inhalation of high and low oxygen concentrations on respiration, pulse rate, ballistocardiogram and arterial oxygen saturation (oximeter) of normal individuals. Am. J. Physiol., 149:277, 1947.

53. Hanson, E. L., O'Connor, N. E., and Drinker, P. A.: Hemodynamic response to controlled ventilation during hypoxia in man and animals. Surg. Forum, 21:207, 1970.

54. Marshall, B. E., and Millar, R. A.: Some factors influencing post-operative hypoxaemia. Anaesthesia, 20:408, 1965.

55. Nunn, J. F., and Payne, J. P.: Hypoxaemia after general anaesthesia. Lancet, 2:631, 1962.

56. Diament, M. L., and Palmer, K. N. V.: Postoperative changes in gas tensions of arterial blood and in ventilatory function. Lancet, 2:180, 1966.

57. Knudsen, J.: Duration of hypoxaemia after uncomplicated upper abdominal and thoracoabdominal operations. Anaesthesia, 25:372, 1970.

58. Siler, J. N., Rosenberg, H., Mull, T. D., et al.: Hypoxemia after upper abdominal surgery: comparisons of venous admixture and ventilation/perfusion inequality components, using a digital computer. Ann. Surg., 179:149, 1974.

59. Georg, J., Hornum, I., and Mellemgaard, K.: The mechanism of hypoxaemia after laparotomy. Thorax, 22:382, 1967.

60. Kitamura, H., Sawa, T., and Ikezono, E.: Postoperative hypoxemia: the contribution of age to the maldistribution of ventilation. Anesthesiology, 36:244, 1972.

61. Beecher, H. K.: Effect of laparotomy on lung volume. Demonstration of a new type of pulmonary collapse. J. Clin. Invest., 12:651, 1933.
62. Alexander, J. I., Spence, A. A., Parikh, R. K., et al.: The role of airway closure in postoperative hypoxaemia. Br. J. Anaesth., 45:34, 1973.
63. Beecher, H. K.: The measured effect of laparotomy on respiration. J. Clin. Invest., 12:639, 1933.
64. Zikria, B. A., Spencer, J. L., Kinney, J. M., et al.: Alterations in ventilatory function and breathing patterns following surgical trauma. Ann. Surg., 179:1, 1974.
65. Fibuch, E. E., Rehder, K., and Sessler, A. D.: Preoperative CC/FRC ratio and postoperative hypoxemia. Anesthesiology, 43:481, 1975.
66. Wahba, W. M., Don, H. F., and Craig, D. B.: Postoperative epidural analgesia: effects on lung volumes. Can. Anaesth. Soc. J., 22:519, 1975.
67. Hollmen, A., and Saukkonen, J.: The effects of postoperative epidural analgesia versus centrally acting opiate on physiological shunt after upper abdominal operation. Acta Anaesth. Scand., 16:147, 1972.
68. Muneyuki, M., Ueda, Y., Urabe, N., et al.: Postoperative pain relief and respiratory function in man: comparison between intermittent intravenous injections of meperidine and continuous lumbar epidural analgesia. Anesthesiology, 29:304, 1968.
69. Cooperman, L. H., and Price, H. L.: Pulmonary edema in the operative and postoperative period: A review of 40 cases. Ann. Surg., 172:883, 1970.
70. Tarhan, S., Moffitt, E. A., Taylor, W. F., et al.: Myocardial infarction after general anesthesia. J.A.M.A., 220:1451, 1972.
71. Levy, R. P., Laus, V. G., and Miraldi, F. D.: The frequency and detection of serious postoperative thromboembolic disease. Surg. Gynecol. Obstet., 140:903, 1975.
72. Lahnborg, G., Bergstrom, K., Friman, L., et al.: Effect of low dose heparin on incidence of postoperative pulmonary embolism detected by photoscanning. Lancet, 1:329, 1974.
73. Mendelson, C. L.: The aspiration of stomach contents into the lungs during obstetric anesthesia. Am. J. Obstet. Gynecol., 52:191, 1946.
74. Philbin, D. M., Sullivan, S. F., Bowman, F. O., et al.: Postoperative hypoxemia: contribution of the cardiac output. Anesthesiology, 32:136, 1970.
75. Spence, A. A., and Smith, G.: Postoperative analgesia and lung function: a comparison of morphine with extradural block. Br. J. Anaesth., 43:144, 1971.
76. Holmdahl, M. H., Modig, J.: The role of regional block versus parenteral analgesics in patient management with special emphasis on the treatment of postoperative pain. Br. J. Anaesth., 47:264, 1975.
77. Salvatore, A. J., Sullivan, S. F., and Papper, E. M.: Postoperative hypoventilation and hypoxemia in man after hyperventilation. N. Engl. J. Med., 280: 467, 1969.
78. Roesch, R., and Stoelting, R.: Duration of hypoxemia during nitrous oxide excretion. Anesth. Analg., 51:851, 1972.
79. Davis, A. G., and Spence, A. A.: Postoperative hypoxemia and age. Anesthesiology, 37:663, 1972.
80. Gibson, R. L., Comer, P. B., Beckham, R. W., et al.: Actual tracheal oxygen concentration with commonly used oxygen equipment. Anesthesiology, 44:71, 1976.
81. Greenbaum, D. M., Millen, J. E., Eross, B., et al.: Continuous positive airway pressure without tracheal intubation in spontaneously breathing patients. Chest, 69:615, 1976.
82. Kirby, R. R., Downs, J. B., Civetta, J. M., et al.: High level positive end expiratory pressure (PEEP) in acute respiratory insufficiency. Chest, 67:156, 1975.
83. Wahba, W. M., Craig, D. B., Don, H. F., et al.: The cardio-respiratory effects of thoracic epidural anaesthesia. Can. Anaesth. Soc. J., 19:8, 1972.
84. Pflug, A. E., Murphy, T. M., Butler, S. H., et al.: The effects of postoperative peridural analgesia or pulmonary therapy and pulmonary complications. Anesthesiology, 41: 8, 1974.
85. Vaughan, R. W., Bauer, S., and Wise, L.: Effect of position (semirecumbent versus supine) on postoperative oxygenation in markedly obese subjects. Anesth. Analg., 55:37, 1976.
86. Bartlett, R. J., Brennan, M. L., Gazzaniga, A. B., et al.: Studies on the pathogenesis and prevention of postoperative pulmonary complications. Surg. Gynecol. Obstet., 137:925, 1973.
87. Cullen, D. J., and Eger, E. I., II: Cardiovascular effects of carbon dioxide in man. Anesthesiology, 41: 345, 1974.
88. Sechzer, P. H., Egbert, L. D., Linde, H. W., et al.: Effect of CO_2 inhalation on arterial pressure, ECG and plasma catecholamines and 17-OH corticosteroids in normal man. J. Appl. Physiol., 15:454, 1960.
89. Cullen, B. F., Eger, E. I., II, Smith, N. T., et al.: The circulatory response to hypercapnia during fluroxene anesthesia in man. Anesthesiology, 34:415, 1971.
90. Prys-Roberts, C., Kelman, G. R., Greenbaum, R., et al.: Circulatory influences of artificial ventilation during nitrous oxide anaesthesia in man. II. Results: the relative influence of mean intrathoracic pressure and arterial carbon dioxide tension. Br. J. Anaesth., 39:533, 1967.
91. Hornbein, T. F., Martin, W. E., Bonica, J. J., et al.: Nitrous oxide effects on the circulatory and ventilatory responses to halothane. Anesthesiology, 31:250, 1969.
92. Marshall, B. E., Cohen, P. J., Klingenmaier, C. H., et al.: Some pulmonary and cardiovascular effects of enflurane (Ethrane) anaesthesia with varying Pa_{CO_2} in man. Br. J. Anaesth., 43:996, 1971.
93. Cromwell, T. H., Stevens, W. C., Eger, E. I., II, et al.: The cardiovascular effects of compound 469 (Forane) during spontaneous ventilation and CO_2 challenge in man. Anesthesiology, 35:17, 1971.
94. Cullen, D. J., Eger, E. I., II, and Gregory G. A.: The cardiovascular effects of carbon dioxide in man, conscious and during cyclopropane anesthesia. Anesthesiology, 31:407, 1969.
95. Gregory, G. A., Eger, E. I., II, Smith, N. T., et al.: The cardiovascular effect on carbon dioxide in man awake and during diethyl ether anesthesia. Anesthesiology, 40:301, 1974.
96. Frumin, J. M., Epstein, R. M., and Cohen, G.: Apneic oxygenation in man. Anesthesiology, 20:789, 1959.
97. Schultz, E. A., Buckley, J. J., Oswald, A. J., et al.: Profound acidosis in an anesthetized human: report of a case. Anesthesiology, 21:285, 1960.
98. Prys-Roberts, C., Smith, W. D. A., and Nunn, J. F.: Accidental severe hypercapnia during anaesthesia. A

case report and review of some physiological effects. Br. J. Anaesth., *39*:257, 1967.

99. Price, H. L.: Effects of carbon dioxide on the cardiovascular system. Anesthesiology, *21*:652, 1960.

100. Fraioli, R. L., Sheffer, L. A., and Steffenson, J. L.: Pulmonary and cardiovascular effects of apneic oxygenation in man. Anesthesiology, *39*:588, 1973.

101. Christian, G., and Greene, N. M.: Blood carbonic anhydrase activity in anesthetized man. Anesthesiology, *23*:179, 1962.

102. West, J. B.: Causes of carbon dioxide retention in lung disease. N. Engl. J. Med., *284*:1232, 1971.

103. Larson, C. P., Jr., Eger, E. I., II, Maullem, M., et al.: The effects of diethyl ether and methoxyflurane on ventilation: II. A comparative study in man. Anesthesiology, *30*:174, 1969.

104. Muallem, M., Larson, C. P., Jr., and Eger, E. I., II: The effects of diethyl ether on Pa_{CO_2} in dogs with and without vagal, somatic and sympathetic block. Anesthesiology, *30*:185, 1969.

105. Davie, I., Scott, D. B., and Stephen, G. W.: Respiratory effects of pentazocine and pethidine in patients anaesthetized with halothane and oxygen. Br. J. Anaesth., *42*:113, 1970.

106. Gal, T. J., and Smith, T. C.: Partial paralysis with *d*-tubocurarine and the ventilatory response to CO_2: an example of respiratory sparing? Anesthesiology, *45*:22, 1976.

107. Don, H. F., Dieppa, R. A., and Taylor, P.: Narcotic analgesics in anuric patients. Anesthesiology, *42*:745, 1975.

108. Norris, J. V., and Don, H. F.: Prolonged depression of respiratory rate following methadone analgesia. Anesthesiology, *45*:361, 1976.

109. Wilson, R. H., Hoseth, W., and Dempsey, M. E.: Respiratory acidosis. I. Effects of decreasing respiratory minute volume in patients with severe chronic pulmonary emphysema, with specific reference to oxygen, morphine and barbiturates. Am. J. Med., *10*:464, 1954.

110. Severinghaus, J. W., and Mitchell, R. A.: Ondine's curse—failure of respiratory center automaticity while awake. Clin. Res., *10*:122, 1962.

111. Krieger, A. J., and Rosomoff, H. L.: Sleep induced apnea. Part 2: respiratory failure after anterior spinal surgery. J. Neurosurg., *39*:181, 1974.

112. Sackner, M. A., Landa, J., and Forrest, T.: Periodic sleep apnea: chronic sleep deprivation related to intermittent upper airway obstruction and central nervous system disturbance. Chest, *67*:164, 1975.

113. Ellison, R. G., Ellison, L. T., and Hamilton, W. F.: Analysis of respiratory acidosis during anesthesia. Ann. Surg., *141*:375, 1955.

114. Birt, C., and Cole, P.: Some physiological effects of closed circuit halothane anaesthesia. Anaesthesia, *20*:258, 1965.

115. Rotherham, E. B., Safar, P., and Robin, E. C.: CNS disorders during mechanical ventilation in chronic pulmonary disease. J.A.M.A., *189*:993, 1964.

116. Lecky, J. H., and Ominsky, A. J.: Postoperative respiratory management. Chest, *62*:50s, 1972.

117. Pontoppidan, H.: Treatment of respiratory failure in nonthoracic trauma. J. Trauma, *8*:938, 1968.

118. Wilson, R. C., and Pontoppidan, H.: Acute respiratory failure: diagnostic and therapeutic criteria. Crit. Care Med., *2*:293, 1974.

119. Hilberman, M., Kamm, B., Lamy, M., et al.: An analysis of potential physiological predictors of respiratory adequacy following cardiac surgery. J. Thorac. Cardiovasc. Surg., *71*:711, 1976.

FURTHER READING

Hedley-Whyte, J., Burgess, G. E., III, Feeley, T. W., et al.: Applied Physiology of Respiratory Care. Boston, Little, Brown, & Co., 1976.

Nunn, J. F.: Applied Respiratory Physiology. ed. 2. London, Butterworth & Co., 1977.

Sykes, M. K., McNicol, M. W., and Campbell, E. J. M.: Respiratory Failure. ed. 2. Oxford, Blackwell Scientific Publications, 1976.

Part Five

The Heart and Blood Vessels

14 Cardiac Dysrhythmias

Marion A. Carnes, M.D.

The primary function of the heart is to receive the venous volume of blood returned from the systemic circulation and, ultimately, to pump that volume of blood back into the systemic circulation. The heart may be viewed, then, as a demand pump.

The demands placed on the pump are determined largely by extracardiac factors. Alterations of general metabolic rate or stress alter tissue demands on the pump by altering the venous return volume of blood. Other alterations of the venous return volume, either excessive from infusion overload or inadequate owing to obstruction or loss, alter the demands on the pump.

The ability of the heart to respond effectively to varying demands is determined by many factors. Cardiac output is the product of heart rate and stroke volume. If there are extremes of heart rate, the efficiency of the heart is impaired, and cardiac output diminishes. Disturbances of electrical rhythm may lead to ineffective or inefficient heart beats, so that the demanded cardiac output may not be delivered.

Stroke volume, another factor determining cardiac output, is influenced by preload, afterload, and myocardial contractility. The term *preload* relates to the pressure or volume within a cardiac chamber at the beginning of a contraction. *Afterload* is the pressure against which a chamber must eject its volume (e.g., the aortic diastolic pressure in the left ventricle). *Myocardial contractility*, the efficiency with which the myocar-

dium contracts to produce work, may be affected by many agents used during anesthesia.

Myocardial contractility is influenced by the electrical activity within the heart. An electrical impulse that is sufficient to cause myocardial cells to contract must be generated within the myocardium. Then this impulse must be conducted throughout the myocardium in a manner that causes an efficiently organized contraction of the myocardium, to eject a certain volume of blood. The generation and conduction of such an electrical impulse must occur regularly, rhythmically, and at an appropriate rate if the heart is to serve efficiently as a demand pump.

In addition to preexisting disease that may be aggravated by anesthesia, physiologic and pharmacologic changes that surpass the heart's ability to compensate may occur.

PHYSIOLOGY OF CARDIAC TISSUE

Disturbances of cardiac rhythm usually result from disorders of electrical impulse formation, disorders of conduction of that electrical impulse, or both. In order to understand these disorders of impulse formation and/or conduction, there must be some knowledge of three electrophysiologic properties of cardiac tissue: automaticity, refractoriness, and conduction velocity.

Automaticity

If one places a microelectrode within a cell of the heart and another microelectrode on the

211

surface of that cell, an electrical potential across the cell membrane can be measured. If changes in this transmembrane potential are plotted on the ordinate of a graph against time on the abscissa, something like a "minielectrocardiogram" is the result. Figure 14-1 is such a graphic depiction of changes in transmembrane electrical potential during the depolarization and repolarization of a cell membrane.

While recognizing the risks of error inherent in oversimplification, the course of events in a cycle of depolarization-repolarization can be described in a naive fashion. Curve A (*solid line*) of Figure 14-1 represents the changes in electrical activity of a myocardial contractile cell membrane. With the cell at rest, an electrical transmembrane potential of about −90 mv. is maintained. Although the cell membrane is slightly permeable to sodium ions, a transport mechanism, the so-called "sodium pump," maintains an extra- to intracellular sodium ratio of about 7 to 1 when the cell membrane is at rest. Potassium ions can cross the cell membrane more readily than sodium ions, but because potassium ions have an electropositive charge, they are retained within the resting cell by the relatively strong electronegative intracellular potential. The electronegative charge within the resting cell is determined largely by ions to which the membrane is not permeable, primarily proteins and nucleic acids, together with the large extracellular concentration of sodium ions. The ratio of intra- to extracellular potassium is about 30 to 1.

If this resting cell membrane is excited appropriately, it becomes sufficiently deranged to allow sodium ions to rush into the cell. This influx of sodium quickly changes the transmembrane potential to about +30 mv., which then allows potassium ions to leave the cell interior. Next, sodium is extruded from the cell by an active transport mechanism, restoring the transmembrane potential to a negative value, which in turn attracts potassium ions into the cell. The process is completed when the transmembrane potential is restored to its normal resting value (membrane resting potential, MRP), and the cell membrane is repolarized.

Purkinje cells are capable of spontaneous depolarization, differing in this respect from other

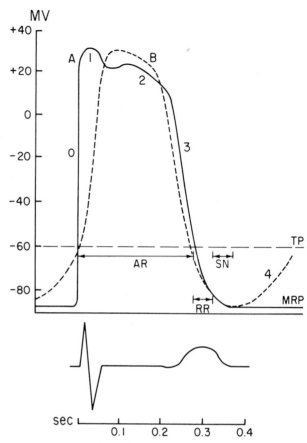

Fig. 14-1. Transmembrane potential of myocardial contractile cell *(A)* and Purkinje cell *(B)*. MRP: membrane resting potential. TP: threshold poential. AR: absolute refractory period. RR: relative refractory period. SN: supernormal period. The numbers 0, 1, 2, 3, and 4 refer to phases of depolarization-repolarization.

myocardial cells. Because of this property, Purkinje cells are also referred to as automatic or pacemaker cells. The electrical events in a cycle of depolarization-repolarization of a Purkinje cell are depicted as Curve B in Figure 14-1. The membrane of a Purkinje cell may be more permeable to sodium ions, or perhaps the sodium pump is less efficient. Whatever the reason, a slow leaking of sodium ions into the Purkinje cell occurs while the cell is in a resting state. The transmembrane potential is changed by this leak of sodium until a threshold potential (TP) of about −60 mv. is reached; at the TP the cell membrane becomes grossly deranged, sodium ions then pour into the cell, potassium is allowed to leave the cell interior, and spontaneous depolarization of the cell membrane has occurred. Repolarization occurs as sodium ions are extruded from the cell and potassium ions are drawn into the cell.

For convenience as well as standardization of terminology, the cycle of depolarization-repolarization has been arbitrarily divided into phases (Fig. 14-1): Phase 0, the almost instantaneous depolarization of the cell membrane; Phase 1, the slight overshoot of electrical potential; Phase 2, the slow beginning of repolarization; Phase 3, the period of rapid progression of repolarization; Phase 4, the period of rest in a myocardial cell or the beginning of diastolic or spontaneous depolarization of a pacemaker (Purkinje) cell.

Automaticity, the spontaneous depolarization of a Purkinje cell, is altered by changes in any or all of three factors: the rate of Phase 4 depolarization, the TP, and the MRP. If the rate of spontaneous depolarization of a Purkinje cell is increased (the slope of Phase 4 becomes more nearly vertical), impulse formation in that affected cell occurs more rapidly. If the MRP is reduced (e.g., −90 mv. to −70 mv.), the cell becomes more excitable, and Phase 4 depolarization can occur more readily. If the TP is lowered (e.g., −60 mv. to −70 mv.), that cell is more irritable, and Phase 4 depolarization occurs more readily.

Physical and chemical influences can alter any or all of these components of automaticity of Purkinje cells. Since Purkinje cells are distributed in varying concentrations throughout the myocardium, their automaticity can be altered enough to allow any of these cells, anywhere in the myocardium, to serve as the pacemaker for the heart. If the pacemaker cell is hypoxic or acidotic, its cell membrane is unstable because of changes in MRP, TP, or both. Additionally, the rate of Phase 4 depolarization is increased. Tachycardia and dysrhythmia commonly result, as seen in the inadequately ventilated patient. Increased sympathetic activity increases the rate of Phase 4 depolarization, as do cyclopropane, methoxyflurane, and cardiac glycosides such as digoxin. A rapid decline in extracellular potassium concentration reduces the MRP and increases the rate of Phase 4 depolarization. Ventricular ectopic beats

or ventricular tachycardia may result from such a change.

Increased vagal activity decreases the rate of Phase 4 depolarization and increases the MRP, slowing the rate of spontaneous depolarization (which reduces automaticity). Sinus activity is affected most, allowing lower pacemaker centers to assume the role of primary pacemaker. Atrial, AV junctional, or idioventricular rhythms may result. Reserpine, in addition to depleting catecholamines, is a parasympathomimetic agent and probably contributes to bradycardia through the mechanism of increased vagal activity. Hypothermia decreases the rate of Phase 4 depolarization, slowing the sinus rate, and allowing "escape" of pacemakers in the atria or AV junctional area. Conversely, hyperthermia increases the rate of Phase 4 depolarization, as one would anticipate. Halothane depresses Phase 4 depolarization and antagonizes the stimulant action of ouabain. This might explain the salutary effects on automaticity seen when halothane is administered to patients in whom digitalis intoxication has produced cardiac dysrhythmia. The opposite is seen when cyclopropane is administered to these patients.

The physical and chemical factors discussed are only some of the many that can influence impulse formation by altering the rate of Phase 4 depolarization, the MRP, or the TP. Whether these factors are malevolent or benevolent depends on the patient's clinical condition at that moment. Such factors may be introduced intentionally to improve the clinical condition of a patient, or they may be allowed to develop inadvertently, to the detriment of the patient's well-being. With understanding of the physiology of automaticity and the physical and chemical influences that alter it, one can anticipate and alter many changes in automaticity that might otherwise threaten the well-being of a patient.

Refractoriness

Once a cell membrane has been stimulated effectively to produce depolarization, no degree of further stimulation will alter the rate or degree of depolarization of that membrane. The membrane is said to be absolutely refractory, and this "absolute refractory period" (AR, Fig. 14-1) persists from the instant of depolarization, until repolarization of the membrane has progressed to the level of the threshold potential. After the electrical potential has been restored at least to TP, the cell membrane can be stimulated to depolarize if an unusually strong stimulus is applied. The cell membrane is said to be only relatively refractory during this period in the cycle. The "relatively refractory period" (RR, Fig. 14-1) begins when the TP is reached during repolarization of the cell membrane and persists until the resting potential for the cell membrane is almost reached. As repolarization of the cell membrane nears completion, just as the resting potential is approached, the cell membrane becomes unusually sensitive to excitation. Since minimal stimulation at this point can produce depolarization of the cell membrane, the period, which lasts only a few milliseconds, is called the *supernormal period* (SN, Fig. 14-1).

The importance of this supernormal period becomes apparent on referring to Figure 14-1. Note that the supernormal period can be temporally superimposed on the T wave of the diagrammatic ECG just beneath. Ectopic depolarization of Purkinje cells anywhere in the myocardium during this brief supernormal period can produce depolarization of other Purkinje cells. The ultimate hazard of such a state is the production of ventricular fibrillation. This is the reason for concern associated with "R-on-T" types of ventricular ectopic beats, which are considered in more detail on page 222.

Conduction Velocity

After pacemaker cells have spontaneously depolarized to generate an impulse, that impulse must be conducted throughout the myocardium in a manner that will trigger an organized contraction of myocardial cells, so that an appropriate volume of blood will be ejected from the ventricular chamber. The velocity with which such an impulse is conducted must be controllable in order to accommodate the various demands on the heart. If greatest efficiency is to be provided, there should be some control over the direction in which impulses are conducted, as well as the character of the impulse accepted for conduction.

The velocity with which an impulse is conducted is intimately and directly related to the manner in which that impulse is generated. Specifically, both the rate of spontaneous depolarization and the amplitude of the action potential produced determine the velocity with which that impulse is conducted. Increasing the rate of Phase 4 depolarization and/or increasing the amplitude of the action potential produced increases the velocity of conduction and vice versa.

If there is a progressive decrease in the rate of depolarization and the action potential amplitude, a progressive impairment of conduction occurs, which is called *decremental conduction.* Such a delay in conduction occurs normally and is the cause of a normal slowing of impulse conduction through the AV node. This delay is measured on the standard ECG as the P-R interval. Decremental conduction can occur in any area of conduction tissue, though it is not normally as marked as that of the AV node. If decremental conduction progresses, failure of conduction may occur. Such failure is usually unidirectional, in that conduction in the normal antegrade direction is blocked, but retrograde conduction is still possible.

Unidirectional failure of conduction is seen in some patients with "coupled" beats, a sequence consisting of a normal beat followed by an ectopic beat, as in some forms of bigeminy. In this condition, a normal impulse conducted through the Purkinje system encounters an area of antegrade block, and conduction failure occurs at that site. However, the impulse traveling through the myocardial cells may reenter the Purkinje system distal to the block and be conducted in a retrograde direction to reenter the conduction system, stimulating the myocardial cells again, but with an abnormal contraction.

Hyperkalemia decreases the rate of depolarization and the amplitude of the action potential, thus reducing the conduction velocity. This is seen on the standard ECG as a widening of the QRS complex, indicating slower than normal conduction of an impulse through the ventricular system. Some antidepressant drugs, such as imipramine and amitriptyline, may impair conduction and produce ECG changes such as prolonged Q-T intervals and depressed S-T segments, and may even suggest acute myocardial infarction. Currently, it is believed that these changes are not merely artifactual in the ECG but are true disturbances of impulse conduction.

A number of physical and chemical factors influence spontaneous depolarization of Purkinje cells (see p. 213). It is apparent that these same factors can indirectly alter conduction velocity by altering the rate and amplitude of impulse formation.

CLINICAL PRESENTATION OF CARDIAC DYSRHYTHMIAS

The incidence of cardiac dysrhythmias occuring in patients during the administration of anesthesia is unknown. While these disturbances are anticipated in patients with preexisting heart disease, transient disturbances in heart rhythm are known to occur in normal, healthy people, at rest, with no known physical or chemical intervention that should contribute to such disturbances. The incidence of cardiac dysrhythmias in patients undergoing anesthesia may be said to vary directly with the diligence with which dysrhythmias are sought. Of more importance than the detection of rhythm disturbances is the evaluation of how such disturbances may affect the efficiency of the demand pump, the heart.

Disturbances of cardiac rhythm are detected by the ordinary methods of monitoring the heart: palpation of an arterial pulse, auscultation of heart sounds, and blood pressure determination by direct or indirect methods. Diagnosis of cardiac dysrhythmias commonly requires the use of the ECG.

Electrocardiography

In this section, it is assumed that the reader has some working knowledge of basic electrocardiography. Under the usual clinical circumstances in anesthetizing areas, only a single lead of the ECG is observed; therefore multichannel electrocardiography is not considered here. Commonly, the single lead that is monitored is lead II, because it usually demonstrates P wave activity better than leads I or III. More recently, the V leads have been monitored, in part because they may indicate the presence of coronary ischemia, if such a state exists.

In observing the ECG, it must be recalled that only the electrical activity of the heart is being monitored, and no direct information is supplied regarding the ability of the myocardium to respond properly to such electrical activity. Standardization of the voltage deflection and the time course of the display are important and should be provided.

The anesthesiologist should ask himself the following questions when observing the ECG: Are P waves present and regular in time, configuration, and voltage? Is each P wave followed by a QRS complex? (Conversely, is each QRS complex preceded by a P-wave?) Is each QRS complex regular in time, configuration, and voltage?

It must be remembered that ectopic impulses can originate in any area of the conduction system: as a single focus or multiple foci; as reentry owing to retrograde conduction; as an "escape" rhythm because of higher failure; and owing to "block" because a properly generated impulse is not conducted.

Because disturbances of ventricular rhythm represent a more serious and immediate threat to circulation than atrial disturbances, anesthesiologists are most concerned about ventricular dysrhythmias.

Examples of Dysrhythmias

The following examples of ECGs represent some commonly seen tracings. Many of them demonstrate slight aberrations from the normal. Several examples of true cardiac dysrhythmias are presented, and some require specific therapy in addition to general supportive care.

Sinus Arrhythmia. P waves appear regular in time, configuration, and voltage (Fig. 14-2). Each P wave is followed by a QRS complex, and each QRS complex is regular in time, configuration, and voltage. On close examination, however, there is variation in the P-P interval. On physical examination of this patient, one observes a variation in the heart rate that ebbs and flows with the patient's respiration. Nonetheless, this is still considered a normal ECG.

Wandering Atrial Pacemaker. P-waves are present but vary in configuration (Fig. 14-3). The P-R

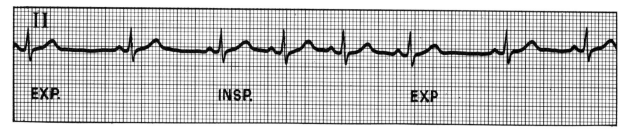

Fig. 14-2. Sinus arrhythmia. Note that the rate increases with inspiration (INSP.) and decreases during expiration (EXP.) when it becomes more regular. (Mangiola, S., and Ritota, M.C.: Cardiac Arrhythmias: Practical ECG Interpretation. Philadelphia, J. B. Lippincott, 1974)

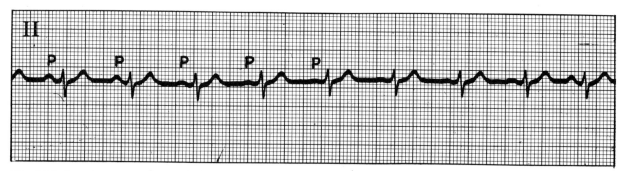

Fig. 14-3. Wandering atrial pacemaker. Note the change in configuration of the P wave as the pacemaker shifts within the sinus node. (Mangiola, S., and Ritota, M.C.: Cardiac Arrhythmias: Practical ECG Interpretation. Philadelphia, J. B. Lippincott, 1974)

interval varies. Each P wave is followed by a QRS complex, and that complex is regular in time, configuration, and voltage. In this tracing, the pacemaker appears in various locations in the atrium. Infrequently, such a change may be caused by digitalis. Usually, no treatment is required.

Wolff-Parkinson-White Syndrome. P waves are regular in time, configuration, and voltage (Fig. 14-4). The apparent abnormality is seen in the much shortened P-R interval and prolonged QRS interval. The P-T interval is normal, however. The impulse arises in the SA node but is conducted aberrantly and quite rapidly either through or around junctional tissue by ectopic Purkinje tissue. No treatment is required unless tachycardia is a part of this process.

Paroxysmal Atrial Tachycardia. P waves are regular in time, but at a much accelerated rate, and they are superimposed upon the T waves (Fig. 14-5). The rate is about twice that of normal. The QRS complexes are regular in time, configura-

tion, and voltage. The arrhythmia is often treated with maneuvers and drugs that increase vagal tone. In the example shown in Figure 14-5, carotid massage was applied and successfully reverted the tachycardia. Beta-adrenergic-blocking agents and digitalis are also used to convert the arrhythmia.

Paroxysmal Atrial Tachycardia With 2:1 Block. The mechanism responsible is the same as in paroxysmal atrial tachycardia (Fig. 14-6). Although this tracing might suggest digitalis intoxication, it must be remembered that this is not diagnosed solely from the ECG. A careful history of digitalis administration is also necessary. In fact, the patient of Figure 14-5 had digitalis intoxication. The patient in Figure 14-6 had not received cardiac glycosides, and his dysrhythmia was corrected by the administration of digoxin.

Atrial Flutter. P waves are difficult to discern, if they are seen at all (Fig. 14-7). QRS complexes appear to be unrelated to P waves and are irregular in time, configuration, and voltage. Patients with

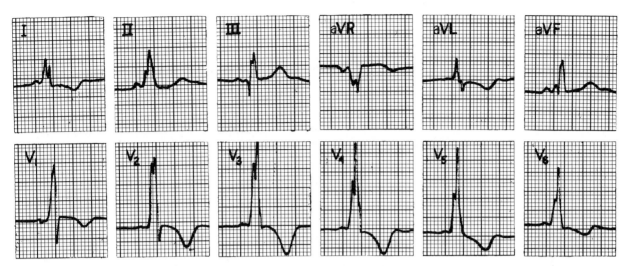

Fig. 14-4. Wolff-Parkinson-White syndrome. The sinus (or atrial) impulse propagates to the ventricles simultaneously through both the normal AV conduction pathway and an aberrant pathway. The impulse spreads more rapidly through the aberrant pathway, reaching the ventricles earlier, causing a short P-R interval and a wide QRS complex, which begins with a slurring resembling the Greek letter delta, Δ (hence, delta wave). (Mangiola, S., and Ritota, M.C.: Cardiac Arrhythmias: Practical ECG Interpretation. Philadelphia, J. B. Lippincott, 1974)

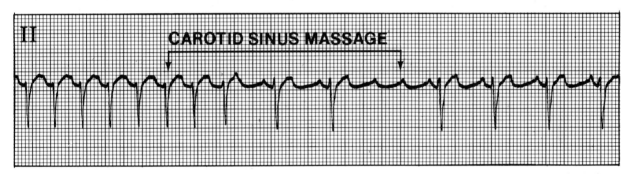

Fig. 14-5. Paroxysmal atrial tachycardia. Carotid sinus massage increases vagal tone, depressing AV conduction and decreasing the ventricular response. (Mangiola, S.: Self-Assessment in Electrocardiography. Philadelphia, J. B. Lippincott, 1977)

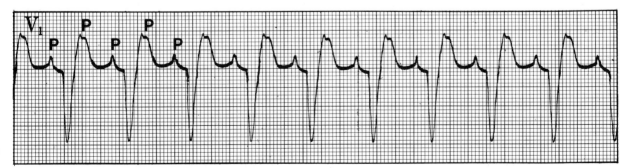

Fig. 14-6. Paroxysmal atrial tachycardia with 2:1 block. (Mangiola, S.: Self-Assessment in Electrocardiography. Philadelphia, J. B. Lippincott, 1977)

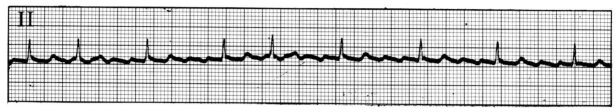

Fig 14-7. Atrial flutter. (Mangiola, S., and Ritota, M.C.: Cardiac Arrhythmias: Practical ECG Interpretation. Philadelphia, J. B. Lippincott, 1974)

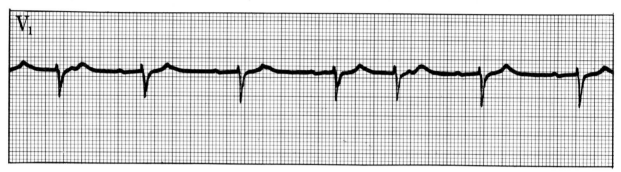

Fig. 14-8. Sinus tachycardia with second degree AV block type I (Wenckebach). (Mangiola, S.: Self-Assessment in Electrocardiography. Philadelphia, J. B. Lippincott, 1977)

atrial flutter usually present with an atrial rate of approximately 300 impulses per min. It usually occurs in aged patients, and is more common in men. Since the AV junction will not accept impulses above 160 to 180 per min. in adults, all atrial impulses are not conducted to the ventricle. Thyrotoxicosis is a commonly overlooked cause of atrial flutter or fibrillation. The importance of this dysrhythmia lies in the rate of ventricular response. Treatment is aimed at reducing the ventricular rate of response to an acceptable level, preferably less than 90 beats per min. Digoxin is the most commonly used drug in treating this dysrhythmia. Propranolol may be used, however, though it may produce asystole by completely blocking AV junctional conduction.

Wenckebach Phenomenon. In examining the tracing in Figure 14-8, two characteristics are noteworthy. One is the appearance of group beating. This always suggests some threatening difficulty in atrioventricular conduction, usually a failure of conduction, or it suggests increased automaticity producing ectopic impulse formation. Next, the P-R interval increases, and the ventricular rate decreases until a beat is dropped

or omitted. Then there is a long pause, followed by resumption of the conduction abnormality. This is the *Wenckebach phenomenon*, a form of second degree AV block, and it suggests digitalis intoxication. These conduction abnormalities are always alarming, since they often worsen to a point of complete atrioventricular block. Atropine may be used to decrease the conduction time from atria to ventricles. However, if there is a history of digitalis ingestion, treatment of digitalis intoxication is appropriate.

Junction (Nodal) Rhythm. P waves are entirely absent (Fig. 14-9). There are QRS complexes, regular in time, configuration, and voltage, though the rate is somewhat slow. Since there is no pacemaker tissue in the atrioventricular node, the term *junctional* is preferred to *nodal*. This is possibly the most common dysrhythmia seen in the operating room. Hyperventilation, especially under anesthesia, accelerates conduction through the AV junctional tissue. Because of this accelerated conduction, the P wave disappears into the QRS complex. The immediate importance of such an ECG change is related only to blood pressure change. Most commonly, one decreases

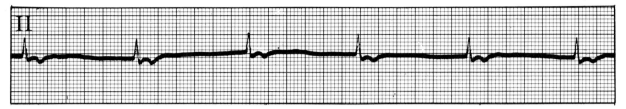

Fig. 14-9. Junctional (nodal) rhythm. In this rhythm, the P wave most often is concealed within the QRS complex but may appear inverted in the S-T segment. (Mangiola, S., and Ritota, M.C.: Cardiac Arrhythmias: Practical ECG Interpretation. Philadelphia, J. B. Lippincott, 1974)

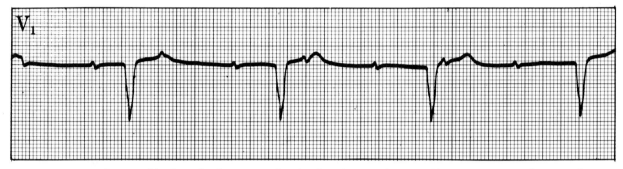

Fig. 14-10. Complete AV block with idioventricular rhythm. (Mangiola, S.: Self-Assessment in Electrocardiography. Philadelphia, J. B. Lippincott, 1977)

the hyperventilation and observes the P wave emerging from the QRS. If a true junctional rhythm exists, both atria and ventricles contract against each other, reducing stroke volume. Commonly, the rate is slower than normal. The result is a decrease in cardiac output. Treatment is directed at increasing atrial automaticity with vagolytic drugs or positive chronotropic drugs.

Complete Heart Block. P waves appear with regularity, maintaining a reasonably uniform configuration and voltage (Fig. 14-10). QRS complexes appear to be reasonably regular, with some variation in configuration and voltage. The striking change is a complete dissociation of atrial and ventricular activity. If at all possible, electrical pacing of this heart should be instituted before anesthesia is contemplated. Attempting to compromise by drug manipulation instead of electrical pacing is likely to end in disaster.

Ventricular Extrasystoles. The outstanding aspect is group beating (Fig. 14-11). P waves are regular in time, configuration, and voltage. Each QRS is not preceded by a P wave, nor is each QRS regular in time, configuration, and voltage. This

is an example of normal electrical activity of the heart with interspersed ventricular ectopic beats. The condition consisting of ventricular ectopic beats that alternate regularly with normal beats is called *bigeminy*. This disturbance is commonly seen early in anesthesia, when intubation is accomplished in the face of inadequate anesthesia. Such a disorder is commonly treated with lidocaine while the amount of sympathetic stimulation is decreased, the depth of anesthesia is increased, and ventilation is improved. If the dysrhythmia appears early in anesthesia, it may be relieved with increased vagal stimulation, like that produced by maintaining pressure on the airway (reservoir bag). Bigeminy may be caused by congestive failure or digitalis intoxication. It may precede fatal dysrhythmia.

A diagnostic paradox may exist in patients with bigeminal rhythm, especially if such a disturbance occurs later in the course of anesthesia. Increased automaticity of one or several Purkinje cells in the ventricle may be the cause of premature impulse formation, causing premature ventricular activity. Usual causes of increased auto-

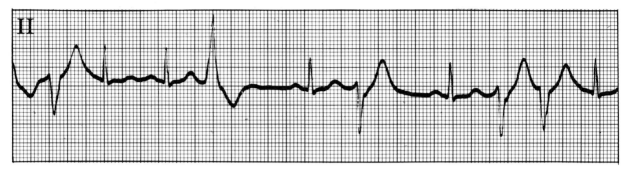

Fig. 14-11. Sinus rhythm with frequent multifocal ventricular extrasystoles, occurring isolated ("bigeminy") or in pairs ("trigeminy"). (Mangiola, S.: Self-Assessment in Electrocardiography. Philadelphia, J. B. Lippincott, 1977)

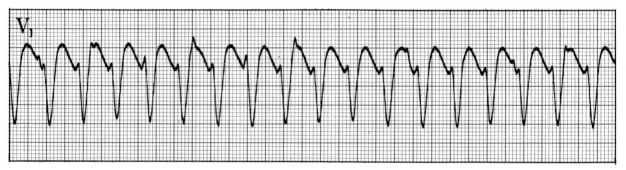

Fig. 14-12. Ventricular tachycardia. (Mangiola, S.: Self-Assessment in Electrocardiography. Philadelphia, J. B. Lippincott, 1977)

maticity (e.g., increased sympathetic activity, hypoxemia) must be excluded or corrected.

Conversely, decreased conduction velocity leading to antegrade conduction block may allow reentry of the electrical signal into the Purkinje system and cause abnormal ventricular contractions. Excessive dosage with some anesthetic agents is not uncommon as a cause of decreased conduction velocity.

Ventricular Tachycardia. No P waves are identified (Fig. 14-12). QRS complexes are abnormal in appearance, configuration, and voltage. The rate is extremely fast and suggests increased automaticity of ventricular pacemaker cells. Ventricular tachycardia may be caused by digitalis intoxication and is often associated with myocardial ischemia or infarction. It is important to notice that toward the end of this tracing the ventricular tachycardia reverts to a reasonably acceptable mechanism. Ventricular tachycardia certainly is an alarming dysrhythmia, but the clinical situa-

tion should be assessed before hasty treatment is undertaken. If treatment is required because of continued ventricular tachycardia, drugs having a membrane effect should be used. The drug of choice is lidocaine, followed by or combined with propranolol or procainamide.

If such a rhythm disturbance appears for the first time during anesthesia, it is reasonable to assume that excessive physiologic trespass has occurred as a result of mismanagement of anesthesia. Surgical stimulation should be halted, and the adequacy of anesthetic level, ventilation, and perfusion should be reassessed. Commonly, by correcting such errors, a reasonably normal rhythm can be restored and surgery completed.

Ventricular fibrillation is completely disordered electrical activity of the heart (Fig. 14-13). This condition must be treated immediately. Electric countershock is required to stop the fibrillation. Fibrillation must be vigorous for countershock to be effective, therefore epineph-

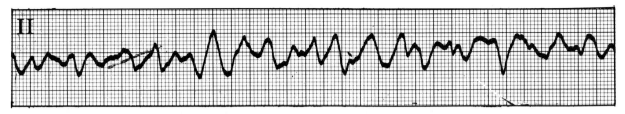

Fig. 14-13. Ventricular fibrillation. (Mangiola, S., and Ritota, M.C.: Cardiac Arrhythmias: Practical ECG Interpretation. Philadelphia, J. B. Lippincott, 1974)

rine in large doses (0.3–0.5 mg.) is administered intravenously. The myocardium must be well oxygenated, requiring good ventilation of the lungs with oxygen and good perfusion of the heart by closed-chest compression. If the myocardium is acidotic, it will not respond to electric countershock, and therefore alkalinizing agents, commonly sodium bicarbonate, are required.

TREATMENT OF CARDIAC DYSRHYTHMIAS

General Considerations

The treatment of cardiac dysrhythmia is usually empirical, often inappropriate, and commonly based on ignorance, lack of understanding, or thoughtless pharmacologic manipulation. All too frequently, the ECG is treated rather than the patient. As suggest on page 211, a clear understanding of the physical and/or chemical factors that alter normal impulse formation and conduction most often leads to the appropriate remedy and, more importantly, to a decision as to whether treatment is necessary or desirable.

A number of changes produced by physiologic and/or pharmacologic means cause, among other clinical aberrations, disturbances of the heart rhythm. Instead of administering an "antiarrhythmic" drug to treat the ECG manifestation of a dysrhythmia, it is better to remedy the disturbed physiology of the patient. The hypoxemic, acidotic patient is better treated with oxygen and alkalinizing agents than with antiarrhythmic drugs. Dysrhythmia caused by congestive heart failure is better treated with cardiac glycosides and diuretics than with antiarrhythmic drugs alone. Other examples of such rational therapy include anticholinergic compounds (atropine) to counteract excessive vagal activity, neostigmine or edrophonium for inadequate vagal activity, exogenous electrical pacing for some cases of ventricular bradycardias, and alpha-adrenergic activators for some cases of hypotension.

Mishaps that may cause disturbances of the patient's cardiac rhythm can occur during the administration of anesthesia. While antiarrhythmic drugs may be necessary to temporize the disturbance, treatment should be directed at the cause of the dysrhythmia.

Errors in Judgment of Depth of Anesthesia. Noxious stimulation perceived through inadequate anesthesia may evoke a strong sympathetic response to produce dysrhythmia and is remedied by deepening anesthesia and/or withdrawing the noxious stimulus.

Errors in Technique, Including Mechanical Failure. Inadequate ventilation to a point of hypoxia and acidosis may result and is remedied by recognizing and correcting respiratory inadequacy.

Inappropriate Intercurrent Drug Therapy. Administration of drugs that alter automaticity (e.g., epinephrine, atropine, potassium) concurrently with agents that sensitize the myocardium (e.g., halothane, cyclopropane) may produce cardiac dysrhythmia. This is prevented by avoiding these combinations or by treating with specific counteractive pharmacologic agents.

Which Arrhythmias Should be Treated?

There is considerable disagreement regarding which cardiac dysrhythmias require treatment; certainly, atrial dysrhythmias that interfere with efficient ventricular function should be treated. Atrial fibrillation, flutter, or tachycardias that result in an inefficiently rapid ventricular response should be treated, with the objective of slowing the ventricular rate, ultimately to an efficient one (usually less than 90 beats/min. in the adult). If the atrial disturbance is chronic, cardiac glycosides (digoxin) or beta-adrenergic-blocking agents may be used. If acute, vagomimetic agents such as neostigmine, vasopressors such as phenylephrine, or electric countershock may be used. Digoxin may also be used to relieve acute supraventricular dysrhythmias, but this requires some judgment. The doses required to correct such atrial activity may be so great that, when reversion to normal atrial activity is produced, digoxin intoxication may develop. If electric countershock is to be attempted, it should precede a trial with digoxin, for digoxin increases refractoriness to electric countershock. If the digitalized patient does respond to electric countershock, a ventricular tachyarrhythmia may soon follow.

Of the ventricular dysrhythmias, the "R-on-T" type is considered to be the most threatening. In this rhythm disturbance, an impulse is generated in the ventricle during the completion of repolarization, during the supernormal period. The danger of this rhythm disturbance is that the ectopic electrical activity may reenter the Purkinje system during the supernormal period to cause a disorganized depolarization of that system, resulting in ventricular fibrillation. Treatment consists of attempting to correct the abnormalities leading to ectopic impulse formation, while an appropriate dose of a membrane-stabilizing drug (discussed below) is administered. Paradoxically, the "R-on-T" type of ectopic activity, while being the most hazardous form of this activity, is most resistant to membrane-stabilizing drugs.

Other types of ventricular activity may require therapy with membrane-stabilizing drugs in addition to efforts to relieve the causes of altered electrical automaticity:

Multiform ectopic ventricular beats occur because a number of ectopic foci exist in the ventricle. Their occurrence suggests that the entire ventricular Purkinje system is becoming deranged, and simultaneous generation of electrical activity in several areas of the ventricle may occur to produce ventricular fibrillation.

Ventricular Ectopic Beats That Occur in "Salvos." The occurrence of three or more ectopic ventricular beats in succession is, by definition, *ventricular tachycardia.* If a focus in the ventricle is so irritable as to spontaneously depolarize rapidly enough to fire a salvo of ectopic impulses, the rate of depolarization of that ectopic focus may progress to produce ventricular fibrillation.

Ventricular Ectopic Beats at a Sustained Frequency Greater Than 5 per min. As above, the threat is that irritability may be increased sufficiently to result in ventricular fibrillation. There is a recognized exception to treating this type of ventricular ectopic activity with membrane-stabilizing drugs, and that is the occurrence of ventricular "parasystoles." In this condition, there is a focus of ectopic depolarization in the ventricle that forms an electrical impulse at a reasonably regular rate, and that rate is quite independent of the normally generated heart rate. Such a focus of ectopic activity is singularly resistant to membrane-stabilizing drugs. By increasing the supraventricular rate with vagolytic agents, positive chronotropic drugs, or electrical pacing to a rate above that inherent in the parasystolic focus, one can suppress the parasystolic focus.

Drug Therapy

Many drugs are available that act directly on the cell membrane. The prototype of such drugs is quinidine.

Quinidine apparently binds itself to the lipoprotein of the cell membrane to alter ion transfer. It slows the rate of depolarization (decreases automaticity) and decreases the action potential, thus slowing conduction. Quinidine is used mainly to prevent supraventricular dysrhythmias, but it can be used to affect atrial automaticity and conduction velocity as well. Quinidine has been said to decrease myocardial contractile force and decrease peripheral resistance, resulting in lowered blood pressure. The best current evidence suggests that no great decrease in myocardial contractility occurs with ordinary doses, and that the decrease in blood pressure results primarily from decreased peripheral resistance. Because of the effect on blood pressure, quinidine is not commonly used during anesthesia.

Procainamide has effects and a mechanism of action similar to quinidine, but, unlike quinidine, it is more effective for ventricular dysrhythmias than for those of atrial origin. Since procainamide also lowers blood pressure, its use as an initial intravenous treatment has been superceded by lidocaine. It is more commonly used if lidocaine fails, or in conjunction with lidocaine.

Disopyramide has been approved recently for oral use as an alternative to quinidine and procainamide. However, in addition to also causing hypotension, disopyramide can aggravate existing heart failure and produce heart block and tachyarrhythmias.

Lidocaine is probably the anesthesiologist's drug of choice for treating ventricular dysrhythmia. It depresses diastolic depolarization and automaticity in ventricular tissue, but it has no effect on conduction velocity. It shortens the action potential and the effective refractory period. Lidocaine is more effective than quinidine or procainamide in treating digitalis-induced ventricular tachyarrhythmias. The major indications for lidocaine are ventricular ectopic beats, especially the "R-on-T" type, those of multiform configuration, in salvos of two or more, or at a sustained frequency greater than 5 per minute. Lidocaine enhances AV conduction to increase the ventricular response to atrial fibrillation in the absence of digitalis. Lidocaine in recommended doses does not depress blood pressure. The recommended dose is 1. mg. per kg.; more commonly, a 50-mg. bolus is given intravenously. The duration of action may be relatively short (2–3 min.). A larger dose of 2 mg. per kg. has a longer duration of effect but has a slightly greater possibility of depressing blood pressure. In practice, one rarely sees significant decreases in blood pressure resulting from bolus injection of lidocaine if the dose is no greater than 2 mg. per kg. Maintenance can be provided with a constant infusion of 2 to 3 mg. per min. (1–5 mg./min.). If breakthrough occurs, another bolus should be given rather than increasing the rate of infusion. Sinus bradycardia and AV block are contradindications to the use of lidocaine, because further slowing of the ventricular rate decreases cardiac output to dangerous levels. Patients with liver disease or renal failure may have problems with distribution, metabolism and excretion of lidocaine. Lidocaine does not relieve the underlying cause of dysrhythmia. It merely "buys time" until the defect can be corrected.

Phenytoin is an interesting drug, though not commonly used. Three mechanisms are proposed for its antiarrhythmic action: centrally, by reducing sympathetic activity; increasing the cell membrane permeability to potassium (much like acetylcholine); and by acting on cardiac muscle like lidocaine or quinidine, which exert a membrane effect. The drug is relatively inefficient in supraventricular dysrhythmia but seems to be of value in ventricular ectopic dysrhythmia. It seems to be especially useful in the ventricular tachyarrhythmias of digitalis toxicity. The usual intravenous dose is 25 to 50 mg. per min. to a total dose of 5 mg. per kg. As a rule, lidocaine is given first; if it is ineffective, then phenytoin in combination with lidocaine may be given. Large intravenous doses may produce AV block. There is a dose-related cardiac depression and decrease in peripheral resistance.

Bretylium has been approved recently for intravenous treatment of life-threatening ventricular tachycardia and fibrillation that is refractory to other therapy. Though efficacious in about half of the patients to whom it is given, bretylium can produce hypotension due to sympathetic blockade, as well as hypersensitivity to vasopressors.

Propranolol is the prototype of beta-adrenergic-blocking agents. Although the most commonly used beta-blocker, it may not be the most desirable. Propranolol slows the sinus rate and the ventricular response to atrial fibrillation through beta-blockade. This slowing seems to be additive to the effect of digitalis. The mechanism involved in abolishing the ectopic beats and tachycardias consists, in part, of beta-blockade and, in part, of a lidocaine-like effect on the cell membrane. This effect produces a delay in AV conduction and can even produce complete AV block. Propranolol decreases oxygen consumption by the myocardium by decreasing cardiac output and contractile force and increases coronary arteriolar resistance, possibly by unopposed alpha-adrenergic activity. Such constriction distributes blood to subendocardial levels, where it is needed in angina. Vasopressors plus propranolol

(80–160 mg./day) cause severe coronary constriction; hence, vasopressors given for hypotension in patients taking large doses of propranolol may be hazardous.

In patients receiving large doses of propranolol (80–160 mg./day), a resting pulse rate below 70 beats per min. that is not increased by exercise indicates severe beta-blockade. Isoproterenol, 0.03 μg. per kg., should increase the pulse rate 6 to 14 beats per min. Calcium chloride, given slowly intravenously, may produce the desired response if isoproterenol fails.

Propranolol is a useful but dangerous drug. It can precipitate and intensify heart failure. The drug blocks secondary manifestations of cardiac stress. If propranolol is to be used intravenously, isoproterenol must be immediately available to counteract its effect. Propranolol is used intravenously, 0.1 to 0.2 mg. every 2 to 3 min., to a total dose of 10 mg. It is usually a second choice to lidocaine and can be used in conjunction with lidocaine.

Digitalis. The term *digitalis* is commonly applied to a number of cardiac glycosides, but digoxin is the glycoside most frequently used in anesthesiology. A full consideration of the pharmacology of digoxin is not appropriate here, but a few generalizations can be made. Digoxin augments the contractile state of normal, non-failing and failing hearts. Digoxin affects the contractile state of all muscles and commonly causes constriction of arteries and veins. Digoxin is frequently recommended to terminate supraventricular tachycardias, but two problems are associated with this use. The supraventricular dysrhythmia (including tachycardia) may be caused by digitalis toxicity. Secondly, if the dysrhythmia is refractory to digoxin, electrical cardioversion is less successful and more hazardous in patients approaching digitalis toxicity.

Part of the antiarrhythmic effect of digoxin is the result of its direct effect on the atrial muscle and the AV node; and, part of this effect is the result of enhancement of vagal stimulation. Two vasoactive drugs have been described as having a "digitalis-like vagal effect." These drugs are methoxamine and phenylephrine. It is true that administration of these drugs usually produces a slowing of the pulse rate, probably reflexly. They are frequently effective in breaking paroxysmal atrial tachycardia.

Potassium. Finally, it is commonly believed that 2 mEq. of potassium can be given safely intravenously to eliminate any cardiac dysrhythmia. Rapid shifts in the extra- to intracellular ratio of potassium can influence automaticity. In patients with normal serum potassium concentrations of around 4 mEq. per L. and a nornal cardiac output of about 5 L. per min., a bolus of 2 mEq. of potassium chloride can be given with relative safety. Because of poor dilution during the first circulation through the coronary arteries, the serum potassium concentration will be equivalent to about 8 mEq. per L. Although this is quite transient, it is sufficient to affect automaticity. If cardiac output is reduced to about 2.5 L. per min., a bolus of 2 mEq. of potassium will produce a transient serum concentration of about 12 mEq. per L., but this is not as transient. In this case of reduced cardiac output, a bolus of 2 mEq. of potassium may disturb impulse formation and conduction velocity to such a degree that the heart will fail to serve its primary function.

FURTHER READING

Bigger, J. T.: Arrhythmias: Mechanisms, diagnosis and treatment. *In* Braunwald, E. (ed.): Heart Disease. Chapters 19 and 20. Philadelphia, W. B. Saunders Company, 1980.

Cranefield, P. F., Wit, A. L., and Hoffman, B. F.: Genesis of cardiac arrhythmias. Circulation, 47:190, 1973.

Fleming, P. R.: Electrocardiography. *In* Scurr, C., and Feldman, S. (eds.): Scientific Foundations of Anaesthesia. ed. 2. pp. 147–160. Philadelphia, F. A. Davis, 1974.

Goldman, M.J.: Principles of Clinical Electrocardiography. ed. 10. Los Altos, Lange Medical Publications, 1979.

Harrison, D. C., Meffin, P. J., and Winkle, R. A.: Clinical pharmacokinetics of antiarrhythmic drugs. Prog. Cardiovasc. Dis., *20*:217, 1977.

Howitt, G.: The pharmacology of the normal and diseased heart in relation to cardiac surgery. Br. J. Anaesth., 43:261, 1971.

Kaplan, J. A., and King, S. B., III: The precordial electrocardiographic lead (V₅) in patients who have coronary-artery disease. Anesthesiology, 45:570, 1976.

Katz, R. L., and Bigger, J. T., Jr.: Cardiac arrhythmias during anesthesia and operation. Anesthesiology, 33:193, 1970.

Pick, A.: Mechanisms of cardiac arrhythmias: from hypothesis to physiologic fact. Am. Heart J., 86:249, 1973.

Pratila, M. G., and Pratilas, V.: Anesthetic agents and cardiac electromechanical activity. Anesthesiology, 49:338, 1978.

Ritota, M. C.: Diagnostic Electrocardiography. ed. 2. Philadelphia, J. B. Lippincott, 1977.

15 Failure of the Peripheral Circulation

David E. Longnecker, M.D.

The primary role of the peripheral circulation is to deliver oxygen and other metabolic substrates to the capillaries, where the essential exchange processes between the blood and the tissue occur. The metabolic processes that produce energy to maintain cellular activity are essentially oxygen-dependent. Although there are anaerobic pathways for energy production, they are stopgap measures, which cannot meet the cellular requirements for energy, except for very brief periods. Thus, any significant impairment of peripheral circulatory function will result in tissue ischemia, and, potentially, cellular damage or death.

Peripheral circulatory failure may be either localized or generalized. Examples of local regional hypoperfusion include the various "steal" syndromes, which result from the shunting of blood away from an organ or circulatory bed, and localized ischemia associated with specific vascular abnormalities (e.g., transient ischemic attacks, myocardial infarctions, vascular trauma). In anesthetic practice, generalized peripheral circulatory failure occurs most commonly in association with anesthetic overdoses and in patients with hypotensive states, especially hypovolemic shock and septic shock. This chapter considers the function of the peripheral circulation, the pathophysiology of the forms of peripheral vascular failure, and the basis for therapy of these disorders.

PHYSIOLOGY OF THE PERIPHERAL CIRCULATION

The principal function of the peripheral circulation is to distribute the cardiac output to all tissues in amounts sufficient to meet the metabolic demands of those tissues. While both the heart and the peripheral circulation determine the absolute amount of cardiac output, the peripheral circulation alone is responsible for the distribution of blood flow. Regulation of peripheral blood flow and, thus, oxygen delivery is accomplished by three distinct regions of the peripheral circulation.

Regions of the Peripheral Circulation

Vessels that Function in Resistance. By far the most important determinants of vascular resistance are the small arterioles. Larger arteries have relatively little vascular smooth muscle in their walls and act primarily as conduits, carrying blood to the site of active control. The walls of small arterioles, ranging in diameter from 10 to 50 μm., contain large amounts of vascular smooth muscle, and alterations in the contractile state of this muscle result in arteriolar constriction or dilatation and, thus, regulation of vascular resistance and blood flow. Since vascular resistance is inversely related exponentially to arteriolar caliber (by approximately the fourth power of the vessel radius), small changes in arteriolar diameter produce major changes in vascular resistance.

Vessels that Function in Exchange. The dense networks of capillaries found in nearly all tissues are primarily responsible for the exchange function within the circulation. Capillaries are thin-walled endothelial tubes that permit the diffusion of gases (O_2 and CO_2) between the tissues and the blood. Blood flow within the capillaries is controlled by precapillary sphincters, located in the terminal arterioles. Local tissue hypoxia results in dilatation of both arterioles and precapillary sphincters. The former reduces vascular resistance to increase overall flow, while the latter opens more capillaries to increase the surface area for gas exchange. Both act to increase the delivery of oxygen to the hypoxic site.

In addition to gas exchange, the capillaries are also sites of solute (e.g., hydrogen ions, electrolytes, proteins) and water exchange between the intravascular compartment and the tissues. Solute exchange across the capillary is determined by capillary permeability and by concentration gradients across the endothelial walls. Fluid movement across the capillary is determined by capillary permeability and by the balance between pressures that force fluid out of the capillary (the capillary hydrostatic pressure and the tissue oncotic pressure) and pressures that hold fluid in the capillary (plasma oncotic pressure plus tissue hydrostatic pressure). Water, solute, and gas exchange are markedly altered by peripheral circulatory failure.

Vessels that Function in Capacitance. The major portion (approximately 70%) of the circulating blood volume is contained in the veins. The small veins act as reservoirs for blood, and changes in venous capacitance are responsible for major changes in venous return and, ultimately, cardiac output. The smaller vessels function as resevoirs, while the large veins act primarily as conduits to return blood to the heart.

Control of Peripheral Circulation

In general, microvascular control may be divided into two categories: remote control and local control. Remote control may be further subdivided into neural control and humoral control. Neural control of the microvasculature is accomplished primarily through the autonomic nervous system, with sympathetic activation resulting in both arteriolar and venular constriction. The microvascular responses to neural stimulation are not uniform among the various vascular beds. Stimulation of the sympathetic nervous system produces only minor changes in vascular resistance in the cerebral and coronary circulations, while the cutaneous, muscle, and renal circulations respond dramatically to sympathetic stimulation. A gradation in response is apparent within a single vascular bed. In general, arterioles are more responsive than veins to sympathetic stimulation, and small arterioles (10–30 μm. in diameter) are more responsive than larger arteries.

Humoral control also serves as a remote mechanism for microvascular regulation. Some of the humoral agents that can alter the microvasculature include epinephrine, norepinephrine, vasopressin, prostaglandins, kinins, and angiotensin. The relative importance of these substances in normal circumstances is not completely defined, although their role in pathologic states, such as hypertension or hemorrhagic shock, is quite evident.

Local microvascular control may be subdivided into metabolic control and myogenic control. Metabolic control implies that some local substance is responsible for moment-to-moment control of the microvasculature. Numerous substances have been implicated as the mediator of this metabolic control; these include oxygen, carbon dioxide, potassium, hydrogen, adenosine, phosphate, and magnesium. While the exact role of each of these substances remains uncertain, it is well established that tissue hypoxia results in the opening of arterioles and precapillary sphincters, presumably in response to some local mediators of vascular control.

Local myogenic control is based on the principle that increased transmural pressure across the vascular wall stimulates vascular smooth muscle to contract, while relaxation occurs when transmural pressure falls. Thus, hypertension and increased microvascular flow would result in arteriolar constriction to reduce flow, while hypotension would cause local arteriolar dilatation to restore flow. While this mechanism may be responsible for the prevention of edema in the legs when humans assume the erect posture, its role in other circumstances is not well known.

COMMON CAUSES OF PERIPHERAL CIRCULATORY FAILURE

Anesthetic Overdose

Premedication. Commonly employed premedicant drugs include the narcotics, the barbiturates, and the benzodiazepine derivates. These drugs can have considerable impact on the cardiovascular system when administered in absolute or relative overdoses.

The cardiovascular effects of typical premedicant doses of morphine are generally quite benign in the supine patient. However, orthostatic hypotension may occur even with modest doses of narcotics.[1] The mechanism of this hypotension is related to the peripheral vascular properties of the drug. Morphine dilates both resistance and capacitance vessels, although these effects are negligible in the supine patient. However, venous dilatation results in pooling of blood in the capacitance vessels and a consequent fall in cardiac output and arterial pressure in the erect individual. The combination of morphine and proper position is a common therapeutic maneuver for the treatment of pulmonary edema, and its effectiveness results from the action of the drug on peripheral capacitance. Obviously, orthostatic hypotension is enhanced by hypovolemia that results from dehydration or acute blood loss.

The treatment of orthostatic hypotension associated with narcotic premedication begins first with awareness and prevention. The premedicated patient should not be allowed to stand without assistance, and the dose of the drug should be reduced in patients who are potentially hypovolemic. More specific therapy should include wrapping the legs with elastic bandages and intravenous fluid therapy. Vasopressors are rarely required to treat this problem.

Barbiturate premedication generally has minimal effects on the cardiovascular system. However, large doses of barbiturates produce cardiovascular failure, again manifested by venous dilatation and pooling of blood in the periphery. The mechanism is at least partially related to the ganglionic-blocking effects of the barbiturates, rather than to a direct effect of the drug on the blood vessels.

Diazepam has relatively little effect on the cardiovascular system per se.[2] The major manifestation of diazepam overdosage is respiratory depression, and cardiovascular depression generally occurs secondary to hypoxia, rather than as a primary event. Obviously, the therapy in these patients should be directed toward correcting the ventilatory problem.

General Anesthesia. Experimentally, barbiturates can depress both the heart and the vascular smooth muscle, but the doses required to produce these effects greatly exceed the usual anesthetic doses of the drugs. More commonly, barbiturates produce only modest changes in blood pressure and blood flow. Of course, hypotension may result from rapid injection of these drugs, which produces quite high but transient blood levels. Autonomic ganglionic blockade and histamine release may also contribute to the development of hypotension in response to barbiturates.

Morphine, even in very large doses, is surprisingly free of cardiovascular effects, provided that two conditions are met: The patient must remain supine; and ventilation must be supported.[3] The frequent use of morphine as a major component of anesthesia for patients with severe myocardial disease attests to the relative lack of effect of this drug on the intact human myocardium.

Ketamine typically results in increases in heart rate, cardiac output, and arterial pressure, without significant alterations in total peripheral resistance.[4] However, the cardiovascular depressant effects of the drug become apparent when relative or absolute overdoses are administered. Thus, large doses of ketamine in animals result in little change in heart rate or cardiac output and a reduction in systemic vascular resistance. The net effect is a tendency toward hypotension. Therapy should be directed at restoring both myocardial performance and peripheral resistance, and therefore a vasopressor drug is more clearly indicated.

The volatile inhalation anesthetics produce cardiovascular depression primarily because of their effects on myocardial performance, rather than peripheral vascular collapse. Deep halothane anesthesia in human volunteers results in profound reductions in cardiac output (nearly 50%) and arterial pressure, but less than a 10-per-cent decrease in systemic vascular resistance.[5] Obviously, the primary treatment for the therapy of arterial hypotension resulting from anesthetic overdose consists of elimination of the drug. When pharmacologic agents are indicated, they should be selected on the basis of the cause of the problem. Peripheral vasoconstrictors should not be employed, but drugs which improve myocardial performance (such as dopamine) are more clearly indicated.

Regional Anesthesia. The local anesthetic drugs produce peripheral vasodilatation by way of two mechanisms: In clinical concentrations, they are direct dilators of vascular smooth muscle (cocaine is an exception); they interrupt neurally mediated adrenergic vasoconstrictor activity by producing a chemical sympathectomy. Since vascular resistance is decreased in the anesthetized area, superficial warmth and venodilation are early signs of regional anesthesia. Alterations in cardiac output, total peripheral resistance, and regional blood flows reflect the balance between vasodilation in the anesthetized area and the compensatory vasoconstriction in the unanesthe-

tized region. Vascular resistance is greatly reduced and capacitance is increased in the lower extremities during spinal or peridural anesthesia, while reflex arteriolar and venous construction occur in the upper extremities to compensate for the decrease in arterial pressure and circulating volume. To a great extent, the circulatory consequences of regional anesthesia may be modified by attempts to correct the alterations in capacitance that accompany regional anesthesia. Wrapping the lower extremities with elastic bandages, the rapid infusion of 500 to 800 ml. of a balanced salt solution immediately prior to anesthesia, and the avoidance of upward tilting of the head usually are effective measures to compensate for the chemical sympathectomy that accompanies spinal or epidural analgesia. Vasopressors are rarely needed when these measures are taken. Obviously, the use of spinal or epidural anesthesia should not be employed in the hypovolemic patient, since the absolute hypovolemia may potentiate the relative hypovolemia produced by the anesthetic procedure, which results in severe reductions in venous return, cardiac output, and arterial pressure.

PATHOPHYSIOLOGY OF HEMORRHAGIC SHOCK

Tissue Perfusion

The fundamental defect in hemorrhagic shock is a decrease in effective circulating blood volume, with a resultant fall in cardiac output. As circulating volume decreases and arterial pressure

Table 15-1. Relative Distribution of Cardiac Output and Regional Vascular Resistance During Normovolemia and During Hemorrhage

REGIONAL CIRCULATION	PER CENT OF CARDIAC OUTPUT (NORMOVOLEMIA)	HEMORRHAGE	
		VASCULAR RESISTANCE	BLOOD FLOW
Brain	14	Slight increase	Slight reduction
Heart	5	No change	Slight reduction
Splanchnic	28	Increase	Decrease
Kidney	23	Marked increase	Marked decrease
Muscle	16	Marked increase	Marked decrease
Skin	8	Marked increase	Marked decrease

falls, the remote and local microvascular regulatory mechanisms are activated to restore tissue perfusion. One of the earliest homeostatic mechanisms is an increase in oxygen extraction from the blood; this results in an increased arteriovenous oxygen difference.[6] Another prompt compensatory factor is the redistribution of cardiac output to favor perfusion of essential organs.

Flow Distribution

With the onset of hemorrhage, there is a prompt increase in vascular resistance in several organs and a consequent redistribution of cardiac output. Table 15-1 summarizes the alterations in vascular resistance and organ blood flow that accompany hemorrhage. The essential features of this redistribution include marked increases in vascular resistance in the renal, skeletal muscle, and cutaneous circulations. Splanchnic vascular resistance is modestly increased, while cerebral and coronary vascular resistance are altered only slightly. The net result is an absolute reduction in blood flow to all organs, but the fraction of blood delivered to the brain and heart is increased at the expense of other organs.[6a] While the short-term effects of this flow distribution are valuable to maintain cerebral and myocardial perfusion, the long-term consequences are failure in other essential organs. The tissue ischemia that occurs in certain critical organs during hypovolemia led to the concept of "target organs" in hemorrhagic shock. Major target organs include the brain, heart, kidneys, and splanchnic viscera.

Target Organs

Although the brain receives an increased percentage of cardiac output during hemorrhage, the absolute amount of cerebral blood flow is reduced. In animal studies, cross-perfusion of the brain from a donor animal increased the survival times of hemorrhaged dogs, suggesting that cerebral ischemia contributes to the lethality of hemorrhage.[7] Myocardial performance ultimately declines during the terminal stages of hemorrhagic shock. Some investigators have attributed this myocardial failure to the release of specific toxic material, "myocardial depressant factor," allegedly liberated from the splanchnic viscera during hemorrhage.[8] Others have been unable to document myocardial depression during hemorrhage in humans[9] or laboratory animals.[10] In fact, it is possible to transplant the hearts of dogs in irreversible hemorrhagic shock into healthy recipients, with excellent survival in the recipient group.[11] Most evidence now supports the concept that myocardial failure during hemorrhage is not a primary event, but rather that it develops terminally as a result of peripheral circulatory failure.

Renal failure is a frequent consequence of profound hemorrhagic hypotension. Hemorrhagic hypotension activates the sympathetic nervous system, and the renal vasculature is especially responsive to this activation and to humoral control. Renal vascular resistance increases promptly in response to hemorrhage, and the combination of reduced perfusion pressure and renal arteriolar constriction severely impairs renal blood flow. The reduction in renal blood flow is especially prominent in the renal cortex of hemorrhaged dogs.[12]

Splanchnic ischemia and consequent tissue hypoxia accompany prolonged hemorrhage, and the prevention of splanchnic ischemia markedly enhances the survival of hemorrhaged dogs. In one study, the mortality of bled dogs was reduced from 90 to 10 per cent by cross-perfusion of the splanchnic circulation from a donor dog.[13] Necrosis of intestinal villi is a common finding in many species after hemorrhagic hypotension, and it has been verified that these lesions result from inadequate oxygen supply to the gut during hemorrhage.[14]

Metabolic Alterations

As tissue ischemia develops during hemorrhage, there is a progressive decline in aerobic metabolism and a resultant increase in anaerobic metabolism. There are two important consequences of the shift to anaerobic metabolism: Energy production is markedly impaired; and metabolic acidosis develops. Under aerobic conditions, glucose is metabolized to pyruvate, which enters the mitochondria, where it is incorporated into the citric acid cycle. This pathway (and the associated respiratory chain) is the principal supplier of adenosine triphosphate (ATP), the major source of energy for cellular activity. However, aerobic metabolism requires molecular oxygen for energy production. In the absence of molecular oxygen, pyruvate is converted to lactic acid, and ATP production is severely restricted (to approximately 5% of the ATP produced by the aerobic metabolism of glucose). The resultant lactic acid accumulation is a major source of the metabolic acidosis that accompanies prolonged hemorrhage. In fact, the severity of the state of shock correlates rather closely with the concentration of lactate in the arterial blood.[15]

Hemodilution

The balance of forces that control fluid transport across the capillary endothelium is markedly altered by hemorrhagic shock. The decrease in capillary hydrostatic pressure that accompanies arterial hypotension favors the net absorption of interstitual fluid into the intravascular compartment.[16] The result is an increase in intravsacular fluid volume and a fall in hematocrit (*i.e.*, hemodilution). The magnitude of hemodilution correlates closely with the volume deficit resulting from hemorrhage,[17] and this is an indicator of the severity of hemorrhage.

Ventilatory Responses

Hemorrhagic shock is a potent stimulus to respiration and results in increases in both respiratory rate and minute ventilation. Airway resistance is slightly reduced, while pulmonary compliance is slightly increased during hemorrhagic shock.[18] The proportion of wasted ventilation (V_D/V_T) is increased during hemorrhage and correlates directly with the fall in pulmonary artery pressure.[19] In uncomplicated hemorrhagic shock, the respiratory stimulation more than compensates for the increase in V_D/V_T, and Pa_{CO_2} is reduced to approximately 25 to 30 torr (3.3–4.0 kPa). Arterial hypoxia is rarely seen until the very late stages of hemorrhage, when generalized circulatory collapse occurs. However, patients with multiple trauma or sepsis frequently manifest arterial hypoxia, resulting from increased pulmonary shunting.[20]

Autonomic Responses to Hemorrhage

The autonomic nervous system plays a key role in the response to hemorrhage. The initial response to hypovolemia is an increase in sympathetic activity, which acts as a compensatory mechanism to provide for perfusion of vital organs (e.g., brain and heart). While the initial sympathetic activation is beneficial, prolonged increases in sympathetic activity result in major reductions in renal and splanchnic perfusion, which ultimately contribute to the demise of the patient. In fact, both survival times and survival rates of hemorrhaged dogs are reduced by the continuous infusion of catecholamines during hemorrhage.[21,22] A number of investigators have demonstrated a marked increase in circulating catecholamines and in plasma renin activity during hemorrhage.[23–24a] Pharmacologic blockade of either system prevents the marked increase in vascular resistance that accompanies hemorrhage in animals and improves survival rates as well.[25–26a]

DIAGNOSIS OF HEMORRHAGIC HYPOTENSION

Clinical Manifestations of Hypovolemia

Hypovolemia is usually quite apparent when it occurs during surgery. The combination of obvious major blood loss plus hypotension leaves little room for doubt concerning a diagnosis. However, blood loss in the pre- or postoperative patient is more difficult to determine. Significant hemorrhage may occur within body cavities without obvious external bleeding. Examples include hemothorax or retroperitoneal hemorrhage accompanying trauma, leaking aortic aneurysm, or postoperative hemorrhage following abdominal or thoracic surgery. Significant blood loss may also occur in the pelvis and thighs in association with fractures in these areas. The major clinical manifestations of hemorrhagic shock result from the reduced blood volume and cardiac output and from the consequent activation of the sympathetic nervous system in response to hypotension.

Hemodynamic manifestations may include arterial hypotension in the supine position, although hypotension is frequently a rather late sign of hemorrhage in the unanesthetized patient. Orthostatic hypotension, produced by moving the patient to the sitting position, will frequently occur in patients who are normotensive in the supine position. Conscious patients often complain of intense thirst.

Sympathetic nervous system activation is manifested by tachycardia, peripheral vasoconstriction, and diaphoresis. Sympathetic activation produces the classic signs of a rapid, thready peripheral pulse, combined with cold, clammy skin. Tachycardia is a key sign and is a compensatory mechanism that is frequently evident well before hypotension ensues.

Monitors for the Hypovolemic Patient

Several monitors can provide valuable assistance in the diagnosis of hypovolemia and serve as sensitive guides to the success of therapy as well. Valuable monitoring techniques include the measurement of central venous (right atrial) pressure, arterial pressure, heart rate, urine output, and blood gases. Measurements of pulmonary artery pressure, pulmonary capillary wedge pressure, and cardiac output are also valuable and may be especially important in patients with myocardial failure, but they are not essential to the proper care of most patients in hemorrhagic shock.

Although arterial pressure is maintained until hypovolemia is quite marked, central venous pressure falls early during hemorrhage. Previous investigations demonstrated that right atrial pressure decreased approximately 7 mm. H_2O (0.69 kPa) for each 100 ml. of blood removed from a 70-kg. adult.[27] Hemorrhage of 500 to 800 ml. in human volunteers resulted in no change in arterial pressure, while central venous pressure was reduced by 70 mm. H_2O (6.9 kPa).[28]

Arterial pressure should be carefully monitored during hypovolemia, but hypotension should be considered a late sign of hemorrhagic shock, especially in the awake patient. In the anesthetized patient with blunted compensatory mechanisms, arterial pressure may fall more rapidly in response to hemorrhage. The Korotkoff sounds become vague and unreliable during profound shock, and either direct measurement of arterial pressure, by way of an arterial cannula and pressure transducer, or estimation of arterial pressure by the Doppler technique is indicated. Direct arterial cannulation has the added advantage of providing a ready source of arterial blood for determination of Pa_{O_2}, Pa_{CO_2}, and *p*H.

Some monitor of organ perfusion is indicated during hemorrhage. Unfortunately, direct measurements of tissue blood flow, or even tissue PO_2, P_{CO_2}, and *p*H, are still investigative techniques at the present time. However, the volume of urine flow is a relative indicator of tissue perfusion, especially since renal hypoperfusion (and consequently decreased urine formation) occurs early during hypovolemia. Urine flow is approximately 1 ml. per kg. per hr. in normotensive, unanesthetized humans. Although anesthesia per se may reduce renal blood flow and urine formation, urine flow rates of less than 0.5 ml. per kg. per hr. are suggestive of poor renal perfusion. Urine flow may stop during moderate to severe hemorrhagic shock.

The measurement of Pa_{O_2}, Pa_{CO_2}, and *p*H can be extremely valuable during hypovolemia. However, arterial blood gas levels are often misleading during hemorrhage. Typically, Pa_{O_2} remains normal, and arterial *p*H is near normal, while Pa_{CO_2} is reduced. With severe hemorrhage, ventilation-perfusion abnormalities result in arterial hypoxemia and metabolic acidosis, manifested by a fall in *p*H, despite hypocapnia. Tissue hypoxia and hypercapnia always accompany hemorrhagic shock, and these alterations are usually not apparent in the arterial blood. Marked tissue hypoxia and hypercapnia have been demonstrated during hemorrhage despite normal arterial blood gases.[29] However, the central venous blood gases do reflect the tissue hypoxia and hypercapnia.[30,31] Normal values for mixed venous oxygen tension and carbon dioxide tension ($P\bar{v}_{O_2}$ and $P\bar{v}_{CO_2}$) are

Table 15-2. Decreases in Cardiac Output and Arterial Pressure During Graded Hemorrhage in Dogs

BLOOD VOLUME REMOVED (%)	CARDIAC OUTPUT (%)	ARTERIAL PRESSURE (%)
10	−21	−7
20	−45	−15

(Hinshaw, D. B., Peterson, M., Huse, W. M., et al.: Regional blood flow in hemorrhagic shock. Am. J. Surg., *102*:224, 1961.)

approximately 43 and 46 torr (5.7 and 6.1 kPa), respectively. $P\bar{v}_{O_2}$ may decrease to approximately 20 torr (2.7 kPa), while $P\bar{v}_{CO_2}$ increases to 55 to 60 torr (7.3–8.0 kPa) during hemorrhage in the absence of major changes in arterial blood gases. Thus, mixed venous blood gases become important monitors of the extent of the microcirculatory impairment accompanying hemorrhage.

Measurement of circulating blood volume should be a useful tool during hypovolemia, since inadequate blood volume is the fundamental defect in hemorrhagic shock. However, the lack of a simple, rapid, reliable method for routine use has hampered the application of this technique in clinical practice. It remains as a useful guide in institutions that are equipped to perform this measurement on a routine basis.

Cardiac output is a helpful guide during hemorrhagic shock. Table 15-2 shows the relationship between cardiac output and arterial pressure in hemorrhaged dogs.[32] Arterial hypotension is a late manifestation of hemorrhage, because an increase in peripheral resistance also accompanies hemorrhage. The availability of balloon-tipped flow-directed catheters allows the measurement of cardiac output (by the thermal dilution technique) and the estimation of left atrial pressure during massive fluid replacement accompanying hemorrhage. However, the total cardiac output gives essentially no information regarding the distribution of blood flow and does not replace the measurement of urine flow, blood gases, or heart rate. While this technique is not essential, it is especially valuable in patients with compromised myocardial function and superimposed hypovolemia.

Several simple and readily available monitors are valuable in the care of the hypovolemic patient. These include heart rate, arterial pressure, urine flow rate, central venous pressure, and arterial and venous blood gases. More involved techniques, including determinations of blood volume, cardiac output, and pulmonary capillary wedge pressure, are also of value, especially in the patient with compromised myocardial function.

THERAPY OF HEMORRHAGIC SHOCK

Therapeutic Goals

The essential feature in hemorrhagic shock is tissue ischemia. Ischemia results both from a reduction in cardiac output and from increased peripheral vascular resistance. Therapy should be directed toward correcting both aspects of the problem. Restoration of effective circulating blood volume is the cornerstone of the treatment of hemorrhagic hypotension. Although drug therapy may increase arterial pressure and/or cardiac output, the only really effective method of restoring arterial pressure, cardiac output, and the normal distribution of blood flow requires the restoration of blood volume. Vasopressors should be regarded as temporizing measures, to be employed only when absolutely essential, and then for the shortest possible time.

Fluid Therapy

Replacement fluids may be categorized according to whether or not they contain red blood cells (RBC). The foundation of volume replacement therapy for hemorrhagic shock is the red blood cell, either in whole blood or as packed cells. Despite the recent popularity of hemodilution, this technique is not recommended in the therapy of hemorrhagic shock. Data in laboratory animals clearly document that oxygen uptake is maintained during isovolemic hemodilution (to a hematocrit of 30%) by increased oxygen extraction.[33] Since oxygen extraction is already increased during hemorrhagic hypotension, this approch can result in significant cellular hypoxia and should be avoided.

The amount of blood to be replaced is difficult to recommend on an absolute basis. Rather, the adequacy of blood replacement therapy should be evaluated by the clinical signs and monitors described. In general, the restoration of arterial pressure, central venous pressure, and urine output and the absence of tachycardia are good indicators that blood volume has been restored. However, it should be remembered that the fluid losses during hemorrhage exceed the visible loss due to the fluid shifts that accompany hemorrhage. Fluid therapy must restore the volume of blood lost from the intravascular compartment and replace the interstitial fluid losses as well.

Replacement fluids that do not contain red blood cells may be categorized into two major groups: crystalloid solutions (electrolyte solutions) and colloid solutions (essentially, solutions with large protein molecules).

Crystalloid solutions may be subdivided into saline solutions and balanced salt solutions. Normal saline does not replace the great number of electrolytes that are contained in extracellular (intravascular and/or interstitial) fluid. Balanced salt solutions are designed to more nearly approximate the electrolyte composition of the extracellular fluid and are the crystalloid fluids of choice for volume replacement during hemorrhage.

Colloid solutions include whole blood, blood components, albumin solutions, and plasma expanders. As indicated, the main colloid replacement therapy should be accomplished with whole blood and packed red blood cells. One of the sequelae of massive fluid therapy is the development of pulmonary complications, especially interstitial pulmonary edema. There is increasing evidence to suggest that concentrated albumin solutions may promote the development of interstitial pulmonary edema by increasing capillary permeability within the lung parenchyma. The infusion of crystalloid or packed red blood cells suspended in crystalloid solution appears to minimize this problem.[34]

Oxygen Therapy

Although arterial hypoxia is uncommon in pure hemorrhagic shock, the administration of supplemental oxygen is advisable to protect against unrecognized pulmonary problems resulting from intrapulmonary shunts or ventilation-perfusion abnormalities. Examples include elderly patients, patients with chronic lung disease, and patients with associated sepsis, pulmonary contusion, or aspiration of gastric contents following multiple trauma. Oxygen therapy may be initiated with an F_{IO_2} of approximately 0.4, and further adjustments should be based on arterial blood gas values.

Acid-Base Therapy

The usual acid-base response to hemorrhage is metabolic acidosis, with superimposed respiratory alkalosis. Generally, the resultant *p*H is not markedly abnormal. However, acidosis may ensue if shock is prolonged. Any significant acid-base disturbance should be corrected promptly. Metabolic acidosis is treated with intravenous sodium bicarbonate (assuming that there is a bicarbonate space of 30% of body weight). If respiratory acidosis (arterial hypercapnia) should occur, this suggests that there is a significant pulmonary abnormality and mandates tracheal intubation and controlled ventilation.

Vasopressors

In general, it is uncommon for a patient to require vasopressors in the treatment of hemorrhagic shock. On occasion it may be necessary to infuse small amounts of vasopressors to temporarily support myocardial and cerebral perfusion until fluid therapy is instituted, but these instances are rare. It should be kept in mind that one of the major pathophysiologic changes during hypovolemia is the development of intense peripheral vasoconstriction, leading to a decrease in capillary blood flow in many tissues. Enhanced peripheral constriction (with catecholamine infusions) increases mortality in hemorrhaged animals, while pharmacologic blockade (with adrenergic blockers) improves survival. Vasopressor therapy should take these findings into consideration. At this time, it would appear that dopamine is the drug of choice when a vasopressor is required. In low doses (3–5 μg./kg./min.), dopamine exhibits a mild positive inotropic effect, with minimal chronotropic effects and no change in peripheral vascular resistance. Stimulation of dopaminergic receptors in the renal vasculature actually increases renal blood flow, a beneficial effect during hypovolemia. High concentrations of dopamine (> 10 μg./kg./min.) result in alpha-adrenergic vasoconstriction in nearly all circulatory beds, including the renal circulation, and should be avoided if at all possible.

Steroids

The use of steroids in the therapy of hemorrhagic shock has been both praised and condemned over the past 20 years. However, recent laboratory and clinical studies suggest that steroids may well have a role in the therapy of hypovolemia. Steroids block the intense arteriolar constriction associated with hypotension, without producing vasodilatation in laboratory animals.[35] This effect is similar to that achieved with alpha-adrenergic blocking drugs, but is without the potential for severe hypotension resulting from arteriolar dilatation. Steroids appear to restore arteriolar diameters (and vascular resistance) to near normal, while alpha-adrenergic blockade changes vasoconstriction to vasodilatation. In addition, survival rates of hemorrhaged animals are considerably improved when steroids are administered shortly after the period of hemorrhage.[35] Finally, the administration of steroids produces significant hemodynamic improvements in hypovolemic patients. In humans, cardiac output increases, and both pulmonary and systemic vascular resistances decrease following steroid administration during hemorrhagic shock.[36] Other beneficial effects attributed to steroids that are administered during hemorrhage include protection against "shock lung," decreased release of lysosomal enzymes, and improved cellular energy production. While many of these are controversial, the effects on vascular resistance and on mortality rates have been indicated. Many of the contradictory findings may be the result of the formulations and doses of the steroids studied. The most favorable results have been obtained with methylprednisolone (30 mg./kg.), and this is the recommended steroid for hemorrhagic shock based on current evidence.

When should steroids be utilized in hemorrhagic shock? The author does not employ this therapy in all patients but reserves them for those who manifest evidence of intense peripheral vasoconstriction. The patient who experiences major hemorrhage in the operating suite but receives prompt and continuous volume replacement and maintains adequate urine flow probably does not need steroids. On the other hand, the patient who arrives in the emergency room in hemorrhagic shock, with intense peripheral constriction and little or no urine output, may benefit considerably from this form of therapy.

Prevention of Renal Failure

One of the most disturbing complications of hemorrhagic shock is the subsequent development of acute renal failure in a patient who survives the initial hypotensive insult. Significant hypotension markedly reduces total renal blood flow and, especially, outer cortical blood flow.[37] While definitive data in humans are lacking, laboratory results indicate that both furosemide[38] and mannitol[39] selectively increase renal cortical blood flow. When oliguria occurs, therapy with one of these diuretics is appropriate. The initial dose of furosemide is 20 to 40 mg., intravenously, and the dose is doubled after 30 minutes if oliguria persists. Mannitol, 25 g., intravenously, may also be employed to attempt to restore renal perfusion and urine output. Since mannitol is a hyperosmolar solution, it should be used with caution in patients with possible myocardial failure.

Anesthetic Management

Again, the principles of therapy rule out administration of drugs that increase peripheal vascular resistance. Thus, cyclopropane, which supports blood pressure primarily by elevating peripheral resistance, should be avoided in hemorrhaged patients. Very little objective evidence has been obtained in humans to support one anesthetic technique over another. However, some data are available comparing various anesthetics during similar degrees of hemorrhage in animals. During graded progressive hemorrhage, animals anesthetized with cyclopropane survive for a markedly

Table 15-3. Cumulative Survival Rates at Various Times After Onset of Hemorrhage

| | Survival Rate (%) | | | |
TIME	PENTOBARBITAL (N=32)	HALOTHANE (N=32)	FLUROXENE (N=32)	KETAMINE (N=32)
60 min	71.9	59.4	78.1	96.9
24 hr	59.4	50.0	56.3	84.4
48 hr	56.3	46.9	37.5	84.4
72 hr	56.3	46.9	25.0	81.3
7 days	53.1	46.9	18.7	81.3

(Longnecker, D. E., and Sturgill, B. C.: Influence of anesthetic agent on survival following hemorrhage. Anesthesiology, *45*:516, 1976.)

shorter time than do those anesthetized with halothane.[40] Table 15-3 depicts cummulative survival rates in rats, subjected to 1 hour of controlled bleeding to a mean arterial pressure of 40 torr (5.3 kPa), while anesthetized with one of four anesthetics.[41] Mortality was greatest in animals receiving fluroxene and least in animals receiving ketamine. The incidence of small bowel and hepatic necrosis following hemorrhage was reduced in animals receiving ketamine in this study. While these results remain to be confirmed in other species (especially primates or humans), they do suggest that ketamine may be a useful drug for anesthesia in the hemorrhaged patient. It is interesting to note that ketamine tends to support blood pressure primarily by increasing cardiac output, with little change in peripheral resistance,[4] and, thus, it follows the proposed therapeutic goals quite appropriately.

SEPTIC SHOCK

Pathophysiology

The majority of cases of septic shock result from bacteremia due to gram-negative enteric bacilli. The specific shock-producing agent is believed to be endotoxin, a lipoprotein-carbohydrate complex present in the bacterial cell wall.

Septic shock may be characterized by at least two distinctly different stages. Early endotoxin shock is manifested by fever, chills, hypotension, and warm extremities. Hemodynamic studies reveal a normal or increased cardiac output and a reduced systemic vascular resistance, despite hypotension. As the stage of shock progresses, vasodilatation is rapidly replaced by peripheral vasoconstriction and reduced cardiac output. This later stage of endotoxin shock closely resembles hemorrhagic shock in most respects, including hemodynamic, respiratory, and metabolic alterations.[42]

Treatment

Elimination of the source of infection is the major goal in endotoxin shock and is accomplished primarily by two methods: appropriate antibiotic therapy and surgical drainage of the infected site. The anesthesiologist frequently encounters these patients during surgery for wound drainage.

Since the late, severe manifestations of septic shock are nearly identical to those of hemorrhagic shock, the same therapeutic principles apply in both conditions. Thus, corticosteroids, fluid replacement, correction of acid-base disturbance, and avoidance of potent peripheral vasoconstrictor drugs are important aspects in the management of septic shock, just as they are in hemorrhagic shock. Obviously, the need for blood replacement is much different in the two conditions, but even in septic shock large volumes of fluid are often required to correct the intravascular volume deficits associated with sequestration of fluid and the fever, vomiting, and diarrhea that often accompany septicemia.

OTHER CAUSES OF PERIPHERAL CIRCULATORY FAILURE

Acidosis and Hypoxia

Surprisingly, the cardiovascular responses to hypoxia, with or without accompanying hypercapnia, are not as clearly defined in humans as one might anticipate. Of necessity, only relatively mild or brief hypoxic periods have been studied in humans. In investigations in animals it is quite apparent that the circulatory responses to hypoxia and hypercapnia are both time-dependent and dose-dependent, and that anesthetics significantly blunt these responses. Overall, the circulatory responses to hypoxia or hypercapnia reflect the integrated responses of the direct vascular effects of the gases plus the neural and humoral responses triggered by their alteration through such mechanisms as the carotid chemoreceptors.

Typically, arterial hypoxemia without hypercapnia produces tachycardia, hypertension, and increased cardiac output. Total systemic vascular resistance is increased, although individual vascular beds may respond quite differently. Vascular beds of renal and skeletal muscle constrict during arterial hypoxemia,[43] while coronary and cerebral arterioles dilate during hypoxia.[44] These changes are consistent with the well established physiologic principle that redistribution of blood flow during cellular hypoxia (resulting from ischemia or hypoxemia) tends to preserve essential organs at the expense of less vital ones. Cardiovascular responses to hypoxia are enhanced by hypercapnia, and intestinal vasodilatation is seen as well when Pa_{CO_2} is elevated.[43]

Hypercapnia in unanesthetized humans and animals results in hypertension, tachycardia, increased cardiac output, and elevated systemic vascular resistance. The fraction of cardiac output distributed to the brain and gut is enhanced by hypercapnia, while renal and skeletal muscle blood flow are reduced due to vasoconstriction.[43] Once again, it should be emphasized that the responses to hypoxia or hypercapnia are markedly reduced by general anesthesia, and, thus, it is considerably more difficult to identify hypoventilation in the anesthetized individual.

Carcinoid Syndrome

Carcinoid tumors occur most commonly in the gastrointestinal tract and the bronchial tree. The tumors contain chromaffin tissue, the secretions of which include serotonin plus other vasoactive polypeptides, including bradykinin and prostaglandins. The carcinoid syndrome consists of marked cutaneous flushing, hypotension, diarrhea, tachycardia, and bronchospasm. The symptoms result from the sudden release of vasoactive substances from the tumors and are often associated with stress or alcohol ingestion. Since the treatment of this syndrome involves surgical excision of the tumors, these patients present special hazards for the anesthetist. Hypotension resulting from peripheral vasodilatation may accompany anesthetic induction and operative manipulation of the tumor. Hypotension may actually be enhanced by many of the vasopressors, which can stimulate the release of vasoactive substances from the tumors. Pure alpha-adrenergic constrictor drugs appear not to enhance tumor secretion, and therefore methoxamine is the recommended vasopressor when the carcinoid syndrome occurs during anesthesia. Obviously, the principles of good anesthetic care, including careful attention to anesthetic depth and fluid balance, are cornerstones in the management of these patients.

Methyl Methacrylate Cement

Arterial hypoxemia, hypotension, and even cardiac arrest have been *associated with* the introduction of acrylic cement into the bone (especially the femoral shaft) during orthopedic surgery, usually for total hip replacement. However, investigations in animals and humans strongly suggest that the cement per se is not the cause of these respiratory and circulatory alterations.[45,46] Intravenous infusions of the monomer do not produce cardiovascular or pulmonary changes, unless the concentration of cement is many times that seen in clinical practice. Rather, these alterations appear to result from embolization produced by the high pressures that occur in the marrow cavities during implantation of the prosthesis. Possible mechanisms include fat and gas embolization and release of tissue-thromboplastic substances.[46] The essentials of anesthetic care include the use of high inspired oxygen concentrations and adequate fluid volume at the time of prosthetic implantation. Venting of the femoral shaft to reduce the amount of embolization is also helpful.[47]

REFERENCES

1. Drew, J. H., Dripps, R. D., Comroe, J. H., Jr.: Clinical studies on morphine. II. The effect of morphine upon the circulation of man and upon the circulatory and respiratory responses to tilting. Anesthesiology, 7:44, 1946.
2. Dalen, J. E., Evans, G. L., Banas, J. S., Jr., et al.: The hemodynamic and respiratory effects of diazepam. Anesthesiology, 30:259, 1969.
3. Lowenstein, E., Hallowell, P., Levine, F. H., et al.: Cardiovascular response to large doses of intravenous morphine in man. N. Engl. J. Med., 281:1389, 1969.
4. Tweed, W. A., Minuck, M., and Mymin, D.: Circulatory responses to ketamine. Anesthesiology, 37:613, 1972.
5. Eger, E. I., II, Smith, N. T., Stoelting, R. K., et al.: Cardiovascular effects of halothane in man. Anesthesiology, 32:396, 1970.
6. Tung, S. H., Bettice, J., Wang, B. O., et al.: Intracellular and extracellular acid-base changes in hemorrhagic shock. Resp. Physiol., 26:229, 1976.
6a. Blahitka, J., and Rakusan, K.: Blood flow in rats during hemorrhagic shock: Differences between surviving and dying animals. Circ. Shock, 4:79, 1977.
7. Kovach, A. G. B., Roheim, P. S., Iranyi, M., et al.: Effect of the isolated perfusion of the head on the development of ischaemic and haemorrhagic shock. Acta Physiol. Hung., 14:231, 1958.
8. Lefer, A. M.: Role of a myocardial depressant factor in the pathogenesis of circulatory shock. Fed. Proc., 29:1836, 1970.
9. Bassin, R., Vladeck, B. C., Kark, A. E., et al.: Rapid and slow hemorrhage in man: sequential hemodynamic responses. Ann. Surg., 173:325, 1971.
10. Hinshaw, L. B., Archer, L. T., Black, M. R., et al.: Myocardial function in shock. Am. J. Physiol., 226:357, 1974.
11. Culpepper, R. D., Kondo, Y., Hardy, J. O., et al.: Successful orthotopic allotransplantation of hearts from dogs in irreversible shock. Surgery, 77:126, 1975.
12. Lavender, J. P., and Sherwood, T.: The renal circulation in haemorrhagic hypotension. Br. Med. Bull., 28:241, 1972.
13. Lillehei, R. C.: The intestinal factor in irreversible hemorrhagic shock. Surgery, 42:1043, 1957.
14. Haglund, U.: The small intestine in hypotension and hemorrhage. Acta Physiol. Scand., 387 [Suppl.]: 3, 1973.
15. Border, G., and Weil, M. H.: Excess lactate: an index of reversibility of shock in human patients. Science, 143:1457, 1964.
16. Haddy, F. J., Scott, J. B., and Molnar, J. I.: Mechanism of volume replacement and vascular constriction following hemorrhage. Am. J. Physiol., 208:169, 1965.
17. Chien, S., Dellenback, R. J., Usami, S., et al.: Blood volume, hemodynamic, and metabolic changes in hemorrhagic shock in normal and splenectomized dogs. Am. J. Physiol., 225:886, 1973.
18. Cahill, J. M., and Byrne, J. J.: Ventilatory mechanics in hypovolemic shock. J. Appl. Physiol., 19:679, 1964.
19. Gerst, P. H., Rattenborg, C., and Holday, D. A.: The effects of hemorrhage on pulmonary circulation and respiratory gas exchange. J. Clin. Invest., 38:524, 1959.
20. Clowes, G. H. A., Jr., Hirsch, E., Williams, L., et al.: Septic lung and shock lung in man. Ann. Surg., 181:681, 1975.
21. Hakstian, R. W., Hampson, L. G., and Gurd, F. N.: Pharmacologic agents in experimental hemorrhagic shock—a controlled comparison of treatment with hydralazine, hydrocortisone, and levarterenol. Arch. Surg., 83:335, 1961.
22. Close, A. S., Wagner, J. A., Klochn, R. A., et al.: The effect of norepinephrine on survival in experimental acute hemorrhagic hypotension. Surg. Forum, 8:22, 1957.
23. Jakschik, B. A., Garland, R. M., Kourik, J. L., et al.: Profile of circulating vasoactive substances in hemorrhagic shock and their pharmacologic manipulation. J. Clin. Invest., 54:842, 1974.
24. Hall, R. C., and Hodge, R. L.: Changes in catecholamine and angiotensin levels in the cat and dog during hemorrhage. Am J. Physiol., 221:1305, 1971.
24a. Miller, E. D., Longnecker, D. E., and Peach, M. J.: Renin response to hemorrhage in awake and anesthetized rats. Circ. Shock, 6:271, 1979.
25. Errington, M. L., and Rocha e Silva, M.: On the role of vasopressin and angiotensin in the development of irreversible hemorrhagic shock. J. Physiol., 242:119, 1974.
26. Halmagyi, D. F. J.: Combined adrenergic receptor blockade in experimental post-hemorrhagic shock. In Forscher, B. K., Lillehei, R. C., and Stubbs, S. S. (eds.): Shock in Low- and High-Flow States. pp. 49–57. Amsterdam, Excerpta Medica, 1972.
26a. Errington, M. L., Rocha, E., and Silva, M.: On the role of vasopressin and angiotensin in the development of irreversible hemorrhagic shock. J. Physiol. (Lond.), 242:119, 1979.
27. Gauer, O. H., Henry, J. P., and Sieker, H. O.: Changes in central venous pressure after moderate hemorrhage and transfusion in man. Circ. Res., 4:79, 1956.
28. Warren, J. V., Brannon, E. S., Stead, E. A., Jr., et al.: The effect of venesection and the pooling of blood in the extremities on the arterial pressure and cardiac output in normal subjects with observations on acute circulatory collapse in three instances. J. Clin. Invest., 24:337, 1945.
29. Brantigan, J. W., Ziegler, E. C., Hynes, K. M., et al.: Tissue gases during hypovolemic shock. J. Appl. Physiol., 37:117, 1974.
30. Halmagyi, D.F.J., Kennedy, M., and Varga, D.: Hidden hypercapnia in hemorrhagic hypotension. Anesthesiology, 33:594, 1970.
31. Lee, J., Wright, F., Barber, R., et al.: Central venous oxygen saturation in shock. Anesthesiology, 36:472, 1972.
32. Hinshaw, D. B., Peterson, M., Huse, W. M., et al.: Regional blood flow in hemorrhagic shock. Am. J. Surg., 102:224, 1961.
33. Pavek, K., and Carey, J. S.: Hemodynamics and oxygen availability during isovolemic hemodilution. Am. J. Physiol., 226:1172, 1974.
34. Siegel, D. C., Moss, G. S., Cochin, A.: Pulmonary changes

following treatment of hemorhagic shock: saline vs. colloid infusion. Surg. Forum, *21*:17, 1970.

35. Altura, B. M., and Altura, B. T.: Peripheral vascular actions of glucocorticoids and their relationship to protection in circulatory shock. J. Pharmacol. Exp. Ther., *190*:300, 1974.

36. Lozman, J., Dutton, R. E., English, M., et al.: Cardiopulmonary adjustments following single high dose administration of methylprednisolone in traumatized man. Ann. Surg., *181*:317, 1975.

37. Selkurt, E. E.: Current status of renal circulation and related nephron function in hemmorhage and experimental shock. I. Vascular mechanisms. Circ. Shock, *1*:3, 1974.

38. Birtch, A. G., Zakheim, R. M., Jones, L. G., et al.: Redistribution of renal blood flow produced by furosemide and ethacrynic acid. Circ. Res., *21*:869, 1967.

39. Abbott, W. M., and Austen, W. G.: The reversal of renal cortical ischemia during aortic occlusion by mannitol. J. Surg. Res., *16*:482, 1974.

40. Theye, R. A., Perry, L. B., and Brzica, S. M., Jr.: Influence of anesthetic agent on response to hemorrhagic hypotension. Anesthesiology, *40*:32, 1974.

41. Longnecker, D. E., and Sturgill, B. C.: Influence of anes-

thetic agent on survival following hemorrhage. Anesthesiology, *45*:516, 1976.

42. Rutherford, R. B., Balis, J. B., Trow, R. S., et al.: Comparison of hemodynamic and regional blood flow changes at equivalent stages of endotoxin and hemorrhagic shock. J. Trauma, *16*:886, 1976.

43. Weissman, M. L., Rubinstein, E. H., and Sonnenschein, R. R.: Vascular responses to short-term systemic hypoxia, hypercapnia, and asphyxia in the cat. Am. J. Physiol., *230*:595, 1976.

44. Wyler, F.: Effects of hypoxia on distribution of cardiac output and organ blood flow in the rabbit. Cardiology, *60*:163, 1975.

45. Modig, J., Busch, C., and Waernbaum, G.: Effects of graded infusions of monomethylmetharylate on coagulation, blood lipids, respiration, and circulation. Clin. Orthop., *113*:187, 1975.

46. Modig, H., Busch, C., Olerud, S., et al.: Arterial hypotension and hypoxaemia during total hip replacement: the importance of thromboplastic products, fat embolism and acrylic monomers. Acta Anaesth. Scand., *19*:28, 1975.

47. Kallos, T.: Impaired arterial oxygenation associated with use of bone cement in the femoral shaft. Anesthesiology, *42*:210, 1975.

16 Cardiac Arrest and Resuscitation

Burton A. Briggs, M.D., and David J. Cullen, M.D.

Hannah Greener, at the age of 15 years, died the 28th of January, 1848, during chloroform anesthesia for removal of a toenail.[1,2] Only 15 months after this, W.T.G. Morton first demonstrated that ether obliterated pain during surgery, and 2 months later, Simpson began using chloroform in his midwifery practice.[3] While Hannah Greener's death was being discussed,[4] a second death occurred during chloroform anesthesia.[5] As other deaths followed, the mixed blessings of general anesthesia were discussed and analyzed by the French Academy of Medicine, Hyderabad Commissions, Royal Medical and Chirurgical Society, British Medical Association, and the Commission on Anesthesia of the American Medical Association.[3] Since these inquiries and studies, the direct relationship between cardiac arrest and anesthesia has continued to be the subject of many subsequent deliberations, including the following: Which anesthetic agents are safest? What is the effect of the patient's preoperative condition? What is the role of adjuvant drugs? How, if at all, does the skill of the surgeon and anesthesiologist influence mortality?

Since Hannah Greener's death, all anesthetic agents and techniques have been associated with cardiac arrests. These disasters have resulted directly or indirectly from errors in patient evaluation, ignorance of anesthetic pharmacology and drug interactions, inattentiveness to the patient, and errors in technique. This chapter discusses the factors contributing to cardiorespiratory arrest and methods for dealing with this crisis.

INCIDENCE OF INTRAOPERATIVE CARDIAC ARREST

In 1956, Briggs, Sheldon, and Beecher reported a retrospective study of operating room deaths and cardiac arrests at the Massachusetts General Hospital during the period of 1925 to 1954.[6] In the first 20 years of that period, there was a steady decrease in such catastrophes; this was attributed to improved patient selection, preoperative patient preparation, and improved surgical and anesthetic techniques. However, during the 3rd decade, the incidence of cardiac arrest increased, because older and sicker patients, who previously would not have been candidates for surgical procedures, were undergoing such procedures. During the 30-year period, the incidence of cardiac arrest was 1 in 1,405 anesthetic administrations. Memery reported that with a group of seven anesthesiologists in community practice, the incidence of cardiac arrest between 1955 and 1964 was 1 in 3,149.[7] In 1957, Pierce cited an incidence of 1 in 1,025,[8] but the rate increased to 1 in 821 during 1963 to 1965. Again, the data suggested that, despite improved monitoring and anesthetic techniques, increasing numbers of poor-risk patients were being subjected to anesthesia and surgery. In 1970, Jude reported an incidence of 1 in 1,216.[9]

HISTORY OF CARDIOPULMONARY RESUSCITATION

The first successful resuscitation of a patient who had suffered intraoperative cardiac arrest occurred in 1867, with the use of a "tracheostomy and the application of galvanism to the cardiac region."[10] In 1891, Naass successfully performed the first cardiac resuscitation with closed chest compression.[11] Ten years later, Igelsrud effectively performed the first open chest cardiac massage.[12] In the study of patients at Massachusetts General Hospital from 1925 to 1954, of 45 who underwent open chest massage within 4 minutes of arrest, 26 (58%) recovered without neurological deficit.[6] In Pierce's report, all successful resuscitations during 1957 and 1963 to 1965 were accomplished with open chest cardiac massage.[8] Yet, the overall rate for successful resuscitation and recovery during both periods was only 35 per cent. In Jude's review in 1970, resuscitation using the closed chest technique was attempted in nine patients, of whom seven (78%) were resuscitated and five (56%) were discharged.[9] Open cardiac compression was used successfully in one of two patients whose chests were already open, and this led to that patient's subsequent discharge. More recently, survival of 41 to 50 per cent, depending upon whether aggravating factors such as hypoxia, hemorrhage, or massive pulmonary embolism were present, has been reported.[13,14]

PATHOPHYSIOLOGY OF CARDIAC ARREST

The ultimate objective of cardiopulmonary function is to provide ample oxygen for mitochondrial respiration.[15] The oxygen cascade, from inspiration of gas to metabolism at the mitochondrial level, can be divided into several steps; the oxygen levels during some of these can be measured readily (Fig. 16-1).[16] At sea level, inspired P_{O_2} ($P_{I_{O_2}}$) is approximately 150 torr (20.0 kPa); alveolar P_{O_2} ($P_{A_{O_2}}$), 100 torr (13.3 kPa); arterial P_{O_2} (Pa_{O_2}), 90 to 95 torr (12.0–12.6 kPa); and mixed venous P_{O_2} ($P\bar{v}_{O_2}$), 47 torr (6.3 kPa). Measurement of Pa_{O_2} (at a known $F_{I_{O_2}}$) indicates only the efficiency of oxygenation by the lungs. During normal oxygen consumption, mean tissue P_{O_2} approximates 51 torr (6.8 kPa).[16] Therefore, if mitochondria operate over a range of P_{O_2} of 1.5 to 10 torr (0.2–1.3 kPa), there is an oxygen partial pressure gradient from tissue to mitochondria of 41 to 49.5 torr (5.5–6.6 kPa). $P\bar{v}_{O_2}$ may indicate adequate oxygen delivery to the tissue, but is influenced by hemoglobin concentration, cardiac output, metabolic rate, and distribution of blood flow.

In addition, the ability of hemoglobin to "unload" oxygen (determined by 2,3-diphosphoglycerate [2,3-DPG]), pH, and temperature effect) will influence the partial pressure gradient driving oxygen from the capillaries to the mitochondria. Increases in 2,3-DPG or temperature, or a decrease in pH, will shift the hemoglobin dissociation curve to the right and will increase the partial pressure gradient (Fig. 16-2, 35-2). Because body oxygen stores are meager at best,[17] any interruption in the normal oxygenation of hemoglobin within the lungs results in a rapid depletion of the available oxygen.

It has been estimated that the mitochondria require an oxygen tension of at least 1.5 torr (0.2 kPa; Pasteur point) to produce ATP aerobically. Aerobic metabolism of one glucosyl unit of glycogen to carbon dioxide and water yields 38 molecules of ATP, while anaerobic metabolism yields only 2 molecules of ATP plus lactic acid.[18] Persistent hypoxia and reduced ATP production result in the disruption of the intracellular lysosomal limiting membranes, enabling release of cellular lytic enzymes. These proteinases, esterases, hydrolases, and phosphotases not only destroy the cell but may form small protein fractions called kinins. Release of kinins into the circulation may initiate organ failure in the kidney, lung, heart, and brain and may also trigger disseminated intravascular coagulation (DIC).[19]

Ames demonstrated that inadequate oxygenation of the brain produces capillary endothelial swelling and interstitial edema.[20] Flores has described the same process within the renal microcirculation.[21] This edema compresses the microvasculature and prevents restoration of tissue

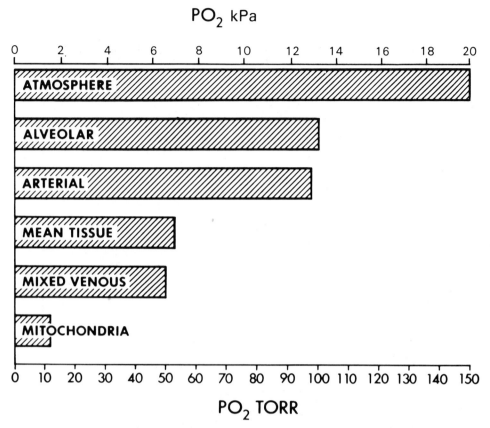

Fig. 16-1. The oxygen cascade in which P_{O_2} falls from the level in ambient air down to the level in mitochondria, the site of utilization.

flow, even if circulation resumes; it is known as the "no-reflow phenomenon." Thus, just as circulation and oxygenation must be maintained within narrow limits at the cellular level, whole body circulation and oxygenation must be provided to maintain tissue blood flow. Herein lies the urgent need to recognize and treat inadequate tissue perfusion in order to prevent the potentially irreversible sequelae of cardiac arrest.

CLINICAL IMPLICATIONS OF CARDIAC ARREST

"If one doesn't see cardiac changes incident to or because of anesthesia, he just is not looking! Or listening! The specific actions of premedications, drugs, and anesthetic agents, mechanical effects of surgery, and the patient's basic disease process may all combine to alter rate, rhythm, and compliance of the heart."[22]

During anesthesia, the patient's ability to compensate and control circulatory changes is altered, and he becomes entirely dependent on the knowledge and skill of the anesthesiologist. For example, establishing a safe and proper level of anesthesia in a patient with a full stomach may further aggravate intravascular volume deficits or cardiovascular disease. These and other considerations, such as the effects of potent inhalation and intravenous agents, the airway and circulatory reflexes that are present or abnormally active under light anesthesia, and the need to rapidly secure the airway, must be kept in mind.

Arrhythmias are present in 60 to 90 per cent of patients during anesthesia and surgery.[23–25] Most frequently they occur at the time of or immedi-

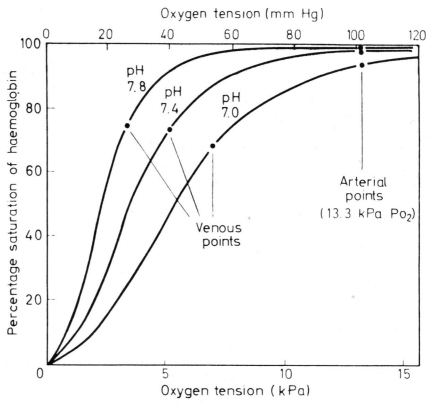

Fig. 16-2. Normal oxyhemoglobin dissociation curve (center) shifts to the right with acidosis and to the left with alkalosis, other factors remaining constant. (Nunn, J.F.: Applied Respiratory Physiology. ed. 2. London, Butterworth & Co. Ltd., 1977)

ately following intubation. These arrhythmias are usually ischemic or reflexive in origin. Myocardial ischemia may be secondary to either hypotension or hypertension (e.g., associated with laryngoscopy and/or intubation). Hypertension increases left ventricular afterload and leads to endocardial ischemia. During some surgical procedures, vagal reflexes secondary to visceral traction or the oculocardiac reflex may occur, usually during light or inadequate anesthesia. The following case reports illustrate these points.

Case 16-1 (Hypovolemia). Mrs. P. was 21 years old and 2 months pregnant. After eating supper, she developed acute left lower abdominal pain and signs of peritoneal irritation. She was brought to the operating room for an abdominal explora-

tion, presumably for a ruptured ectopic pregnancy. Her blood pressure was 100/60, pulse, 120, respirations, 30, height, 168 cm., weight, 55 kg., and hematocrit, 30 per cent; the chest radiograph was clear. Because she had recently eaten, spinal anesthesia (tetracaine, 10 mg., with epinephrine, 0.2 mg.) was selected and administered with the patient in the lateral position. When the patient was turned supine, her blood pressure was unobtainable.

Case 16-2 (Myocardial Ischemia). While mowing his lawn after supper, Mr. F., an active 63-year-old, sustained several lacerations of his left hand, requiring operative repair estimated to last 3 to 4 hours. Past history included two myocardial infarctions, the last of which occurred the previous year. Because he had a full stomach, anesthesia was induced rapidly with thiopental (300 mg.) and succinylcholine (80 mg.). Following intubation, systolic blood pressure was 70 torr and then became unobtainable over the next 2 minutes. After a successful resuscitation, additional history revealed that he had been taking alpha-methyldopa and hydrochlorothiazide to control his hypertension and mild congestive heart failure.

Case 16-3 (Visceral Traction). Miss L., 59 years of age, was undergoing an elective cholecystectomy performed under narcotic, nitrous oxide, relaxant anesthesia. During dissection of the gall bladder, traction was applied to the cystic duct, immediately initiating bradycardia (88 to 40 beats/min.) and decreasing the systolic blood pressure from 140 to 60 torr. Upon release of traction, the pulse rose to 70 beats per min., and systolic blood pressure, to 110 torr. Moments later, when the cystic duct was clamped, pulse and blood pressure were unobtainable.

In critically ill patients, blood gas and electrolyte or metabolic abnormalities plus anesthesia are most often responsible for potentially fatal arrhythmias. This may be observed in the uremic patient, who becomes more acidotic after being anesthetized and develops a hyperkalemic arrest. Respiratory compensation (respiratory alkalosis) for metabolic acidosis is prevented by the respiratory depressant effects of anesthesia and/or inadequate controlled ventilation. Superimposing respiratory acidosis upon metabolic acidosis drives potassium from the cell, leading to hyperkalemia and arrest. Prevention of these arrhythmias depends on adequate oxygenation and minimal changes in pH.[26] "Normal" electroeyte values measured before anesthesia and surgery may not reflect the electrolyte status of the patient during surgery. Extensive bowel preparations, diuretic usage, inanition, or recent administration of digitalis glycosides may predispose the patient to significant changes in electrolyte values. The administration of succinylcholine to patients with extensive burns,[27] uremia,[28] tetanus, massive

trauma,[29,30] and denervation injuries[31] may produce hyperkalemic arrest. Cardiac arrests have been reported following anaphylactic and allergic reactions to drugs such as thiopental[32] and succinycholine[33] and to blood products.

DIAGNOSIS OF CARDIAC ARREST

A precordial or esophageal stethoscope, ECG, temperature, and blood pressure cuff are basic monitoring equipment and should be used routinely for all patients undergoing anesthesia. Critically ill patients will benefit from additional measurements of intra-arterial blood pressure, central venous pressure, serial arterial blood gases, electrolytes, and, when appropriate, pulmonary artery and pulmonary capillary wedge pressure. Reliance on monitoring should add to but not replace careful and thoughtful personal attention to the patient. Both continuous close observation and monitoring are mandatory for detecting any changes in vital signs.

Cardiac arrest is usually diagnosed by the absence of a pulse or blood pressure. Occasionally, "false arrests" occur in the operating room due to malfunction of monitoring equipment (i.e., the precordial or esophageal stethoscope disconnects, the blood pressure cuff slips, or an ECG lead detaches). However, faulty monitoring equipment should not blind the anesthesiologist to a true cardiac arrest. There are other visual or tactile signs that aid in making a rapid diagnosis. Inspection of the surgical field will reveal whether or not the patient's blood is well oxygenated. If the abdomen is open, palpation of the aorta or other major vessels by the surgeon will then confirm or exclude a diagnosis of cardiac arrest.

A change in respiratory patterns should alert the anesthesiologist to the possibility of cardiovascular deterioration (assuming muscle relaxants were not used). Again, a thorough but quick check of the anesthesia apparatus for leaks or obstruction is imperative. The flowmeters should be scanned to exclude the possibility of delivery of a hypoxic gas mixture.[34] Hypoxia normally stimulates respiration and cardiac activity. However, in dogs (and, presumably, in humans) receiving surgical concentrations of halothane, hypoxia profoundly depresses circulation and respiratory activity, which swiftly leads to arrest.[35] One should also check for an excessive concentration of inhalation agents in the breathing circuit; this is caused by spillage of liquid agents into the inspired gas line.[36,37] If spillage has occurred, the anesthesia machine must be disconnected, or resuscitation will not be successful. Symmetrical chest expansion during inflation suggests that there is no major airway obstruction, but aeration should be verified by auscultation. Difficulties encountered while attempting to inflate the lungs may be unrelated to airway obstruction. The presence of a tension pneumothorax should always be suspected whenever compliance worsens (see Chap. 12).

If indeed a cardiac arrest has occurred, the list of steps below should be followed in rapid sequence.

Resuscitation of Patients in Cardiac Arrest

1. Turn off all anesthetic agents.
2. Call for help!
3. Flush the anesthetic circuit with oxygen, and give 100% oxygen to the patient.
4. Ensure that there is a patent airway (preferably by intubation).
5. Smell the anesthetic circuit to check for excessive concentrations of anesthetic agents.
6. Give a precordial thump (if an ECG monitor is being used), and then begin external cardiac massage.
7. Obtain equipment to display the ECG, if it is not already available.
8. Obtain and charge the defibrillator, if it is not already available.
9. Obtain emergency drugs.

If external cardiac massage is unsuccessful in restoring circulation after 10 to 15 minutes, the chest should be opened, particularly when tension pneumothorax, intrathoracic bleeding, or cardiac tamponade is suspected.

After beginning resuscitation, the size of the pupils should be noted. A marked change in pupillary size or reactivity may reflect the adequacy of circulation. Normal pupils dilate 10 to 15 seconds after the onset of cerebral anoxia. Dilated pupils may seem ominous but do not contraindicate cardiopulmonary resuscitation (CPR). When, after circulatory assistance, the pupils become smaller, cerebral circulation is at least marginally improved, and perhaps some improvement in the prognosis for cerebral recovery may be expected.

However, dilation of the pupils may also be influenced by the anesthetic. If deep anesthesia with methoxyflurane, ether, or cyclopropane was instituted prior to cardiac arrest, the pupils will probably be dilated. Narcotics may produce pupillary constriction. Halothane and isoflurane do not in themselves dilate the pupils (at normal anesthetic concentrations), but nitrous oxide either alone or in combination with other inhalation agents will enhance pupillary dilation.[38]

The object of cardiopulmonary resuscitation (CPR) is to prevent cerebral anoxia. If resuscitation is not attempted, irreversible changes begin approximately 3 to 4 minutes following cessation of cerebral perfusion; this is probably related to the "no-reflow phenomenon" (see p. 248). For CPR to be even partially successful, it must be initiated and performed adequately within the first 1 or 2 minutes of arrest.

IMPLEMENTATION OF CPR

The current standards for CPR have been established by the American Heart Association and the National Academy of Sciences National Research Council.[39] The standards include the familiar A-B-C steps of CPR:

A. Airway
B. Breathing — artificial ventilation
C. Circulation — artificial circulation

CPR

The Airway

The upper airway of an unconscious person can become obstructed when supporting structures surrounding the airway relax. By extending the head and elevating the jaw, a patent airway can be established. In some "cardiac arrests," this maneuver is all that is necessary for resuscitation. One hand is positioned under the neck, which is then lifted, while the other hand is placed on the forehead to extend the head. The tongue is thereby elevated away from the posterior pharynx, which relieves the most common cause of airway obstruction. If proper extension fails to clear the airway, it may be necessary to curl the fingers bilaterally around the angles of the mandible and displace the mandible forward (even to the point of dislocating the temporomandibular joint). This sometimes opens the airway, so that ventilation can continue. If obstruction persists, other causes must be sought, such as misplaced dentures or regurgitation of gastric contents into the oropharynx. Large items can be removed manually, but liquid and stomach contents must be suctioned (see Chap. 8).

Once the airway is secured, oxygen should be administered. However, increased pressure may be required to ventilate the patient between cardiac compressions. Such pressure may promote gastric distention, which raises the diaphragm and interferes with adequate inflation of the lung. Moreover, gastric distention promotes regurgitation and possible pulmonary aspiration. Hence, to protect the airway and enable the delivery of a high concentration of oxygen to the lungs, the trachea should be intubated as soon as practical. To facilitate intubation, it is necessary to politely call "time out" from cardiac compression and swiftly insert the endotracheal tube. (The anesthesiologist should ensure that the laryngoscope light and endotracheal tube cuff work before calling "time out"!) A belching or gurgling sound, associated with a rapidly enlarging abdominal mass and no breath sounds, demands immediate and proper replacement of the tracheal tube. If esophageal intubation has been avoided, the chest wall should move well and breath sounds should be present. The position of the tube within the trachea must be checked to avoid endobroncial intubation. Frequently, success at intubating the trachea overwhelms the operator, who is so relieved at accomplishing this technical feat under adverse conditions that he inserts the tube full length, to ensure that it will never slip out. The tip of the endotracheal tube then enters the right mainstem bronchus and occludes both the left mainstem and right upper lobe bronchi.

Breathing

Within the operating room, ventilation is achieved by using a mask or endotracheal tube, attached to a semiopen or semiclosed system with reservoir bag. Occasionally, mouth-to-mouth or mouth-to-tube ventilation may be necessitated by defective equipment, contamination of the anesthesia circuit from spilled inhalation agents, or the development of a respiratory arrest while the patient is in transit from the operating room to the recovery room. Respiratory assistance should be provided for all inadequately perfused patients. Manual respiratory assistance is mandatory for patients undergoing external cardiac compression, since sternal compression significantly interferes with spontaneous ventilation. In patients with decreased cardiac output (50% of normal at best), oxygen supplementation is required.

The recommended initial ventilatory maneuver is four rapid, full inflations that do not permit full lung deflation between breaths. Thereafter, there should be one inflation every 5 seconds (one every 3 seconds in a child).

Circulation

At the first instant cardiac arrest is recognized in the monitored patient, a sharp blow to the midsternum (precordial thump) may be all that is necessary to reestablish electromechanical activity of the heart. In the well oxygenated patient, the precordial thump may reverse sudden ventricular fibrillation, asystole, or ventricular tachycardia associated with inadequate circulation.[39] However, precordial thump is not effective in the patient with anoxic arrest. If pulse and blood pressure do not return immediately, CPR should be instituted promptly. Application of successive precordial thumps, in the hope that the third or fourth blow will produce an effective cardiac rhythm, is discouraged.

To obtain effective external cardiac compression, the patient must be horizontal, on a hard surface[40]; the operating room table is ideal, although a board, tray, or floor serves well outside the operating room. The heel of one hand is placed parallel to and over the lower half of the sternum. The heel of the second hand rests on top of the first. Application of pressure over the xyphoid is avoided, because of danger to the liver or spleen from lacerations. With elbows extended, the weight of the shoulders should be directly perpendicular to the patient's chest. Rhythmic compression of the sternum (1.5 to 2 in. in adults) is accomplished by exerting a straight downward force, thus compressing the heart between the sternum and vertebral column. Compression should be smooth and firm, with a frequency of 60 to 80 compressions per minute.

The most common errors in technique are the following: placing the heel of the hand too low over the xyphoid; flexing the elbows, thereby reducing the force generated by the trunk and shoulders; not lifting the fingers off of the ribs, so that the ribs break or costochondral separations occur; removing the hands from the sternum during relaxation, which leads to a tendency to "bounce" and to physically damage the thoracic cage when the compression is not applied directly over the sternum; and not compressing the sternum at a regular and continuous rate. The force required to depress the sternum will vary from mere finger pressure in the newborn, to hand and arm weight in the child, to full shoulder and trunk weight in the athletic adult. In older individuals with arthritis and brittle ribs, extreme care should be exercised to avoid cracking or disarticulation of the ribs. The usual ratio for cardiac compression and ventilation is 5 to 1, at a cardiac rate of 60 compressions per minute. Increasing the frequency of cardiac massage to 80 per minute results in improvement in cardiac output.[41]

As soon as possible, the cardiac rhythm should be determined by ECG. If ventricular fibrillation is present, external defibrillation should be attempted, using a DC defibrillator, set at approximately 400 joules in adults (5 joules/kg.). The power output of each individual defibrillator may vary, so that the anesthesiologist must be acquainted with the output characteristics of the equipment available. The defibrillator paddles should be covered well with electrode paste or, preferably, with saline-soaked gauze pads. One paddle should be lateral to the cardiac apex in the midaxillary line, and the other, to the right of the upper sternum, below the clavicle.[42] The ECG machine is disconnected before defibrillation, unless it is protected against a large flow of current. After defibrillation is attempted, ventilation and external cardiac compression are continued until a functional rhythm has been restored.

If an effective rhythm greater than 60 beats per minute is obtained, the anesthesiologist may stop and palpate for carotid or femoral pulses. If both a pulse and adequate blood pressure are found, observation and assisted ventilation are indicated. Blood pressure should be measured frequently to evaluate cardiovascular trends and to help determine the need for catecholamine support. If pulses are not present, CPR is resumed immediately, while further attempts at defibrillation are made. If an ECG is not immediately available to determine rhythm, electrical defibrillation may be attempted. If there is ventricular fibrillation, defibrillation is the appropriate therapy of choice. However, if the rhythm is asystolic, defibrillation may be employed in an attempt to restore a functional rhythm.

PHARMACOLOGY AND DEFINITIVE THERAPY IN CARDIAC ARREST

True cardiac arrest involves either asystole or ventricular fibrillation. In asystole, the therapeutic objective is to initiate electrical activity, either by inducing ventricular fibrillation with drugs or by promoting ventricular contractions with electrical pacing.

Drugs commonly used for asystolic cardiac arrest are epinephrine (0.5–1.0 mg.) and sodium bicarbonate (1 mEq./kg.), given intravenously. When these are unsuccessful in converting asystole to ventricular fibrillation, epinephrine administration may be repeated, perhaps with an intravenous bolus of isoproterenol (0.25–0.5 mg.). If the arrest is secondary to hyperkalemia, then calcium chloride (1 g.) should be given. Additional doses of sodium bicarbonate (0.5 mEq./kg.) are used only if substantial acidosis is revealed by blood gas analysis. Once ventricular fibrillation is observed, defibrillation with 300 to 400 joules is indicated. Sometimes two "shocks" in quick succession are necessary to convert ventricular fibrillation to a functional rhythm. When the chest is open and intrathoracic cardiac compression is performed, only 50 to 100 joules are required for internal defibrillation.

Ventricular pacing wires are usually passed transthoracically through a needle into the right ventricle. After the needle is removed, the wire is attached to the pacemaker and gently withdrawn, until a pacing complex is obtained on the ECG. Once proper positioning of the wire is established, the pacemaker voltage may be reduced to that just above threshold, and the rate is adjusted to 90 to 110 beats per minute. (Pulse and blood pressure are checked again). It is very difficult to insert transvenous pacing wires during CPR. However, when the chest is open, pacing wires may be attached directly to the epicardium.

If the patient is in ventricular fibrillation but does not respond to countershock, the heart must be made more receptive to the defibrillation current. Epinephrine (0.5–1.0 mg.), given intravenously, and/or calcium chloride (1 g.) usually convert a fine ventricular fibrillation pattern (low voltage on the ECG pattern) to a coarser, higher voltage pattern that is more likely to respond to "countershock."

During resuscitation, efforts to improve coronary perfusion are necessary, particularly in the patient with a history of coronary vascular disease. This may be accomplished by increasing peripheral resistance with norepinephrine infusion. Although defibrillation has been achieved, coronary perfusion must be maintained, even temporarily at the expense of other tissue, or fibrillation is likely to recur. If ventricular fibrillation resumes in spite of adequate coronary perfusion, it is probably caused by an irritable focus within the heart. Ventricular irritability can usually be suppressed with lidocaine (40–100 mg., I.V. bolus, up to 5 mg./kg. total dosage) without affecting cardiac output. When irritability persists after a reasonable cardiac output has been established, a continuous infusion of lidocaine is indicated to suppress the irritable focus.

During and after successful resuscitation, arterial blood gases, measured at frequent intervals, are necessary to evaluate oxygenation, ventilation, and acid-base balance. These serve as guides to respiratory therapy and to further administration of bicarbonate.

Complications of CPR

Even with properly performed CPR, certain complications may occur.[43–46a] These include costochondral separations, fractured ribs, pneumothorax or hemothorax, lung contusions, lacerated liver or spleen, aspiration pneumonitis, hyperosmolality, hypercapnia, and fat embolism. Careful attention to detail will keep complications to a minimum.

EVALUATION OF RESUSCITATION

When cardiac arrest occurs during an anesthetic that includes the use of muscle relaxants, the usual signs of brain death (e.g., areflexia and lack of respiratory effort) may not apply. Also, pupillary signs may be modified, but to a lesser extent, by the anesthetic drugs. If ventricular activity is inadequate after 30 to 60 minutes of maximal resuscitative effort, resuscitation should be stopped. When resuscitation has been successful, appropriate steps must be taken to carefully monitor and support the patient's vital functions.

There is adequate evidence to support the use of pharmacological doses of corticosteroids in an attempt to prevent some of the sequelae of cardiovascular collapse, such as "shock lung" and cerebral edema. Initial doses of 3 to 5 mg./per kg. of methylprednisolone or 1 mg./per kg. of dexamethasone have been recommended for use in an attempt to prevent cellular swelling. Maintenance doses of methylprednisolone (60–100 mg. q6 hours) may be beneficial in the treatment of cerebral edema. In addition to the use of corticosteroids, other measures, such as administration of potent diuretic agents, controlled hyperventilation, and hypothermia, are used to reduce cerebral edema and decrease metabolic demands.[47]

Incidence of Sudden Unexpected Death

In 1964, Himmelhoch reported results of 65 resuscitations at the Peter Bent Brigham Hospital.[48] Only three cases occurred in the operating room, although nine occurred in the recovery room. None of them were attributed to anesthetic-related problems. Only four patients (6%) survived to leave the hospital. These dismal results were hard to accept.

Recently Meltzer, at the Presbyterian Hospital in Philadelphia, studied the incidence and cause of sudden hospital death. Each death was carefully analyzed.[49] In a 31-month period, there were 20,000 admissions and 1,206 deaths. Of these, 79 per cent were expected, and 253, or 21 per cent, were unexpected. A total of 96 were considered irreversible at the time of diagnosis; therefore, 157 of 1,206, or 13 per cent, were unexpected but potentially reversible sudden deaths. Extrapolating these data to the average hospital which admits 10,000 patients per year leads to the following conclusion: 79 patients per 10,000 hospital admissions die unnecessarily each year. Approximately 35 million patients are admitted annually to hospitals; this means that 274,750 sudden and reversible deaths occur each year. Meltzer asked the following question: "Is cardiopulmonary resuscitation an overall solution to the problem?" In his study, 38 per cent of resuscitation efforts occurred in special care areas, with an 18-per-cent survival rate. But 62 per cent of resuscitations occurred in general ward areas, with only a 4-per-cent survival rate. The results of resuscitation in Meltzer's recent study are no better than those of Himmelhoch's study; this suggests that poor resuscitation in the general hospital setting is due to an unacceptable time lapse between the onset of cardiac arrest and the discovery and institution of appropriate therapy. Some of Meltzer's recommendations include the following:

Recognition of High-Risk Categories. Ninety per cent of sudden death patients had an abnormal ECG on admission; 92 per cent were admitted for a medical illness; 69 per cent had known heart disease; and 47 per cent were over 70 years of age.

Prophylactic Monitoring of the Patient at Risk. Meltzer's study demonstrated a better survival in patients given CPR in intensive care units rather than in the general ward. Is this because their arrest was noted and effective therapy was instituted sooner?

Neurologic Recovery in Cardiac Arrest

Finally, we must consider the evaluation of neurologic recovery, as reported by Plum in a group of 65 patients who suffered cardiac arrest.[50] Using bedside evaluation and clinical studies, he attempted to predict the outcome of coma. Of patients who began to awaken within 6 hours following arrest, 60 per cent experienced a good recovery. Of patients who showed no response to noxious stimuli after 6 hours, 87 per cent died and

10 per cent made a good recovery. Of patients who had no oculovestibular reflex after 12 hours, most died; a few recovered with severe neurologic disability. All of them had an arrest during anesthesia.

The figures above must be remembered when one is considering heroic measures in the first few hours of coma. The results with current therapy are so poor that these measures, if applied early enough, are indicated in an attempt to improve neurologic recovery. Safar and colleagues have been studying neurologic recovery in detail, attempting to introduce certain therapeutic maneuvers, following arrest, that will improve survival.[51] They subjected dogs to 12 minutes of circulatory arrest by inducing ventricular fibrillation. Among dogs which they successfully resuscitated by closed chest massage, they treated 60 with routine post-CPR care and five by a combination of the following measures: elevation of mean arterial pressure to 150 to 180 torr with norepinephrine for 6 hours; administration of 1.5 mg. per kg. of heparin; flushing the cerebral circulation with a 10-per-cent solution of dextran-40 through a catheter in the ascending aorta; normovolemic hemodilution with 10 ml. per kg. of dextran-40. All of their untreated dogs remained comatose until death, and most of them developed muscle spasticity prior to recovery of electroencephalogram (EEG) activity. Some exhibited opisthotonos or running movements for days. Among the treated group, all five were awake within 24 hours, none were spastic, all were standing, walking, and eating by 48 hours, and all were normal or nearly normal with slight ataxia. In contrast, in the untreated group, none of the dogs awakened, all were spastic, none stood, walked, or ate, and all were comatose. Three died within 36 hours, and the other three were sacrificed on the 7th day.

It is postulated that the institution of hypertension, heparinization, and hemodilution are all directed toward reversing the "no-reflow phenomenon" and restoring capillary flow in vessels that previously were obstructed. Much experimental work remains before this therapy can be recommended for humans. Obviously, the therapeutic modalities used in experimental studies would have to be modified according to the cause of cardiac arrest. If ischemic heart disease is the basis for arrest, then hypertension of 150 to 180 torr (mean arterial pressure) is contraindicated, because of the effect of afterload and increasing myocardial work. The administration of heparin depends upon the clinical situation. However, in a young person who suffers an unexpected, sudden catastrophe and whose circulation and gas exchange can be restored rapidly, these maneuvers may be very useful; a neurologic recovery, an infrequent occurrence in the past, may thereby be achieved.

Barbiturate Treatment in Cardiac Arrest

Another mode of therapy that is now being investigated involves high-dose barbiturate anesthesia, given shortly after the ischemic insult. Hoff has shown that pentobarbital (19 mg./kg.), administered before or after middle cerebral artery occlusion in baboons, reduces the degree of brain infarction.[52] Bleyaert performed a long-term study using a monkey model: 16 minutes of global brain ischemia was produced by inflating a high pressure neck tourniquet; this was followed by 7 days of neurologic intensive care. The efficacy of barbiturate therapy in reducing the neurologic deficit was evaluated. The investigators administered 90 mg. per kg. of thiopental, beginning 5 minutes after circulation to the brain was restored; one-third of the dose was given in the first 5 minutes, and the remainder, over the next hour. The control group of monkeys developed severe neurologic deficits. Thiopental produced remarkable recovery in the treated group, so that after 5 days the monkeys were essentially normal when given a detailed examination.

The results of this study contrast with those of the study by Plum.[50] However, Plum waited 6 hours to retest patients for response to noxious stimuli, which then separated those likely to recover from those likely to die. On the other hand, Bleyaert's study suggests that to have a beneficial effect, barbiturate therapy must be administered within 60 minutes following restoration of circulation.[53] Similarly, Marshall and colleagues have recently reported markedly improved neurological status in patients with severe head injuries, who received pentobarbital infusions to a total dose of 3 to 5 mg. per kg., within a few hours of injury.[54]

TEAM APPROACH

The smooth, cooperative performance of cardiopulmonary resuscitation by a team does not happen by chance. Time must be devoted to education and practice, so that each individual knows what is expected of him. The physicians and nurses in the operating room must be acquainted with equipment function and availability. After each resuscitation, the participants should discuss the procedure, ascertain errors in technique or diagnosis, or account for the success of therapy. This will improve the quality of care provided for the next patient.[55] The burden of improving patient care falls upon both the surgeon, who must perfect the preoperative preparation of the patient, and the anesthesiologist, who must skillfully administer the anesthetic and recognize that not all patients respond similarly to stresses that occur in the operating room.

REFERENCES

1. Fatal application of chloroform. Edinburgh Med. Surg. J., *69*:409, 1848.
2. Sibson, H.: London Med Gaz, *42*:108, 1848.
3. Beecher, H. K.: The first anesthesia death with some remarks suggested by it on the fields of the laboratory and the clinic in the appraisal of new anesthetic agents. Anesthesiology, *2*:443, 1941.
4. Editorial. Lancet, *1*:161, 1848.
5. Mussey, R. D.: Chloroform in surgical operations. Boston Med. Surg. J., *38*:194, 1848.
6. Briggs, B. D., Sheldon, D. B., and Beecher, H. K.: Study of a thirty-year period of operating room deaths at the Massachusetts General Hospital, 1925-1954. J.A.M.A., *160*: 1439, 1956.
7. Memery, H. N.: Anesthesia mortality in private practice. A ten year study. J.A.M.A., *194*:1185, 1965.
8. Pierce, J. A.: Cardiac arrests and deaths associated with anesthesia. Anesth. Analg., *45*:407, 1966.
9. Jude, J. R., Bolooki, H., and Nagel, E.: Cardiac resuscitation in the operating room: Current status. Ann. Surg., *171*:948, 1970.
10. Stetson, J. B.: Resuscitation under anesthesia—some interesting early reports. Anesthesiology *20*:62, 1959.
11. Maass, D.: Die Methode den wiederbelebung ber herztod nach chloroformeinathmung. Ber. Klin. Wschr., *12*:265, 1892.
12. Keen, W. W.: Case of total laryngectomy (unsuccessful) in which massage of the heart for chloroform collapse was employed with notes of 25 other cases of cardiac massage. Ther. Gaz., *28*:217, 1904.
13. McLure, J. N., Skardasis, G. M., and Brown, J. M.: Cardiac arrest in the operating area. Am. Surg., *38*:241, 1972.
14. Minuck, M.: Cardiac arrest in the operating room—Part I (1965–1974). Can. Anaesth. Soc. J., *23*:357, 1976.
15. Finch, C. A., and Lenfant, C.: Oxygen transport in man. N. Engl. J. Med., *286*:407, 1972.

16. Flenley, D. C.: The rationale of oxygen therapy. Lancet, *1*:270, 1967.
17. Farhi, L. E.: Gas stores of the body. *In* Handbook of Physiology, Section 3, Vol. 1, p. 873, 1964.
18. Nunn, J. F.: Applied Respiratory Physiology. ed. 2. London, Butterworth & Co. Ltd., 1977.
19. Principles of Emergency Respiratory Care for the Anesthesiologist. In Sladen, A. (ed.): American Society of Anesthesiologists Workshop, 1971.
20. Ames, A., III, Wright, R. L., Kowada, N., et al.: Cerebral ischemia. II. The no-reflow phenomenon. Am J. Path., *52*:437, 1968.
21. Flores, J., DiBona, D. R., Beck, C. H., et al.: The role of cell swelling in ischemic renal damage and the protective effect of hypertonic solute. J. Clin. Invest., *51*:118, 1972.
22. Jenkins, M. T.: Editor's Note In Petty, L. D., and Giesecke, A. H.: Cardiac considerations in anesthesia. Clin. Anesth., *3*:168, 1968.
23. Bertrand, C. A., Steiner, N. V., Jameson, A. G., et al.: Disturbances of cardiac rhythm during anesthesia and surgery. J.A.M.A., *216*:1615, 1971.
24. Kuner, J.: Cardiac arrhythmias during anesthesia. Dis. Chest, *52*:580, 1967.
25. Wheeler, J.: Cardiac rhythm disorders during anesthesia. Mo. Med. J., *62*:680, 1965.
26. Camarata, S. J., Weil, M. H., Hanashiro, P. K., et al.: Cardiac arrest in the critically ill. Circulation, *44*:688, 1971.
27. Tolmie, J. D., Joyce, T. H., and Mitchell, G. D.: Succinylcholine danger in burned patients. Anesthesiology, *28*:467, 1967.
28. Cook, D. R., and Cosimi, A. B.: Potassium release after succinyl-choline in acutely uremic monkeys. Anesthesiology, *36*:297, 1972.
29. Kopriva, C., Ratliff, J., Fletcher, J. R., et al.: Serum potassium changes after succinyl-choline in patients with acute massive muscle trauma. Anesthesiology, *34*:246, 1971.
30. Mazze, R. I., Escue, H. M., and Houston, J. B.: Hyperkalemia and cardiovascular collapse following administration of succinylcholine in traumatized patients. Anesthesiology, *31*:540, 1969.
31. Smelt, R. B.: Hyperkalemia following succinylcholine administration in neurological disorders. A review. Can. Anaesth. Soc. J., *18*:199, 1971.
32. Fox, G. S., Wilkinson, R. D., and Rabow, F. I.: Thiopental anaphylaxis: a case and a method for diagnosis. Anesthesiology, *35*:655, 1971.
33. Jerums, G., et al.: Anaphylaxis to suxamethonium: A case report. Br. J. Anaesth., *39*:73, 1967.
34. Eger, E. I., II, and Epstein, R. M.: Hazards of anesthesia equipment. Anesthesiology, *25*:490, 1964.
35. Cullen, D. J., and Eger, E. I., II: The effect of anesthetic depth on the respiratory response to hypoxia in dogs: a dose response study. Anesthesiology, *33*:487, 1970.
36. Kopriva, C. J., and Lowenstein, E.: An anesthetic accident: cardiovascular collapse from liquid halothane delivery. Anesthesiology, *30*:246, 1969.
37. Munson, W. M.: Cardiac arrest: hazard of tipping a vaporizer. Anesthesiology, *26*:235, 1965.
38. Cullen, D. J., and Eger, E. I., II: Clinical signs of anesthesia. Anesthesiology, *36*:21, 1972.
39. Standards for cardiopulmonary resuscitation (CPR) and emergency cardiac care (ECC). J.A.M.A., *227*(Suppl.):833, 1974.
40. Kouwenhoven, W. B., Jude, J. P., and Knickerbocker, G. G.: Closed-chest massage, J.A.M.A., *173*:1064, 1960.
41. Goldberg, A. H.: Cardiopulmonary arrest. N. Engl. J. Med., *290*:381, 1974.
42. Kouwenhoven, W. B., Milnor, W. R., Knickerbocker, G. G., et al.: Closed-chest defibrillation of the heart. Surgery, *42*:550, 1957.
43. Bishop, R. L., and Weisfeld, M. L.: Sodium bicarbonate administration during cardiac arrest: effect on arterial *p*H, P , and osmolality. J.A.M.A., *235*:506, 1976.
44. Jackson, C. T., and Greendyke, R. M.: Pulmonary and cerebral fat embolism after closed chest massage. Surg. Gynecol. Obstet., *120*:25, 1965.
45. Mattar, J. A., Weil, M. H., Shubin, H., et al.: Cardiac arrest in the critically ill. II. Hyperosmolal states following cardiac arrest. Am. J. Med., *56*:162, 1974.
46. Patterson, R. H., Burns, W. A., and Jannotta, F. S.: Complications of external cardiac resuscitation: a retrospective review and survey of the literature. Med. Ann. D.C., *43*:389, 1974.
46a. McIntyre, K. M., Parisi, A. F., Benfari, R., et al.: Pathophysiological syndromes of cardiopulmonary resuscitation. Arch. Intern. Med., *138*:1130, 1978.
47. Marsh, M. L., Marshall, L. F., and Shapiro, H. M.: Neurosurgical intensive care. Anesthesiology, *47*:149, 1977.
48. Himmelhoch, S. R., Dekker, A., Gazzaniga, A. B., et al.: Closed chest cardiac resuscitation: a prospective clinical and pathological study. N. Engl. J. Med., *270*:118, 1964.
49. Meltzer, L. E.: The incidence of sudden unexpected death among hospitalized patients. Presented at American Association for the Advancement of Science, Boston, 1976.
50. Plum, F.: Presented at Society of Critical Care Medicine, Pittsburgh, 1976.
51. Safar, P., Stezoski, S. W., and Nemoto, E. M.: Amelioration of brain damage after 12 minutes of cardiac arrest in dogs. Arch. Neurol., *33*:91, 1976.
52. Hoff, J. T., Smith, A. L., Hankinson, H. L., et al.: Barbiturate protection from cerebral infarction in primates. Stroke, *6*:28, 1975.
53. Bleyaert, A. L., Nemoto, E. M., Stezoski, S. W., et al.: Amelioration of post ischemic encephalopathy by sodium thiopental after 16 minutes of global brain ischemia in monkeys. The Physiologist, *18*:145, 1975.
54. Marshall, L. F., Smith, R. W., and Shapiro, H. M.: The outcome with aggressive treatment in severe head injuries. Part II. Acute and chronic barbiturate administration in the management of head injury. J. Neurosurg., *50*:26, 1979.
55. Harley, H. R. S.: Reflections on cardiopulmonary resuscitation. Lancet, *2*:1, 1966.

FURTHER READING

Standards and guidelines for cardiopulmonary resuscitation (CPR) and emergency cardiac care (ECC). J.A.M.A., *244*, No. 5:453 1980.

17 Perioperative Myocardial Infarction

Emerson A. Moffitt, M.D., and Lawrence K. Harris, M.D., F.R.C.P.(C)

Over 1 million people experience heart attacks each year in the United States,[1] and another 5 to 6 million people have known or suspected coronary artery disease.[2] Every practicing anesthesiologist must anesthetize some of this high-risk population regularly; we studied a series of patients and found that there were 13 with a history of previous myocardial infarction in every 1000 patients requiring anesthesia.[3] Thus, the prevalence of the potentially lethal perioperative complication of infarction warrants a better understanding of its occurrence. This should result in a reduced incidence of perioperative infarction and an increased survival rate when the complication occurs.

Myocardial infarction related to anesthesia has three chronological frames of reference: patients who require anesthesia and who have had an infarction (recently or in the past); the risk and incidence of infarction occurring during anesthesia; and primary or recurrent infarction postoperatively. This chapter, however, is not organized in a chronological fashion but, rather, considers various facets of myocardial infarction through the whole perioperative period. The diagnosis, evaluation, and management of infarction, during and after anesthesia, and its incidence and prevention are presented.

ANATOMY AND PATHOPHYSIOLOGY

The myocardium is supplied with blood by two coronary arteries arising from the aorta within the sinuses of Valsalva (Fig. 17-1). The right coronary artery runs along the right atrioventricular (AV) groove and gives rise to vessels that course to the right ventricle. In approximately 90 per cent of human hearts, the right coronary artery crosses the crux and then divides into branches that supply the diaphragmatic surface of the left ventricle. Branches from the right coronary artery anastamose with branches from the left anterior descending branch of the left coronary artery near the apex, and posterolaterally with branches from the circumflex branch of the left coronary artery. Branches of the right coronary artery supply the sinoatrial (SA) node in 55 per cent of hearts, and the AV node, in 90 per cent. The frequent association of sinus and nodal bradydysrhythmias in inferior myocardial infarction is due to ischemia of nodal cells secondary to obstruction of the right coronary artery.

The left coronary artery arises within the left sinus of Valsalva and after a short distance divides into the left anterior descending and circumflex branches. The left anterior descending branch courses inferiorly along the anterior interventricular groove and frequently winds around the apex and anastamoses with posterior descending branches of the right coronary artery. Along its course, the left anterior descending branch gives off septal perforating branches that penetrate the interventricular septum, plus diagonal branches that supply the anterolateral left ventricular wall.

The circumflex branch of the left coronary

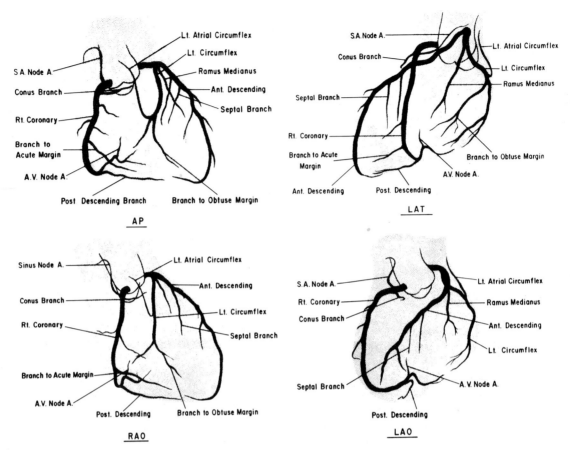

Fig. 17-1. Anatomic representation of the coronary arteries. (Abrams, H.L., and Adams, D.F.: The coronary arteriogram. N. Engl. J. Med., *281*:1276, 1336, 1969)

artery courses laterally in the AV groove and gives off branches that supply the lateral wall of the left ventricle and branches that course posterolaterally to anastomose with the right coronary artery. Branches to the SA node and AV node arise from the circumflex branch in 45 per cent and 10 per cent of hearts, respectively,[4,5]

Coronary blood flow occurs primarily during diastole, and therefore flow is dependent not only upon arteriolar resistance, but also upon diastolic filling time. In the normal resting heart, approximately 120 to 150 ml. per minute flow through the left ventricle, and, unlike other organs, the heart extracts most of the oxygen (70%) from the blood passing through itself.[6]

Myocardial ischemia occurs whenever oxygen demand exceeds supply. Myocardial metabolism is uniquely aerobic, and ischemia leads to anaerobic metabolism, resulting in an accumulation of metabolites, less efficient function, decreased contractility, and dysrhythmias.

By definition, *myocardial infarction* means necrosis of myocardial tissue. This is usually secondary to obstructive coronary artery disease; however, the patient may not have experienced exertional angina prior to the acute event. Following infarction, complications may be related to rhythm disturbances, disordered pump function, or both.

Ventricular dysrhythmias arise as a result of accumulation of toxic products of necrosis and anaerobic metabolism, especially products that result from disordered intracellular–extracellular potassium ratios in the infarcted area secondary to release of intracellular potassium from the necrosed cells. Also, ischemia of the SA node and AV node secondary to right coronary obstruction may result in bradydysrhythmias. These may be due directly to ischemia or to vagal influences secondary to ischemia.

Pump failure, or severely decreased cardiac output secondary to infarction, correlates with the amount of muscle damage. Page has shown that in most cases of cardiogenic shock following infarction, at least 30 per cent of the left ventricle is involved.[7] Generally, the degree of pump failure is directly related to the size of the infarct, and new infarcts are additive when superimposed upon previous damage.

CLINICAL PRESENTATION OF MYOCARDIAL INFARCTION

Classically, acute myocardial infarction presents with severe, steady substernal chest distress, accompanied by nausea, dyspnea, and diaphoresis. There is little doubt that a myocardial infarction has occurred if the patient presents primarily with these complaints. Unfortunately, these classic manifestations may be masked in the immediate postoperative period by sedation, residua of anesthesia, and pain from the operative site. Therefore, if the subjective symptoms are not reliable, suspicion must be based on objective clinical data.

Dysrhythmias

The large majority of patients with acute myocardial infarction have ventricular ectopic beats. In at least one study, 100 per cent of patients with myocardial infarction had ectopic beats or premature ventricular contractions (PVCs).[8] PVCs are the most common dysrhythmias in humans with or without infarction,[9] but PVCs in the postoperative period may be due to other factors that produce increased cardiac irritability (*e.g.*, hypoxia, acidosis). However, the presence of ventricular irritability in the postoperative period suggests that it may have been precipitated by an acute ischemic event. Dysrhythmias are discussed in Chapter 14. In the acutely ischemic (or infarcted) heart, PVCs should be treated immedi-

ately if they are multifocal or paired, fall on the T wave of the preceding sinus beat, or are more frequent than six per minute. In these situations, PVCs are often forerunners of more malignant ventricular arrhythmias. Naturally, in the postoperative period, ventricular tachycardia or ventricular fibrillation must also be treated immediately. After the myocardium and circulation have stabilized, further investigation should be undertaken to document a possible acute myocardial infarction.

Left Ventricular Failure

Acute left ventricular failure is a common complication of myocardial infarction. In our study of 451 consecutive admissions to a coronary care unit, 20 per cent of patients with myocardial infarction had either radiological or clinical evidence of left ventricular failure. Therefore, the development of hypoxemia or symptoms of dyspnea or orthopnea, with or without râles, and an elevated jugular venous presure, may represent acute myocardial infarction rather than an overload of blood volume. Persistent hypoxemia may be due to acute myocardial infarction, even without acute pulmonary edema, providing that respiratory depression is not present.

Hypotension

Subnormal arterial pressure in the postoperative period has a variety of causes. When there is no circulating volume deficit or persisting anesthetic effect, acute myocardial infarction must be excluded. In patients who suddenly develop cardiovascular collapse with shock, infarction is the likely cause. Even persistent mild hypotension with an adequate blood volume should suggest the presence of myocardial infarction, but further investigation is indicated before the blood volume is augmented.

DIFFERENTIAL DIAGNOSIS OF MYOCARDIAL INFARCTION

The diagnosis of myocardial infarction during anesthesia is even more difficult than in the postoperative period. In addition to the patient's insensitivity to pain, a host of other complicating factors may confuse the issue by frequently causing the same abnormal findings. However, an acute ischemic episode is initially suggested by a fall in blood pressure, with or without a rate and rhythm change. While infarction can occur in patients without known heart disease, likely candidates during anesthesia are those with a history of previous infarction, coronary artery disease, diabetes mellitus, and hypertension.

Hypotension during anesthesia usually is caused by the combination of myocardial depression, arteriolar and venous dilatation from the anesthetic agents, and the effects of positive pressure ventilation, particularly if the patient also experiences hypovolemia. Surgical events such as impeded vena caval flow and mesenteric traction are regular offenders. Hypoxemic impairment of cardiac function can occur insidiously if too high a concentration of nitrous oxide is given to a patient with increased shunting in the lungs. All of these must be excluded as potential causes before attributing persisting hypotension with elevated venous pressure to myocardial failure from an infarction.

Since the anesthesiologist must make a decision quickly regarding the seriousness of the problem, a tentative diagnosis must be made from the ECG. Until a 12-lead tracing can be obtained, he must rely upon the standard leads. Careful placement of leads is essential for accurate diagnosis; a lead placed in the V5 position on the chest wall is the most sensitive indicator.[10] As in the awake patient, frequent PVCs, bigeminy, and S-T segment elevation are highly suggestive of an ischemic myocardium, even if Q waves are absent. However, these signs regularly occur during anesthesia in patients with coronary artery disease. If they persist after elimination of hypoxemia, hypotension, hypercapnia, and anesthetic-induced cardiac depression, the presence of an infarcted segment is suggested. If new Q waves develop, the ECG becomes diagnostic.

Changes in the pulse rate are not diagnostic, since many other factors, such as changes in vagal tone, have the same effects. Tachycardia can result from surgical stimulation during light anesthesia, or it may be due to ventricular failure. Ventricular hyperirritability, as evidenced by PVCs and bigeminy, may be due to an acutely ischemic area of myocardium, but, again, there may be other causes. Decreased concentrations of myocardial and whole body potassium, stemming from long-term diuretic therapy, may be involved; digitalis toxicity is still another possible complication. The migration of potassium into myocardial cells during respiratory alkalosis can also produce hyperirritability.

DIAGNOSTIC AIDS IN CLINICAL EVALUATION OF MYOCARDIAL INFARCTION

Acute myocardial infarction can be diagnosed from the 12-lead ECG in approximately 70 to 80 per cent of cases. The classical ECG of a patient with acute transmural infarction has Q waves greater than 0.04 seconds and S-T segment elevation in leads over the involved ares, with reciprocal changes reflecting the opposite wall. The earliest changes, however, may be only S-T segment elevation or tall T waves in leads over the involved area. In an anterior infarction, changes will be seen in the chest leads, lead 1 and lead aVL (Fig. 17-2), and with inferior infarction, in leads II, III, and aVF (Fig. 17-3). Approximately 30 per cent of infarctions cannot be diagnosed by ECG, either because of left bundle branch block or nontransmural infarction that does not result in a Q wave.[11] Non-transmural infarction usually presents only with S-T segment and T wave abnormalities. Since typical changes of infarction may not be present in the first ECG obtained, serial tracings should be obtained for three days in any patient with suspected ischemic changes. The development of flattening or depression of S-T segments, with or without T wave inversion, indicates the occurrence of an acute ischemic event and possible infarction. The mortality and complications of acute non-transmural myocardial infarction are not different from those for patients sustaining an acute transmural infarction.[12]

Serum Enzymes

Serum enzyme elevations have been used in the diagnosis of acute myocardial infarction for many years.[13] Serum levels of glutamic-oxaloacetic

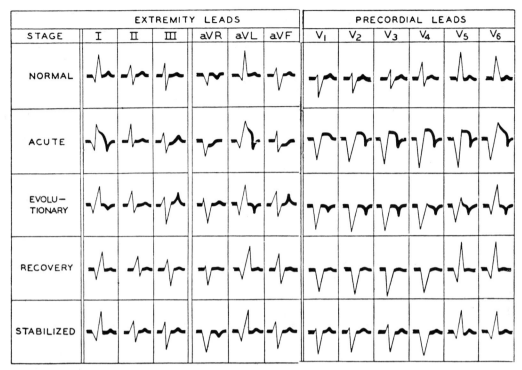

Fig. 17-2. Anterior myocardial infarction. Acute Stage: Abnormal Q wave is shown, with elevated S-T segment and inverted T wave in leads I, aVL, and V_1 through V_6. S-T segment depression (a reciprocal change occurring on the opposite side of the heart) is present in leads III, aVR, and aVF. Evolutionary Stage: S-T segment is isoelectric; inverted, symmetrical T wave is shown in leads I, aVL, and precordial leads; tall symmetrical T wave, in leads III and aVF. Recovery Stage: T waves are returning to normal. Stabilized Stage: T waves are normal; the only evidence of old infarction is the Q wave in leads I, aVL, V_4, V_5, and V_6. (Modified from Lipman, B.S., and Massie, E.: Clinical Scalar Electrocardiography. ed. 5. pp. 246–247, Chicago, Year Book Medical Publishers, 1965)

transaminase (GOT), lactic dehydrogenase (LDH), and creatine phosphokinase (CPK) are determined most commonly.[14] Unfortunately, the ubiquitous nature of these enzymes (e.g., their presence in many tissues other than cardiac muscle) has reduced their diagnostic specificity for acute myocardial infarction in the presence of other organ injury.[15–18] The usual enzymatic changes with acute infarction consist of a rise in GOT and CPK within the first 24 hours and a later rise in LDH (Fig. 17-4). However, hepatic disease, muscle trauma (as in a major operation), hemolysis, and intramuscular injections also result in a release of one or more of these enzymes into the blood, so that evaluation of the enzyme rise becomes difficult or impossible in these cases.[15,16,18]

In recent years, the ability to separate enzymes according to their origin has increased their usefulness and specificity in making an enzymatically based diagnosis. Both CPK and LDH can be fractionated into their various components (or isoenzymes): LDH, by either electrophoresis or heat, and CPK, by electrophoretic or chromatographic techniques. LDH isoenzyme terminology is confusing, however, since the five fractions have been numbered differently by the Europeans and the Americans (Fig. 17-5). Figure 17-6 displays a profile of LDH isoenzymes as they occur in both skeletal and cardiac muscle injury.[19] With regard to LDH, heart muscle damage results primarily in rise of the alpha-1 fraction (No. 1 in American terminology), but since this fraction is

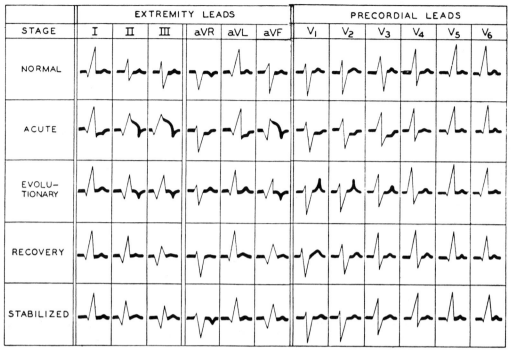

Fig. 17-3. Inferior myocardial infarction. Acute Stage: Abnormal Q wave is shown with elevated S-T segment and inverted T wave in leads II, III, and aVF; a depressed S-T segment (reciprocal change), in leads I, aVR, aVL, V_1, V_2, and V_3. Leads facing the uninjured anterior wall may show reciprocal changes in right precordial leads (as here) or no changes. Evolutionary Stage: inverted symmetrical T wave is shown in leads II, III, and aVF; tall symmetrical T wave, in leads I, aVL, V_1, V_2, V_3, and V_4. Recovery Stage: T waves are returning to normal. Stabilized Stage: T waves are normal; Q wave, in leads II, III, an aVF. (Modified from Lipman, B.S., and Massie, E.: Clinical Scalar Electrocardiography. ed. 5. pp. 248–249. Chicago, Year Book Medical Publishers, 1965)

also present in red cells, hemolysis of the specimen can give a false positive.

CPK fractionation is used mostly to distinguish skeletal injury from cardiac muscle injury. CPK has three isoenzymes: MM, MB, and BB. MM is the principal isoenzyme in both skeletal and cardiac muscle; in injured patients, most of the CPK consists of MM isoenzymes,[20] from both the heart and skeletal muscle. However, since the heart is the only organ that contains the isoenzyme MB, the presence of an MB fraction shows that at least some of the CPK originated in the myocardium. If the MB fraction peaks, this is even more indicative of acute myocardial infarction.[21]

INCIDENCE OF MYOCARDIAL INFARCTION

What is the incidence of coronary disease and of previous infarction in the population hospitalized for anesthesia and operation? In the United States, there are over 5 million people with known or suspected coronary disease,[3] and more than 1 million people have a myocardial infarction every year.[1] Annually, approximately 700,000 people die of coronary disease; 400,000 of these die suddenly.[1] A myocardial infarction or "coronary" is likely to occur in 20 per cent of all North American men before the age of 65.[1] Of these, 20 percent die within 3 hours of the onset of their first attack, and another 10 per cent die

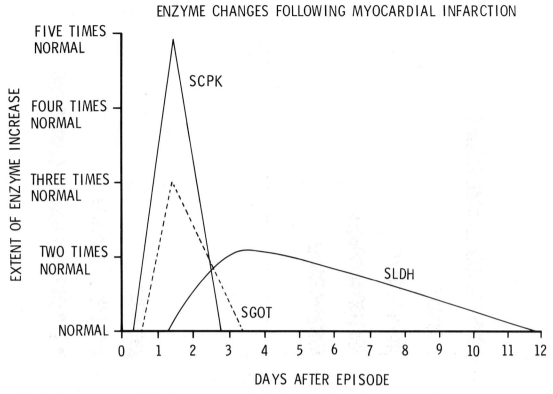

Fig. 17-4. Enzymatic profile of acute myocardial infarction. (Coodley, E.L.: Enzymes in cardiac disease. *In* Coodley, E.A.: Diagnostic Enzymology. ed. 2. pp. 39–69. Philadelphia, Lea & Febiger, 1970)

	ANODE (+)		SPECIMEN APPLICATION POINT ↘		CATHODE (−)
AMERICAN NUMERAL	LDH_1	LDH_2	LDH_3	LDH_4	LDH_5
EUROPEAN NUMERAL	LDH_5	LDH_4	LDH_3	LDH_2	LDH_1
ELECTROPHORETIC	α_1	α_2	β	γ_1	γ_2
TYPICAL TISSUE SOURCE	MYOCARDIUM			LIVER	

Fig. 17-5. Modified classification of three isoenzyme nomenclatures based on electrophoretic mobility. (Louderback, A.L., and Shanbran, E.: Lactic dehydrogenase isoenzyme electrophoresis. J.A.M.A., *205*:294, 1968)

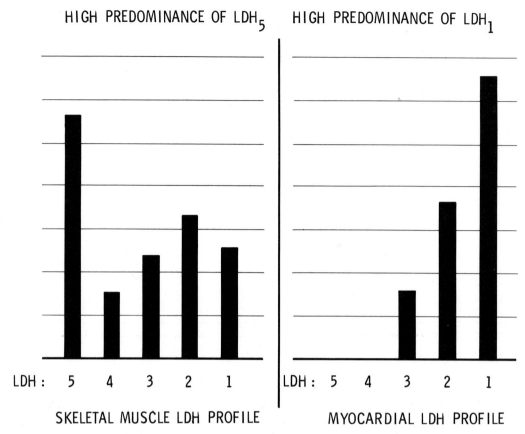

Fig. 17-6. Isoenzyme profiles for LDH in suspected myocardial infarction. (After Coodley, E.L.: Enzymes in cardiac disease. *In* Coodley, E.A.: Diagnostic Enzymology. ed. 2. pp. 39–69. Philadelphia, Lea & Febiger, 1970)

within the first week.[1] The long-term prognosis is also rather grim. Survivors of a myocardial infarction who return to full-time work have a 5-year death rate that is five times that of men without known heart disease.[1] Another heart attack is the usual cause of death.

In our series of nearly 33,000 surgical patients over 30 years of age, there were 12.8 in 1,000 with a known history of infarction.[3] The prevalence increases by decade with age, from 0.7 in 1,000 in people 30 to 39 years of age, to a high of 27.9 in 1,000 in the 70- to 79-year-old age-group (Table 17-1). Considering the large number of people with heart disease, every anesthesiologist should

expect to manage these high-risk patients often during major surgery.

Given the relatively high prevalence of prior infarction in the surgical population, how much is the risk increased during and after anesthesia in such patients? Four large series have supplied answers. Tarhan and co-workers found that 28 of 422 patients (6.6%) with a previous infarction, operated upon during 1967 and 1968, re-infarcted within one week of surgery.[3] Of 32,455 patients without known infarction, 43 (0.13%) had an infarction in the first postoperative week. Analysis of patients operated upon during 1974 and 1975 at the same institution yielded similar re-

Table 17-1. Relation of Myocardial Infarction to Previous Infarction and to Surgical Population*

			MYOCARDIAL INFARCTION IN MEN		MYOCARDIAL INFARCTION IN WOMEN	
AGE, YR.	GENERAL ANESTHESIA (No.)	TOTAL PREVIOUS MYOCARDIAL INFARCTION PER 1,000 ANESTHETIZED	PREVIOUSLY	AGAIN, POST-OPERATIVELY	PREVIOUSLY	AGAIN, POST-OPERATIVELY
30–39	4,081	0.7	3	. . .	. . .	. . .
40–49	6,906	3.6	24	2	1	. . .
50–59	8,825	10.5	75	5	18	. . .
60–69	8,375	20.9	147	13	28	. . .
70–79	4,051	27.9	90	6	23	1
80+	639	20.3	10	1	3	. . .
Total	32,877	12.8	349	27	73	1

*Tarhan, S., Moffitt, E. A., Taylor, W. F., et al.: Myocardial infarction after general anesthesia. J.A.M.A., *220*:1451, 1972

sults[21a]. Thus, patients who have had a prior infarction appear to be 50 times more likely to experience a postoperative infarction than those who have not. Plumlee and Boettner reported that 24 of 18,018 patients (0.13%) in their study had an infarction during or soon after anesthesia and operation.[22] Five of the 24 had preoperative ECG evidence of an infarction. More recently, Goldman and associates documented the importance of an infarction within six months of surgery in their elegant formulation of a cardiac risk index: 22 of 1001 patients (2.2%) studied prospectively who had had an infarction accounted for 5 of the 19 cardiac deaths (26.3%).[22a,22b] Therefore, with the high incidence of infarction and death in patients with coronary disease not associated with surgery, it is indeed surprising that there are not more infarctions during anesthesia or postoperatively.

Factors Involved in the Occurrence of Intraoperative or Postoperative Infarction

Studies of Tarhan and co-workers and Plumlee and Boettner also suggest that the following factors must be considered, to avoid an intraoperative or postoperative infarction:

Preoperative Cardiac State. Seventeen of 24 patients who infarcted had preexisting heart disease; 11 of them were categorized in Class III or IV (New York Heart Association, functional classification).[22] Seven patients in this series had diabetes. Of 43 patients who had a primary infarction postoperatively,[3] 16 had preoperative angina, six others were diabetic, and ten had hypertension requiring treatment. All patients with cardiovascular disease are in a class of increased risk by themselves. Too often in the past, they have been given only routine care and attention.

Preoperative Hypertension. Intuition and several small series have suggested that preoperative hypertension, especially if untreated, may be a contributing factor in the etiology of perioperative myocardial infarction.[22c] Yet, only one of the large series has noted such a correlation, and a weak one at that.[21a] Even when Goldman intensively evaluated preoperative hypertension as a predictor of intra- and postoperative cardiovascular complications, he could find no statistically significant relationships.[22a,22b,22d] Importantly, he concludes,

. . . elective surgery in the absence of ideal antihypertensive therapy need not subject patients to an added clinical risk provided a) diastolic pressure is stable and not higher than 110 torr, and b) intraoperative and recovery room blood pressure values are closely monitored and treated to prevent hypertensive or hypotensive episodes . . .[22d]

That is, *intra*operative management of the patient with mild to moderate hypertension may be

Table 17-2. Relation of Myocardial Infarction to Anesthetic Agents*

| | MYOCARDIAL INFARCTION | | |
AGENTS AND MIXTURES	PREVIOUSLY	AGAIN, POST-OPERATIVELY	AGAIN, %
Thiopental, O_2, N_2O, tubocurarine			
With methoxyflurane	57	5	8.8
With halothane	268	18	6.7
With ether	66	4	6.1
With pentazocine	3	. . .	. . .
Thiopental, O_2, N_2O	21	. . .	. . .
With halothane, gallamine	1	1	. . .
With gallamine	1	. . .	. . .
With cyclopropane	1	. . .	. . .
Thiopental, diazepam	2	. . .	. . .
Thiopental, O_2, surgical infiltrate	1	. . .	. . .
Innovar,† O_2, N_2O, tubocurarine	1	. . .	. . .
Total	422	28	6.6

*Tarhan, S., Moffitt, E. A., Taylor, W. F., et al.: Myocardial infarction after general anesthesia. J.A.M.A., 220:1451, 1972

†Mixture containing droperidol and fentanyl citrate

more important than preoperative antihypertensive therapy.

Type of Anesthesia. Tarhan and associates studied a wide range of agents and found that there was no correlation between the occurrence of myocardial infarction and the type of anesthesia used (Table 17-2).[3,21a]

Duration of Anesthesia. A correlation between duration of anesthesia and infarction was found in the first study by Tarhan[3] but not the second,[21a] although one would expect a longer exposure to depressant drugs to be more hazardous. Yet, during the anesthetic, the patient is more carefully monitored and managed than at any other time; this possibly explains why the duration of anesthesia is not necessarily significant.

Site of Operation. Operations in the thorax and upper abdomen are followed by a much greater number of infarctions (Table 17-3). This is not surprising, since there is greater impairment of ventilation and a likelihood of more severe shunting and atelectasis after such procedures.

Circulatory State During Anesthesia. A pattern of unstable blood pressure was seen in almost all patients in Plumlee's series[22]; such instability consisted of changes of more than 25 per cent during anesthesia as compared to the conscious state, or changes lasting more than 10 minutes. They concluded that infarction took place during anesthesia in ten patients and that hypotension or wide swings in blood pressure were either causative or resulted from the acute ischemic episode. The importance of intraoperative and early postoperative hypotension has also been noted by other investigators.[23]

Oxygenation During Anesthesia and Postoperatively. Plumlee and Boettner noted that nitrous oxide was the major agent used in nine of the 24

Table 17-3. Relation of Myocardial Infarction to Site and Type of Operation*

	MYOCARDIAL INFARCTION				
	IN MEN		IN WOMEN		AGAIN (%)
SITE AND TYPE OF OPERATION	PREVIOUSLY	AGAIN, POST-OPERATIVELY	PREVIOUSLY	AGAIN, POST-OPERATIVELY	(MEN & WOMEN)
Thorax and upper abdomen	(113)	(15)	(18)	(1)	(12.2)†
Great vessels	49	5	5	. . .	9.0
Lung	14	5	. . .	. . .	36.0
Other intrathoracic	4	3	. . .	. . .	75.0
Biliary, upper abdomen	46	2	13	1	5.0
Other	(236)	(12)	(55)	. . .	(4.1)†
Extraperitoneal abdominal	5	1	2	. . .	14.0
Endoscopic: oral	8	2	. . .	. . .	25.0
perineal	5	2	. . .	. . .	40.0
Perineal GU‡	48	2	. . .	. . .	4.0
Anorectal	7	1	. . .	. . .	14.0
Vertebral column	14	1	2	. . .	6.0
Extremities, bone	18	2	5	. . .	9.0
Head and neck	13	1	5	. . .	6.0
Miscellaneous	118	. . .	41	. . .	. . .
Total	349	27	73	1	6.6

*Tarhan, S., Moffitt, E. A., Taylor, W. F., et al.: Myocardial infarction after general anesthesia. J.A.M.A., *220*:1451, 1972
†Difference between groups is significant (P<.001).
‡Genitourinary

patients who infarcted; 75-per-cent nitrous oxide was used in six cases. In Tarhan's series, on the 3rd postoperative day there was a significantly greater incidence of infarcts, which implied that arterial oxygen desaturation from miliary atelectasis is greatest at this time. Patients with cardiovascular disease need an inspired concentration of 40 to 50 per cent during anesthesia and a similarly elevated inspired concentration after the operation.

Interval from Previous Infarction to Anesthesia and Operation. A major operation within 3 months of an infarction is followed by reinfarction in 37 per cent of cases (Table 17-4). Within the next 3 months, the incidence falls to 16 per cent, and beyond that time it stabilizes at 4 to 5 per cent. Arkins similarly noted that 11 of 40 patients, or 40 per cent, re-infarcted when operated on within 3 months of infarction.[24] Therefore, only operations for life-threatening conditions should be performed within 6 months after a heart attack.

Mortality of Patients with Perioperative Infarction. In Tarhan's first series[3], 54 per cent of patients (69% in the second series[21a]) died following postoperative re-infarction, and 87 per cent of patients with known coronary artery disease died as a result of their first infarction. Three-fourths of these deaths occurred within 48 hours of the infarction; this contrasts with a corresponding figure of approximately one-third for patients with nonsurgical infarctions. In Plumlee's series, 83 per cent, or 20 of 24 patients, died of postoperative infarction.[22]

TREATMENT OF MYOCARDIAL INFARCTION DURING ANESTHESIA

If a combination of typical dysrhythmias and hypotension persists during anesthesia, the anesthesiologist must assume that a major infarction has occurred, until it is disproved. First, the operation must be terminated as rapidly as proper surgical judgment allows.

Table 17-4. Relation of Myocardial Infarction to Interval from Previous Myocardial Infarction*

| | MYOCARDIAL INFARCTION | | | | |
| | IN MEN | | IN WOMEN | | AGAIN (%) |
MONTHS	PREVIOUSLY	AGAIN, POST-OPERATIVELY	PREVIOUSLY	AGAIN, POST-OPERATIVELY	(MEN & WOMEN)
0–3	8	3	. . .	. . .	37
4–6	15	3	4	. . .	16
7–12	31	2	11	. . .	5
13–18	26	1	1	. . .	4
19–24	19	1	2	. . .	5
25+	186	10	46	1	5
Old	64	7	9	. . .	10
Other†	. . .	. . .	. . .	. . .	. . .
Total	349	27	73	1	6.6

*Tarhan, S., Moffitt, E. A., Taylor, W. F., et al.: Myocardial infarction after general anesthesia. J.A.M.A., *220:* 1451, 1972
†Age not recorded for myocardial infarction.

Concomitantly, the anesthesiologist must examine every aspect of the maintenance of the patient. The cardiac output and circulation must be restored to preanesthetic levels, as closely as possible.

The major considerations of treatment are as follows:

Attain optimal blood volume by administering colloid or whole blood, up to a central venous pressure of about 15 torr or to a pulmonary artery wedge or end-disastolic pressure of 20 torr.

Lighten the anesthestic level to decrease cardiac depression from potent agents.

Use peripheral vasoconstrictors, such as methoxamine, if hypotension is present with evidence of vasodilatation.

Maintain a high arterial oxygen tension; discontinue nitrous oxide; draw an arterial blood gas sample.

Treat acute left ventricular failure with a rapidly acting diuretic, such as furosemide (40 mg.) or ethacrynic acid (50–100 mg.), administered intravenously. If, however, hypotension is also present, a flow-directed pulmonary artery catheter should be inserted, and blood volume should be augmented if the pulmonary artery wedge pressure or end-diastolic pressure is low. Inotropic agents, such as calcium chloride, in incremental doses of 1 to 3 g., or dopamine infusion[25,26] is indicated if pulmonary artery wedge

or pulmonary artery end-diastolic pressure is normal or elevated. Vasodilatating agents, such as intravenous nitroprusside or phentolamine, also may be beneificial in increasing cardiac output by reducing afterload (peripheral resistance).[27] There is a risk that catecholamines may induce hyperirritability in the presence of injured, hypoxic myocardium, but cardiac output must be maintained.

Correct-acid-base abnormalities, such as respiratory alkalosis and metabolic acidosis, that may impair cardiac function.

Correct electrolyte changes, such as hypokalemia.

Reduce the detrimental effect of controlled (positive pressure) ventilation on cardiac output by using a slow rate (10–12/min.) and an appropriate tidal volume; avoid hyperventilation.

Set up additional monitoring not already present: an ECG tracing of high quality, a central venous or, preferably, a pulmonary artery catheter, direct arterial pressure catheter, and blood gas and electrolyte analyses.

TREATMENT OF POSTOPERATIVE MYOCARDIAL INFARCTION

The large majority of deaths following myocardial infarction are due to arrhythmias. Therefore, it is mandatory that any patient who is suspected of having had an acute cardiac ischemic episode should be monitored in an intensive care area, where developing arrhythmias can be promptly diagnosed and appropriately treated. Generally, the management of the patient who develops a postoperative infarction should be no different from that of any patient with a new infarction. This includes analgesics, sedatives, and an elevated inspired concentration of oxygen.

Acute left left ventricular failure is best managed initially by rapidly acting diuretics, such as furosemide or ethacrynic acid, given intravenously. Digitalis preparations should be reserved for patients who do not respond to diuretics and should also be administered intravenously. Digoxin is preferred because of its rapid onset of action. Since the acutely ischemic myocardium is more sensitive to the arrhythmogenic effects of digitalis, less than the usual digitalizing dose should be given. The average patient requires between 0.75 and 1.5 mg. of digoxin as a digitalizing dose[28]; in patients with an acute infarct, approximately two-thirds should be given in divided doses over 24 hours.

Continuing hypotension requires insertion of a flow-directed pulmonary artery catheter. A pulmonary artery wedge or end-diastolic pressure of 15 torr or less is an indication for careful volume replacement. Cardiac output may increase simply by increasing left ventricular filling pressure, and a filling pressure of 18 to 20 torr is optimum. Post-infarction hypotension with an elevated pulmonary artery or end-diastolic pressure is best managed with catecholamine infusion, such as dopamine (2–20 μg./kg./min.); when this is unsuccessful, consideration should be given to intra-aortic balloon pumping, if available. Vasodilator therapy with nitroprusside, phentolamine, or nitroglycerin may improve cardiac output as well, in selected cases. Isoproterenol should be avoided in the patient with acute myocardial infarction, because the drug not only stimulates arrhythmias but also inappropriately increases myocardial oxygen consumption.

Analgesics should be given intravenously to avoid further interference with serum enzyme determinations and for careful titration of effective dose. Initially, morphine (2.5 mg.) or meperidine (10 mg.) is an appropriate analgesic; adminis-

tration can be repeated until pain is relieved, while the patient is watched for respiratory depression.

The use of anticoagulants following myocardial infarction is still controversial.[29] Peripheral embolism from an endocardial clot is a small but definite risk, and pulmonary embolism is an even greater hazard. Recent operation may preclude both anticoagulation therapy and early ambulation, placing the patient at increased risk from pulmonary embolism. Conversely, blood coagulability is increased early postoperatively,[30] and men with previous infarction tend toward excess thrombus formation.[31] Hence, prophylactic short-term anticoagulation may be justified to reduce embolization in this high-risk group.

Major operation plus an acute infarction are additive stresses, and convalescence will be longer than for either event alone. The rapidity of mobilization after myocardial infarction has undergone major conceptual changes, with increasing evidence favoring early mobilization and discharge after the uncomplicated infarction. Uncomplicated postoperative infarctions should be managed similarly. Following the initial period of monitoring and stabilization, mobilization should proceed so that the patient is ready for discharge in about 2 weeks. Naturally, the speed of mobilization depends on the size and complications of the infarction (*e.g.*, failure), in addition to any limitations owing to the operation.

PREVENTION OF INFARCTION DURING AND AFTER ANESTHESIA

As discussed on page 259, the risk of another infarction occurring during or after anesthesia for a major operation is 50 times greater for patients who have had an infarction than for those who have not.[3] The important consideration is the time interval between the infarction and the operation. Clearly, only life-threatening emergencies should be treated surgically within 6 months of a heart attack.

After the infarcted area has had 6 months to heal and form firm scar tissue, the incidence of postoperative re-infarction stabilizes at 4 to 5 per cent, which still classifies it as a major risk. The primary aim in such a patient is to manage the anesthetic and postoperative period so as to avoid another infarction and its lethal outcome.

In addition, patients who have not had an infarction but who have hypertension, diabetes mellitus, and ischemic heart disease, are also at increased risk. This is particularly true of patients with *unstable angina pectoris,* defined as angina pectoris that has occurred for the first time within the past 3 months, or angina that has been progressing in severity (*e.g.,* precipitated with less effort, new sites of radiation of pain, or episodes of pain poorly or incompletely relieved by nitroglycerin). From retrospective studies, it appears that approximately 40 per cent of patients with myocardial infarction have had a recent change in their anginal pattern prior to the infarction. While this cannot be applied to other patients, it is reasonable to assume that the patient with unstable angina has a higher risk of primary infarction perioperatively.

Most patients with angina are now treated with propranolol. Recently, it has become evident that stopping propranolol abruptly risks precipitating an acute infarction.[32-34] Moreover, although continued administration of the drug has been associated with intraoperative cardiac depression,[35] other investigators have reported that propranolol does not increase the risk of complications.[36,37] Therefore, the drug should be administered until the operation and should be reinstituted as soon as possible postoperatively. Particularly large doses can be tapered to smaller doses over a 2- to 3-day period prior to surgery[38]; if these patients become symptomatic upon reduction of propranolol, however, the need for elective surgery should be reassessed.

Every patient who has had a previous infarction should have an ECG on the 1st and 3rd postoperative days for comparison with the preoperative pattern, to assist in the early diagnosis and treatment of ischemia and impending infarction.

Anesthesia After Recent Infarction

Prevention of circulatory depression and further enlargement of the infarcted segment are primary aims in the patient who needs an emergency operation in the first weeks after an acute infarction. In addition, the most frequent life-threatening event in this period is embolization of an endocardial thrombus from the left ventricle. The less hazardous sites for such emboli to lodge are in the limbs, where the embolus can be removed relatively easily. If mesenteric arteries are blocked, intervention by laparotomy is associated with a much higher risk and is one of the greatest anesthetic challenges. The patient with a massive pulmonary embolus from a peripheral vein is one of the most difficult to keep alive; the anesthesiologist must maintain the circulation until cardiopulmonary bypass can be instituted.

Preoperative Assessment. Recently infarcted patients usually have an unstable circulation, and the state of myocardial function needs critical assessment: Is there congestive failure even to the point of basal rales or pulmonary edema? Is cardiogenic shock present with severe hypotension, peripheral constriction, and cyanosis? If dyspnea and hypoxemia are present, are they primarily pulmonary or cardiac in origin? If there is hypotension, is it accompanied by normal or low venous pressure, or by high jugular venous, central venous, or pulmonary artery pressure? What is the state of cerebral perfusion and function? Are drugs such as isoproterenol, dopamine, or digitalis being given to support the circulation? The risk associated with surgery is directly related to the number of these complications, and the length of the operation should be determined by these factors.

Anesthetic Considerations. In recently infarcted patients, the essential obligation is to maintain their precarious circulation and tissue oxygenation during the operation. This involves close management of the three essential components of the circulation: blood volume, cardiac output, and peripheral resistance.[39] The anesthesiologist must increase the blood volume to produce a left ventricular end-diastolic, left atrial, or pulmonary arterial wedge pressure of 15–22 torr, if these pressures are lower initially. Pressures of this magnitude are associated with the maximum safe sarcomere length and ventricular volume for the greatest stroke and cardiac output. If these pressures are greater than 22 to 25 torr, the myocardium is already "overstretched" and myocardial failure occurs; pharmacological efforts to reverse the failure are required.

Cardiac output and peripheral resistance are the other determinants of a satisfactory circulation. The output is quite likely to be reduced in the acute infarction period. The compensatory response is increased arteriolar resistance, thus avoiding or reversing hypotension. Since all potent anesthetic drugs depress the myocardium and decrease peripheral resistance, general anesthesia is likely to cause further hypotension in the compromised, infarcted heart. Mild hypotension is acceptable because it reduces cardiac work,[40] but coronary perfusion must be maintained. Controlled positive pressure ventilation reduces cardiac output by reducing venous return.

Hence, in the first few weeks after infarction, the anesthesiologist should avoid general anesthesia, if at all possible. To minimize depression of circulation, the best approach is as follows:

INFILTRATION OF A LOCAL ANESTHETIC is done over the operative site, keeping below the toxic dose;

SMALL INCREMENTS OF AN OPIATE AND DIAZEPAM, intravenously, are used for analgesia and to cloud the sensorium. The patient in cardiogenic shock often is not alert. Doses of opiate and Innovar[41] sufficient to produce arteriolar dilatation (*i.e.*, significant hypotension) should be avoided.

OXYGEN ADMINISTRATION BY MASK is used to maintain an arterial tension of over 150 torr (20.0 kPa). If spontaneous respiration and Pa_{O_2} are not adequate, assisted ventilation with an endotracheal tube is needed.

INSERTION OF AN INTRA-ARTERIAL NEEDLE OR CATHETER allows continuous measurement of blood pressure and intermittent determination of oxygen tension and acid-base balance. The circulation can be more precisely and successfully managed with a flow-directed pulmonary artery catheter.

If the patient has a stable circulation and more than 2 weeks have elapsed since infarction, a light level of general anesthesia with a diazepam induction will not unduly depress the blood pressure. No more than 50-per-cent nitrous oxide

should be used, if it is used at all; that is, assure a Pa_{O_2} of at least 150 torr (20.0 kPa).

Management of Problems During Operation. Arterial hypotension and abnormalities of rate and rhythm are the most frequent problems during surgery.

When hypotension occurs, one must determine the cause: blood loss, vasodilatation, decreased cardiac output, or a combination of these. Blood loss should be treated early by augmentation. Since peripheral resistance is usually elevated when cardiac output is low, if any drug has caused dilatation leading to severe hypotension, the treatment is to reimpose peripheral tone with methoxamine. Severe vasoconstriction is detrimental, but arterial pressure must be maintained.

A more likely cause of hypotension is further decrease in cardiac output from deterioration of contractility. While positive inotropic drugs, such as digitalis and isoproterenol, are more likely to initiate ventricular dysrhythmias in a hyperirritable heart with dead and injured muscle, their judicious use may be necessary to maintain even a minimally adequate circulation. Isoproterenol or dopamine administered by continuous infusion often can increase cardiac output without producing tachycardia that is severe enough to negate the beneficial effect. Intermittent doses of calcium chloride (100 mg.) also improve contractility, since calcium chloride is one of the most effective stimulants to the myocardium.

Abnormalities of heart rate, particularly bradycardia, are frequent after infarction. While there is controversy regarding the danger of post-infarction bradycardia and the value of atropine in abolishing it, rates remaining below 60 beats per min. during operation are usually accompanied by hypotension. Small doses of intravenous atropine increase the rate and elevate the blood pressure. The other consideration in severe bradycardia is that ectopic foci from injured muscle predispose the heart to premature beats during the prolonged intervals between sinus beats, with the risk of ventricular fibrillation. One excellent practice in the infarcted surgical patient with bradycardia is to insert a transvenous pacemaker to obtain precise control of rate. Certainly, if various degrees of AV block are present, the capability of pacing is essential before anesthesia. Both gallamine[42] and pancuronium[43] tend to increase heart rate and are useful in preventing bradycardia during anesthesia.

Dysrhythmias are frequently a problem, particularly those that are hyperirritable in nature. Ectopic activity occurring early after infarction may have several causes that act together: reduced arterial oxygen tension in arterial blood, abnormal electrical activity from the hypoxic and infarcted tissue, elevated or decreased plasma potassium or carbon dioxide levels, elevated or exogenous plasma catecholamine concentrations, digitalis toxicity, and the presence of a high concentration of quinidine or procaineamide. Management of ectopic beats and rhythms should be prompt and vigorous to reduce the detrimental effect on cardiac output and avoid the highly lethal complication of ventriculatlar fibrillation. First, all possible contributing causes, such as hypoxemia or carbon dioxide or potassium abnormalities (usually hypocapnia and hypokalemia), are controlled. Following this, the need for isoproterenol, if it is being given, is reassessed. Lidocaine administered by bolus (1 mg./kg.) and by drip (2–4 mg./min.) depresses ectopic foci. Procaineamide (100 mg./5 min. to a maximum of 1 g.) is usually effective in controlling ventricular dysrhythmias resistant to lidocaine. Propranolol during anesthesia should be avoided early after infarction, if possible, because it is a myocardial depressant. The ability to control the rate at 90 to 100 beats per minute, rather than allowing a slower sinus rate, is an effective way of reducing the incidence of PVCs. Both ventricular fibrillation and persisting ventricular tachycardia should be treated by closed chest DC countershock.

REFERENCES

1. Stamler, J.: The primary prevention of coronary heart disease. *In* Braunwald, E. (ed.): The Myocardium: Failure and Infarction. pp. 219–236. New York, H. P. Publishing Co., 1974.
2. Vital Health Statistics: Coronary Heart Disease in Adults. United States, 1960–62. Series 11, No. 10. U.S. National Center for Health Statistics, September 1965.
3. Tarhan, S., Moffitt, E. A., Taylor, W. F., et al.: Myocardial infarction after general anesthesia. J.A.M.A., *220*:1451, 1972.
4. James, T.: Anatomy of the Coronary Arteries. New York, Hoeber, 1961.
5. Abrams, H. L., and Adams, D. F.: The coronary arteriogram. N. Engl. J. Med., *281*:1276, 1336, 1969.
6. Marshall, R. J., and Shepherd, J. T.: Cardiac Function in Health and Disease. p. 193. Philadelphia, W. B. Saunders, 1968.
7. Page, D. L., Caulfield, J. B., Kastor, J. A., et al.: Myocardial changes associated with cardiogenic shock. N. Engl. J. Med., *285*:133, 1971.
8. Romhilt, D. W., Bloomfield, S. S., Chou, T., et al.: Unreliability of conventional electrocardiographic monitoring for arrhythmia detection in coronary care units. Am. J. Cardiol., *31*:457, 1973.
9. Chung, E. K.: Ventricular arrhythmias. *In* Chung, E. K.: Principles of Cardiac Arrhythmias. Baltimore, Williams & Wilkins, 1971.
10. Kaplan, J. A., and King, S. B., III: The precordial electrocardiographic lead (V5) in patients who have coronary-artery disease. Anesthesiology, *45*:570, 1976.
11. Lipman, B. S., Massie, E., and Kleiger, R. E.: Clinical Scalar Electrocardiography, ed. 6. pp. 218–225. Chicago, Year Book Medical Publishers, 1972.
12. Scheinman, M. M., and Abbott, M. A.: Clinical significance of transmural versus non-transmural electrocardiographic changes in patients with acute myocardial infarction. Am. J. Med., *55*:602, 1973.
13. LaDuc, J. S., Wroblewski, F., and Karmen, A.: Serum glutamic oxalacetic transaminase activity in human acute transmural myocardial infarction. Science, *120*:497, 1954.
14. Batsakis, J. G., and Briere, R. O.: Enzymatic profile of myocardial infarct. Am. Heart J., *72*:274, 1966.
15. Coodley, E. L.: Enzymes in cardiac disease. *In* Coodley, E. A.: Diagnostic Enzymology. ed 2. pp. 39–69. Philadelphia, Lea & Febiger, 1970.
16. Hobson, R. W., Conant, C., Mahoney, W. D., et al.: Serum creatine phosphokinase. Analysis of postoperative changes. Am. J. Surg., *124*:625, 1972.
17. Sobel, B. E., and Shell, W. E.: Serum enzyme determination in the diagnosis and assessment of myocardial infarction. Circulation, *45*:471, 1972.
18. Killen, D. A.: Serum enzyme elevations, a diagnostic test for acute myocardial infarction during the early postoperative period. Arch. Surg., *96*:200, 1968.
19. Louderback, A. L., and Shanbran, E.: Lactic dehydrogenase isoenzyme electrophoresis. J.A.M.A., *205*:294, 1968.
20. Konttinen, A., and Somer, H.: Determination of serum creatine kinase isoenzymes in myocardial infarction. Am. J. Cardiol., *29*:817, 1972.
21. Varat, M. A., and Mercer, D. W.: Cardiac specific creatine phosphokinase isoenzyme in the diagnosis of acute myocardial infarction. Circulation, *51*:855, 1975.
21a. Steen, P. A., Tinker, J. H., and Tarhan, S.: Myocardial reinfarction after anesthesia and surgery. J.A.M.A., *239*:2566, 1978.
22. Plumlee, J. E., and Boettner, R. B.: Myocardial infarction during and following anesthesia and operation. South Med. J., *65*:886, 1972.
22a. Goldman, L., Caldera, D. L., Nussbaum, S. R., et al.: Multifactorial index of cardiac risk in noncardiac surgical procedures. N. Engl. J. Med., *297*:845, 1977.
22b. Goldman, L., Caldera, D. L., Southwick, F. S., et al.:

Cardiac risk factors and complications in non-cardiac surgery. Medicine, *57*:357, 1978.

22c. Prys-Roberts, C.: Hypertension and anesthesia—Fifty years on. Anesthesiology, *50*:281, 1979.

22d. Goldman, L., and Caldera, D. L.: Risks of general anesthesia and elective operation in the hypertensive patient. Anesthesiology, *50*:285, 1979.

23. Wasserman, F., Bellet, S., and Saichek, R. P.: Postoperative myocardial infarction. N. Engl. J. Med., *252*:967, 1955.

24. Arkins, R., Smessaert, A. A., and Hicks, R. G.: Mortality and morbidity in surgical patients with coronary disease. J.A.M.A., *190*:485, 1964.

25. Dopamine for treatment of shock. Med. Lett. Drug Ther., *17*:13, 1975.

26. Terazi, R. C.: Sympathomimetic agents in the treatment of shock. Ann. Intern. Med., *81*:364, 1974.

27. Chatterjee, K., and Swan, H. J. C.: Vasodilatation therapy in acute myocardial infarction. Mod. Concepts Cardiovasc. Dis., *43*:119, 1974.

28. Jelliffe, R. W.: An improved method of digoxin therapy. Ann. Intern. Med., *69*:703, 1968.

29. Feinstein, A. R.: More blood for the anticoagulant battle. N. Engl. J. Med., *292*:1400, 1975.

30. Grigoryan, N. A., and Alimov, T. U.: Changes in the coagulating and anti-coagulating system of the blood during endotracheal anesthesia. Eksp. Khir. Anest., *14*:64, 1969.

31. Goldenfarb, P. B., Cathey, M. H., Zucker, S., et al.: Changes in the hemostatic mechanism after myocardial infarction. Circulation, *43*:538, 1971.

32. Diaz, R. G., Somberg, J., Freeman, E., et al.: Myocardial infarction after propranolol withdrawal. Am. Heart J., *88*:257, 1974.

33. Alderman, E. L., Coltart, J., Wettach, G. E., et al.: Coronary artery syndromes after sudden propranolol withdrawal. Ann. Intern. Med., *81*:625, 1974.

34. Miller, R. R., Olson, H. G., Amsterdam, E. A., et al.: Propranolol-withdrawal rebound phenomenon. Exacerbation of coronary events after abrupt cessation of antianginal therapy. N. Engl. J. Med., *293*:416, 1975.

35. Viljoen, J. F., Estafanous, G., and Kellner, G. A.: Propranolol and cardiac surgery. J. Thorac. Cardiovasc. Surg., *64*:826, 1972.

36. Caralps, J. M., Mulet, J., Wienke, H. R., et al.: Results of coronary artery surgery in patients receiving propranolol. J. Thorac. Cardiovasc. Surg., *67*:526, 1974.

37. Kaplan, J. A., Dunbar, R. W., Bland, J. W., et al.: Propranolol and cardiac surgery: a problem for the anesthesiologist. Anesth. Analg., *54*:571, 1975.

38. Should propranolol be stopped before surgery? Med. Lett. Drugs. Ther., *18*:41, 1976.

39. Moffitt, E. A., and Sessler, A. D.: The circulation in anaesthesia. Can. Anaesth. Soc. J., *11*:173, 1964.

40. Bland, J. H. L., and Lowenstein, E.: Halothane-induced decrease in experimental myocardial ischemia in the non-failing canine heart. Anesthesiology, *45*:287, 1976.

41. Tarhan, S., Moffitt, E. A., Lundborg, R. O., et al.: Hemodynamic and blood-gas effects of Innovar in patients with acquired heart disease. Anesthesiology, *34*:250, 1971.

42. Smith, N. T., and Whitcher, C. E.: Hemodynamic effects of gallamine and tubocurarine during halothane anesthesia. J.A.M.A., *199*:114, 1967.

43. Miller, R. D., Eger, E. I., II, Stevens, W. S., et al.: Pancuronium-induced tachycardia in relation to alveolar halothane, dose of pancuronium and prior atropine. Anesthesiology, *42*:352, 1975.

FURTHER READING

Bigger, J. T., Jr., and Giardina, E. V.: The pharmacology and clinical use of lidocaine and procaineamide. Med. Coll. Virginia Quart., *9*:65, 1973.

Goldman, L., Caldera, D. L., Nussbaum, S. R., et al.: Multifactorial index of cardiac risk in noncardiac surgical procedures. N. Engl. J. Med., *297*:845, 1977.

Goldman, L., Caldera, D. L., Southwick, F. S., et al.: Cardiac risk factors and complications in non-cardiac surgery. Medicine, *57*:357, 1978.

Prys-Roberts, C.: Hypertension and anesthesia—Fifty years on. Anesthesiology, *50*:281, 1979.

Tarazi, R. C.: Sympathomimetic agents in the treatment of shock. Ann. Intern. Med., *81*:364, 1974.

18 Air Embolism

John D. Michenfelder, M.D.

Air embolism is a recognized potential complication of a number of surgical, diagnostic, therapeutic, and traumatic circumstances. A partial list of events reported in the literature as precipitating factors includes any surgical procedure in which the surgical field is above the level of the heart (for example, neurosurgery with the patient in an upright position); any procedure that requires externalization of the circulatory system (open heart surgery[1] and hemodialysis[2]); any procedure that requires gas insufflation (Rubin's test,[3] pneumoperitoneoscopy,[4] therapeutic pneumothorax, pneumoencephalography,[5] pneumocystometry,[6] arthrography,[7] and pressurized blood transfusions); any procedure that provides continuity between atmosphere and the low pressure venous circulation[8] (subclavian vein puncture, central venous cannulation); thoracic trauma[9] (e.g., blast injury, thoracentesis, excessive positive airway pressure, open chest wounds); and miscellaneous events (e.g., equipment failure during vacuum abortion,[10] cunnilingus[11]).

TYPES OF AIR EMBOLI

For diagnosis, treatment, and prognosis, it is important to differentiate between embolization of air to the venous-pulmonary circulation and to the systemic arterial circulation, although the simultaneous occurrence of embolization to both circulations is a distinct possibility (so-called paradoxical embolization). For the most part, systemic arterial embolization is a complication of either extracorporeal bypass procedures or thoracic trauma. Venous air embolization is by far more common, but entry to the venous system does not preclude the possibility of air then crossing to the systemic arterial system. This may obviously occur in the presence of a patent foramen ovale or other intracardiac septal defects but may also occur by direct passage of air by way of the pulmonary circulation. The latter possibility is controversial to a degree, since intrapulmonary AV shunts have not been demonstrated convincingly in man, and the possibility of air crossing the pulmonary capillary system is debated.

The primary threat of air in the systemic arterial system is the possibility of embolization to either the coronary or cerebral circulations. Embolization to the coronary circulation may be rapidly fatal because of ischemia-induced terminal arrhythmias, and even with survival, myocardial infarction is a distinct possibility. Embolization to the cerebral circulation is followed by variable degrees of neurologic deficit, which, not uncommonly, are transient in nature (lasting several days), although cerebral infarction with permanent deficit may occur. Recognition of these complications is primarily by alertness to their possible occurrence and, during extracorporeal circulation, by either direct visualization of air bubbles or monitoring blood flow with air-detecting devices (for example, Doppler flowmeter[12]). Nonetheless, diagnosis is commonly made only in retrospect, particularly with regards neurologic complications. Specific therapy after embolization occurs is not usually possible, since, with the exception of immediate pressurization to several atmospheres in a hyperbaric chamber,[13] none is available.

By contrast, venous air embolization is accompanied by a number of diagnostic signs and is amenable to specific therapeutic measures. Progress in techniques of diagnosis and management has been considerable in the past 10 years, due in large part to developing subspecialization in fields such as neuroanesthesia, which results in an accumulated experience by a small group of individuals. Because of the common use of the sitting or upright position in certain neurosurgical procedures (posterior fossa exploration and cervical laminectomy), the incidence of venous air embolism is, by far, greater than that seen in any other surgical practice. The combination of a surgical wound at the highest possible level above the heart and the likelihood of opening noncollapsible venous channels (dural sinuses and diploic veins) accounts for this. Nonetheless, any vein, if opened at a level above the heart (depending on the venous pressure), may aspirate air if it cannot collapse. The literature abounds with individual case reports attesting to this fact.

CLINICAL CORRELATES

The immediate consequences of venous air embolism are several and are a function of both the volume of air embolized and the rate of embolization. Studies of morbidity and mortality in laboratory animals have attempted to quantitate the volume per unit time of air required to produce clinical signs. These studies have limited value, since there is no meaningful way to translate the results to humans. However, the following qualitative information has been documented and does apply to humans. Small volumes of air, injected slowly, are tolerated without clinical signs. Large volumes (3–8 ml./kg.) injected rapidly may be quickly fatal, presumably because of obstruction of the pulmonary outflow tract. Between these extremes, many pathological events may occur: partial outflow obstruction (with acute cor pulmonale and systemic hypotension); arrhythmias (usually ectopic ventricular); acute pulmonary dysfunction due to embolization to the pulmonary vasculature resulting in hypercapnia, hypoxia, and tachypnea; and embolization to the systemic arterial system. In addition, two cases of post-embolic pulmonary dysfunction have been reported,[14,15] and other cases have been alluded to, but not formally reported. This suggests that air embolized to the pulmonary circulation may result in prolonged vascular obstruction, possibly as the result of activation of clotting mechanisms. This syndrome is, however, not well-defined and will require animal investigation for documentation.

DIAGNOSIS OF AIR EMBOLISM

Air in volumes (and at a rate) sufficient to produce any of the above clinical effects will be accompanied by a fairly definitive diagnostic sign, the appearance of a characteristic heart murmur. In the less recent literature, this is commonly referred to as a "mill-wheel" murmur, which is described as a loud, coarse, continuous murmur that may obliterate both the first and second heart sounds and can, at times, be heard without the aid of a stethoscope. This murmur is now recognized as a late sign of a large air embolus. It is almost always preceded by more subtle changes in the heart sounds, which can be easily detected with an esophageal stethoscope. With small volumes of air (1–4 ml.), the initial change is the development of a tympanic quality to the normal heart sounds ("drum sign").[16] This is followed by the appearance of a soft but coarse systolic murmur, which can be simulated by squeezing a mixture of air and water in a balloon. With increasing volumes of air, the murmur becomes progressively louder (assuming adequate myocardial contractions) and eventually is heard in diastole as well as systole. If there are no specific monitoring devices available, the appearance of these heart sounds should provide the first diagnostic sign of air embolus.

It is now generally accepted that in surgical

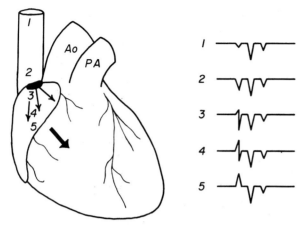

Fig. 18-1. Diagramatic changes in V lead of an ECG recorded when the tip of the catheter enters the right heart. At positions *1* and *2*, the P, QRS, and T vectors (*arrows*) point away from the catheter, and all waves are predominately negative (with greater amplitude at position *2*). Just beyond the SA node (position *3*), the initial deflection of the P save is positive, since the first portion of the vector points toward the catheter tip. At position *4*, the P wave is equally biphasic, and at position *5*, the P wave is positive.

procedures in which the risk of air embolus is known to be relatively high, additional monitoring devices should be used.[17] To date, the most valuable of these appear to be placement of a right atrial catheter,[18,19] monitoring end-expired carbon-dioxide,[20] and monitoring heart sounds produced by the reflection of ultrasound (Doppler flowmeter).[21,22]

Right Atrial Catheter

A right atrial catheter is useful both as a diagnostic and therapeutic tool. Aspiration of even a single air bubble from the right atrium confirms a suspected diagnosis, and in the event of a massive embolus, the ability to aspirate part of the intracardiac air contributes to overall management. Accurate placement of a right atrial catheter should be done preoperatively (or following induction of anesthesia) and can be accomplished by several means. Attachment of the saline-filled catheter to the V lead of a standard ECG permits recording of the ECG from the tip of the catheter. Characteristic ECG changes are

easily recognized as the catheter descends in the superior vena cava and enters the right atrium (Fig. 18-1). The abrupt change of the P wave from a negative to a biphasic complex signals entry into the right atrium and passage by the SA node.[23] Alternatively, a pressure transducer may be attached to the catheter, which is advanced until a typical right ventricular pressure wave is recorded; the catheter is then withdrawn until the pressure tracing abruptly changes to that of a central venous (atrial) pressure. Finally, the approximate location of the catheter can be ascertained by injection of a radiopaque material and serial chest radiographs, as needed. Reliance upon diagnosis of air embolus by aspiration of air from a catheter has resulted in a reported incidence of approximately 7 per cent in posterior fossa surgery.[19]

End-Expired Carbon Dioxide

Monitoring of end-expired carbon dioxide is an indirect but useful means of diagnosing air embolus. This approach is based upon the assumption that embolized air will be rapidly ejected into the pulmonary circulation, resulting in transient arteriolar-capillary obstruction. This will result in an abrupt reduction in the concentration of exhaled carbon dioxide, which usually can be differentiated from the less abrupt reduction in expired carbon dioxide that occurs with a decrease in cardiac output. Relying upon this monitor, Brechner reported an incidence of air embolism of approximately 7 per cent in posterior fossa surgery.[20]

Ultrasound

Monitoring of reflected ultrasound (Doppler flowmeter) is now recognized as the most sensitive diagnostic device for detecting intracardiac air.[23a] With this technique, injected air volumes of as little as 0.25 ml. can be detected by an abrupt alteration in the quality, intensity, and rhythm of the sound as the air enters the heart. Placement of the Doppler transducer is critical, for one must be certain it is monitoring movement of right heart structures. On the chest wall this is a relatively discrete area, usually at the right parasternal region, between the third and fifth intercostal spaces. However, on occasion, proper placement may be midsternal or, rarely, left parasternal. In most subjects, a second area that detects primarily left heart movement can be localized over the left chest wall. Monitoring of these Doppler sounds will not permit recognition of air embolus and will compound the problem by producing a false sense of security. Proper placement of the Doppler transducer can be tested by the injection of small volumes of carbon dioxide by way of the right atrial catheter or by forceful injection of saline through the catheter. The latter test produces an abrupt "swishing" sound, which is caused presumably by both turbulent flow and a whipping action of the catheter tip.[24] A positive test confirms the proper placement of both the right atrial catheter and the Doppler transducer. With Doppler monitoring, the true incidence of air embolism in patients who undergo surgery in the sitting position is 25 to 40 per cent.[21,22] Because of its extreme sensitivity, it is argued that the Doppler transducer produces unnecessary alarm, since it is obvious that most of the air emboli detected are clinically insignificant. This is certainly true, since in general, Doppler monitoring cannot quantitate the amount of air embolized but can only detect its presence. Nonetheless, it is apparent that the serious consequences of air embolism can be prevented only by early detection and vigorous therapy. Since the therapeutic measures employed are of themselves relatively innocuous, the possibly needless application of these measures seems a small price to pay.

Nonspecific Diagnostic Signs

In addition to the fairly specific diagnostic signs provided by monitoring esophageal heart sounds, by aspirating the right atrial catheter, by monitoring end-expired carbon dioxide, and by monitoring Doppler heart sounds, there are a number of suggestive but nonspecific, diagnostic signs of venous air embolism. Hypotension and cardiac arrhythmias commonly accompany a significant episode of air embolism; indeed, the degree of clinical significance is commonly defined by the magnitude of the hypotension and

the seriousness of the arrhythmia. Additionally, tachypnea and cyanosis may ensue as a direct result of embolization of air to the pulmonary circulation. Central venous pressure always increases with a significant embolus secondary to air obstruction in the pulmonary circulation. This, in turn, might be reflected by ECG changes compatible with acute cor pulmonale. The appearance of any of these secondary signs should suggest air embolism in patients known to be at risk.

THERAPY OF AIR EMBOLISM

When air embolism is recognized, treatment is directed toward two goals: prevention of further air entry into the various sytem, and evacuation of the air already embolized from the heart. Prevention of further entry of air can be accomplished immediately by elevating the venous pressure in the surgical wound. If successful, this will not only prevent air entry, but will also identify for the surgeon the source of the embolism (by venous bleeding), which he can occlude immediately. Measures to elevate the venous pressure include jugular vein compression, continuous positive pressure ventilation, abrupt inflation of a previously placed Gardner G-suit,[25] rapid infusions of fluids and/or blood, and lowering of the patient's head. (Obviously, jugular compression and lowering of the head specifically refer to neurosurgery in the sitting position; however, the principles are the same regardless of the source of air embolism.)

Jugular vein compression is an easy and rapidly effective technique. This maneuver should only be used with the knowledge and agreement of the neurosurgeon. It commonly is accompanied by bradycardia (carotid sinus stimulation) and may be hazardous in patients with carotid artery disease. Continuous positive pressure ventilation, infusion of fluids, and inflation of a Gardner G-suit will result in an increase in central venous pressure. This effect may be transient with a Gardner G-suit, since compensation for the translocated blood volume can be expected. Placing the surgical wound in a dependent position is effective, but if this maneuver denies the surgeon access to the wound, it is, to a degree, self-defeating.

Evacuation of the air from the heart can be accomplished directly, in part, by aspirating and manipulating the right atrial catheter. The percentage of embolized air recovered by this technique is unknown and probably quite variable but is apparently sufficient to prevent obstruction of the pulmonary outflow tract. The air not aspirated will embolize eventually to the pulmonary circulation, where absorption (and possible systemic embolization) can be expected. In the event of hypotension, vasopressors with a positive inotropic action should be administered to encourage movement of air out of the heart. If nitrous oxide is being used, it should be discontinued immediately in order to prevent volume expansion of the embolized air due to the different solubilities of nitrous oxide and nitrogen.[26] In patients in whom air embolism is suspected but unproven, the volume expansion effect of nitrous oxide can be used as a test to unmask small volumes of air in the heart or pulmonary vasculature.[27]

Other therapeutic techniques have been recommended and applied with variable results. In theory, reducing blood surface tension should discourage the formation of large gas bubbles and, hence, encourage dispersal of embolized air and minimize vascular obstructive effects. In practice, this appears effective if surface-tension-reducing agents are administered prior to the embolization of air but are ineffective after the event.[28] Placing the patient with his head down in a left lateral position (Durant's position)[29] has been recommended as a means of displacing air from the pulmonary outflow tract and may be life-saving in the event of a massive air embolism. Direct transthoracic aspiration of air from the heart has been used but is obviously a potential hazard and probably not indicated if a right atrial catheter is in place.

PREVENTION OF AIR EMBOLISM

It is now generally recognized that with appropriate monitoring and vigorous therapy the morbidity and mortality from venous air embolism can be dramatically reduced. Whereas the majority of cases reported prior to 1965 were fatal[30] (and often recognized only postmortem), death due to air embolism is now relatively rare in those surgical procedures known to be associated with this complication. Fatal episodes of air embolism are now reported primarily in unusual or unexpected surgical, therapeutic, or diagnostic circumstances that are not commonly associated with air embolism, and, hence, not monitored by the aforementioned techniques.

REFERENCES

1. Lawrence, F. G., McKay, H. A., and Sherensky, R. T.: Effective measures in the prevention of intraoperative aeroembolus. J. Thorac. Cardiovasc. Surg., 62:731, 1971.
2. Manuel, M. A., Stewart, W. K., Tulley, F. M., et al.: Air embolism monitor for use in hemodialysis. Lancet, 2:1356, 1971.
3. Rubin, I. C.: Uterotubal Insufflation. p. 354. St. Louis, C. V. Mosby, 1947.
4. McQuaide, J. R.: Air embolism during peritoneoscopy. S. Afr. Med. J., 46:422, 1972.
5. Jacoby, J., Jones, J. R., Ziegler, J., et al.: Pneumonecephalography and air embolism: simulated anesthetic death. Anesthesiology, 20:336, 1959.
6. Merrill, D. C.: Air cystometry and embolism. Urology, 4:495, 1974.
7. Saha, A. K.: Air embolism during anaesthesia for arthrography in a child. Anaesthesia, 31:1231, 1976.
8. Ordway, C. B.: Air embolus via CVP catheter without positive pressure: presentation of case and review. Ann. Surg., 179:479, 1974.
9. Thomas, A. N., and Stephens, B. G.: Air embolism: a cause of morbidity and death after penetrating chest trauma. J. Trauma, 14:633, 1974.
10. Munsick, R. A.: Air embolism and maternal death from therapeutic abortion. Obstet. Gynecol., 39:688, 1972.
11. Fatteh, A., Leach, W. B., and Wilkinson, C. A.: Fatal air embolism in pregnancy resulting from orogenital sex play. Forensic Sci., 2:247, 1973.
12. Gallagher, E. G., and Pearson, D. T.: Ultrasonic identification of sources of gaseous microemboli during open heart surgery. Thorax, 28:295, 1973.
13. Kindwall, E. P.: Massive surgical air embolism treated with brief recompression to six atmospheres followed by hyperbaric oxygen. Aerosp. Med., 44:663, 1973.
14. Chandler, W. F., Dimsheff, D. G., and Taren, J. A.: Acute pulmonary edema following venous air embolism during a neurosurgical procedure. J. Neurosurg., 40:400, 1974.
15. Still, J. A., Lederman, D. S., and Renn, W. H.: Pulmonary edema following air embolism. Anesthesiology, 40:194, 1974.
16. Shivpuri, D. N., Viswanathan, R., and Sharma, M. L.: A pre-symptomatic diagnostic sign of venous air embolism. J. Indian Med. Assoc., 33:86, 1959.
17. Buckland, R. W., and Manners, J. M.: Venous air embo-

lism during neurosurgery—a comparison of various methods of detection in man. Anaesthesia, *31*:633, 1976.

18. Michenfelder, J. D., Terry, H. R., Daw, E. F., et al.: Air embolism during neurosurgery. Anesth. Analg., *45*:390, 1966.

19. Michenfelder J. D., Martin, J. T., Altenburg, B. M., et al.: Air embolism during neurosurgery. An evaluation of right-atrial catheters for diagnosis and treatment. J.A.M.A., *208*:1353, 1969.

20. Brechner, V. L., and Bethune, R. W. M.: Recent advances in monitoring pulmonary air embolism. Anesth. Analg., *50*:255, 1971.

21. Maroon, J. C., Edmonds-Seal, J., and Campbell, R. L.: An ultrasound method for detecting air embolism. J. Neurosurg., *31*:196, 1969.

22. Michenfelder, J. D., Miller, R. H., and Gronert, G. A.: Evaluation of an ultrasonic device (Doppler) for the diagnosis of venous air embolism. Anesthesiology, *36*:164, 1972.

23. Robertson, J. T., Schick, R. W., Morgan, F., et al.: Accurate placement of ventriculo-atrial shunt for hydrocephalus under electrocardiographic control. J. Neurosurg., *18*:255, 1961.

23a. Gildenberg, P. L., O'Brien, R. P., Britt, W. J., et al.: The efficacy of Doppler monitoring for the detection of venous air embolism. J. Neurosurg., *54*:75, 1981.

24. Tinker, J. H., Gronert, G. A., Messick, J. M., et al.: Detection of air embolism: a test for positioning of right atrial catheter and Doppler probe. Anesthesiology, *43*:104, 1975.

25. Garner, W. J., and Dohn, D. F.: The antigravity suit (G-suit) in surgery: control of blood pressure in the sitting position and in hypotensive anesthesia. J.A.M.A., *162*: 274, 1956.

26. Munson, E. S., and Merrick, H. C.: Effect of nitrous oxide on venous air embolism. Anesthesiology, *27*:783, 1966.

27. Munson, E. S., Paul, W. L., Perry, J. C., et al.: Early detection of venous air embolism using a Swan-Ganz catheter. Anesthesiology, *42*:223, 1975.

28. Holt, E. P., Jr., Webb, W., Cook, W. A., et al.: Air embolism, hemodynamics and therapy. Ann. Thorac. Surg., *2*:551, 1966.

29. Durant, T. M., Long, J., and Oppenheimer, M. J.: Pulmonary (venous) air embolism. Am. Heart J., *33*:269, 1947.

30. Ericsson, J. A., Gottlieb, J. D., and Sweet, R. B.: Closed-chest cardiac massage in the treatment of venous air embolism. N. Engl. J. Med., *270*:1353, 1964.

Part Six

The Nervous System

19 Altered Temperature Regulation

Werner E. Flacke, M.D., Joan W. Flacke, M.D., John F. Ryan, M.D., and Beverley A. Britt, M.D.

Section One: Normal Homeostasis

Werner E. Flacke, M.D., and Joan W. Flacke, M.D.

Unlike other chapters in this book, Section 1 of this chapter deals not with specific complications, but rather with normal physiology, and will serve as an introduction to abnormal temperature regulation, described in Sections 2 and 3.

Temperature regulation in mammals, including humans, involves two types of physiological functions: behavioral or "voluntary," usually conscious; and autonomic, usually "involuntary" and/or "subconscious."[1,2]

BEHAVIORAL RESPONSES IN THERMOREGULATION

Behavioral responses include changes of body posture, locomotion, and more complicated processes, such as nest building in animals and construction of houses in man, including technological extensions like heating and air-conditioning. Behavioral activities are most important for temperature homeostasis. The fact that behavioral mechanisms or activities are so important may surprise many readers, because,

accustomed as we are to seeing them in everyday life, we usually do not consider their significance in thermoregulation. Man and beast "come in from the cold" if they can, and many languages have expressions meaning that not to do so exemplifies lack of intelligence. There are characteristic body postures for heat conservation and heat dissipation. A patient whose body temperature is below that of his *set point* (see p. 281) curls up with knees flexed, in a fetal position, with extremities close to the body. Alternately, a patient whose body temperature is higher than the set point stretches out, with extremities widely extended. The obvious "purpose" of these postures is to minimize or maximize surface area and, thus, heat dissipation. These postures do not indicate body temperature per se; they indicate only its relation to the set point.[3] If a patient has an elevated temperature, posture permits instantaneous analysis regarding whether the peak temperature has already been reached or whether the temperature is still rising. Although it is interesting to examine these behavioral

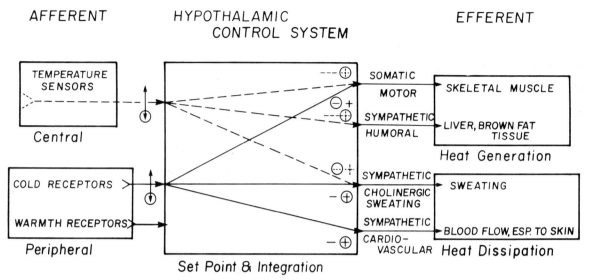

Fig. 19-1. Schematic representation of the main components of the thermoregulatory system.

The diagram shows the three components of the temperature-regulating system: *(A)* afferent, sensory input from the periphery (cold and warmth receptors) and from the anterior hypothalamus; *(B)* the "integrating and regulating" central system with its main neuronal networks located in the anterior and the posterior hypothalamus; *(C)* the efferent or motor systems, subserving heat generation and heat dissipation. No attempt is being made to indicate details of the network that must possess feedback circuits and involve several neurohumoral systems, as described in the text.

The only attempt that has been made is to indicate the effects of changes in afferent inputs upon various parts of the efferent systems. Increase or decrease in afferent input is shown by arrows pointing upward or downward. The down arrows are encircled for easier identification of changes on the efferent side brought about by afferent changes. Solid and interrupted lines are used to connect inputs and outputs to facilitate recognition of related changes. In the interest of avoiding too much crowding, no connections have been drawn between the input from warmth receptors and efferents.

temperature-related activities, it may not be productive, because anesthetics, of course, obliterate patient volition.

INVOLUNTARY RESPONSES IN THERMOREGULATION

Involuntary responses involve autonomic functions, such as cutaneous vasoconstriction and non-muscular thermogenesis or skin vasodilatation and increased sweating. They also include some processes usually not considered to be autonomic, such as the use of skeletal muscles for heat production by increasing muscle tone and by shivering. Obviously, this "voluntary" use of muscle is not really voluntary, and is often even subconscious.

THE THERMOREGULATORY SYSTEM

The basic components of the thermoregulatory system are given in Figure 19-1. Like any control system, it comprises three parts:

Parts of the Thermoregulatory System

Afferent or temperature "sensors"
    Peripheral (in skin, mucosa, and deep tissues)
    Central (located in the anterior hypothalamus and other CNS structures)
Efferent or "motor systems"
    Heat-generating mechanisms
    Heat-dissipating mechanisms
A control system (a neuronal network in the posterior hypothalamus)

AFFERENT SYSTEMS

Peripheral "Sensors"

Until relatively recently, it was assumed that peripheral temperature receptors did not play any significant role in the maintenance of constant body temperature. This assumption was based upon studies in which the properties of these receptors were deduced only from subjective sensations of temperature described by human subjects. Of course, humans have no built-in "thermometer" calibrated on an absolute scale. Temperature sensation changes with time and is influenced by other factors (attention, experience, emotions). It is clear that such subjective sensations do not reflect directly the magnitude of the signal coming from the sensors; they are likely to be modulated by central processing. That this is indeed the case was proven first by Hensel and Zotterman in 1949, when they measured the frequency of firing of single afferent nerve fibers, while controlling the temperature at the site where the corresponding receptor was located.[4] It became clear immediately that temperature receptors are calibrated on an absolute scale, and that they "report" without change the local temperature, as long as this temperature remains constant. (The fact that there is a transient "overshoot" when local temperature is changed rapidly is unimportant in this context.) It was also found that there are both cold and warm receptors; the former respond with increased frequency of discharge to decreasing temperature, and the latter respond in the reverse.

These observations, confirmed and greatly enlarged since 1949, have made it possible (indeed, mandatory) to assign a role in body temperature homeostasis to these peripheral sensors.[1,2] It should be noted that the density of temperature receptors in different parts of the body is unequal. Some skin areas (fingertips, circumoral areas) are much more richly endowed than most, while others have less than the average. It has not yet been possible to assign a "weighing factor" to different peripheral areas, but it can be postulated that the weighted, integrated peripheral temperature input is one of the most important inputs for temperature regulation.

Central "Sensors"

It has been known since about 1885 that certain areas of the brain play a prominent role in temperature regulation; for example, electrical or mechanical stimulation of the corpus striatum causes marked increases in body temperature in many species. Barbour, in 1912, discovered that a distinct area in the anterior hypothalamus is temperature-sensitive. Localized cooling of this area causes an increase in body temperature; heating has the opposite effect. Again, this observation has been confirmed and refined since that time. Recently, the electrical activity of single neurons has been recorded in the same area[5,6,7] and was found to change systematically, either with only local temperature or with both local and peripheral temperature.[5,7] Controversy continues over whether at least some of these neurons are, indeed, sensory endorgans for temperature or whether they are simply interneurons with a high temperature coefficient (Q_{10}). It is important that the temperature in the anterior hypothalamus is the dominant factor in the regulation of body temperature.

EFFERENT SYSTEMS

The efferent mechanisms serve as effector systems for temperature regulation and consist of heat-generating and heat-dissipating components, though none serve exclusively for thermoregulation.

Heat-Generating Mechanisms

All chemical processes in the body release heat as a by-product. The magnitude of the chemical process is usually determined by factors other than thermoregulation. There are, however, chemical processes other than those in skeletal muscles that can be activated specifically for thermoregulatory purposes. These processes involve mainly the liver and brown fat tissues and are probably mediated by beta-adrenergic hormones.[8] Nevertheless, the main "engine" for heat generation is the skeletal muscle, which can increase heat generation by a factor of four to five.

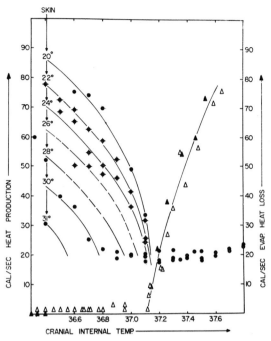

Fig. 19-2. Influence of changes in central and peripheral temperature on heat production and evaporative heat dissipation. The figure summarizes the observations made in one human volunteer. Central temperature was measured by a tympanic thermometer and skin temperature and heat dissipation were measured by a rapidly responding calorimeter. Heat generation was calculated from continuously recorded oxygen uptake. Temperature "loads" consisted of ingestion of cold water and served to drive central and peripheral temperature apart. For further explanation, see text. (Benzinger, T. H., et al.: The thermostatic control of human metabolic heat production. Proc. Natl. Acad. Sci. U.S.A., *47:* 730, 1961)

Heat-Dissipating Mechanisms

Heat dissipation is accomplished by vasodilatation of skin vessels, with resultant heat loss to the environment (radiation, conduction), and by evaporation of water.[1,2] Some water diffuses through the intact skin, but the major proportion is produced from sweat glands innervated by cholinergic nerves that belong anatomically to the sympathetic nervous system. Evaporation of moisture from the airways also plays a role, but man is unique among primates in that he does not use respiration to any recognizable extent for thermoregulatory purposes. Overall, the total heat-dissipating capacity roughly equals the heat-generating capacity.[9] (This is not surprising; any engineer who designs a temperature control system with unequal overall heating and cooling capacities would not have his job for long.) It should be noted that the cardiovascular system plays a far greater role in temperature regulation than just that of regulating skin perfusion. The cardiovascular system is responsible for heat distribution from sites of generation to other tissues and for transport from the body core to the surfaces, where dissipation takes place.

CONTROL SYSTEM

Occasionally, the term *center* is used to describe an anatomical locations in the CNS where mechanical, electrical, and/or chemical interventions can affect the central thermoregulatory system. It does not always seem clear that the term *center* cannot be taken literally, to mean the anatomical locations where nerve cells or, at least, the bodies of nerve cells that are involved in thermoregulatory functions are concentrated. Actually, a *center* is simply a location where it has been found possible to "make contact" with these neurons. In the case of biochemical or pharmacological observations, it seems likely that the contact areas represent the location of synaptic junctions in the neuronal network that makes up the regulatory system. For electrophysiological observations, especially for single-unit recordings, the contact site may be near the neuronal cell body or close to axonal or dendritic extensions. Thus, one should remember that all "centers" are only one part of a neuronal network, with connections reaching into many parts of the CNS that are never mentioned in conjunction with temperature regulation.

The operation of the entire temperature-regulating system is depicted in Figure 23-2.[9] This figure describes heat generation on the left ordinate and evaporative heat dissipation on the right ordinate, against tympanic (central) temperature plotted on the abscissa. Points of equal skin temperature are connected by lines. All points are derived from one typical experiment in an unclothed human volunteer.

Heat dissipation begins only when the central temperature rises above 37.1°C but increases very sharply with increasing central temperature and is apparently insensitive to skin temperature. For an increase of 0.5°C in central temperature, from 37.1 to 37.6°C, heat loss is quadrupled, from about 20 to nearly 80 cal. per sec. Throughout this range, heat generation remains at or near the lowest observed level. Heat generation is presumably at a basal level, with an increment due to the increased enzyme activity resulting from increased body temperature (van't Hoff's law). The increased metabolism required to support activation of the evaporative heat dissipating system, (e.g., increased blood flow and sweat gland activity) also raises heat generation above the basal level.

However, when central temperature falls or, rather, is forced by experimental measures below 37.1°C, heat generation rises nearly as sharply with falling central temperature as does heat dissipation with rising central temperature. Unlike heat dissipation, there is a clear input from skin temperature that affects both the internal temperature at which heat generation begins and the magnitude of increase in heat generation per degree of fall of central temperature. The value to which the central temperature is permitted to drop, before the regulatory system begins counteracting the fall is directly proportional to the level of the skin temperature. In other words, the integrated skin temperature determines the sensitivity of the central regulatory system. Thus, the critical central temperature for initiation of either heat generation or heat dissipation is the *set point* temperature. A central temperature above the set point value results in heat dissipation, whereas a lower central temperature results in heat generation.[1,6,9,10]

Humoral Agents

Several humoral agents have been implicated as central mediators in thermoregulation. However, two points should be kept in mind regarding research in this area: Even "localized" application of these substances to specific areas often involves quantities and volumes that guarantee that a large number of synaptic junctions will be affected; and it is very likely, indeed, that even closely spaced synapses mediate processes or events of opposite functional significance. Also, although the "wiring diagram" of the temperature control system of different species is likely to be rather similar in principle, it is quite possible that the transmitters or mediators employed differ from one species to another. This is so in the periphery and may be true in the CNS, as well. Thus, it is risky to extrapolate findings from one species to another, especially to humans.

Catecholamines. High concentrations of norepinephrine (NE) and other catecholamines are found throughout the hypothalamus. Histochemical studies indicate that their location is predominantly presynaptic (i.e., in axonal terminals or nerve endings). Local injection in the anterior hypothalamus causes *hypothermia* in a neutral or cold environment.[2,7] This is true for several species, including monkeys. Drugs like the tricyclic antidepressants, which inhibit re-uptake of norepinephrine into the nerve endings (the major mechanism for terminating the effect of free norepinephrine after release), imitate injection of the amine. Thus, norepinephrine may play a role in activating heat-dissipating processes.

5-Hydroxytryptamine (5-HT). The effects of norepinephrine are opposed by those of 5-HT. Microinjection into the anterior hypothalamus causes increased body temperature in several species, including monkeys.[2,8] When unanesthetized animals are exposed to cold (when investigators try to increase their heat generation), increased concentrations of 5-HT are found in fluid perfusing through the same CNS area where 5-HT injection is effective.

Acetylcholine (ACh). Carbachol, the acetylcholine analog that is not as rapidly hydrolyzed as acetylcholine itself, has been found to prompt thermoregulatory responses when microinjections were made in several sites throughout the hypothalamus. These effects are blocked by atropine and are, thus, "cholinergic muscarinic" in nature. Atropine, given locally or injected into the ventricular system, causes hypothermia in a cold environment.[3] Acetylcholine itself is effective only when given with or after physostigmine, which decreases cholinesterase activity. These findings suggest that acetylcholine is the transmitter at several synaptic junctions of neuronal pathways involved in temperature regulation. If all of these sites are blocked by atropine, hypothermia follows when the ambient temperature is low. Clinically, it is well known that hyperthermia is often seen in atropine or scopolamine poisoning. Little information about ambient temperature is usually available in such cases, but as hyperthermia is not invariably reported, it may be safe to suspect that hyperthermia is seen only when ambient temperature is high.

Prostaglandin E₁ (PGE₁). When injected in minute amounts (20–30 μg.) into the anterior hypothalamus, PGE_1 causes marked hyperthermia,[2,3,8] which has all the hallmarks of a temperature increase secondary to an increase in the set point. As a result, when ambient temperature is high enough to raise body temperature, there is vasoconstriction rather than vasodilatation and heat loss. Shivering occurs when active heat generation is needed to raise body temperature in a cold environment. Also, thermal stimuli at the new elevated temperature, such as ingestion of cold water, elicit a thermoregulatory response, just as they would at normal temperature. In other words, the body is regulated with respect to the set point raised by PGE_1 with intact thermoregulation, a characteristic of the febrile state. Therefore, it has been suggested that PGE_1 is a mediator in the fever production elicited by exotoxins, endotoxins, or other pyrogens.[3] This thesis, although very attractive because it would account for the temperature-lowering effect of anti-inflammatory antipyretics (e.g., aspirin), which are known to inhibit formation of prostaglandins,[11] has not been confirmed by all investigators.

These humoral agents, with the exception of acetylcholine, act only when they are making contact with sites in the *anterior* hypothalamus. They have therefore been proposed as "transmitters" in synaptic junctions between temperature sensors (peripheral or central) and the neuronal network subserving temperature regulation (e.g., the set point).[2,5,8]

Sodium-Calcium Balance. Perfusing the posterior hypothalamus near the mammillary bodies with an artificial cerebrospinal fluid that has high concentrations of either sodium or calcium ions or contains a calcium-chelating agent like ethylenediamine tetraacetate (EDTA) effects a temperature change.[8,12] No temperature changes occur when the anterior hypothalamus is thus perfused. High calcium concentration reduces body temperature while leaving thermoregulation intact, and high sodium concentration or reduction of ionized calcium by chelating agents increases body temperature in the same fashion. Thus, these conditions of the extracellular ionic environment may also be described as "resetting the set point," but in a different location in the CNS. Incomplete reports have appeared indicating that fever induced by toxins or pyrogens is accompanied by appropriate ionic changes in the hypothalamic extracellular fluid.

Regardless of the many details involved in temperature regulation that have been described (mediators, ion ratios), in fact we have no real understanding of the nature of the underlying biological mechanisms. How is the set point temperature defined? How are deviations of body temperatures from the set point detected? And, how are these differences translated into efferent signals to thermoregulatory "motor" systems that serve to return body temperature to the set point level? It is possible to suggest mechanisms, but we do not even know if these mechanisms are mainly electrophysiological or biochemical. Thus, we are still a long way from understanding the thermoregulatory central mechanisms.

DRUG EFFECTS ON BODY TEMPERATURE

It is most convenient to consider the actions of drugs in the same sequence as the physiological aspects of body temperature regulation are discussed: that is, in terms of their actions on the afferent or sensory system, the efferent or motor system, and the central processing apparatus. Of course, any drug may have effects on more than one site, but in general, a drug's actions on body temperature is most prominent and important at one site.

Afferent Effects

We do not know whether centrally acting drugs act upon the temperature-sensitive structures ("sensors") in the anterior hypothalamus. With regard to the peripheral sensors, menthol, locally applied, increases ("sensitizes") the frequency of firing of cold receptors. Systemic administration of large doses of menthol also increases body temperature, as theory suggests. On the other hand, increased local carbon dioxide concentration reduces the activity of cold receptors, and it has been known for some time that carbon dioxide baths induce a sensation of warmth out of proportion to the bath temperature. We are not aware of any reliable studies of the effect of carbon dioxide baths on body temperature.

Efferent Effects

Drugs acting on the efferent thermoregulatory mechanisms *limit the range* of temperature loads that the body can tolerate (without recourse to behavioral actions). For example, neuromuscular blocking agents, so commonly used by anesthesiologists, block only the for heat generation by muscle. Their quaternary ammonium structure prevents penetration of the blood-brain barrier; thus, these agents have no "central" effect. Not unexpectedly, such drugs do not alter body temperature unless heat generation by muscle is needed to maintain normal temperature. On the other hand, the central effects of another drug much used in anesthesia, atropine, are discussed elsewhere. The peripheral effect of atropine, block of sweating, greatly decreases the capacity of the body to dissipate heat. Hence, this peripheral effect reduces the ability of the body to endure high heat loads, and this effect must be considered in high ambient temperatures or when heat generation is large. The thermal effects of most drugs can be explained similarly, once the general pharmacological actions are known.

Central Effects

General anesthetic agents probably act centrally, although we are not aware of a single complete analysis of the mechanism and site of action of a general anesthetic agent. The action may be specific for thermoregulatory systems, affecting the "sensor" mechanism in the anterior hypothalamus or the "regulatory" mechanisms in the posterior hypothalamus, or may mainly influence the central mechanisms subserving the efferent thermoregulatory peripheral systems.[8] General anesthetics induce neither hypothermia nor hyperthermia; they only depress the regulatory system. The direction of change in body temperature depends upon the environment: In our "air-cooled" operating rooms, hypothermia is, of course, the usual problem, but in tropical countries where modern air conditioning is not prevalent, hyperthermia is still the most common and most serious problem during general anesthesia.

A clinical example of the use of centrally acting drugs is deliberate hypothermia. The important point to be remembered during induction of hypothermia is the need to attenuate or block thermoregulation. If this is not done sufficiently, activation of the powerful heat-generating mechanisms will result in increased oxygen consumption and, therefore, additional loads on the respiratory and circulatory systems. Since deliberate hypothermia is most commonly employed in critically ill patients, this additional stress is hardly inconsequential. Thus, induction of hypothermia should not begin until the patient's central temperature regulation has been sufficiently blocked. This requires deep anesthesia, if only general anesthetic agents are used, or lighter levels of anesthesia, if more specific inhibitors of central thermoregulation are employed. One such drug is chlorpromazine or one of its analogs. From about 1950 to 1955, the French pioneers of "hibernation artificiel" used a mixture of agents, commonly referred to as "cocktail lytique," consisting of promethazine, meperidine, and chlorpromazine. It is likely that the central actions of the phenothiazines and the action of the narcotic analgesic were additive or more than additive in the thermoregulatory-blocking action of the mixture.

A few comments might be made regarding the mechanism of action of the antipyretic agents,[8] the prototype of which is acetylsalicylic acid (aspirin). It is well established that these agents do not induce hypothermia but act only to reduce an elevated body temperature; they "reset the set point."[13] Recent observations in monkeys demonstrate that high doses of salicylates also reduce the magnitude of body temperature increase when such increase is brought about by exposure to very high ambient temperature.[14] These observations demonstrate an effect in the presence of a normal set point. However, one should not overlook the fact that the doses required were very much larger (> 25 mg./kg.) than the clinically used antipyretic doses. The appearance of a "new" type of effect at higher doses is very common in pharmacology and should not lead us to question the selectivity of action of a drug at lower dose levels.

Of mainly theoretical interest is the action of several so-called analeptic agents, such as pentylenetetrazole and picrotoxin.[8] These agents actively induce hypothermia, and the effect is blocked by small doses of barbiturates. The usual CNS stimulatory effects of these agents and the blocking effect of the hypnotics suggest that analeptics stimulate heat-dissipating central mechanisms.

A study of drug action on body temperature and on temperature-regulating mechanisms reveals a surprising degree of consistency with physiological theory.

Section Two: Unintentional Hypothermia

John F. Ryan, M. D.

Mild to moderate hypothermia is often an accepted concomitant to general anesthesia. To assess the value or harm of this decrease in our patient's body temperature, a review of the fundamentals of temperature regulation seems appropriate.

TEMPERATURE REGULATION

The principles of temperature control have only recently been elucidated (see p. 277). Though thermoregulation is a basic homeostatic mechanism, it is only in the last 20 years that these regulatory principles have been demonstrated. In the decade from 1959 to 1969, Theodore Benzinger, working for the U.S. Navy, utilized the total body gradient calorimeter and measurements of direct oxygen consumption to explain the principles by which the human body maintains a given temperature.[15] In the course of his studies, he perfected tympanic thermometry. Many investigators have studied temperature homeostasis,[16-28]

but our understanding of temperature control is a result of Benzinger's meticulous efforts.

Homeostatic Mechanisms

Benzinger identified two mechanisms that are activated by a fall in body temperature and three mechanisms activated by an increase in body temperature (see below). He further noted that the body zealously maintains the blood that perfuses the posterior hypothalamus at a precise temperature. Any deviation from this activates the appropriate mechanisms to bring the temperature of the blood back to the pre-set level (set point). This temperature that the central thermostat maintains is affected by a number of variables, such as local hypothalamic concentrations of sodium,[29] calcium,[30] norepinephrine,[26] tryptophan,[26] hormones,[26] and pyrogens.[31-35] Fever sets the thermostat at a higher level, and the body attempts to reach that new set point by increasing metabolism. Aspirin resets the thermostat to a lower level in the febrile state and thus decreases the metabolic demands.

Five Principal Mechanisms of Human Thermoregulation

Response to temperature fall
    The excitation of metabolic heat production by cold-reception at the skin
    The central warm-inhibition of thermoregulatory heat production

Response to temperature elevation
    The excitation of sweating by central warm-reception
    Vasodilatation elicited by central warm-reception
    The inhibition of thermoregulatory sweating by cold-reception at the skin

As body temperature falls below the set point of the hypothalamic center, heat production increases. The increase in heat production is regulated by the integration of total body skin temperature and is weighted in favor of exposed areas. Above a skin temperature of 33°C, heat production is minimal. As the integrated skin temperature decreases below 33°C, the heat production at a given hypothermic level increases in a stepwise manner, to a maximum that is reached at 20°C; below 20°C, heat production decreases. These stepwise changes are caused by an increase in the frequency and amplitude of firing of cold sensors in the skin as temperature decreases.[20] The maximum response at 20°C defines critical ambient temperature.[36,37] An awake, undraped person will maintain body temperature to an ambient temperature of 20°C; below this level, central temperature falls.

The only situation in which the skin temperature cannot stimulate increased heat production is when the central or core temperature (the temperature of the blood perfusing the hypothalamus) is at or above the set point. Loss of skin temperature regulation has been noted in paraplegic patients with spinal cord section,[38] which interrupts the central ingress of information, and in massively burned patients,[39] in whom sensors have been destroyed. Other areas, such as the muscle spindles and parts of the hypothalamus itself,[40] act as sensors stimulating the hypothalamic center, but these are approximately 1,000 times less sensitive than skin cold receptors.

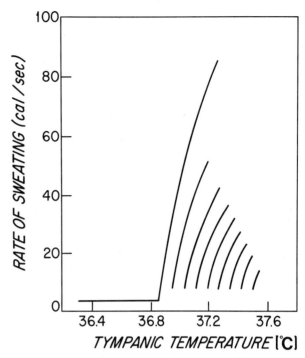

Fig. 19-3. Inhibition of sweating by cold-reception at the skin. At skin temperatures below 33° C, increasing inhibition takes place, represented by slanting tympanic isotherms *(right).* Inhibition is complete at skin temperatures below 29° C. (Benzinger, T. H.: Heat regulation: homeostasis of central temperature in man. Physiol. Rev., *49*: 671, 1969)

The rise in body temperature is followed by a change in blood flow from a central to a more peripheral distribution, and the initiation of sweating: The evaporation of sweat leads to cooling of the blood. A rise of 0.7°C above the set point of a person will lead to a four-fold increase in sweat rate. At or below the set point of the hypothalamic thermostat, sweating does not occur. Inhibition of sweating can occur at a cold ambient temperature.[41] The athlete perspiring from exercise stops sweating when he steps out into the chill winter air. In this situation, evaporation does not occur, and the layer of perspiration acts as insulation to the raised temperature of the blood. Therefore, skin temperature, if decreased sufficiently (29°C), can shut off sweating (Fig. 19-3).

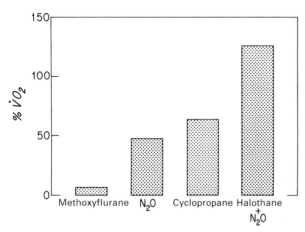

Fig. 19-4. The effect of different anesthetics on postoperative oxygen consumption in the presence of hypothermia. (Roe, C. F., Goldberg, M. J., Blair, C. S., et al.: The influence of body temperature on early postoperative oxygen consumption. Surgery, *60:* 85, 1966)

ANESTHESIA AND THERMOREGULATION

What is the effect of anesthesia on thermoregulation? At present, there is no definitive answer to this question. Typically, oxygen consumption decreases slightly during general anesthesia at normothermia. However, we have found a twofold *increase* in oxygen consumption during anesthesia and surgery in children during mild hypothermia (34.0°–36.5°C).[42] Deep hypothermia has been well studied during anesthesia, but there is little data on mild hypothermia, during which compensatory heat production may occur. Another study revealed a similar but less exaggerated change in oxygen consumption.[43] Both of these studies parallel the work of Dawkins and Scopes in awake neonates.[44] As a result, most investigators should maintain body temperature at 37°C during their measurements of oxygen consumption during anesthesia.[45–47] Except for lack of shivering, there is no evidence to denote that thermoregulation ceases during anesthesia. The syndrome of malignant hyperthermia has demonstrated that shivering is not necessary for marked heat production and temperature elevation (see p. 295).[48–50]

The hypothermic patient in the recovery room strives to return to normothermia at a metabolic cost. We have all seen the shivering patient who increases heat production at the end of anesthesia. Usually the shivering can be halted immediately by covering the patient with a warm blanket, which decreases the severity of the body's response to hypothermia. Roe demonstrated increased oxygen consumption in patients with temperature falls of 0.3°C and more.[51] The largest increase in oxygen consumption was noted after halothane anesthesia compared to other anesthetics (Fig. 19-4). Aged patients were not able to increase their oxygen consumption in response to decreased temperature and, thus, developed peripheral hypoxemia. Roe concluded that the sickest (often the oldest) patients were at greatest risk for mild hypothermia in the immediate postoperative period.

PREVENTION OF HYPOTHERMIA

If it is true that a cold patient is at risk, how do we maintain normothermia in the operating room? Factors that assist in preventing hypothermia are listed below. The most important variable is room temperature. Morris and Wilkey have defined 21°C as a critical ambient operating room temperature at or above which body temperature is maintained.[52] All patients studied had an initial temperature fall in the first 15 min., irrespective of room temperature. This fall is attributed to

---

Prevention of Hypothermia

Monitor temperature.
Keep room temperature warm:
   > 25.6°C, newborns
   > 24.4°C, neonates
   21.1°C, adults
Cover the patient.
Warm any blood transfusions.
Apply these techniques to infants:*
   Use a heating blanket.
   Apply steri-drapes, wrap extremities.
   Use a radiant heat source.
   Heat fluids (especially for cystoscopy).
   Use heated, humidified anesthetics.

---

*These techniques are useful in warming a cold adult, also.

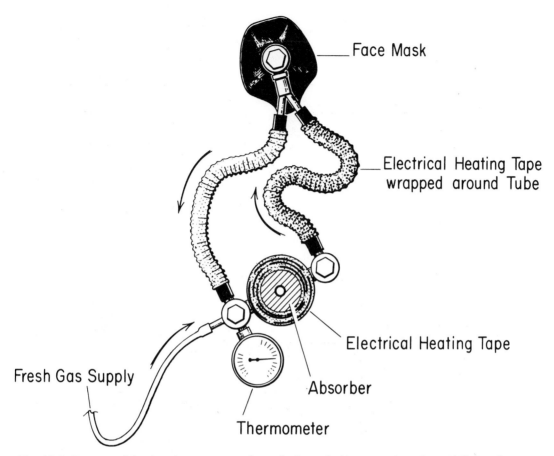

Face Mask

Electrical Heating Tape
wrapped around Tube

Electrical Heating Tape

Fresh Gas Supply

Absorber

Thermometer

Fig. 19-5. Passage of dry inspiratory gases through the soda lime cannister humidifies and warms
the anesthetics. The process is enhanced by heating the cannister with either a heating tape or a
warming blanket. This technique functions best with low flows and by wrapping the inspiratory
limb with an electrical heating tape.

undraping, cool skin cleansing solutions, and lack of motion of the anesthetized patient. Heat loss occurs by radiation, convection, conduction, and evaporation. In neonates, radiant heat loss is particularly important.[53] Even in a warmed iso-lette, an infant can become hypothermic if he is uncovered and the walls of the isolette are cool because of low ambient temperature. The operating room is an isolette, and to maintain our patient's temperature, we first need a warm environment to prevent radiant heat loss.

The importance of air flow in convective loss has received little attention. Certainly in modern air-conditioned operating rooms, air flow velocity is sufficiently high to cool patients, especially infants and small children whose surface area is large relative to their weight. The orthopedic patient, cared for in the high-flow sterile chamber used in some institutions for total hip repair, can cool markedly because of the wind chill factor from high air flow and convective loss.

Conductive loss to cool sheets and drapes does occur. Prevention of heat loss by use of a heating blanket is not of value in adults or children with a surface area above 0.5m.[2] (normally equivalent to 15 months of age or 10 kg. in weight) and adds the responsibility of protecting the patient from burns owing to pooled cleansing solution or a faulty thermostat.[54]

Evaporative heat loss may occur in the operat-

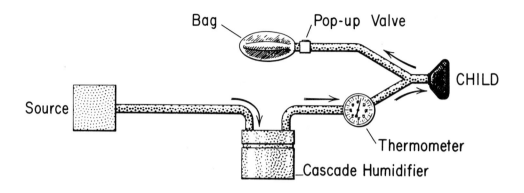

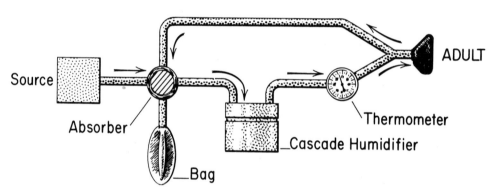

Fig. 19-6. Humidification of anesthetic gases. The relatively dry anesthetic gases are passed through a heated humidifier and, in this case, into a Jackson-Rees modification of Mapleson D anesthesia system. The temperature of the warmed, humidified anesthetics is monitored in the inspiratory limb close to the patient. This temperature is kept between 30 to 35° C[82] and is closely monitored. The temperature of the sterile water within the humidifier is not as important as the temperature of the anesthetics bathing the tracheobronchial tree.

ing room above 23°C as outlined by Clark,[55] but more commonly, sweating is related to problems in anesthetic management.[56]

Heated Humidification

Intraoperative use of heated, humidified inspired gas is a useful method of maintaining or restoring temperature. Various methods have been advocated, such as the following: heating the carbon dioxide absorber,[57] and passing inspiratory gases through it (Fig. 19-5); using a heated humidifier in the circle system (Fig. 19-6)[58,59]; and

tory gases through it (Fig. 23-5); using a heated humidifier in the circle system (Fig. 23–6)[58,59]; and using an ultrasonic nebulizer.[60,61] This last method has the limitation of administration of a significant fluid load to the patient. With the first two methods, it is reasonable to measure the temperature of the heated gases prior to their administration to prevent overheating. Use of a system that warms adequately and humidifies anesthetic gases prevents caloric expenditure for these functions. Also, cooling of the aortic blood does not occur from the cool dry gases flowing into the trachea. Two problems, however, may arise from the use of heated, humidified gases:

While attempting to eliminate insensible fluid loss, with replacement of fluids, the anesthesiologist should take into account that fluid requirements will be markedly diminished; and, there is a potential for cross-infection, unless a reliable system of gas sterilization of individual units is maintained.

Radiant Heat

The use of radiant heat lamps to prevent heat loss in premature infants, neonates, and burned patients is effective.[62,63] The lamp should be kept at least 70 cm. from the skin of the patient. The skin temperature should be monitored by a covered probe to prevent overheating (Fig. 19-7), for a decrease of 25 cm. in the distance from the heat source to the patient increases skin temperature to 38°C. During abdominal surgery, the relationship of radiant infrared heating to the development of adhesions has recently been questioned in a preliminary study in rabbits.[64]

In infants, radiant heat loss has been reduced by use of a silver swaddle.[65] This body wrap consists of an inner layer of polyethylene and an outer layer of aluminum foil. Areas are peeled open to insert monitors and intravenous lines. Although this is an effective deterrent to heat loss, care must be taken to prevent pooling of cleansing solutions inside the wrap.

Warming of Transfused Blood

Warming blood has become common practice during transfusion, particularly when infusing massive volumes.[66] To bring 500 ml. of bank blood (4°C) to body temperature requires 32 kcal. per hour, approximately 50 per cent of basal metabolic heating output by a 70-kg. person. Warming of cleansing solutions, intravenous fluids, and drugs and warming of cystoscopy fluids in children are important adjuncts to maintaining body temperature.

TEMPERATURE MONITORS

What is the best method of monitoring temperature? Two approaches are available: determina-

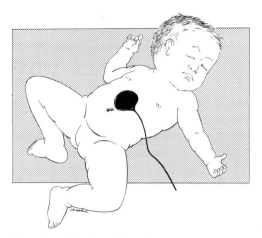

Fig. 19-7. The skin thermometer is monitoring the heat from a radiant heat source. The thick adhesive cover that holds the thermistor in place also shields it from direct heating by the lamp. This ensures that the temperature recorded is that of the skin surface.

tion of central temperature and monitoring of non-central temperature.

Core Temperature

The term *central* refers to the fact that the temperature recorded reflects the temperature of the blood flowing by the temperature-sensitive center of the hypothalamus (Aronsohn-Sachs center[16]). Temperature sensors placed on the tympanic membrane,[67] in the lower third of the esophagus,[68] or in the nasopharynx[52] measure central temperature during anesthesia. Morris corroborated the close relationship of these parameters.[52]

The blood coursing adjacent to the tympanic membrane is similar in temperature to blood flowing in the branches of the internal carotid artery to the hypothalamic center. The sensor placed in the lower third of the esophagus measures the temperature of aortic blood and escapes the cooling influences of dry anesthetic gases in the endotracheal tube. The nasotracheal sensor is warmed by branches of the internal carotid artery. If the sensor is moved into the pharynx, cool air will lower the reading, and this illustrates the importance of proper placement.

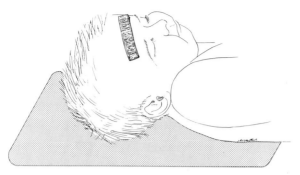

Fig. 19-8. The disposable strip has an adhesive backing that is applied to the forehead. Individual calibrated crystals become visible in response to heat. A blue color signifies the appropriate temperature.

Peripheral Temperature

Non-central monitors measure local changes in temperature that depend on regional blood flow and other factors. They do not measure core temperature but are useful and convenient monitors of relative changes in body temperature. For example, a rapidly falling rectal temperature not explained by peritoneal lavage, prolonged cystoscopy, or replacement of cold bowel[69] into the abdomen reflects decreased temperature in the tissues perfused by the inferior hemorrhoidal artery.

Axillary temperature monitoring is also simple to perform. If the arm can be abducted to prevent air cooling of the probe, and if cold intravenous fluids do not distort the response of the probe, this method is a useful guide to changes in temperature.

A sensing device that uses temperature-sensitive liquid crystals calibrated to yield digital images at the appropriate temperatures is available. (Fig. 19-8).[70] This adhesive-backed disposable strip can be placed on the forehead of most patients. This location is advantageous from a physiologic and anatomic standpoint. Vasoconstriction is delayed in this area, despite hypothermia.[71,72] Twenty-three per cent of heat loss down to 15.5°C ambient temperature occurs from the head. Below 15.5°C, up to 40 per cent of heat loss occurs from the head. Thus, the skin in this area remains relatively well perfused under ther-

mal stress. Therefore, these strips should track closely central or core temperature. In mild hypothermia, these strips typically give readings 2 to 3°C below tympanic temperature on adults and track changes within approximately 0.5°C.[70]

The most important factors in the choice of a temperature sensor are the location of the surgical incision and the experience of the anesthesiologist with a particular probe. All temperature sensors can inadvertently perforate the body cavity into which they are introduced, and obvious care must be taken to prevent perforation of the eardrum, esophagus, or rectum.

THE IMPORTANCE OF MONITORING TEMPERATURE

Measures taken to monitor temperature and prevent hypothermia are outlined on page 286. Data presented by Steward,[43] our own findings,[42] and our knowledge of thermoregulatory principles should make us wary of mild hypothermia. Until there is evidence that complete abolition of compensatory increased heat production is the response to a fall in core temperature, it seems reasonable to assume that thermoregulatory responses are present during general anesthesia.

It is vital to avoid "cold stress" in the newborn and sick premature neonate. Evidence of increased mortality, marked metabolic acidosis, and apnea (see chap. 44) compels the anesthesiologist to pay stringent attention to maintaining normothermia.[73–78] Relatively simple methods, such as control of ambient operating room temperature[79] and humidification of inspired gases[80] are effective in maintaining normothermia.

Roe's findings of increased postoperative oxygen consumption following intraoperative mild hypothermia also indicate that it is necessary to monitor and maintain temperature at or near 37°C.[51] In addition, preliminary studies by Roe suggest that hypothermia during anesthesia is followed by a rebound hyperthermia, at least in the 20 patients they studied.[81] If these data were shown to be true for a large population, it could have important clinical implications.

Finally, the possibility of the pathophysiologic syndrome of malignant hyperthermia has made temperature monitoring particularly important (see Section 3). The early recognition of a rise in temperature of 0.5°C or more during surgery is important in controlling febrile responses in septic patients; recognizing possible iatrogenic pyrogenic responses[82] during anesthesia (seven of the last eight cases of increases in temperature above 42°C witnessed by the author were not due to malignant hyperthermia); and confirming the diagnosis of malignant hyperthermia early (a temperature elevation from 35°C to 37°C aids in the diagnosis of an unexplained tachycardia).

Because of our lack of understanding of the principles of temperature control until recently, monitoring of temperature during anesthesia has held little importance. The simplest way to make temperature monitoring routine is to place our monitoring device on the anesthesia machine. Today, the compulsion to monitor temperature often stems from a fear of vulnerability. In the future it is hoped that the motivation to attach the sensor to the patient will depend upon an increased understanding of the fundamentals of temperature regulation.

Section Three: Malignant Hyperthermia

Beverley A. Britt, M.D.

Malignant hyperthermia (MH) is a myopathic disorder that occurs in humans[83–85] and pigs.[86,87] The incidence in children, adolescents, and young adults is about 1 in 15,000 anesthetic administrations, and in middle-aged adults, about 1 in 50,000 or less.[83] In adults, particularly, the incidence varies geographically, is more common in a few smaller and relatively isolated communities, where some genetic loading and illegitimate cross-fertilization has occurred. MH is rare in adults over the age of 50 years and in infants under the age of 2 years. The reasons for these differences are not entirely clear but appear to be related to muscle bulk, strength, and activity.[88] Nearly half of all MH-susceptible patients have been given one or more apparently uneventful general anesthetics.

EPIDEMIOLOGY OF MALIGNANT HYPERTHERMIA

Hereditary Aspects

The first person to recognize MH as a hereditary disease was Denborough.[89] In 1960, a young

man came under his care who had previously developed fever, cyanosis, sweating, and tachycardia during halothane anesthesia. Denborough noted that ten of this patient's relatives had died after manifesting similar symptoms during anesthesia with diethyl ether. Subsequent investigations by Denborough showed that the mode of inheritance of the disorder in this family was autosomal dominant. Thus, there was transmission through three successive generations; both men and women were affected, and on the average, half of the offspring of an affected parent were themselves afflicted.[90]

A few years later in Wisconsin, an investigation of an even larger family of 20 members who had had acute MH reactions suggested autosomal dominant inheritance.[91] In this study it was found that an affected father passed the trait on to his son, and this excluded sex linkage (Fig. 19-9).[83]

More recent investigations, however, suggest that in some families MH susceptibility may depend on two or more genes. Thus, in some patients, MH has been observed in the families of both parents (Fig. 19-10). Their parents have each

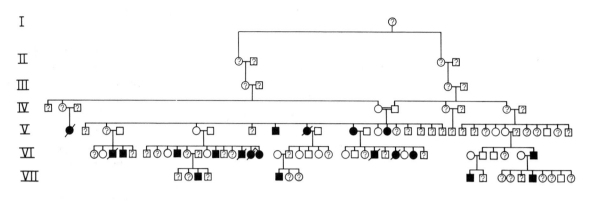

Fig. 19-9. A pedigree of a Wisconsin family in which 20 members had had malignant hyperthermic reactions. (Henschel, E. O. (ed.): Malignant Hyperthermia: Current Concepts. New York, Appleton-Century-Crofts, 1977.)

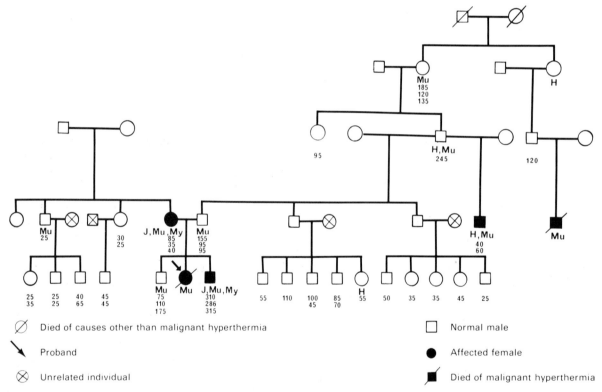

Fig. 19-10. Pedigree of an MH family exhibiting atypical inheritance. The proband died during a rigid MH reaction. The mother survived a similar rigid MH reaction. A second cousin of the proband's father died during a rigid MH crisis. The mother, the proband's brother, and paternal step-uncle all had muscle biopsies positive for malignant hyperthermia. The mother exhibited a moderate elevation of the serum CPK on one occasion. Both brothers, the father, the grandfather and the great-grandmother of the proband displayed significant elevations of the serum CPK. Numerals refer to CPK in international units; H, congenital inguinal hernia; J, joint hypermobility; Mu, excessive muscularity; My, muscle biopsy positive for malignant hyperthermia. (Henschel, E. O. (ed.): Malignant Hyperthermia. Current Concepts. New York, Appleton-Century-Crofts, 1977)

displayed the various stigmata of malignant hyperthermic myopathy.[92] With regard to MH reactions and muscle defects, the offspring of susceptible pigs exhibit a mean severity equal to that of their parents and have more than three phenotypes.

While there is no sex linkage, there does appear to be sex influence. Thus, throughout life, MH crises occur more commonly in men than in women. This difference is particularly marked in the prime years following puberty, between the ages of 16 and 30. Adult women thus appear to possess some characteristic that inhibits the hyperthermic trait. It is of interest that only two MH reactions have ever been described during pregnancy.[4] After the age of 29, the incidence of MH reactions progressively falls in both sexes.

Reduced penetrance is a feature of MH: A person who is clinically normal can pass the trait onto his or her offspring. People who have been anesthetized uneventfully with a great variety of agents, nevertheless, have had descendants who have developed acute MH reactions during anesthesia. Another characteristic of the MH trait is variable expressivity: The severity of the defect varies among different families. For example, the mortality rate in the Wisconsin family (Fig. 19-9) is about 40 per cent,[91] while in the family studied by Denborough, the mortality is in excess of 90 per cent.[89]

The racial distribution of MH is worldwide. In the majority of cases reported, the patients were Caucasian. However, the disorder also occurs in Oriental populations (Chinese, Filipino, Ceylonese, and Japanese). It is rare but not unknown among other racial groups, including Blacks.[90] However, nearly all afflicted Blacks studied have exhibited some phenotypic characteristics suggesting partial Caucasian ancestry.

Environmental Factors

Some environmental factor is usually necessary for the development of an acute MH crisis. In susceptible humans, this is most often a drug; these "triggering" drugs are almost entirely confined to anesthetic practice. They include the potent inhalation agents, most of the skeletal muscle relaxants (with the possible exception of pancuronium), and, rarely, some of the amide type of local anesthetics. With regard to mortality and rigidity during MH reactions, a review of 425 patients showed halothane and methoxyflurane to be the most potent, while cyclopropane and enflurane are weaker triggers.[90] Nitrous oxide may also be a very weak inducer of MH crisis.[93] Nevertheless, use of this agent by us in over 200 MH-susceptible patients has not induced an MH reaction. Succinylcholine is a potent precipitator of rigidity, but a weak inducer of fever, and by itself, it is not lethal. Curare alone occasionally can cause a nonfatal fever in susceptible patients.[94] In conjunction with inhalation agents, curare can aggravate an already established reaction.[95] The author and other investigators have found that lidocaine and mepivacaine have rarely precipitated MH in severely afflicted patients and not infrequently have worsened a crisis triggered by other agents.*

Malignant hyperthermic crises can also be precipitated outside the operating room by high environmental temperatures, mild infections, extreme emotional excitement, muscle injury, or exercise. We have found that muscle exercise on a hot day is especially likely to induce an MH reaction in an emotionally tense individual (e.g., a competitive football game in the middle of summer).†[88,96]

CLINICAL PRESENTATION OF MALIGNANT HYPERTHERMIA

Early Signs of MH

The clinical sign that most consistently is first observed in MH is tachycardia or a rapid ventricular arrhythmia,[86,90] such as ventricular extrasystoles, nodal tachycardia, multiple foci, bigeminy, or ventricular tachycardia (Table 23-1). Such an arrhythmia is present in nearly all cases of MH, with and without rigidity, and usually occurs prior to the detection of fever and, occasionally, even prior to the onset of muscle rigidity. Unless

---

*Personal communication, M. Mendenhall.
†Personal communication, R. Cichosz.

**Table 19-1. Early Clinical Signs
of Malignant Hyperthermia**

CLINICAL SIGNS PRESENT WITHIN 30 MIN. OF INDUCTION	NO. OF PATIENTS		% OF PATIENTS WITH SIGNS
	NOT PRESENT	PRESENT	
Tachycardia	13	324	96.1
Rigidity	56	286	83.6
Altered blood pressure	32	189	85.5
Tachypnea	27	159	85.5
Cyanosis	72	177	71.1
Fever	219	97	30.7

(Henschel, E. O. (ed.): Malignant Hyperthermia: Current Concepts. New York, Appleton-Century-Crofts, 1977)

there is some obvious explanation of arrhythmia, one must suspect MH. Many fatal cases of MH have occurred because triggering agents were used for long periods, even though arrhythmias were present almost from the beginning of the anesthetic. The tachycardia is not only a result of an MH rigor of the heart muscle but is also probably secondary to fever, acidosis, and electrolyte abnormalities. Somewhat later, tall, peaked T waves and slurred, bizarre QRS complexes typical of hyperkalemia may occur. S-T segment depression, T wave inversion, and prominent U waves characteristic of hypocalcemia may be observed. Terminally, ventricular fibrillation supervenes. The assumption that these arrhythmias are caused by inadequate anesthesia can have only the most unfortunate consequence for the patient.[88,90]

Another common early sign of MH is instability of the systolic blood pressure (Table 19-1). The levels vary more than usual between readings, and generally there is an overall moderate rise until shortly before arrest, when profound hypotension and bradycardia occur.[88,90]

If the patient is breathing spontaneously, rapid and deep respirations and excess of heat and discoloration of the soda lime cannister may be observed (Table 19-1). This hyperventilation represents an attempt of the body to excrete excess carbon dioxide being produced by the hypermetabolizing muscles. Because of the increased carbon dioxide production, the soda lime becomes hot and discolored earlier than usual.[90]

The surgeon may complain of dark blood in the wound. The skin may acquire a peculiar mottled cyanotic appearance (Table 19-1). Initially, the cyanotic areas may be interspersed with patches of bright red flushing. Gradually, as the microcirculation fails, these red areas also become cyanosed. The cyanosis is a reflection both of accelerated oxygen consumption by the rapidly metabolizing muscles and of peripheral vasoconstriction.

Rigidity may be marked or, occasionally, may not occur at all. It is sometimes first observed in the muscles of the extremities, the jaws, or the chest. Rigidity is most characteristically noticed after the infusion of succinylcholine. Thus, the fasciculations are either grossly exaggerated or, strangely, may not occur. Then, instead of paralysis, a rigor-mortis-like muscle stiffness begins in the jaw muscles, and this makes intubation difficult or impossible. Repeated doses of succinylcholine worsen rather than relieve stiffness. Rigidity spreads to the remainder of the skeletal muscles after a variable time. The use of a belladonna alkaloid in addition to succinylcholine tends to increase the incidence and severity of the rigidity.[97] When nondepolarizing relaxants are given in an attempt to relieve muscle stiffness, the rigidity usually becomes worse, instead of abating. In patients who have not received succinylcholine, the onset of muscle stiffness may be delayed, and its development is more insidious.

Cyclopropane and enflurane, which are possibly less lethal agents, may be also less likely to induce rigidity than halothane and methoxyflurane. A person who has been exercising vigorously or who has suffered muscle trauma immediately prior to anesthesia (e.g., a patient who arrives from the sports field with a fracture and a surrounding muscle contusion) is somewhat more likely to develop rigidity than is the patient undergoing elective surgery, who has been bedridden for several days prior to anesthesia.[90] Patients with certain coexisting diseases, such as polymyositis[98] and conditions that elevate serum calcium (e.g., sarcoma,[99] Paget's disease, or hyperparathyroidism, are likely to have a high incidence of intense rigidity. Patients with a severe inherent defect are more likely to become rigid than those with a mild defect.

About 20 per cent of patients never manifest any perceptible increase in muscle tone. While some of these patients may have a different skeletal muscle defect, most appear to be etiologically similar to those who display rigidity: They have a mild inherent defect, undergo anesthesia with weak triggering agents, and lack muscle exercise or muscle injury immediately prior to anesthesia.

Fever, the clinical hallmark of an MH reaction[*83–85,90,95,100] is a *result and not a cause* of the various biochemical derangements that occur in skeletal muscle in an MH crisis. It is, therefore, of relatively late onset. *By the time elevation in body temperature is observed, the patient's future is already very seriously compromised.* The maximum temperature level obtained is quite variable. As a rule, the mortality rate is directly related to the highness of the maximum temperature.[90] Death has occurred, however, in patients whose maximum temperature elevations have been relatively low,[*85] while on the other hand, patients with a fever of 44°C have survived.[101] A rise in temperature, particularly if it occurs rapidly, may enable the anesthesiologist to diagnose MH while the patient's temperature is still within the normal range. For instance, suppose that an MH-susceptible patient does not react in the 1st hour of anesthesia. During this period, the temperature may decrease to about 35°C, as it does in normal patients not infrequently. At the beginning of the 2nd hour, the MH reaction commences, and the temperature starts to rise. At this point, the anesthesiologist is observing a patient who is experiencing the early stages of an MH reaction but has a temperature within the normal range. Nevertheless, the fact that the thermistor reading is rising should suggest MH. This is one of the several reasons that routine thermometry of all patients undergoing anesthesia is so important. Other evidence of the fever of MH includes hot, flushed skin, excessive heat of

Table 19-2. Mortality Associated With Inhalation Anesthetic Agents and Muscle Relaxants

Drug	% Died	% Rigidity Present	% Maximum Temperature (>39.4°C)
Halothane	71.9	86.3	81.0
Methoxyflurane	71.4	83.3	82.0
Enflurane	33.3	59.1	90.0
Diethyl Ether	72.7	66.6	100.0
Cyclopropane	36.6	16.7	93.8
Succinylcholine	0.0	81.8	30.8
d-Tubocurarine	0.0	0.0	33.3

the anesthetic rebreathing bag, and hot tissues at the wound site.[*83–85,90] The liver tends to be especially hyperthermic.[102] Inhalation agents induce a higher maximal temperature than do muscle relaxants (Table 19-2). Although succinylcholine alone does not cause a high maximal temperature, it does induce an early onset of MH fever. On the other hand, the higher maximum temperature that follows the use of an inhalation agent alone usually has a somewhat later onset. Employment of both succinylcholine and an inhalation agent initiates an early onset of fever and leads to a very high maximum temperature. The highest so far recorded is 45°C.[†] One reason these high temperatures have not been described more frequently is that most clinical mercury thermometers or electronic thermistors can not be read in this range. A number of reports have stated that the temperature was "off scale."[90]

Laboratory Findings in MH Patients

The *p*H falls to profoundly low values in MH, not only because of respiratory acidosis, but also because of metabolic acidosis. The metabolic acidosis is mainly a reflection of accelerated lactic acid formation in the muscles. When considered separately, no significant relationship exists between mortality and either respiratory or metabolic acidosis. When considered together, however, a relationship does exist: As *p*H falls, mortality rises.

---

*Personal communication, J. DeKrey.
*Personal communication, M. K. Mendenhall.

†Personal communication, J. Sax.

Arterial oxygen tensions are often reduced, but not always as much as one might expect. Not infrequently, Pa_{O_2} is above 100 torr, even when frank cyanosis is also present. Nevertheless, $P_{(A-a)O_2}$ is often grossly exaggerated. There is a significant relationship between the level of the arterial oxygen tension and survival.

A variety of electrolyte abnormalities occur. These are thought to be due to loss of integrity of the sarcolemma, increased mobilization of ions in the muscle cell, and various therapeutic maneuvers. For instance, the serum calcium may rise transiently early and then fall to subnormal levels within 1 or 2 hours of induction of anesthesia. Similarly, serum potassium initially rises markedly and then several hours later falls equally markedly. Total body potassium depletion may continue for several days. Rises in serum phosphorous, magnesium, glucose (without ketone body formation), lactate, and pyruvate also occur. For all blood gas and electrolyte parameters measured, the mortality is higher when the values are grossly abnormal than when they are normal.[90]

Somewhat later (several hours to several days), large molecules escape from the muscle cell, such as creatine phosphokinase (CPK), lactate dehydrogenase, glutamic oxalic transaminase, aldolase, and myoglobin.[90]

Late Complications of MH

Though only one-fourth the size of hemoglobin, myoglobin is able to penetrate into the renal parenchyma and therefore has a more deleterious effect on renal function than does hemoglobin. Myoglobin may also directly constrict the afferent arterioles. Thus, the appearance of red or brown urine is usually followed by oliguria and anuria, with few or no red cells in the urine and a progressively rising blood urea nitrogen (BUN). Myoglobinuria alone does not worsen the prognosis; the development of an elevated BUN or oliguria does significantly lower the survival rate.[90]

Impaired coagulation, sometimes associated with hemolysis, is another untoward development, and presently death occurs in two-thirds of these cases.[90] Marked reduction in platelets, fibrinogen, and factor VIII occurs. The reason for the consumption coagulopathy is not certain. It may be secondary to the biochemical disturbances, though the primary defect may involve some blood element. For instance, the ATP–hypoxanthine ratio of the platelets is less than normal.* The ouabain-sensitive ATPase activity of the red cell membrane of MH-susceptible patients is reduced.[103] There is also an unusually high correlation of MH susceptibility with a von Willebrand's-like coagulation defect. Clinically, there are multiple hematomata and bleeding from body orifices and wound and needle sites.

Acute pulmonary edema secondary to left ventricular failure is a complication that is usually followed shortly by death. Coarse, moist rales are audible and rattling sounds can be heard emanating from the anesthetic tubing. Pink, frothy sputum regurgitates through the endotracheal tube. Edema occurs because the heart muscle appears to be afflicted with MH rigor in a manner similar to that of the skeletal muscle. Blood is, therefore, unable to leave the lungs and enter the left ventricle.[90]

Some patients, usually those who have received heroic treatment, survive through all these complications. After they linger for several days without regaining consciousness, death finally occurs. These patients may have localized twitches, grand mal convulsions, fixed and dilated pupils, no tendon reflexes, and a body temperature that always corresponds to the environmental temperature. The latter may be a result of failure of the central temperature-regulating mechanism. The cause of brain death is obscure. It may be secondary to temperature and biochemical abnormalities, or the primary defect might also affect the brain cells.[104]

Prognosis of MH

The overall mortality from MH is presently about 53 per cent. If the patient dies early, within 1 or 2 hours, the immediate cause is usually ventricular fibrillation arising from the preceding

---

*Personal communication, C. C. Solomons.

rapid ventricular nodal rhythm. If demise occurs after many hours, death is often associated with pulmonary edema or consumption coagulopathy. Death occurring after several days is usually a result of acute renal failure or progressive neurological deterioration.[88]

Convalescence of MH Patients

Hopeful prognostic signs are a progressive lightening of coma often associated with restlessness; a return of normal reflexes, temperature, and blood pressure; slowing and strengthening of the heart beat; improvement of renal function; and disappearance of clinical bleeding. When the patient is well enough to communicate, he frequently complains of severe pain and tenderness in his muscles, especially in the muscles of the thigh, which are sometimes grossly swollen. These signs and symptoms are particularly likely to occur if the reaction has been associated with rigidity. (87.9% of patients who experience rigidity show them.) This rhabdomyolysis has often been misdiagnosed as phlebitis. As the swelling disappears, the muscle may occasionally seem wasted and even weak. The patient may also complain of generalized easy fatigability that may continue for several months. Eventually, these residual effects almost completely disappear.[90]

The rare patient who has been resuscitated from a cardiac arrest may have severe neurological deficits, such as paralysis and loss of special senses, that apparently result from the hypoxia precipitated by the arrest itself.

ETIOLOGY OF MALIGNANT HYPERTHERMIA

What defect could possibly cause these bizarre clinical and biochemical derangements? In spite of several years of intensive investigation, the etiology and pathophysiology of malignant hyperthermia have not been entirely clarified. Two facts contribute to this deficiency. First, MH appears to be caused by several different primary defects in different families. Second, the defects of MH, like many other genetic syndromes transmitted by dominant inheritance, are probably

structural abnormalities within cell membranes, and, therefore, are much more difficult to investigate than are the recessive conditions that are usually caused by deficiencies in circulating proteins or enzymes.[104]

The most probable immediate cause of the acute catabolic crisis of MH appears to be a sudden rise in the concentration of myoplasmic calcium (Fig. 19-11). This hypothesis is supported by the observation that drugs that raise myoplasmic calcium, such as lidocaine, cardiac glycosides, and caffeine, worsen the prognosis of MH reactions in vivo.[105] Caffeine, in addition, causes contractures in vitro that are greater in MH-susceptible than in normal muscle.[106–109] On the other hand, drugs that lower myoplasmic calcium, (e.g., dantrolene[110,111] and procaineamide[112–114]) improve survival in vivo.[105,115] In vitro, these also attenuate contractures induced by caffeine in MH-susceptible muscle.[116,117] The abnormality that accounts for this rapid rise of myoplasmic calcium has yet to be established. Some possibilities that are not necessarily mutually exclusive are as follows: inhibition of calcium uptake in sarcoplasmic reticulum[107–121]; defective accumulation of calcium in the mitochondria[122–128]; an excessively fragile sarcolemma, with resultant passive diffusion of calcium into the myoplasm from the extracellular fluid;*[129] and exaggeration of adrenergic innervation with, therefore, multiple indirect effects.[96,130–147] The resulting elevated myoplasmic calcium has a number of heat-producing effects.[148–152] Moderate rises, for example, activate phosphorylase,[142–147] thereby increasing the catabolism of glycogen to lactic acid, carbon dioxide, and heat. This activation of phosphorylase is reinforced further by another protein kinase, phosphorylase kinase (Fig. 19-11)[142–147] Thus, a patient with a mild MH defect that causes only a small rise in myoplasmic calcium can be expected to manifest fever and respiratory and metabolic acidosis, but not muscle rigidity.

Still higher concentrations of calcium activate

---

*Personal communication, T. G. Nelson, E. W. Jones, and D. Holbert.

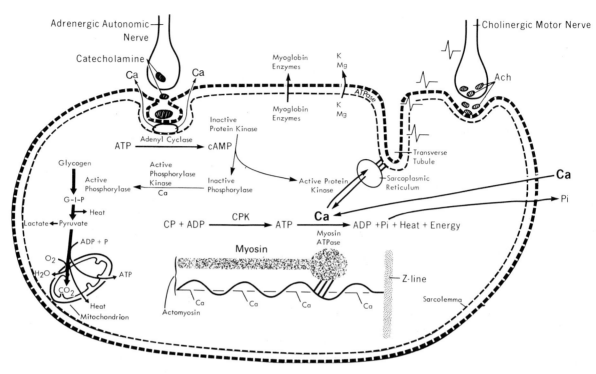

Fig. 19-11. Schematic diagram of proposed mechanism underlying malignant hyperthermia.

myosin ATPase, which then hydrolyzes ATP to ADP plus phosphate, heat, and free energy, which is utilized in the formation of actomyosin (Fig. 19-11).[103,153–158]

Finally, highly elevated myoplasmic calcium combines with troponin, the long thread-like myofibril that lies within the helices of actin (Fig. 19-12). During relaxation, troponin prevents myosin from combining with actin. The calcium, however, induces a conformational change in the troponin, so that instead of being one long strand, the calcium-troponin complex becomes a series of small segments between which are gaps. Through these gaps the cross-bridges on the myosin combine with the receptors on the actin. This enables myosin to slide over actin and form short and rigid actomyosin.[159-164] Yet another protein kinase is known to potentiate directly the formation of this calcium-troponin complex; this further increases the ease with which myosin can combine with actin (Fig. 19-12). As the muscle temperature rises, these events become self-sustaining, since increased temperature eliminates the calcium requirement for myosin-actin interaction.[165] Thus, a patient with a severe MH defect that causes a marked rise in concentrations of myoplasmic calcium can be expected to exhibit muscle rigidity as well as fever and acidosis.

In normal muscle, once the acetylcholine-induced muscle action potential ceases, calcium is taken back into the sarcoplasmic reticulum, and the muscle returns to its resting state. During an MH crisis, however, the myoplasmic calcium concentration remains permanently elevated, so that muscle contracture continues unabated. Some of the excess calcium may be absorbed by the mitochondria. Within the mitochondria, the resulting toxic calcium concentrations uncouple oxidative phosphorylation from electron transport, thereby decreasing ATP production but further exacerbating oxygen consumption and lactate, carbon dioxide, and heat output.[166–171] Early in the reaction, ATP levels in the muscle are maintained through conversion of high-

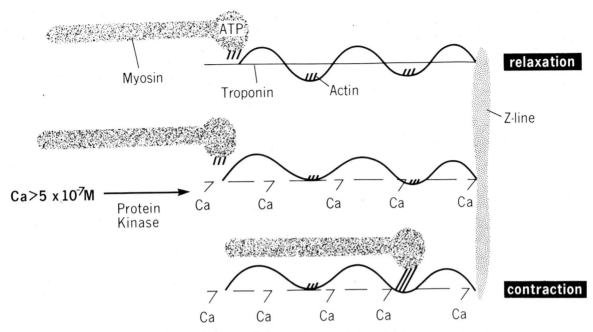

Fig. 19-12. A combination of myoplasmic calcium and treponin results in contraction.

energy creatine phosphate and ADP to creatine and ATP.[172] Once, however, the store of high energy creatine phosphate has been exhausted, ATP levels in the muscle decline rapidly[173] and membrane ATPases fail through lack of their substrate ATP. As a result, ions and molecules simply diffuse according to the natural concentration gradients. Thus, potassium, magnesium, and phosphate and, somewhat later, large molecules, such as enzymes and myoglobin, "leak" outward. The myoglobin obstructs the renal tubules and thereby induces an acute renal failure. Because the concentration gradient favors diffusion of calcium in the opposite direction, it flows into the myoplasm, thereby exacerbating the already existing calcium-dependent biochemical derangements (Fig. 19-11).[104]

MH appears to involve a widespread membrane defect. Similar abnormal biochemical disturbances also seem to occur in other types of cells, including nerve or brain cells, platelets and red blood cells, and cardiac muscle. Thus, the severe neurological deterioration, consumption coagulopathy, hemolysis, and bizarre arrhythmias that are characteristic features of fulminant MH reactions probably result more from activation of primary defects in the membranes of these tissues than from damage secondarily induced by acid-base, electrolyte, and temperature disturbances. Furthermore, in MH-susceptible people undergoing elective investigation, abnormalities of red blood cells,[174] platelets,[131] peripheral nerves,[175] personality,[96] and bone[176] can be detected infrequently.

PREANESTHETIC DIAGNOSIS OF MALIGNANT HYPERTHERMIA

Identification of patients susceptible to MH prior to anesthesia is critical in the prevention of acute MH reactions. Extensive investigation of all available relatives of a suspected family is first conducted, including serum CPK estimations, clinical examination for evidence of muscle abnormalities, and previous anesthetic history. These studies are inexpensive and not too time-consuming or excessively uncomfortable for the patient. They are, unfortunately, not very accurate. Nevertheless, serum CPK measurements do enable us to select people who are most likely to

Table 19-3. Number of Patients and Their Relatives With Musculoskeletal Abnormalities Most Commonly Seen in Malignant Hyperthermia

Type of Muscle Abnormality	Muscle Abnormalities in Patient	Muscle Abnormalities in Relatives
Generalized muscularity	88	93
Muscle cramps	30	55
Muscle weakness	11	15
Abnormal muscle biopsy	27	55
Joint hypermobility	43	51
Thoracic kyphosis, kyphoscoliosis, lumbar lordosis	26	29
Hernia	25	43
Squint	19	16
Ptosis	18	7
Other	10	18
None	102	87

(Henschel, O. E. (ed.): Malignant Hyperthermia: Current Concepts. New York, Appleton-Century-Crofts, 1977)

be at risk. Intensive electrophysiological and muscle biopsy studies are then performed on these high-risk people. Although accurate, these intensive studies are time-consuming, uncomfortable, and expensive.[88]

Clinical Abnormalities of MH-Susceptible Patients

Prior to or after recovery from anesthesia, there may be some difficulty with temperature control in MH-susceptible patients. The normal diurnal variation in temperature may not occur. Excessively high temperatures may develop during mild infections. Severe exercise may induce what appears to be a hyperthermic reaction with fever, muscle cramps, and brown urine.[90]

Muscle anomalies are present in 67 per cent of these patients and in about 36 per cent of first-degree relatives.[88,90,177] The most commonly found musculoskeletal abnormalities are enumerated in Table 19-3. The muscles, although strong, are sometimes not well coordinated. The patients, therefore, while active in sports, are generally not very proficient unless the sport requires great physical strength but minimal coordination (e.g., weight lifting). Many patients complain of muscle cramps that occur spontaneously, during or after exercise[177] or following coffee drinking. A muscle weakness or a history of MH during anesthesia may also be noted in the patient's relatives.

Noninvasive Laboratory Techniques

High concentrations of serum CPK in MH patients and their relatives were first described by Denborough[178] and by Isaacs in 1970.[179] Somewhat conflicting studies of CPK in MH families have been reported since 1970 by other investigators.[103,131,179–187] Thus, while this test is a useful diagnostic parameter, relying on it too heavily is likely to lead to diagnostic error. Although many patients do have elevated serum CPK levels, others occasionally or always have values within the normal range.

There are many problems in using CPK elevation as a marker for MH susceptibility.[177] Values may be falsely low if the sample is exposed to light or is not frozen promptly in dry ice or liquid nitrogen. Normal individuals may have elevated serum CPK levels if they have exercised within 1 or 2 weeks of sampling. Excessive tourniquet pressure, forcible suction of blood through the needle, or vigorous squirting of blood against the wall of the syringe also lead to higher than expected values. Finally, many other conditions associated with muscle damage also elevate the serum CPK, such as a recent myocardial infarct,[188] muscular dystrophy and other myopathies,[188] paranoid schizophrenia,[189] various neurological disorders,[190–194] hypothyroidism,[195] acute and chronic alcoholism,[196] a recent intramuscular injection,[197] and muscle trauma or exercise.[177]

In spite of these problems, in about 45 per cent of families, the serum CPK level is higher than normal in the probands and in some of their relatives. In 20 per cent of families, no CPK elevation can be detected either in those who have had previous MH reactions or in any of their relatives. In the remaining 35 per cent of families, the CPK levels are elevated in some members, but the elevations tend to be small, not always reproducible, and do not always occur in the proband. Therefore, CPK measurement cannot be relied upon as the sole diagnostic criterion. There is, however, a significant positive correlation between a high serum CPK level and a clinical muscle abnormality in members of MH-susceptible families.[177] Thus, the presence of both a high CPK level and a muscle abnormality in the same person is a much better marker of the MH trait than is the presence of either alone.[88,90,177]

Measurement of CPK isoenzymes in serum has been proposed as another test useful in the diagnosis of MH.[185] However, a number of human and porcine MH-susceptible families have been found to have normal CPK isoenzyme patterns.[198–200] The use of column chromatography as opposed to electrophoresis appears to increase the sensitivity of this test and the incidence of detection of an abnormal isoenzyme pattern.*[199]

Serum pyrophosphate levels are higher than normal in some MH-susceptible patients.[131] Such a test, however, poses technical problems, and most routine hospital laboratories are probably not equipped for it.

Neuroelectrophysiological studies may also assist in diagnosis because many patients susceptible to the rigid variant of MH have a reduction of motor neuron counts in several muscle groups. Motor unit counting is more accurate than concentric-needle electromyography (EMG) in the diagnosis of rigid MH susceptibility, though slightly less accurate than the caffeine contracture test (see below).[200] Upon routine EMG, there is an increased incidence of polyphasic action potentials of short duration in a few patients.

Finally, neutron activation analysis reveals total body calcium to be less in some adult MH-susceptible patients than in normal people.[176] In addition, the author has noted that MH-susceptible people have a slightly increased incidence of fractures.

Invasive Laboratory Techniques: Muscle Biopsy

Noninvasive studies discussed above are all subject to gross errors. The only accurate method

---

*Personal communication, D. Nealon.

presently available of diagnosing MH susceptibility is a skeletal muscle biopsy. The most commonly measured and the most accurate is the caffeine contracture test.[106] A small, carefully excised fascicle of muscle from the vastus lateralis is prepared isometrically and attached by means of a force transducer to a polygraph. The muscle on its frame is placed in a bath of Krebs' Ringer solution and bubbled with carbogen and various doses of caffeine and caffeine plus halothane (Fig. 19-13). Caffeine induces in rigid MH-susceptible muscle a greater than normal increase in resting muscle tension (contracture). The addition of halothane further increases the contracture in both normal and MH-susceptible muscle, but particularly in the latter.[106] In some very rigid MH-susceptible muscle, halothane even without the prior addition of caffeine precipitates a contracture that never occurs with normal muscle.[108,152,187]

Moulds has found that procaine relieves the contracture,[201,202] and that calcium and potassium accentuate the contracture.[108] In addition, a few MH-susceptible patients identified by biopsy belong to families whose members never manifest rigidity during anesthesia. Their excised muscle (without halothane) is resistant to caffeine; that is, a greater than normal dose of caffeine is required to raise the resting muscle tension by 1.0 g.[92,203]

Equilibration with halothane results in greater ATP depletion in MH-susceptible porcine muscle than in normal muscle.[204] This test has been adapted for use in humans belonging to rigid MH families.[203] Although not quite as reliable as the caffeine contracture test, the ATP depletion test does not require as much skill and equipment as the former. The ATP depletion test cannot be used, however, for patients belonging to MH-susceptible families that do not exhibit rigidity during anesthesia.[90]

Muscle biopsied from MH-susceptible people has lower concentrations of creatine phosphate and higher concentrations of glucose-6-phosphate than normal.[205] Their deviation from normal can be increased by prior equilibration with halothane, as in the ATP depletion test. Similarly, the author has observed that lactic acid concentra-

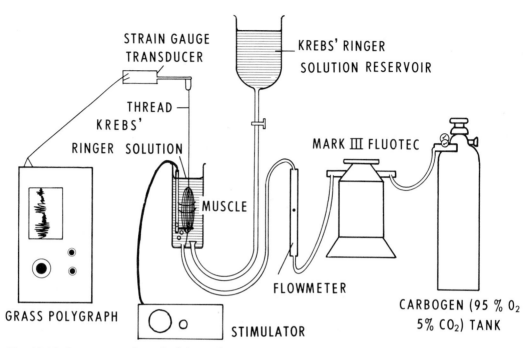

Fig. 19-13. Experimental method for isolated isometric muscle contraction study.

tions rise and pyruvate concentrations fall in MH-susceptible muscle equilibrated with halothane.

A number of microscopic abnormalities are fairly common in MH-susceptible muscle. These are less helpful in diagnosis than the caffeine contracture or ATP depletion tests because the alterations are not specific for MH susceptibility and are lacking in a few probands, even in some who show regidity. Generally, however, there is an increased variation in fiber diameter, with small angular fibers that contain clumps of pyknotic nuclei (Fig. 19-14) and large round fibers that have increased numbers of internal nuclei. Some of the more grossly abnormal muscle revealed by NADase stains exhibit disorganized round areas that on electron microscopy are found to be devoid of mitochondria. These areas have been characterized variously as central cores,[206] target or targetoid cells,[107] or simply as moth-eaten cells.[207] Abnormal ratios of Type I–II fiber may also be seen on ATPase stains.[206,207]

Electron microscopy may reveal a rare, degenerated, frankly necrotic cell, Z-line streaming, and occasional aggregations of mitochondria, or greatly increased size and numbers of mitochondria.[107,204,205,207]

In a very few patients, the intramuscular nerves contain thickened epineurium and thinned myelin.[107] Silver stains reveal that in some areas the intramuscular neurons are degenerating in a bead-like fashion and in other areas are regenerating and sprouting many new and abnormal endings.[208] There may be areas with elongated motor end-plates that contain excessively large mitochondria.[207]

COUNSELING PATIENTS SUSCEPTIBLE TO MALIGNANT HYPERTHERMIA

If on the basis of the foregoing investigations a diagnosis of MH is made, what can be done for such a patient and his family? First, a pedigree of

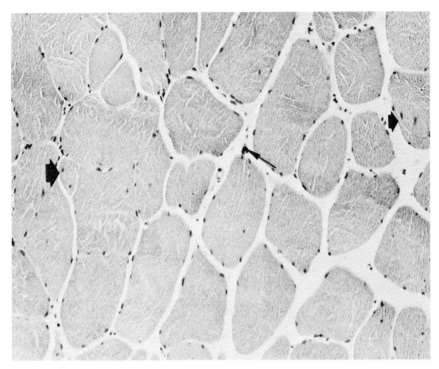

Fig. 19-14. Great variability in fiber size is noted with normal, small, and large fibers in MH-susceptible muscle. There are occasional tiny fibers with clumps of dark pyknotic nuclei (thin arrow), as well as large and small fibers with internal nuclei (thick arrows). (Henschel, E. D. (ed.): Malignant Hyperthermia: Current Concepts. New York, Appleton-Century-Crofts, 1977)

the family is prepared. For each member, the date of birth, muscle abnormalities, previous normal and hyperthermic general anesthetics, and serum CPK levels are itemized. The pedigree is sent to the parents of each family group and to their attending physicians and interested anesthesiologists in the local community. The patients are warned about the danger to them of potent inhalational agents, skeletal muscle relaxants, and amide types of local anesthetics. They are reassured that there are safe and effective agents available for them. Reassurance is important, because MH-susceptible patients naturally are apprehensive about possible future anesthetics. The patients are given a monograph, written in layman's language, entitled "Answers to Some Questions About Malignant Hyperthermia," and they are given a Medic Alert Bracelet that is lettered as follows: *Malig. Hyperthermia, No Potent Inhal. Anes. Agents or Musc. Relaxants.*

These bracelets are recommended for people who have had a previous MH crisis or a positive biopsy; first-degree relatives of a person who has had a previous malignant hyperthermic crisis or a positive muscle biopsy; people who have a clinical muscle abnormality and who are also members of families suspected to be MH-susceptible; and people who have had high levels of CPK on one or more occasions. These bracelets have been an important factor in reducing mortality from MH. It is, of course, essential to ensure that the patient actually wears the bracelet at all times.[177]

MANAGEMENT OF ELECTIVE ANESTHETICS IN PATIENTS SUSCEPTIBLE TO MALIGNANT HYPERTHERMIA

A patient suspected to be at risk for MH should not be denied anesthesia, not even purely elective anesthesia. Safe and effective analgesia and reasonably adequate operating conditions can be achieved through some combination of barbiturates, narcotics, neuroleptanalgesics, and tranquilizers, or by local anesthetic of the ester group, such as procaine or tetracaine.[88] Although nitrous oxide has been considered safe in the past, a recent report casts some doubt on its use.[93] However, we still anesthetize all of our MH-susceptible patients undergoing elective surgery with nitrous oxide and have not encountered difficulties.

One of the several anesthetic techniques that we employ for MH-susceptible patients is as follows: If the patient is apprehensive, a night sedative, either an intermediate-acting barbiturate (e.g., secobarbital) or flurazepam, is prescribed the evening prior to surgery. An intravenous infusion of Ringer's solution with 5-per-cent glucose is started 4 hours preoperatively and administered at the rate of 3 ml. per kg. per hour. The purpose of the infusion is to prevent hypotension, since the agents that are employed during the anesthetic tend to induce vasodilatation. Pantopon (0.25 mg./kg.) and diazepam (0.25 mg./kg.) are administered intramuscularly 1 hour postoperatively, thus ensuring that the patient arrives in the operating theatre in a reasonably tranquil state. Belladonna alkaloids are not given because they are associated with an increased incidence of rigidity[97] and death. On arrival in the operating theatre, the patient is placed on a hypothermia blanket, which is turned on only if the body temperature rises. A second over-blanket is available in the room. Temperature probes are placed in the axilla and rectum, and ECG leads are attached to the patient. A box available in the room contains emergency drugs (e.g., sodium bicarbonate, dantrolene sodium, procaineamide, furosemide, mannitol, insulin, glucose, potassium chloride, chlorpromazine, and intravenous solutions). The gas machine contains no vaporizers and its rubber tubing and bags are new and, therefore, vapor-free. Blood is taken for electrolyte (including potassium, phosphorus, calcium, and magnesium) and serum enzyme (CPK, LDH, and GOT) determinations.

Induction is commenced with nitrous oxide and oxygen by means of a face mask for 5 minutes. Droperidol (1 mg./kg.) and fentanyl (0.3 μg./kg.) are infused followed by a sleep-inducing dose of thiopental. After brief manual hyperventilation with nitrous oxide and oxygen, the trachea is intubated without muscle relaxant or throat spray. If tracheal analgesia is desired, cocaine or tetracaine spray may be used; however, lidocaine should not be used because it is a weak trigger of MH. Anesthesia is maintained with nitrous oxide, oxygen, fentanyl, and, if necessary, intermittent doses of thiopental or diazepam. For surgical procedures requiring muscle relaxation, an appropriate local or regional anesthetic is added, using procaine or tetracaine.

A number of procedures can be undertaken with a local or regional anesthetic without accompanying general anesthesia. Again, the agents chosen may be procaine, chloroprocaine, or tetracaine, but not lidocaine, mepivacaine, dibucaine, prilocaine, bupivacaine, or etidocaine. These patients always should be well sedated to overcome apprehension. This apprehension is caused partly by the natural fear of death during anesthesia that MH-susceptible patients have, but it also appears to result from an inherent tendency of MH-susceptible people to have tense hyperactive personalities.

At the end of the anesthetic, a second sample of blood is drawn for the same biochemical analyses that were performed at the beginning of the anesthetic. The patient is then transferred very gently to the recovery room, still on the cooling blanket and with all monitoring devices still attached. In the recovery room, measurements of all vital signs are made at least once every 5 minutes. The patient remains there until there is no danger of an MH reaction, when all vital signs have been normal and stable for at least 4 hours, and when all the laboratory tests ordered at the end of the anesthetic have been reported to be normal. Just before leaving the recovery room, a third set of blood samples is obtained for determination of serum electrolytes and enzymes.

On return to the ward, vital signs are measured at least once each hour for the first 4 hours and then once every 4 hours for 24 hours. For the first 4 days, serum enzymes (CPK, LDH, GOT) are determined each day, and 24-hour samples of urine are collected for myoglobin analysis.

MANAGEMENT OF ACUTE MALIGNANT HYPERTHERMIC REACTIONS

In spite of meticulous efforts to diagnose MH prior to anesthesia, it is inevitable in the foreseeable future that some susceptible patients will be anesthetized inadvertently with triggering agents. The key to success in the management of resultant crises is the immediate cessation of all potent inhalational anesthetics and/or muscle relaxants. Every patient who has been anesthetized for less than 10 min. has survived, while the majority of patients who have rigid reactions and who have been anesthetized for more than 2 hours have expired. Thus, since one of the most important aspects of management of the acute crisis is prompt discontinuance of the anesthetic, the ability to recognize the condition early is essential. Routine temperature monitoring and frequent checks for skin warmth, cyanosis, and excessive heat and discoloration of the soda lime cannister are essential. The anesthesiologist should remember that lack of rigidity does not rule out the occurrence of an MH reaction.[95] If in doubt, the anesthesiologist should stop all triggering anesthetic agents. Since awakening, even from a fairly mild reaction is likely to be considerably delayed, the surgeon will probably be able to adequately close the wound in most instances. If the surgical condition is life-threatening and requires prolonged anesthesia, it may be reasonable to complete the procedure with the aid of non-triggering agents, such as droperidol or thiopental, once the acute manifestations have been controlled.[105]

If possible, all rubber anesthetic tubes and bags ought to be changed to new and unused ones, since lipid-soluble agents such as halothane and especially methoxyflurane are absorbed in significant quantities by this equipment and are then given off over a considerable period of time.[88,209]

A drug that lowers myoplasmic calcium should be of benefit for both cardiac and skeletal muscle rigors during an MH reaction. Procaine and procaineamide have such an effect on the myoplasm

of the heart muscle cell. Because of their potential for depressing the myocardium, such drugs must be administered under continuous ECG monitoring at a rate not exceeding 1 mg. per kg. per min. Infusion should be discontinued as soon as arrhythmias are relieved. The total dosage should probably not exceed 10 mg. per kg.

A drug that has proven to be superior to procaine or procaineamide is dantrolene, which is thought to prevent release of calcium into the skeletal muscle myoplasm.[110,111,115,117] It is uncertain whether this excess calcium is released from the sarcoplasmic reticulum or the extracellular fluid. Dantrolene has no effect on the CNS, motor neuron, myoneural junction, or electrical excitability of the sarcolemma.[111,112,210–212] It is presently being used in oral form to treat spasms associated with cerebral palsy, athetosis, quadriplegia, Parkinson's disease, and multiple sclerosis.[213–215] Dantrolene has been used successfully to treat acute MH crises in swine in doses of 7 to 10 mg. per kg.[115,116] Since dantrolene has little or no effect on cardiac muscle, concomitant administration of procaineamide may be necessary, though in doses smaller than those recommended when it is used by itself.

Lidocaine has no role in the treatment of malignant hyperthermia. This drug has the opposite action of procaine on the sarcoplasmic reticulum[112–114]; that is, lidocaine accelerates calcium loss from and prevents reuptake of calcium into the sarcoplasmic reticulum.[216] It significantly increases mortality. Cardiac glycosides also accelerate calcium release from the sarcoplasmic reticulum and radically increase the death rate.[217,218] Thus, even though tachycardia and acute pulmonary edema are present, cardiac glycosides are contraindicated during an MH reaction.[105]

To achieve significant temperature reduction in fulminant cases, not only must the patient be cooled externally by water baths, but internal cooling is also necessary. This can be accomplished by intravenous infusions and lavage of the stomach, rectum, and open body cavities with cold solutions. Extracorporeal cooling[119] may also be employed if readily available, but it should not be attempted to the exclusion of other, simpler techniques that can usually be instituted much more rapidly. Although cooling should be prompt and vigorous, it must not be prolonged, or malignant hyperthermia may be succeeded by an equally malignant *hypo*thermia; the patient then appears to lose all control over central temperature regulation, so that it passively adjusts to the environmental temperature. It is, therefore, advisable to discontinue cooling when the temperature has fallen to about 38°C. Secondary temperature rises may recur, but these tend to be milder and more easily managed by reapplication of external cooling. The fairly low rate of survival that follows the application of cooling is probably due to the delay in instruction and incompleteness of the technique in many patients.[105]

High inspired oxygen concentration is of uncertain value. MH pigs ventilated with oxygen have a slightly lower survival rate than MH pigs ventilated with room air.[219] Some investigators argue that oxygen leaks across the damaged mitochondrial membrane and within the mitochondria induces uncoupling of oxidative phosphorylation.[220–222] The data obtained in human patients usually support this hypothesis, although they are probably biased because some of the more fulminantly ill patients receive 100-per-cent oxygen, while less severely ill patients are more frequently managed without such therapy.[105]

One would expect a better survival rate in patients who have been hyperventilated, to increase excretion of the excess carbon dioxide being produced by the hypercatabolic muscle (i.e., 3 times the value given in the Radford nomogram). Statistically, however, the opposite appears to be true. The reasons for this paradox are not clear; data obtained from studies of ventilation may be biased, like data of studies of high inspired oxygen concentrations.[105]

Buffers to correct the lactic acidosis have been recommended by many investigators.[83–85,88,100,101,105,223] Survival rates are better in patients who receive sodium bicarbonate than in those who receive trimethamine (THAM). Even sodium bicarbonate does not significantly raise the survival rate above the average of 47 per cent. Assessment of individual cases suggests, however, that partial correction of the *pH* to about 7.2 to 7.3 gives better results than does complete correction to 7.3 to 7.4.[105]

Furosemide is used not only to prevent sodium overload, but also, along with mannitol, helps to dislodge myoglobin casts from the renal tubules. Recommended doses are about 1.0 mg. per kg. of furosemide and 7 to 10 ml. per kg. of 20-per-cent mannitol. The rather poor survival rates associated with the use of these two diuretics has, however, been disappointing. This may be the result of delayed administration of these agents. Once acute renal shutdown has occurred, diuretics should be discontinued and renal dialysis instituted. Thus, although not quite statistically significant, the patients in renal failure seem to have an improved survival when dialysis has been employed.[105]

The treatment of potassium abnormalities in MH crises is similar to their management in acute diabetic coma. The initial hyperkalemia can be corrected with regular insulin in glucose (e.g., 50 units of regular insulin in 50 ml. of 50% glucose in a 70-kg. adult). The subsequent hypokalemia is treated with infusions of potassium chloride. Serum potassium levels should be measured frequently, because the change from a high to a low serum potassium concentration may occur quite suddenly. Survival is slightly (although not statistically significantly) better if both insulin and potassium chloride are infused than if only insulin is given.[105]

There is some controversy over the use of calcium gluconate, which has been employed during a number of MH crises to treat the neurogenic tetany that results from the very low serum calcium concentrations. Exogenous calcium, however, undoubtedly moves in significant quantities into the muscle cells across the damaged sarcolemma and thereby further elevates myoplasmic calcium. This exacerbates the acute catabolic state of the muscle cell. Transient improvement of tetany does occur after calcium infusion, but the overall survival rate, nevertheless, decreases.[105]

Tranquilizers such as chlorpromazine have been employed in a number of patients to accelerate heat loss through vasodilation. They may also play a role by inhibition of catecholamine transmission.[224,225] Use of these agents has been gratifying, particularly because transquilizers are usually employed only in the more desperately ill patients.[105] It is of interest that the survival rate does not decrease following use of other intravenous anesthetics, such as narcotics and barbiturates.[105]

Steroid infusion has also been recommended, because these agents exert a membrane-stabilizing effect.[93] This recommendation is based upon experience with one patient who developed fever following the administration of nitrous oxide on two different occasions. The crises were apparently relieved by the administration of dexamethasone. Subsequently, a muscle fascicle was removed from the patient. The excised muscle developed a greater than normal contracture in the presence of halothane. The contracture was relieved by the addition of dexamethasone. Observations in 290 patients, however, suggest that their use significantly increases mortality.[105]

Catecholamine-like drugs are absolutely contraindicated during an MH reaction, even though the patient may be hypotensive. Use of these agents is associated with a mortality rate of about 85 per cent. These agents further impair the already compromised microcirculation and thus aggravate tissue hypoxia and acidosis. They may also hyperactivate skeletal muscle adenyl cyclase (Fig. 19-11). Experience with beta-blockers such as propranolol is so far inconclusive, possible because of the small sample size.[105]

Treatment of consumption coagulopathy has usually consisted of that recommended by consultant hematologists (e.g., heparin, fresh frozen plasma, platelets, and other clotting factors). This therapy has been ineffective. These agents, however, are usually only given to the most critical cases.

Patients in acute MH crisis should be moved as little as possible, since any physical stimulus tends to convert a ventricular arrhythmia into ventricular fibrillation. A number of arrests in ventricular fibrillation have occurred just when the patient is being moved from the operating table onto the stretcher.

Monitoring should include temperature, blood pressure, pulse and heart rate, central venous pressure, ECG, and frequent determination of blood gases and electrolytes. Evaluation of serum enzymes is necessary only once each day. Urine color and volume must be observed frequently, as long as danger of acute renal failure exists.

Treatment is aided by availability of the following in the operating room: a protocol outlining for each member of the team (anesthesiologist, nurse, orderly, and recovery room nurses) his or her responsibilities; a box containing all necessary emergency equipment and drugs needed to treat MH; ice cold intravenous solutions in the operating room refrigerator; an immediate source of large quantities of crushed ice; and personnel who are aware of the clinical signs of MH, who have studied the contents of the protocol, who know where the MH emergency box, the cold intravenous solutions, and the crushed ice are located, and who are able to work harmoniously together as an effective team.[105]

Careful attention to the details of diagnosis and treatment of acute MH crisis has produced a gratifying reduction in mortality: from 76 per cent before 1965 to 28 per cent after 1972. Thus, malignant hyperthermia is not the lethal syndrome that we previously considered it to be.

REFERENCES

1. Benzinger, T. H., Kitzinger, C., and Pratt, A. W.: The human thermostat. *In* Hardy, D. J. (ed.): Temperature—Its Measurement and Control in Science and Industry. vol. 3. pp. 637–665. New York, Reinhold, 1963.
2. Bligh, J.: Temperature Regulation in Mammals and Other Vertebrates. New York, American Elsevier, 1973.
3. Cooper, K. E., Preston, E., and Veale, W. L.: Effects of atropine, injected into a lateral cerebral ventricle of the rabbit, on fevers due to i.v. leucocyte pyrogen and hypothalamic and intraventricular injection of PGE$_1$. J. Physiol. (Lond), *254*:729, 1976.
4. Hensel, H., and Zotterman, Y.: The response of the cold receptors to constant cooling. Acta Physiol. Scand., *22*:96, 1951.
5. Boulant, J. A., and Hardy, J. D.: The effect of spinal and skin temperatures on the firing rate and the thermosensitivity of preoptic neurones. J. Physiol. (Lond), *240*:639, 1974.
6. Boulant, J. A.: The effect of firing rate on preoptical neuronal thermosensitivity. J. Physiol. (Lond), *240*:661, 1974.
7. Jell, R. M.: Responses of rostral hypothalamic neurones to peripheral temperatures and to amines. J. Physiol. (Lond), *240*:295, 1974.

8. Lomax, P., Schonbaum, E., and Jacobs, J.: Temperature Regulation and Drug Action. Basel, Karger, 1975.

9. Benzinger, T. H., Pratt, A. W., and Kitzinger, C.: The thermostatic control of human metabolic heat production. Proc. Natl. Acad. Sci. U.S.A., 47:730, 1961.

10. Cranston, W. I., Duff, G. W., Hellman, R. F., et al.: Thermoregulation in rabbits during fever. J. Physiol. (Lond), 257:767, 1976.

11. Clark, W. G., and Cumby, H. R.: Antagonism by antipyretics of the hyperthermic effect of a prostaglandin precursor, sodium arachidonate, in the cat. J. Physiol. (Lond), 257:581, 1976.

12. Myers, R. D., and Yaksh, T. L.: Thermoregulation around a new 'set-point' established in the monkey by altering the ratio of sodium to calcium ions within the hypothalamus. J. Physiol., 218:609, 1971.

13. Cabanal, M., and Massonet, B.: Temperature regulation during fever. Change of set-point or change of gain? Tentative answer from behavioural studies in man. J. Physiol. (Lond), 238:561, 1974.

14. Lin, M. T., and Chai, C. Y.: Effect of sodium acetylsalicylate on body temperature of monkeys during heat exposure. J. Pharmacol. Exp. Ther., 194:165, 1975.

15. Benzinger, T. H.: Heat regulation: homeostasis of central temperature in man. Physiol. Rev., 49:671, 1969.

16. Aronsohn, E., and Sach, J.: Die beziehungen des gehirns zur korperwarme and zum fieber. Arch. Ges. Physiol., 37:232, 1885.

17. Isenschmidt, R., and Krehl, L.: Uber den einfluss des gehirns auf die warmeregulation. Arch. Exptl. Pathol. Pharmakol., 70:109, 1912.

18. Barbour, H. G.: Die wirkung unmittelbarer erwarmung and abkuhlung der warmezentra auf die korperperatur. Arch. Exptl. Pathol. Pharmakol., 70:1, 1912.

19. Ranson, S. W.: The hypothalamus as a thermostat regulating body temperature. Psychosomat. Med., 1:186, 1939.

20. Hensel, H., and Zotterman, Y.: Quantitative beziehunges zwischen der entladung einzelner katlefasern und der temperatur. Acta Physiol. Scand., 23:291, 1951.

21. Hensel, H., and Boman, K. K. A.: Afferent impulses in cutaneous sensory nerves in human subjects. J. Neurophysiol., 23:564, 1960.

22. von Euler, C.: Physiology and pharmacology of temperature regulation. Pharmacol. Rev., 13:361, 1961.

23. Hardy, J. D.: Physiology of temperature regulation. Physiol. Rev., 41:521, 1961.

24. Belding, H. S., and Hertig, B. A.: Sweating and body temperatures following abrupt changes in envrionmental temperature. J. Appl. Physiol., 17:103, 1962.

25. Bayliss, L. E., Dicker, S. E., and Eggleton, M. G.: Some factors concerned in temperature regulation in man. J. Physiol. (Lond.), 172:8P, 1964.

26. Feldberg, W., and Myers, R. D.: Effects of temperature of amines injected into the cerebral ventricles. A new concept of temperature regulation. J. Physiol. (Lond.), 173:226, 1964.

27. Adamsons, K., Jr., and Towell, M. E.: Thermal homeostasis in the fetus and newborn. Anesthesiology, 26:531, 1965.

28. Hall, J. F., and Klemm, F. K.: Thermoregulatory responses to disparate thermal environments. Fed. Proc., 26:556, 1967.

29. Myers, R. D., and Yaksh, T. L.: Thermoregulation around a new "set-point" established in the monkey by altering the ratio of sodium to calcium ions within the hypothalamus. J. Physiol. (Lond.), 218:609, 1971.

30. Hanegan, J. L., and Williams, W. A.: Brain calcium: role in temperature regulation. Science, 181:663, 1973.

31. Cabanac, M., and Hardy, J. D.: Effect of temperature and pyrogen on unit activity in the rabit's brain stem. Fed. Proc., 26:555, 1967.

32. Eisenman, J. S.: Pyrogen induced changes in thermoresponsiveness of septal, preoptic and hypothalamic neurons. Physiologist, 10:160, 1967.

33. Wit, A., and Wang, S. C.: Temperature-sensitive neurons in preoptic/anterior hypothalamic region: actions of pyrogen and acetylsalicylate. Am. J. Physiol., 215:1160, 1968.

34. Nakayama, T., and Hovi, T.: Effects of anesthetic and pyrogen on thermally sensitive neurons in the brainstem. J. Appl. Physiol., 34:351, 1973.

35. Myers, R. D., and Tytell, M.: Fever: reciprocal shift in brain sodium to calcium ratio as the set-point temperature rises. Science, 178:765, 1972.

36. Wyndham, C. H., Williams, C. G., and Loots, H.: Reactions to cold. J. Appl. Physiol., 24:282, 1968.

37. Wyndham, C. H., Ward, J. S., Strydom, N. B., et al.: Physiologic reactions of caucasian and Bantu males on acute cold exposure. J. Appl. Physiol., 19:583, 1964.

38. Downey, J. A., Chiodi, H. P., and Darling, R. C.: Central temperature regulation in the spinal man. J. Appl. Physiol., 22:91, 1967.

39. Szyfelbein, S. K., and Ryan, J. F.: Thermoregulatory responses in burned children. International Congress on Burn Injuries, Buenos Aires, 1974.

40. Thauer, R.: Der mechanismus der warmeregulation. Ergeb. Physiol., 41:607, 1939.

41. Benzinger, T. H.: The diminution of thermoregulatory sweating during cold-reception at the skin. Proc. Natl. Acad. Sci. U.S.A., 47:1683, 1961.

42. Ryan, J. F., Wilson, R. S., Goudsouzian, N. G., et al.: Body temperature and oxygen consumption in children during anaesthesia. Br. J. Anaesth. [In Press].

43. Steward, D. J.: Oxygen consumption during anesthesia in infants. 14th Clinical Conference in Pediatric Anesthesiology, Los Angeles, January 24, 1976.

44. Dawkins, M. J. R., and Scopes, J. W.: Non-shivering thermogenesis and brown adipose tissue in the human newborn infant. Nature, 206:201, 1965.

45. Owen-Thomas, J. B., Meade, F., Jones, R. S. et al.: The measurement of oxygen uptake in infants with congenital heart disease during general anaesthesia and intermittent positive pressure ventilation. Br. J. Anaesth., 43:746, 1971.

46. Nisbet, H. I. A., Dobbison, T. L., Thomas, T. A., et al.: Oxygen uptake in ventilated children during methoxyflurane anaesthesia. Can. Anaesth. Soc. J., 20:334, 1973.

47. Jones, R. S., Meade, F., and Owen-Thomas, J. B.: Oxygen and nitrous oxide uptake during general anaesthesia for cardiac catheterization in infants with congenital heart disease. Br. Heart J., 34:52, 1972.

48. Britt, B. A., and Kalow, W.: Malignant hyperthermia, a statistical review. Can. Anaesth. Soc. J., 17:293, 1970.

49. Ryan, J. F., and Papper, E. M.: Malignant fever during and following anesthesia. Anesthesiology, 32:196, 1970.

50. Ryan, J. F., Donlon, J. V., Malt, R. A., et al.: Cardiopulmonary bypass in the treatment of malignant hyperthermia. N. Engl. J. Med., *290*:1121, 1974.

51. Roe, C. F., Goldberg, M. J., Blair, C. S., et al.: The influence of body temperature on early postoperative oxygen consumption. Surgery, *60*:85, 1966.

52. Morris, R. H., and Wilkey, B. R.: The effects of ambient temperature on patient temperature during surgery not involving body cavities. Anesthesiology, *32*:102, 1970.

53. Rackow, H., and Salanitre, E.: Modern concepts in pediatric anesthesiology. Anesthesiology, *30*:208, 1969.

54. Goudsouzian, N. G., Morris, R. H., and Ryan, J. F.: The effects of a warming blanket on the maintenance of body temperature in anesthetized infants and children. Anesthesiology, *39*:351, 1973.

55. Clark, R. E., Orkin, L. R., and Rovenstein, E. A.: Body temperature studies in anesthetized man. Effect of environmental temperature, humidity and anesthesia system. J.A.M.A., *154*:311, 1954.

56. Linton, C. D.: Sweating and anesthesia: a consideration of cause and effects. Anesthesiology, *22*:56, 1961.

57. Berry, F. A., and Hughes-Davies, D. I.: Method of increasing the humidity and temperature of the inspired gases in the infant circle system. Anesthesiology, *37*:456, 1972.

58. Tovell, R. M., Lion, K. S., Lovell, B. S.: Recent advances in inhalation therapy utilizing high humidity. Anesth. Analg., *40*:105, 1961.

59. Pflug, A. G., Aasheim, G. M., Foster, C., et al.: Prevention of post-anaesthetia shivering. Can. Anaesth. Soc. J., *25*:43, 1978.

60. Avery, M. E., Galina, M., and Nachman, R.: Mist therapy. Pediatrics, *39*:160, 1967.

61. Sara, C., and Currie, T.: Humidification by neubulization. Med. J. Aust., *1*:174, 1965.

62. Smith, R. M.: Temperature monitoring and regulation. Pediatr. Clin. North. Am., *16*:643, 1969.

63. Friedman, F., Adams, F. H., and Emmanouilides, G.: Regulation of body temperature of premature infants with low energy radiant heat. J. Pediatr. *70*:270, 1967.

64. Arima, E., and Fonkalsrud, E. W.: The relationship of intestinal adhesions to infrared heating lamp exposure. J. Pediatr. Surg., *10*:231, 1975.

65. Dick, W., Kreuscher, H., and Luhker, D.: Prevention of heat loss during anesthesia and operation in the newborn baby and small infant. Acta Anaesthesiol. Scand. *37*[Suppl.]:134, 1970.

66. Boyan, C. P.: Cold or warm blood for massive transfusions? Ann. Surg., *160*:282, 1964.

67. Benzinger, M.: Tympanic thermometry in surgery and anesthesia. J.A.M.A., *209*:1207, 1969.

68. Whitby, J. D., and Dunkin, L. J.: Cerebral, oesophageal and nasopharyngeal temperatures. Br. J. Anaesth., *43*:673, 1971.

69. Roe, C. F.: Effect of bowel exposure on body temperature during surgical operations. Am. J. Surg., *122*:13, 1971.

70. Newbower, R. S., Cooper, J. B., Ryan, J. F., et al.: Monitoring temperature: a new method (abstr). p. 391. American Society of Anesthesiologists, Annual Meeting, 1974.

71. Marcus, P.: Some effects of cooling and heating areas of the head and neck on body temperature measurement in the ear. Aerosp. Med., *44*:397, 1973.

72. Marcus, P.: Some effects of radiant heating of the head on body temperature measurement at the ear. Aerosp. Med., *44*:403, 1973.

73. Bigler, J. A., and McQuiston, W. O.: Body temperatures during anesthesia in infants and children. J.A.M.A., *146*:551, 1951.

74. France, G. G.: Hypothermia in the newborn: body temperatures following anaesthesia. Br. J. Anaesth., *29*:390, 1957.

75. Harrison, G. G., Bull, A. B., and Schmidt, H. J.: Temperature changes in children during general anaesthesia. Br. J. Anaesth., *32*:60, 1960.

76. Hercus, V.: Temperature changes during thoracotomy in children, infants and the newborn. Br. J. Anaesth., *32*:476, 1960.

77. Calvert, D. G.: Inadvertent hypothermia in paediatric surgery and a method for its prevention. Anaesthesia, *17*:29, 1962.

78. Farman, J. V.: Heat loss in infants undergoing surgery in air-conditioned theatres. Br. J. Anaesth., *34*:543, 1962.

79. Bennett, E. J., Patel, K. P., and Grundy, E. M.: Neonatal temperature and surgery. Anesthesiology, *46*:303, 1977.

80. Epstein, R. A.: Humidification during positive-pressure ventilation in infants. Anesthesiology, *35*:532, 1971.

81. Roe, C. F.: Benign postoperative fever. Surg. Forum, *21*:65, 1970.

82. Modell, J. H.: Septicemia as a cause of immediate postoperative hyperthermia. Anesthesiology, *27*:329, 1966.

83. Gordon, R. A., Britt, B. A., and Kalow, W. (eds.): International Symposium on Malignant Hyperthermia. Springfield, Charles C. Thomas, 1973.

84. Henschel, E. O. (ed.): Malignant Hyperthermia: Current Concepts New York, Appleton-Century-Crofts, 1977.

85. Symposium on Malignant Hyperthermia, Hiroshima J. Anesth., *7*(2, 3, 4):1971.

86. Jones, E. W., Kerr, D. D., and Nelson, T. E.: Malignant hyperthermia—observations in Poland China pigs. *In* Gordon, R. A., Britt, B. A., Kalow, W. (Eds.): International Symposium on Malignant Hyperthermia. pp. 198–207. Springfield, Charles C. Thomas, 1973.

87. Jones, E. W., Nelson, T. E., Anderson, I. L., et al.: Malignant hyperthermia of swine. Anesthesiology, *36*:42, 1972.

88. Britt, B. A.: Malignant hyperthermia. Modern Medicine of Canada, June, 1976.

89. Denborough, M. A., Forster, J. F. A., Lovell, R. R. H., et al.: Anaesthetic deaths in a family. Br. J. Anaesth., *34*:395, 1962.

90. Britt, B. A., Kwong, F. H-F., and Endrenyi, L.: The clinical and laboratory features of malignant hyperthermia management—a review. *In* Henschel, E. O. (ed.): Malignant hyperthermia syndrome. pp. 9–45. New York, Appleton-Century-Croft, 1977.

91. Britt, B. A., Locher, W. G., and Kalow, W.: Hereditary aspects of malignant hyperthermia. Can. Anaesth. Soc. J., *16*:89, 1969.

92. Kalow, W., Britt, B. A., and Richter, A.: Individuality in human skeletal muscle as revealed by studies on malignant hyperthermia. Can. J. Genet. Cytol., *18*:565, 1976.

93. Ellis, F. R., Clarke, I. M. C., Appleyard, T. N., et al.: Malignant hyperpyrexia induced by nitrous oxide and treated with dexamethasone. Br. Med. J., *4*:270, 1974.

94. Britt, B. A., Webb, G., and Leduc, C.: Mild malignant hyperthermia induced by curare. Can. Anaesth. Soc. J., *21*:371, 1974.

95. Britt, B. A., and Kalow, W.: Malignant hyperthermia: a statistical review. Can. Anaesth. Soc. J., *17*:293, 1970.

96. Wingard, D. W.: Malignant hyperthermia—acute stress syndrome of the human? In Henschel, E. O. (ed.): Malignant Hyperthermia: Current Concepts. pp. 79–98. New York, Appleton-Century-Croft, 1977.

97. Kalow, W., and Britt, B. A.: Drugs causing rigidity in malignant hyperthermia. Lancet, *2*:390, 1973.

98. Davies, D. D. Hypertonic syndrome associated with suxamethonium administration. Br. J. Anaesth., *42*:656, 1970.

99. Schweizer, O., Howland, W. S., Ryan, G. M., et al.: Hyperprexia in the operative and immediate postoperative period. Anesth. Analg., *50*:906, 1971.

100. Bergmann, H., and Blauhut, B. (eds.): Maligne Hyperthermie Akupunktur Biomedizinische Technick Abdominelle Intensivtherapie. Berlin, Springer-Verlag, 1975.

101. Beldavs, J., Small, V., Cooper, D. A., et al.: Postoperative malignant hyperthermia: a case report. Can. Anaesth. Soc. J., *18*:202, 1971.

102. Harrison, G. G., Berman, M. C., Hickman, R., et al.: Anaesthetic induced malignant hyperpyrexia—some observations of the syndrome in Landrace pigs. p. 158. Australasian Congress of Anaesthesiology, Melbourne, Australia, 1970.

103. Kelstrup, J., Reske-Nielsen, E., Haase, J., et al.: Malignant hyperthermia in a family: a clinical and serological investigation of 139 members. Acta Anaesth. Scand., *18*:58, 1974.

104. Britt, B. A.: Malignant hyperthermia: aetiology and pathophysiology. Presented at the VI World Congress of Anesthesiology, Mexico City, 1976.

105. Britt, B. A., Kwong, F. H-F, and Endrenyi, L.: Management of malignant hyperthermia susceptible (MHS) patients—a review. In Henschel, E. O. (ed.): Malignant Hyperthermia: Current Concepts. pp. 63–78. New York, Appleton-Century-Croft, 1977.

106. Kalow, W., Britt, B. A., Terreau, M. E., et al.: Metabolic error of muscle metabolism after recovery from malignant hyperthermia. Lancet, *2*:895, 1970.

107. Britt, B. A., Kalow, W., Gordon, A., et al.: Malignant hyperthermia: an investigation of five patients. Can. Anaesth. Soc. J., *20*:431, 1973.

108. Moulds, R. F. W., and Denborough, M. A.: Biochemical basis of malignant hyperpyrexia. Br. Med. J., *2*:245, 1974.

109. Nelson, T. E., Bedell, D. M., and Jones, E. W.: Porcine malignant hyperthermia: effects of temperature and extracellular calcium concentration on halothane-induced contracture of susceptible skeletal muscle. Anesthesiology, *42*:301, 1975.

110. Ellis, K. O., and Bryant, S. H.:Excitation-contraction uncoupling in skeletal muscle by dantrolene sodium. Naumyn-Schmiedebergs Arch. Pharmacol. *274*:107, 1972.

111. Ellis, K. O., and Carpenter, J. F.: Studies on the mechanism of action of dantrolene sodium, a skeletal muscle relaxant. Nauyn-Schmiedeberg's Arch. Pharmacol., *275*:83, 1972.

112. Inesi, G., and Watanabe, S.: Temperature dependence of ATP hydrolysis and calcium uptake by fragmented sarcoplasmic membranes. Arch. Biochem. Biophys., *121*:665, 1967.

113. Johnson, P. N., and Inesi, G.: The effect of methylxanthines and local anaesthetics on fragmented sarcoplasmic reticulum. J. Pharmacol. Exp. Therap., *169*:308, 1969.

114. Thorpe, W., and Seeman, P.: Drug-induced contracture of muscle. In Gordon, R. A., Britt, B. A., and Kalow, W. (eds.): International Symposium on Malignant Hyperthermia. pp. 152–162. Springfield, Charles C. Thomas, 1973.

115. Harrison, G. G.: Control of the malignant hyperprexic syndrome in MHS swine by dantrolene sodium. Br. J. Anaesth., *47*:62, 1975.

116. Gronert, G. A., Milde, J. H., and Theye, R. A.: Dantrolene in porcine malignant hyperthermia. Anesthesiology, *44*:488, 1976.

117. Anderson, I. L., and Jones, E. W.: Porcine malignant hyperthermia: effect of dantrolene sodium on in-vitro halothane-induced contraction of susceptible muscle. Anesthesiology, *44*:57, 1976.

118. Britt, B. A., Endrenyi, L., and Cadman, D. L.: Calcium uptake into muscle of pigs susceptible to malignant hyperthermia: in vitro and in vivo studies with and without halothane. Br. J. Anaesth., *47*:650, 1975.

119. Ryan, J. F., Donlon, J. V., Malt, R. A., et al.: Cardiopulmonary bypass in the treatment of malignant hyperthermia. N. Engl. J. Med., *290*:1121, 1974.

120. Porter, K. R., and Franzini-Armstrong, C.: The sarcoplasmic reticulum. Sci. Am., *212*:73, 1965.

121. Bianchi, C. P.: Cell calcium and malignant hyperthermia. In Gordon, R. A., Britt, B. A., and Kalow, W. (eds.): International Symposium on Malignant Hyperthermia. pp. 147–151. Springfield, Charles C. Thomas, 1973.

122. Britt, B. A., Endrenyi, L., Cadman, D. L., et al.: Porcine malignant hyperthermia: effects of halothane on mitochondrial respiration and calcium accumulation. Anesthesiology, *42*:292, 1975.

123. Green, D. E.: The mitochondrion. Sci. Am., *210*:63, 1964.

124. Green, D. E., and Hatefi, Y.: The mitochondrion and biochemical machines. Science, *133*:13, 1961.

125. Chance, B., Mela, L., and Harris, E. J.: Interaction of ion movments and local anesthetics in mitochondrial membranes. Fed. Proc., *27*:902, 1968.

126. Lehninger, A. L.: The Mitochondrion. New York, W. A. Benjamin Inc., 1965.

127. Batra, S.: The effect of drugs on calcium uptake and calcium release by mitochondria and sarcoplasmic reticulum of frog skeletal muscle. Biochem. Pharmacol., *23*:89, 1974.

128. Dransfeld, H., Greeff, K., Schorn, A., et al.: Calcium uptake in mitochondria and vesicles of heart and skeletal muscle in presence of potassium, sodium, k-strophanthin and pentobarbital. Biochem. Pharmacol., *18*:1335, 1969.

129. McIntosch, D., and Berman, M. C.: Neutral lipid and phospholipid composition of normal and myopathic skeletal muscle of pigs. S. Afr. Med. J., *48*:1221, 1974.

130. Pollock, R. A., and Watson, R. L.: Malignant hyperthermia associated with hypocalcemia. Anesthesiology, *34*:188, 1971.

131. Solomons, C. C., and Myers, C. N.: Hyperthermia of

osteogenesis imperfecta and its relationship to malignant hyperthermia. *In* Gordon, R. A., Britt, B. A., and Kalow, W. (eds.): International Symposium on Malignant Hyperthermia. pp. 319–330. Springfield, Charles C. Thomas, 1973.

132. Hall, G. M., Lucke, J. N., and Lister, D.: Treatment of porcine malignant hyperthermia. A review based on experimental studies. Anaesthesia, 30:308, 1975.

133. Bowman, W. C., and Nott, M. W.: Actions of sympathomimetic amines and their antagonists on skeletal muscle. Pharmacol. Rev., 21:27, 1969.

134. Jenkinson, D. H.: Classification and properties of peripheral adrenergic receptors. Br. Med. Bull., 29:142, 1973.

135. Mayer, S. E., and Stull, J. T.: Cyclic AMP in skeletal muscle. Ann. N.Y. Acad. Sci., 185:433, 1971.

136. Steer, M. L., Atlas, D., and Levitzki, A.: Inter-relations between β-adrenergic receptors, adenylate cyclase and calcium. N. Engl. J. Med., 292:409, 1975.

137. Severson, D. L., Drummond, G. E., and Sulakhe, P. V.: Adenylate cyclase in skeletal muscle. J. Biol. Chem., 247:2949, 1972.

138. Sutherland, E. W., Rall, R. W., and Menon, T.: Adenyl cyclase. I. Distribution, preparation and properties. J. Biol. Chem., 237:1220, 1962.

139. Entman, M. L., Levey, G. S., and Epstein, S. E.: Demonstration of adenyl cyclase activity in canine cardiac sarcoplasmic reticulum. Biochem. Biophys. Res. Comm., 35:728, 1969.

140. Wray, H. L., Gray, R. R., and Olsson, R. A.: Cyclic adenosine 3',5'-monophosphate-stimulated protein kinase and a substrate associated with cardiac sarcoplasmic reticulum. J. Biol. Chem., 248:1496, 1973.

141. Rabinowitz, M., Desalles, L., Meisler, J., et al.: Distribution of adenyl cyclase activity in rabbit skeletal muscle fractions. Biochim. Biophys. Acta, 97:29, 1965.

142. Drummond, G. I., Valdares, J. R. E., and Duncan, L.: Cardiac phosphorylase and phosphorylase kinase. *In* Paul, W. M., Daniel, E. E., Kay, C. M., et al. (eds.): Muscle, pp. 111–124. Oxford, Pergamon Press, 1965.

143. Ozawa, E., and Ebashi, S.: Requirements of Ca ion for the stimulating effect of cyclic 3'5'-AMP on muscle phosphorylase b kinase. J. Biochem., 62:285, 1967.

144. Ozawa, E., Hosoi, K., and Ebashi, S.: Reversible stimulation of muscle phosphorylase b kinase by low concentrations of calcium ions. J. Biochem., 61:531, 1967.

145. Krebs, E. G., Graves, D. J., and Fischer, E. H.: Factors affecting the activity of muscle phosphorylase b kinase. J. Biol. Chem., 234:2867, 1959.

146. Krebs, E. G., DeLange, R. J., Kemp, R. G., et al.: Metabolic effects of catecholamines B. Activation of skeletal muscle phosphorylase. Pharmacol. Rev., 18:163, 1966.

147. Sutherland, E. W., and Rall, T. W.: The relation of adenosine-3—adenosine-3',5'-phosphate and phosphorylase to the actions of catecholamines and other hormones. Pharmacol. Rev., 12:265, 1960.

148. Sandow, A.: Skeletal muscle. Ann. Rev. Physiol., 32:1040, 1970.

149. Hoyle, G.: How is muscle turned on and off? Sci. Am., 222:85, 1970.

150. Hasselbach, W.: Relaxing factor and the relaxation of muscle. Prog. Biophys. Mol. Biol., 14:167, 1964.

151. Huxley, H. E.: Structural evidence concerning the mechanism of contraction in striated muscle. *In* Paul, W. M., Daniel, E. E., Kay, C. M., et al. (eds.): pp. 3–28. Oxford, Pergamon Press, 1965.

152. Mitchelson, K. R.: Investigations of Malignant Hyperprexia. [Unpublished Ph.D. Thesis] University of Melbourne, Australia, 1974.

153. Perry, S. V.: Muscle proteins in contraction. *In* Paul, W. M., Daniel, E. E., Kay, C. M., et al. (eds.) Muscle. pp. 29–42. Oxford, Pergamon, Press, 1965.

154. Perry, S. V.: The role of myosin in muscular contraction. Aspects of Cell Motility, 22:1, 1968.

155. Ebashi, S.: Calcium binding activity of vesicular relaxing factor. J. Biochem., 50:236, 1961.

156. Weber, A., and Winicur, S.: Dependence of superprecipitation of actomyosin on the concentration of ionized calcium. Fed. Proc., 20:300, 1961.

157. Weber, A., and Herz, R.: Requirement for calcium in the synaeresis of myofibrils. Biochem. Biophys. Res. Comm., 6:364, 1961.

158. McCarl, R. L., Margossian, S. S., Jackman, L. M., et al.: Characterization of rat heart myosin. II. Enzymatic properties. Biochemistry, 8:3659, 1969.

159. Winegrad, S.: The location of muscle calcium with respect to the myofibrils. J. Gen. Physiol., 48:997, 1965.

160. Yasui, B., Fuchs, F., and Briggs, F. M.: The role of the sulfhydryl groups of tropomyosin and troponin in the calcium control of actomyosin contractility. J. Biol. Chem., 243:735, 1968.

161. Han, M. H., and Benson, E. S.: Conformational changes in troponin induced by Ca++. Biochem. Biophys. Res. Comm., 38:378, 1970.

162. Wakabayashi, T., and Ebashi, S.: Reversible change in physical state of troponin induced by calcium ion. J. Biochem., 64:731, 1968.

163. Ebashi, S., Ebashi, F., and Kodama, A.: Troponin as the Ca++ receptive protein in the contractile system. J. Biochem., 62:137, 1967.

164. Murray, J. M., and Weber, A.: The cooperative action of muscle proteins. Sci. Am., 230:59, 1974.

165. Fuchs, F.: Thermal inactivation of the calcium regulatory mechanism of human skeletal muscle actomyosin: a possible contributing factor in the rigidity of malignant hyperthermia. Anesthesiology, 42:584, 1975.

166. Lehninger, A. L.: Physiology of mitochondria. *In* Gaebler, O. H. (ed.): Enzymes, Units of Biological Structure and Function. New York, Academic Press, 1956.

167. Lehninger, A. L.: Biochemistry. Part II. New York, Worth Publishers, Inc. 1970.

168. Rosenberg, H., and Haugaard, N.: The effects of halothane on metabolism and calcium uptake in mitochondria of the rat liver and brain. Anesthesiology, 39:44, 1973.

169. Thaker, J. H., Wrogemann, K., and Blanchaer, M. C.: Effect of ruthenium red on oxidative phosphorylation and the calcium and magnesium content of skeletal muscle mitochondria of normal and bio 14.6 dystrophic hamsters. Biochim. Biophys. Acta, 314:8, 1973.

170. Chance, B.: The energy-linked reaction of calcium with mitochondria. J. Biol. Chem., 240:2729, 1965.

171. Rasmussen, H.: Mitochondrial ion transport: mechanism and physiological significance. Fed. Proc., 25:903, 1966.

172. Lohmann, K.: Uber die enzymatische aufspeltung der kreatinphosphosaure; zugleich ein beitrag zum chemis-

mus der muskelkontraktion. Biochem. Zeit., *271*:264, 1934.

173. Berman, M. C., and Kench, J. E.: Biochemical features of malignant hyperthermia in landrace pigs. *In* Gordon, R. A., Britt, B. A., and Kalow, W. (eds.): International Symposium on Malignant Hyperthermia, pp. 287–306. Charles C. Thomas, 1973.

174. Harrison, G. G., and Verburg, C.: Erythrocyte osmotic fragility in hyperthermia-susceptible swine. Br. J. Anaesth., *45*:131, 1973.

175. La Cour, D., Juul-Jensen, P., and Reske-Nielsen, E.: Malignant hyperthermia during anaesthesia. Acta Anaesth. Scand., *15*:299, 1971.

176. Harrison, J. E.: I.V.N.A.A. experience with idiopathic osteoporosis and with osteoporosis secondary to hyperthyroidism and malignant hyperthermia. Presented at the 2nd Conference on I.V.N.A.A., Glasglow, Scotland, 1976.

177. Britt, B. A., Endrenyi, L., Peters, P. L., et al.: Screening of malignant hyperthermic susceptible families by CPK measurement and other clinical investigations. Can. Anaesth. Soc. J., *23*:263, 1976.

178. Denborough, M. A., Hudson, M. C., Forster, J. F. A., et al.: Biochemical changes in malignant hyperpyrexia. Lancet, *2*:1137, 1970.

179. Isaacs, H., and Barlow, M. B.: The genetic background to malignant hyperpyrexia revealed by serum creatine phosphokinase estimations in asymptomatic relatives. Br. J. Anaesth., *42*:1073, 1970.

180. King, J. O., Denborough, M. A., and Zapf, P. W.: Inheritance of malignant hyperpyrexia. Lancet, *1*:365, 1972.

181. Aldrete, J. A., Padfield, A., and Solomons, C. C.: Possible predicitve tests for malignant hyperthermia during anesthesia. J.A.M.A., *215*:1465, 1971.

182. Barlow, M. B., and Isaacs, H.: Malignant hyperpyrexial deaths in a family. Reports of three cases. Br. J. Anaesth., *42*:1072, 1970.

183. Parikh, R. K., and Thomson, W. H. S.: Malignant hyperthermia: a fatal case and his family. Br. J. Anaesth., *44*:742, 1972.

184. Kyei-Mensah, K., Lockwood, R., Tyrell, J. H., et al.: Malignant hyperpyrexia: a study of a family. Br. J. Anaesth., *43*:811, 1971.

185. Zsigmond, E. K., Starkweather, W. H., Duboff, G. S., et al.: CPK and malignant hyperthermia. Anesth. Analg., *51*:220, 1972.

186. Larard, D. G., Rice, C. P., Robinson, R. W., et al.: Malignant hyperthermia: a study of an affected family. Br. J. Anaesth., *44*:93, 1972.

187. Ellis, F. R., Keaney, N. P., and Harriman, D. G. F.: Histopathological and neuropharmacological aspects of malignant hyperpyrexia. Proc. R. Soc. Med., *66*:66, 1973.

188. Hess, J. W., MacDonald, R. P., Frederick, R. J., et al.: Serum creatine phosphokinase (CPK) activity in disorders of heart and skeletal muscle. Ann. Intern. Med., *61*:1015, 1964.

189. Meltzer, H.: Muscle enzyme release in the acute psychoses. Arch. Gen. Psychiat., *21*:102, 1969.

190. King, J. O., and Zapf, P.: A review of the value of creatine phosphokinase estimations in clinical medicine. Med. J. Aust., *1*:699, 1972.

191. Pearce, J. M. S., Pennington, R. J., and Walter, J. N.: Scrum enzyme studies in muscle disease. Part II. Serum creatine kinase activity in muscular dystrophy and other myopathic and neuropathic disorders. J. Neurol. Neurosurg. Psychiat., *27*:96, 1964.

192. Williams, E. R., and Bruford, A.: Creatine phosphokinase in motor neurone disease. Clin. Chim. Acta, *69*:53, 1967.

193. Cao, A., DeVirgiliis, S., Lippi, C., et al.: Creatine kinase isoenzymes in serum of children with neurological disorders. Clin. Chim. Acta., *23*:475, 1969.

194. Sherwin, A. L., Norris, J. W., and Bulcke, J. A.: Spinal fluid creatine kinase in neurological disease. Neurology, *19*:993, 1969.

195. Graig, F. A., and Smith, C. J.: Serum creatine phosphokinase activity in altered thyroid states. J. Clin. Endocrinol., *25*:723, 1965.

196. Nygren, A.: Muscular involvement in acutely intoxicated alcoholics revealed by elevated serum CPK activity. Opusc. Med. Bd., *10*:329, 1965.

197. Meltzer, H. Y., and Margulies, P.: Release of creatine phosphokinase from muscle. I. Effect of polymyxin B., compound 48/80, and serotonin. Biochem. Pharmacol., *20*:3501, 1971.

198. Bernhardt, D., and Schiller, H.: Maligne hyperthermie in allgemeinanaesthesie. Abnorme histochemische und elektronenoptische muskelbefunde in kombination mit pathologischen serum-CPK-wertern als beweis fur das vorliegen einer primaren myopathic. Anaesthesist, *22*:367, 1973.

199. Addis, P. B., Britt, B. A., Henderson, A. R., et al.: CPK isoenzymes in human and porcine subjects susceptible to malignant hyperthermia. *In* Aldrete, J. A., and Britt, B. A. (eds.): Malignant Hyperthermia: Second Inernational Symposium on Malignant Hyperthermia. New York, Grune & Stratton, 1978.

200. Britt, B. A., McComas, A. J., Endrenyi, L., et al.: Motor unit counting and the caffeine contracture test in malignant hyperthermia. Anesthesiology, *47*:49, 1977.

201. Moulds, R. F. W.: Studies on Malignant Hyperpyrexia. [Unpublished Ph.D. Thesis] University of, Melbourne, Australia, 1974.

202. Moulds, R. F. W., and Denborough, M. A.: Procaine in malignant hyperpyrexia. Br. Med. J., *4*:526, 1972.

203. Britt, B. A., Endrenyi, L., Kalow, W., et al.: The ATP depletion test: comparison with the caffeine contracture test as a method of diagnosing malignant hyperthermia susceptibility. Can. Anaesth. Soc. J. *23*:624, 1976.

204. Harrison, G. G., Saunders, S. J., Biebuyck, J. F., et al.: Anaesthetic-induced malignant hyperpyrexia and a method for its prediction. Br. J. Anaesth., *41*:844, 1969.

205. Isaacs, H., and Heffron, J. J. A.: Morphological and biochemical defects in muscles of human carriers of the malignant hyperthermia syndrome. Br. J. Anaesth., *47*:475, 1975.

206. Denborough, M. A., Dennett, X., and Anderson, R. M.: Central-core disease and malignant hyperpyrexia. Br. Med. J., *1*:272, 1973.

207. Harriman, D. G. F., Sumner, D. W., and Ellis, F. R.: Malignant hyperpyrexia myopathy. Q. J. Med., New Series XLII, 639, 1973.

208. LaCour, D., Juul-Jensen, P., and Reske-Nielsen, E.: Central and peripheral mechanisms in malignant hyperthermia. *In* Gordon, R. A., Britt, B. A., Kalow, W. (eds.): International Symposium on Malignant Hyperthermia. pp. 380–386. Springfield, Charles C. Thomas, 1973.

209. Samulska, H. M., Samala, R., and Noble, W. H.: Unintended exposure to halothane in surgical patients: halothane wash-out studies. Can. Anaesth. Soc. J., *19*:35, 1972.
210. Putney, J. W., and Biachi, C. P.: Effect of dantrolene on E-C coupling in skeletal muscle. Fed. Proc., *32*:772, 1973.
211. Ellis, K. O., and Carpenter, J. F.: The effects of dantrolene sodium (F-440) on skeletal muscle. Fed. Proc., *32*:772, 1973.
212. Butterfield, J. L., and Ellis, K. O.: Effects of dantrolene sodium, a skeletal muscle relaxant, on the contractility of cardiac and smooth muscle. Fed. Proc., *32*:772, 1973.
213. Chyatte, S. B., and Birdsong, J. H.: The use of dantrolene sodium in disorders of the central nervous system. S. Med. J., *64*:830, 1971.
214. Gelenberg, A. J., and Poskanzer, D. C.: The effect of dantrolene sodium on spasticity in multiple sclerosis. Neurology, *23*:1313, 1973.
215. Chyatte, S. B., Birdsong, J. H., and Roberson, D. L.: Dantrolene sodium in athetoid cerebral palsy. Arch. Phys. Med. Rehab., *54*:365, 1973.
216. Bianchi, C. P., and Bolton, T. C.: Action of local anaesthetics on coupling systems in muscle. J. Pharmacol. Exp. Therap., *157*:388, 1967.
217. Fozzard, H. A.: Excitation-contraction coupling and digitalis. Circulation, *47*:5, 1973.
218. Koch-Weser, J.: Mechanism of digitalis action on the heart. N. Engl. J. Med., *277*:469, 1967.
219. Kerr, D. D., Jones, E. W., Nelson, T. E., et al.: Treatment of malignant hyperthermia in swine. Anesth. Analg., *52*:734, 1973.
220. Gatz, E. E., Hill, M. J., Bennett, W. G., et al.: Effects of pentobarbital upon 2,4-dinitrophenol-induced hyperpyrexia during halothane anaesthesia. Fed. Proc., *29*:356, 1970.
221. Gatz, E. E., and Jones, J. R.: Effects of six general anesthetics upon mitochondrial oxidative phosphorylation: possible site and mechanism of malignant hyperpyrexia. Fed. Proc., *28*:356, 1969.
222. Gatz, E. E.: The mechanism of induction of malignant hyperpyrexia based on in vitro to in vivo correlative studies. *In* Gordon, R. A., Britt, B. A., and Kalow, W. (eds.): International Symposium on Malignant Hyperthermia, pp. 399–408. Springfield, Charles C. Thomas, 1973.
223. Frey, R., Kern, F., and Mayrhofer, O., (eds.): Maligne Hyperthermie Akupunktur Biomedizinische Technik Abdominelle Intensivtherapie. Berlin Springer-Verlag, 1975.
224. Short, C. E., Paddleford, R. R., McGrath, C. J., et al.: Advances in preanaesthetic evaluation and management of malignant hyperthermia in the experimental model. Presented at the International Anesthesia Research Society Meeting, Miami Beach, Florida, 1975.
225. Seeman, P., Chau-Wong, M., Tedesco, J., et al.: Brain receptor for antipsychotic drugs and dopamine: direct binding assays. Proc. Natl. Acad. Sci. U.S.A., *72*:4376, 1975.

FURTHER READING

Aldrete, J. A., and Britt, B. A. (eds.): Malignant Hyperthermia: Second International Symposium. New York, Grune & Stratton, 1978.
Bligh, J.: Temperature Regulation in Mammals and Other Vertebrates. New York, Elsevier North-Holland, Inc., 1973.
Gronert, G. A.: Malignant hyperthermia. Anesthesiology, *53*:395, 1980.
Hall, G. M.: Body temperature and anaesthesia. Br. J. Anesth., *50*:39, 1978.
Henschel, E. O. (ed.): Malignant Hyperthermia: Current Concepts. New York, Appleton-Century-Crofts, 1977.
Holdcroft, A.: Body Temperature Control. New York, Macmillan Publishing, 1980.
Lomax, P., Schonbaum, E., and Jacobs, J.: Temperature Regulation and Drug Action. Basil, S., Karger, A. G., 1975.
Maclean, D., and Emslie-Smith, D.: Accidental Hypothermia. Oxford, Blackwell-Scientific Publications, 1977.

20 Increased Intracranial Pressure

Jerry D. Levitt, M. D.

Increased intracranial pressure is a common finding in patients with a wide variety of neoplastic, congenital, vascular, metabolic, infectious, and traumatic lesions of the central nervous system. Inappropriate anesthetic management can increase brain damage and make neurologic surgery more difficult or impossible. But the appropriate anesthetic drugs and techniques for these patients will lower intracranial pressure, maintain cerebral perfusion, and expedite the surgical procedure. This chapter considers how anesthetic drugs and techniques influence intracranial pressure.

ANATOMY AND PATHOPHYSIOLOGY OF INCREASED INTRACRANIAL PRESSURE

The skull can be considered to be an almost rigid box that contains, in an adult, about 1400 g. of brain tissue, 70 ml. of cerebrospinal fluid (CSF),[1] and 130 ml. of blood.[2] As a general rule, the capacity of the cranium is fixed and any increase in the volume of one component will lead to an increase in intracranial pressure (ICP) unless there is a reciprocal decrease in the volume of the other components.

Under normal circumstances, ICP is a function of the production and absorption of CSF. About 70 per cent of CSF production occurs in the choroid plexus of the lateral ventricles, while the balance is derived from the brain interstitial fluid. In the adult, CSF is produced at a rate of 0.4 ml. per min. and this rate is constant at pressures up to 20 torr.[3] CSF flows from the lateral ventricles through the foramina of Monro to the third ventricle and then through the aqueduct of Sylvius to the fourth ventricle. It then flows through the foramina of Luschka and Magendie and into the spinal and cerebral subarachnoid spaces. Absorption occurs through unidirectional tubules in the arachnoid villi into the large dural venous sinuses.[4] The rate of CSF absorption varies directly with the pressure gradient between the subarachnoid space and the dural sinuses. Absorption ceases when the gradient is less than 5 torr. Although the CSF circulation clears particulate material and large molecules from the brain, CSF is not simply an ultrafiltrate of plasma. Rather it is a fluid whose chemical composition is narrowly regulated.[3]

Intracranial pressure is generally considered to be the hydrostatic pressure of the cerebrospinal fluid within the ventricular system or in the subarachnoid space over the cerebral hemispheres. Pressures above 150 mm. CSF or 11 torr are usually considered abnormal. The instantaneous intracranial pressure reflects each heart beat and the respiratory cycle. ICP increases about 2 torr with each cardiac cycle owing to an increase in cerebral blood volume with arterial pulsation. Changes in ICP during the respiratory cycle are similar to the changes in central venous pressure with respiration. During spontaneous ventilation, ICP decreases a few torr upon inspiration and

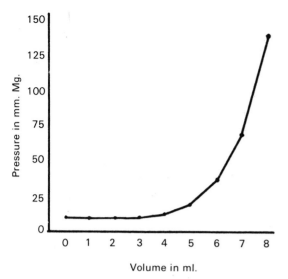

Fig. 20-1. The intracranial volume-pressure curve. This curve was compiled from the intracranial-pressure responses of six monkeys in which a supratentorial extradural balloon was inflated. (Langfitt, T. W.: Clin. Neurosurg., *16*: 436, 1969)

increases at the onset of expiration. With intermittent positive pressure ventilation, ICP increases upon inspiration.

The intracranial pressure response to a mass lesion depends on the nature of the lesion, its location, and its rate of expansion. The conventional representation of the intracranial volume-pressure curve is shown in Fig. 20-1. The form of this curve was originally derived from experiments in which the intracranial pressure of a monkey was recorded during the constant, slow inflation with saline of a supratentorial extradural balloon.[5] The curve has three phases. In the first, there is little pressure change as the balloon is inflated. In the second, increases in balloon volume cause larger increases in pressure. In the third, the baseline pressure is elevated and small increases in volume cause very large increases in pressure. In these experiments, the balloon was inflated at the rate of 1 ml. per hr., and phase 2 of the curve was reached when the volume was 5 ml. Injection of the eighth milliliter of saline produced a 70 torr increase in pressure. This curve is relevant clinically because patients with expanding lesions seem to follow the same

course, but with different time scales. For example, a patient with a slowly growing meningioma might not reach phase 2 for many years, but a patient with an intracranial hemorrhage could reach phase 2 within an hour.

There are several mechanisms by which volume compensation occurs during the initial phase of expansion of a mass lesion. Cerebrospinal fluid is translocated through the foramen magnum into the spinal subarachnoid space. When any increase in ICP has occurred, the absorption of CSF increases. These two mechanisms will, if there is no obstruction to the flow of CSF from the third or fourth ventricles, lead to a decrease in the size of the ventricular system. As ICP increases more, thin-walled cerebral veins are compressed, reducing cerebral venous blood volume and providing additional spatial compensation for the expanding mass. Phase 2 is reached when these compensating mechanisms are exhausted. As the volume of the mass lesion increases, obstruction of CSF channels may occur. In addition, chronically increased ICP eventually leads to compression of dural sinuses and increased dural venous pressure,[6] reducing the pressure gradient across the arachnoid villi and decreasing CSF absorption.

Intracranial Compliance

Hence, when ICP increases, small changes in volume lead to progressively greater changes in pressure. The function which describes this property is called elastance of the CSF space (E_{CSF}), and is defined as follows:[7]

$$E_{CSF} = \frac{dP}{dV},$$

where dP is the change in ICP that occurs immediately upon a small change in intracranial volume, dV. The reciprocal of elastance, intracranial compliance (C_{CSF}), is the change in volume that will result in a unit change in ICP:

$$C_{CSF} = \frac{1}{E_{CSF}} = \frac{dV}{dP}.$$

Conventionally it is said that compliance decreases as a mass lesion expands; that is, as the patient moves to the right along the intracranial volume-pressure curve. If ICP is being monitored by a catheter in a lateral ventricle, compliance may be measured by injecting a small volume of saline (up to 1 ml.) or by withdrawing a similar volume of CSF through the catheter and recording the change in ICP.[8] A change in pressure greater than 2 torr per ml. indicates decreased compliance. Without injecting or withdrawing fluid, one can use the change in ICP with each heart beat as an indication of compliance. The increase in intracranial blood volume that occurs with arterial pulsation is analogous to the saline injection, and an increase in the ICP pulse pressure indicates a decrease in compliance. Cerebral vasodilation by hypercarbia, hypoxia, volatile anesthetics, and other interventions discussed below also increases cerebral blood volume. Similarly, the ICP responses to these depend upon intracranial compliance.

Various groups have derived mathematical models to describe the pressure-volume relationships of the intracranial contents, and some have attempted to verify their models by comparing experimental results with computer predictions.[7,9] These experiments suggest that evaluating compliance or elastance alone will not predict how close a patient is to decompensation. Another quantity that can be followed is the rate of return of ICP to baseline following a saline injection.[10] This is a function of CSF absorption and may be a better predictor of a patient's capacity for further spatial compensation. Finally, some authors have stated that elastance itself is a function of ICP and, therefore, measurement of elastance does not provide any more clinically useful information than does measurement of ICP.[11] In the presence of a normal ICP, compliance testing can demonstrate how near a patient is to phase 2 on his volume-pressure curve, but when ICP is elevated, one can assume that compliance is decreased.

CONSEQUENCES OF INCREASED INTRACRANIAL PRESSURE

The effects of increased ICP depend on the magnitude of the pressure and on the nature of the lesion. In general, five consequences are recognized.

1. Increased ICP leads to a decrease in cerebral perfusion pressure (CPP) and may cause cerebral ischemia. Cerebral perfusion pressure equals mean arterial pressure (MAP) minus cerebral venous pressure. However, in the presence of increased ICP, CPP = MAP − ICP. Brain blood flow in maintained until CPP falls below 50 torr in a patient previously normotensive. Chronic hypertensives require a higher CPP.[12] Uncontrolled ICP leading to cerebral ischemia is a common cause of brain death following head injury.

2. Increased ICP can cause *regional* ischemia in an area of the brain already subjected to pressure from a mass lesion.

3. Increased ICP can induce a state of *vasomotor paralysis*, in which cerebral blood flow becomes a passive function of arterial blood pressure.[13] In this state, areterial hypertension leads to increased cerebral blood volume and cerebral edema, which further increase ICP.

4. Increased ICP can cause any of the brain herniation syndromes illustrated in Fig. 20-2.[14]

5. Increased ICP in the presence of a space-occupying lesion can lead to neurologic dysfunction secondary to distortion of the brain.

It is important to realize that the falx cerebri and the tentorium are rather rigid structures and that an expanding lesion or localized brain edema results first in a local pressure increase. Generally, there will be a pressure gradient between the affected and adjacent intracranial compartments. For example, increases in cerebral blood volume by volatile anesthetics can magnify these pressure gradients and cause brain distortion or herniation.

RELATIONSHIP BETWEEN CBF AND ICP

Any anesthetic drug or technique that increases CBF is capable of increasing ICP. Cerebral blood flow is regulated by the radius of the cerebral arterioles. Generally, an increase in CBF

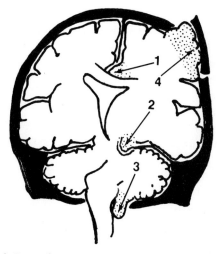

Fig. 20-2. Brain herniations: *(1)* Cingulate. The cingulate gyrus and a portion of the affected hemisphere are displaced beneath the falx, causing pressure on the anterior cerebral artery and vein. *(2)* Temporal, tentorial, or unical. The medial aspect of the temporal lobe is displaced through the tentorial notch, compressing the oculomotor nerve (III) and the midbrain, causing ipsilateral pupillary dilatation. *(3)* Cerebellar or tonsillar. The cerebellar tonsils are displaced through the foramen magnum, compressing the cervicomedullary junction and causing respiratory and then cardiac arrest. *(4)* Transcalvarial. Brain tissue herniates through an operative or traumatic opening in the cranium. (Fishman, R. A.: N. Engl. J. Med., *293:* 706, 1975)

leads to an increase in cerebral blood volume (CBV) and an increase in ICP. How much ICP increases depends upon the magnitude of the blood volume increase and the position of the patient on his intracranial volume-pressure curve. Cerebral blood flow is regulated by multiple factors, which include chemical (Pa_{CO_2}, Pa_{O_2}, metabolic (cerebral metabolic rate for oxygen ($CMRO_2$)), autoregulatory, and neurogenic. Also, many anesthetic drugs affect CBF.

Chemical Regulation of CBF. Although other mechanisms may be involved, the final common pathway of chemical regulation of CBF is believed to be the hydrogen ion concentration of the brain interstitial space. Increased hydrogen ion concentration (acidosis) causes vasodilitation, while decreased hydrogen ion concentration causes vasoconstriction.[15] The effect of Pa_{CO_2} on CBF is considered in detail in Chapter 25. For this

discussion, it is important to note that in the Pa_{CO_2} range of 20 to 60 torr, CBF varies directly with Pa_{CO_2} and changes by a factor of at least 3 (20 to 60 ml./100g./min.).[16,88] Changes in Pa_{O_2} affect CBF very little at Pa_{O_2} levels above 50 torr. As Pa_{O_2} falls lower, there is a large, progressive increase in CBF.[17] Tissue lactic acid is believed to mediate this response.

Metabolic Regulation of CBF. Normally, cortical blood flow is coupled to neuronal activity on a millimeter by millimeter and second to second basis.[18] Opening the eyes, for example, increases blood flow in the visual cortex. Probably through metabolic regulation, seizures and painful stimulation increase CBF. The mediator of this response is not known, but local hypoxia and hydrogen ion concentration do not seem to be involved.

Autoregulation of CBF. This is the process whereby CBF normally remains constant over the range of mean arterial pressure from 60 to 130 torr.[19] Below the lower limit of autoregulation, cerebrovascular resistance is minimal and CBF is a function of arterial pressure. As arterial pressure is raised toward the upper limit of autoregulation, the cerebral vessels constrict maximally until the "breakthrough point" is reached. CBF then increases as the arterial pressure increases. These high flows are associated with opening of tight junctions in the vascular endothelium and with vasogenic cerebral edema.[20] In chronic hypertensives, the lower and upper limits of autoregulation are both higher than in normals.[12] This affords some protection against hypertensive cerebral edema, but renders the brain more sensitive to ischemic damage during hypotension. Autoregulatory changes in cerebrovascular tone require up to 2 minutes to complete. Therefore, sudden changes in blood pressure may change CBF and ICP temporarily. Head trauma, hypoxia, hypercarbia, tumors, certain drugs, and increased ICP may produce a state of "vasomotor paralysis," in which CBF varies with blood pressure in the range where autoregulation normally occurs.

Neurogenic Regulation of CBF. Neurogenic mechanisms have been thought to exert little influence on the resting level of CBF. Stimulation or interruption of the cervical sympathetic chain lowers or raises CBF by only about 10 per cent.

However, hypovolemic hypotension (shock) lowers CBF, whereas a similar level of induced hypotension does not,[21] and stimulation of the cervical sympathetic chain lowers CBF during hypercarbia.[22] Recent work in baboons suggests that the increase in CBF during hypoxia is a function of the carotid body chemoreceptors.[23] Similarly, the cerebrovascular response to hypercarbia may be mediated by a catecholamine system that originates in the locus ceruleus in the brain stem. In the rat, sedative doses of diazepam block the response to hypercarbia.[24] The clinical implications of these observations are not clear at this time.

EFFECT OF ANESTHETIC DRUGS AND TECHNIQUES ON ICP

Drug-induced hypercarbia increases CBF and ICP. In this discussion of drug effects, we assume that ventilation is controlled and consider the changes in ICP that occur during normo- and hypocarbia. The discussion is limited to non-explosive drugs currently in use.

Inhalation Anesthetics

Halothane increases CBF and ICP. In patients without intracranial pathology, these increases are small and of no clinical importance. In thirteen patients with space-occupying intracranial lesions anesthetized with nitrous oxide at normocapnia, the addition of halothane 1 per cent caused a mean increase in ICP of 20 torr. The ICP of one patient in that series increased by 37 torr, and the ICP of most of the patients was still increasing when the halothane was discontinued 10 minutes after it was started.[25] These and similar observations and the experience of seeing massive brain swelling during some neurosurgical procedures in which halothane anesthesia was used has prompted some anesthesiologists to question whether halothane has any place in neurosurgical anesthesia. On the other hand, for some, halothane is the principal anesthetic for neurosurgical patients. One group, for example, has reported that hyperventilation with nitrous oxide and oxygen to a Pa_{CO_2} of less than 30 torr for 10 minutes before the introduction of halothane

and the restriction of inspired halothane concentration to 0.5 per cent prevents dangerous increases in ICP.[26] When halothane was administered at the same time as hyperventilation was begun, some patients had large increases in ICP, but in every case the ICP returned to the pre-halothane level in 30 minutes.

I suggest the following precautions when halothane is administered to patients with intracranial pathology:

1. Hyperventilate the patient and limit the halothane concentration, as described above.
2. Do not administer halothane to patients with clear evidence of increased ICP (e.g., papilledema, large masses, severe injury) unless ICP is being measured or the bone flap has been removed and the brain is in view.
3. Be prepared to discontinue halothane if brain swelling increases or is not controlled by hyperventilation or osmotic diuretics.

Halothane may be most useful in those neurosurgical patients with oxygenation problems, which would limit the use of nitrous oxide, and in patients with intracranial aneurysms, in whom control of blood pressure is usually more important than control of ICP.

Methoxyflurane, in inspired concentrations of 0.5 and 1.5 per cent, causes dose-related increases in ICP in patients with space-occupying lesions.[25] Methoxyflurane might be useful at lower concentrations, but this has not been investigated.

Enflurane. An early study in man suggested that enflurane had no effect on CBF.[27] This work was criticized because the systemic blood pressures of the subjects had decreased as a result of the anesthetic. In subsequent studies in which blood pressure was supported with phenylephrine, enflurane was found to cause large increases in CBF.[28] This suggests that enflurane can increase ICP. In fact, we have observed alarming brain swelling when enflurane was administered to a neurosurgical patient in order to lower blood pressure. Since the electroencephalographic seizure activity that occurs during enflurane anesthesia is potentiated by hypocarbia, enflurane may be less useful than halothane for patients with increased ICP.

Isoflurane, in inspired concentrations of up to about 1.3 per cent, has no effect on CBF. Increasing the concentration to 2.0 per cent results in a doubling of the CBF; however, equipotent concentrations of enflurane (2.7%) and, especially, halothane (1.2%) produce even greater increases in CBF. As is true with other halogenated agents, the increased intracranial pressure occurring with isoflurane can be abolished by hyperventilation.[28a]

Nitrous Oxide. In a study of 12 patients with intracranial pathology, induction of anesthesia with 66 per cent nitrous oxide in oxygen increased ICP by 27 torr (mean) in the absence of changes in arterial blood pressure or Pa_{CO_2}. Hyperventilation (mean $Pa_{CO_2} = 29$) reduced ICP to control levels in all cases.[29] In two reports in which nitrous oxide was not associated with increases in CBF or ICP, short-acting barbiturates had been used to induce anesthesia.[30,31] Two studies of dogs anesthetized with 0.1–0.2-per cent halothane in 60–70-per cent nitrogen in oxygen demonstrated increases in CBF and $CMRO_2$ when nitrous oxide was substituted for the nitrogen.[32,33]

Clearly, nitrous oxide can increase ICP, and this increase can be prevented by prior barbiturate administration and treated by hyperventilation. Few anesthesiologists would use only nitrous oxide to induce anesthesia in an alert patient, but some might attempt this in a lethargic or obtunded patient. If increased ICP or intracranial mass lesion is suspected, a barbiturate should be used for the induction of anesthesia, and hyperventilation to Pa_{CO_2} of 30 torr or lower should be part of the anesthetic technique.

Intravenous Agents

Barbiturates. Thiopental (1.5–3.0 mg./kg.) in bolus doses causes rapid introperative reduction of ICP in neurosurgical patients. This effect occurs both in patients with chronically increased ICP during induction of anesthesia and in those with ICP increases secondary to painful stimulation, such as tracheal intubation.[34] Pentobarbital coma has been used over periods of several days or weeks to control ICP in patients with severe head injury[35] or Reye's syndrome.[36] The dosage of pentobarbital is 3 to 5 mg./kg.

initially, followed by hourly doses to maintain a blood barbiturate concentration of about 3 mg. per dl. In some centers, maintenance of a burst-suppression EEG pattern, rather than the blood barbiturate concentration, is used to determine barbiturate dose. These techniques are used only in patients whose ventilation is controlled.

Barbiturates cause dose-related decreases in CBF and $CMRO_2$. Sedative doses are without effect, but light thiopental anesthesia results in a 35 per cent decrease in CBF and $CMRO_2$, and deep thiopental anesthesia, in a 50 per cent decrease.[37] Several studies have shown that after a dose of barbiturate sufficient to silence the EEG, additional barbiturate causes no further reduction in CBF and $CMRO_2$.[38] It is most likely that the primary effect of barbiturates is to reduce neuronal activity and oxygen demand. Metabolic regulation then reduces CBF proportionally. Barbiturates may also constrict cerebral vessels directly, but in either case the resulting decrease in CBF lowers ICP.

Barbiturates play a key role in the management of patients with increased ICP. First, they can be used to attenuate the ICP response to tracheal intubation and other painful manipulations in the emergency care of head-injured patients and in the induction of anesthesia in patients with increased ICP.[39] Second, they can be used to treat increases in ICP that occur intraoperatively.[34] Third, they are useful for the long-term management of increased ICP in patients in intensive care units.[40]

Diazepam, 0.5 mg./kg., administered intravenously to induce anesthesia, reduced lumbar CSF pressure in patients without brain pathology.[41] This is consistent with a study of comatose head-injured patients in whom diazepam, 15 mg., decreased CBF and $CMRO_2$ by 25 per cent.[42] However, in a study of paralyzed and ventilated rats, sedative doses of diazepam reduced CBF, but not $CMRO_2$.[43] When 70 per cent nitrous oxide was added, both CBF and $CMRO_2$ decreased by 40 per cent. Although diazepam can decrease ICP, one should observe two precautions in using it. First, diazepam has a long plasma half-life and, if given prior to surgery, may result in a somnolent patient postoperatively. If this is suspected, physostigmine may reverse the somnolence.[44]

Second, patients with intracranial pathology may be very sensitive to depressant drugs, and respiratory arrest has occurred following intravenously administered diazepam.[45] This complication would be particularly serious in a patient with increased ICP.

Narcotics. At normocarbia in man, morphine causes no change in ICP.[46] The effects of morphine on CBF and $CMRO_2$ in man are not known with certainty. A recent study in which morphine (3 mg./kg.) and 70 per cent nitrous oxide were given to normocarbia volunteers showed no change from awake controls in either CBF or $CMRO_2$.[47] However, it is possible that in this study, any effect of morphine to lower CBF and $CMRO_2$ was masked by the opposite effects of nitrous oxide, which were discussed above.

Neuroleptic Drugs. In a study of nine patients who had been given muscle relaxants and were being ventilated with nitrous oxide at normocarbia, droperidol, 5 mg., and fentanyl, 0.1 mg., given intravenously resulted in a mean reduction in ICP from 23 to 18 torr.[48] Although the mean arterial pressure decreased, there was no significant change in cerebral perfusion pressure. The mechanism for this reduction in ICP was suggested by a study in which dogs were ventilated at normocapnia with nitrous oxide.[49] Droperidol (0.3 mg./kg.) caused a persistant 40 per cent decrease in CBF, with little change in $CMRO_2$. Fentanyl (0.006 mg./kg.) decreased both CBF and $CMRO_2$ by 45 per cent, but both returned to control in 30 minutes. When droperidol and fentanyl were given together, the initial decreases in CBF and $CMRO_2$ were similar to those following fentanyl alone, but 40 minutes after injection, CBF and $CMRO_2$ were similar to those following droperidol alone. These studies suggest that droperidol is a potent, long-acting cerebral vasoconstrictor that should be useful in the anesthetic management of patients with increased ICP. However, in a more recent study of nine patients with intracranial pathology who were anesthetized with barbiturate and nitrous oxide, droperidol (7.5–12.5 mg.) increased ICP in four, although the mean ICP of the group did not change. Cerebral perfusion pressure decreased in all patients after droperidol administration and decreased further when fentanyl (0.2–0.3 mg.) was injected.[50] There are two additional precautions that one should keep in mind when using droperidol in patients with intracranial pathology. First, the sedative properties of droperidol may last 18 hours and may cause concern in the postoperative period. This effect may be antagonized with physostigmine.[51] Second, as droperidol decreases CBF out of proportion to $CMRO_2$, it may critically decrease the cerebral perfusion pressure (CPP).[50] It is advisable to include drugs that decrease $CMRO_2$ (e.g., barbiturates) when droperidol is used.

Ketamine increases CBF and has caused alarming increases in ICP in patients with intracranial disease.[52,53] It is of interest that the increase in CBF is not related to a global increase in $CMRO_2$. Although ketamine anesthesia has been used in neuroradiology, it is difficult at this time to see a place for this agent in neuroanesthesia.

Muscle Relaxants

Succinylcholine, administered to patients with intracranial pathology to facilitate tracheal intubation, can cause large increases in ICP.[54] This is probably secondary to the increases in intraabdominal, intrathoracic, and venous pressures that occur with succinylcholine-induced fasciculations and may be prevented by the prior administration of a small dose of a non-depolarizing muscle relaxant.[55] Succinylcholine, when administered to patients with a variety of neurologic lesions, can cause arrhythmias and cardiac arrest secondary to acute hyperkalemia.[56,57] Although the increase in serum potassium can be modififed by prior administration of a non-depolarizing agent,[58,59] I prefer to avoid the use of succinylcholine in neurosurgical patients. After inducing anesthesia and demonstrating that the patient can be hyperventilated with a mask, I inject an "intubating dose" of a non-depolarizing muscle relaxant. Smaller doses of the same drug maintain paralysis during the surgical procedure.

d-Tubocurarine and Pancuronium. Large doses of d-tubocurarine administered rapidly may increase ICP[60] and can cause blood pressure to decrease, leading to a decreased CPP. This response lasts less than 2 minutes and can be prevented by thiopental administration.[39] Pancuronium is not known to release histamine and would seem, therefore, to be the muscle relaxant of choice for patients whose ICP is likely to be elevated. However some patients anesthetized with a barbiturate-narcotic-nitrous oxide technique and given pancuronium (0.1 mg./kg.) develop tachycardia and hypertension. These and other patients who are given pancuronium require larger doses of narcotics and hypotensive drugs to control their blood pressures during surgery. For this reason, I prefer d-tubocurarine for muscular relaxation of patients in whom an increase in blood pressure would be more dangerous than an increase in ICP. This would include patients with aneurysms and other vascular malformations, patients about to have transsphenoidal hypophysectomies (who will receive submucous injections of epinephrine), patients with traumatic lesions characterized by hyperemia and normal ICP, and patients whose mass lesions are small.

Hypotensive Agents

There are three distinct indications in neuroanesthesia for drugs that decrease blood pressure. The first is to reduce blood pressure below the upper limit of autoregulation to prevent cerebral edema, vascular congestion, and a concomitant increase in ICP. The second is to lower blood pressure slightly below the patient's usual pressure in order to improve operating conditions. The third is to lower the blood pressure profoundly in order to increase the ease and safety of surgery on aneurysms and arteriovenous malformations.

Sodium Nitroprusside is a direct dilator of the cerebral vasculature in the goat and interferes with autoregulation of CBF.[61] It is not surprising therefore that some authors have observed increases in ICP and decreases in CPP when sodium nitroprusside is administered to patients with intracranial mass lesions.[62] Probably these patients should not receive sodium nitroprusside before the skull is open. Another group has found that the increase in ICP occurred only at the start of the sodium nitroprusside infusion and that ICP returned to baseline when the mean arterial pressure was reduced to 70 per cent of the initial pressure.[63] The clinical significance of these studies is controversial at the present time and the observations themselves pose unanswered

questions. For example, in one of the studies,[63] ICP did not increase in hyperventilated patients, but in the other study,[62] all patients were hyperventilated and the increase in ICP occurred in spite of hyperventilation. Other studies have demonstrated that the interference with autoregulation persists after sodium nitroprusside hypotension is terminated so that abrupt increases in blood pressure during that period may cause large increases in CBF.[64] However, sodium nitroprusside is most useful for inducing profound hypotension during surgery for aneurysms or arteriovenous malformations and for controlling bleeding during dissections of vascular tumors.

Trimethaphan, a short-acting ganglionic-blocking drug with some direct vasodilating properties, caused no vasodilatation when injected directly into the cerebral vasculature of the goat.[65] In a group of neurosurgical patients rendered hypotensive with trimethaphan, the mean ICP did not change, but two individual patients had modest ICP increases of 9.3 and 5.7 torr, respectively.[63] Within the autoregulatory range, trimethaphan seems less likely to cause increases in ICP than sodium nitroprusside. I use trimethaphan in bolus doses of 3 to 5 mg. to control blood pressure when necessary during the induction of anesthesia, and as a constant infusion to effect moderate decreases of blood pressure during neurosurgery. There is some evidence that *profound* hypotension induced by trimethaphan in dogs causes more disturbance of cerebral metabolism than does hypotension produced by sodium nitroprusside, if the dose of the latter can be kept less than 1 mg. per kg.[66]

Other Hypotensive Agents. *Nitroglycerin* is a potent vasodilator when injected into the cerebral circulation of the goat,[65] but it may not cause cerebral dilatation when administered intravenously.[67] More information is needed in order to determine the usefulness of this agent in patients with increased ICP. *Hydralazine* is used commonly to control hypertension in postoperative neurosurgical patients, but it may increase ICP.[68] Again, more information is needed. *Pentolinium tartrate* is a long-acting (approximately 3 hours) ganglionic blocking agent whose actions should be qualitatively similar to trimethaphan, although there are no studies that examine the effect of this drug on ICP. I use pentolinium (2–16 mg.) to lower blood pressure somewhat below the patient's usual pressure early in a neurosurgical procedure, without incurring the task of attending to a constant infusion. Subsequently, profound hypotension can be induced with exceedingly small amounts of sodium nitroprusside because of the potentiation by pentolinium.

EFFECTS OF ANESTHETIC TECHNIQUES ON ICP

Maneuvers performed during anesthesia and intensive care can influence ICP and CPP by effecting changes in arterial oxygen and carbon dioxide tensions, cerebral venous return, cerebral metabolic rate, and systemic blood pressure.

Pa_{O_2} and Pa_{CO_2}

Through chemical regulation, hypoxia and hypercarbia increase CBF, CBV, and, in susceptible patients, ICP. Both hypercarbia and hypoxia can result from the hypoventilation that follows respiratory obstruction or insufficient manual or mechanical ventilation. Because control of the airway may be lost temporarily when anesthesia is induced, I encourage patients with increased ICP to hyperventilate while oxygen is administered immediately before anesthetic induction. Ventilation should be interrupted for only the briefest periods necessary for intubating the trachea, suctioning secretions, and positioning the patient. Patients with increased ICP may require higher than expected inspiratory oxygen concentrations (F_IO_2) to prevent hypoxia because of neurogenic pulmonary edema.[69] During induced hypotension, it may be necessary to increase both F_IO_2 and minute ventilation because of the increased ventilatory dead space[70] and ventilation-perfusion mismatch[71] that occur with this technique. Frequent blood-gas determinations are important in the management of patients with increased ICP.

Cerebral Venous Return

Impeding the drainage of venous blood from the brain increases intracranial pressure by engorging cerebral veins.[72,73] Maneuvers that impede cerebral venous drainage include forcing the neck into

any extreme position,[73] increasing intrathoracic pressure (and venous pressure), and placing the patient in a head-down position. Head position is critically important, because the head-up position will modify the transmission of intrathoracic venous pressure into the intracranial compartment. Positive end-expiratory pressure (PEEP) has increased ICP in some patients with severe head injuries. In some of these patients, blood pressure and cerebral perfusion pressure decreased and neurologic deterioration occurred.[74] Interestingly, the magnitude of the increase in ICP frequently exceeded the level of PEEP. The application of PEEP probably increases ICP only in patients with decreased intracranial compliance.[75] Some investigators have found no increase in ICP following the application of very high levels of PEEP.[76] Nevertheless, ICP monitoring is indicated in comatose head-injured patients who are treated with PEEP.

Coughing can increase ICP. The abrupt increase in intra-abdominal and intrathoracic pressures is transmitted via the epidural veins to the spinal subarachnoid space, where it initiates a pressure wave that rises to the foramen magnum.[77] Lumbar CSF pressures in excess of 100 torr have been recorded during coughing. When a patient "bucks" on an endotracheal tube, it is likely that the same mechanism acts in concert with impeded cerebral venous drainage to increase ICP.

It follows that a patient with increased ICP should be maintained in a head-up position, more so if PEEP is necessary. The neck should be kept in a neurtral position, the tidal volumes should be the smallest that will prevent atelectasis, and coughing, straining, and bucking should be prevented by the administration of adequate doses of non-depolarizing muscle relaxants.

Cerebral Metabolic Rate

Regional cerebral blood flow is coupled to regional $CMRO_2$ through metabolic regulation of CBF. Therefore, factors that increase brain activity increase CBV and ICP in susceptible patients. Anxiety has been shown to increase CBF,[78] and pain is known to increase ICP.[79] Adequate anesthesia, usually in the form of barbiturates and narcotics, should precede painful stimulation, such as laryngoscopy, tracheal intubation, surgical incision, or application of a head clamp. It is of interest that ICP can increase following painful stimulation even when blood pressure does not increase.[79]

Blood Pressure

Blood pressures above the upper limit of autoregulation increase CBV and ICP and promote cerebral edema that further increases ICP. In a normal brain, this occurs at a mean blood pressure above 130 torr, but a diseased brain is more vulnerable.[80] Cerebral ischemia, and in some patients, head injury, cause diffuse hyperemia, which may represent impaired autoregulation. Any increase in blood pressure in these patients may increase ICP and cerebral edema. Intracranial mass lesions and infarcts may be surrounded by an area of hyperemia that has been called luxury perfusion and may represent regional vasomotor paralysis.[5] Hypertension can increase the blood volume in these areas, promote edema formation, and cause a local increase in pressure. Of course, hypertension can increase ICP by causing bleeding from an intracranial aneurysm or arteriovenous malformation.

For these reasons, the blood pressure of patients with intracranial pathology should be controlled. During surgery, control may be achieved by adequate anesthesia with barbiturates, narcotics, or inhalational agents. If these are not sufficient, the anesthesiologist should use a hypotensive drug, as described above, taking care not to reduce CPP to less than 50 torr. Following a period of profound hypotension, autoregulation may be impaired for 1.5 hours,[64,81] so that blood pressure control should be continued postoperatively for patients treated with deliberate hypotension.

PREOPERATIVE CONSIDERATIONS REGARDING INTRACRANIAL HYPERTENSION

Patients at Risk

Patients with head trauma, large space-occupying lesions, rapidly enlarging lesions, recent hemorrhage, or hydrocephalus are likely to have increased ICP. The signs and symptoms of acutely increased ICP may be limited to altered consciousness and one of the herniation syndromes. In chronic conditions, papilledema and radiographic changes consisting of a "beaten silver" appearance of the cranial vault and erosion of the posterior clinoids of the sella may be seen. When ICP has increased sufficiently to cause medullary ischemia, the patient will demonstrate the "Cushing triad," which consists of systemic hypertension, bradycardia, and respiratory irregularities.[82]

Measurement of ICP

ICP is measured most commonly through either an intraventricular catheter or a subarachnoid bolt connected by a fluid path to an electronic pressure transducer external to the patient.[83,84] By convention, pressure is referenced to the level of the external auditory meatus. The bolt is simply screwed into a drill hole in the skull after a small incision is made in the dura. The catheter is introduced into a lateral ventricle through a burr hole and passes through the substance of the brain. CSF can be drained from the catheter, but not from the bolt, making the catheter a therapeutic tool. Also, saline can be injected into the catheter to measure intracranial compliance. Systems utilizing intracranial transducers have been developed but are not in general use. Recording the pressure on slowly moving paper simplifies recognition of pressure waves, but is not necessary for adequate monitoring. Measurement of pressure in the *spinal* subarachnoid space does not provide information about ICP if there is obstruction to CSF flow. Furthermore, in the presence of a mass lesion, loss of CSF from a lumbar puncture may lead to brain stem herniation, so that the lumbar space is not used for continuous measurement of CSF pressure.

At the present time, there is no general agreement on the indications for ICP monitoring. In an alert patient, changes in the level of consciousness, headache, and signs elicited by neurological examination should provide adequate warning of increasing ICP. In patients with impaired consciousness, especially those being treated for hydrocephalus or for cerebral edema from trauma, mass lesion, or infarct, ICP monitoring provides important information for managing therapy. Should these patients come to surgery, ICP monitoring intraoperatively elminates any speculation about the effects on ICP and CPP of drugs, manipulations, ventilation, blood pressure changes, and position. In patients being treated with barbiturate coma for increased ICP, continuous monitoring of ICP is the only practical method for determining the efficacy of treatment.

Lundberg, in 1960, was the first to perform long-term monitoring of ICP in patients with intracranial pathology.[85] He described A, B, and C waves, but the clinical significance of the B and C waves is uncertain. Lundberg's A waves, which are now called plateau waves, consist of abrupt increases in ICP above 50 torr lasting from 5 to 20 minutes. Plateau waves occur when intracranial compliance is seriously decreased. If treatment is not successful, ICP may increase to the level of systemic blood pressure, and blood flow to the brain will cease. This event is called a terminal wave and leads rapidly to brain death.

INTRAPOPERATIVE SIGNS OF INCREASED ICP

Since many of the cardipulmonary signs of intracranial hypertension are nonspecific, it is unlikely that this complication will be diagnosed intraoperatively in a patient in whom it was not suspected before operation. Hypertension and bradycardia may not appear because of the administration of anesthetic and adjunctive drugs. Respiratory irregularities will not be seen if the patient is ventilated mechanically or manually. A large alveolar-arterial gradient for oxygen (A-aDO_2) may be an expression of neurogenic pulmonary edema secondary to intracranial hypertension.[69,86] But, because there are more likely causes of a large A-aDO_2 during anesthesia, this cannot be considered an important sign. Similarly, the eye signs of transtentorial herniation may be obscured by anesthesia. Trimethaphan or pentolinium administration or very deep halothane anesthesia can dilate the pupils widely and render them unresponsive. However, *unilateral* pupillary dilatation during anesthesia, particularly in a patient with a supratentorial mass lesion, is evidence of transtentorial herniation, if there is no other obvious cause. In unanesthetized patients, prominent U-waves, S-T segment elevation and depression, notched T-waves, and short-

ening or prolongation of the Q-T interval are among the electrocardiographic changes associated with increased ICP.[87]

During a neurosurgical operation, ICP becomes zero when the dura is open. If the dura is tense before being opened, ICP is probably increased. If the brain itself is tense or herniates through the dural opening, then the brain is obviously swollen. The causes of a swollen brain in an open skull are the same as the causes of increased ICP in a closed skull: mass lesion, hydrocephalus, edema, or increased blood volume.

TREATMENT OF INCREASED ICP

Intracranial hypertension occurs in many different circumstances, and the treatment indicated depends upon the urgency of the situation. For example, an oral corticosteroid could be used to treat increased ICP in a patient with a brain tumor and papilledema but lacking other neurologic signs. On the other hand, controlled hyperventilation and intravenous mannitol might be life-saving for a patient whose pupils were dilating following a head injury. The discussion that follows focuses on the operating room and intensive care unit settings.

In addition to the specific therapies discussed below, the following general measures should be observed:

1. Assure adequate ventilation and oxygenation to prevent hypoxia and hypercarbia (see *Hyperventilation*, below).
2. Assure unimpeded cerebral venous drainage by elevating the head, placing the neck in a neutral position, correcting obstructions in the breathing circuit, and providing adequate muscular relaxation.
3. Assure that adequate sedation or narcosis precedes painful stimulation.
4. Discontinue halogenated anesthetic agents and substitute barbiturates and/or narcotics.
5. Control systemic arterial pressure to provide an adequate CPP and to minimize formation of cerebral edema.

Hyperventilation

This reduces Pa_{CO_2} and this decreases CBF and CBV through chemical regulation. In an adult,

CBV can be reduced by about 5.6 ml. through a 10 torr decrease in Pa_{CO_2}.[88] In a patient with decreased intracranial compliance, this small decrease in volume can cause a large decrease in ICP. During hyperventilation, the arterioles in relatively normal areas of the brain constrict and "make room" for a mass lesion. Hyperventilation may be less effective in diffuse lesions. In normal man, the effect of sustained hyperventilation on CBF diminishes dramatically after 4 hours, probably because of compensatory changes in CSF and blood acid-base status.[89] The time course of these changes in head-injured patients is not known. The effect of hyperventilation is very rapid and this treatment alone may reverse a herniation syndrome. Harp presents evidence in Chapter 25 that suggests that Pa_{CO_2} should not be decreased to less than 20 torr.

Osmotic Agents

Many agents, when administered in hypertonic solution, increase plasma osmolality and, in the presence of an intact blood-brain barrier, cause the movement of water from the brain to the plasma, decreasing the bulk of the brain. Intravenous mannitol and oral glycerol are in common use. In the past, urea was used, but is now used infrequently because of a "rebound" increase in ICP about 12 hours after administration.[90] When the blood urea concentration is high, some urea diffuses across the blood-brain barrier and enters the intracellular space. When the blood urea concentration decreases as a result of renal excretion, the blood osmolality becomes lower than that of the brain, and water diffuses into the brain.

Mannitol, the most commonly used osmotic agent, is administered intravenously as a 20 or 25 per cent solution. The usual acute dose of 1 to 1.5 g. per kg. is given during a 10–20-minute period. More rapid administration can cause hypotension by increasing blood flow to skeletal muscle.[91] The cerebral dehydrating effect depends upon the osmotic gradient between the brain and plasma and not upon the volume of the diuresis. The effect is maximal in 45 minutes and lasts 4 or 5 hours. If it is necessary to control ICP for a prolonged period, repeated doses or a continuous infusion[92] of mannitol can be administered, but

fluid and electrolyte losses should be replaced and the plasma osmolality must be used as a guide. At a plasma osmolality above 310 mOsm, the blood-brain barrier threshold for mannitol is exceeded, and mannitol gradually accumulates in the brain.[93] Above a plasma osmolality of 350 mOsm, renal failure and progressive systemic acidosis occur.[92] If ICP cannot be controlled with mannitol at a plasma osmolality less than 310 mOsm, another technique (barbiturate coma, for example) should be added to the treatment.

Mannitol is a carbohydrate that is not metabolized. It has no toxicity itself, but the increase in intravascular volume that occurs following acute administration and preceeding the diuresis may precipitate congestive heart failure in susceptible patients. Fluid and electrolyte abnormalities may result if the diuresis is profound.

Glycerol, 1.5 g. per kg., is administered orally or by nasogastric tube.[94] Attempts to use glycerol intravenously have resulted in hemolysis and hemoglobinuria.[95] Glycerol is metabolized and, therefore, may be the osmotic agent of choice in patients with renal failure and increased ICP.[96]

Loop Diuretics

Furosemide, 1 mg. per kg., is as effective as mannitol, 1 g. per kg., in reducing brain volume during elective craniotomy in patients with no signs of increased ICP.[97] This is accomplished with a small decrease in serum sodium and potassium and presumably no increase in intravascular volume, so that it may be safer than mannitol for patients who are susceptible to congestive heart failure.[97] Furosemide has been shown also to decrease ICP after head trauma in patients treated previously with a corticosteroid and mannitol.[98] The mechanism of the furosemide effect on ICP is not known with certainty, but probably it is not limited to the diuretic effect. Furosemide is known to reduce CSF production in animals[99] and may also prevent swelling of glial cells through an inhibition of ion transport.[98] Furosemide has not been tested for its ability to treat herniation syndromes or to decrease severe intracranial hypertension in the absence of other agents. In these situations, it appears to be a useful adjunct to mannitol.

Barbiturates

The use of barbiturates for the treatment of increased ICP has been discussed above. It should be noted that barbiturates lower ICP more rapidly than do any other drugs. Thiopental, for example, is effective within 1 minute after intravenous administration. Because of this property and the fact that an adequate dose of thiopental can prevent ICP from increasing following tracheal intubation, in the absence of hypovolemia or other contraindications barbiturate administration should precede emergency intubation of brain-injured patients who require ventilatory support. Additional barbiturate administration may be indicated during subsequent diagnostic and surgical procedures and in the intensive care unit, if steroids, mannitol, and surgical decompression do not control ICP.[40] However, recent studies question whether barbiturates provide any unusual cerebral protection beyond their effect on ICP. Mortality and morbidity in head trauma[40a] and in Reye's syndrome[40b,40c] may be unchanged by barbiturate administration.

Corticosteroids

Of the available corticosteroids, the one most commonly used for treating intracranial hypertension is dexamethasone, which essentially lacks any mineralocorticoid effect. Steroids reduce the amount of edema surrounding intracranial lesions preoperatively and diminish the amount of edema that occurs in manipulated neural tissue postoperatively.[100,101] Dexamethasone is administered in doses up to 10 mg. q.i.d. for these indications. Recently, two controlled studies have reported that the fraction of patients surviving head trauma increases dramatically following the administration of very high doses of dexamethasone.[102,103] Although more information about dosage is needed, one group suggests giving 50 to 100 mg. intravenously during the initial stabilization of patients with severe head injuries.[40] The well known side effects of steroid therapy[104]—gastrointestinal hemorrhage, suscep-

tibility to infection, adrenal suppression, psychosis, and others—may occur. It takes several hours for steroids to reduce ICP, and the full effect may not occur before 24 hours. Therefore, steroids are not useful in the emergency treatment of intracranial hypertension. Steroid therapy, however, appears ineffective when the ICP is greater than 25 torr.[104a,104b]

CSF Drainage

Lumbar CSF drainage is used occasionally to improve access to aneurysms of the circle of Willis. Because of the danger of herniation of the cerebellar tonsils, lumbar drainage is seldom performed when ICP is increased. Intracranial hypertension resulting from obstructive hydrocephalus can be treated by draining CSF through a burr hole from a catheter placed in a lateral ventricle. Increased ICP from cerebral edema can be treated in a similar fashion, but withdrawal of CSF may lead to collapse of the ventricular system.

Hypothermia

Hypothermia reduces ICP, probably by reducing CBF and $CMRO_2$. When hypothermia is used to lower ICP in the absence of barbiturates, the maximum effect is achieved at temperatures below 27°C.[105] At these temperatures, hypotension and ventricular fibrillation are common, and management is complicated by changes in the viscosity, coagulability, and acid-base status of the blood. Shapiro and colleagues[106] found that hypothermia to 30°C further reduced the ICP of patients being treated with pentobarbital coma for intracranial hypertension. Currently, Shapiro allows the temperatures of similar patients to drift between 33°C and 35°C.[35] However, there are no clinical data that demonstrate that patients treated with barbiturates and mild hypothermia have a better outcome than patients treated with barbiturates alone.

Prolonged hypothermia (1–3 days) introduces additional problems that include a progressive reduction in both cardiac output and oxygen consumption, with severe metabolic acidosis upon rewarming. Hemodynamic collapse and death ensue in animal models.[207,108] (See Chap. 49.)

REFERENCES

1. Youmans, J.R., (ed.): Neurological Surgery. p. 316. Philadelphia, W. B. Saunders, 1973.
2. Hedlund, S., and Nylin, G.: Cerebral blood flow and circulation time, studied with labelled erythrocytes. Arch. Inter. Pharmacodyn. Ther., *139*:503, 1962.
3. Plum, F., and Siesjö, B. K.: Recent advances in CSF physiology. Anesthesiology, *42*:708, 1975.
4. Cutler, R. W. P., Page, L., Galicich, J., *et al.*: Formation and absorption of cerebrospinal fluid in man. Brain, *91*:707, 1968.
5. Langfitt, T. W.: Increased intracranial pressure. Clin. Neurosurg. *16*:436, 1969.
6. Shulman, K., Yarnell, P., and Ransohoff, J.: Dural sinus pressure in normal and hydrocephalic dog. Arch. Neurosurg. *10*:575, 1964.
7. Sullivan, H. G., Miller, J. D., Becker, D. P., *et al:.*,The physiological basis of intracranial pressure change with progressive epidural brain compression. J. Neurosurg., *47*:532, 1977.
8. Miller, J. D., Garibi, J., and Pickard, J. Q.: Induced changes of cerebrospinal fluid volume. Arch. Neurol., *28*:265, 1973.
9. Marmarou, A., Shulman, K., and Rosende, R. M.: A non linear analysis of the cerebrospinal fluid system and intracranial pressure dynamics. J. Neurosurg. *48*:332, 1978.
10. Marmarou, A., Shulman, K., and LaMorgese, J.: Compartmental analysis of compliance and outflow resistance of the cerebrospinal fluid system. J. Neurosurg. *43*:523, 1975.
11. Sklar, F. H., and Elashvili, I.: The pressure-volume function of brain elasticity—physiological considerations and clinical applications. J. Neurosurg., *47*:670, 1977.
12. Strangaard, S., Olesen, J., Skinhoj, E., *et al.*: Autoregulations of brain circulation in severe arterial hypertension. Br. Med. J., *1*:507, 1973.
13. Langfitt, T. W., Weinstein, J. D., and Kassell, N. F.: Cerebral vasomotor paralysis produced by intracranial hypertension. Neurology (Minneap.), *15*:622, 1965.
14. Fishman, R. A.: Brain edema. N. Engl. J. Med., *293*:706, 1975.
15. Wahl, M., Deetjen, P., Thurau, K., *et al.*: Micropuncture evaluation of the importance of perivascular pH for the arteriolar diameter on the brain surface. Pfluegers Arch. *316*:152, 1970.
16. Reivich, M.: Arterial P_{CO_2} and cerebral hemodynamics. Am. J. Physiol., *206*:25, 1964.
17. Kogure, K., Scheinberg, P., Reinmuth, O. M., *et al.*: Mechanisms of cerebral vasodilatation in hypoxia. J. Appl. Physiol., *29*:223, 1970.
18. Ingvar, D. H., and Lassen, N. A. (eds.): Brain work: The Coupling of Function, Metabolism, and Blood Flow in the Brain. Copenhagen, Munksgaard, 1975.
19. Lassen, N. A., and Christensen, M. S.: Physiology of cerebral blood flow. Br. J. Anaesth., *48*:719, 1976.
20. Johansson, B., Strandgaard, S., and Lassen, N. A.: On the pathogenesis of hypertensive encephalopathy—the hypertensive ''break through'' of autoregulation of cerebral blood flow with forced vasodilation, flow increase, and blood-brain barrier damage. Circ. Res. (Suppl. I), *34*:I-167,: 1974.
21. Fitch, W., Ferguson, G. G., Sengupta, D., *et al.*,: Autoregulation of cerebral blood flow during controlled hypotension. Stroke, *4*:324, 1973.
22. James, I. M., Millar, R. A., and Purves, M. J.: Observations on the extrinsic neural control of cerebral blood flow in the baboon. Circ. Res., *25*:77, 1969.
23. Ponte, J., and Purves, M. J.: The role of the carotid body chemoreceptors and carotid sinus baroreceptors in the control of cerebral blood vessels. J. Physiol. (Lond.), *237*:315, 1974.
24. Berntam, L., Dahlgren, N., and Siesjö, B. K.: Cerebral blood flow and oxygen consumption in the rat brain during extreme hypercarbia. Anesthesiology, *50*:299, 1979.
25. Jennett, W. B., Barker, J., Fitch, W., *et al.*: Effect of anaesthesia on intracranial pressure in patients with space-occupying lesions. Lancet, *1*:61, 1969.
26. Adams, R. W., Gronert, G. A., Sundt, T. M., *et al.*: Halothane, hypocapnia, and cerebrospinal fluid pressure in neurosurgery. Anesthesiology, *37*:510, 1972.
27. Wollman, H., Smith, A. L., and Hoffman, J. C.: Cerebral blood flow and oxygen consumption in man during electroencephalographic seizure patterns induced by anesthesia with ethrane. Fed. Proc., *28*:356, 1969.
28. Murphy, F. L., Kennell, E. M., Johnstone, R. E., *et al.*: The effects of enflurane, isoflurane, and halothane on cerebral blood flow and metabolism in man. Abstracts of Scientific Papers, Annual Meeting of the American Society of Anesthesiologists, pp. 61–62, 1974.
28a. Adams, R. W., Cucchiara, R. F., Gronert, G. A., *et al.*: Isoflurane and cerebrospinal fluid pressure in neurosurgical patients. Anesthesiology, *54*:97, 1981.
29. Henriksen, H. T., and Jörgensen, P. B.: The effect of nitrous oxide on intracranial pressure in patients with intracranial disorders. Br. J. Anaesth., *45*:486, 1973.
30. Wollman, H., Alexander, S. C., Cohen, P. J., *et al.*: Cerebral circulation during general anesthesia and hyperventilation in man. Anesthesiology, *26*:329, 1965.
31. Phirman, J. R., and Shapiro, H. M.: Modification of nitrous oxide-induced intracranial hypertension by prior induction of anesthesia. Anesthesiology, *46*:150, 1977.
32. Theye, R. A., and Michenfelder, J. D.: The effect of nitrous oxide on canine cerebral metabolism. Anesthesiology, *29*:1119, 1968.
33. Sakabe, T., Kuramoto, T., Inove, S., *et al.*: Cerebral effects of nitrous oxide in the dog. Anesthesiology, *48*:195, 1978.
34. Shapiro, H. M., Galindo, A., Wyte, S. R., *et al.*: Rapid intraoperative reduction of intracranial pressure with thiopentone. Br. J. Anaesth., *45*:1057, 1973.
35. Marshall, L. F., Smith, R. W., and Shapiro, H. M.: The outcome with agressive treatment in severe head injuries. Part II: Acute and chronic barbiturate administration in the management of head injury. J. Neurosurg., *50*:26, 1979.
36. Marshall, L. F., Shapiro, H. M., Rauscher, A., *et al.*: Pentobarbital therapy for intracranial hypertension in metabolic coma—Reye's syndrome. Crit. Care Med., *6*:1, 1978.
37. Smith, A. L.: Barbiturate protection in cerebral hypoxia. Anesthesiology, *47*:285, 1977.
38. Michenfelder, J. D.: The interdependency of cerebral functional and metabolic effects following massive doses of thiopental in the dog. Anesthesiology, *41*:231, 1974.

39. Moss, E., Powell, D., Gibson, R. M., et al.: Effects of tracheal intubation on intracranial pressure following induction of anaesthesia with thiopentone or althesin in patients undergoing neurosurgery. Br. J. Anaesth., 50:353, 1978.

40. Marsh, M. L., Marshall, L. F., and Shapiro, H. M.: Neurosurgical intensive care. Anesthesiology, 47:149, 1977.

40a. Miller, J. D.: Barbiturates and raised intracranial pressure. Ann. Neurol., 6:189, 1979.

40b. Rockoff, M. A., Marshall, L. F., and Shapiro, H. M.: High-dose barbiturate therapy in humans: A clinical review of 60 patients. Ann. Neurol, 6:194, 1979.

40c. Trauner, D. A.: Treatment of Reye syndrome. Ann. Neurol, 7:2, 1980.

41. Bali, I. M., and Dundee, J. W.: The effect of induction agents on cerebrospinal fluid pressure. Br. J. Anaesth., 49:1169, 1977.

42. Cotev, S., and Shalit, M. N.: Effects of diazepam on cerebral blood flow and oxygen uptake after head injury. Anesthesiology, 43:117, 1975.

43. Carlsson, C., Hägerdal, M., Kaasik, A. E., et al.: The effects of dizaepam on cerebral blood flow and oxygen consumption in rats and its synergistic interaction with nitrous oxide. Anesthesiology, 45:319, 1976.

44. Larson, G. F., Hurlbert, B. J., and Wingard, D. W.: Physostigmine reversal of diazepam-induced depression. Anesth. Analg., 56:348, 1977.

45. Hall, S. C., and Ovassapian, A.: Apnea after intravenous diazepam therapy. J. A. M. A., 238:1052, 1977.

46. Weitzner, S. W., McCoy, G. T., and Binder, L. S.: Effects of morphine, levallorphan, and respiratory gases on increased intracranial pressure. Anesthesiology, 24:291, 1963.

47. Jobes, D. R., Kennell, E. M., Bush, G. L., et al.: Cerebral blood flow and metabolism during morphine-nitrous oxide anesthesia in man. Anesthesiology, 47:16, 1977.

48. Fitch, W., Barker, J., Jennett, W. B., et al.: The influence of neuroleptanalgesic drugs on cerebrospinal fluid pressure. Br. J. Anaesth., 41:800, 1969.

49. Michenfelder, J. D., and Theye, R. A.: Effects of fentanyl, droperidol, and Innovar on canine cerebral metabolism and blood flow. Br. J. Anaesth., 43:630, 1971.

50. Misfeldt, B. B., Jörgensen, P. B., Spotoft, H., et. al.: The effects of droperidol and fentanyl on intracranial pressure and cerebral perfusion pressure in neurosurgical patients. Br. J. Anaesth., 48:963, 1976.

51. Bidwai, A. V., Cornelius, L. R., and Stanley, T. H.: Reversal of Innovar-induced postanesthetic somnolence and disorientation with physostigmine. Anesthesiology, 44:249, 1976.

52. Shapiro, H. M., Wyte, S. R., and Harris, A. B.: Ketamine anaesthesia in patients with intracranial pathology. Br. J. Anaesth., 44:1200, 1972.

53. Takeshita, H., Okuda, Y., and Sari, A.: The effects of ketamine on cerebral circulation and metabolism in man. Anesthesiology, 36:69, 1972.

54. Sondergard, W.: Intracranial pressure during general anesthesia. Dan. Med. Bull., 8:18, 1961.

55. Cullen, D. J.: The effect of pretreatment with nondepolarizing muscle relaxants on the neuromuscular blocking action of succinylcholine. Anesthesiology, 35:572, 1971.

56. Cooperman, L. H., Strobel, G. E., and Kennell, E. M.: Massive hyperkalemia after administration of succinylcholine. Anesthesiology, 32:161, 1970.

57. Cowgill, D. B., Mostello, L. A., and Shapiro, H. M.: Encephalitis and a hyperkalemic response to succinylcholine. Anesthesiology, 40:409, 1974.

58. Weintraub, H. D., Heisterkamp, D. V., and Cooperman, L. H.: Changes in plasma potassium concentration after depolarizing blockers in anesthetized man. Br. J. Anaesth., 41:1048, 1969.

59. Konchigeri H. N., and Tay C. H.: Influence of pancuronium on potassium efflux produced by succinylcholine. Anesth. Analg., 55:474, 1976.

60. Tarkkanen, L., Laitinen, L., and Johansson, G.: Effects of d-tubocurarine on intracranial pressure and thalamic electrical impedance. Anesthesiology, 40:247, 1974.

61. Ivankovich, A. D., Miletich, D. J., Albrecht, R. F., et al.: Sodium nitroprusside and cerebral blood flow in the anesthetized and unanesthetized goat. Anesthesiology, 44:21, 1976.

62. Cottrell, J. E., Patel, K., Turndorf, H., et al.: Intracranial pressure changes induced by sodium nitroprusside in patients with intracranial mass lesions. J. Neurosurg., 48:329, 1978.

63. Turner, J. M., Powell, D., Gibson, R. M., et al.: Intracranial pressure changes in neurosurgical patients during hypotension induced with sodium nitroprusside or trimethaphan. Br. J. Anaesth., 49:419, 1977.

64. Keaney, N. P., McDowall, D. G., Turner, J. M., et al.: The effects of profound hypotension induced with sodium nitroprusside on cerebral blood flow and metabolism in the baboon. Br. J. Anaesth., 45:639, 1973.

65. Ivankovich, A. D., Sheth, D. J., Shulman, M., et al.: Autoregulation of cerebral blood flow during infusion of trimethaphan or nitroglycerin in the goat. Abstracts of Scientific Papers, American Society of Anesthesiologists Annual Meeting, pp. 77–78, 1978.

66. Michenfelder, J. D., and Theye, R. A.: Canine systemic and cerebral effects of hypotension induced by hemorrhage, trimethaphan, halothane, or nitroprusside. Anesthesiology, 46:188, 1977.

67. Chestnut, J. S., Albin, M. S., Gonzalez-Abola, E., et al.: Clinical evaluation of intravenous nitroglycerin for neurosurgery. J. Neurosurg., 48:704, 1978.

68. Overgaard, J., and Skinhoj, E.: A paradoxical cerebral hemodynamic effect of hydralazine. Stroke, 6:402, 1975.

69. Shapiro, H. M.: Intracranial hypertension: Therapeutic and anesthetic considerations. Anesthesiology, 43:445, 1975.

70. Eckenhoff, J. E., Enderby, G. E. H., Larson, A.. et al.: Pulmonary gas exchange during deliberate hypotension. Br. J. Anaesth., 35:750, 1963.

71. Wildsmith, J. A. W., Drummond, G. B., and MacRae, W. R.: Blood gas changes during induced hypotension with sodium nitroprusside. Br. J. Anaesth., 47:1205, 1975.

72. Cuypers, J., Matakas, F., and Potolicchio, S. J., Jr.: Effect of central venous pressure on brain tissue and brain volume. J. Neurosurg., 45:89, 1976.

73. Hulme, A., and Cooper, R.: The effects of head position and jugular vein compression (JVC) on intracranial pressure (ICP). A clinical study. In Beks, J. W. F., Bosch, D. A., Brock, M. (eds.): Intracranial Pressure III, pp. 259–263. Berlin, Springer-Verlag, 1976.

74. Shapiro, H. M., and Marshall, L. F.: Intracranial pressure responses to PEEP in head-injured patients. Trauma, *18*:254, 1978.

75. Apuzzo, M. L. J., Weiss, M. H., Petersons, V., *et al.*: Effect of positive end expiratory pressure ventilation on intracranial pressure in man. J. Neurosurg., *46*:227, 1977.

76. Frost, E. M.: Effects of positive end-expiratory pressure on intracranial pressure and compliance in brain-injured patients. J. Neurosurg., *47*:195, 1977.

77. Williams, B.: Cerebrospinal fluid pressure changes in response to coughing. Brain, *99*:331, 1976.

78. Kety, S. S.: Circulation and metabolism of the human brain in health and disease. Am. J. Med., *8*:205, 1950.

79. Shapiro, H. M., Wyte, S. R., Harris, A. B., *et al.*: Acute intraoperative intracranial hypertension in neurosurgical patients: mechanical and pharmacologic factors. Anesthesiology, *37*:399, 1972.

80. Alexander, S. C., and Lassen, N. A.: Cerebral circulatory response to acute brain disease: implications for anesthetic practice. Anesthesiology, *32*:60, 1970.

81. Keaney, N. P., Pickerodt, V. W., McDowall, D. G., *et al.*: Cerebral circulatory and metabolic effects of hypotension produced by deep halothane anaesthesia. J. Neurol. Neurosurg. Psychiatry, *36*:898, 1973.

82. Youmans, J. R., (ed.): Neurological Surgery. p. .1467. Philadelphia, W. B. Saunders, 1973.

83. McDowall, D. G.: Monitoring the brain. Anesthesiology, *45*:117, 1976.

84. Shapiro, H. M.: Monitoring in neurosurgical anesthesia. In Saidman, L. J., and Smith, N. T. (eds.): Monitoring in Anesthesia, pp. 171-204. John Wiley & Sons, Inc., 1978.

85. Lundberg, N.: Continuous recording and control of ventricular fluid pressure in neurosurgical practice. Acta Psychiatr. Scand., [Suppl.] *36*:I-193, 1960.

86. Parks, L. K., and Bergman, N. A.: Hypoxia as a manifestation of neurogenic pulmonary dysfunction. Anesthesiology, *45*:93, 1976.

87. Jachuck, S. J., Ramani, P. S., Clark, F., *et al.*: Electrocardiographic abnormalities associated with raised intracranial pressure. Br. Med. J., *1*:242, 1975.

88. Grubb, R. L., Raichle, M. E., Eichling, J. O., *et al.*: The effects of changes in Pa_{CO_2} on cerebral blood volume, blood flow, and vascular mean transit time. Stroke, *5*:630, 1974.

89. Raichle, M. E., Posner, J. B., and Plum, F.: Cerebral blood flow during and after hyperventilation. Arch. Neurol., *23*:394, 1970.

90. Rosomoff, H. L.: Distribution of intracranial contents after hypertonic urea. J. Neurosurg., *19*:859, 1962.

91. Coté, C. J., Greenhow, D. E., and Marshall, B. E.: The hypotensive response to rapid administration of hypertonic solutions in man and in the rabbit. Anesthesiology, *50*:30, 1979.

92. Becker, D. P., and Vries, J. K.: The alleviation of increased intracranial pressure by the chronic administration of osmotic agents. In Brock, M., and Dietz, H. (eds.): Intracranial Pressure—Experimental and Clinical Aspects. pp. 309–315. Berling Springer-Verlag, 1972.

93. Silber, S. J., and Thompson, N.: Mannitol induced central nervous system toxicity in renal failure. Invest. Urol., *9*:310, 1972.

94. Cantore, G., Guidetti, B., and Virno, M.: Oral glycerol for the reduction of intracranial pressure. J. Neurosurg., *21*:278, 1964.

95. Hägnevik, K., Gordon, E., Lins, L. E., *et al.*: Glycerol-induced haemolysis with haemoglobinuria and acute renal failure. Lancet, *1*:75, 1974.

96. Arieff, A. I., Lazarowitz, V. C., and Guisado, R.: Experimental dialysis disequilibrium syndrome: Prevention with glycerol. Kidney Int., *14*:270, 1978.

97. Cottrell, J. E., Robustelli, A., Post, K., et al.: Furosemide- and mannitol-induced changes in intracranial pressure and serum osmolality and electrolytes. Anesthesiology, *47*:28, 1977.

98. Cottrell, J. E., Marx, W., Marlin, A., *et al.*: Furosemide reduces increased intracranial pressure after head trauma. Abstracts of Scientific Papers, American Society of Anesthesiologists Annual Meeting, pp. 161–162, 1978.

99. McCarthy, K. O., and Reed, D. J.: The effect of acetazolamide and furosemide on cerebrospinal fluid production and choroid plexus carbonic anhydrase activity. J. Pharmacol. Exp. Ther., *189*:194, 1974.

100. Galilich, J. H., and French, L. A.: Use of dexamethasone in treatment of cerebral edema resulting from brain tumors and brain surgery. Am. Prac., *12*:169, 1961.

101. Maxwell, R. E., Long, D. M., and French, L. A.: The clinical effects of a synthetic gluco-corticoid used for brain edema in the practice of neurosurgery. In Reulen, H. J., and Schürmann, K. (eds.): Steroids and Brain Edema. pp. 219–232. Heidelberg, Springer-Verlag, 1972.

102. Gobiet, W., Bock, W. J., Liesegang, J. *et al.*: Treatment of acute cerebral edema with high dose of dexamethasone. In Beks, J. W. F., Bosch, D. A., and Brock, M. (eds.): Intracranial Pressure III. pp. 232–235. Berlin, Springer-Verlag, 1976.

103. Faupel, G., Reulen, H. J., Müller, D., *et al.*: Double-blind study on the effects of dexamethasone on severe closed head injury. In Pappius, H. M., and Reulen, W. (eds.), Dynamics of Brain Edema. pp. 337–343. Berlin, Springer-Verlag, 1976.

104. Marshall, L. F., King, J., and Langfitt, T. W.: The complications of high-dose corticosteroid therapy in neurosurgical patients: A prospective study. Ann. Neurol., *1*:201, 1977.

104a. Gudeman, S. K., Miller, J. D., and Becker, D. P.: Failure of high-dose steroid therapy to influence intracranial pressure in patients with severe head injury. J. Neurosurg., *51*:301, 1979.

104b. Saul, T. G., Ducker, T. B., Salcman, M., et al.: Steroids in severe head injury: A prospective randomized clinical trail. J. Neurosurg., *54*:596, 1981.

105. Rosomoff, H. J., Shulman, K., Raynor, R., *et al.*: Experimental brain injury and delayed hypothermia. Surg. Gynecol. Obstet., *110*:27, 1960.

106. Shapiro, H. M., Wyte, S. R., and Loeser, J.: Barbiturate-augmented hypothermia for reduction of persistent intracranial hypertension. J. Neurosurg., *40*:90, 1974.

107. Steen, P. A., Soule, E. H., and Michenfelder, J. D.: Detrimental effect of prolonged hypothermia in cats and monkeys with and without regional cerebral ischemia. Stroke, *10*:522, 1979.

108. Steen, P. A., Milde, J. H., and Michenfelder, J. D.: The detrimental effects of prolonged hypothermia and rewarming the the dog. Anesthesiology, *52*:224, 1980.

FURTHER READING

Fishman, R. A.: Brain edema. N. Engl. J. Med., *293*:706, 1975.

Gordon, E. (ed.): A basis and practice of neuroanesthesia. Monographs in Anesthesiology, Vol. 2. Amsterdam, Experta Medica, 1975.

Langfitt, T. W.: Increased intracranial pressure. Clin. Neurosurg., *16*:436, 1969.

Lassen, N. A., and Christensen, M. S.: Physiology of cerebral blood flow. Br. J. Anaesth., *48*:719, 1976.

Plum, F., and Siesjö, B. K.: Recent advances in CSF physiology. Anesthesiology, *42*:708, 1975.

Shapiro, H. M.: Intracranial hypertension: therapeutic and anesthetic considerations. Anesthesiology, *43*:445, 1975.

21 Cerebral Hypoxia With Hyperventilation

James R. Harp, M.D., and Harry Wollman, M.D.

Cerebral ischemia occurs whenever blood flow becomes inadequate to maintain normal brain function and metabolism. Functional abnormality may range from minimal changes in reaction time to irreversible coma. A corresponding range of alterations in cerebral metabolism can be identified. One might arbitrarily define clinically significant cerebral ischemia in terms of irreversibility of functional or metabolic change—that is, the point at which permanent brain tissue injury occurs. This chapter questions whether hypocapnic ischemic injury is likely to occur in normal humans, and whether hypocapnic cerebral vasoconstriction is likely to reduce brain tissue tolerance to other forms of circulatory compromise, such as vascular stenosis or hypotension.

RELATIONSHIP BETWEEN VENTILATION AND Pa_{CO_2}

Hyperventilation affects cerebral blood flow (CBF) by lowering cerebral arteriolar P_{CO_2} and hydrogen ion concentration. If one doubles alveolar ventilation, Pa_{CO_2} will fall within minutes to half its initial value.[1] For example, if $(\dot{V}_A)$, equals 4 L. per min., and Pa_{CO_2} equals 40 torr, increasing $\dot{V}_A$ to 8 L. per min. lowers Pa_{CO_2} to 20 torr. From a practical point of view, attainment of $\dot{V}_A$ of 8 L. per min. requires an increase in minute ventilation in healthy young adults from 6 to 14 L. per min.[2] To produce $\dot{V}_A$ of 16 L. per min. and a Pa_{CO_2} of 10 torr, minute ventilation must be increased

to 27 L. per min.[2] Thus, while a Pa_{CO_2} of 20 torr may be achieved readily in a clinical setting, it seems unlikely that a Pa_{CO_2} of 10 torr will occur. As discussed below, a Pa_{CO_2} of 20 torr approaches the limits of safety in healthy patients.

EFFECT OF Pa_{CO_2} ON BRAIN BLOOD FLOW

Pa_{CO_2} and Cerebral Blood Flow in Normal Subjects

The response of CBF to variations of Pa_{CO_2} in the absence of intracranial pathology has been well documented in animals[3] (Fig. 21-1) and humans (Fig. 21-2).[4–8] Between a Pa_{CO_2} of 20 and 80 torr, an increase of 1 torr produces a 2- to 4-per-cent increase in CBF. In anesthetized humans, volatile agents which themselves produce some degree of cerebral vasodilation may reduce the effect of Pa_{CO_2} at levels above 50 torr, while hypocapnic cerebral vasoconstriction remains unaltered.[2,7] This means that the range of Pa_{CO_2} occurring in anesthetized patients—that is, from 20 torr to 60 torr—can effect a threefold change in CBF, from 20 to 60 ml. per 100 g. brain per min. In clinical anesthesia, Pa_{CO_2} is the most potent single determinant of CBF.

Pa_{CO_2} and Cerebral Blood Flow in Patients with Intracranial Pathology

Focal areas of cerebral hyperemia have been described in apoplexy,[9–11] brain tumor,[12] subarach-

331

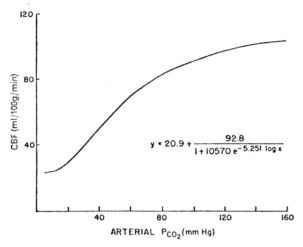

Fig. 21-1. The relationship between cerebral blood flow and Pa_{CO_2} in monkeys. (Redrawn from Reivich, M.: Arterial P_{CO_2} and cerebral hemodynamics. Am. J. Physiol., *206*:25, 1964, *In* Harp, J.R., and Wollman, H.: Cerebral metabolic effects of hyperventilation and deliberate hypotension. Br. J. Anaesth., *45*:256, 1973)

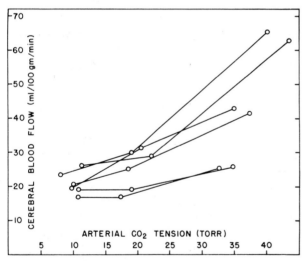

Fig. 21-2. Cerebral blood flow as a function of Pa_{CO_2} in six men. (Wollman, H., Smith, T. C., and Stephen, G.W.: Effects of extremes of respiratory and metabolic alkalosis on cerebral blood flow in man. J. Appl. Physiol., *24*:60, 1968)

mic brain tissue. Within hyperemic areas, there is no vascular autoregulation to blood pressure changes, and CBF is directly dependent upon cerebral perfusion pressure. It has been predicted that hypocapnia, by increasing vascular resistance in normal cerebral arterioles, might increase perfusion pressure and blood flow in these hyperemic foci, and that this should lead to improved blood flow in adjacent ischemic brain tissue. This phenomenon, called an *inverse steal*, has been documented in some instances[15] but is not by any means predictable. For example, hypocapnic reduction of regional cerebral blood flow (rCBF) in ischemic brain has been shown to occur in a 9-year-old girl with acute occlusion of the middle cerebral artery.[16] Because of this unpredictability, institution of hypocapnia in an attempt to increase flow to ischemic brain is not justified, except in patients in whom measurement of rCBF can be made.

When Pa_{CO_2} is increased in patients who exhibit focal abnormalities of CBF, rCBF may decrease in hyperemic foci as well as in ischemic regions. This phenomenon has been called the *intracerebral steal*. In one 16-year-old patient with an acute subdural hematoma, increase of Pa_{CO_2} from 24 to 36 torr produced a significant reduction in rCBF in an ischemic frontal region.[17] In a second patient, a 67-year-old man with 95-per-cent stenosis of the right carotid artery and a 7-day-old right cerebral infarction, increase of Pa_{CO_2} from 33 to 39 torr reduced focal rCBF in the area of the middle cerebral artery from 17 to 12 ml. per 100 g. per min.[18] These are exceptional cases, for intracerebral steal does not regularly occur at Pa_{CO_2} of less than 60 torr. The common response of CBF to hypercapnia in patients with intracranial disease is a smaller increase than that which occurs in normal humans.[10,19]

POSSIBLE HARMFUL EFFECTS OF HYPERVENTILATION

Evidence for Ischemia Secondary to Hyperventilation in Normal Humans

The rate of fall of CBF decreases at a Pa_{CO_2} of less than 20 torr (Fig. 21-2).[2,3,5,20,21] Perhaps brain

noid hemorrhage,[13] and head injury.[14] It is believed that these areas of increased flow are produced by diffusion of vasodilator substances, such as lactate or potassium, from adjacent ische-

ischemia at this degree of CBF reduction (40%) may preclude additional hypocapnic cerebral vasoconstriction. There are greater degrees of cerebral vasoconstriction when hypocapnia is combined with hyperbaric oxygenation,[22] which permits the brain to remain adequately oxygenated during severe vasoconstriction. A similar phenomenon occurs when hypothermic animals are hyperventilated.[21]

EEG Changes During Hyperventilation

Early electroencephalographers described reductions in EEG frequency in association with hyperventilation that are very similar to those appearing when Pa_{CO_2} is lower than 20 torr,[23-27] a level at which the cerebral vasoconstrictor response has begun to diminish. Elevation of blood sugar levels[28] and inhalation of 100-per-cent oxygen[24,29] reduce the severity of EEG slowing with hyperventilation, while exposure to hyperbaric oxygen totally abolishes these changes.[30] Hypoxia[28,29] and carotid artery compression[31] exaggerate EEG slowing during hyperventilation. All of these observations suggest that production of cerebral ischemia secondary to reduced brain blood flow is the mechanism by which hyperventilation produces EEG slowing. Additional support for this hypothesis is that EEG slowing correlates better with jugular Pv_{O_2} (20 ± 1 torr) than with jugular Pv_{CO_2} or pH.[32]

CEREBRAL METABOLIC CHANGES DURING HYPERVENTILATION

Carbohydrate Metabolism During Hyperventilation

Alterations of intracellular pH alone may produce marked changes in cerebral carbohydrate metabolism. Alkalosis has been shown to increase lactate production in brain in vitro by two- to threefold.[33] During hyperventilation, brain tissue lactate increases gradually as Pa_{CO_2} is lowered from 40 to 20 torr; at this point lactate levels begin to increase very rapidly, and excess lactate levels appear for the first time.[34] In humans, hyperventilation to Pa_{CO_2} of 10 torr produces a 10-per-cent reduction of cerebral oxygen consumption, accompanied by an increase in cerebral glucose consumption and a marked increase in the fraction of glucose undergoing anaerobic metabolism.[35] These changes are similar to those seen during hypoxia.[36]

Measurement of NADH During Hyperventilation

Studies of cellular oxygenation have focused on the measurement of NAD and its reduced form, NADH. NAD is a coenzyme essential for the electron transport coincident with cellular respiration. When there is sufficient cellular oxygen, NADH levels are low. But, should the cell become hypoxic, the amount of intracellular (mitochondrial) NADH increases, thus serving as a marker for the state of cellular oxygenation. In rats, for example, hyperventilation to Pa_{CO_2} of 12 torr produces a significant increase in mitochondrial NADH, and this increase is totally reversed by carbon dioxide inhalation and partially reversed by inhalation of 100 per-cent oxygen.[37] Similar levels of NADH are present in brain mitochondrial preparations at P_{O_2} of 0.5 torr, while oxygen consumption, a less sensitive index of cellular oxygenation, is not reduced until P_{O_2} of 0.2 torr.[38]

Adenosinetriphosphate (ATP) and Phosphocreatine in Hyperventilation

High-energy phosphates may be considered the coin of the metabolic realm, since they represent the means by which energy is captured in catabolism for use in anabolic processes. Cerebral tissue contains scanty stores of phosphocreatine and ATP. Total interruption of CBF depletes these stores within 1 min. in mice[39] and within 3 to 6 min. in dogs.[40] During partial ischemia, cerebral ATP levels decline gradually, over a period of hours.[41]

Earlier investigations failed to demonstrate reduction in brain ATP or phosphocreatine during acute hyperventilation in cats and rats,[34] and only minimal declines in ATP were observed in the dog.[42] Hyperventilation to Pa_{CO_2} of 10 torr in the rat has recently been found to produce slight reduction in brain phosphocreatine and slight increases in brain ADP,[43] suggesting a reduction in brain ATP. None of these studies have produced convincing evidence of cerebral energy store reduction owing to hyperventilation. However, following middle cerebral artery occlusion in squirrel monkeys, prolonged hyperventilation (2 hours) has been shown to increase the rate of ATP depletion and lactate accumulation.[41]

Regulation of Intracellular pH During Hyperventilation

It is possible to determine experimentally brain intracellular pH from measurements of P_{CO_2} of cisternal cerebrospinal fluid (which is equal, at steady state, to brain tissue P_{CO_2}), and total carbon dioxide content of brain tissue (obtained from a brain biopsy specimen), using the Henderson-Hasselbach relationship. Brain intracellular pH is closely regulated during hyperventilation. In the rat, reduction of Pa_{CO_2} from 38.6 torr to 14.9 torr increased arterial pH from 7.429 to 7.677 in one study, while brain intracellular pH increased from 7.044 to 7.088, in spite of a fall in P_{CO_2} tissue tension from 44.9 to 23.6 torr.[44] The relative constancy of intracellular pH is caused by the accumulation of acid metabolites, the most significant being lactate and glutamate.

EVIDENCE FOR ISCHEMIA SECONDARY TO HYPERVENTILATION IN PATIENTS WITH INTRACRANIAL PATHOLOGY

Except for one rare study in humans,[16] it is necessary to review animal studies for evidence of ischemia secondary to hyperventilation. Hypocapnia has been shown to produce additional reduction of CBF in ischemic brain following acute occlusion of intracranial vessels in various species.[45–50] An early study by Soloway showed that hyperventilation markedly reduced the extent of infarction following transtemporal clipping of the internal carotid and middle cerebral artery in dogs, though control and experimental groups were not entirely comparable.[51] In this study, hyperventilation to Pa_{CO_2} of 20 to 25 torr was begun 60 min. before vascular clipping and continued for 2 hours following clipping.

In a subsequent study in which hypocapnia was instituted 30 min. following vascular clipping, no "hypocapnic protection" could be identified.[49] Yamamoto and Feindel occluded a distal branch

of the middle cerebral artery in dogs following wide craniectomy under pentobarbital anesthesia.[50] Effects of changed Pa_{CO_2} upon blood flow in the resulting ischemic area were evaluated by ^{133}Xe flow measurement and by fluorescein angiography. Hypocapnia uniformly reduced flow, and hypercapnia increased flow in the ischemic brain. Yamaguchi and Waltz occluded the middle cerebral artery of cats transorbitally and measured rCBF response to altered Pa_{CO_2} using ^{14}C-antipyrine.[47] Again, hypocapnia reduced blood flow in ischemic regions. In contrast to Yamamoto's findings, hypercapnia also produced reduced flow in ischemic brain. A possible explanation of this difference is that hypercapnia increased intracranial pressure in animals without craniotomy, reducing perfusion pressure in ischemic areas, an effect which would be less marked when wide craniectomy permitted expansion of brain tissue.

These studies and the others previously cited provide no evidence for the occurrence of "inverse intracerebral steal" or the so-called Robin Hood syndrome.

Michenfelder determined the effect of hyperventilation upon metabolism in ischemic brain of squirrel monkeys following transorbital occlusion of the middle cerebral artery.[41] Cerebral levels of lactate and pyruvate were higher and ATP levels significantly lower in hypocapnic animals than in spontaneously ventilating animals. Much of this effect may have been secondary to reduction of mean arterial pressure from 114 to 89 torr in ventilated animals, especially since metabolite levels nearly identical to those of hypocapnia appeared when animals were mechanically ventilated and made normocapnic by adding carbon dioxide to inspired gases.

While additional studies are needed in this area, present evidence indicates that normocapnia is probably more desirable than hypocapnia or hypercapnia in management of acute stroke.

POSSIBLE BENEFITS OF HYPERVENTILATION

Benefits of Hyperventilation in Normal Subjects

The clinical impression that hyperventilation reduces anesthetic requirement has not been tested in controlled conditions. Reduction in abdominal electromyogram intensity during hyperventilation has been noted, suggesting to some physicians that there is a reduced requirement for relaxant drugs. Increased alveolar ventilation increases alveolar anesthetic concentration, increasing the anesthetic effect of any given inspired concentration. In addition, hypocapnia decreases or abolishes ventilatory drive. Yet, careful studies find no change in MAC with hyperventilation.[52–54] Hence, at present, evidence for this "advantage" of hyperventilation during anesthesia is not convincing.

Benefits of Hyperventilation in Patients With Intracranial Pathology

Carotid Endarterectomy. Distal carotid artery pressure measured during endarterectomy is frequently increased during hypocapnia,[55,56] though this does not necessarily indicate increased CBF.[18,56] However, in patients having focal abnormalities of CBF, mild hypocapnia (Pa_{CO_2} = 35 torr) and its attendant increase in carotid artery pressure may be desirable. Unfortunately this group, comprising 15 to 20 per cent of patients undergoing endarterectomy, can be identified only through measurement of rCBF. Since Pa_{CO_2} of 35 torr is not likely to be harmful to most patients, this level seems most desirable for management of carotid endarterectomy.

Intracranial Hypertension. Brain tissue reacts to injury by swelling, and in general, the degree of swelling relates to the severity of injury. Within the cranial vault, unoccupied space is limited, and marked brain swelling invariably leads to intracranial hypertension or increased intracranial pressure. Intracranial hypertension reduces cerebral perfusion pressure. Autoregulation maintains CBF until cerebral perfusion pressure falls to about 60 torr; beyond this point, CBF becomes directly proportional to perfusion pressure.

Intracranial pressure may fluctuate in brain injury, suddenly increasing to levels beyond the autoregulatory range and falling again after a period of minutes. These fluctuations are called *pressure waves*, and may be accompanied by symptoms of CNS deterioration.

Finally, with extreme brain edema, intracranial pressure rises to equal mean arterial pressure.

CBF ceases. This state of cerebral vasomotor paralysis defines brain death.

Hyperventilation can modify the circulatory component of brain tissue reaction to injury. Pressure waves can be aborted as Pa_{CO_2} is lowered.[57] Elevated intracranial pressure may be dramatically reduced. For this reason, hyperventilation, as well as direct measurement of intracranial pressure,[58] has been recommended in treatment of brain swelling.[59] Carefully controlled clinical trials measuring rCBF, intracranial pressure, EEG, and neurologic status are in progress and should be able to document the usefulness of hyperventilation in the treatment of cerebral edema.

CLINICAL RECOMMENDATIONS

Hyperventilation is capable of producing significant transient cerebral ischemia in normal man.[36] However, no permanent harm should result when Pa_{CO_2} is reduced to 20 torr for a period of hours in normal patients. Normocapnia appears more desirable than either hypercapnia or hypocapnia in acute stroke, while mild hypocapnia (Pa_{CO_2} = 35 torr) appears most desirable in patients undergoing carotid endarterectomy. When there is marked brain swelling, hyperventilation may be helpful in controlling intracranial pressure. It is practical and desirable that intracranial pressure be monitored when hyperventilation is used to treat brain swelling.[58]

REFERENCES

1. Severinghaus, J. W., and Lassen, N.: Step hypocapnea to separate arterial from tissue P_{CO_2} in the regulation of cerebral blood flow. Circ. Res., 20:272, 1967.
2. Wollman, H., Smith, T. C., Stephen, G. W., et al.: Effects of extremes of respiratory and metabolic alkalosis on cerebral blood flow in man. J. Appl. Physiol., 24:60, 1968.
3. Reivich, M.: Arterial P_{CO_2} and cerebral hemodynamics. Am. J. Physiol., 206:25, 1964.
4. Kety, S. S., and Schmidt, C. F.: The effects of altered arterial tensions of carbon dioxide and oxygen on cerebral blood flow and cerebral oxygen consumption of normal young men. J. Clin. Invest., 27:484, 1968.
5. Wasserman, A. J., and Patterson, J. L., Jr.: The cerebrovascular response to reduction in arterial carbon dioxide tension. J. Clin. Invest., 40:1297, 1961.
6. Pierce, E. C., Jr., Lambertsen, C. J., Deutsch, S., et al.: Cerebral circulation and metabolism during thiopental anesthesia and hyperventilation in man. J. Clin. Invest., 41:1664, 1962.

7. Alexander, S. C., Wollman, H., Cohen, P. J., et al.: Cerebrovascular response to Pa$_{CO_2}$ during halothane anesthesia in man. J. Appl. Physiol., *19*:561, 1964.

8. McHenry, L. C., Slocum, H. C., Bivins, H. E., et al.: Hyperventilation in awake and anesthetized man. Effects on cerebral blood flow and cerebral metabolism. Arch. Neurol., *12*:270, 1965.

9. Hoedt-Rasmussen, K., Skinhöj, E., Paulson, O, et al.: Regional cerebral blood flow in acute apoplexy. Arch. Neurol., *17*:271, 1967.

10. McHenry, L. C., Goldberg, H. I., Jaffe, M. E., et al.: Regional cerebral blood flow's response to carbon dioxide inhalation in cerebrovascular disease. Arch. Neurol., *27*:403, 1972.

11. Paulson, O. B.: Cerebral apoplexy (stroke). Pathogenesis, pathophysiology and therapy as illustrated by regional blood flow measurements in the brain. Stroke, *2*:327, 1971.

12. Paulson, O. B., Olesen, M. D., and Christensen, M. S.: Restoration of autoregulation of cerebral blood flow by hypocapnea. Neurology, *22*:286, 1972.

13. Heilbrun, M. P., Olesen, J., and Lassen, N. A.: Regional cerebral blood flow studies in subarachnoid hemorrhage. J. Neurosurg., *37*:36, 1972.

14. Kasoff, S., Zingesser, L. H., and Shulman, K.: Compartmental abnormalities of regional cerebral blood flow in children with head trauma. J. Neurosurg., *36*:463, 1972.

15. Paulson, O. B.: Regional cerebral blood flow in apoplexy due to occlusion of the middle cerebral artery. Neurology, *20*:63, 1970.

16. Brock, M., Hadjidmos, A. A., and Schürmann, K.: Possible adverse effects of hyperventilation on rCBF during the acute phase of total proximal occlusion of a main cerebral artery. *In* Brock, M., Fieschi, C., Inguar, D. H., et al. (eds.): Cerebral Blood Flow: Clinical and Experimental Results. pp. 254–257. Berlin, Springer-Verlag, 1969.

17. Heilbrun, M. P., Jorgensen, P. B., and Boysen, G.: Relationships between perfusion pressure and regional cerebral blood flow in patients with intracranial mass lesions. Eur. Neurol., *8*:11, 1972.

18. Waltz, A. G., Sundt, T. M., and Michenfelder, J. D.: Cerebral blood flow during carotid endarterectomy. Circulation, *45*:1091, 1972.

19. Dyken, M. L.: Intracranial steal in complete occlusion of the internal carotid artery. Eur. Neurol., *7*:301, 1971.

20. Noell, W., and Schneider, M.: Uber die durchblutung und die sauerstoff versorgung des gehirns. Pflügers Arch., *250*:35, 1948.

21. Hägerdahl, M., Harp, J. R., and Siesjö, B. K.: Influence of changes in arterial P$_{CO_2}$ on cerebral blood flow and cerebral energy state during hypothermia in the rat. Acta Anesth. Scand. 57:(Suppl.) 25, 1975.

22. Reivich, M., Dickson, J., Clark, J., et al.: Role of hypoxia in cerebral circulatory and metabolic changes during hypocarbia in man: studies in hyperbaric milieu. Scand. J. Clin. Lab. Invest., *102*[Supp.] IV B, 1968.

23. Gibbs, F. A., Williams, D., and Gibbs, E. L.: Modification of the cortical frequency spectrum by changes in CO_2, blood sugar, and O_2. J. Neurophysiol., *3*:49, 1940.

24. Davis, H., and Wallace, W. M.: Factors affecting changes produced in the electroencephalogram by standardized hyperventilation. Arch. Neurol. Psychiat., *47*:606, 1942.

25. Alexander, S. C., Cohen, P. J., Wollman, H., et al.: Cerebral carbohydrate metabolism in man: studies during nitrous oxide anesthesia. Anesthesiology, *26*: 624, 1965.

26. Morgan, P., and Ward, B.: Hyperventilation and changes in electroencephalogram and electroretinogram. Neurology, *20*:1009, 1970.

27. Paulson, O. B., and Sharbough, F. W.: Physiologic and pathophysiologic relationship between the electroencephalogram and the regional cerebral blood flow. Acta. Neurol. Scand., *50*:194, 1974.

28. Engel, G. L., Ferris, E. B., and Logan, M.: Hyperventilation: analysis of clinical symptomatology. Ann. Intern. Med., *27*:683, 1947.

29. Holmberg, G.: The electroencephalogram during hypoxia and hyperventilation. Electroencephalogr. Clin. Neurophysiol., *5*:371, 1953.

30. Cohen, P. J., Reivich, M., and Grenbaum, L. J., Jr.: Electroencephalographic changes induced by 100% oxygen breathing at 3 ATA in awake man. Proceedings of the Third International Conference on Hyperbaric Medicine, p. 323–328. Washington D.C., National Academy of Science, 1966.

31. Meyers, J. S., Gotoh, F., and Favale, F.: Effects of carotid compression on cerebral metabolism and electroencephalogram. Electroencephalogr. Clin. Neurophysiol., *19*:362, 1965.

32. Gotoh, F., Meyers, J. S., and Takagi, Y.: Cerebral effects of hyperventilation in man. Arch. Neurol., *12*:410, 1965.

33. Domonkos, J., and Huszak, I.: Effect of hydrogen ion concentration on the carbohydrate metabolism of brain tissue. J. Neurochem., *4*:238, 1959.

34. Granholm, L., Lukjanova, L., and Siesjö, B. K.: The effect of marked hyperventilation upon tissue levels of NADH, lactate, pyruvate, phosphocreatine, and adenosine phosphates of rat brain. Acta Physiol. Scand., *77*:179, 1969.

35. Alexander, S. C., Smith, T. C., Strobel, G., et al.: Cerebral carbohydrate metabolism of man during respiratory and metabolic alkalosis. J. Appl. Physiol., *24*:66, 1968.

36. Harp., J. R., and Wollman, H.: Cerebral metabolic effects of hyperventilation and deliberate hypotension. Br. J. Anaesth., *45*:256, 1973.

37. Granholm, L., and Siesjö, B. K.: The effects of hypocapnea upon the cerebrospinal lactate and pyruvate concentrations and upon the lactate, pyruvate, ATP, ADP, phosphocreatine and creatine concentrations of cat brain. Acta Physiol. Scand., *75*:257, 1969.

38. Chance, B., Schoener, B., and Schindler, F.: The intracellular oxidation-reduction state in oxygen. *In* Dickens, F., and Niel, E. (eds.): Oxygen in the Animal Organism. pp. 367–392. New York, Macmillan, 1964.

39. Duffy, T. E., Nelson, S. R., and Lowry, O. H.: Cerebral carbohydrate metabolism during acute hypoxia and recovery. J. Neurochem., *19*:959, 1972.

40. Michenfelder, J. D., and Theye, R. A.: The effects of anesthesia and hypothermia on canine cerebral ATP and lactate during anoxia produced by decapitation. Anesthesiology, *33*:430, 1970.

41. Michenfelder, J. D., and Sundt, T. M.: The effect of hypocapnia on the metabolism of ischemic brain in squirrel monkeys. Anesthesiology, *38*:445, 1973.

42. Michenfelder, J. D., VanDyke, R. A., and Theye, R. A.: The effect of anesthetic agents and techniques on canine ATP and lactate levels. Anesthesiology, *33*:315, 1970.

43. McMillan, V., and Siesjö, B. K.: The influences of hypo-

capnea upon intracellular pH and upon some carbohydrate substrates, amino acids and organic phosphates in brain. J. Neurochem, 21:1283, 1973.

44. Siesjö, B. K.: Acid-base balance and energy metabolism in the brain. International Congress Series No. 292. Anaesthesiology: Proceedings of Fifth World Congress of Anaesthesiologists, Kyoto, September 19–23, 1972. pp. 121–127. Amsterdam, Exerpta Medica, 1972.

45. Harrington, T. M., and DiChiro, G.: Effect of hypocarbia and hypercarbia in experimental brain infarction. Neurology, 23:294, 1973.

46. Sundt, T. M., and Waltz, A. G.: Cerebral ischemia and reactive hypermia. Studies of cortical blood flow and microcirculation before, during and after occlusion of middle cerebral artery of squirrel monkeys. Circ. Res., 28:426, 1971.

47. Yamaguchi, T. Y., Regli, R., and Waltz, A. G.: Effect of Pa_{CO_2} on hyperemia and ischemia in experimental cerebral infarction. Stroke, 2:139, 1971.

48. Brawley, B. W., Strandness, P., and Kelly, W. A.: The physiologic response to therapy in experimental cerebral ischemia. Arch. Neurol., 17:180, 1962.

49. Soloway, M., Moriarty, G., and White, R. J.: Effect on delayed hyperventilation in the treatment of experimental vascular occlusion. Neurology, 21:479, 1971.

50. Yamamoto, Y. L., Phillips, K. M., Hodge, C. P., et al.: Microregional blood flow changes in experimental cerebral ischemia. J. Neurosurg., 35:155, 1971.

51. Soloway, M., Nadel, W., and Albin, M. S.: The effect of hyperventilation on subsequent cerebral infarction. Anesthesiology, 29:975, 1968.

52. Bridges, B. E., Jr., and Eger, E. I., II: The effect of hypocapnia on the level of halothane anesthesia in man. Anesthesiology, 27:634, 1966.

53. Eisele, J. H., Eger, E. I. II, and Muallem, M.: Narcotic properties of carbon dioxide in the dog. Anesthesiology, 28:856, 1967.

54. Shim, C. U., and Anderson, N. B.: The effect of oxygen on minimal anesthetic requirements in the toad. Anesthesiology, 34:333, 1971.

55. Ehrenfeld, W. K., Hamilton, W. K., Larson, C. P., et al.: Effect of CO_2 and systemic hypertension on downstream arterial pressure during carotid endarterectomy. Surgery, 67:87, 1970.

56. Boysen, G., Ladegaard-Pedersen, J., Henriksen, H., et al.: The effects of P_{CO_2} on regional cerebral blood flow and internal carotid arterial pressure during carotid clamping. Anesthesiology, 35:286, 1971.

57. Lundberg, N., Kjallavist, A., and Bien, C.: Reduction of increased intracranial pressure by hyperventilation. A therapeutic aid in neurological surgery. Acta Psychiat. Scand., 36 [Suppl 139], 1964.

58. Marsh, M. L., Marshall, L. F., and Shapiro, H. M.: Neurosurgical intensive care. Anesthesiology, 47:149, 1977.

59. Gordon, E.: Controlled respiration in the management of patients with traumatic brain injuries. Acta Anesth. Scand., 15:193, 1971.

22 Cranial Nerve Injury Following Trichloroethylene

Jonathan M. Kelley, M.D.

Widely used in industry as a degreasant and also as a dry-cleaning solvent, trichloroethylene is used as an inhalation anesthetic occasionally by its few adherents in medicine. Many anesthesiologists are particularly deterred from using this agent, because of reports of patients developing postanesthetic cranial nerve injuries. These result from exposure to toxic decomposition products of trichloroethylene and are discussed in this chapter.

PHYSICAL AND CHEMICAL PROPERTIES OF TRICHLOROETHYLENE

Among volatile liquid anesthetics, trichloroethylene has several unique properties that form the basis of its neurotoxicity. The vapor pressure of trichloroethylene at 20°C is 57 torr,[1] blood–gas solubility coefficient, 9.15 to 9.85, and oil–gas solubility coefficient, 960.[2] Hence, as the most lipid-soluble of all the inhalation anesthetics, it should be the most potent, theoretically,[3] but is actually the least potent, as observed clinically. The high lipid solubility and the concentrations used clinically, then, result in the sequestering of considerable volumes of the agent in body tissues. Thus, trichloroethylene may be released over a period of several days. Given the presence of a capable hepatic microsomal enzyme system, it is not surprising that trichloroethylene is the most extensively metabolized inhalation anesthetic.[4] In fact, it is the only inhalation anesthetic to be metabolized to sedative-hypnotic products, chloral hydrate and trichloroethanol.[4]

Trichloroethylene is manufactured by chlorination of acetylene[5] or by boiling tetrachloroethylene with lime.[6] Though relatively stable at temperatures of up to 45°C,[7] above that temperature, particularly in the presence of light and soda lime, trichloroethylene decomposes to dichloroacetylene:[7–11]

$$\underset{\text{Cl}}{\overset{\text{Cl}}{}}\!\!C\!\!=\!\!C\underset{\text{Cl}}{\overset{\text{H}}{}} + \text{NaOH} \rightarrow$$

$$\text{Cl}\!-\!\text{C}\!\equiv\!\text{C}\!-\!\text{Cl} + \text{NaCl} + \text{H}_2\text{O}$$

Dichloroacetylene is highly toxic to nervous tissue and is produced in increasing amounts as the soda lime becomes warmer (because the absorption of carbon dioxide by soda lime is an exothermic reaction). The reaction accelerates markedly above 60°C, the temperature that is reached within one-half hour with a closed-circuit system containing poor quality soda lime; at 100°C, for example, 2.5 per cent of trichloroethylene vapor decomposes to dichloroacetylene.[7]

Dichloroacetylene combusts spontaneously in air or oxygen to form phosgene and carbon monoxide:

$$Cl—C{\equiv}C—Cl + O_2 \rightarrow O{=}C\begin{smallmatrix}Cl\\ \\ Cl\end{smallmatrix} + CO$$

In the presence of moisture (as in an anesthetic circuit), a variety of other decomposition products, such as dichloroacetylchloride and trichloroacetylchloride, appear. Further hydrolysis yields the corresponding acids. These acids, as well as phosgene, are also highly toxic to both nervous tissue and lung.

Besides temperature, several other factors affect the production of dichloroacetylene and the secondary decomposition products.[7] The more hygroscopic is the soda lime, the higher is the caustic soda (NaOH) content; and, the smaller are the granules of soda lime, the greater is the amount of trichloroethylene decomposition. However, decomposition is retarded by the presence of excess trichloroethylene and, particularly, by the addition of 10-per-cent silica to the soda lime.[12]

CLINICAL PRESENTATION OF NERVE INJURIES AND RELATION TO TRICHLOROETHYLENE

Two dozen cases of cranial nerve injuries associated with trichloroethylene anesthesia were reported in 1943 and 1944.[8,9,13–16] Duration of anesthesia was as brief one-half hour. The ages of the patients and their surgical procedures were unrelated to the subsequent development of neurological injuries. The patients awakened from anesthesia with more than the usual amount of nausea and vomiting, often with concomitant headache. On the 1st or 2nd postoperative day, they showed the onset of signs and symptoms of cranial nerve injury, manifested by bilateral facial numbness, especially around the lips (cranial nerve V). Cranial nerve involvement increased during the next several days to include, in decreasing frequency of occurrence, loss of corneal reflexes (V), facial weakness (VII), oculo-motor palsy with anisocoria (III), hoarseness (X), weakness of the tongue (XII), paralysis of lateral gaze (VI), diminished hearing (VIII), and constriction of visual fields (II). Within a few days of onset, nearly half of the patients developed transient corneal or facial herpetic vesicles. Although all signs and symptoms in some patients vanished during a period of several months, most had permanent facial numbness and weakness. Two severely affected patients died with encephalitis. No effective therapy was devised.

Initially, the presence of contaminants known to produce neuritis in some samples of trichloroethylene seemed like an adequate explanation for the syndrome.[17] However, as more cases occurred and the chemistry of the agent was reviewed, the relationship between the neurological deficits and the instability of trichloroethylene in the presence of alkali and heat became recognized. Indeed, two common factors differentiated affected from unaffected patients. All affected patients had been anesthetized using anesthesia circuits containing soda lime, and all had either received trichloroethylene or followed patients who had received the agent through the same circuit, usually but not necessarily on the same day.

More recently, reports of similar cranial nerve injuries have come from industries in which trichloroethylene is used as a degreasant.[18,19] Workers exposed to the fumes of the heated liquid have suffered injury to every cranial nerve except the olfactory (I) and accessory (XI) nerves. Electrophysiological evidence of asymptomatic slowed conduction time in the ulnar and facial nerves has been demonstrated for 34 and 80 weeks following industrial exposure. Neuropathological examination of a fatally exposed industrial worker showed extensive myelin and axon degeneration of the trigeminal (V) nerve tracts and nuclei, especially in the sensory areas. Herpetic vesicles also often appeared following the onset of cranial nerve injury but probably do not denote a primary illness, as had been hypothesized.[14] It is very likely that herpetic vesicles indicate the occurrence of a process similar to activation of latent herpes simplex, known to occur after trigeminal sensory-root section.[20]

Although the intentional use of trichloroethylene in circle absorbing systems ended with the publicity given to the syndrome in 1944, and although this agent has been largely abandoned for surgical anesthesia, complications related to toxic decomposition products may still occur. For example, trichloroethylene analgesia is still used for obstetrical labor. Hence, a patient who self-administers trichloroethylene by hand-held inhaler during labor may receive general anesthesia later that day, perhaps for removal of retained placental fragments, and exhale residual amounts of the agent into the soda lime. One such case has been described.[21] Additionally, trichloroethylene may be inadvertently substituted for another volatile agent when filling a vaporizer. Such an error resulted in a fulminant case of acute necrotizing tracheobronchitis and focal alveolar hemorrhages. It is very likely that these were caused by the phosgene and hydrochloric acid liberated by the decomposition of the agent during a 4.5-hour anesthetic.[22]

CLINICAL RECOMMENDATIONS

These neural complications, other aspects of its clinical pharmacology (e.g., delayed recovery following prolonged administration, sensitization of the myocardium to catecholamines, and tachypnea), and the availability of more satisfactory anesthetics have forced the abandonment of trichloroethylene in most clinical settings. Nonetheless, this agent is still used in English-speaking countries, especially during obstetrical labor.

Given the gravity of these complications and, in particular, the lack of effective therapy, attention must be directed to preventing the circumstances in which trichloroethylene may decompose. Cranial nerve injuries and chemical burns of the respiratory tract can occur *only* when trichloroethylene has decomposed to dichloroacetylene, or phosgene and hydrochloric acid, in the presence of heat, light, or soda lime. For this reason, the agent is supplied in amber bottles containing the acid-accepting stabilizer thymol and should be removed from the bottle only at the time of use. Furthermore, trichloroethylene

should never be stored near heat sources, such as hot water pipes, radiators, or warm electrical equipment. The agent should *never* be used in the presence of soda lime, even though the temperatures generated by the soda lime currently in use probably do not rise much above 40°C.[23]

As a result, one may ask: When is it safe to administer anesthesia through a system containing soda lime to a patient who has recently received trichloroethylene? The agent has been detected in blood as long as 48 hours after anesthesia.[24] It is prudent to use anesthesia equipment without soda lime when one anesthetizes any patient who has received trichloroethylene within the previous 24 hours.

REFERENCES

1. Churchill-Davison, H. C. (ed.): A Practice of Anaesthesia. ed. 4. p. 269. London, Lloyd-Luke, 1978.
2. Eger, E. I., II, and Larson, C. P., Jr.: Anesthetic solubility in blood and tissues: values and significance. Br. J. Anaesth., 36:140, 1964.
3. Saidman, L. J., Eger, E. I., II, Munson, E. S., et al.: Minimum alveolar concentrations of methoxyflurane, halothane, ether and cyclopropane in man. Correlation with theories of anesthesia. Anesthesiology, 28:994, 1967.
4. Kelley, J. M., Brown, B. R., Jr.: Biotransformation of trichloroethylene. Int. Anesthesiol. Clin., 12:85, 1974.
5. Smith, G. F.: Trichloroethylene. A review. Br. J. Ind. Med., 23:249, 1966.
6. Cohen, E. N., and Brewer, H. W.: Toxicity of impurities. *In* Chenoweth, M. B. (ed.): Modern Inhalation Anesthetics. p. 479. New York, Springer-Verlag, 1972.
7. Firth, J. B., and Stuckey, R. E.: Decomposition of Trilene in closed circuit anaesthesia. Lancet, 1:814, 1945.
8. Humphrey, J. H., and McClelland, M.: Cranial nerve palsies with herpes following general anaesthesia. A report from the Central Middlesex County Hospital. Br. Med. J., 1:315, 1944.
9. Carden, S.: Hazards in the use of closed circuit technique for Trilene anaesthesia. Br. Med. J., 1:319, 1944.
10. Hunter, A. R.: Trilene hazards. Br. Med. J., 1:341, 1944.
11. Morton, H. J. V.: Trigeminal paralysis after trichloroethylene anaesthesia. Br. Med. J., 2:828, 1943.
12. Carney, T. P., and Gillespie, N. A.: Correspondence, Br. J. Anaesth., 19:139, 1945.
13. McAuley, J.: Trichloroethylene and trigeminal anaesthesia. Br. Med. J., 2:713, 1943.
14. Enderby, G. E. H.: The use and abuse of trichloroethylene. Br. Med. J., 2:300, 1944.
15. Dangers of Trilene anaesthesia. Lancet, 1:379, 1944.
16. Goldschmidt, M. W.: Two complications with trichloroethylene anaesthesia. Lancet, 2:414, 1943.
17. Hewer, C. L.: Further observations on trichloroethylene. Proc. R. Soc. Med., 36:463, 1944.
18. Buxton, P. H., and Hayward, M.: Polyneuritis cranialis

associated with industrial trichloroethylene poisoning. J. Neurol. Neurosurg. Psychiatry, *30*:511, 1967.

19. Feldman, R. G., Mayer, R. M., and Taub, A.: Evidence for peripheral neurotoxic effect of trichloroethylene. Neurology, *20*:599, 1970.

20. Carton, C. A., and Kilbourne, E. D.: Activation of latent herpes simplex by trigeminal sensory-root section. N. Engl. J. Med., *246*:172, 1952.

21. Ostlere, G.: Trichloroethylene Anaesthesia. Edinburgh, Livingstone, 1953.

22. Case history No. 39: Accidental use of trichloroethylene (Trilene, Trimar) in a closed system. Anesth. Analg., *43*:740, 1964.

23. Kilpatrick, L. C.: Rubber soda-lime cannister. Anaesthesia, *6*:236, 1951.

24. Powell, J. F.: Trichloroethylene: absorption, elimination and metabolism. Br. J. Ind. Med., *2*:142, 1945.

FURTHER READING

Atkinson, R. S.: Trichloroethylene anaesthesia. Anesthesiology, *21*:67, 1960.

Defalque, R. J.: Pharmacology and toxicology of trichloroethylene: a critical review of the world literature. Clin. Pharmacol. Ther., *2*:665, 1961.

23 Ophthalmological Complications

Richard L. Bitner, M.D.

There are few patients undergoing surgery who present as great a challenge and who command such precise requirements for successful completion as do patients undergoing ophthalmic surgery. The choice between local and general anesthesia is not always straightforward and may depend on many factors other than the physical condition of the patient. Care in selection of agents and techniques for safe management of general anesthesia is essential, since the risk of anesthesia to life is always greater than that of ophthalmic surgery. This type of surgery primarily involves the very young and the very old. A poorly managed anesthetic can contribute to loss of vision when the eye is opened due to accident or surgery. The interaction of ophthalmic drugs with anesthetic drugs must be considered. Moreover, anesthetics have definite effects on the physiology of the eye. Additional problems include the preparation of the young child for his first experience with anesthesia and dealing with an aged patient's anxiety over loss of vision. Since eye surgery is performed in almost every community hospital, an understanding of these matters is essential for everyone who administers anesthesia.

Communication and rapport among the physicians caring for these patients is of utmost importance if the anesthesiologist is to provide the exacting conditions required for safe ophthalmic surgery (see the list below).

Conditions Required for Safe Ophthalmic Surgery

A still, fixed eye
Minimal bleeding
Decreased oculocardiac reflexes
Decreased intraocular pressure
Smooth emergence without nausea, vomiting, or retching
Postoperative analgesia

There is little doubt that during operations in which the globe is not opened, there can be more flexibility in surgical conditions; but, for intraocular procedures, perfection is required.

LOCAL VERSUS GENERAL ANESTHESIA

Normally, when local anesthesia is selected, the ophthalmologist is responsible for the management of the patient and will utilize his favorite routine, although the anesthesiologist may be consulted in matters of premedication of specific patients and may be asked to monitor the patients during the procedure. With attention to details and rapport between surgeon and patient, local anesthesia is entirely satisfactory for practically any ophthalmic operation. Indeed, many ophthalmologists claim that only the exceptional case should be done under general anesthesia.

Considerations affecting the choice of anesthesia include the following: duration of surgery; the patient's age; the patient's mental and emotional status; the surgeon's mental and emotional status; and communication problems, such as language barriers or deafness.[1]

Because of the high risk involved, the patient undergoing an ophthalmic procedure must trust his surgeon, and the surgeon's habits and personality must be such that he can work with a patient under local anesthesia; otherwise, serious consideration must be given to the use of general anesthesia.

Attention to the patient's physical comfort is important regardless of the type of anesthesia selected, but it is essential if the anesthesiologist hopes for cooperation under local anesthesia. Patients with arthritis or skeletal deformities require attention to positioning and padding on the operating table. Ventilation about the patient's face must be adequate, and the patient must be kept warm. Of course, close monitoring of the patient is mandatory.

Although complications of general anesthesia comprise the majority of this chapter, local anesthesia is not without its hazards:

Hazards of Local Anesthesia

Excessive premedication
Incomplete block of muscles with compression of the globe and extrusion of intraocular contents
Retrobulbar hemorrhage
Penetration of the ocular nerve
Intraocular injection

GENERAL ANESTHESIA: PHYSIOLOGICAL CONSIDERATIONS AND COMPLICATIONS

The Oculocardiac Reflex

It has been observed for decades that ocular surgical maneuvers can provoke changes in cardiac rate and rhythm. The afferent arc of the reflex is mediated by the ophthalmic division of the trigeminal nerve; the efferent pathway is the vagus nerve. A variety of stimuli applied to and about the eye can initiate these changes. Pressure on the globe and extraocular muscle stretch, especially of the medial rectus muscle, are the most dependable exciting stimuli.[2] In addition, eye trauma, retrobulbar hematomas, retrobulbar

block itself,[3] and direct pressure on tissue remaining in the orbital apex after enucleating[4] will elicit the reflex. This reflex may occur during both local and general anesthesia, regardless of whether general anesthesia is deep or light. Arrhythmias reported include sinus bradycardia, nodal rhythms, SA block, wandering pacemaker, and ventricular bigeminy. The normal heart rate returns generally within 20 seconds after the release of pressure. Berler's survey of the literature revealed an overall incidence of 50 per cent,[3] although the incidence varies from 16 to 82 per cent.[2-5] Often, reports of high incidence involved subjects in young age-groups, who have greater vagal tone.

If the described mechanism of the oculocardiac reflex is correct, then complete anesthesia of the orbital contents should block the afferent pathway and prevent the reflex. Thus, Berler and Kirsch and colleagues found that retrobulbar block abolished the reflex in 100 per cent of patients who demonstrated it.[3,4] In fact, Kirsch recommended routine retrobulbar block after he was able to demonstrate complete abolition of the reflex in every patient who demonstrated ECG changes.[4] Retrobulbar block can take several minutes to reach full effectiveness; therefore, the surgeon should wait 1 to 2 minutes after the block is administered before he begins the surgical procedure.

Routine subcutaneous or intramuscular premedication with atropine is recommended by no one and can be considered useless as an effective prevention of this reflex.[3,4,6] However, intravenous atropine in doses of 0.5 to 1 mg. has been found to be effective by Bosomworth,[2] Sorenson,[6] Reed,[7] and Moonie.[8] Taylor cleverly studied a group of children undergoing bilateral eye surgery by "protecting" the first eye with retrobulbar block and the second eye, with atropine given intravenously.[5] Although 58 per cent of controls demonstrated the reflex, no patient manifested oculocardiac reflex after retrobulbar block, while 28 per cent did so after atropine. Prophylactic use of glycopyrrolate may be justified in pediatric patients having strabismus correction because of the more active vagal reflexes in children (making bradycardia more common) and the absence of tachycardia (and tachyarrhythmias) following use of glycopyrrolate.[5a]

Deacock and Oxer suggested the selection of an anesthetic technique involving the use of gallamine after they found that it afforded considerable protection against the oculocardiac reflex.[9]

There remains, however, considerable difference of opinion regarding the importance of the reflex. Berler questions whether the reflex should be prevented at all.[3] Moonie and colleagues found that continuous eye traction caused fatigue of the reflex; a return to normal rate and rhythm occurred in an average time of about 50 seconds, with a range of 8 to 228 seconds.[8] They suggested that fatigue of the reflex might explain the apparent beneficial effect of retrobulbar block.

There remains little doubt that continuous monitoring by the anesthesiologist is essential during eye surgery to detect serious or potentially fatal rhythm changes.

Increase in Intraocular Pressure

Normal intraocular pressure is 10 to 22 torr and varies daily by 2 to 3 torr. It is highest in the morning and lowest at night. Intraocular pressure is greater than the pressure in any other tissue; even intracranial pressure is only 7 to 8 torr. Position also plays a role: Intraocular pressure is 2 to 3 torr higher during recumbency than during standing. A pressure above 25 torr is definitely abnormal.

Soon after succinylcholine was introduced, Hoffman and Holzer reported that it increased the intraocular pressure in unanesthetized humans as much as 18 torr.[10] Shortly thereafter, reports appeared of vitreous expulsion in patients receiving succinylcholine during open eye surgery. The maximal effect of a single dose of succinylcholine on intraocular pressure occurs within 20 to 30 seconds and lasts 2 to 5 minutes.[11,12] There is, of course, some variation in response, depending on dose and elapsed time between succinylcholine administration and induction with the thiopental.[13] The rise in pressure follows continuous intravenous and single intravenous injection and is also evident following intramuscular injection of succinylcholine in the pediatric patient.[12,14] An actual increase in extraocular muscle tension is believed to be a factor in this increase,[11,14–16] since cutting all the extraocular muscles virtually eliminates the pressure response to succinylcholine. Furthermore, Katz,[17] Miller,[18] and others[19,20] have found that prior administration of *d*-tubocurarine or gallamine markedly suppresses or completely abolishes extraocular muscle contraction and the increase in intraocular pressure produced by succinylcholine. Hexafluorenium is also effective if given just before succinylcholine.[17] Carballo suggests that the prior administration of acetazolamide is effective in avoiding the increased intra-ocular pressure produced by succinylcholine (see Chap. 45).[21]

Clearly, succinylcholine should not be used as the sole muscle relaxant during anesthesia in a patient with glaucoma or an open eye injury, or in the course of surgery when the eye has been opened.

The control of intraocular pressure is not unlike the control of intracranial pressure in neurosurgery, because the sclera, like the skull, is inelastic.[22] Carballo[21] and Duncalf[23] have presented the factors at length that influence intraocular pressure There is no rise in intraocular pressure with elevated arterial pressure, although low systemic arterial pressure results in a lowering of the intraocular pressure.

The normal pressure can be raised as much as 60 per cent by forced breathing against an obstruction (Valsalva's maneuver). A mild cough can double the pressure. There is rapid return to normal values after cessation of the stress.[24,25] Hypoventilation, hypoxia, and hypercapnia all elevate the pressure in the eye,[26,27] while hyperventilation, high oxygen tension, and hypocapnia lower the intraocular tension.[21,26] Tracheal intubation alone can elevate the pressure. Finally, increased venous pressure, regardless of the cause, is reflected by an increase in intraocular pressure.

Nearly all general anesthetic agents cause a decrease in intraocular pressure; thus, diethyl ether, cyclopropane, vinyl ether, thiopental,[13,24,28] chloroform, halothane, trichloroethylene,[29] methoxyflurane,[30,31] and neuroleptanalgesia[30] all cause significant reductions in intraocular pressure. On the other hand, ketamine produces a rise in intraocular pressure for as long as 30 minutes following intramuscular administration.[32]

Although one might expect to lower intraocular pressure with the proper choice of anesthetic agents and avoidance of succinylcholine, a particular method of ventilation or the level of arterial blood pressure interact with the effects of anesthesia to influence the final value.

Recently, marijuana has also been reported to produce lowering of the intraocular pressure.[33]

Interactions of Ophthalmic Drugs With Anesthetic Drugs

Ophthalmic drugs can alter responses to anesthetic agents. Echothiophate iodide is a long-acting cholinesterase inhibitor used in the treatment of gluacoma and sometimes in the therapy of esotropia in children. Although it is administered topically, there is systemic absorption sufficient to produce a considerable decrease in pseudocholinesterase activity. Levels of less than 5 per cent of normal activity have been reported in patients who have been receiving echothiophate iodide eye drops chronically.[34] It can take up to 4 weeks for the depressed pseudocholinesterase level to return to normal following the cessation of prolonged therapy. In view of the fact that the short duration of action of succinylcholine results from its rapid destruction by the enzyme pseudocholinesterase, one should expect that patients on chronic echothiophate therapy might demonstrate prolongation of effects of succinylcholine because of impaired metabolism. Numerous reports of this complication exist.[35–38] It is, therefore, imperative that, during the preoperative interview of the patient who is about to undergo anesthesia for any surgical procedure, the anesthesiologist ask about the recent use of eye drops. One should administer succinylcholine with caution to patients who have received echothiophate within several weeks of anesthesia, and a nerve stimulator should be used to gauge the duration of the neuromuscular blockade.

More commonly encountered than echothiophate now in the patient with open-angle glaucoma is timolol, a recently introduced beta-adrenergic receptor blocking agent. Among the problems noted are bradycardia,[38a,38b] hypotension,[38b] syncope,[38b] exacerbation of bronchial asthma,[38c] and worsening of congestive heart failure. Although anesthetics and anesthetic adjuvants have not been implicated in the affected patients, it is clear that drugs used during anesthesia can exacerbate any of these problems.

Because 10-per-cent phenylephrine is commonly used by eye surgeons preoperatively and at the conclusion of ophthalmic procedures for pupillary dilatation and decongestion of the sclera, anesthesiologists should be aware that adverse systemic effects of this topical drug have been noted. Solosko and Smith reported severe hypertension in several patients.[39] They considered this side effect to be especially hazardous in aged patients, who may suffer vascular accidents, and in infants, who might absorb as much as 10 mg. from topical instillation. It is not clear whether the main site of absorption is the conjunctiva or the nasal mucosa after drainage by way of the tear ducts. Phenylephrine should never be administered topically after eye surgery has commenced and venous channels are open to permit rapid absorption. Aviado recommends that 10-per-cent phenylephrine be avoided, because of its potentially hazardous cardiovascular side effects.[40] It has been suggested that there is very little increase of mydriatic effects in concentrations above 5 per cent.[41] However, for severe hypertensive responses, intravenous trimethaphan, nitroprusside, or phentolamine may be necessary.

OCULAR COMPLICATIONS OF ANESTHESIA FOR GENERAL SURGERY

Corneal Abrasion

The most common ocular complication of general anesthesia, corneal abrasion from the anesthetic mask or surgical drapes,[42] can be avoided easily by proper selection of mask size and attention to detail during laryngoscopy, intubation, and positioning. This problem is especially likely to arise during head and neck surgery, when the face is draped, or during procedures in which the patient must be placed in a prone position. Injuries can be sustained by pressure on the eyes by a surgical assistant, instruments, or the surgical drapes. Indeed, the corneal epithelium can be damaged simply through drying while it remains open for a protracted period.[43] Many anesthesiologists routinely apply an ophthalmic ointment, such as boric acid, for protection of the eye. However, this method permits introduction of possibly contaminated material into the eye, and patients often complain of postoperative blurring of vision. Simple application of adhesive tape, gently, over the closed lids provides satisfactory protection of the cornea.

Chemical injuries of the eye can occur from spillage of solutions during skin preparation or from volatile agents, such as ether or chloroform, when open drop methods are used.

The patient who sustains a corneal abrasion will complain of feeling a foreign body, tearing, photophobia, and pain that is aggravated by blinking and eye movement. Following gross examination, a local anesthetic should be instilled, and the eye should be examined with fluorescein staining, utilizing a slit lamp if possible.

Although the complication can be managed effectively by the anesthesiologist, it is highly desirable to have an ophthalmologist see the patient in consultation, preferably while the patient is still in the recovery room. Corneal abrasions are usually treated by patching the injured eye and applying a prophylactic antibiotic ointment. Healing normally occurs within 24 hours. However, since permanent sequelae are possible, attention should be paid to every detail to avoid these problems.

Retinal Ischemia

Compression of the central retinal artery from pressure exerted on the globe by an improperly fitting anesthetic mask or head support can occur, especially during periods of hypotension that is deliberate or the result of deep anesthesia, blood loss or reflex. Ischemia of the retina and optic nerve can result (see Chap. 48). Ischemia and infarction of the retina caused by types of embolism have been reported following cardiac surgery.[44] An increase in intraocular pressure sufficient to compromise retinal blood flow can occur

if, during repair of retinal detachment, more than 40 per cent of the vitreous is replaced with SF_6 and nitrous oxide administration is continued.[44a–44c]

Precipitation of Acute Glaucoma

There has been concern that acute (narrow-angle) glaucoma may be aggravated as a result of the pupillary dilatation caused by anticholinergic drugs given during anesthesia. In fact, atropine and scopolamine, when instilled into the conjunctival sac, are mydriatics. Thus, they are contraindicated, when given in this manner, in patients with glaucoma. However, when administered parenterally in usual doses, an acute attack of intraocular hypertension will not be precipitated by anticholinergics, although patients with known glaucoma should continue to receive their drug therapy (e.g., pilocarpine or physostigmine eye drops) in the perioperative period.[45]

OCULAR COMPLICATIONS OF OXYGEN ADMINISTRATION

Following exposure to supplemental oxygen, the newborn infant can develop retrolental fibroplasia, a proliferative retinal vascularization, which may resolve with time or progress to fibrosis and blindness. Although many factors may be involved in its development,[46–51] retrolental fibroplasia most commonly occurs in the premature infant who breathes in excessive concentration of oxygen for a prolonged period.[52,53] Infants weighing less than 1500 g. or having a gestational age of less than 32 weeks are particularly prone to develop this retinal lesion. In fact, infants continue to be at risk until they have reached a *post-conception* age of 44 weeks.[54] Individual susceptibility is so great that some infants can be blinded by only a few hours of exposure to an enriched oxygen mixture during anesthesia,[55] whereas others suffer no eye injury following much longer exposures.[48,49,56]

The measures that the anesthesiologist should take are clear:[57] When supplemental oxygen must be administered to an infant whose *post-conception* age is less than 44 weeks for respiratory care or general anesthesia, Pa_{O_2} must be maintained at a level no higher than the newborn's normal range (60–100 torr or 8.0–13.3 kPa) to *minimize* the likelihood of eye damage. In both the intensive care unit and the operating room, an oxygen–air blender may be required to avoid delivering excessive oxygen concentrations, and the inspired mixture should be verified with an oxygen analyzer. Frequent determinations of Pa_{O_2} should be made, particularly in infants with cardiorespiratory disease, in whom therapy causes prompt and marked changes in pulmonary perfusion and ventilation and, thus, Pa_{O_2}. Ideally, blood for determination Pa_{O_2} should be obtained from a radial or temporal artery, rather than from an umbilical artery catheter. The latter, because of its placement distal to the ductus arteriosus, can yield lower Pa_{O_2} values as a result of pulmonary-to-aorta shunting during periods of hypotension. Finally, given the ease with which hyperventilation may be achieved and the fact that $P_{A_{O_2}}$ rises as a result, Pa_{O_2} should be monitored whenever assisted or controlled ventilation is used.

REFERENCES

1. Donlon, J. V., Jr.: Local anethesia for opthalmic surgery: Patient preparation and management. Ann. Ophthalmol., 12:1183, 1980.
2. Bosomworth, P. P., Ziegler, C. H., and Jacoby, J.: The oculo-cardiac reflex in eye muscle surgery. Anesthesiology, 19:7, 1958.
3. Berler, D. K.: The oculocardiac reflex. Am. J. Ophthalmol., 56:954, 1963.
4. Kirsch, R. E., Samet, P., Kugel, V., et al.: Electrocardiographic changes during ocular surgery and their prevention by retrobulbar injection. Arch. Ophthalmol., 58:348, 1957.
5. Taylor, C., Wilson, F. M., Roesch, R., et al.: Prevention of the oculo-cardiac reflex in children. Comparison of retrobulbar block and intravenous atropine. Anesthesiology, 24:646, 1963.
5a. Meyers, E. F., and Tomeldan, S. A.: Glycopyrrolate compared with atropine in prevention of the oculocardiac reflex during eye-muscle surgery. Anesthesiology, 51:350, 1979.
6. Sorenson, E. J., and Gilmore, J. E.: Cardiac arrest during strabismus surgery. A preliminary report. Am. J. Ophthalmol., 41:748, 1956.
7. Reed, H., and McCaughey, T.: Cardiac slowing during strabismus surgery. Br. J. Ophthalmol., 46:112, 1962.
8. Moonie, G. T., Rees, D. L., and Elton, D.: The oculocardiac reflex during strabismus surgery. Can. Anaesth. Soc. J., 11:621, 1964.
9. Deacock, A. C., and Oxer, H. F.: The prevention of reflex bradycardia during ophthalmic surgery. Br. J. Anaesth., 34:451, 1962.
10. Hoffman, H., and Holtzer, H.: Die wirkung von muskelralaxantien auf den intraokularen druck. Klin. Monatsbl. Augenbheilkd., 123:1, 1953.
11. Lincoff, H. A., Breinin, G. M., and DeVoe, A. G.: The effect of succinylcholine on the extraocular muscles. Am. J. Ophthalmol., 43:440, 1957.
12. Schwartz, H., and de Roetth, A., Jr.: Effect of succinylcholine on intraocular pressure in human beings. Anesthesiology, 19:112, 1958.
13. Joshi, C., and Bruce, D. L.: Thiopental and succinylcholine: action on intraocular pressure. Anesth. Analg., 54:471, 1975.
14. Craythorne, N. W. B., Rottenstein, H. S., and Dripps, R. D.: The effect of succinylcholine on intraocular pressure in adults, infants and children during general anesthesia. Anesthesiology, 21:59, 1960.
15. Cullen, D. J., Eger, E. I., II, Stevens, W. C., et al.: Clinical signs of anesthesia. Anesthesiology, 36:21, 1972.
16. Dillon, J. B., Sabawala, P., Taylor, D. B., et al.: Depolarizing neuromuscular blocking agents and intraocular pressure in vivo. Anesthesiology, 18:439, 1957.
17. Kirby, D. B.: Use of curare in cataract surgery. Arch. Ophthalmol. 43:678, 1950.
18. Miller, R. D., Way, W. L., and Hickey, R. F.: Inhibition of succinylcholine-induced intraocular pressure by nondepolarizing muscle relaxants. Anesthesiology, 29:123, 1968.
19. Dillon, J. B., Sabawala, P., Taylor, D. B., et al.: Action of succinylcholine on extraocular muscles and intraocular pressure. Anesthesiology, 18:44, 1957.
20. Macri, F. J., and Grimes, P. A.: The effects of succinylcholine on the extraocular striate muscles and on the intraocular pressure. Am. J. Ophthalmol., 44:221, 1957.
21. Carballo, A. S.: Succinylcholine and acetazolamide (Diamox) in anaesthesia for ocular surgery. Can. Anaesth. Soc. J., 12:486, 1965.
22. Farmati, O.: Fundoscopic, ophthalmodynamometric, and tonometric observations during cardiopulmonary bypass in man. Can. Anaesth. Soc. J., 14:584, 1967.
23. Duncalf, D.: Anesthesia and intraocular pressure. Bull. N.Y. Acad. Med., 51:374, 1975.
24. Kornblueth, W., Aladjemoff, L., Magora, F., et al.: Influence of general anesthesia on intraocular pressure in man. The effect of diethyl ether, cyclopropane, vinyl ether, and thiopental sodium. Arch. Ophthalmol., 61:84, 1959.
25. Macri, F. J.: Interdependence of venous and eye pressure. Arch. Ophthalmol., 65:150, 1961.
26. Duncalf, D., and Weitzner, S. W.: The influence of ventilation and hypercapnea on intraocular pressure during anesthesia. Anesth. Analg., 42:232, 1963.
27. Han, Y. H., Lowe, H. J., and Evers, J. L.: Effect of carbon dioxide on intraocular pressure in anesthetized man. Anesthesiology, 25:99, 1964.
28. Epstein, H. M., Fagman, W., Bruce, D. L., et al.: Intraocular pressure changes during anesthesia for electroshock therapy. Anesth. Analg., 54:479, 1975.
29. Magora, F., and Collins, V. J.: The influence of general anesthetic agents on intraocular pressure in man. The effect of common nonexplosive agents. Arch. Ophthalmol., 66:64, 1961.
30. Ivankovic, A. D., and Lowe, H. J.: The influence of

methoxyflurane and neuroleptanesthesia on intraocular pressure in man. Anesth. Analg., *48*:933, 1970.

31. Schettini, A., Owre, E. S., and Fink, A. I.: Effect of methoxyflurane anaesthesia on intraocular pressure. Can. Anaesth. Soc. J., *15*:172, 1968.

32. Yoshikawa, K., and Murai, Y.: The effect of ketamine on intraocular pressure in children. Anesth. Analg., *50*:199, 1971.

33. Hepler, R. S., and Frank, I. R.: Marihuana smoking and intraocular pressure. J.A.M.A, *217*:1392, 1971.

34. DeRoetth, A., Detbarn, W., Rosenberg, P., et al.: Effect of phospholine iodide on blood cholinesterase levels of normal and glaucoma subjects. Am. J. Ophthalmol., *59*:586, 1965.

35. Cavallaro, R. J., Krumperman, L. W., and Kugler, F.: Effect of echothiophate therapy on the metabolism of succinylcholine in man. Anesth. Analg., *47*:570, 1968.

36. Eilderton, T. E., Farmati, O., and Zsigmond, E. K.: Reduction in plasma cholinesterase levels after prolonged administration of echothiophate iodide eyedrops. Can. Anaesth. Soc. J., *15*:291, 1968.

37. Gesztes, T.: Prolonged apnoea after suxamethonium injection associated with eye drops containing an anticholinesterase agent. A case report. Br. J. Anaesth., *38*:408, 1966.

38. Pantuck, E. J.: Echothiophate iodide eye drops and prolonged response to suxamethonium. A case report. Br. J. Anaesth., *38*:406, 1966.

38a. Kim, J. W., and Smith, P. H.: Timolol-induced bradycardia. Anesth. Analg., *59*:301, 1980.

38b. McMahon, C. D., Schaffer, F. N., Hoskins, H. D., et al.: Adverse effects experienced by patients taking timolol. Am. J. Ophthalmol., *88*:736, 1979.

38c. Jones, F. L., Jr., and Ekberg, N. L.: Exacerbation of asthma by timolol. N. Engl. J. Med., *301*:270, 1979.

39. Solosko, D., and Smith, R. B.: Hypertension following 10 per cent phenylephrine ophthalmic. Anesthesiology, *36*:187, 1972.

40. Aviado, D. M.: Sympathomimetic Drugs. p. 289. Springfield, Charles C Thomas, 1970.

41. Haddah, N. J., Moyer, N. J., and Riley, F. C.: Mydriatic effect of phenylephrine hydrochloride. Am. J. Ophthalmol., *70*:729, 1970.

42. Snow, J. C., Kripke, B. J., Norton, M. L., et al.: Corneal injuries during general anesthesia. Anesth. Analg., *54*:465, 1975.

43. Batra, Y. K., and Bali, M.: Corneal abrasions during general anesthesia. Anesth. Analg., *56*:363, 1977.

44. Gutman, F. A., and Zegarra, H.: Ocular complications in cardiac surgery. Surg. Clin. North Am., *51*:1095, 1971.

44a. Smith, R. B., Carl, B., Linn, J. G., et al.: Effect of nitrous oxide on air in vitreous. Am. J. Ophthalmol., *78*:314, 1974.

44b. Fineberg, E., Macheimer, R., Sullivan, P.: Sulfur hexafluoride in owl monkey vitreous cavity. Am. J. Ophthalmol., *79*:67, 1975.

44c. Stinson, T. W., and Donlon, J. W., Jr.: Interaction of intraocular SF_6 and air with nitrous oxide. Anesthesiology, *51*:516, 1979.

45. Schwartz, H., de Roeth, A., Jr., and Papper, E. M.: Anesthetic use of atropine and scopolamine in patients with glaucoma. J.A.M.A., *165*:144, 1957.

46. James, L. S., and Lanman, J. T. (eds.): History of oxygen therapy and retrolental fibroplasia. Pediatrics, *57* [Suppl.]:591, 1976.

47. Johnson, L., Schaffer, D., and Boggs, T. R.: The premature infant, vitamin E deficiency and retrolental fibroplasia. Am. J. Clin. Nutr., *27*:1158, 1974.

48. Kalina, R. E., Hodson, W. A., and Morgan, B. C.: Retrolental fibroplasia in a cyanotic infant. Pediatrics, *50*:765, 1972.

49. Bruckner, H. L.: Retrolental fibroplasia—associated with intrauterine anoxia? Arch. Ophthalmol., *80*:504, 1968.

50. Ashton, N., and Henkind, P.: Experimental occlusion of retinal arterioles. B. J. Ophthalmol., *49*:225, 1965.

51. Adamkin, D. H., Shott, R. J., Cook, L. N., et al.: Nonhyperoxic retrolental fibroplasia. Pediatrics, *60*:828, 1977.

52. Kinsey, V. E., Arnold, H. J., Kalina, R. E., et al.: Pa_{O_2} levels and retrolental fibroplasia: a report of the cooperative study. Pediatrics, *60*:655, 1977.

53. Shahinian, L., Jr., and Malachowski, N.: Retrolental fibroplasia. A new analysis of risk factors based on recent cases. Arch. Ophthalmol., *96*:70, 1978.

54. Patz, A.: Retrolental fibroplasia. Surv. Ophthalmol., *14*:1, 1969.

55. Betts, E. K., Downes, J. J., Schaffer, D. B., et al.: Retrolental fibroplasia and oxygen administration during general anesthesia. Anesthesiology, *47*:518, 1977.

56. Aranda, J., and Sweet, A.: Sustained hyperoxemia without cicatricial retrolental fibroplasia. Pediatrics, *54*:434, 1974.

57. Phibbs, R. H.: Oxygen therapy: a continuing hazard to the premature infant. Anesthesiology, *47*:486, 1977.

FURTHER READING

Aboul-eish, E.: Physiology of the eye pertinent to anesthesia. Int. Anesthesiol. Clin., *13*:1, 1973.

Linn, J. G., Jr., and Smith, R. B.: Intraoperative complications and their management. Int. Anesthesiol. Clin., *13*:149, 1973.

Symposium on anaesthesia and the eye. Br. J. Anaesth., *52*:641, 1980.

24 Awareness During Anesthesia

Richard L. Bitner, M.D.

"Is the patient asleep?" is often asked by operating room personnel as they converse during surgery. There has developed, however, a deep concern on the part of many anesthesiologists that careless talk in the operating room is not only less than professional but is to be strictly avoided. One of the first accounts of "awareness" during apparent anesthesia appeared in 1950,[1] and since then numerous reports and editorials have appeared in anesthesia, surgery, and medical hypnosis journals.[2–26]

Some reports, like that of Sia,[14] describe patients who were aware of events occurring in the operating room but experienced no pain. Others document patients who suffered extreme discomfort. A syndrome of traumatic neurosis following awareness has been described.[25] Certainly, most cases occurred during nitrous oxide-relaxant anesthesia, but the complication has been reported following administration of most anesthetic agents. Awareness during anesthesia has, no doubt, presented itself during the practice of every experienced anesthesiologist.

AN AFFAIR OF MODERN ANESTHESIA

Prior to the introduction of muscle relaxant drugs, potent inhalation agents were the mainstay of anesthetic practice, and the depth of anesthesia could be readily monitored while their continued administration caused a progressive depression of major body systems. The introduction of curare as a neuromuscular blocking agent into clinical anesthesia by Griffith and Johnson in 1942 radically changed surgical anesthesia. Relatively light levels of inhalation anesthesia could then be used, sinced curare produced profound muscle relaxation. Until this period, no serious consideration was given to the possibility that a patient would be aware of his surroundings during a general anesthetic. Thereafter, paradoxically, it was possible for a patient to be motionless but conscious, or to move reflexly but be unconscious.

ETIOLOGY OF AWARENESS DURING ANESTHESIA

The problem of awareness during adequate anesthesia must always be distinguished from patient recall caused by an inadvertently lightened level of anesthesia.[27] There are a number of known causes of awareness, and these can therefore be avoided.[9] It must be emphasized that none of these have to be present for awareness to occur,[2] yet they must not be ignored during administration of anesthesia, since hearing is considered the first function to return with lightening of anesthesia.[29]

Concomitant Induction and Muscular Relaxation. The use of an ultra-short-acting induction agent that has a clinical effect which dissipates before the inhalation agent reaches adequate levels is a frequent cause of awareness early in an anesthetic.

Efficiency of Nitrous Oxide Administration. All too often, the calibration of flowmeters is not correct and is seldom checked for accuracy. The unwary anesthesiologist can therefore unknowingly deliver to his patient a lower concentration of nitrous oxide than desired.

Failure of Nitrous Oxide Flow. Whether it is caused by empty machine tanks or a line failure, an undetected failure of nitrous oxide delivery that lasts for only a few minutes can lead to patient awareness.

Hypoventilation or Interruption of Ventilation. Discussions of nitrous oxide-relaxant anesthesia have emphasized the importance of the apparent hypnotic effect of hypocapnia.[9] This effect results from hyperventilation, which increases the rate of rise of the alveolar anesthetic concentration, decreases or removes the ventilatory drive, and causes cerebral blood flow to decrease. There is, however, no alteration in the MAC (see Chap. 21).

"Resistance" to Anesthesia. One cannot predict exactly how a particular patient will respond to the usual concentration of pharmacologic agents.

Inadequate Supplementation of Nitrous Oxide. Subtle signs of light anesthesia should not be ignored. They include eyelid movement, wrinkling of the forehead, slight movements of upper extremities, sweating, tearing, and an elevation of pulse or blood pressure. It is very important for the anesthesiologist to have access to the patient and for the patient's face to be adequately lighted. When this is not possible, inhalation agents should be considered.

Mechanical Ventilator Maladjustment. Certain ventilators can mix air or oxygen with the anesthetic mixture when they are not adjusted properly or when the inflow rate is insufficient. Waters has reviewed this matter at length.[28]

STUDIES OF AWARENESS DURING ANESTHESIA

Numerous studies on awareness during anesthesia have appeared in the past decade; investigators have reported an incidence that varies from 0 to 10 per cent.[9,17-21,24,26]

Prospective Studies

One of the most intriguing prospective studies of awareness during anesthesia is that of Levinson.[30] In 1965, he reported on ten volunteer patients who were good hypnotic subjects and who were about to undergo dental surgery. They received a thiopental-nitrous oxide-ether anesthetic, which was monitored by EEG. When the EEG consisted entirely of irregular, slow, high voltage waves, indicating a very deep level of anesthesia, the anesthetist stopped the operation by saying, "Just a moment! I don't like the patient's color. Much too blue. His lips are very blue. I'm going to give a little more oxygen." At an interview 1 month later, none of the patients could remember consciously any events that occurred during the operation. Their first memories were of awakening in the ward. They were then hypnotized and regressed to the time of the actual surgery. Of the ten patients, four were able to repeat, almost exactly, the words used by the anesthetist. Four patients remembered hearing something or somebody talking, and some identified the speaker as the anesthetist. Everyone in this group displayed marked anxiety and either awoke from hypnosis or were resistant to further investigation. The other two patients denied hearing anything.

Many investigators have played prerecorded tapes into patients' ears during anesthesia. McIntyre reported that none of 17 patients who had undergone nitrous oxide anesthesia recalled a story told to them during surgery.[11] Terrell studied 37 patients: One-half of the patients listened to a tape recording of words intended to be nonsensical, such as riddles and telephone numbers, which a patient might not remember afterwards; a second tape, played for the other half of the patients, consisted of possibly stressful words that might be meaningful to anyone. Only general statements were used; they did not refer to the patient's specific history or physical condition. In none was it possible to elicit by the techniques employed, including hypnosis, any recall of what transpired during anesthesia.[16]

As a result of this study, Terrell believed that

anesthesiologists and surgeons should not be held accountable for anything said during surgical anesthesia. Likewise, he did not believe that personnel in the operating room could give the anesthetized patient positive suggestions.

Brice studied recall and dreaming during anesthesia.[31] He presented patients with tape recordings of choir or piano music and found no evidence that they were able to hear. However, dreaming occurred in 44 per cent of patients in his series, most often in those who moved during the procedure. In Brice's un-premedicated group of patients, nearly half described waiting for surgery as the most unpleasant feature of the surgical experience, and postoperative pain was the major complaint in 20 per cent. The third most common complaint was related to requests that the patient lift his head when he was unable to do so immediately after operation. This finding seems to have some practical significance.

Other investigators have exposed anesthetized patients to a series of recordings of positive suggestions. Abramson played tapes to 45 patients: Some tapes contained positive suggestions or music, and some were blank for periods of deep anesthesia.[32] No differences postoperatively were detected between the groups and their requirements for analgesics, sedatives, or tranquilizers, the number of catheterizations performed, or the length of immediate postoperative hospitalization. However, this was a small group, and the author wonders if the suggestions might have been more likely to be effective if they had been given during induction or recovery phases of anesthesia.

In contrast to Abramson's series, Pearson arranged a double-blind trial, in which tape recordings were played to 81 anesthetized patients; some of the tapes contained positive suggestions of postoperative well-being, while others contained music or were blank.[33] Assessment of these patients in the postoperative period by an independent observer, blind to the content of the tapes, showed that those who had listened to the positive suggestions had a smoother postoperative course and were discharged sooner than the patients who had not.

A series by Hutchinson involved 200 consecutive surgical patients who had been given positive suggestions by the anesthesiologist while they were anesthetized.[9] Of those patients, 70 per cent required no analgesic drugs postoperatively, and only 4 per cent required more than 100 mg. of meperidine. In 1960 Wolfe and Millet reached a similar conclusion from a trial involving 1,500 patients.[34] In 1959, Rosea showed that hearing persists in patients under anesthesia with nitrous oxide and gallamine, even with a nitrous oxide concentration as high as 71 to 73 per cent.[35]

Retrospective Studies

Wilson investigated a series of 150 unpremedicated obstetrical patients, most of whom underwent caesarean section.[17] Three patients in this group recalled facts from the anesthetic period, and 46 recalled some form of dream. Ten patients experienced pain during anesthesia; two of these also had factual recall, while seven had dreams. Half of the dreams were pleasant and half unpleasant, but the occurrence of pain during the dream was invariably associated with distress. There was no relationship between the dose of thiopental for induction (100–150 mg.) and recall of dreams. Wilson suggests that potent premedication may play an important role in administration of nitrous oxide-relaxant anesthesia.

A follow-up study of 656 general surgical, gynecologic, and neurosurgical patients was reported by Hutchinson.[9] Inquiry was made into each patient's recall of the operative period and dreams during anesthesia. Eight patients in this series either remembered some part of the procedure or had a dream suggestive of a partial return to consciousness.

Overview

There is little doubt that clinical cases of awareness during apparent surgical anesthesia do occur, even though these investigations (some of which were carefully controlled) did not uniformly confirm this. One must decide, therefore, whether there is a difference between an experimental situation, in which tapes of music or "words" are played to a patient, and the environment in the operating room.

Only in Levison's study were the patients challenged with a simulated but convincingly threatening conversation that was connected to the operative procedure; even then there was no recall at the conscious level, but the use of hypnosis produced the startling results reported. One should not be surprised that the innocuous material presented to patients in the other prospective studies failed to be revealing, since they were artificial stimuli of no apparent interest to the patients and irrelevant to their surgical conditions. In the retrospective studies and the numerous case reports, the material heard and to which patients responded on a conscious level always was related to the patient's welfare or comfort. Most often, the patients reported threatening or offensive comments made by operating room personnel.

CONTRIBUTIONS OF MEDICAL HYPNOSIS

Many physicians claim that patients do not hear under general anesthesia, because they have conscious amnesia; yet, Levinson's study suggests that this belief represents specious thinking.[30] Psychoanalytic treatment assumes that the causes of neurotic disorders lie deep in the subconscious. Thus, medical hypnosis, which is said to act at the level of the subconscious, is a valuable technique in the study of the phenomenon of awareness during anesthesia. Unfortunately, few anesthesiologists have had formal training in its use. The contributions of Cheek, who has investigated more than 800 surgical operations utilizing hypnosis, have emphasized repeatedly that the sense of hearing may be preserved in anesthetized patients, although below the level of conscious awareness. His works include many case histories documenting recollections that have been reported in detail under hypnosis.[4,36-42] He notes that the side of the table from which the voice comes and the attitude of the speaker are always distinct. The understanding of anesthetized patients is literal and childlike. Statements that would otherwise be innocuous may take on a different meaning to anesthetized patients. A remark like "This thing isn't working" that actually refers to the suction apparatus may fill the anesthetized patient with fears about his

anatomy. Cheek's explorations further indicate that statements heard during anesthesia and retained in a patient's subconscious have a bearing on his attitude toward the surgeons and may affect his proper recovery. Awareness can also have far reaching potential effects on a patient's psychological state. Psychoanalysts tell us that while conscious memory of traumatic events can be repressed, the accompanying emotion is not repressed and can contribute to anxiety and depression. Cheek calls these "the invisible scars of surgery."

The reader may conclude that if the subconscious is occasionally alert during clinical anesthesia, patients might be open to positive suggestions, as well as to pessimistic comments made in the operating room.[33,43-45] This topic is discussed further by Cheek[4,36-42] as well as other investigators.[33,43-45]

CLINICAL RECOMMENDATIONS

It is difficult to offer the reader sound advice on the best treatment for signs of awareness under general anesthesia. Many clinicians advise the administration of additional narcotics. Indeed, the work of Wilson and Turner suggests that there was a lesser frequency of unpleasant recall in nitrous oxide-relaxant anesthesia when patients were premedicated with a narcotic.[17] However, the study of Agarwal and Sikh failed to confirm this.[24] Merely changing to an inhalation anesthetic technique does not necessarily solve the problem.[18]

By word of mouth, the anesthesiologist is advised to administer scopolamine, but in Crawford's series the incidence of awareness was not significantly altered.[20] However, in this study of obstetrical patients, the addition of 0.1-per-cent methoxyflurane after delivery of the infant reduced the incidence of recall from 6.9 to 0.6 per cent.

A drug that ensures amnesia when it is administered during occurrence of disturbing signs of lightness of anesthesia would be helpful. Many clinicians use diazepam in this way. Yet, it is difficult to find sound clinical studies to confirm the efficacy of this practice. Two recent studies were unable to demonstrate any *retrograde* amnesic effect of diazepam or lorazepam,[21,46] although both drugs can produce anterograde amnesia. Lorazepam is associated with considerably more drowsiness following anesthesia.

Many investigators are convinced that meaningful sounds, meaningful silence, and meaningful conversation are registered and can have a profound influence upon the behavior of a patient during surgery and for many years thereafter. Therefore, the anesthesiologist should treat the unconscious patient with the same respect that he shows for patients in full possession of their senses. In recent years, the number of patients undergoing surgery under superficial chemical anesthesia has increased, and it is prudent to treat every operative patient as though he is capable of hearing. Hypnosis provides us with a better understanding of reactions to surgery and anesthesia. Our specialty should include instruction on ways in which the subconscious mind of patients can be protected and aided in their struggle with the stresses of life. In the future, anesthesiologists may be forced to decide whether the risk of consciousness during surgery does not outweigh the risk of using potent inhalation drugs. Patients must be unconscious of their surroundings and free of pain. In the meantime, while the anesthesiologist watches the ordinary clinical signs of anesthesia and notes the variations that indicate lightness, all personnel in the operating room should be guarded in their conversations, so that they do not adversely affect the patient at the subconscious level. Furthermore, it may not be unreasonable to offer encouraging suggestions to the patient while he is apparently anesthetized.

REFERENCES

1. Winterbottom, E. H.: Insufficient anaesthesia. Br. Med. J., 1:247, 1950.
2. Bahl, C. P., and Wadwa, S.: Consciousness during apparent surgical anaesthesia. Br. J. Anaesth., 40:289, 1968.
3. Brunn, J. T.: The capacity to hear, understand and to remember experiences during chemo-anesthesia: a personal experience. Am. J. Clin. Hypn., 6:27, 1963.
4. Cheek, D. B.: Further evidence of persistence of hearing under chemoanesthesia: detailed case report. Am. J. Clin. Hypn., 7:55, 1964.
5. Clutton-Brock, J.: Some aspects of the problem of consciousness and anaesthesia. Anaesthesia, 19:115, 1964.
6. Erickson, M. H.: Chemo-anesthesia in relation to hearing and memory. Am. J. Clin. Hypn., 6:31, 1963.
7. Graff, T. D., and Phillips, O. C.: Consciousness and pain during apparent surgical anesthesia. J.A.M.A., 170:2069, 1959.
8. Holmes, C. M.: "Perchance to Dream": The paradox of awareness during general anaesthesia. Aust. N.Z. J. Surg., 40:200, 1970.
9. Hutchinson, R.: Awareness during surgery. Br. J. Anaesth., 33:463, 1960.
10. Marx, G. F., Steen, S. N., Schapira, M., et al.: Pain and awareness during surgical anesthesia. N.Y. State J. Med., 67:2623, 1967.
11. McIntyre, J. W. R.: Awareness during general anaesthesia: preliminary observations. Can. Anaesth. Soc. J., 13:495, 1966.
12. Parkhouse, J.: Awareness during surgery. Postgrad. Med. J., 36:674, 1960.
13. Scott, D. L.: Awareness during general anaesthesia. Can. Anaesth. Soc. J., 19:173, 1972.
14. Sia, R. L.: Consciousness during general anesthesia. Anesth. Analg., 48:363, 1969.
15. Stephen, C. R.: Awareness during anesthesia. Clin. Anesth., 3:113, 1968.
16. Terrell, R. K., Sweet, W. O., Gladfelter, J. H., et al.: Study of recall during anesthesia. Anesth. Analg., 48:86, 1969.
17. Wilson, J., and Turner, D. J.: Awareness during caesarean section under general anaesthesia. Br. Med. J., 1:281, 1969.
18. Wilson, S. L., Vaughan, R. W., and Stephen, C. R.: Awareness, dreams and hallucinations associated with general anesthesia. Anesth. Analg., 54:609, 1975.
19. Famewo, C. E.: Awareness and dreams during general anaesthesia for Caesarean section. Can. Anaesth. Soc. J., 23:636, 1976.
20. Crawford, J. S.: Awareness during operative obstetrics under general anaesthesia. Br. J. Anaesth., 43:179, 1971.
21. Barr, A. M., Moxon, A., Woollam, C. H. M., et al.: The effect of diazepam and lorazepam on awareness during anaesthesia for Caesarean section. Anaesthesia, 32:873, 1977.
22. Dunnett, I. A. R.: Awareness during endotracheal intubation. Br. J. Anaesth., 49:491, 1977.
23. Mostert, J. W.: States of awareness during general anesthesia. Perspect. Biol. Med., 19:68, 1975.
24. Agarwal, G., and Sikh, S. S.: Awareness during anaesthesia. Br. J. Anaesth., 49:835, 1977.
25. Blacher, S. S.: On awakening paralyzed during surgery. J.A.M.A., 234:67, 1975.
26. McKenna, T., and Wilton, T. N. P.: Awareness during endotracheal intubation. Anaesthesia, 28:599, 1973.
27. Robson, J. G.: Measurement of depth of anaesthesia. Br. J. Anaesth., 41:785, 1969.
28. Waters, D. J.: Factors causing awareness during surgery. Br. J. Anaesth., 40:259, 1968.
29. Trustman, R., Dubovsky, S., and Titley, R.: Auditory perception during general anesthesia—myth or fact? Int. J. Clin. Exp. Hypn., 25:88, 1977.
30. Levinson, B. W.: States of awareness during general anaesthesia. Br. J. Anaesth., 37:544, 1965.
31. Brice, D. D., Hetherington, R. R., and Utting, J. E.: A simple study of awareness and dreaming during anaesthesia. Br. J. Anaesth., 42:535, 1970.

32. Abramson, M., Greenfield, I., and Heron, W. T.: Response to or perception of auditory stimuli under deep surgical anesthesia. Am. J. Obstet. Gynecol., *96*:584, 1966.
33. Pearson, R. E.: Response to suggestions given under general anesthesia. Am. J. Clin. Hypn., *4*:106. 1961.
34. Wolfe, L. S., and Millet, J. B.: Control of post-operative pain by suggestion under general anesthesia. Am. J. Clin. Hypn., *3*:109, 1960.
35. Rosen, J.: Hearing tests during anaesthesia with nitrous oxide and relaxants. Acta Anaesth. Scand., *3*:1, 1959.
36. Cheek, D. B.: Unconscious perception of meaningful sounds during surgical anesthesia as revealed under hypnosis. Am. J. Clin. Hypn., *1*:101, 1959.
37. Cheek, D. B.: Use of preoperative hypnosis to protect patients from careless conversation. Am. J. Clin. Hypn., *3*:101, 1960.
38. Cheek, D. B.: What does the surgically anesthetized patient hear? Rocky Mt. Med. J., *57*:49, 1960.
39. Cheek, D. B.: The anesthetized patient can hear and can remember. Am. J. Proctol., *13*:287, 1962.
40. Cheek, D. B.: Importance of recognizing that surgical patients behave as though hypnotized. Am. J. Clin. Hypn., *4*:227, 1962.
41. Cheek, D. B.: Surgical memory and reaction to careless conversation. Am. J. Clin. Hypn., *6*:237, 1964.
42. Cheek, D. B.: The meaning of continued hearing sense under general chemo-anesthesia: a progress report and report of a case. Am. J. Clin. Hypn., *8*:275, 1966.
43. Bensen, V. B.: One hundred cases of post-anesthetic suggestion in the recovery room. Am. J. Clin. Hypn., *14*:9, 1971.
44. Hutchings, D. D.: The value of suggestion given under anesthesia. A report and evaluation of 200 consecutive cases. Am. J. Clin. Hypn., *4*:26, 1961.
45. Koluch, F. T.: Role of suggestion in surgical convalescence. Arch. Surg., *85*:304, 1962.
46. Pandit, S. K., Heisterkamp, D. V., and Cohen, P. J.: Further studies of the anti-recall effect of lorazepam: a dose-effect relationship. Anesthesiology, *45*:495, 1976.

25 Postoperative Emotional Responses

Henry Rosenberg, M.D.

Theodore L. Badger, M.D., discussing his personal experience after open heart surgery, stated the following:[1] "It is the utter helplessness of recovery that seeks a humanizing of relationships with those around you. Were it possible for the recovery room residents to see and know their patients preoperatively, much confidence would be instilled into these patients . . ."

That personality changes may occur following surgery is well known, having been first described by Dupuytren in 1819.[2] The initial discussions of disorientation, combativeness, depression, and other inappropriate behavior that develops postoperatively usually ascribed the etiology of such problems to sepsis or drug toxicity.[3–6] However, with the development of psychiatric concepts, it was realized that in addition to organic causes, emotional upheavals following surgery were often rooted in the complex reactions of the mind-body schema that occur with stress in general and consequent to surgery and anesthesia in particular.

At first, many physicians believed that postoperative psychosis was a distinct, clinically definable entity deriving from a specific etiology.[7,8] By the 1940s, however, the fallacy of such a view was apparent. In the 1950s, when open heart surgery began to be performed extensively, the high incidence of "post-cardiotomy" delirium (up to 70%) prompted intense study and reflection about postoperative emotional changes. It was realized that "postoperative psychosis," like "postpartum psychosis," is a multifactorial syndrome in terms of etiology, manifestation, and prognosis.

The role of anesthetic agents and the anesthesiologist in the occurrence and manifestations of postoperative personality changes is difficult to evaluate. This is so because anesthesia is only one of several emotionally charged interventions in the surgical period.

CLINICAL PRESENTATION OF POSTOPERATIVE EMOTIONAL RESPONSES

In general, in adults, disruptive or disturbing behavior changes occur immediately on emergence from anesthesia or after a lucid interval of 24 to 48 hours (often occurring first in the intensive care unit).[9,10] Less overt but just as disturbing personality changes, such as depression, bad dreams, and, in children, regressive behavior, may last for days to weeks after surgery. The form and severity of such changes are varied.

Postanesthetic excitement as it occurs on emergence from anesthesia is ". . . usually characterized by restlessness, disorientation, crying, moaning, or irrational talking. In its extreme form there is wild thrashing about together with shouting or screaming."[11] Although several studies have examined the etiology of emergence excitement, more subtle personality changes such as quiet confusion, depression, and other affective disorders occurring in the recovery room have received few comments.[12]

In contrast, postoperative psychologic changes beginning after a lucid interval have been the subject of many comments and studies. The changes that may occur at this time are varied and include brain syndrome, neurotic emotional responses, and psychotic behavior.[7,13]

Brain syndrome is basically a sensorial defect, consisting of disorientation, impairment of memory, judgment, and intellectual functions and illusions,* as well as lability of affect. The syndrome is usually reversible, especially when associated with correctable toxic or metabolic etiologies.

Neurotic emotional responses may take the form of an anxiety state, depression, and conversion reaction (converting anxiety into bodily symptoms).

Psychotic behavior may be expressed as psychotic depression, with suicidal tendencies, manic depressive reactions, schizophrenic reactions, hallucinations, and grossly inappropriate behavior and moods.

Only rarely do these syndromes become severe enough to require psychiatric hospitalization.[14] More often they may be controlled by psychotherapy, minor and major tranquillizers, and correction of organic problems.

Yet another mode of expression of personality change is a hypokinetic, withdrawn state, which is often described after sudden major catastrophes. This type of reaction is usually evident soon after operation and may persist for days or weeks.[1,10]

These reactions pose severe problems in nursing care and may jeopardize recovery. Often they are manifestations of the patient's inability to cope with the psychologic stress represented by the threat of loss of life and limb and change of body image, or simply sensory deprivation.[15]

---

*The misinterpretation of sensory stimuli is termed an illusion. Hallucinations are responses to nonexistent external stimuli.

However, behavioral changes may also be the result of, or aggravated by, physiologic insults. Of course, preoperative identification of the patient who is vulnerable to such psychologic deterioration is important in management (see p. 00).

Psychologic and emotional problems extending into the late postoperative period (after patient discharge) are of concern as well, especially with the increasing popularity of outpatient surgery. These problems may take the form of recurring bad dreams, the experience of deja vu, inability to concentrate, diminution of attention span, general malaise, and regressive behavior. Such symptoms have been shown to follow even brief surgical procedures.[16] The patient's attitude toward subsequent surgery is influenced by these experiences.

Although evaluation of the etiology of postoperative and postanesthetic responses is complex, certain organic and psychologic factors are known to predispose patients to emotional problems. A working knowledge of these factors is essential for prevention and treatment. Since most studies deal with either observations in the recovery room during emergence from anesthesia or the period beginning 24 or more hours postoperatively, the discussion below generally follows this division.

IMMEDIATE EMOTIONAL RESPONSES TO ANESTHESIA AND SURGERY

Only 3 to 5 per cent of patients exhibit emergence excitement, based on studies performed when cyclopropane and diethyl ether were still in general use.[11,17,18] More subtle changes were found by Winkelstein in a far greater percentage of patients.[12] His group observed that patients awakening from general anesthesia—thiopental followed by halothane, cyclopropane, ether, or nitrous oxide—were lucid but exhibited a lack of concern about the surgical procedure and a lack of appropriate affective responses. Although patients undergoing procedures with spinal anesthesia showed a more appropriate affect, the investigators nevertheless attributed the changes following general anesthesia to psychogenic rather than pharmacologic factors.

Table 25-1. Operations and Emergence Excitement*

OPERATION	NUMBER OF PATIENTS	NUMBER WITH EXCITEMENT	INCIDENCE (%)
Tonsillectomy	406	67	14.0
Thyroid	406	55	13.6
Circumcision	82	9	11.0
Hysterectomy	1157	90	7.8
Perineal plastic	299	21	7.0
Abdominal wall	502	35	7.0
Eye	83	5	6.0
Breast	915	55	6.0
Upper abdominal	1006	51	5.0
Extremity	1055	50	4.7
Face	737	29	3.9
Intrathoracic	608	23	3.8
Transurethral resection	187	7	3.4
Dilatation and curettage	2554	72	2.9
Neck	232	6	2.5
Appendectomy	119	4	2.5
Dental	303	7	2.2
Intracranial	181	3	1.6
Spinal fusion	266	4	1.5
Other	1196	61	5.1

*(Eckenhoff, J.E., Kneale, D.H., and Dripps, R.D.: The incidence and etiology of postanesthetic excitement. Anesthesiology, *22*: 667, 1961)

Influence of the Operative Site

Eckenhoff, Kneale, and Dripps retrospectively evaluated 14,000 surgical procedures in patients 3 years of age or older and found that tonsillectomy, thyroid surgery, and circumcision were most frequently associated with emergence excitement (Table 25-1).[11] In general, surgery, on the airway, the breast, and the organs of reproduction, as well as procedures associated with strong emotional significance, are likely to be accompanied by a high incidence of emergence excitement.

Intrathoracic and upper abdominal operations are most often accompanied by emergence excitement according to the surveys of Smessaert,[18] Coppolino,[17] and Knox.[14] The discrepancies may be related to influences that were not controlled, such as premedication and anesthetic agents.

Anesthetic Agent

Clearly, the inhalation agents most often associated with emergence delirium are cyclopropane and ether. Thiopental, nitrous oxide, and narcotic nitrous oxide are least often implicated. Halo-thane (and presumably enflurane) are intermediate.[11]

Smessaert found that with a barbiturate anticholinergic premedication, delirium was present in 2 per cent of patients anesthetized with diethyl ether, 4 per cent of those anesthetized with cyclopropane, 2.5 per cent of those having cyclopropane-ether, and 1 per cent of those anesthetized with thiopental-nitrous oxide.[18] Eckenhoff found a 6.1-per-cent incidence of excitement with cyclopropane, and 7 per cent with ether (Table 25-2).[11]

The interaction of other factors with anesthetic agents is evident in Table 25-3. After breast biopsy, there was no difference in the incidence of excitement with cyclopropane-ether compared to all other agents. (Neither group received narcotic premedication.) After thyroid surgery, however, one-quarter of the patients anesthetized with cyclopropane-ether were excited, while none of those receiving "all other anesthetics" were agitated, even though the same preanesthetic medications had been given.

In one of the few studies examining the psycho-

Table 25-2. Anesthetic Agents and Postoperative Excitement*

AGENT	NUMBER OF PATIENTS	NUMBER WITH EXCITEMENT	INCIDENCE (%)
Cyclopropane + ether	1732	139	7.9
Thiopental + cyclopropane	2073	149	7.2
Ether†	877	62	7.0
Cyclopropane	3725	227	6.1
N_2O + halothane	193	7	3.6
Other combinations	523	14	2.5
Thiopental + N_2O	1548	35	2.3
Spinal + supplement	935	16	1.7
Thiopental + N_2O + halothane	184	3	1.6
Thiopental + N_2O + narcotic	504	2	0.4

*Eckenhoff, J.E., Kneale, D.H., and Dripps, R.D.: The incidence and etiology of postanesthetic excitement. Anesthesiology, *22*: 667, 1961
†Induction with any other agent

logic effects of anesthesia without surgery, James evaluated the effects of 90 to 180 min. of cyclopropane-oxygen anesthesia in young healthy volunteers undergoing studies of cerebral blood flow.[19] No postanesthetic excitement was seen. However, a variety of subjective complaints were common up to 6 days after anesthesia (Table 25-4). A decrease in the ability to learn and sustain mental effort was revealed by psychologic testing for several days.

A recent evaluation of the effects of 4.4 to 7.2 hours of halothane or isoflurane anesthesia, again in healthy male volunteers not undergoing surgery, disclosed similar results.[20] Subjective dysphoric complaints persisted for up to 8 days. Halothane was associated with more complaints than isoflurane. This difference was thought to be related to the greater fat solubility of halothane compared to isoflurane and/or the metabolites of halothane. Indeed, bromide levels after prolonged halothane anesthesia may attain levels known to cause behavioral changes.[21]

Ketamine is associated with a high incidence of emotional reactions in the recovery room and, possibly, for long periods after its administration. In the recovery room, vivid dreams, often unpleasant, are quite common, and their incidence ranges from 9 to over 40 per cent.[10,22] Droperidol and the benzodiazepines purportedly mitigate these reactions.[23] although there is not uniform agreement concerning their effectiveness.[24] Apparently, the more psychologically stressful is the surgical procedure, the more likely it is that there will be an unpleasant emotional reaction. Krestow found that 30 of 50 patients undergoing therapeutic abortions had unpleasant dreams, and 17 of them subsequently rejected ketamine for other procedures.[24] However, Garfield, studying soldiers in a burn ward undergoing skin grafts and minor orthopaedic procedures, found a low incidence of unpleasant dreams and a more ready acceptance of the agent.[25] Several case reports have also incriminated ketamine as the cause of recurrent bad dreams, experiences of déjà vu, and dysphoric reactions for weeks postoperatively.[26,27]

Meyer and Blacher have implicated the *lack* of anesthesia in the production of personality changes.[28,29] In several cases in which succinylcholine and light anesthesia were used for mitral commissurotomy, patients recalled fragments of conversation and noises in the operating room. They were aware of being unable to move or talk intraoperatively. Whereas preoperatively these

Table 25-3. Anesthetic Agents and Percentage of Postoperative Excitement

	CYCLOPROPANE-ETHER ANESTHESIA		ALL OTHER ANESTHETICS	
	NO NARCOTIC IN PREMEDICATION	NARCOTIC IN PREMEDICATION	NO NARCOTIC IN PREMEDICATION	NARCOTICS IN PREMEDICATION
Group C-breast 531 patients (excitement 14%)	14.5	12.5	14.8	3.1
Group D-thyroid 493 patients (excitement 16.2%)	24.7	11.0	0	2.4

(Eckenhoff, J. E., Kneale, D.H., and Dripps, R.D.: The incidence and etiology of postanesthetic excitement. Anesthesiology, *22:* 667, 1961)

patients had displayed only appropriate signs of anxiety, postoperatively they were either expressionless, mute, and apathetic or sometimes excited and hallucinating. Harrowing repetitive dreams and fantasies were common for several days. Further studies are needed regarding the relation between intraoperative awareness and psychologic changes postoperatively.[30,31]

Preanesthetic Medication

Premedication also influences the incidence of emotional reactions on emergence from anesthesia. In both adults[16,32] and children,[33] a barbiturate-anticholinergic premedicant (especially scopolamine) is associated with a high incidence of excitement. Addition of a narcotic to this combination or administering a narcotic shortly before the termination of the procedure results in a smoother, calmer awakening. Pain owing to surgery itself or prolonged immobilization leading to muscle soreness is believed to be an important contributing factor in the production of emergence excitement.[11]

Premedicant drugs reported to be associated with emergence excitement or delirium include the phenothiazines[33] and pentazocine.[34] In cases in which scopolamine has been implicated as a cause of delirium, physostigmine, the tertiary amine cholinesterase inhibitor, in a dose of 1 to 2 mg. intravenously, dramatically and rapidly reverses the delirium.[35,36] Even when delirium occurs several hours after scopolamine, the response to physostigmine may be dramatic.

Age, Sex, and Physical Status

Sex does not appear to influence the incidence of emergence delirium. Age, however, is a more significant factor. Eckenhoff found that younger, more vigorous patients were more often excited in the recovery room;[11] aged patients rarely displayed emergence excitement.

Other Factors

A host of other influences bear on the appearance of emergence excitement. Drug-dependent patients, particularly alcoholics, may display the first signs of withdrawal after the abstinence enforced by surgery.[37]

The duration of anesthesia is also related to emergence excitement. A significantly increased incidence of delirium occurs with procedures that last for over 4 hours.[7] This may be related to the complexity of the surgery, to the likelihood of fluid shifts,[38] or, perhaps, to the dysphoria that Davison and coworkers showed was likely to occur after 4 to 8 hours of anesthesia.[20] In open heart surgery, pump time rather than operative time is correlated with emotional upsets.[32]

Important organic causes of behavioral disorders are hypoxia, hypercapnia, electrolyte disorders, and acid-base changes (Table 25-5).[39,40] Electrolyte changes that may occur postoperatively and lead to behavioral changes are hyponatremia (e.g., after transurethral surgery), hypochloremia (e.g., after intestinal drainage), and hyperosmolar states (see Chap. 26).

Table 25-4. Subjective Changes in the First 24 Hours in 18 Subjects

% OF SUBJECTS	SUBJECTIVE CHANGE
82	Decreased desire to smoke
78	Weakness
78	Tiredness, listlessness, decreased energy
72	Sore throat
67	Decreased ability to think and concentrate
61	Poor coordination
61	Dizziness, particularly when standing
50	Nauseated with motion
44	*Abnormal thoughts or depression*
39	Vomiting associated with motion
39	Poor appetite
33	Increased cough or sputum production
28	*Nervousness and restlessness*
28	*Sleep disturbances*
28	Nausea without motion
22	Smelled odor of cyclopropane intermittently
22	Vomiting without motion
6	Tasted cyclopropane

(James, F.M.: The effects of cyclopropane anesthesia without operation on mental functions of normal man. Anesthesiology, *30:* 264, 1969)

Table 25-5. Organic Causes of Postoperative Disturbances of Consciousness

CEREBRAL-ORGANIC	RESPIRATORY	HEMODYNAMIC	INFECTIOUS-TOXIC	METABOLIC
Trauma, primary-secondary (edema, conditioning)	Hypoxemia and hypercapnia (compensated respiratory acidosis)	Dimished O_2 content of arterial blood (anemia, hypoxemia)	Inflammation	Hydration
Elimination of cerebral cortex	Decompensated respiratory acidosis and alkalosis	Diminished minute volume (hypovolemia, circulatory collapse, heart and vascular insufficiency, pulmonary embolism)	Endogenous intoxication (burns, ileus)	Electrolyte disturbance
Disregualtion of sleep-awakening function		Circulatory arrest (Adams-Stokes disease or syncope, asystole, ventricular fibrillation)	Bacterial endotoxin, peritonitis, empyema, septicemia	Acid-base imbalance
			Exogenous intoxication	Hepato-renal collapse
			Iatrogenic (anesthesia, drugs)	Endocrine imbalance

(Kaufer, C.: Etiology of consciousness disturbances in surgery. Minn. Med., *51:*1509, 1968)

Patients undergoing emergency surgery are also more likely to be excited postoperatively.[41] The same is true of patients with delirium or organic brain syndrome that exists preoperatively.[42]

Personality and psychologic makeup are important determinants of the expression of emotional problems. Their role is discussed below.

The treatment of excitement and delirium in the recovery room consists of restraint, small doses of intravenous narcotics, and repetitive reassurance, orientation, and explanation.[11] Physostigmine may also be used. Of course, a search for respiratory, circulatory, and other organic problems is in order as well. Hypnosis has also been used with some success.

EMOTIONAL CHANGES THAT OCCUR 24 HOURS OR MORE AFTER SURGERY

On occasion, despite uneventful awakening from anesthesia, disorientation, confusion, and psychotic behavior become manifest 24 to 48 hours after surgery. Although anesthetic concentrations may persist at low levels for several days postoperatively and may alter behavior as discussed, the anesthetic agent is of lesser consideration in the evaluation of the etiology of these behavioral disturbances.

A great deal has been written about certain aspects of the psychiatric and emotional problems that develop following this lucid interval. Patients having open heart procedures are particularly susceptible. The incidence of postoperative emotional changes ranges from 30 to 70 per cent, depending on the series. "Post-cardiotomy psychosis," however, is very uncommon in those under the age of 16.[43]

Tufo and colleagues believe that neurologic deficits from cerebral emboli, hypoxia, and hypoperfusion are responsible for most, if not all, behavioral changes after open heart surgery.[44-47] In their studies, a high positive correlation was demonstrated between delirium and abnormal neurologic signs with long pump runs and time during which bypass mean perfusion pressure is below 50 torr.

Other workers disagree, pointing to the significant reduction of post-cardiotomy delirium by careful attention to preoperative psychiatric support and changes in the intensive care routine.[22,48,49] Specifically, intensive care nurses were trained to communicate with their patients, explain procedures, and provide sleep-wake cycles; clocks, calendars, and radios were introduced to provide contact with reality. Psychiatric support was provided by preoperative exploration of patients' fears, fantasies, and expectations regarding surgery. The resultant reduction in emotional disturbances was impressive.[50,51]

A recent study showed a rather low incidence of postoperative emotional problems in patients undergoing coronary artery bypass procedures.[52] This may be the result of improvements in operative technique, or the difference in personalities of patients with coronary artery disease compared to patients with rheumatic heart disease. However, even when similar surgical populations were compared, there was an overall decline in the incidence of post-cardiotomy delirium.[48] This is associated with both shorter pump runs and changes in intensive care procedures.

Following general surgery, patients most likely to experience gross personality difficulties 24 to 48 hours after surgery are the aged,[53] the 6-month-to 5-year-old child,[54,55] people with preexisting personality disturbances,[53] addicted or habitual drug users, and people having little emotional support from family and friends.[53]

Again, organic factors are not to be overlooked. Medical and surgical complications must always be suspected in patients showing mental deteriorations over a short period of time. It has often been noted that mild confusion, illusions, and disorientation precede significant medical or surgical problems by 12 to 24 hours.[10,53]

Although patients over 70 are less likely to exhibit emergence excitement,[11] they frequently deteriorate emotionally postoperatively.[56] Factors involved are a poor ability to cope with unfamiliar surroundings and situations[8] and the prevalence of cardiovascular and respiratory abnormalities in this age-group. In particular, immobility is tolerated poorly. Changes in mental status and orientation may be induced by sedatives and narcotics and often precipitate confusion and delirium. The treatment for these states is frequently the *withdrawal* of such medication, rather than administration of additional drugs.[57]

Nonetheless, from the psychologic standpoint, the aged tolerate elective surgery rather well.[58,59] In a detailed study of psychologic and social deterioration in patients over 65, Simpson found a low incidence of such deterioration attributable to surgery and anesthesia.[60] He concluded that "... anesthesia has no effect on the physical activity, mental ability, personality or social integration ..." in this age-group when studied several months after surgery.

Personality changes may occur after surgery or hospitalization alone in children.[61] Nightmares, bedwetting, fear of strangers, fear of the dark, temper tantrums, aggressive behavior, and fears of separation are some of the common symptoms. They are most likely to follow surgery in children of age 6 months to 4 years, in whom separation anxiety figures prominently in psychic development.

The incidence of behavior disturbances in children appears to be related to the efficacy of premedication and preoperative preparation in reducing anxiety and, in particular, to the smoothness of induction of anesthesia.[54,62] The following have been suggested to reduce anxiety and achieve smooth induction: narcotic-barbiturate premedication[33]; intensive psychological preparation of the child directly and by the parents[62]; induction of anesthesia with an ultra-short-acting barbiturate rather than a gas[55]; ketamine premedication followed by pentazocine prior to emergence[63]; and minimizing hospitalization, primarily through day surgery programs.[55]

In addition to cardiac surgery, a variety of other procedures are associated with a significant incidence of postoperative emotional problems: orthopaedic procedures, especially in the aged (immobilization)[7,41]; plastic surgery (disappointment that occurs when surgery fails to correct personality problems?); cancer surgery[64]; vasectomy[65]; and ophthalmic surgery (lack of sensory input).[66]

Medications, particularly barbiturates, begun or withdrawn abruptly in the postoperative period may cause bad dreams and emotional upset.

Tranquilizers and barbiturates are prescribed freely for the hospitalized patient. Sudden withdrawal of medication that inhibits the REM dreaming phases of sleep may cause vivid and often unpleasant dreams for several nights.[67] Such dreams may be wrongly attributed to residual anesthetic effects. Similarly, alcoholics and people taking mood-altering medications regularly should not discontinue use of their drugs abruptly.

PSYCHOLOGICAL FACTORS AND THE ROLE OF THE ANESTHESIOLOGIST IN THE MANAGEMENT OF POSTOPERATIVE EMOTIONAL PROBLEMS

As already indicated, attitudes, fears, ego strengths, and emotional makeup affect the patient's emotional responses to surgery and anesthesia. Titchner found that 86 per cent of 200 surgical patients displayed psychological symptoms or behavior disturbance to the extent that a psychiatric illness could be diagnosed preoperatively.[42] His sample was drawn from a low socioeconomic group of deprived and underprivileged people with a high incidence of broken homes. Corman also noted the same trends in a similar population.[68]

The incidence of postoperative psychosis or disorders was 22 per cent in Titchner's study[42] and 39 per cent in Corman's study.[68] When reactions did occur, they were often explainable "... in the light of the dynamic life history of the patient." However, not all neurotic people have emotional upsets postoperatively. Indeed, psychotics often show temporary improvement in their behavior after surgery. Abram and Gill, two psychiatrists, were unable to predict accurately a patient's postoperative psychologic course based on preoperative interviews.[69]

However, on a statistical basis, certain psychiatric "factors" were found significantly more frequently in patients manifesting postoperative delirium (Table 25-6).[41] Titchner found that alcoholics, patients entering the hospital in delirium, immobilized aged patients, and aged and lonely patients were at greatest risk for psychologic aberrations after surgery.[42,53,70] Their findings also showed that close attention and emotional sup-

Table 25-6. Psychiatric Factors that Influence Postoperative Delirium*

	NO DELIRIUM (n=60)		DELIRIUM (n=57)	
ITEM	NUMBER	%	NUMBER	%
Alcholism†	2	3	15	25
Depression†	6	11	35	58
Family history of psychosis‡	1	2	7	12
Gastrointestinal disorder	13	23	24	40
Insomnia‡	7	12	19	32
Organic brain syndrome†	0	0	22	37
Paranoid personality‡	2	4	11	18
Postoperative psychosis†	3	5	14	23
Psychiatric treatment‡	2	4	11	18
Psychosis‡	1	2	7	12
Retirement problems‡	3	5	12	20

*Morse, F.M., and Litin, E.M.: Postoperative delirium: a study of etiologic factors. Am. J. Psychiatry, *126:* 388, 1969. Copyright ©1969, American Psychiatric Association.
†Statistically significant: $P<.01$.
‡Statistically significant: $P<.05$.

port by family, friends, and hospital personnel were of value in the prevention of psychotic reactions. Other studies have found the same to be true of cancer patients.[64]

A detailed psychiatric evaluation of 26 patients undergoing routine surgical procedures led Janis to conclude that a certain amount of preoperative anxiety and tension is imperative for psychologic stability postoperatively.[71] This "work of worrying" alerts the patient's psychological defense to impending stress. Inadequate time for such "worrying" predisposes patients undergoing emergency surgery to postoperative delirium. The neurotic, although his defenses may be weaker than a normally adjusted patient, nevertheless activates psychological defenses prior to surgery. Deutsch observed the following over 30 years ago:[72]

. . . the factor of greatest importance for the successful conquest of operation anxiety and its results is the amount of preoperative preparation; that is, whether the operation was performed as an emergency without the patient having a chance to prepare himself or whether . . . the patient had an opportunity for a longer or shorter time of inner preparation. In the first case we have to expect a psychic shock reaction in the patient and its influence on the postoperative situation. The conditions developed in such a shock reaction are very closely related to the so-called traumatic neuroses, which usually are called forth by serious accidents, unexpected attacks, train wrecks, and other situations of sudden and unheralded invasions of danger . . . Symptoms developed in such a condition are those of general irritability, sleeplessness, anxiety dreams and nightmares, attacks of anxiety with cardiac and respiratory distress, with vasomotor and secretory disturbances, etc.

Janis found that patients who showed no anxiety prior to major surgery and patients who displayed great anticipatory fear were most liable to behavior problems postoperatively.[71] These patients who show no anxiety must be made aware of the reality of surgery; otherwise, they will be angry, hostile, and resentful postoperatively. Patients who show great anxiety need to have their emotional excitement toned down. Many investigators have warned the physician to beware of the patient who claims to have no fears regarding impending surgery.[13,73] While it may not be possible to achieve full therapeutic results in a short time, a realistic exploration of the events surrounding surgery and anesthesia is usually helpful. Preoperative psychiatric consultation may be indicated when the emotional preparations for surgery seem grossly unrealistic.

THE PREOPERATIVE VISIT

The value of the anesthesiologist's preoperative visit has been widely emphasized. The visit is of importance from a physiologic as well as psychologic point of view. Several studies show that preoperative psychologic preparation reduces the incidence of postoperative emotional disturbance in the cardiac patient.[48,50,51] Thus, intensive preparation by nurses, anesthesiologists, surgeons, and psychiatrists are employed. Such preparation usually consists of detailed descriptions of mechanical ventilation, monitoring, and physiotherapy procedures, as well as psychiatric interviews. The interviews are directed to exploring anxieties and fantasies, providing realistic explanations, and correcting misconceptions. These procedures dramatically reduce the incidence of postcardiotomy psychosis.

In children, Jackson, an anesthesiologist, showed that through honest, detailed preoperative explanation to 5-, 6-, and 7-year-olds, a mask induction of anesthesia was rarely stormy or complicated.[62] Unfortunately, follow-up evaluation of problems in the recovery room and delayed abnormal behavior was not explored. Eckenhoff, however, showed that postoperative behavior problems were more likely to occur in children who had a stormy induction of anesthesia.[54]

In adults undergoing general surgery, Egbert and colleagues evaluated the preoperative visit. His group found that a preoperative discussion of ". . . the patient's condition, the time of operation, and the nature of the anesthetic, informing the patient about what would happen the next day as well as questioning him about previous experiences with anesthetics . . ." in combination with pentobarbital and atropine, "adequately" (calm and drowsy) prepared 71 per cent of patients.[74] In contrast, 48 per cent of patients receiving pentobarbital without interview and 35 per cent receiving atropine and no interview were adequately prepared. Psychologic benefits were noted for as long as 18 hours after interview. Again, unfortunately, postoperative behavior was not investigated. However, in another study, Egbert found that detailed preoperative instructions concerning maneuvers to relieve pain de-creased morphine requirements postoperatively.[75] Kolouch comments on the use of posthypnotic suggestion to promote a speedy uneventful recovery from surgery.[76]

Unfortunately, there is no study that directly documents the effect of a "routine" preanesthetic visit on postoperative emotional response. However, based on evidence cited as well as comments of psychiatrists,[4,31,59] it is reasonable to believe that the anesthesiologist may exert significant beneficial effects on a patient's postoperative emotional responses. Too often it is assumed that the surgeon discusses and assesses the patient's attitudes toward surgery. Even if this were the case, most patients have specific questions and fears concerning anesthesia. More than 92 per cent of 100 patients interviewed postoperatively by Sheffer and Greifenstein had apprehension and fear of anesthesia.[59] Sometimes patients voiced specific fears: 43 per cent desired complete withdrawal from the environment during surgery; 29 per cent found general anesthesia unpleasant; and 15 per cent were distressed by spinal anesthesia, and 11 per cent by regional or local anesthesia. Often, however, the fears were displayed by various changes in behavior (Table 25-7). Almost all patients expressed a "healthy active interest and curiosity" in the anesthetic. Unfortunately, in most cases ". . . the attitudes revealed that the anesthetists failed to establish rapport with [them] . . ." Most patients desired not only information but reassurance as well.

What can the anesthesiologist reasonably hope to accomplish in the brief preoperative visit? Direct answers to simple questions are of great value. Most patients are concerned about the type of anesthesia: general, spinal, or other; induction of anesthesia; extent of pain; state of wakefulness; the chances of arousal during anesthesia; whether they might say things that would embarrass them; and the chances of not awakening from anesthesia.

These are quite meaningful, even though seemingly naive questions, and are loaded with emotional significance. Anesthesia is equated on a subconscious or conscious level with death.[4,13] As such, even though many will ask these questions in a jocular tone, they are to be answered honest-

Table 25-7. Number of Patients With Conversion Symptoms Prior to Surgery

MOTOR		AUTONOMIC	
Restlessness	35	Loss of appetite	13
Pacing the floor	16	Urinary frequency	23
Tense muscles	18	Increased sweating	36
Compulsive biting	7		
Tension tapping of fingers	14		
Compulsive hair rubbing	12		
Total motor	102	Total autonomic	72

(Sheffer, M.B., and Greifenstein, F.E.: The emotional responses of patients to surgery and anesthesia. Anesthesiology, *21:* 502, 1960)

ly. Even though they may not be brought up directly, they are of concern to all patients and may be answered as part of the description of the events that will occur prior to, during, and after surgery. The physician may give the patient a feeling of reassurance by describing the events surrounding surgery and anesthesia, including details like scrub suits, intravenous, the number of people in the operating room, the circumstances in which the patient will find himself on awakening from anesthesia, oxygen administration, *pain*, the taking of vital signs, and the recovery room. Other supportive or predictive statements will, thereby, attain added weight.

Above all, though, the anesthesiologist's goal should be to establish a relationship with the patient and to present himself as a person who is interested in the patient as a human being.[13]

In some hospitals, a recovery room nurse visits the preoperative patient with the hope of giving him a further psychologic anchor during the transition from clouded consciousness to arousal.

All patients, particularly those at greatest risk to postoperative psychiatric disturbance, should, if possible, be encouraged to voice their fears and concerns. It is valuable to correct misapprehensions and unrealistic expectations regarding anesthesia and, particularly, arousal from anesthesia.

Optimally, the anesthesiologist's support should continue in the recovery room and postoperatively. Although the patient's affect on emergence may be blunted, "a salutory influence" is created by continuation of the physician-patient relationship even there.[12] Even in the case of recovery from ketamine, where it is generally recommended to leave patients undisturbed until fully awake, Garfield found that most patients appreciated the reassurance and human contact during emergence.[25] An early postoperative visit may permit the patient to discuss unpleasant experiences, permit adequate explanations of untoward events, and answer questions remaining concerning anesthesia. Perhaps explanation of fears and anxieties during this time will prevent them from being transformed into psychological defense mechanisms that may be reactivated during similar stressful situations in the future.

Patients who experience repetitive nightmares and preoccupation with death postoperatively should be suspected of having been aware during anesthesia. These patients often are reluctant to discuss their awareness because of fear that they might be thought insane. However, Blacher has recently shown that direct discussion of their awareness during anesthesia often cures the symptoms dramatically (see Chap. 24).[29]

REFERENCES

1. Badger, T. L.: The physician-patient in the recovery and intensive care units. Arch. Surg., *109*:359, 1974.
2. Dupuytren, B.: Clinical records of surgery. Lancet, *2*:919, 1834.
3. Miller, H. H.: Acute psychoses following surgical procedures. Br. Med. J., *1*:558, 1938.

4. Straker, M.: Surgical procedures and neurotic illness. Can. Med. Assoc. J., *65*:128, 1951.

5. Cobb, S., and McDermott, N. T.: Postoperative psychosis. Med. Clin. North Am., May, 569, 1938.

6. Savage, G. H.: Insanity following the use of anaesthetics in operations. Br. Med. J., *2*:1199, 1887.

7. Morse, R. M., and Litin, E. M.: The anatomy of a delirium. Am. J. Psychiatry, *128*:143, 1971.

8. Oltman, J. E., and Friedman, S.: The role of operative procedure in the etiology of psychosis. Psychiatr. Q., *17*:405, 1943.

9. Baxter, S.: Psychological problems on intensive care. Br. J. of Hosp. Med., *11*:875, 1966.

10. Katz, N. M., Agle, D. P., DePalma, R. G., et al.: Delirium in surgical patients under intensive care. Arch. Surg., *104*:310, 1972.

11. Eckenhoff, J. E., Kneale, D. H., and Dripps, R. D.: The incidence and etiology of postanesthetic excitement. Anesthesiology, *22*:667, 1961.

12. Winkelstein, C., Blacher, R. S., and Meyer, B. C.: Psychiatric observations on surgical patients in recovery room. N.Y. State J. Med., *65*:865, 1965.

13. Schnaper, N.: Postanesthetic (postoperative) emotional responses. Anesthesiology, *22*:674, 1961.

14. Knox, J. W. D., Bovill, J. G., Clarke, R. S. J., et al.: Clinical studies of induction agents. XXXVI: Ketamine. Br. J. Anaesth., *42*: 875, 1970.

15. Zubek, V. P.: Effects of prolonged sensory and perceptual deprivation. Br. Med. Bull., *20*:38, 1964.

16. Fahy, A., and Marshall, M.: Postanaesthetic morbidity in out-patients. Br. J. Anaesth., *41*:433, 1969.

17. Coppolino, C. A.: Incidence of postanesthetic delirium in a community hospital: a statistical survey. Milit. Med., *128*:238, 1963.

18. Smessaert, A., Schehr, C. A., and Artusio, J. F.: Observations in the immediate post-anaesthesia period: II Mode of Recovery. Br. J. Anaesth., *332*:181, 1960.

19. James, F. M.: The effects of cyclopropane anesthesia without surgical operation on mental functions of normal man. Anesthesiology, *30*:264, 1969.

20. Davison, L. A., Steinhelber, J. C., Eger, E. I., II, et al.: Psychological effects of halothane and isoflurane anesthesia. Anesthesiology. *43*:313, 1975.

21. Johnstone, R. E., Kennel, E. M., Behar, M. G., et al.: Increased serum bromide concentrations after halothane anesthesia in man. Anesthesiology, *42*:598, 1975.

22. Kornfeld, D. S.: Open heart surgery and the psyche. J.A.M.A., *213*:1343, 1970.

23. Sadove, M. S., Hartano, S., Redlin, T., et al.: Clinical study of droperidol in the prevention of the side effects of ketamine anesthesia: a progress report. Anesth. Analg., *50*:526, 1971.

24. Krestow, M.: The effect of post-anaesthetic dreaming on patient acceptance of Ketamine anaesthesia: a comparison with thiopentane-nitrous oxide anaesthesia. Can. Anaesth. Soc. J., *21*:385, 1974.

25. Garfield, J. M., Garfield, F. B., Stone, J. G., et al.: A comparison of psychological responses to ketamine and thiopental-nitrous oxide-halothane anesthesia. Anesthesiology, *36*:329, 1972.

26. Fine, J., and Finestone, S. C.: Sensory disturbances following ketamine anesthesia: recurrent hallucinations. Anesth. Analg., *52*:428, 1973.

27. Meyers, E. F., and Charles, P.: Prolonged adverse reactions to ketamine in children. Anesthesiology, *49*:39, 1978.

28. Meyer, B. C., and Blacher, R. S.: A traumatic reaction induced by succinylcholine chloride. N.Y. State J. Med., *61*:1255, 1961.

29. Blacher, R. S.: On awakening paralyzed during surgery. J.A.M.A., *234*:67, 1975.

30. Cheek, D. B.: Further evidence of persistence of hearing under chemoanesthesia: detailed case report. Am. J. Clin. Hypn. 7:55, 1964.

31. Terrell, R. K., Sweet, W. O., Gladfelter, J. M., et al.: Study of recall during anesthesia. Anesth. Analg., *48*:86, 1969.

32. Nadelson, T.: The psychiatrist in the surgical intensive care unit. I. Postoperative delirium. Arch. Surg., *111*:113, 1976.

33. Freeman, A., and Bachman, L.: Pediatric anesthesia: an evaluation of preoperative medication. Anesth. Analg., *38*:429, 1959.

34. Hamilton, R. C., Dundee, J. W., Clarke, R. S. J., et al.: Studies of drugs given before anaesthesia. XIII: pentazocine and other opiate antagonists. Br. J. Anaesth., *39*:647, 1967.

35. Bernards, W.: Case history number 74: reversal of phenothiazine induced coma with physostigmine. Anesth. Analg., *52*:938, 1973.

36. Greene, L. T.: Physostigmine treatment of anticholinergic-drug depression in postoperative patients. Anesth. Analg., *50*:222, 1971.

37. Mays, E. T., Ransdell, H., and DeWuse, B. M.: Metabolic changes in surgical delirium termors. Surgery, *67*:780, 1970.

38. McMurrey, J. D., and Law, S. W.: Postoperative changes in electrolyte balance. Anesthesiology, *22*:819, 1961.

39. Atlschule, M. D.: Postoperative psychosis. Surg. Clin. North. Am. *49*:677, 1969.

40. Kaufer, C.: Etiology of consciousness disturbances in surgery. Minn. Med., *51*:1509, 1968.

41. Morse, R. M., and Litin, E. M.: Postoperative delirium: A study of etiologic factors. Am. J. Psychiatry, *126*:388, 1969.

42. Titchner, J. L., Zwerling, I., Gottschalk, L., et al.: Psychosis in surgical patients. Surg. Gynecol. Obstet., *102*:59, 1956.

43. Kornfeld, D. S., Zimberg, S., and Malm, J. R.: Psychiatric complications of open heart surgery. N. Engl. J. Med., *273*:287, 1965.

44. Silverstein, A., and Kreiger, H. P.: Neurologic complications of cardiac surgery. Arch. Neurol., *5*:601, 1960.

45. Gilman, S.: Cerebral disorders after open heart surgery. N. Engl. J. Med., *272*:489, 1965.

46. Tufo, H. M., Muslin, H., and Ostfeld, A. M.: Central nervous system: complications in the surgical patient. Disease-A-Month: November, 1968. Chicago, Year Book Medical Publishers, 1968.

47. Tufo, H. M., Ostfeld, A. M., and Shekelle, R.: Central venous system: dysfunction following open-heart surgery. J.A.M.A., *212*:1333, 1970.

48. Abram, H. S.: Psychotic reactions after cardiac surgery—a critical review. Semin. Psychiatry, *3*:70, 1971.

49. Heller, S. S., Frank, K. A., Malm, J. R., et al.: Psychiatric complications of open heart surgery. N. Engl. J. Med., *283*:1015, 1970.

50. Layne, O. L., Jr., and Yudofsky, S. C.: Psychosis in

cardiotomy patients: the role or organic and psychiatric factors. N. Engl. J. Med., *284*:518, 1971.

51. Lazarus, H. R., and Hagens, J. H.: Prevention of psychosis following open heart surgery. Am. J. Psychiatry, *124*:1190, 1968.
52. Rabiner, C. J., Willner, A. E., and Fishman, J.: Psychiatric complications following coronary bypass surgery. J. Nerv. Ment. Dis., *160*:342, 1975.
53. Titchner, J. L., and Levine, M.: Surgery as a human experience. New York, Oxford University Press, 1960.
54. Eckenhoff, J. E.: Relationship of anesthesia to postoperative personality changes in children. Am. J. Dis. Child., *86*:587, 1951.
55. Steward, D. J.: Experiences with an out-patient anesthesia service for children. Anesth. Analg., *52*:877, 1973.
56. Bedford, P. D.: Adverse cerebral effects of anaesthesia in old people. Lancet, *2*:259, 1955.
57. Patkin, M.: Postoperative confusion. Med. J. Aust., *2*:559, 1973.
58. Brander, P., Kjellberg, M., and Tammisto, T.: The effects of anaesthesia and general surgery on geriatric patients. Ann. Chiriag. Fenn., *59*:138, 1970.
59. Sheffer, M. B., and Greifenstein, F. E.: The emotional responses of patients to surgery and anesthesia. Anesthesiology, *21*:502, 1960.
60. Simpson, B. R., Williams, M., Scott, J. F., et al.: The effects of anaesthesia and elective surgery on old people. Lancet, *2*:887, 1961.
61. Vernon, D. T. A., Schulman, J. L., and Foley, J. M.: Changes in children's behavior after hospitalization. Am. J. Dis. Child., *111*:581, 1966.
62. Jackson, K.: Psychologic preparation as a method of reducing the emotional trauma of anesthesia in children. Anesthesiology, *12*:293, 1951.
63. Rita, L., Cox, J. M., Seleny, F. L., et al.: Ketamine hydrochloride for pediatric premedication: I. Comparison with pentazocine. Anesth. Analg., *53*:375, 1974.
64. Abrams, R. D., and Funisinger, J. E.: Guilt reactions in patients with cancer. Cancer, *6*:474, 1953.
65. Wolfers, H.: Psychological aspects of vasectomy. Br. Med. J., *4*:297, 1970.
66. Preu, P. W., and Gueda, F. P.: Psychoses complicating recovery from extraction of cataract. Arch. Neurol. Psychiat., *38*:818, 1937.
67. Quinlan, D. M., Kimball, C. P., and Osborne, F.: The experience of open heart surgery. IV Assessment of disorientation and dysphoria following cardiac surgery. Arch. Gen. Psychiatry, *31*:241, 1974.
68. Corman, H. H., Hornick, E. J., Kritchman, M., et al.: Emotional reactions of surgical patients to hospitalization, anesthesia and surgery. Am. J. Surg., *96*:646, 1958.
69. Abram, H. S., and Gill, B. F.: Predictions of postoperative psychiatric complications. N. Engl. J. Med., *265*:1123, 1961.
70. Zwerling, I., Titchner, J., Gottschalk, L., et al.: Personality disorder and the relationships of emotion to surgical illness in 200 surgical patients. Am. J. Psychiatry, *112*:270, 1955.
71. Janis, I. L.: Psychological stress. New York, John Wiley & Sons, Inc., 1958.
72. Deutsch, H.: Some psychoanalytic observations in surgery. Psychosom. Med., *4*:105, 1942.
73. Schnaper, N.: What preanesthetic visit? Anesthesiology, *22*:486, 1961.
74. Egbert, L. D., Battit, G. E., Turndorf, H., et al.: The value of the preoperative visit by an anesthetist. J.A.M.A., *185*:553, 1963.
75. Egbert, L. D., Battit, G. E., Welch, C. E., et al.: Reduction in postoperative pain by encouragement and instruction in patients. N. Engl. J. Med., *270*:825, 1964.
76. Kolouch, F. T.: Role of suggestion in surgical convalescence. Arch. Surg., *85*:304, 1962.

FURTHER READING

Eckenhoff, J. E., Kneale, D. H., and Dripps, R. D.: The incidence and etiology of postanesthetic excitement. Anesthesiology, *22*:667, 1961.

McEvoy, J. P.: Organic brain syndromes. Ann. Intern. Med., *95*:212, 1981.

26 Prolonged Emergence and Failure to Regain Consciousness

J. Kenneth Denlinger, M.D.

Although many factors are known to prolong anesthetic effect, reports of prolonged emergence in man are largely anecdotal. This chapter categorizes the various causes of postoperative coma and cites clinical reports of prolonged emergence. Metabolic disturbances, such as the hyperosmolar syndrome, are reviewed in some detail, because anesthesia may mask the cerebral manifestations of these potentially lethal disturbances and thereby delay their recognition.

THE MECHANISM OF CORTICAL AROUSAL

Classical studies by Moruzzi and Magoun showed that wakefulness depends on diffuse cortical activation by the reticular formation of the brain stem.[1] It has been generally accepted that cortical arousal and focus of attention elicited by afferent sensory stimuli are mediated by the reticular activating system (RAS). Furthermore, it is known that barbiturates produce early depression of this multisynaptic ascending pathway.[2] Certain metabolic disorders associated with CNS depression, such as hypoglycemia and hypoxia, also result in early depression of auditory-evoked potentials in the reticular formation of the brain stem at a time when cortical-evoked potentials are minimally depressed.[3] Selective vulnerability of the reticular activating system to certain anesthetic and metabolic disturbances may be related to the multisynaptic nature of this ascending pathway. According to this concept, functional depression of a neural pathway is directly proportional to the number of synapses involved in that pathway.[4]

Although selective depression of the reticular activating system may be of some significance in the delayed awakening of certain patients following anesthesia, many other cortical and subcortical neural pathways are also involved. Recent evidence in humans and experimental animals has shown that general anesthesia is produced by a variety of neurophysiologic mechanisms. For example, ether produces early cortical depression, and ketamine results in neural excitation, both at cortical and subcortical levels.[5,6] Thus, the neurophysiologic mechanism of prolonged narcosis following anesthesia is drug-dependent and may involve neural stimulation or depression at cortical or subcortical levels.

Although acetylcholine is not the primary excitatory cortical neurotransmitter, the ascending cholinergic arousal system may be the pharmacologic equivalent of the reticular activating system.[7] Stimulation of this neural pathway at the level of the midbrain causes cortical electrographic arousal, as well as release of acetylcholine in the cortex. Direct application of acetylcholine to acetylcholine-sensitive cortical neurons results in prolonged excitation, a pharmacological effect that is potentiated by anticholinesterases and blocked by atropine in experimental animals.[8] Although atropine is capable of producing CNS depression in humans when used in massive doses, the central anticholinergic syndrome is more frequently seen following premedicant doses of scopolamine. Physostigmine is chosen as the pharmacologic antagonist, because this anticholinesterase readily crosses the blood-brain barrier, in contrast to its analogue, neostigmine, which possesses a quaternary amine group and penetrates the blood-brain barrier poorly.[9]

DIFFERENTIAL DIAGNOSIS OF POSTOPERATIVE COMA

Failure to awaken promptly after general anesthesia may be related to three basic causes: prolonged action of anesthetic drugs, metabolic encephalopathy, and neurologic injury (see the list below).

Differential Diagnosis of Prolonged Recovery and Failure to Regain Consciousness

Prolonged drug action
  Overdose
  Increased central sensitivity
    Age
    Biologic variation
    Metabolic effects
  Decreased protein binding
  Delayed anesthetic excretion
  Anesthetic redistribution
  Decreased hepatic metabolism, drug interaction, and biotransformation
Metabolic encephalopathy
  Hepatic, renal, endocrine, and neurologic disorders
  Hypoxia and hypercapnia
  Acidosis
  Hypoglycemia
  The hyperosmolar syndrome
  Electrolyte imbalance (Na+, Ca++, Mg++), water intoxication
  Hypothermia and hyperthermia
  Neurotoxic drugs
Neurologic injury
  Cerebral ischemia
  Intracranial hemorrhage
  Cerebral embolus (air, calcium, fibrin, fat)
  Hypoxia and cerebral edema

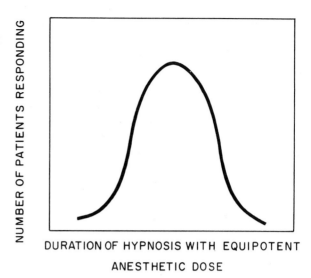

Fig. 26-1. Biologic variation in central sensitivity to anesthetic action.

PROLONGED ACTION OF ANESTHETIC DRUGS

Overdose

Delayed awakening after general anesthesia is most commonly caused by anesthetic overdose. Such overdose can occur when anesthetics are administered for the wrong reason. For example, elevated perfusion pressure during cardiopulmonary bypass or intraoperative hypertension due to a catecholamine-secreting tumor might be treated with large doses of barbiturate in an attempt to deepen anesthesia. Failure to employ specific vasodilators or adrenergic blocking agents in such circumstances can lead to anesthetic overdose and delayed recovery.

Increased Central Sensitivity

The duration of hypnotic effect of a general anesthetic is dependent upon both the concentration of anesthetic in the brain and the sensitivity of the brain receptor site to the particular anesthetic agent. Biologic variation in sensitivity is expressed by the bell-shaped Gaussian curve, which relates frequency of response to duration of hypnotic effect (Fig. 26-1). Sensitivity of the brain to hypnotic drug action may be influenced by a number of physiologic and pharmacologic factors. Circadian rhythm affects halothane anesthetic requirement in rats. MAC is decreased 10 to 14 per cent during the inactive phase of a cycle induced by alternating periods of light and darkness.[10] It is possible that such a cyclic variation may also apply to the duration of hypnotic effect in anesthetized man. Anesthetic requirement is also reduced by advanced age, hypothermia, and hypothyroidism.[11] It would seem likely that these factors also increase the duration of hypnotic drug action, in part, by increasing CNS sensitivity. Reserpine, methyldopa, and chronic administration of dextro-amphetamine reduce anesthetic requirement in experimental animals.[12,13] However, significant prolongation of anesthesia has not been reported in humans following the use of catecholamine-depleting drugs. While variation in CNS sensitivity is a valid explanation for some cases of prolonged emergence from anesthesia, this diagnosis is usually made by exclusion and cannot be substantiated until all other factors that influence drug action and level of consciousness are considered.

Decreased Protein Binding

Drugs that compete with barbiturates for common binding sites increase barbiturate sleeping time by displacement of barbiturate from plasma protein. For example, administration of sodium acetrizoate (a radiographic contrast material) increases the duration of pentobarbital narcosis by way of this mechanism.[14] Thiopental concentration in the brain and heart following intravenous administration is markedly increased by pretreatment with sulfadimethoxine, a drug that undergoes extensive protein binding.[15] Hypoproteinemia may prolong the duration of barbiturate anesthesia by a reduction in the delivery of barbiturate to the liver.[16]

Delayed Anesthetic Excretion

The decrease in brain anesthetic concentration, which is evidenced clinically by emergence or awakening from anesthesia, is dependent upon factors similar to those that govern anesthesia uptake and distribution. Clinical experience shows that emergence from anesthesia is slow when high concentrations of soluble agents, such as methoxyflurane or diethyl ether, are employed for long surgical procedures. The degree of solubility of an anesthetic agent is directly proportional to the effect of anesthetic duration on speed of recovery.[17] High fat solubility provides an anesthetic reservoir from which the agent is released after termination of anesthesia.

Increased cardiac output delays emergence from anesthesia by reducing anesthetic clearance from the brain in the early phases of recovery.[17] Postoperative hypoventilation also delays emergence from anesthesia by decreasing the alveolar–venous blood anesthetic tension gradient. Stoelting and Eger compared the effect of four-fold variation in ventilation on the rate of fall of alveolar concentration for three anesthetic agents of differing solubility.[18] The effect of increasing ventilation was found to be greatest for halothane, an agent of moderate solubility, whereas it had a less significant effect for nitrous oxide and methoxyflurane.

Anesthetic Redistribution

It is well known that awakening after a single intravenous dose of thiopental is dependent primarily upon redistribution of this drug in lean body tissue.[19] In fact, it has been suggested that redistribution may be the major factor responsible for the termination of hypnotic action of all clinically useful barbiturates, as well as other hypnotic drugs, such as diazepam.[20] However, there is considerable experimental evidence that hepatic metabolism may also be of some importance in the duration of sleep produced by a single intravenous dose of thiopental. Gross alteration in hepatic function (hepatectomy, portal vein diversion) is associated with significantly prolonged barbiturate sleeping time in animals.[16] While it may be controversial whether or not metabolism is of clinical importance in the recovery following a single intravenous dose of barbiturate,[19,21] it is certain that the metabolic effect is significant when multiple doses of barbiturate or other intravenous hypnotic drugs are administered over a prolonged period of time. Saturation of body tissues limits the magnitude of redistribution and, thus, prolongs the CNS action of an otherwise short-acting agent.

Decreased Hepatic Metabolism

Extremes of age, malnutrition, hypothermia, and simultaneous administration of multiple drugs that are detoxified by the hepatic microsomal system (e.g., ethanol, barbiturates) are factors associated with decreased hepatic metabolism and prolonged anesthetic emergence. Alteration in hepatic microsomal metabolism has been demonstrated to influence the uptake and elimination of methoxyflurane in rats.[22] Monoamine oxidase (MAO) inhibitors also inhibit hepatic microsomal enzymes. However, the mechanism by which MAO inhibitors potentiate narcotics, barbiturates, and other sedative drugs has not been established.[23] Bis-[p-nitrophenyl] phosphate prolongs the anesthetic action of propanidid by inhibition of the hepatic enzyme system responsible for rapid hydrolysis of this agent.[24]

Combination of ketamine anesthesia with various tranquilizers for the purpose of reducing hallucinatory phenomena upon emergence may delay anesthetic emergence. Recent evidence suggests that hepatic biotransformation of ketamine plays a significant role in the termination of its CNS action even after a single intravenous dose.[25] Ketamine may be quite different from thiopental in this respect, and therefore some degree of caution is advised when ketamine is administered to patients with gross hepatic dysfunction. Since the halothane anesthetic requirement is significantly reduced 6 hours after ketamine administration in the rat,[26] ketamine can no longer be regarded as a short-acting agent and may contribute to prolonged recovery from anesthesia.

Biotransformation of halothane is associated with release of free bromide ion in concentrations sufficient to produce postoperative drowsiness and lethargy in humans.[27,28] Preoperative ingestion of bromide-containing drugs, impaired renal function, and hepatic enzyme induction are factors that might predispose patients to higher bromide levels in the postoperative period. Increased plasma bromide levels may have contributed to one case of prolonged coma following successful repair of an intracranial aneurysm.[27]

METABOLIC ENCEPHALOPATHY

A number of systemic metabolic disturbances resulting in CNS depression can occur in the postanesthetic period and must be distinguished from residual effects of anesthesia. Such metabolic encephalopathy often increases the sensitivity of the brain to depressant drugs.

Liver Disease

Patients with severe liver disease and a history of hepatic coma develop EEG slowing and CNS depression following small doses of morphine, whereas healthy volunteers or patients without a history of hepatic coma do not develop EEG changes.[29] Narcotics have been implicated as a causative factor in many cases of hepatic coma and should be used with caution in patients with severe liver disease. Although barbiturate sleeping time is markedly prolonged in animals after hepatectomy or drug-induced hepatic damage, studies in patients with severe liver disease have not shown increased sensitivity to single or multiple doses of thiopental.[16,30] Enhanced CNS penetration of cimetidine in liver disease results in mental confusion that may be mistaken for hepatic encephalopathy.[30a]

Kidney Disease

Prolongation of barbiturate anesthesia has been reported in patients with renal failure and azotemia.[31] This effect is probably a result of enhanced CNS sensitivity to barbiturates, although other factors such as decreased protein binding, electrolyte disturbances, and acid-base imbalance may also be involved. It has been suggested that increased sensitivity to hypnotic drugs in uremic patients is the result of changes in permeability of the blood-brain barrier.[32]

Endocrine and Neurologic Disorders

Hypothyroidism is associated with decreased anesthetic requirement in experimental animals.[33] Clinical reports suggest that patients with severe adrenal insufficiency may demonstrate prolonged unconsciousness in the postanesthetic period.[34,35,36] Delayed emergence after thiopental anesthesia has been reported in a patient with Huntington's chorea, although this patient subsequently responded in a normal fashion to nitrous oxide-ether anesthesia.[37]

Hypoxia and Hypercapnia

Postoperative respiratory failure may also result in prolonged emergence from anesthesia. Hypoventilation not only causes respiratory acidosis and hypoxia but also retards excretion of inhalation anesthetics. Carbon dioxide narcosis in the absence of hypoxia may occur in patients with severe chronic lung disease who receive high concentrations of inspired oxygen. Studies in dogs indicate that carbon dioxide produces narcosis primarily by inducing cerebral tissue acidosis.[38] However, narcosis is frequently observed in patients with respiratory failure who have less severe degrees of hypercapnia. This discrepancy may be explained by factors other than hypercapnia, such as concomitant hypoxia, drug therapy, and cerebrovascular disease.

Acidosis

Clinical studies in patients with cerebral acidosis of various causes show that mental confusion, delirium, or coma invariably occurs when cerebrospinal fluid pH falls to 7.25 or lower ($[H^+] \geq$ 56.2 nmol./L.).[39] Cerebrospinal fluid (CSF) acidosis and central depression is more severe when hypercapnia is acute, since carbon dioxide diffuses rapidly into the extracellular fluid of the brain, whereas bicarbonate ion crosses the blood-brain barrier much more slowly. The combination of acute respiratory acidosis and chronic metabolic alkalosis may be associated with profound cerebral acidosis and coma, despite normal arterial pH. In a comatose patient with pneumonia and chronic lung disease, during mechanical ventilation with 40-per-cent inspired oxygen, Bulger obtained the following measurements:[40] pH of cerebrospinal fluid, 7.15 ($[H^+] = 70.8$ nmol./L.); arterial pH, 7.45 ($[H^+] = 35.5$ nmol./L.); Pa_{CO_2}, 72

torr (9.6 kPa); and Pa_{O_2}, 63 torr (8.4 kPa). Ventilation was increased; the patient's mental status steadily improved as a result, and the pH of the cerebrospinal fluid returned to normal.

A paradoxical increase in cerebral acidosis with progressive deterioration in the level of consciousness has been reported in diabetic patients with severe ketoacidosis who are given therapeutic doses of sodium bicarbonate.[41] The increase in arterial pH produced by bicarbonate administration results in decreased alveolar ventilation, producing an increase in arterial and brain carbon dioxide tension. The net result is a decrease in brain pH at a time when arterial pH is increasing. Measurement of the pH of cerebrospinal fluid is of value in explaining why some patients with serum acidosis are awake and alert, whereas others with similar serum pH values are stuporous or comatose. That systemic acidosis per se does not invariably cause coma is substantiated by arterial pH measurements of 6.8 ($[H^+] = 158.0$ nmol./L.), obtained in two laboratories independently, in a patient who was fully alert and oriented.[39] Severe metabolic acidosis in this patient resulted from chronic bicarbonate loss from the gastrointestinal tract, and concurrent cerebrospinal fluid measurements were as follows: pH, 7.36 ($[H^+] = 43.7$ nmol./L.), P_{CO_2}, 15 torr (2.0 kPa), and bicarbonate, 8.5 mEq./L. (8.5 mmol./L.).

Hypoglycemia

Although anesthesia and surgical stress generally increase blood glucose, dangerous hypoglycemia can occur intraoperatively in rare instances, such as during manipulation of insulin-producing tumors of the pancreas or retroperitoneal carcinomas.[42] Fatal postoperative hypoglycemic coma has been reported in diabetic patients given insulin and/or chlorpropamide preoperatively.[43,44] Several unusual drug interactions also predispose to hypoglycemia. Salicylates, sulfonamides, and ethanol have known hypoglycemic effects. Propoxyphene has been reported to produce severe hypoglycemia manifested by hemiparesis and mental confusion.[45] The hypoglycemic action of tolbutamide and chlorpropamide is enhanced in patients who receive chloramphenicol.[46,47] The combination of chlorpromazine and orphenadrine also has been reported to produce hypoglycemic coma.[48] Severe liver dysfunction can also contribute to hypoglycemia by impairment of gluconeogenesis. Aldrete reported several instances of severe hypoglycemia following hepatic transplantation; arterial hypotension, loss of consciousness, and metabolic acidosis resulted.[49]

The Hyperosmolar Syndrome

Recent clinical reports of hyperosmolar, hyperglycemic, non-ketotic coma occurring in the perioperative period have established this syndrome as a cause of prolonged unconsciousness following general anesthesia.[50,51,52] In view of the 40- to 60-per-cent mortality rate in patients with this disorder, the importance of early recognition and treatment is apparent. Approximately half of these patients have no prior history of diabetes, but in most cases a severe concomitant illness, such as sepsis, pneumonia, pancreatitis, uremia, cerebrovascular accident, or large surface-area burns, is present. Severe dehydration, exacerbated by the osmotic diuretic effect of hyperglycemia, contributes to the hyperosmolarity. Administration of hypertonic solutions (e.g., hyperalimentation, mannitol administration) may also lead to hyperosmolarity. As might be expected, this disorder can occur following peritoneal dialysis, hemodialysis, and cardiac surgery. Factors that tend to elevate the blood sugar, such as massive steroid therapy and intravenous administration of dextrose, may also precipitate it. (Marked hyperglycemia has been observed during extracorporeal circulation and profound hypothermia in infants.) Although not directly implicated as a causative factor, the hyperglycemic response to surgical stress and certain anesthetic agents may be an important etiologic consideration.

The diagnosis of hyperosmolar, hyperglycemic, non-ketotic coma is confirmed by measurement of blood glucose greater than 600 mg. per dl. and elevated serum osmolarity in the absence of ketoacidosis.[53] Azotemia and hypokalemia are also commonly seen. Although this disorder may develop slowly over several days, a case described in the immediate postanesthetic period was characterized by a very rapid, fulminant course. Regular insulin, 50 units, intravenously, has been recommended as the initial step in lowering blood glucose; subsequent insulin dosage depends on the rate of decline in blood glucose.[54] Lowering of blood glucose too rapidly may precipitate hypovolemic shock and cerebral edema. Large quantities of 0.45-per-cent saline are usually required to correct dehydration, and hypovolemic shock may be corrected with saline and albumin. Potassium supplementation is also required, as large amounts of potassium are transported intracellularly with increased glucose utilization. Coma that accompanies the hyperosmolar syndrome is thought to result from cerebral intracellular dehydration. Damage to intracranial "bridging" veins may occur as a result of brain shrinkage. Brain edema also may occur during the treatment phase if the blood glucose level is allowed to decrease too rapidly. Water diffuses intracellularly along a gradient established by lowered extracellular glucose and elevated intracellular sorbitol concentration.[55] Caution must be exercised, therefore, to prevent lowering of blood glucose too rapidly.

Electrolyte Imbalance

Severe electrolyte disturbance in the postoperative period can also contribute to prolonged emergence from anesthesia. Dilutional hyponatremia can result from water absorption during transurethral prostatic surgery. Coma, hemiparesis, and other alarming neurological sequelae can accompany water intoxication or hyponatremia due to inappropriate release of antidiuretic hormone. Severe hypercalcemia and hypermagnesemia, similarly, produce CNS depression and can lead to coma. The hypocalcemia of hypoparathyroidism is frequently associated with mental changes, diffuse EEG abnormalities, and increased intracranial pressure.

Hypothermia and Hyperthermia

Hypothermia can also contribute to prolonged postoperative unconsciousness by reducing the rate of biotransformation of depressant drugs, by increasing the solubility of inhalation anesthetics, and by a direct hypothermic effect on the brain (cold narcosis). Anesthetic requirement in dogs is decreased 50 per-cent when body temperature is lowered from 38° C to 28° C.[56] However, moderate hypothermia alone (30° – 32° C) does not produce loss of consciousness in normal humans.[57] Severe hyperthermia (>40° C), on the other hand, does result in loss of consiousness ("heat stroke").

Neurotoxic Drugs

CNS depression can also result from the toxic effect of certain drugs. For example, certain cancer chemotherapeutic agents, such as L-asparaginase and vincristine, frequently produce CNS depression with EEG changes.[58] Although rarely seen in patients emerging from anesthesia, the toxic potential of such chemotherapeutic agents must be considered in the differential diagnosis.

NEUROLOGIC INJURY

Failure to regain consciousness after general anesthesia may result from neurologic damage caused by cerebral ischemia, hemorrhage, or embolism.

Cerebral Ischemia

The safety of deliberate, controlled hypotension in most patients without cerebrovascular disease has been well substantiated (see Chap. 48).[43,59] Normal recovery of consciousness has been reported in patients undergoing deliberate hypotension, with brachial blood pressures ranging from 40 to 65 torr and with the head tilted upward 27 degrees for periods of up to 90 minutes.[59] Measurement of jugular venous oxygen tension in normal patients undergoing deliberate hypotension, induced by a combination of ganglionic blockade, head-up tilt, positive airway pressure, and halothane, revealed no evidence of cerebral hypoxia.[60] However, prolonged unconsciousness due to ischemic brain damage has complicated the technique of deliberate hypotension in rare cases.[61] Brierley and Cooper reported pathological brain lesions in a previously healthy 45-year-old woman who demonstrated prolonged

postoperative unconsciousness and organic dementia following deliberate hypotensive anesthesia.[62] Hypotension is more likely to produce cerebral ischemia in patients with cerebrovascular disease. Thus, hypotension can be particularly harmful in the diabetic, hypertensive, and geriatric patient. Obstruction of blood flow in the vertebral or carotid circulation may occur when the anesthetized patient is positioned improperly (e.g., extremes of cervical flexion, extension or rotation, carotid compression from retractors or other mechanical apparatus).[63]

Hemorrhage

Intracranial hemorrhage with an expanding supratentorial hematoma can produce loss of consciousness by brain stem compression and herniation. Hypertension evoked by laryngoscopy and tracheal intubation can result in cerebral hemorrhage during anesthesia. A recent study has shown that the magnitude of this hypertensive response can be decreased by spraying the trachea with lidocaine.[64] Cerebral hemorrhage is also a feared complication in patients who require anticoagulation for extended periods of time (e.g., prolonged extracorporeal circulation).

Cerebral Embolism

Failure to regain consciousness after cardiac surgery may result from cerebral embolism (see Chap. 18). Intravenous infusion of very small amounts of air is dangerous in patients with right-to-left shunt and should be avoided especially in pediatric patients with congenital, cyanotic heart disease. Entrainment of air into the arterial circulation may occur at many sites during cardiac surgery, and meticulous care is required to prevent this complication. Other sources of cerebral embolus in the cardiac patient include calcified mitral and aortic valves, atherosclerotic plaques, left atrial or ventricular thrombus, and bacterial endocarditis. Irrigation of radial arterial cannulae can result in retrograde brachial arterial flow and cause cerebral embolism.[65] Arterial cannulae should be irrigated by continuous infusion or with 1 or 2 ml. of saline to prevent this complication.

CNS depression accompanying fat embolism

typically occurs 12 to 48 hours after fracture of a long bone or massive tissue trauma. Therefore, fat embolism can present as prolonged unconsciousness following general anesthesia for reduction of skeletal fractures.[66] Fat embolism has also been reported after closed-chest cardiac massage and after massive corticosteroid therapy. Jones described a patient who was receiving massive doses of steroids as immunosuppressive therapy following renal homotransplantation; the patient failed to regain consciousness after general anesthesia for laparotomy.[67] Coma and death in this patient was attributed to systemic fat embolism, probably arising from corticoid-induced fatty liver.

Clinical experience indicates that anesthetic requirement is markedly reduced after cardiopulmonary bypass. Lack of pulsatile blood flow; disruption of the blood-brain barrier; microembolism of air, fibrin, thrombus, calcium, or fat; and hypoperfusion of the brain are all factors that may contribute to cerebral depression in the post-perfusion period. Removal of particulate material by microfiltration may reduce the incidence of embolic complications. Continuous monitoring of arterial perfusion pressure and the EEG may result in earlier detection of cerebral ischemia.

Hypoxia

In the past, the most common cause of postoperative unconsciousness was the delivery of hypoxic gas mixtures during induction of anesthesia with nitrous oxide.[68] Today, cerebral hypoxia remains an important hazard, despite technologic improvements in anesthesia delivery systems and oxygen monitoring devices. When intraoperative hypoxia is suspected to be the cause of prolonged postoperative unconsciousness, and when other structural, metabolic, and pharmacological causes have been reasonably excluded by clinical and laboratory examination, neurologic consultation should be obtained for further evaluation and an organized approach to therapy. Serial EEG evaluation may be of some prognostic value in establishing the likelihood of recovery.[69] Deliberate hypothermia may reduce cerebral edema and prevent further cerebral damage if instituted promptly. Even though the patient may seem to recover fully, neurologic deterioration has been reported days to weeks postoperatively.[70] The cause of this delayed postanoxic encephalopathy is unknown.

CLINICAL EVALUATION AND TREATMENT

Because of the many and varied causes of prolonged postoperative unconsciousness, an orderly, systematic approach to clinical evaluation is mandatory. Consideration of the patient's drug history, preexisting systemic disease, and the nature of the operative procedure frequently provides evidence that allows the anesthesiologist to select the most likely causes of prolonged CNS depression. Intelligent action may then be taken to make or exclude a specific diagnosis.

The importance of a thorough preoperative medical history and physical examination is emphasized by the following clinical narrative:

Case 26-1. Unilateral pupillary dilatation was observed in a young, healthy patient who remained unconscious following cardiotomy for repair of an atrial septal defect. Because of the unequal pupil size as well as unconsciousness in the early postoperative period, it was greatly feared that this patient might have suffered cerebral embolism or hemorrhage. However, there were no other focal neurologic signs, and the patient awakened within a reasonable period of time. Careful examination of the patient's hospital record revealed that anisocoria had been present since birth. A thorough knowledge of the patient's preoperative physical findings would have obviated the case for concern.

When the anesthesiologist is faced with an unconscious patient in the recovery room, and there is no obvious explanation for CNS depression, careful assessment of ventilation and oxygenation is of immediate importance. Measurements of minute ventilation, arterial blood gases, *p*H, and blood glucose should be obtained promptly. Body temperature should be measured and circulatory function should be assessed in order to evaluate cerebral perfusion. Additional laboratory studies may indicate the presence of previously undiagnosed hepatic, renal, or endocrine disease. Determination of serum electrolytes, calcium, magnesium, and osmolarity should be considered. The changes in EEG patterns are of some diagnostic value in predicting the likelihood of eventual recovery.[69]

Systemic metabolic encephalopathy may produce loss of consciousness with or without focal neurologic signs. For example, insulin coma in the diabetic patient may present as hemiplegia that is accompanied by the signs of a unilateral upper motoneuron lesion; the result may be an incorrect diagnosis of a cerebral vascular accident. Treatment with intravenous glucose in such cases results in rapid arousal and disappearance of the abnormal neurologic signs. Plum and Posner reported dissimilar neurologic signs accompanying successive instances of hypoglycemic coma in the same patient.[71] Explanations for this variation in neurophysiologic response to a metabolic insult in a certain patient are speculative, at best. Focal neurologic signs accompanying prolonged recovery from anesthesia must therefore be interpreted in the context of anesthetic drug action and metabolic effects on the CNS.

CNS depression secondary to narcotics and anticholinergic drugs may be reversed by the use of specific drug antagonists. Narcotic-induced somnolence may be excluded from the differential diagnosis by administration of naloxone. Prolonged unconsciousness due to the anticholinergic action of scopolamine may also be excluded by administration of physostigmine. Although scopolamine may have been administered many hours previously, physostigmine, in an equal milligram dose, administered intravenously, sometimes produces a striking arousal response. There is evidence, too, that physostigmine can reverse somnolence due to tranquilizers and, perhaps, even general anesthetics.[72] This dose of physostigmine rarely produces other side effects. However, atropine should be available to treat bradycardia, should it occur from increased vagal tone.

Whereas the value of specific drug antagonists such as naloxone and physostigmine is well established in the evaluation and treatment of postoperative depression, this does not apply to the use of nonspecific analeptic agents. The use of these is to be discouraged, because their diagnostic benefit is probably outweighed by attendant risks (*e.g.*, convulsions, relapse into unconsciousness).

REFERENCES

1. Magoun, H. W.: The Waking Brain, pp. 74–97. Springfield, Charles C Thomas, 1964.
2. French, J. D., Verzeano, M., and Magoun H. W.: A neural basis for the anesthetic state. Arch. Neurol. Psychiat., 69:519, 1953.
3. Arduini, A., and Arduini, M. G.: Effect of drugs and metabolic alterations on brain stem arousal mechanism. J. Pharmacol. Exper. Ther., 110:76, 1954.
4. Larabee, M. G., and Posternak, J. M.: Selective action of anesthetics on synapses and axons in mammalian sympathetic ganglia. J. Neurophysiol., 15:91, 1952.
5. Darbinjan, T. M., Golovchinsky, V. B., and Plehotkina, S. T.: The effects of anesthetics on reticular and cortical activity. Anesthesiology, 34:219, 1971.
6. Ferrer-Allado, T., Brechner, V. L., Dymond, A., et al.: Ketamine-induced electroconvulsive phenomena in the human limbic and thalmic regions. Anesthesiology, 38:333, 1973.
7. Krnjevic, K.: Central cholinergic pathways. Fed. Proc., 28:113, 1969.
8. Krnjevic, K.: Chemical transmission and cortical arousal. Anesthesiology, 28:100, 1967.
9. Duvoisin, R. C., and Katz, R.: Reversal of central anticholinergic syndrome in man by physostigmine. J.A.M.A., 206:1963, 1968.
10. Munson, E. S., Martucci, R. W., and Smith, R. E.: Circadian variations in anesthetic requirement and toxicity in rats. Anesthesiology, 32:507, 1970.
11. Eger, E. I., II: MAC. *In* Eger, E. I., II (ed.): Anesthetic Uptake & Action. pp. 1–25. Baltimore, Williams & Wilkins, 1974.
12. Miller, R. D., Way, W. L., Eger, E. I., II: The effects of alpha-methyldopa, reserpine, guanethidine and iproniazid on minimum alveolar anesthetic requirement (MAC). Anesthesiology, 29:1153, 1968.
13. Johnston, R. R., Way, W. L., and Miller, R. D.: Alteration of anesthetic requirement by amphetamine. Anesthesiology, 36:357, 1972.
14. Lasser, E. C., Elizondo-Martel, G., Granke, R. C.: Potentiation of pentobarbital anesthesia by competitive protein binding. Anesthesiology, 24:665, 1963.
15. Ghonein, M. M., Pandya, H. B., and Kelley, S. E.: Binding of thiopental to plasma proteins: effects on distribution in the brain and heart. Anesthesiology, 45:635, 1976.
16. Saidman, L. J.: Uptake, distribution and elimination of barbiturates. *In* Eger, E. I., II (ed.): Anesthetic Uptake & Action. pp. 264–284. Baltimore, Williams & Wilkins, 1974.
17. Eger, E. I., II: Recovery from anesthesia. *In* Eger, E. I., II (ed.): Anesthesia Uptake & Action. pp. 228–248. Baltimore, Williams & Wilkins, 1974.
18. Stoelting, R. K., and Eger, E. I., II: The effects of ventilation and anesthetic solubility on recovery from anesthesia. Anesthesiology, 30: 290, 1969.

19. Price, H. L., Kovnat, P. J., Safer, J. N., et al.: The uptake of thiopental by body tissues and its relation to the duration of narcosis. Clin. Pharm. Ther., *1*:16, 1960.

20. Way, W. L., and Trevor, A. J.: Sedative-hypnotics. Anesthesiology, *34*:170, 1971.

21. Saidman, L. J., and Eger, E. I., II: The effect of thiopental metabolism on duration of anesthesia. Anesthesiology, *27*:118, 1966.

22. Berman, M. L., Lowe, H. J., Bochantin, J., et al.: Uptake and elimination of methoxyflurane as influenced by enzyme induction in the rat. Anesthesiology, *38*:352, 1973.

23. Schmidt, K. F., and Roth, R. H., Jr.: Interaction of psychotropic drugs with agents employed in clinical anesthesia. Clin. Anesth., *3*:60, 1967.

24. Boyce, J. R., Wright, F. J., Cervenko, F. W., et al.: Prolongation of anesthetic action by BNPP [Bis-[p-nitrophenyl] phosphate]. Anesthesiology, *45*:629, 1976.

25. Cohen, M. L., Chan, S., Way, W. L., et al.: Distribution in the brain and metabolism of ketamine in the rat after intravenous administration. Anesthesiology, *39*:370, 1973.

26. White, P. F., Johnston, R. R., and Pudwill, C. R.: Interaction of ketamine and halothane in rats. Anesthesiology, *42*:179, 1975.

27. Tinker, J. H., Gandolfi, A. J., and Van Dyke, R. A.: Elevation of plasma bromide levels in patients following halothane anesthesia. Anesthesiology, *44*:194, 1976.

28. Johnstone, R. E., Kennell, E. M., Behar, M., et al.: Increased serum bromide concentration after halothane anesthesia in man. Anesthesiology, *42*:598, 1975.

29. Laidlaw, J., Read, A. E., and Sherlock, S.: Morphine tolerance in hepatic cirrhosis. Gastroenterology, *40*:389, 1961.

30. Haseluhn, D. H.: The use of pentothal in the presence of severe hepatic disease. Anesth. Analg., *36*:73, 1957.

30a. Schentag, J. J., Cerra, F. B., Calleri, G. M., et al.: Age, disease, and cimetidine disposition in healthy subjects and chronically ill patients. Clin. Pharmacol. Therp., *29*:737, 1981.

31. Dundee, J. W., and Richards, R. K.: Effect of azotemia upon the action intravenous barbiturate anesthesia. Anesthesiology, *15*:333, 1954.

32. Freeman, R. B., Sheff, M. G., Maher, J. F., et al.: The blood-cerebrospinal fluid barrier in uremia. Ann. Intern. Med., *56*:233, 1962.

33. Babad, A. A., and Eger, E. I., II: The effects of hyperthyroidism and hypothyroidism on halothane and oxygen requirements in dogs. Anesthesiology, *29*:1087, 1968.

34. Salam, A. A., and Davies, D. M.: Acute adrenal insufficiency during surgery. Br. J. Anaesth., *46*:619, 1974.

35. Morss, H. L., and Baillie, T. W.: A case of postoperative respiratory insufficiency and prolonged unconsciousness. Br. J. Anaesth., *30*:19, 1958.

36. Dundee, J. W.: Anaesthesia and surgery in adrenocortical insufficiency. Br. J. Anaesth., *29*:166, 1957.

37. Davies, D. D.: Abnormal response to anesthesia in a case of Huntington's Chorea. Br. J. Anaesth., *38*:490, 1966.

38. Eisele, J. H., Eger, E. I., II, and Muallem, M.: Narcotic properties of carbon dioxide in the dog. Anesthesiology, *28*:856, 1967.

39. Posner, J. B., and Plum, F.: Spinal-fluid *p*H and neurologic symptoms in systemic acidosis. N. Engl. J. Med., *277*:605, 1967.

40. Bulger, R. J., Schrier, R. W., Arend., W. P., et al.: Spinal-fluid acidosis and the diagnosis of pulmonary encephalopathy. N. Engl. J. Med., *274*:433, 1966.

41. Ohman, J. L., Jr., Marliss, E. B., Aoki, T. T., et al.: The cerebrospinal fluid in diabetic ketoacidosis. N. Engl. J. Med., *284*:283, 1971.

42. Schnelle, N., Molnar, G, D., Ferris, D. O., et al.: Circulating glucose and insulin in surgery for insulomas. J.A.M.A., *217*:1072, 1971.

43. Enderby, G. E. H.: A report on mortality and morbidity following 9,107 hypotensive anaesthetics. Br. J. Anaesth., *33*:109, 1961.

44. Schen, R. J., and Khazzam, A. S.: Postoperative hypoglycemic coma associated with chlorpropamide. Br. J. Anaesth., *47*:899, 1975.

45. Wiederholt, I. C., Genco, M., and Foley, J. M.: Recurrent episodes of hypoglycemia induced by propoxyphene. Neurology, *17*:703, 1967.

46. Christensen, L. K., and Skovsted, L.: Inhibition of drug metabolism by chloramphenicol. Lancet, *2*:1397, 1969.

47. Petitpierre, B., and Fabre, J.: Chlorpropamide and chloramphenicol. Lancet, *1*:789, 1970.

48. Buckle, R. M., and Guillebaud, J.: Hypoglycemic coma occurring during treatment with chlorpromazine and orphenadrine. Br. Med. J., *4*:599, 1967.

49. Aldrete, J. A., LeVine, D. S., and Gingrich, T. F.: Experience in anesthesia for liver transplantation. Anesth. Analg., *48*:802, 1969.

50. Bedford, R. F.: Hyperosmolar hyperglycemic non-ketotic coma following general anesthesia: report of a case. Anesthesiology, *35*:652, 1971.

51. Wulfson, H. D., and Dalton, B.: Hyperosmolar hyperglycemic nonketotic coma in a patient undergoing emergency cholecystectomy. Anesthesiology, *41*:286, 1974.

52. Toker, P.: Hyperosmolar hyperglycemic nonketotic coma, a case of delayed recovery from anesthesia. Anesthesiology, *41*:284, 1974.

53. Arieff, A. I., and Carroll, H. J.: Nonketotic hyperosmolar coma with hyperglycemia: clinical features, pathophysiology, renal function, acid-base balance, plasma-cerebrospinal fluid equilibria and the effects of therapy in 37 cases. Medicine, *51*:73, 1972.

54. Gerich, J. E., Martin, M. N., and Recant, L.: Clinical and metabolic characteristics of hyperosmolar nonketotic coma. Diabetes, *20*:228, 1971.

55. Clements, R. S., Blumenthal, S. A., Morrison, A. D., et al.: Increased cerebrospinal-fluid pressure during treatment of diabetic ketosis. Lancet, *2*:671, 1971.

56. Eger, E. I. II, Saidman, L. J., and Brandstater, B.: Temperature dependence of halothane and cyclopropane anesthesia in dogs: correlation with some theories of anesthetic action. Anesthesiology, *26*:764, 1965.

57. Cooper, K. E., and Kenyon, J. R.: A comparison of temperatures measured in the rectum, oesophagus, and on the surface of the aorta during hypothermia in man. Br. J. Surg., *44*:616, 1957.

58. Weiss, H. D., Walker, M. D., and Wiernik, P. H.: Neurotoxicity of commonly used antineoplastic agents. N. Engl. J. Med., *291*:75, 127, 1974.

59. Editorial: Cerebral complications of hypotensive anaesthesia. Br. Med. J., *2*:1523, 1962.

60. Eckenhoff, J. E., Enderby, G. E. H., Larson, A., et al.: Human cerebral circulation during deliberate hypotension and head-up tilt. J. Appl. Physiol., *18*:1130, 1963.

61. Miller, R., and Tausk, H. C.: Prolonged anesthesia associated with hypotension induced by trimethaphan. Anesth. Rev., *1*:36, 1974.
62. Brierley, J. B., and Cooper, J. E.: Cerebral complications of hypotensive anesthesia in a healthy adult. J. Neurol. Neurosurg. Pyschiat., *25*:24, 1962.
63. Toole, J. F.: Effects of change of head, limb and body position on cephalic circulation. N. Engl. J. Med., *279*:307, 1968.
64. Denlinger, J. K., Ellison, N., and Ominsky, A. J.: Effects of intratracheal lidocaine on circulatory responses to tracheal intubation. Anesthesiology, *41*:409, 1974.
65. Lowenstein, E., Little, J. W., III, and Lo, H. H.: Prevention of cerebral embolism from flushing radial-artery cannulas. N. Engl. J. Med., *285*:1414, 1971.
66. Patrick, R. T., and Devloo, R. A.: Embolic phenomena of the operative and postoperative period. Anesthesiology, *22*:715, 1961.
67. Jones, J. P., Jr., Engleman, E. P., and Najarian, J. S.: Systemic fat embolism after renal homotransplantation and treatment with corticosteroids. N. Engl. J. Med., *273*:1453, 1965.
68. Haugen, F. P.: The failure to regain consciousness after general anesthesia. Anesthesiology, *22*:657, 1961.
69. Binnie, C. D., Prior, P. F., Lloyd, D. S. L., et al.: Electroencephalographic prediction of fatal anoxic brain damage after resuscitation from cardiac arrest. Br. Med. J., *4*:265, 1970.
70. Plum, F., Posner, J. B., and Hain, R. R.: Delayed neurological deterioration after anoxia. Arch. Intern. Med., *110*:56, 1962.
71. Plum, F., and Posner, J. B.: The Diagnosis of Stupor and Coma. ed. 2. p. 39, 176–179. Philadelphia, F. A. Davis, 1972.
72. Hill, G. E., Stanley, T. H., and Sentker, C. R.: Physostigmine reversal of postoperative somnolence. Can. Anaesth. Soc. J., *24*:707, 1977.

FURTHER READING

Eger, E. I. II: Anesthetic Uptake and Action. Baltimore, Williams and Wilkins, 1974.
Harmel, M. H. (ed.): Neurologic considerations. Clin. Anesth. *3*, 1968.
Plum, F., and Posner, J. B.: The Diagnosis of Stupor and Coma. ed. 3. Philadelphia, F. A. Davis, 1981.

Part Seven

The Kidney and Electrolytes

27 Fluid and Electrolyte Problems

Robert S. Wharton, M.D.,
and Richard I. Mazze, M.D.

Section One: Normal Fluid and Electrolyte Physiology

The successful outcome of major operative procedures on seriously ill patients often requires expert management of fluid and electrolyte therapy and the early recognition and treatment of complications. In order to accomplish this, the physician must have a thorough knowledge of the composition and distribution of fluids and electrolytes within the body; of the normal homeostatic mechanisms for fluid and electrolyte handling; and of the ways in which anesthetic drugs and surgical intervention affect these. By understanding these factors, the clinician can prevent most problems; moreover, complications that do occur can be accurately and rapidly characterized, so that appropriate treatment can be started. In this chapter, an approach to intraoperative fluid management is developed based upon basic physiological principles, the nature of the operation, and the type and severity of the patient's illness.

COMPOSITION OF BODY FLUIDS

Volumes and Distribution

In the average young adult man, total body water (TBW) makes up approximately 60 per cent of body weight, and in the young adult female, 55 per cent.[1-6] This may vary greatly among individuals, primarily because of differences in the ratio of lean body mass to adipose tissue. The percentage of total body water is inversely proportional to the degree of obesity. Also, with increasing age, there is a steady decline in total body water as a proportion of body weight; it reaches a low value in geriatric patients of about 52 per cent in men and 46 per cent in women (Table 27-1). In contrast to the large variation in water content between different people, the water content of each person remains remarkably constant, owing to extremely effective homeostatic mechanisms.

Total body water may be divided into two

Table 27-1. Variation in Total Body Water in Normal Humans

AGE	SEX	TBW (% BODY WEIGHT)
0–1 (months)		75.7
1–12		64.5
1–10 (years)		61.7
10–16	M	58.9
	F	57.3
17–39	M	60.6
	F	50.2
40–59	M	54.7
	F	46.7
60+	M	51.5
	F	45.5

(Edelman, I. S., and Leibman, J.: Anatomy of body water and electrolytes. Am. J. Med., 27:256, 1959)

Total Body Water (TBW) = 60% of 70-kg Man = 42 Liters					
Intracellular (ICF) = 23 L (55% TBW)		Extracellular (ECF) = 19 L (45% TBW)			
Other Cells 21 L, 50% TBW	RBC 2 L, 5% TBW	FECV=11.5 L, 27% TBW			Bone, Connective Tissue, Cartilage, Transcellular = 7.5 L, 18% TBW
		Plasma 3 L, 7% TBW	Interstitial Fluid=8.5 L, 20% TBW		

Fig. 27-1. Distribution of body water in a normal 70-kg. man (FECV = Functional extracellular volume).

major functional compartments (Fig 27-1); the intracellular compartment accounts for 55 per cent of body water, and the extracellular, 45 per cent. Extracellular water is further divided into a rapidly equilibrating compartment, the functional extracellular fluid space, and a very slowly equilibrating space. The former is composed of plasma and interstitial fluid, which together represent approximately 27 per cent of total body water, or 16 per cent of body weight. In a healthy, 70-kg. man, this is approximately 12 L. Conservation of functional extracellular fluid volume is one of the main priorities of body homeostatic mechanisms. Slowly equilibrating extracellular water is found in bone, cartilage, connective tissues, and transcellular spaces, where it is present as cerebrospinal fluid, synovial fluid, and intraluminal fluid of the gastrointestinal tract. Practically speaking, slowly equilibrating extracellular water does not equilibrate with plasma, so it does not enter into problems of fluid and electrolyte balance.

Electrolyte Content

Extracellular Fluid. The predominant cation of extracellular fluid is sodium. Total body stores of sodium are about 4500 mEq. (103 g.),* of which about 2800 mEq. are exchangeable (e.g., not incorporated within the crystalline phase of bone).[3] Normal extracellular sodium concentra-

tion is 135 to 145 mEq. per L. (135–145 mmol./L.). Other cations present in significant concentrations are potassium, 3.5 to 5.0 mEq. per L. (3.5–5.0 mmol./L.); magnesium, 1.5 to 2.5 mEq. per L. (0.8–1.3 mmol./L.); and calcium, 4.5 to 5.5 mEq. per L. (2.3–2.7 mmol./L.). By comparison, hydrogen ion concentration in extracellular fluid is only 3.5 to 4.5 × 10^{-5} mEq. per L. (3.5–4.5 × 10^{-5} mmol./L.); however, it is vital to maintain it to close tolerance. Major corresponding anions in extracellular fluid are chloride, 95 to 106 mEq. per L. (95–106 mmol./L.); and bicarbonate, 22 to 28 mEq. per L. (22–28 mmol./L.).

Intracellular Fluid. Potassium and magnesium are the major cations of intracellular fluid and are present in concentrations of approximately 160 mEq. per L. (160 mmol./L.), and 25 mEq. per L. (12.5 mmol./L.), respectively; sodium concentration is only about 10 mEq. per L.(10 mmol./L.). The predominant intracellular anions are phosphate and sulfate, approximately 100 and 20 mEq. per L., respectively; bicarbonate and chloride together contribute about 10 mEq. per L. Intracellular proteins exert a net negative charge of 55 mEq. per L. and makes up most of the difference between cation and anion content.[3] An estimated 10 to 15 per cent of intracellular ions are osmotically inactive, presumably bound to intracellular lipids, proteins, or nucleic acids.

Osmotic Pressure, Osmolality, and Tonicity

Extremely important to the understanding of fluid and electrolyte homeostasis is the phenome-

---

*For conversion of milligrams to milliequivalents:

$$mEq: = \frac{mg.}{mol.\ wt.} \times valence$$

non *osmotic pressure*, defined as the tendency of water to move across a semipermeable membrane from a more dilute to a more concentrated solution. It is measured as the difference in hydrostatic pressure necessary to prevent such movement. Osmotic concentration can be expressed in units of osmolality or osmolarity. A 1-osmolal solution contains 1 osmol of solute per kilogram of water; a 1-osmolar solution contains 1 osmol of solute to which sufficient water has been added to result in a final volume of 1 L. The total number of osmols in a solution is equal to the sum of the number of moles of unionized solute plus the number of equivalents of each ion divided by its valence. Osmolarity is frequently referred to in clinical discussions, although osmolality would be more precise, since laboratory measurements are almost invariably made in milliosmols per kilogram. In practice, there is little difference between the two.

The normal osmolality of both extracellular and intracellular fluid is about 285 to 295 mOsm. per kg. Sodium salts account for 90 to 95 per cent of the osmolality of plasma interstitial fluid, and potassium salts contribute a majority of intracellular osmotic forces. The osmotic concentration of intracellular fluid is subject to very precise homeostatic regulation.

All solutions that have the same osmolality are isosmotic. An isotonic solution is one that is physiologically isosmotic with cell fluid; when it is substituted for extracellular fluid, there is no net transfer of water into or out of cells. For example, 1.8-per-cent urea is isosmotic but is not isotonic, because it diffuses across cell membranes. To be isotonic, a solute must be nondiffusible, as is 0.9-per-cent sodium chloride.

No significant steady-state difference in osmolality can exist across water-permeable cell membranes. If extracellular fluid is made hypotonic or hypertonic, there will be a net movement of water into or out of cells until osmotic concentrations are equal. However, only water, and not sodium or potassium ions, is free to move into and out of cells in order to restore osmotic equilibrium. Thus, when plasma osmolality is low, intracellular fluid volume will expand at the expense of functional extracellular fluid volume,

whether the latter is low or high; when plasma osmolality is high, intracellular fluid volume will contract, irrespective of extracellular fluid volume. The terms *volume depletion* and *volume overload*, as used clinically, refer only to extracellular fluid volume; changes in intracellular fluid volume may actually be in a direction opposite that of extracellular volume.

There is a slight difference in osmotic pressure between the intravascular and interstitial fluid compartments, owing to the higher concentration of protein within the intravascular space. This pressure is referred to as the *colloid osmotic* or *oncotic pressure* and is about 28 torr; it is this difference in pressure that prevents excessive fluid loss from capillaries. In states of protein deficiency or abnormal capillary permeability to protein, plasma oncotic pressure is decreased.

NORMAL HOMEOSTATIC MECHANISMS

Renal Mechanisms for Water and Electrolyte Regulation

Maintenance of volume and composition of the internal fluid environment is one of the primary functions of the kidney. Together, the kidneys comprise only 0.4 per cent of total body weight, yet they receive 20 to 25 per cent of cardiac output, or about 1200 ml. of blood each minute. Every 24 hours, the 2 million renal glomeruli filter about 160 L. of water, containing 24,000 mEq. of sodium, 700 mEq. of potassium, 5,000 mEq. of bicarbonate, and 20,000 mEq. of chloride. As glomerular filtrate flows through the proximal convoluted tubule, its volume is reduced by approximately 80 per cent because of the active reabsorption of sodium accompanied by passive reabsorption of chloride and water (Fig. 27-2). Since water diffuses freely across proximal tubular epithelium, tubular fluid remains isosmotic with plasma. About 90 per cent of filtered bicarbonate is absorbed in the proximal tubule after combining with actively secreted hydrogen ion to form carbonic acid; the latter is rapidly dehydrated to carbon dioxide by carbonic anhydrase, present in the brush border of proximal tubular epithelium. Essentially all filtered potassium is

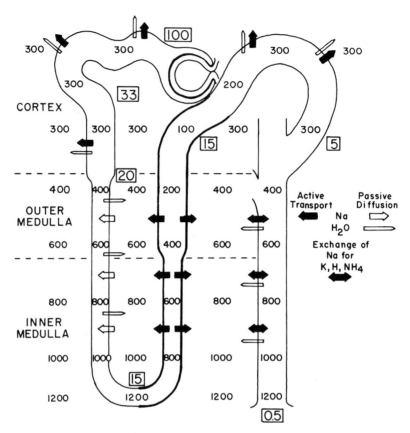

Fig. 27-2. Summary of passive and active exchanges of water and ions in the nephron in the course of elaboration of hypertonic urine. Concentrations of tubular urine and peritubular fluid are given in milliosmols per liter; large, boxed numerals indicate the estimated per cent of glomerular filtrate remaining within the tubule at each level. (Adapted from Pitts, R. F.: Physiology of the Kidney and Body Fluids. ed. 3. Chicago, Year Book Medical Publishers, 1974. Copyright © 1974 by Year Book Medical Publishers. Used by permission)

actively reabsorbed in the proximal tubule, as are glucose and most amino acids. The fraction of filtered water and electrolytes reabsorbed in the proximal tubule remains relatively constant, despite changes in glomerular filtration rate. This phenomenon, referred to as *glomerulo-tubular balance*, prevents fluctuations in glomerular filtration rate from causing large shifts in sodium balance.

As the remaining tubular fluid flows through the loop of Henle, two important events occur that are essential to the ability of the kidney to concentrate and dilute urine: Tubular fluid in the ascending limb of the loop of Henle is rendered hypotonic to plasma by virtue of the active transport of sodium (or perhaps, chloride) across the tubular epithelium, which is uniquely impermeable to water; and, an osmotic gradient is established in the renal medullary and papillary interstitium, as a direct result of the anatomic configuration of the loop of Henle and its associated capillaries. Osmolality of the papillary interstitium in a healthy young person can be as high as 1200 to 1300 mOsm. per kg., or four to five times that of plasma. The mechanisms by which this gradient is established and maintained are commonly referred to as *countercurrent multiplication* and *countercurrent exchange.*

Tubular fluid in the distal convoluted tubule is hypotonic to the surrounding cortical interstitium. Its volume is approximately 15 per cent of that of the initial glomerular filtrate, and its composition is largely unaffected by the volume or osmotic status of the patient. From this point on, however, handling of tubular fluid is variable and is subject to numerous regulatory mechanisms. Sodium ions can be either reabsorbed or excreted, largely in exchange for potassium. Hydrogen ions are secreted as required, mostly as titratable acid and ammonium. Nearly all of the water can be passively reabsorbed into the hypertonic medullary interstitium from the collecting ducts, if the latter have been made permeable by the action of antidiuretic hormone (ADH). Conversely, in the absence of ADH, the epithelium of the collecting ducts remains impermeable to water, so that virtually all of the water reaching the distal tubule is excreted. The net result of these processes is the maintenance of volume, osmolality, and composition of body fluids within very close tolerances, in spite of highly variable dietary and metabolic loads.

Conservation of Functional Extracellular Fluid Volume (Sodium Regulation)

Functional extracellular fluid volume is one of the best defended parameters of fluid and electrolyte physiology; its conservation is accomplished primarily by regulation of sodium excretion. Volume depletion mediated by arterial and possibly left atrial baroreceptors leads to retention of sodium. As sodium is retained, other mechanisms act to maintain normal osmolality. In all probability, there are several mechanisms for the regulation of sodium excretion; their hierarchy has not been delineated. A brief description of several of these follows:

Aldosterone Release. In the presence of aldosterone, sodium is exchanged for potassium in the distal tubule. The first step in this complex process is the release of renin by the renal juxtaglomerular apparatus, probably as a result of reduced renal perfusion pressure or decreased sodium delivery to the macula densa of the distal tubule. Renin mediates the conversion of circulating angiotensinogen to angiotensin I, which undergoes cleavage in the lung to form angiotensin II; the latter is a potent stimulator of aldosterone release. In addition, baroreceptors in the carotid sinus, and possibly elsewhere, are thought to mediate aldosterone release in response to depletion of intravascular and/or extracellular fluid volume.

Until recently, aldosterone was widely believed to be the principal regulator of sodium balance. However, it has been observed that sodium excretion is well regulated in situations in which circulating aldosterone levels are constant and, therefore, not subject to feedback mechanisms. Hence, factors other than aldosterone release may be equally important in the regulation of sodium excretion.

Alterations in Glomerular Filtration. It has been suggested that changes in glomerular filtration rate might lead to parallel changes in sodium excretion. Although major changes in glomerular filtration rate may affect sodium excretion, it is unlikely that this mechanism would be precise enough to be a major regulator of sodium balance.

Redistribution of Intrarenal Blood Flow. Redistribution of renal blood flow between cortical and juxtamedullary nephrons has been shown experimentally to alter sodium excretion.[7] Juxtamedullary nephrons have a longer proximal tubule and loop of Henle than do cortical nephrons and, therefore, are better able to conserve sodium; it appears that they are preferentially perfused in states of sodium depletion. In states of severe volume depletion, cortical blood flow may be critically impaired.[8] As yet, there is insufficient evidence to establish whether neural, humoral, or intrarenal mechanisms or a combination of these mediate redistribution of intrarenal blood flow.[9]

Peritubular Hydrostatic and Oncotic Pressure. Physical changes in the peritubular environment may significantly affect sodium excretion.[6] Specifically, decreased intracapillary hydrostatic pressure or increased capillary colloid osmotic pressure should facilitate sodium and water reabsorption across tubular epithelium. This theory is supported by the observation that volume replacement with colloid-free solutions results in a greater diuresis than with plasma substitutes.[10]

Natriuretic Hormone. The existence of a humoral factor, other than aldosterone, that may regulate sodium excretion has been suspected for several years and is supported, in part, by animal experimentation.[11] It is postulated that volume expansion, mediated by one or more baroreceptors, may induce the release of a natriuretic hormone, which inhibits sodium reabsorption at the proximal tubule. However, this factor has not been isolated, and its existence is disputed.

Maintenance of Osmolality (Water Regulation)

In contrast to the poorly understood and undoubtedly complex mechanisms for control of functional extracellular fluid volume, control of body fluid osmolality is mediated by a single substance, ADH.[1,12] When osmolality is increased by more than 2 per cent, ADH is released from the posterior pituitary gland. ADH acts at the collecting duct and, to a lesser extent, at the distal convoluted tubule, rendering them permeable to water, which then passes into the hypertonic medullary interstitium. Vasa recta carry this water back to the renal venous circulation; in the process, a small volume of concentrated urine is excreted. Secretion of ADH persists until sufficient water is retained to restore plasma osmolality to normal values. Conversely, when osmolality falls, ADH secretion is suppressed. The distal tubules and collecting ducts become impermeable to water, so that tubular fluid reaches the calyceal system with reabsorption of little or no water. The net result is a loss of free water and an increase in plasma osmolality. The mechanism by which increased osmolality triggers ADH secretion is thought to relate to a decrease in intracellular volume of the neurons of the hypothalamic supraoptic nuclei.

Non-osmotic Regulation of ADH Secretion. Many non-osmotic factors are known to stimulate or inhibit ADH release, and several of these are important to fluid homeostasis of surgical patients.[12,13] The most significant is the release of ADH in response to isosmotic contraction of extracellular water and/or plasma volume. ADH secretion in response to volume depletion may be maintained despite significant reductions in plasma osmolality. Although functional extracellular fluid volume will be restored toward normal by retention of free water, the resulting hyponatremia has potentially serious consequences. The effector mechanisms responsible for the non-osmotic release of ADH are thought to be located either in the carotid sinus baroreceptors (high pressure system) or left atrial volume receptors (low pressure system).

Many drugs used during anesthesia, including narcotics, barbiturates, and inhalation anesthetics, are associated with ADH-like effects.[12,13] It is not known if these drugs act directly on the pituitary-hypophyseal axis or indirectly through hemodynamic alterations; the latter is the most likely. Pain, emotional stress, positive pressure respiration, beta-adrenergic agents, such as isoproterenol, and cholinergic agents, such as acetylcholine, also are known to stimulate ADH secretion. The importance of non-osmotic stimuli to ADH secretion during the perioperative period should not be underestimated.

Potassium Regulation

Virtually all of the 700 mEq. of potassium filtered daily by the glomeruli is actively reabsorbed in the proximal tubule. In the distal tubule, potassium appears to be passively secreted into the tubular lumen, in exchange for sodium, along a transepithelial electrical gradient. Following intake of a potassium load, aldosterone facilitates increased distal tubular secretion of potassium. Tubular secretion of potassium also is increased in alkalosis; the mechanism probably involves changes in electrical gradients rather than competition between potassium and hydrogen ions for a single excretory pump.[1] Additionally, increased tubular secretion of potassium may occur when large sodium loads are presented to the distal tubule (e.g., when diuretic therapy interferes with sodium reabsorption in the proximal tubule and loop of Henle). An obligatory renal potassium loss of about 20 mEq. per day occurs even in states of potassium depletion. In patients with renal disease, potassium balance is usually well maintained until kidney function is severely compromised.[14]

DYNAMICS OF WATER AND SOLUTE BALANCE

Because surgical patients are frequently (albeit inadvertently) subjected to the stresses of water and/or sodium deprivation or excess, it is important to examine the dynamics of fluid and electrolyte balance in normal subjects as well as in patients with renal or cardiac disease.

Normal Fluid and Electrolyte Balance

A healthy 70-kg. man on an unrestricted diet usually will consume 1500 to 2000 ml. of water and from 50 to 150 mEq. each of sodium, potassium, and chloride. Intermediary metabolism generates approximately 300 ml. of water (mostly from oxidation), 40 to 80 mEq. of nonvolatile acids, and 30 g. (500 mOsm.) of urea.[1,15,16] About 800 ml. of water is lost by way of insensible routes, such as through the lungs and skin, so that each day, the kidneys are required to excrete approximately 1000 to 1500 ml. of water, 200 to 400 mEq. of electrolytes, 40 to 80 mEq. of nonvolatile acid, and 500 mOsm. of urea.[5] This represents a total osmotic load of 750 to 1000 mOsm. Since most people concentrate urine to a maximum osmolality of 750 to 1250 mOsm. per kg. (the peak value decreases with age), a 24-hour urine volume of 600 to 1000 ml. is required to excrete this amount of solute. When insensible water loss and water generated by metabolism are included in these calculations, it can be seen that there is a daily obligatory water requirement of 1100 to 1500 ml. If less than this amount of water is provided, the total osmotic load cannot be excreted, and solute will be retained.

Water excess is tolerated far better than water restriction by most people. Urine flow can increase to 20 ml. per min., accompanied by a decrease in osmolality to as low as 35 mOsm. per kg. Thus, a water intake of 20 L. per day can be tolerated without the development of significant fluid or electrolyte abnormalities.

Variations in sodium intake within a range of about 1 to 4 g. per day (40–175 mEq./day) are tolerated with minimal change in extracellular fluid volume. Even a steady sodium load of 10 to 15 g. per day may be tolerated, although ultimately, such a diet probably would lead to expansion of extracellular fluid volume by 1 L. or more. At the other extreme, a normal person can adapt to a diet almost totally devoid of sodium by reabsorbing almost all filtered sodium.

Fluid and Electrolyte Balance in Intrinsic Renal Disease

Patients with renal disease are less able to tolerate extremes of water and sodium intake. Urine-concentrating mechanisms are affected before diluting mechanisms, so that patients with renal disease are less able to tolerate water restriction than are normal patients.[17] The ability to concentrate urine or excrete a sodium load is decreased roughly in proportion to the decrease in glomerular filtration rate. Some degree of sodium wasting is found in most types of renal disease, and losses of 100 mEq. per day or more are not uncommon.[18]

Fluid and Electrolyte Balance in Congestive Heart Failure and Cirrhosis

Certain disease states, notably congestive heart failure and hepatic cirrhosis, are associated with an overexpanded extracellular volume and impairment of mechanisms for sodium and water excretion. In the case of congestive heart failure, expansion of functional extracellular fluid volume is most likely a compensatory mechanism, mediated by carotid sinus baroreceptors.[13] The mechanism for the impairment of sodium and water excretion associated with advanced liver failure is less clear, although a similar baroreceptor mechanism has been postulated.

EFFECTS OF ANESTHESIA ON RENAL FUNCTION

In surgical patients without renal disease, all general anesthetics temporarily depress renal function, including urine flow, glomerular filtration rate, renal blood flow, and electrolyte excretion.[19–21] This consistent and generalized depression of renal function can be attributed to many factors, such as type and duration of the surgical procedure; physical status of the patient, especially that of the cardiovascular and renal systems; preoperative and intraoperative blood volume, and fluid and electrolyte balance[22,23]; anesthetic agent[19]; and depth of anesthesia.[24] Depression of renal function induced by anesthetic agents is though to be caused by their indirect effects on the circulatory, sympathetic nervous, and endocrine systems, rather than by their direct effects on the nephron. A brief consideration of the indirect effects of anesthetic agents on renal function follows.

Circulatory Effects of Anesthesia

During general anesthesia, renal blood flow and glomerular filtration may be depressed as a consequence of cardiovascular depression, renal vasoconstriction, or both. Cyclopropane and diethyl ether are associated with marked increases in renal vascular resistance as a result of increased levels of circulating catecholamines.[25,26] Halothane and thiopental, although they do not evoke a significant catecholamine response, are associated with a moderate increase in renal vascular resistance as blood is shunted away from the kidney to compensate for hypotension induced by myocardial depression and peripheral vasodilation.[27] Balanced anesthetic techniques employing drugs with alpha-adrenergic-blocking activity, such as droperidol, have been reported to cause no depression in renal blood flow in well hydrated patients.[28]

Sympathetic Nervous System Effects of Anesthesia

The renal vasculature is richly supplied with sympathetic constrictor fibers but is devoid of sympathetic dilator or parasympathetic innervation. In the resting, unanesthetized, supine patient subject to no physical or psychic stress, there is little sympathetic tone. A great variety of normal and abnormal physiologic conditions cause mild to moderate increases in sympathetic tone. In patients with these conditions, there is a relatively greater decrease in renal blood flow than in glomerular filtration; that is, filtration fraction increases, and the glomerular filtration rate is maintained.[29] In patients with conditions causing severe stress, such as fear, pain, hypotension, hemorrhage, and general anesthesia, sympathetic tone is greatly increased, renal blood flow markedly decreases, and glomerular filtration rate declines as well. The role of the sympathetic nervous system in the renal effects of anesthesia is supported by experiments in dogs with one normal and one denervated kidney.[30] Induction of pentobarbital or chloralose anesthesia in these animals is associated with a decrease in renal blood flow and glomerular filtration to the normal kidney, whereas no change is seen on the denervated side.

Endocrine Effects of Anesthesia

ADH. Antidiuresis associated with anesthesia and surgery is, at least in part, caused by an increase in circulating ADH. The numerous nonosmotic stimuli to ADH secretion that are of importance to surgical patients are discussed above.

Renin-Angiotensin. At present, we cannot define the precise role of renin-angiotensin in the renal alterations that occur during anesthesia. Renin levels (and presumably angiotensin II levels as well) increase during anesthesia.[26] These elevated levels may explain the redistribution of intrarenal blood flow that is believed to occur during anesthesia.[9]

Aldosterone. Increased aldosterone secretion is, undoubtedly, partly responsible for the decreased sodium excretion that occurs during and after operation. It has been suggested that anesthetics cause aldosterone secretion by changing the circulatory pressures that activate baroreceptors or by acting on the afferent or efferent limb of the baroreceptor reflex arc.[31] Alternatively, aldosterone release during anesthesia may result from activation of the renin-angiotensin pathway.

Section Two: Disorders of Fluids and Electrolytes

Body fluid and electrolyte homeostasis is discussed in terms of three aspects: volumes of distribution, osmolality, and electrolyte composition. It is convenient to analyze disorders of fluid and electrolyte balance in the same terms. While some clinical disorders involve only one of these variables, many are complex. Treatment of complex disorders is facilitated if the simple underlying disturbances are first identified and then corrected either sequentially or simultaneously, depending on their relative urgency.

DISTURBANCES OF FUNCTIONAL EXTRACELLULAR FLUID VOLUME

A simple volume disturbance is a deviation from normal functional extracellular fluid volume with maintenance of normal osmolality. Since water and electrolytes diffuse freely across capillary endothelium, changes in intravascular volume are reflected throughout the interstitial space, so that the usual ratio of 3 to 1 for interstitial fluid volume and plasma volume remains relatively constant in most disturbances. However, in markedly hypoalbuminemic states, decreased plasma oncotic pressure results in a disproportionately high interstitial fluid volume. Isolated disturbances of functional extracellular fluid volume do not significantly alter intracellular fluid volume or composition.

Functional Extracellular Volume Deficit

Contraction of extracellular fluid volume is the most common fluid disorder in the surgical patient.[16,32,33] Nevertheless, mild or moderate degrees of hypovolemia frequently go unrecognized. There are two reasons for this: Major losses of fluid from the extracellular space can occur through internal fluid shifts, without any visible evidence of fluid loss[32,33]; and, no single set of physical signs or clinical biochemical determinations accurately measures the functional extracellular fluid space. In the patient undergoing major surgery, the difficulty in assessing extracel-

lular fluid volume is compounded by the effects of preoperative medications and surgical manipulation and the combined cardiovascular, renal, autonomic nervous system, and hormonal effects of the anesthetic agents. Isotope dilution techniques for the determination of functional extracellular fluid volume have been used as a research tool but are not practical in clinical situations.[32–35] The complications of severe extracellular fluid volume deficits such as hypovolemic shock with progressive lactic acidosis, acute renal failure, myocardial infarction, and cerebral ischemia, may be prevented by prompt and adequate volume replacement.

Signs of volume depletion vary with the severity and rapidity of onset of the disturbance. When volume loss is acute, circulatory signs predominate. These include some or all of the following: tachycardia; hypotension; decreased pulse pressure; peripheral vasoconstriction; diminished heart sounds; weak, thready, or undetectable peripheral pulses; collapsed neck veins; low central venous pressure and left atrial pressure; and oliguria. In the awake patient, neurologic signs, including drowsiness, apathy, lassitude, and stupor, may be seen with increasing degrees of volume depletion. Dryness of mucous membranes and the tongue is observed relatively early, but other tissue signs, such as sunken eyes, furrowed tongue, and decreased skin turgor are usually not apparent until significant deficits have continued for many hours.[15,16] Laboratory evidence of volume depletion includes elevated hematocrit and, after 24 hours or more, elevated blood urea nitrogen (BUN). If tissue perfusion is inadequate, metabolic acidosis results from increased production of lactate.

Deficits in isosmotic extracellular fluid volume may occur as a result of either measurable external fluid losses or unmeasurable internal redistribution of fluid into nonequilibrating compartments. Internally sequestered fluid is completely nonfunctional as extracellular fluid and may be considered temporarily lost from the body. In addition, effective extracellular fluid volume deficits occur when the capacitance of the vascular system is increased by the vasodilatory action of anesthetic agents or adjuvant drugs, or when myocardial function is depressed, to the extent that existing left atrial pressure (preload) is less than that required for optimal cardiac output.

Clinically significant external losses may be caused by the following: hemorrhage; excessive urine output resulting from intrinsic renal disease, diuretic therapy, inorganic fluoride nephropathy, or osmotic diuresis associated with diabetes mellitus or administration of radiographic contrast solutions; or increased gastrointestinal output resulting from vomiting, diarrhea, nasogastric suction, fistula drainage, or preoperative bowel purgation.

Internal fluid sequestration to a clinically significant degree is seen in a high percentage of surgical patients and may result from either the primary disease or the surgery itself. Proper preoperative and intraoperative volume replacement in such patients requires an appreciation of the magnitude of these losses. Rapid shifts of large volumes of extracellular fluid into a nonfunctional "third space" can result from acute abdominal lesions, such as acute pancreatitis, perforated gastric ulcer with chemical peritonitis, generalized bacterial peritonitis from any cause, volvulus, and intestinal obstruction. Volume deficits of greater than 3 L. occur frequently and result from accumulation of fluid in the intestinal lumen and free peritoneal cavity, as well as in thickened, inflamed bowel wall, mesentery, and peritoneum. Crush injuries, burns, thrombophlebitis, and fractures, especially of the femur or pelvis, also are associated with major internal fluid sequestration.

Intraoperative "third space" shifts generally are related to the degree of tissue dissection and manipulation. Major abdominal surgery, extensive retroperitoneal dissection, and bowel manipulation may result in sequestration of 3 L. of fluid.[32,33] Less extensive surgery is associated with lesser fluid shifts.

Prevention and Treatment. Preoperatively, the volume status of every patient should be thoroughly assessed. The recent clinical history is likely to indicate possible causes of volume depletion or internal fluid shifts. Fluid balance records, serial measurements of body weight, and determinations of hematocrit and BUN at intervals yield valuable information. Finally, physical examination may reveal signs of volume deficit, although clinical signs of fluid depletion may not be present until losses exceed 2 L. Whenever possible, existing deficits should be fully replaced before induction of anesthesia. Excessive hypotension during induction usually indicates less than adequate preoperative fluid replacements. The best indication of adequate fluid replacement is the reversal of clinical signs of volume deficit and establishment of a urine output of 50 to 100 ml. per hour.

In patients with significant cardiac or renal impairment or in whom large fluid shifts are expected, continuous measurement of urine output with an indwelling catheter is essential. In patients without significant cardiac or pulmonary disease, central venous pressure is usually a good indirect measure of left atrial pressure, or left ventricular preload; as such, it can be used to gauge adequacy of volume replacement, especially when very rapid infusions are employed. It has been shown, however, that in patients with marked impairment of myocardial function or severe pulmonary disease, central venous pressure may not correlate with left atrial pressure.[36] In such patients, when volume status is uncertain or rapid infusions may be required, the only way to adequately measure left ventricular filling pressure is by determination of pulmonary artery wedge pressure using a balloon-tipped pulmonary artery catheter.[37,38]

Careful estimation of blood loss and internal fluid shifts and prompt replacement with appropriate solutions usually prevent intraoperative hypovolemia. Deterioration of circulatory performance together with diminution of urine output usually means that fluid losses have been underestimated and should be reassessed.

Selection of Replacement Fluid. Except for insensible losses, virtually all intraoperative losses are isosmotic and should be replaced with isosmotic solutions. The question of which solution to use (e.g., normal saline, balanced salt solution, albumin, plasma substitute, whole blood, or packed erythrocytes, is still debated. The physiologic approach presented here is that losses should be replaced with fluid of the same composition: Blood lost should be replaced with whole blood; protein-rich exudates should be replaced with a plasma equivalent; and fluid sequestered as soft-tissue edema should be replaced with balanced salt solution. However, it has·been proposed that blood loss not expected to result in a hematocrit of less than 30 per cent should not be replaced with blood, but rather with electrolyte solutions with or without added colloid.[39,40] It is argued that, aside from eliminating the risk of hepatitis, oxygen transport to the tissues is well maintained with a hematocrit as low as 30 per cent; decreased oxygen-carrying capacity is compensated by a lowered blood viscosity and a higher cardiac output, without increased myocardial oxygen consumption.

It has been suggested that colloid-free balanced salt solution plus packed erythrocytes be employed for fluid resuscitation following extensive blood loss; this is said to result in morbidity that is no higher than that after resuscitation with whole blood and colloid-containing solutions.[10,41] Since colloid-free solutions equilibrate throughout the functional extracellular compartment, the volume of balanced salt solution required to replace a given blood or plasma loss is three or four times greater than the volume lost. This approach, although well tolerated by most patients, is not physiologic, may be associated with greater perioperative morbidity in patients with decreased cardiopulmonary reserve.

Functional Extracellular Volume Excess

Isosmotic overload of the functional extracellular compartment is encountered far less frequently in surgical patients than is hypovolemia. In nearly all cases, acute volume overload is iatrogenic and results from the intravenous administration of salt-containing solutions at a rate that exceeds the patient's ability to excrete them. Chronic isosmotic volume expansion is seen in congestive heart failure, cirrhosis, and advanced renal insufficiency. All three conditions result

from disordered homeostatic mechanisms for sodium excretion.

Clinical signs are related to the degree of overload of the systemic and pulmonary circulation, the rapidity with which overload occurs, and the amount of cardiovascular reserve. Early signs include distention of peripheral veins, increased right and left heart filling pressures (central venous and left atrial pressures, respectively), increased pulse pressure, and bounding peripheral pulses. More severe degrees of overload may precipitate heart failure or pulmonary edema, heralded by the development of an S_3 gallop, decreased pulmonary compliance, pulmonary auscultatory changes, including wheezes and/or rales, and increasing $P_{(A-a)_{O_2}}$.

Prevention and Treatment. The ability of healthy people to excrete a large solute load is decreased during anesthesia and operation. This is related to anesthetic-induced depression of renal blood flow and glomerular filtration rate, as well as to the numerous factors that result in ADH release. Still, patients with normal cardiac and renal reserve develop symptomatic volume overload only when large excesses of fluid have been rapidly administered. In most patients volume overload may be avoided by monitoring circulatory function and by auscultation of heart and breath sounds. When it can be anticipated that large volumes of fluid will be administered, monitoring of urine output and/or central venous pressure is advisable.

Patients with decreased cardiac reserve or renal disease are less able to excrete a volume load during anesthesia than are other patients. Even a mild excess in fluid administration can precipitate congestive heart failure or pulmonary edema; therefore, volume replacement must be approached with great caution. Urine output and central venous pressure should be monitored, but both may be misleading in patients with severely depressed left ventricular function. Oliguria may reflect critically low cardiac output despite administration of the maximum tolerated fluid load. Ideal management of patients with extremely poor myocardial reserve undergoing extensive surgical procedures requires direct measurement of arterial pressure perioperatively, as well as measurement of pulmonary artery wedge pressure.

Treatment of volume overload should vary with the severity of symptoms. The healthy patient with mild overload may require only fluid restriction. The patient with pulmonary edema may require treatment with diuretics, digitalis, high inspired oxygen tension, and mechanical ventilation, including positive end-expiratory pressure. Inotropic agents, such as dopamine, are useful if myocardial depression has contributed to pulmonary edema.

Fluid Shifts into the "Third Space"

Fluid sequestered in traumatized tissues does not constitute a part of the functional extracellular fluid volume. Therefore, a patient should not be considered to be volume overloaded on the basis of fluid shifts into the "third space," even when *total* extracellular fluid volume is expanded by several liters. The return of sequestered fluid into the functional extracellular fluid volume occurs gradually during the first 5 or 6 postoperative days and usually causes no problems. In fact, reinfusion may occur so gradually that it is undetectable except by serial weight determinations. However, among patients who have a marked tendency to retain sodium, reentry of "third space" fluid into the functional extracellular fluid volume can impose a significant volume overload, so that diuretic administration may become necessary.

DISTURBANCES OF OSMOLALITY OF BODY FLUID

Primary disturbances of serum osmolality are characterized by net total body gains or losses of free water in excess of sodium and may result from either inappropriate perioperative fluid therapy or primary derangements of normal osmoregulatory mechanisms. Associated volume disturbances may be present.

In contrast to isosmotic volume disturbances, which affect only the extracellular fluid compartment, osmotic disorders principally alter the intracellular environment. An excess of extracellular free water results in a rapid redistribution of

water into cells, increasing intracellular volume and lowering intracellular osmolality until it again equals that of extracellular fluid. Extracellular free water deficits have the opposite effect.

Since sodium salts normally account for over 90 per cent of the osmotic activity of extracellular fluid, alterations in osmolality are usually paralleled by alterations in serum sodium concentration. However, osmotic disturbances cannot be diagnosed on the basis of changes in serum sodium concentration alone. Increased concentrations of other extracellular solutes, most notably glucose, may contribute significantly to plasma osmolality. A plasma glucose concentration of 500 mg. per dL., for example, contributes approximately 28 mOsm. per kg. to plasma osmolality.* Thus, plasma osmolality is increased by 1 mOsm. per kg. for every 18 mg. per dL. increase in plasma glucose concentration (mol. wt. of glucose = 180). Accordingly, a hyperglycemic patient may have a depressed serum sodium concentration, but a normal or high serum osmolality and a normal or contracted intracellular volume. Positive diagnosis of osmotic disorders requires that the osmotic contribution of all extracellular particles be estimated or, ideally, that serum osmolality be determined.

Hyponatremia and Water Intoxication

Variable degrees of hyponatremia commonly occur following surgery, usually as a result of the intravenous administration of sodium-free or hypo-osmotic solutions.[15,16,42] Less common causes of hypo-osmolar states include overhydration during transurethral surgery of the prostate and the syndrome of inappropriate ADH secretion; they are discussed below separately. The terms *hyponatremia* and *hypo-osmolality* are often used synonymously, although the difference between the two should be kept in mind.

Hyponatremia, defined as a serum sodium concentration of less than 135 mEq. per L. (135 mmol./L.), results when water is retained in

---

*For conversion of milligrams per deciliter to milliosmols per kilogram:

$$\text{mOsm./kg.} = \frac{\text{mg./dl.} \times 10}{\text{mol. wt.}}$$

excess of sodium; there is a net positive free water balance. Several factors may predispose the operative patient to a positive free water balance: Inappropriately large volumes of sodium-free or hypo-osmotic parenteral fluids may be administered during the perioperative period; pain and emotional stress, administration of narcotics, barbiturates and inhalation anesthetics, and positive pressure respiration may result in the secretion of ADH and the retention of free water; reduction of functional extracellular fluid volume may occur due to "third space" formation, despite intraoperative volume replacement that is otherwise adequate, and this will directly and potently stimulate ADH release; renal blood flow and glomerular filtration rate may be depressed by as much as 70 per cent during anesthesia and surgery, and the ability to excrete a water load is equally depressed; formation of endogenous free water from oxidation of fats and lysis of lean tissue is substantially increased in catabolic patients and may add 600 ml. or more of water per day to the free water load.

Mild hyponatremia may not be associated with clinically recognizable symptoms or signs. However, when serum sodium falls to approximately 125 mEq. per L. (125 mmol./L.) or lower, *water intoxication*, characterized by disorientation, confusion, muscle twitching, and hyperactive deep tendon reflexes, usually will be observed. *Severe hyponatremia*, serum sodium less than 120 mEq. per L. (120 mmol./L.) may result in convulsions, stupor, coma, or death. The neurologic manifestations reflect a derangement of cerebral function secondary to decreased intracellular osmolality and expanded intracellular volume, which leads to cerebral edema and increased intracranial pressure.

For many years it was thought that postoperative patients have an absolute inability to tolerate water loads. It has been demonstrated that postoperative water intolerance can be significantly ameliorated or even prevented by proper intraoperative volume replacement.[22,43,44] However, when even relatively modest deficits of functional extracellular fluid volume are allowed to persist postoperatively, normal homeostatic mechanisms become operative, resulting in significant retention of free water and marked hyponatremia. The following example may serve to illustrate this important point:

Hypothetical Case Report. A healthy 70-kg. man (total body water, 42 L.; functional extracellular fluid volume, 12 L.), undergoing an uncomplicated cholecystectomy, may sustain intraoperative "third space" fluid shifts of approximately 2 L. A volume deficit of this magnitude will stimulate ADH secretion, resulting in near maximal renal water conservation; thus, urine output might decrease to approximately 500 ml. per day. Assuming insensible water losses of 800 ml. per day and endogenous water production of 500 ml. per day, the patient's daily net obligatory water losses would total approximately 800 ml. If the patient were to receive daily parenteral fluid therapy consisting of 3 L. of 5-per-cent glucose in water, he would have a net positive water balance of over 4 L. 48 hours following operation. Serum osmolality would drop to 260 to 270 mOsm. per kg., and serum sodium concentration, to about 125 to 130 mEq. per L. (125–130 mmol./L.). Only about one-quarter of the net water gain, or about 1 L., would be expected to remain in the extracellular compartment; hence, a functional extracellular fluid volume deficit of approximately 1 L. still would exist, even though total body water increased by 4 L. Had the 2-L. intraoperative volume deficit been replaced with a corresponding volume of balanced salt solution, there would not have been a volume stimulus to ADH secretion; the patient's ability to handle the postoperative free water load would have been greatly improved, if not normal, and a significant osmotic disturbance might not have occurred. A word of caution: Care must be exercised when infusing large volumes of salt containing solutions to patients with decreased cardiac reserve; the amount of salt necessary to prevent an osmotic disturbance may be in excess of that required to precipitate congestive heart failure. An appropriate balance must be struck in this situation.

Prevention and Treatment. Most cases of serious hyponatremia and water intoxication can be avoided by adherence to basic principles of fluid therapy. Intraoperative and postoperative administration of electrolyte-free water should be based upon calculated free water losses; normally, they will not exceed 1000 to 1500 ml. per day. Fluid losses and fluid shifts should be fully replaced with isotonic solutions like normal saline, balanced salt solutions, and blood or plasma substitutes. Finally, parenteral fluid therapy should be guided by frequent determination of serum electrolyte concentrations and, when indicated, serum osmolality.

Treatment of hyponatremia and water intoxication will depend on the severity of signs and symptoms and the volume status of the patient. If symptoms are mild and functional extracellular fluid volume is normal or elevated, water restriction alone will be sufficient to correct the problem. When hypovolemia exists as well, correction of the volume deficit with isotonic saline should result in a steady water diuresis and a return of osmolality to normal. Administration of hypertonic saline (3–5%) or 1 M sodium bicarbonate solution is advisable only when hyponatremia is severe and signs of water intoxication are life-threatening, (e.g., in patients in coma or in whom seizures have occurred). The total sodium deficit can be determined by multiplying estimated total body water in liters, by the deficit in serum sodium, in millequivalents per liter (millimoles/liter). Total body water, rather than functional extracellular fluid volume, is used in this calculation, since the osmotic deficit is distributed throughout intracellular as well as extracellular water. However, it is only necessary to administer a fraction of the total deficit in order to correct signs of severe hyponatremia. One-third of the calculated sodium deficit should be administered as hypertonic saline, at a rate of 150 to 200 mEq. per hour, and during this time the condition of the patient must be continuously assessed. Complete correction of large sodium deficits using hypertonic saline should not be attempted, and no other fluids should be administered while hypertonic saline is being infused. Rapid intravascular shifts of water in response to the high osmotic load can result in dangerous volume overload, congestive heart failure, and pulmonary edema, particularly in patients with reduced cardiac and/or renal reserve. Furosemide or ethacrynic acid may be of value in treating

patients showing signs of fluid overload, but it must be remembered that these agents increase sodium loss, particularly at high dosage levels.

Inappropriate Secretion of ADH

Occasionally, aged patients and patients with pulmonary neoplasms have developed prolonged severe antidiuresis after major surgery.[45,46] One or more days following operation they exhibit a variety of diffuse neurologic signs, including confusion, restlessness, disorientation, and somnolence; in severe cases, there may be profound stupor and seizures. Laboratory examination reveals a low serum concentration of sodium, frequently less than 120 mEq. per L. (120 mmol./L.) and a correspondingly low serum osmolality; however, urine is inappropriately hypertonic and frequently contains large amounts of sodium. These patients do not appear to have deficits of extracellular fluid volume, although there is little data to substantiate this impression. Renal function, including creatinine clearance, is normal or near normal, as is adrenal function. Administration of isotonic saline aggravates the condition, since water is selectively retained and sodium is excreted. Fluid restriction leads to improvement in the hyponatremia; free water is excreted, sodium is retained, and neurologic status returns to normal.

The etiology of the syndrome of inappropriate ADH secretion is unknown. A likely factor is prolonged administration of hypotonic salt solutions to patients subjected to the many non-osmotic stimuli for ADH release.

Prevention and Treatment. In aged patients undergoing major surgery, stimuli to ADH secretion should be minimized. Dehydration should be corrected in advance of operation, if possible. Periods of hypovolemia and hypotension during and after surgery should be avoided, volume deficits should be corrected with isotonic solutions, and administration of narcotics should be discontinued, when possible. Finally, urine output must be monitored, and serum electrolytes, checked early in the postoperative period.

If the syndrome develops, it should be treated by restricting all oral and parenteral water intake.

This will result in a negative water balance, primarily through insensible water losses, with correction of hyponatremia. Infusion of hypertonic saline is not effective, since nearly all administered sodium may be excreted without producing a net negative water balance. Furthermore, expansion of an aged patient's extracellular volume may result in pulmonary edema.

An alternative treatment has been proposed for use in patients with life-threatening neurologic signs.[47] This involves first establishing a steady diuresis by the intravenous administration of furosemide and then measuring and replacing urinary electrolyte losses with appropriate amounts of hypertonic (3%) saline and potassium. Severe hyponatremia can be corrected in several hours by this method, although the underlying problem may take several more days to resolve.

Hypo-osmolar Volume Overload During Transurethral Prostatectomy

Continuous bladder irrigation during transurethral resection of the prostate frequently results in rapid absorption of large amounts of irrigating solution by venous sinuses opened during surgery.[48-53] The amount of fluid absorbed depends upon three factors: the duration of the surgery; the number and size of the venous sinuses opened; and the hydrostatic pressure of the irrigating solution. During prostatectomy, an average of 1200 to 2000 ml. of irrigating solution may be absorbed; however, absorption of over 4 L. has been documented.[51] The consequences of absorption of a fluid load of this magnitude are dependent not only upon the volume that is absorbed, but upon the osmolality of the irrigating fluid and the cardiovascular and renal status of the patient. Presently used irrigation fluids are of two types: distilled water; and isosmolar, nonelectrolytic solutions, such as 1.2-per-cent glycine, or Cytal, a mixture of sorbitol and mannitol. Solutions are nonelectrolytic so that they inhibit the dispersion of high voltage electrocautery current.

Distilled water is sometimes preferred by the urologist, because blood in the bladder is rapidly hemolyzed, and superior visibility is provided. However, its use is more hazardous, because in addition to acute volume overload, there are also the risks of dilutional hyponatremia and intravascular hemolysis. The signs and symptoms of hypo-osmolar volume overload include restlessness, confusion, nausea, chills, tachypnea, and increased blood pressure, pulse pressure, and central venous pressure. Later, coma, convulsions, cyanosis, pulmonary edema, and cardiovascular collapse may occur.[52] The diagnosis is established by determining lowered serum sodium concentration (<125 mEq./L. or 125 mmol./L.) and serum osmolality (<260 mOsm./kg.); intravascular hemolysis also occurs at these levels. Not all patients exhibit the complete constellation of symptoms. Patients with little cardiovascular reserve, for example, may develop congestive heart failure and pulmonary edema before body fluid osmolality is depressed enough to cause major signs of water intoxication. Alternatively, patients who initially were volume depleted may tolerate substantial increases in intravascular volume without circulatory overloads and may develop only signs of water intoxication.

The use of isosmotic irrigation solutions is safer than that of distilled water, since intravascular absorption does not depress plasma osmolality. Thus, gross intravascular hemolysis and the disordered intracellular physiology and CNS effects of water intoxication rarely occur, although serum sodium concentration may be markedly depressed. The risk of hypervolemia, congestive heart failure, and pulmonary edema, however, is just as great with the use of isosmotic irrigants.

Prevention and Treatment. Efforts of the surgical team should be directed toward minimizing the absorption of irrigation fluid and detecting complications as early as possible. The duration of surgery should be limited; a maximum of 1 hour has been recommended.[48] Dissection should not be carried into the venous sinuses lying deep in the prostatic capsule, and the hydrostatic pressure of the irrigating fluid should be as low as is compatible with adequate surgical visibility. Urologists should be encouraged to abandon the use of distilled water as an irrigating fluid. Most agree that although visibility is better with distilled water compared to isosmotic solutions, isosmotic solutions are satisfactory when the urologist is trained to use them.

Early diagnosis is based on observation of the aforementioned signs. This is best accomplished with anesthetic techniques that neither alter the patient's sensorium nor significantly interfere with his cardiovascular compensatory mechanisms. Spinal anesthesia best meets these requirements and should be employed unless contraindicated. Lumbar and caudal epidural anesthesia are acceptable alternative techniques. A sensory block to a level of T10 is optimal. If general anesthesia is administered, as sometimes it must be, the opportunity to monitor changes in sensorium is lost, and some degree of cardiovascular depression will occur. Diagnosis then depends upon demonstration of progressive signs of increasing intravascular volume. If signs of hyponatremia and/or volume overload develop, surgery should be terminated as rapidly as possible, and corrective therapy should be instituted.

Hypernatremia

Hypernatremia is an uncommon but potentially lethal disturbance, characterized by serum sodium concentrations greater than 150 to 155 mEq. per L. (150–155 mmol./L.), increased osmolality of body fluids, and decreased intracellular volume.[15,16,42] In many cases, an associated functional extracellular fluid volume deficit exists. Clinical manifestations in the nonanesthetized patient are predominantly neurologic and include delirium, stupor, fever, and occasional athetoid and choreiform movements. Cardiovascular signs are related to the degree of intravascular volume depletion. Mucous membranes are characteristically dry and sticky.

Hypernatremia arises whenever free water losses exceed water replacement. The disorder is most frequently seen in surgical patients who are receiving parenteral or enteric hyperalimentation with high-calorie, high-protein solutions. The increased solute load results in obligatory urinary excretion of large volumes of water; this leads to hypernatremia unless sufficient sodium-free water is administered with the alimentation fluid. A similar mechanism is responsible for the hypernatremia seen in association with the osmotic diuresis produced by urea, mannitol, or even excess glucose administration.

Excessive non-osmotic renal water loss is characteristic of the ADH-resistant polyuria seen in methoxyflurane nephrotoxicity.[54,55] Diabetes insipidus, high output renal failure, and the diuretic phase following acute oliguric renal failure all are marked by the inability to conserve free water. Finally, increased insensible water loss, if not replaced, can result in the syndrome of hypernatremia. Increased evaporative water losses occur in patients with fever or abnormal sweating, in patients with extensive burns or large, open granulating wounds, and in patients with tracheostomies breathing unhumidified air. In these situations, evaporative water losses may amount to several liters per day.

Prevention and Treatment. An awareness of clinical situations likely to result in abnormal renal and extrarenal water loss is the key to prevention of hypernatremia. Replacement of free water losses, as indicated by fluid balance records, serial weight measurements, and frequent determination of serum electrolyte concentrations, effectively prevents this complication. If hypernatremia does occur, treatment consists of correcting the free water deficit with 5-per-cent dextrose. Assuming total body sodium content is normal, the existing total body water can be calculated as follows:

$$\text{Existing TBW} = \frac{\text{normal [Na}^+]}{\text{existing [Na}^+]} \times \text{normal TBW}$$

The free water deficit, the difference between existing and normal total body water, should be slowly replaced over a period of 24 hours or more. It is not desirable to correct hyperosmolar disturbances too rapidly. Serum sodium should be determined after partial correction of the disturbance, and therapy should be reevaluated.[56]

DISTURBANCES OF ELECTROLYTE COMPOSITION

Hypokalemia

Hypokalemia, defined as a serum potassium concentration less than 3.5 mEq. per L. (3.5

mmol./L.), is common in surgical patients. Signs and symptoms of hypokalemia are related to disordered muscle physiology that results from alterations in transmembrane potassium gradients. Generalized muscular weakness and muscle cramps are the predominant symptoms of hypokalemia. Paralytic ileus frequently occurs. Of most concern to anesthesiologists are the cardiac effects of hypokalemia. Myocardial contractility may be depressed. Alterations in resting membrane potential and spontaneous rates of depolarization may result in life-threatening ventricular arrhythmias. Additionally, digitalis toxicity is markedly enhanced by hypokalemia. ECG abnormalities include flattened T waves, sagging S-T segments, and the appearance of U waves.[15,16,57] Diagnosis is made by measurement of serum potassium but may be suggested by clinical signs and ECG findings.

Low serum potassium levels can result either from total body depletion or from factors that promote potassium influx into cells, such as alkalosis or the simultaneous administration of glucose and insulin. Abnormally high gastrointestinal losses of potassium (>40 mEq./day) may result from vomiting, diarrhea, nasogastric drainage, or draining enteric fistulae. Excessive renal potassium losses also are seen following diuretic therapy with furosemide, ethacrynic acid, or the thiazides; during the diuretic phase of acute tubular necrosis; in patients with renal tubular acidosis and hyperaldosteronism; and following glucocorticoid treatment. Severe serum potassium deficits are frequently seen following cardiopulmonary bypass; the reason for this is not well understood.

Prevention and Treatment. The risk of potentially fatal arrhythmias in patients with significant hypokalemia makes it desirable to postpone elective surgery until deficits can be corrected, either by oral or by intravenous administration of potassium chloride. Routine intravenous replacement of potassium deficits in asymptomatic patients ordinarily should not exceed a rate of 10 mEq. per hour. Dangerously low serum potassium levels should be treated aggressively, especially when accompanied by cardiac arrhythmias. In these cases, potassium chloride may be administered at a rate of up to 20 to 30 mEq. per hour,

with continuous ECG monitoring of the patient. Adequate renal function must be assured prior to potassium infusion.

Hyperkalemia

Hyperkalemia, defined as a serum potassium concentration greater than 5.5 mEq. per L. (5.5 mmol./L.), is a much less common problem in surgical patients than hypokalemia. However, when a significant elevation of serum potassium occurs, it may be rapidly fatal, and therefore it constitutes a major emergency. Severe disturbances in cardiac rhythm, including heart block, idioventricular rhythm, ventricular fibrillation, and cardiac arrest in asystole, may develop when serum potassium exceeds 7.0 mEq. per L. (7.0 mmol./L.).[57] ECG changes associated with hyperkalemia include tall, peaked T waves, widened QRS complexes, A-V block, and loss of P waves. The definitive diagnosis of hyperkalemia depends upon laboratory determination of serum potassium concentration. However, a presumptive diagnosis can be made and therapy can be begun on the basis of characteristic ECG changes in a clinical situation in which hyperkalemia is suspected.

Serum potassium may become elevated due to decreased renal potassium excretion, excessively rapid intravenous administration, or abnormal release of intracellular stores.[2,58] Singly or in combination, these factors may result in a fatal elevation of serum potassium concentration. Excretion of potassium is decreased in renal failure, hypoaldosteronism, and after administration of aldosterone-inhibiting diuretics, such as spironolactone and triamterene. High serum potassium levels may follow rapid intravenous administration of potassium supplements or of old, stored blood. Serum potassium concentration increases in stored blood at a rate of about 1 mEq. per day, so that 21-day-old blood may have a potassium concentration of 25 to 30 mEq. per L. (25–30 mmol./L.; see Chap. 35). Major trauma, hypoxia, or severe tissue acidosis may result in the release of large amounts of potassium from damaged cells.

Of unique concern to the anesthesiologist is the marked, sometimes fatal rise in serum potassium that follows the administration of succinylcholine to patients who have sustained major trauma, burns, or spinal cord injuries or who have developed progressive neuromuscular diseases.[59-63] This is discussed in detail in Chapter 45.

Prevention and Treatment. Patients with hyperkalemia secondary to decreased renal excretion should be dialyzed prior to elective surgery in order to lower serum potassium concentration to normal levels. When massive amounts of blood are transfused, careful attention should be paid to the ECG in order to detect early signs of hyperkalemia. Finally, administration of succinylcholine should be avoided for a period of several days to 6 months after major trauma, burns, or spinal cord injury.

Emergency treatment of hyperkalemia involves three steps:[14,17] Immediately antagonizing the adverse cardiac effects of potassium by intravenous administration of 10-per-cent calcium chloride, in 1-ml. increments, or 10-per-cent calcium gluconate, in 2- to 3-ml. increments, until the characteristic ECG changes of hyperkalemia have reverted to normal; promoting the intracellular shift of circulating potassium by intravenous administration of glucose, 50 g., regular insulin, 20 units, and sodium bicarbonate, 100 mEq.; and removing potassium from the body by the rectal administration of a cation exchange resin, such as sodium polystyrenesulfonate (Kayexalate), 25 g., in 200 ml. of 10-per-cent dextrose. If serum potassium cannot be lowered effectively by these methods, emergency hemodialysis or peritoneal dialysis is indicated.

REFERENCES

1. Pitts, R. F: Physiology of the Kidney and Body Fluids', ed. 3. Chicago, Year Book Medical Publishers, 1974.
2. Bradbury, M. W. B.: Physiology of body fluids and electrolytes. Br. J. Anaesth., 45:937, 1973.
3. Hays, R. M.: Dynamics of body water and electrolytes. In Maxwell, M. H., and Kleeman, C. R. (eds.): Clinical Disorders of Fluid and Electrolyte Metabolism. pp. 1–43. New York, McGraw-Hill, 1972.
4. Edelman, I. S., and Leibman, J.: Anatomy of body water and electrolytes. Am. J. Med., 27:256, 1959.
5. Atherton, J. C.: Renal physiology. Br. J. Anaesth., 44:236, 1972.
6. Bricker, N. S., and Schultze, R. G.: Renal function: general concepts. In Maxwell, M. H., and Kleeman, C.R. (eds.): Clinical Disorders of Fluid and Electrolyte Metabolism. pp. 663–696. New York, McGraw-Hill, 1972.
7. Barger, A. C.: Renal hemodynamic factors in congestive heart failure. Ann. N.Y. Acad. Sci., 139:276, 1966.
8. Hollenberg, N. K., Epstein, M., Rosen, S. M., et al.: Acute oliguric renal failure in man: evidence for preferential renal cortical ischemia. Medicine, 47:455, 1968.
9. Hollenberg, N. K., Adams, D. F., Soloman, H. S., et al.: What mediates the renal vascular response to a salt load in normal man? J. Appl. Physiol., 33:491, 1972.
10. Siegel, D. C., Cochin, A., Geocaris, T., et al.: Effects of saline and colloid resuscitation on renal function. Ann. Surg., 177:51, 1973.
11. DeWardener, H. E.: Control of sodium resorption. Br. Med. J., 3:611, 1969.
12. Kleeman, C. R.: Water metabolism. In Maxwell, M. H., and Kleeman, C. R. (eds.): Clinical Disorders of Fluid and Electrolyte Metabolism. pp. 215–295. New York, McGraw-Hill, 1972.
13. Schrier, R. W., and Berl, T.: Nonosmolar factors affecting renal water excretion. N. Engl. J. Med., 292:81, 1975.
14. Goldsmith, H. J.: The chemical pathology of renal failure. Br. J. Anaesth., 44:259, 1972.
15. Dougan, L. R., and Finlay, W. E. I.: Fluid and electrolyte balance: assessment of the patient. Br. J. Anaesth., 45:945, 1973.
16. Shires, G. T., and Canizaro, P. C.: Fluid, electrolye, and nutritional management of the surgical patient. In Schwartz, S. T., Lillehei, R. C., Shires, G. T., et al. (eds.): Principles of Surgery, ed. 2. pp. 65–96. New York, McGraw-Hill, 1974.
17. Petrie, J. J. B.: The clinical features, complications and treatment of chronic renal failure. Br. J. Anaesth., 44:266, 1972.
18. Cove-Smith, J. R., and Knapp, M. S.: Sodium handling in analgesic nephropathy. Lancet, 2:70, 1973.
19. Cousins, M. J., and Mazze, R. I.: Anaesthesia, surgery, and renal function: immediate and delayed effects. Anaesth. Int. Care, 1:355, 1973.
20. Larson, C. P., Mazze, R. I., Cooperman, L. H., et al.: Effects of anesthetics on cerebral, renal and splanchnic circulations: recent developments. Anesthesiology, 41:169, 1974.
21. Mazze, R. I., and Barry, K. G.: Prevention of functional renal failure during anesthesia and surgery by sustained hydration and mannitol infusion. Anesth. Analg. 46:61, 1967.
22. Abel, R. M., Buckley, M. J., Austen, W. G., et al.: Etiology, incidence and prognosis of renal failure following cardiac operations. J. Thorac. Cardiovasc. Surg., 71:323, 1976.
23. Boba, A., and Landmesser, C. M.: Renal complications after anesthesia and operation. Anesthesiology, 22:781, 1961.
24. Mazze, R. I., Schwartz, F. D., Slocum, H. C., et al.: Renal function during anesthesia and surgery: I. The effects of halothane anesthesia. Anesthesiology, 24:279, 1963.
25. Price, H. L., Linde, H. W., Jones, R. E., et al.: Sympathoadrenal responses to general anesthesia in man and their relation to haemodynamics. Anesthesiology, 20:563, 1959.
26. Deutsch, S., Pierce, E. C., and Vandam, L. D.: Cyclopropane effects on renal function in normal man. Anesthesiology, 28:547, 1967.
27. ———: Effects of anesthesia with thiopental, nitrous oxide and neuromuscular blocks on renal function in normal man. Anesthesiology, 20:184, 1968.

28. Gorman, H. M., and Craythorne, N. W. B.: The effects of a new neuroleptanalgesic agent (Innovar) on renal function in man. Acta Anaesth. Scand., 24[Suppl.]:111, 1966.

29. Smith, H. W.: Physiology of the renal circulation. Harvey Lect., 35:166, 1939.

30. Berne, R. M.: Hemodynamics and sodium excretion of denervated kidney in anesthetized and unanesthetized dog. Am. J. Physiol., 171:148, 1952.

31. Robertson, J. D., Swan, A. A., and Whitteridge, D.: Effects of anaesthetics on systemic baroreceptors. J. Physiol. (Lond.), 131:463, 1956.

32. Shires, T., Williams, J., and Brown, F.: Acute change in extracellular fluids associated with major surgical procedures. Ann. Surg., 154:803, 1961.

33. Hoye, R. C., Bennett, S. H., Geelhoed, G. W., et al.: Fluid volume and albumin kinetics occurring with major surgery. J.A.M.A., 222:1255, 1972.

34. Virtue, R. W., LeVine, D. S., and Aikawa, J. K.: Fluid shifts during the surgical period: RISA and S^{35} determinations following glucose, saline or lactate infusion. Ann. Surg., 163:523, 1966.

35. Roth, E., Lax, L. C., and Maloney, J. V.: Ringer's lactate solution and extracellular fluid volume in the surgical patient: a critical analysis. Ann. Surg., 169:149, 1969.

36. Forrester, J. S., Diamond, G., McHugh, T. J., et al.: Filling pressures in the right and left sides of the heart in acute myocardial infarction. N. Engl. J. Med., 285:190, 1971.

37. Swan, H. J. C., Ganz, W., Forrester, J., et al.: Catheterization of the heart in man with the use of a flow-directed baloon-tipped catheter. N. Engl. J. Med., 283:447, 1970.

38. Lappas, D., Lell, W. A., Gabel, J. C., et al.: Indirect measurement of the left-atrial pressure in surgical patients: pulmonary-capillary wedge and pulmonary artery diastolic pressures compared with left atrial pressure. Anesthesiology, 38:394, 1973.

39. Rush, B. F., and Stewart, R. A.: More liberal use of a plasma expander: impact on a hospital blood bank. N. Engl. J. Med., 280:1202, 1969.

40. Gollub, S., Svigals, R., Bailey, C. P., et al.: Electrolyte solution in surgical patients refusing transfusion. J.A.M.A., 215:2077, 1971.

41. Moss, G. S., Siegel, D. C., Cockin, A., et al.: Effects of saline and colloid solutions on pulmonary function in hemorrhagic shock. Surg. Gynecol. Obstet., 133:53, 1971.

42. Orloff, M. J., and Hutchin, P.: Fluid and electrolyte response to trauma and surgery. *In* Maxwell, M. H., and Kleeman, C. R. (eds.): Clinical Disorders of Fluid and Electrolyte Metabolish. pp. 1063–1088. New York, McGraw-Hill, 1972.

43. Shires, T., and Jackson, D. E.: Postoperative salt tolerance. Arch. Surg., 84:703, 1962.

44. Crandell, W. B.: Parenteral fluid therapy. Surg. Clin. North Am., 48:707, 1968.

45. Deutsch, S., Goldberg, M., and Dripps, R. D.: Postoperative hyponatremia with the inappropriate release of antidiuretic hormone. Anesthesiology, 27:250, 1966.

46. Bartter, F. C., and Schwartz, W. B.: The syndrome of inappropriate secretion of ADH. Am. J. Med., 42:790, 1967.

47. Hantman, D., Rossier, B., Zohlman, R., et al.: Rapid correction of hyponatremia in the syndrome of inappropriate secretion of antidiuretic hormone: an alternative treatment to hypertonic saline. Ann. Intern. Med., 78:870, 1973.

48. Marx, G. F., and Orkin, L. R.: Complications associated with transurethral surgery. Anesthesiology, 23:802, 1962.

49. Desmond, J.: Complications of transurethral prostatic surgery. Can. Anaesth. Soc. J., 17:25, 1970.

50. Taylor, R. O., Maxson, E. S., Carter, F. H., et al.: Volumetric, gravimetric, and radioisotopic determination of fluid transfer in transurethral prostatectomy. J. Urol., 79:490, 1958.

51. Maluf, N. S., Boren, J. S., and Brandes, Q. E.: Absorption of irrigating solution and associated changes upon transurethral electroresection of the prostrate. J. Urol., 75:824, 1956.

52. Still, J. A., and Modell, J. H.: Acute water intoxication during transurethral resection of the prostate, using glycine solution for irrigation. Anesthesiology, 38:98, 1973.

53. Pennisi, S. A., Rowland, H. S., Vinson, C. E., et al.: Hyponatremia as affected by various irrigants used during transurethral electroresection of the prostate. J. Urol., 86:249, 1961.

54. Mazze, R. I., Shue, G. L., and Jackson, S. H.: Renal dysfunction associated with methoxyflurane anesthesia: a randomized prospective clinical evaluation. J.A.M.A., 216:278, 1971.

55. Mazze, R. I., Trudell, J. R., and Cousins, M. J.: Methoxyflurane metabolism and renal dysfunction: clinical correlation in man. Anesthesiology, 35:247, 1971.

56. Levinsky, N. G.: Fluid and electrolytes. *In* Thorn, G. W., Adams, R. D., Braunwald, E., et al. (eds.): Harrison's Principles of Internal Medicine. ed 8. pp. 364–375. New York, McGraw-Hill, 1977.

57. Vaughan, R. S., and Lunn, J. N.: Potassium and the anaesthetist. Anaesthesia, 28:18, 1972.

58. Tanaka, K., and Pettinger, W. A.: Pharmacokinetics of bolus potassium injections for cardiac arrhythmias. Anesthesiology, 38:587, 1973.

59. Mazze, R. I., Escue, H. M., and Houston, J. B.: Hyperkalemia and cardiovascular collapse following administration of succinylcholine to the traumatized patient. Anesthesiology, 31:540, 1969.

60. Gronert, G. A., Dotin, L. N., Ritchey, C. R., et al.: Succinylcholine induced hyperkalemia in burned patients, Parts I and II. Anesth. Analg., 48:764, 958, 1969.

61. Gronert, G. A., and Theye, R. A.: Pathophysiology of hyperkalemia induced by succinylcholine. Anesthesiology, 43:89, 1975.

62. Cooperman, L. H.: Succinylcholine-induced hyperkalemia in neuromuscular disease. J.A.M.A., 213:1867, 1970.

63. Stone, W. A., Beach, T. P., and Hamelberg, W.: Succinylcholine—danger in the spinal cord injured patient. Anesthesiology, 32:168, 1970.

FURTHER READING

Andreoli, T. E., Grantham, J. J., Rector, F. C., Jr. (eds.): Disturbances in Body Fluid Osmolality. Bethesda, American Physiological Society, 1977.

Brenner, B. M., and Stein, J. H. (eds.): Sodium and Water Homeostasis. Edinburgh, Churchill Livingston, 1978.

Leaf, A., and Cotran, R.: Renal Pathophysiology. New York, Oxford University Press, 1976.

Schrier, R. W. (ed.): Renal and Electrolyte Disorders. ed 2. Boston, Little Brown, 1980.

28 Oliguria

James R. Dooley, M.D., and Richard I. Mazze, M.D.

One of the most ominous signs in clinical practice is the marked reduction or cessation of urinary output in a surgical patient during or after operation. Such a decrease in urine output can occur suddenly or over a period of several hours or days. It may be the harbinger of the syndrome of acute renal failure, a disorder which, when well established, is still associated with a mortality rate in excess of 50 per cent.[1] Fortunately, oliguria in most surgical patients is readily reversed if promptly treated. Anesthesiologists, therefore, must be aware that oliguria may occur in many clinical settings, and they must be able to correctly diagnose and treat its underlying causes.

FUNCTIONAL DEFINITION OF OLIGURIA

Nephrologists usually define *oliguria* as a urine output of less than 20 ml. per hour or 400 ml. per day in a 70-kg. adult. *Renal insufficiency* is defined as a measurable reduction in renal function with normal serum biochemical values. *Renal failure* is an advanced stage of renal insufficiency, in which renal function has deteriorated to such an extent that there is impairment of homeostatic mechanisms, and abnormal serum biochemical values are present. Thus, the definition of oliguria implies a state of renal failure, since a urine output of 400 ml. per day is usually less than that required to excrete the average daily solute load of 650 to 750 mOsm., given a maximally concentrated urine (1.2 mOsm./ml.). However, renal failure may also be present in spite of a high urine output if normal water, electrolyte, and acid-base balances are not maintained, and accumulation of metabolic waste products occur. It is clear, then, that the criteria for appropriateness of urine output must include the quality as well as the quantity of urine that is formed. Therefore, states of renal dysfunction described in terms of the amount of urine voided in a given period, such as oliguric renal failure, non-oliguric renal failure, and polyuric renal failure, should not be viewed as separate disease entities but as part of the continuum of renal failure.

Before discussing the clinical presentation and significance of states of low urine output, a review of the mechanisms for concentration and dilution of urine is appropriate. Two energy-conserving principles are involved in the concentration of urine: countercurrent multiplication and countercurrent exchange.

CONCENTRATION OF URINE

Countercurrent Multiplication

Countercurrent multiplication was first suggested by Kuhn and Ryffel[2] and is illustrated in Figure 28-1.[3] The principle of countercurrent

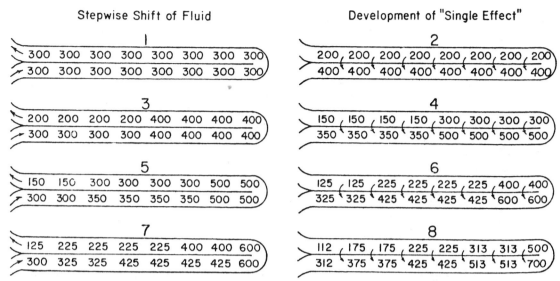

Fig. 28-1. The principle of countercurrent multiplication of concentration is based on the assumption that at any level along the loop of Henle, a gradient of 200 mOsm. per L. can be established between ascending and descending limbs by active transport of ions. (Pitts, R. F.: Physiology of the Kidney and Body Fluid, ed. 3. Chicago, Year Book Medical Publishers, 1974. Copyright © 1974 by Year Book Medical Publishers. Used by permission)

multiplication of concentration is based on the assumption that at any level along the loop of Henle, a gradient of 200 mOsm. per L. can be established between ascending and descending limbs by active transport of ions. In Step 1, the loop is filled with fluid containing 300 mOsm. per L. of sodium chloride. A gradient of 200 mOsm. per L. is established in Step 2, the development of the "single effect." Fluid moves down the tubule in Step 3, because of the introduction of additional fluid with an osmolality of 200 mOsm. per L. The 200-mOsm. gradient is again developed in Step 4. The process continues, so that by Step 8 there is a longitudinal gradient of 400 mOsm. per L. This can reach a value as high as 900 to 1200 mOsm. per L. in humans, 2500 mOsm. per L. in dogs, and 5,000 mOsm in kangaroo rats. Longitudinal gradients of this magnitude are possible in spite of the fact that the system expends only the amount of energy necessary to produce a vertical gradient of 200 mOsm. per L. at any single level. During the development of a gradient, the outgoing fluid is always hypotonic to the inflowing fluid at the same level. It should also be noted

that the solute pumped from the ascending limb is progressively concentrated in the interstitial fluid contained in the loop and reaches its greatest concentration at the point of reversal of flow. Also, for the system to work, the ascending limb of the loop must be impermeable to water. If it were not, the transport of solute between the two ends would be accompanied by the diffusion of an osmotically equivalent amount of water, and a concentration gradient could not be developed. Finally, the system depicted in Figure 28-1 can do no osmotic work unless an osmotic-equilibrating device is added; the collecting duct plays this role.

The formation of concentrated urine by countercurrent multiplication is illustrated in Figure 28-2. Isotonic fluid from the proximal tubule enters the descending limb of the loop of Henle. From the corresponding level of the thick part of the ascending limb, chloride is actively excreted into the interstitium, and its concentration is thereby reduced in the ascending limb and increased in the interstitium; sodium follows passively. Water passively diffuses out of the de-

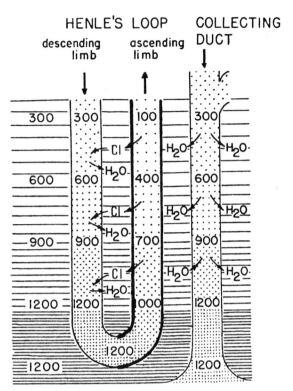

Fig. 28-2. The operation of countercurrent multiplication of concentration in the formation of hypertonic urine. (Adapted from Pitts, R. F.: Physiology of the Kidney and Body Fluids. Ed. 3. Chicago, Year Book Medical Publishers, 1974. Copyright © 1974 by Year Book Medical Publishers. Used by permission. [Adapted from Pitts, R. F.: The Physiological Basis of Diuretic Therapy. Springfield, Charles C. Thomas, 1959])

scending limb into the interstitium, and sodium and chloride passively diffuse into the descending limb. Impermeability of the ascending limb to water is indicated in Figure 28-2 by the heavily outlined walls. The collecting duct serves as an osmotic exchanger, permitting osmotic equilibration of the final urine with the hypertonic interstitium of the medulla and papilla. In states of dehydration, there is a high titer of circulating antidiuretic hormone (ADH) and the permeability of the collecting ducts to water is high. Isotonic tubular fluid entering the collecting ducts from the distal tubules loses water to the hypertonic interstitium. The final urine attains an osmolar concentration equal to that in the interstitium. During antidiuresis, urea, the major end product of protein metabolism, constitutes about 40 per cent of total medullary and papillary solute concentration; sodium and chloride make up most of the balance.

To form dilute urine, the countercurrent mechanism continues to function qualitatively in the same manner. However, when there is no ADH, the distal tubule and collecting ducts become relatively impermeable to water. Thus, hyposmotic urine is excreted, despite the existence of osmotic gradients.

Countercurrent Exchange

The principle of countercurrent exchange is illustrated in Figure 28-3A and B as it applies to a thermal model; in Figure 28-3C, the application to conservation of medullary hyperosmolality is demonstrated.[4] In Figure 28-3A, a tube is shown through which water flows at the constant rate of 10 ml. per min. A heat source supplies 100 cal. per min., so that the fluid entering the system has a temperature of 30°C, and fluid leaving the system has a temperature of 40°C. If, as shown in Figure 28-3B, the tube is bent upon itself and insulated to prevent heat loss to the outside but arranged to allow free exchange of heat between the inflowing and the outflowing streams, certain aspects of its performance will change. Although the temperature of the outflowing stream will be the same, the temperature at the heat source will be much higher in the countercurrent system, for heat will be transferred from the outflowing to the inflowing streams. If the function of the fluid stream is considered to be that of cooling the heat source, then the system in Figure 28-3A is much more efficient than the system in Figure 28-3B. Stated from the opposing point of view, the countercurrent system in Figure 28-3B has reduced the effective flow needed to cool the heat source to a small fraction of the true flow.

The vasa recta capillary shown in Figure 28-3C illustrates the operation of the countercurrent vascular loops in terms of its effect in maintaining the osmotic gradient in the renal medulla. Blood enters the loop at a concentration of 300

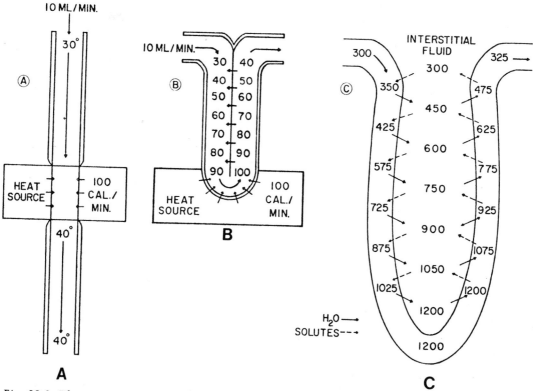

Fig. 28-3. The principle of countercurrent exchange. (*A, B*) Thermal models. (*C*) Operation of countercurrent exchange across the vasa recta reduces the rate of dissipation of the osmolar gradient between cortex and medulla. (Redrawn from Berliner, R. W. Levinsky, N. G., Davidson, D. G., et al.: Dilution and concentration of the urine and the action of antidiuretic hormone. Am. J. Med., *24*: 730, 1958)

mOsm. per L. As the capillary dips into the medullary and papillary interstitium, water diffuses out from the blood, and osmotically active particles diffuse into the blood. As blood traverses the loop and ascends, the reverse process occurs. Water short circuits the loop and passes directly to the emerging capillary. Red cells and plasma protein become more concentrated at the tip of the capillary loop because of this "short circuiting" of water. Thus, the loop operates to reduce the effect of blood flow with respect to the dissipation of the interstitial osmotic gradient.

The two countercurrent systems differ: Countercurrent multiplication of concentration is an active process that requires transport of solute from the ascending limb of the loop of Henle into the medullary interstitium; countercurrent ex-

change is a passive process and depends on the diffusion of solutes and water in both directions across the permeable walls of the vasa recta. Countercurrent multiplication alone establishes and maintains the gradient of osmolar concentration between the cortex and the tip of the papillae. Countercurrent exchange plays no role in establishing this gradient; indeed, countercurrent exchange can only dissipate a gradient if that gradient is not actively maintained. However, countercurrent exchange reduces the rate of dissipation of the gradient and, hence, reduces the rate at which the countercurrent multiplier must pump solute to maintain any given gradient. Together, countercurrent multiplication and exchange permit the formation of a concentrated urine with a minimum expenditure of energy.

Summary of the Urinary Concentrating and Diluting Mechanism

Each day, 160 to 180 L. of water is filtered through the glomeruli of the healthy adult. Each liter of filtrate contains 300 mOsm. of solute, consisting primarily of sodium, chloride, and bicarbonate ions. As the filtrate passes through the proximal convoluted tubules, sodium is actively extruded into the renal cortical interstitium. Chloride follows sodium passively, and water is reabsorbed by osmosis. The ions and water deposited in the interstitium are rapidly removed by blood perfusing the cortical capillaries. Although the volume of fluid in the proximal tubule is reduced by approximately 75 per cent, the osmolar concentration remains unchanged at 300 mOsm. per L. (see Fig. 27-2). As the tubular fluid flows along the thin descending limbs of Henle's loops, water diffuses out into the hypertonic interstitium of the medulla and papilla, and sodium and chloride diffuse in. The volume of tubular fluid decreases, and the osmotic pressure increases progressively, to the point of reversal of flow. In the thick part of the ascending limb of Henle's loops, chloride is extruded into the interstitium. Because water cannot pass through the ascending limbs, the osmolar concentration of the tubular fluid is reduced. At each level, a gradient of about 200 mOsm. per L. is established between tubular contents and hypertonic interstitium.

The fluid that enters the distal convoluted tubules is hypotonic to the surrounding cortical interstitial fluid; its volume is reduced to 15 per cent of that of the original glomerular filtrate. In states of water deprivation, the titer of circulating ADH is high. This causes the epithelium of the distal tubules and collecting ducts to become freely permeable to water, so that tubular fluid is isotonic with cortical interstitial fluid by the middle of the distal segment. The active extrusion of sodium and the passive osmotic diffusion of water are resumed in the distal tubule, and tubular fluid volume entering the collecting duct is thus reduced to a few per cent of that of the original glomerular filtrate. Collecting duct fluid, initially isosmotic, gives up water and becomes progressively concentrated as it descends through the hypertonic medullary and papillary interstitium. Concentration of the final urine entering the renal pelvis reflects the osmotic milieu of the interstitial tissue at the tips of the papillae.

The water, which diffuses out of the descending limbs of Henle's loops and out of the collecting ducts, is removed by blood perfusing the vasa recti of the medulla and papilla. These vessels act as countercurrent exchangers, reducing the loss of osmotically active solutes from the medulla and papilla. In water diuresis, the titer of circulating ADH is so low that the epithelium of the distal tubules and collecting ducts is impermeable to water. Tubular fluid, normally hypotonic as it leaves the loops of Henle, is maintained dilute or is even further diluted throughout the remainder of the nephron by the continued active extrusion of ions. In this manner, the final urine is dilute and its volume large.

CLINICAL ASPECTS OF OLIGURIA

Clinical Presentation of Oliguria

Intraoperative oliguria cannot be diagnosed unless there is a means of monitoring urine production. Thus, the use of an indwelling urethral catheter is justified in surgical procedures when it is anticipated that large blood loss may occur, that deliberate hypotensive techniques will be used, that osmotic diuretics will be given, that the ureters may be damaged, that operating time will be prolonged, that the aorta will be cross-clamped, or that cardiopulmonary bypass will be used. Additionally, if the patient has suffered extensive tissue damage from trauma or burns, it is important to monitor urine output during surgery.

During operation, urinary output should be noted frequently and charted on the anesthesia record, at least hourly. A sudden decrease in urine output is cause for concern. A review of vital signs, blood loss, "third space" loss, surgical manipulation and placement of packs, and the tally of intake and output usually reveals the cause. It should be remembered that a mechanical problem with the catheter may be the reason for an apparently low urine volume. Mucus plugs, bladder wall tissue, and blood clots may obstruct drainage holes at the catheter tip. Also, if the patient is placed in a steep head-down position, urine may pool in the bladder dome or kidneys and cause subsequent scant drainage from the catheter.

If there is reason to suspect decreased urinary output, palpation of the bladder may be helpful. However, a full bladder under these circumstances may merely reflect urine formed prior to operation or prior to the oliguric insult. To make a definitive diagnosis, an indwelling catheter must be inserted, and the rate of urine formation must be determined.

Postoperatively, uncatheterized patients who have not voided for a prolonged period must be watched carefully, particularly if they have had pelvic surgery; reoperation may be necessary. By contrast, when a catheter is in place, the clinical presentation of oliguria is quite obvious. Its treatment, however, necessitates a review of the many possible causes of low urine output, so that by exclusion, the appropriate therapy can be instituted.

Classification and Differential Diagnosis of Oliguria

One approach to the differential diagnosis of oliguria is to establish the anatomical location of the initiating disturbance. For conveneince, the three categories used to classify acute renal failure may be used to describe oliguria, although it must be kept in mind that several types may exist simultaneously (Table 28-1).[5] The categories are postrenal (obstruction and/or extravasation), prerenal (inadequate renal perfusion), and renal (intrinsic). This classification is important because specific therapy for both prerenal and postrenal disorders is often completely corrective, whereas the therapy for intrinsic renal disease is only 50-per-cent effective.[6]

In many cases, it is not difficult to determine the cause of oliguria and azotemia from the clinical presentation alone. Observation of the pattern of urine flow offers the first clue. For example, complete anuria is rare; it occurred in only one of 85 patients in a series reported by Swann and Merrill.[7] Cortical necrosis, vascular accidents, the glomerulitides, and the vasculitides are the likely causes of anuria. Obstruction, at times, may result in anuria, but with this disorder there also may be large fluctuations in urine flow as the obstructing body changes position.

Determination of urine composition is helpful in distinguishing oliguria of prerenal origin from that due to established acute tubular necrosis, as shown in Table 28-2.

The urinary sediment is also of diagnostic value in distinguishing between the causes of oliguria. If oliguria is prerenal in origin, there is a preponderance of hyaline and finely granular casts in the sediment, and coarse and cellular casts are seen only rarely. When oliguria is caused by acute tubular necrosis, there are frequent dirty, brown cellular casts and numerous epithelial cells, both free and in casts. A paucity of formed elements in the urine suggests that obstruction may be present. Red blood cells or heme-pigmented casts are rare, except when hemoglobinuria or myoglobinuria is present. Proteinuria is of little diagnostic value, for it may be associated with a wide variety of disorders.

A supine radiograph of the abdomen helps to determine kidney size and visualize calcified stones. The kidneys are normal or increased in size in acute renal failure, while they are frequently small in patients with chronic renal disease. Urographic studies are used to exclude obstruction and, with modern techniques, are safe even in acute oliguric renal failure. Intravenous pyelography will reveal an immediate, dense, and persistent nephrogram in patients with acute tubular necrosis and pyelonephritis, but not with other forms of oliguria. In oliguria of prerenal origin, a normal pyelogram is seen. In established oliguric renal failure, the pyelogram is not seen, but the nephrogram often is dense enough to allow detection of the calyceal system and observation of filling defects. However, retrograde urography may still be necessary in some cases to localize obstructing lesions precisely.

The remainder of this chapter discusses the many conditions that may result in a urine flow of less than 400 ml. per day.

POSTRENAL OLIGURIA

The category of postrenal oliguria comprises only a small percentage of oliguric disorders (Table 28-1). Obstruction, hindrance of normal urinary outflow, is the significant disorder in this category. Extravasation of urine from a ruptured bladder is also included. Obstruction of urine flow leads to an increase in hydrostatic pressure in the urinary tract proximal to the obstruction; ultimately, a marked decrease in glomerular filtration rate ensues. Morphologic damage to renal parenchyma occurs in proportion to the degree and duration of obstruction and also depends on related factors, such as the virulence of the associated pyelonephritis, which often develops in the presence of urinary stasis. Obstruction of urine flow is a far more frequent cause of postrenal oliguria than is extravasation.

Table 28-1. Major Causes of Oliguria

CLASSIFICATION	CAUSE	CLASSIFICATION	CAUSE
Postrenal		Renal	
Obstruction	Calculi, neoplasms of bladder and pelvic organs, prostatism, surgical accidents, ureteral instrumentation	Heme pigments Intravascular hemolysis	Transfusion reactions, hemolysis due to toxins or immunologic damage, malaria
Extravasation	Rupture of bladder	Rhabdomyolysis and myoglobinuria	Trauma, muscle disease, prolonged coma, seizures, heat stroke, severe exercise
Prerenal			
Hypovolemia	Skin losses (sweating, burns)	Nephrotoxins	
	Fluid losses (diuretics, osmotic diuresis in diabetes mellitus)	Pregnancy-related	Toxic abortifacients, septic abortion, uterine hemorrhage, eclampsia, postpartum renal failure
	Hemorrhage		
	Sequestration (burns, peritonitis)	Glomerulitis	Post-streptococcal, lupus erythematosus
Cardiovascular failure			
Myocardial failure	Infarction, tamponade, dysrhythmias	Vasculitis	Periarteritis, hypersensitivity angiitis
Vascular pooling	Sepsis, septic abortion, anaphylaxis, extreme acidosis	Malignant nephrosclerosis	
		Acute diffuse pyelonephritis, papillary necrosis	
Vascular obstruction		Severe hypercalcemia	
Arterial	Thrombosis, embolism, aneurysm	Intratubular precipitation	Myeloma, urates after cytotoxic drugs, sulfonamides
Venous	Thrombosis, vena caval obstruction, diffuse small vein thrombosis in amyloidosis	Hepatorenal syndrome	

(Modified from Levinsky, N. G., Alexander, E. A., and Venkatachalam, M. A.: Acute renal failure. *In* Brenner, B. M., and Rector, F. C. (eds.): The Kidney. Philadelphia, W. B. Saunders, 1981)

Table 28-2. Urine Composition in Oliguria of Prerenal Origin and Acute Tubular Necrosis

	PRERENAL OLIGURIA	ACUTE TUBULAR NECROSIS
Urinary sodium	<10 mEq./L. (<10 mmol./L.)	>25 mEq./L. (>25 mmol./L.)
Urinary specific gravity	>1.015	1.010–1.015
Urinary/plasma osmolality	>1.1	1.1 or less
Urinary/plasma urea	>20:1	3:1, rarely >10:1
Urinary/plasma creatinine	40:1 or more, rarely <10:1	<10:1

The passage of urine depends upon the patency of compressible structures, so that obstruction can be further divided into that resulting from extrinsic or intrinsic causes. Extrinsic obstruction with oliguria may be caused by rapidly growing pelvic tumors or by retroperitoneal fibrosis. This category includes retroperitoneal malignancies, rapidly growing cervical carcinomas, and massive uterine fibromyomata. Complete bilateral ureteral obstruction owing to lymphomatous or leukemic involvement of the lymph nodes also may occur. Iatrogenic oliguria may follow inadvertent placement of surgical ligatures or trauma to the ureters. The incidence of these mishaps among patients undergoing gynecologic surgery is reported to be 0.1 to 0.25 per cent.[8,9] A review of 161 patients with ureteral injuries showed that 72 per cent followed gynecologic surgery, and an additional 12 per cent followed obstetrical procedures.[10] Approximately 20 to 25 per cent of ureteral injuries are bilateral, resulting in immediate anuria. A common non-iatrogenic problem in aged patients is obstructive uropathy and oliguria secondary to fecal impaction.

Intrinsic obstruction can be caused by blood clots, calculi, prostatic obstruction, and various neoplasms. Bladder carcinoma accounts for 32 per cent of cases of obstructive uremia with oliguria, while prostatic carcinoma is half as frequent.[11] Only 700 cases of primary ureteral tumors have been reported, and metastatic tumors of the ureter are even rarer.[12] Patients with calculi of the genitourinary tract may have sudden oliguria if stones are bilateral or present in the bladder. Patients with bladder stones often present with intermittent anuria or oliguria, as the calculus may act as a ball valve. Benign prostatic enlargement is a frequent cause of impaired urinary flow in aged patients, following operations around the groin or rectum when pain prevents the relaxation of voluntary sphincters. Overflow incontinence may occur after anesthesia in aged men, with a total urinary output of less than 400 ml. per day. This may be a particular problem if belladonna alkaloids have been administered for premedication or during the course of the anesthetic (see Chap. 30). Oliguria also may follow ureteral catheterization, owing to edema that obstructs the ureteral orifices.

Extravasation of urine outside of the bladder may occur after trauma to the pelvis and may be associated with oliguria. Damage to the bladder rarely occurs if it is relatively empty at the time of injury; however, pelvic fractures are associated with a 9- to 15-per-cent incidence of ruptured bladder.[13] Since the ureters are thin retroperitoneal structures, they are rarely injured, except from direct trauma during surgery.

Treatment of Postrenal Oliguria

For simple cases of urinary retention, encouraging the postoperative patient to stand may induce urination. If this is not possible, if the patient is in severe pain, or if the bladder appears to be overdistended, then a single catheterization with a type of urethral catheter other than indwelling is the appropriate treatment. A note of caution: If too much time is permitted to elapse before the first postoperative voiding and the bladder becomes grossly overdistended and atonic, an indwelling catheter will have to be inserted for 5 to 7 days (see Chap. 30).

The definitive treatment of more complicated cases of postrenal oliguria is usually surgery. If the obstruction is high in the genitourinary tract, cutaneous nephrostomy may be necessary in order to provide urinary drainage. If bladder calculi cause obstruction, suprapubic cystostomy or urethral catheterization is the first therapeutic maneuver. Massive diuresis occasionally follows relief of obstruction, so the patient must be observed for signs of hypovolemia and electrolyte imbalance. Hypotension also has occurred following rapid decompression of an overdistended bladder. If obstruction is recognized and treated promptly, normal renal function returns rapidly.

PRERENAL OLIGURIA

Oliguria in surgical patients is most commonly prerenal in origin; that is, it is caused by inadequate renal perfusion. Renal hypoperfusion may be caused by cardiac failure or, rarely, renal artery thrombosis. However, the most likely causes of renal hypoperfusion in surgical patients are inadequate circulating blood volume and, during operation, administration of anesthetic agents. Systemic hypotension may be associated with both of these, but need not be, as there may be reflex shunting of blood away from the kidneys to more "vital organs." When renal blood flow is only minimally or moderately depressed, there is a compensatory increase in filtration fraction, so that glomerular filtration rate and urine formation remain relatively unaffected. However, when depression of renal blood flow is marked, glomerular filtration rate, urine formation, and electrolyte excretion also are significantly reduced. These changes are particularly likely to occur with anesthetic agents, such as diethyl ether and cyclopropane, that evoke a strong catecholamine response. Anesthetic-induced changes are reversed readily when administration of the agent is discontinued.[14-18]

Oliguria secondary to decreased circulating blood volume, whether originally caused by blood loss, sequestration into a surgical "third space," dehydration, or gastrointestinal loss, is amenable to treatment, but not as readily as oliguria secondary to anesthetic administration. This is particularly true if hypovolemia is severe and persistent, so that renal ischemia is present as well. Under these circumstances, functional lesions develop a renal morphological component; carried to an extreme, simple prerenal oliguria is converted into oliguric renal failure. The importance of time in the progression of functional renal insufficiency to organic renal failure is illustrated in Figure 28-4.[19]

There is little disagreement that renal insufficiency owing to prerenal causes may develop into classical acute renal failure unless promptly treated. The mechanism by which this occurs has become better understood only recently. Renal micropuncture experiments indicate that intratubular obstruction by interstitial edema or intratubular casts may be a contributing factor and that excessive back flow of filtrate across denuded or damaged tubules also may be involved.[20] However, the most common factor in the pathogenesis of the syndrome of acute renal failure appears to be suppression of glomerular filtration.[21] Since light and electron microscopy of glomeruli generally fail to reveal structural abnormalities, it is likely that reduced glomerular filtration is caused by vasomotor phenomena.[22]

Hollenberg and colleagues have employed the krypton isotope-washout technique and renal arteriography to measure intrarenal distribution of blood flow in patients with renal failure.[23] They demonstrated that the rapid flow compartment, thought to represent superficial cortical blood flow, is markedly reduced or absent in patients with acute oliguric renal failure secondary to hypotension but is reduced only in proportion to total renal blood flow in patients with chronic renal failure.[23] In other studies, they showed similar disproportionate decreases in superficial cortical blood flow in patients with acute renal failure due to nephrotoxins,[24] in patients undergoing acute renal allograft rejection,[25] and in a patient with irreversible acute renal failure following methoxyflurane anesthesia.[26] They suggested that sustained preglomerular vasoconstriction, causing persistent homogeneous reductions in renal cortical perfusion sufficient to induce the cessation of glomerular filtration, may be the pathogenetic final common pathway in acute renal failure.

It is not clear from their studies how the reduction in cortical perfusion is induced or sustained. There is evidence to suggest that a local intrarenal vasomotor mechanism, controlled by a vasoactive mediator, such as the renin-angiotensin system, is the predominant factor in the changes in distribution of renal perfusion. As long as 30 years ago, hypertrophy of cellular elements of the juxtaglomerular apparatus was observed in the kidney tissue of patients with acute renal failure related to the crush syndrome. It was postulated that a vasopressor substance was released from this area, resulting in altered renal blood flow, decreased glomerular filtration rate, and, finally, renal failure.[27] More

recently, elevations in plasma renin levels have been observed in both clinical[28] and experimental[29] acute renal failure. However, the finding of increased renin levels in acute renal failure has not been a consistent one, and it is not known whether increased renin activity, when it occurs, is a consequence rather than a cause of acute renal failure. Perhaps, the most serious defect of the concept of increased renin-angiotensin activity as the common mediator of renal vascular changes in acute renal failure is the inability to reverse adverse changes in renal function with drugs, such as hydralazine and acetylcholine, that block the effects of angiotensin, despite producing improvements in renal blood flow and cortical perfusion.[30]

It is easier to prevent renal ischemia than to treat it once it is established. This is particularly true of surgical patients with reduced circulating blood volume, in whom the added insult of

Fig. 28-4. Schematic representation of the importance of time in the progression of functional to organic or parenchymal renal failure. Systemic hypotension may be used as an example of an extra-renal precipitating factor. Reflex spasm of the renal arteries occurs, and renal blood flow is severely decreased. Glomerular filtration rate and urine flow fall rapidly. Finally, anuria occurs. If renal response to the hypotension is not arrested before time X, renal lesions are initiated. During the interval between time X and Y, therapy will be effective in alleviating the functional component of renal failure and preventing further progression of organic lesions. At time Y, however, organic lesions are of such severity that total organic failure is present, pathologically characterized (in this example) by acute tubular necrosis. At this point, arresting the renal effect of hypotension can have no immediate salutory effect, since the patient is suffering classical, organic renal shutdown. (Barry, K. G., and Malloy, J. P: Oliguric renal failure. J.A.M.A., *179*: 510, 1962. Copyright © 1962, American Medical Association)

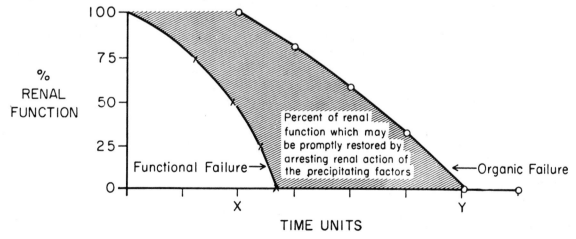

general anesthesia, with its attendant myocardial depression and peripheral vasodilation, may accelerate the renal ischemic process. Barry demonstrated the advantages of preoperative hydration with 15 ml. per kg. of 0.3-per-cent saline and replacement of urine output, in a group of six patients anesthetized with both light (0.5–1.0%) and deep (1.2–3.0%) halothane.[31] A control group of six patients were anesthetized with similar halothane concentrations but were not given fluids from the night before operation until the conclusion of anesthesia. Premedication with morphine-scopolamine produced a significant decrease in effective renal blood flow (p-aminohippurate (PAH) clearance), glomerular filtration rate (inulin clearance), and urine flow in the non-hydrated control patients, but not in the hydrated patients Fig. 28-5. Anesthesia with light halothane resulted in greater decreases in these variables in non-hydrated patients than in the hydrated patients. However, the advantage of hydration was lost with deeper levels of halothane. Thus, in healthy young patients, dehydration and halothane anesthesia resulted in moderate changes in renal hemodynamics and function. In patients with reduced circulating blood volume, these changes are likely to be of even greater magnitude and could lead to the development of acute renal failure if not properly treated.

Restoration of circulating blood volume to values as near normal as possible, then, is a major goal of the preoperative therapy of hypovolemic patients, regardless of the etiology of the deficit. During operation, there may be additional fluid losses owing to hemorrhage, formation of a surgical "third space," pooling of fluids in the intestines, or evaporative loss from exposed intestinal surfaces; these must be corrected. Finally, hypovolemia during the postoperative period must be avoided as carefully as during the preoperative or intraoperative periods. In addition to the obvious causes of hypovolemia, such as hemorrhage and gastrointestinal drainage, more unusual events, such as gram-negative bacterial sepsis, are likely to occur after operation, particularly when extensive procedures have been undertaken in debilitated patients. Release of endotoxins from cell walls of dying bacteria, usually

Escherichia coli, results in pooling of blood in the microcirculation. Relaxation of precapillary sphincters combined with intense constriction of post-capillary sphincters results in stagnation of blood with hypovolemia, hypotension, hypoxemia, and acidosis. Activation of complement by the endotoxin that initiated the process also may lead to intravascular coagulation.[32]

Finally, persistent oliguria and renal failure following open heart surgery may be of prerenal origin. Abel studied 500 consecutive patients who underwent cardiopulmonary bypass and found that 35 developed moderate or severe acute renal failure.[33] The mortality rate for this group was 88.8 per-cent, and there were no survivors among patients requiring dialysis. The development of renal failure could be correlated with the duration of cardiopulmonary bypass and the length of time that mean arterial blood pressure remained below 80 torr. The etiology of renal failure in these patients was not always clear. Possible causes included prolonged duration of a low cardiac output state, multiple renal emboli from atrial thrombi or valvular calcifications, renal artery or venous occlusion, subclinical aortic dissection following retrograde aortic perfusion, and the administration of nephrotoxic drugs.[34,34a]

Treatment of Prerenal Oliguria

Correction of hypovolemia will, in many cases, increase cardiac output, enhance renal perfusion, and prevent parenchymal ischemic changes. A diagnostic and therapeutic maneuver is the rapid infusion of 500 ml. of balanced salt solution and the determination of the response of the kidneys to this challenge. If there is an increase in urine flow, then the additional fluids must be administered, since significant oliguria usually will not occur unless extracellular fluid volume is depleted by 25 per cent or more. Generally, replacement fluid should match the type of fluid that has been lost, although organ perfusion may be enhanced by hemodilution. Central venous pressure measurements are invaluable in determining the total volume of fluid to be administered. However, in patients with marked impairment of myocardial function or severe pulmonary disease, central venous pressure may not correlate with left atrial

PAH CLEARANCE

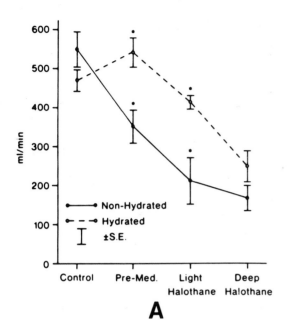

A

INULIN CLEARANCE

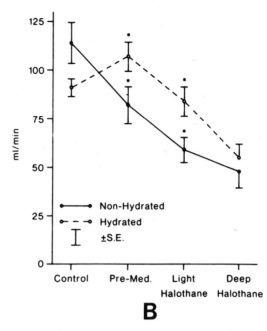

B

URINE FLOW

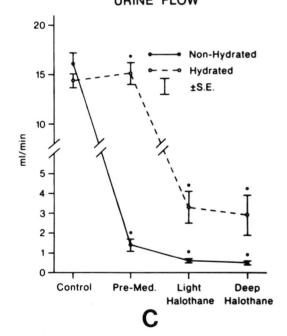

C

Fig. 28-5. (*A, B, C*) Effective renal blood flow (PAH clearance), glomerular filtration rate (inulin clearance), and urine flow in non-hydrated and hydrated patients. Premedication consisted of morphine (10 mg.) and scopolamine (0.4 mg.). Light halothane (0.5–1.0%) and deep halothane concentrations (1.2–3.0%) were used. Hydrated patients and patients anesthetized with light halothane had less depression of renal hemodynamics and function than non-hydrated and deeply anesthetized patients.

pressure. In such patients, when volume status is uncertain or rapid infusions are required, the only effective way to clinically measure left ventricular filling pressure is by determination of pulmonary artery wedge pressure using a balloon-tipped, pulmonary artery catheter.[35]

If replacement of fluid losses does not reverse oliguria, it is possible that cardiac failure may be present. In these patients, inotropic agents, such as dopamine or isoproterenol, should be administered, as indicated. The use of digitalis in the operating room is now uncommon owing to the greater simplicity and lesser hazard of inotrope administration.

The question of the efficacy of diuretic administration in the treatment of oliguria is still debated. Because these agents are potentially harmful, their mechanism of action must be understood if they are to be employed in the treatment of oliguria. Osmotic diuretics such as mannitol produce a diuresis because they are filtered by the glomerulus but not reabsorbed in the renal tubule; thus, they obligate the excretion of water. Additionally, they increase intravascular volume, and they may block renin release.[36] Because they increase blood volume, they are contraindicated in patients with oliguria secondary to congestive heart failure. Loop diuretics, such as furosemide and ethacrynic acid, produce a diuresis by blocking sodium reabsorption in the loop of Henle and distal convoluted tubule. When administered to patients with congestive heart failure, they promote a profuse natriuresis with increased urine flow. This results in a decrease in intravascular volume and, ultimately, an improvement in cardiac performance. The use of loop diuretics is clearly beneficial to these patients.[37,38] However, these agents are contraindicated in oliguria of hypovolemic origin, because they may promote diuresis despite a reduced intravascular volume and thereby aggravate renal ischemic changes. If, after an initial positive response to diuretic treatment, urine flow again decreases below 1 ml. per kg. per hour, diuretic treatment should be continued while fluid and electrolyte balance are carefully maintained. If used in this manner, diuretics may prevent functional renal failure from progressing to organic renal disease.[38–40] If diuretics are not completely effective, they still may improve the clinical situation by converting oliguric renal failure to high output renal failure, which is more easily managed than the former.[1,38] However, some nephrologists believe that, except when oliguria is secondary to heart failure, diuretics are not indicated. They cite the increased salt and water loss and ototoxicity associated with the loop diuretics and the osmotic nephrosis that may occur after mannitol administration as significant disadvantages of this type of therapy. In general, we believe that diuretic agents are useful in treating oliguria in some patients; their administration should be associated with few complications if basic physiologic principles are followed and dosage is not excessive. A trial with the appropriate diuretic agent is indicated in most cases of oliguria. Transient hypotension due to vasodilatation in skeletal muscle may occur following rapid intravenous administration of hyperosmotic solutions such as mannitol.[41]

Finally, if oliguria is caused by bacterial endotoxin shock, antibiotics, vasopressors, inotropic agents, and, perhaps, steroids are indicated for treatment.

PRIMARY RENAL OLIGURIA

Approximately 50 per cent of patients admitted to renal dialysis units have nonsurgical diseases; oliguria is part of the complex of symptoms in most of these cases. The causes of oliguria of primary renal origin are indicated in Table 28-1. Few of these patients come under the care of the anesthesiologist, and the differential diagnosis and treatment of their diseases is not discussed here.

An exception is oliguria and renal failure owing to release of hemoglobin from lysed red blood cells, secondary to blood transfusion reaction or to mechanical trauma inflicted by a pump-oxygenator. Hemoglobin appears in the urine after all binding sites to plasma haptoglobin are occupied and the resorptive capacity of proximal tubular cells is exceeded. Additionally, renal tubular cells are sloughed, and heme pigment obstructs the tubular lumens. Micropuncture studies have shown that obstruction of renal tubules is not the major pathophysiologic event in the development of experimental oliguric renal failure, rather, the primary factor is a major reduction in glomerular filtration rate.[20,21] It also has been observed that the transfusion of incompatible blood leads to disseminated intravascular coagulation, with deposition of fibrin in renal tubules. Red cell membranes are thought to initiate the coagulation process, ultimately leading to a decrease in platelets, fibrinogen, and factors II, V, and VII.[42] Myoglobinuria following extensive, crushing-type muscle injuries also may lead to oliguric renal failure. The mechanism is probably the same as that following hemoglobin administration.

Treatment of Primary Renal Oliguria

There is evidence that treatment with mannitol, if instituted prior to hemolysis or shortly thereafter, will ameliorate or prevent renal failure.[19] This, in fact, is the basis for the widely used practice of including 12.5 to 25 g. of mannitol with the solutions used for priming pump-oxygenators for cardiopulmonary bypass. However, when oliguric renal failure is established, hemodialysis is the treatment of choice.

If medical management of the patient is meticulous and complications such as infection, hemorrhage, or cardiac arrhythmias do not supervene, then return of renal function, in most cases, will be complete. On the other hand, if oliguria is caused by renal cortical necrosis, and there is no hope of return of renal function, then chronic dialysis or renal transplantation must be employed to maintain life.

REFERENCES

1. Brown, C. B.: Established Acute Renal Failure Following Surgical Operations. *In* Friedman, E. A., and Eliahou, H. E. (eds.): Proceedings, Conference on Acute Renal Failure. pp. 187–208. DHEW Publication No. (NIH) 74-608, 1973.
2. Kuhn, W., and Ryffel, K.: Herstellung konzentrierter losungen aus verdunnten durch blosse membranwirkung. Ein modellversuch zur funktion der niere. Z. Physiol. Chem., 276:145, 1942.
3. Pitts, R. F.: Physiology of the Kidney and Body Fluids ed. 3. Chicago, Year Book Medical Publishers, 1974.
4. Berliner, R. W., Levinsky, N. G., Davidson, D. G., et al.: Dilution and concentration of the urine and the action of antidiuretic hormone. Am. J. Med., 24:730, 1958.
5. Levinsky, N. G., Alexander, E. A., and Venkatachalam, M. A.: Acute renal failure. *In* Brenner, B. M. and Rector, F. C. (eds.): The Kidney. ed 2. pp. 1181–1236. Philadelphia, W. B. Saunders, 1981.
6. Harrington, J. T., and Cohen, J. C.: Current concepts: Acute oliguria. N. Engl. J. Med., 292:89, 1975.
7. Swann, R. C., and Merrill, J. P.: The clinical course of acute renal failure. Medicine, 32:215, 1953.
8. Smith, A.: Injuries of pelvic ureter. Surg. Gynecol. Obstet., 140:761, 1975.
9. Charles, A. H.: Some hazards of pelvic surgery. Proc. R. Soc. Med., 60:656, 1967.
10. Wesolowski, S.: Ureteral injuries. Int. Urol. Nephrol., 5:39, 1973.
11. Chisholm, G. D., and Shackman, R.: Malignant obstructive uraemia. Br. J. Urol., 40:720, 1968.
12. Wanrick, S.: Carcinoma of pancreas causing ureteral obstruction. J. Urol., 110:395, 1973.
13. Derrick, F., and Kretkowski, R.: Trauma to kidney, ureter, bladder and urethra. Postgrad. Med., 55:183, 1974.
14. Burnett, C. H., Bloomberg, E. L., Shortz, G., et al.: A comparison of the effects of ether and cyclopropane anesthesia on renal function of man. J. Pharmacol. Exp. Ther., 96:380, 1949.
15. Habif, D. V., Papper, E. M., Fitzpatrick, H. F., et al.: The renal and hepatic blood flow, glomerular filtration rate, and urinary output of electrolytes during cyclopropane, ether, and thiopental anesthesia, operation, and the immediate postoperative period. Surgery, 30:241, 1951.
16. Deutsch, S., Goldberg, M., Stephen, G. W., et al.: Effects of halothane anesthesia on renal function in normal man. Anesthesiology, 27:793, 1966.
17. Mazze, R. I., Cousins, M. J., and Barr, G. A.: Renal effects and metabolism of isoflurane in man. Anesthesiology, 40:536, 1974.
18. Cousins, M. J., Greenstein, L. R., Hitt, B. A., et al.: Metabolism and renal effects of enflurane in man. Anesthesiology, 44:44, 1976.
19. Barry, K. G., and Malloy, J. P.: Oliguric renal failure. J.A.M.A., 179:510, 1962.
20. Ruiz-Guinazu, A., Coelho, J. B., and Paz, R. A.: Methemoglobin-induced acute renal failure in the rat: in vivo observation, histology and micropuncture measures. Nephron, 4:257, 1967.
21. Flanigan, W. J., and Oken, D. E.: Renal micropuncture study of the development of anuria in the rat with mercury-induced renal failure. J. Clin. Invest., 44:449, 1965.
22. Olsen, T. S., and Skjoldborg, H.: The fine structure of the renal glomerulus in acute anuria. Acta. Pathol. Microbiol. Scand., 70:205, 1967.
23. Hollenberg, N. K., Epstein, M., Rosen, S. M., et al.: Acute oliguric renal failure in man: evidence for preferential renal cortical ischemia. Medicine, 47:455, 1968.
24. Hollenberg, N. K., Adams, D. F., Oken, D. E., et al.: Acute renal failure due to nephrotoxins: renal hemodynamic and angiographic studies in man. N. Engl. J. Med., 282:1329, 1970.
25. Hollenberg, N. K., Birtch, A., Rashid, A., et al.: Relationships between intrarenal perfusion and function: serial hemodynamic studies in the transplanted human kidney. Medicine, 51:95, 1972.

26. Hollenberg, N. K., McDonald, F. D., Cotran, R., et al.: Irreversible acute oliguric renal failure: a complication of methoxyflurane anesthesia. N. Engl. J. Med., *286*:877, 1972.

27. Goormaghtigh, N.: Vascular and circulatory changes in renal cortex in anuric crush syndrome. Proc. Soc. Exp. Biol. Med., *59*:303, 1945.

28. Tu, W. H.: Plasma renin activity in acute tubular necrosis and other renal disease associated with hypertension. Circulation, *31*:686, 1965.

29. Di Bona, G. E., and Sawin, L. L.: The renin-angiotensin system in acute renal failure in the rat. Lab. Invest., *25*:528, 1971.

30. Ladefoged, T., and Winkler, K.: Effect of dihydralizine and acetylcholine on renal blood flow, mean circulation time for plasma and renal resistance in acute renal failure. *In* Gessler, U., Schroder, K., and Weidinger, H. (eds.): Pathogenesis and Clinical Findings with Renal Failure. pp. 7–15. Stuttgart, Georg Thieme Verlag, 1971.

31. Barry, K. G., Mazze, R. I., and Schwartz, F. D.: Prevention of surgical oliguria and renal-hemodynamic suppression by sustained hydration. N. Engl. J. Med., *270*:1371, 1964.

32. Mergenhagen, S. E., Synderman, R., Gewurz, H., et al.: Significance of complement to the mechanism of action of endotoxin. Curr. Top. Microbiol. Immunol., *50*:37, 1971.

33. Abel, R.: Etiology, incidence, and prognosis of renal failure following cardiac operations. J. Thorac. Cardiovasc. Surg., *71*:323, 1976.

34. ———: Renal dysfunction following open heart surgery. Arch. Surg., *108*:175, 1974.

34a. Hilberman, M., Derby, G. C., Spencer, R. J., et al: Sequential pathophysiological changes characterizing the progression from renal dysfunction to acute renal failure following cardiac operation. J. Thorac. Cardiovasc. Surg., *79*:838, 1980.

35. Lappas, D., Lell, W. A., Gabel, J. C., et al.: Indirect measurement of the left-atrial pressure in surgical patients: pulmonary-capillary wedge and pulmonary artery diastolic pressures compared with left atrial pressure. Anesthesiology, *38*:394, 1973.

36. Barry, K. G., and Berman, A. R.: The acute effects of the intravenous infusion of mannitol on blood and plasma volumes. N. Engl. J. Med., *264*:1085, 1961.

37. Cantarovich, F., Locatelli, A., Fernandez, J. C., et al.: Furosemide in high doses in the treatment of acute renal failure. Postgrad. Med. J., *47*[Suppl.]:13, 1971.

38. Muth, R. G.: Furusemide in Acute Renal Failure. *In* Friedman, E. A., and Eliahou, H. E. (eds.): Proceedings, Conference on Acute Renal Failure. pp. 245–263. Bethesda, DHEW Publication No. (NIH) 74-608, 1973.

39. Barry, K. G., Cohen, A., and LeBlanc, P.: Mannitolization: 1. The prevention and therapy of oliguria associated with cross-clamping of the abdominal aorta. Surgery, *50*:335, 1961.

40. Stahl, W. M., and Stone, A. M.: Prophylactic diuresis with ethacrynic acid. Ann. Surg., *172*:361, 1970.

41. Coté, C. J., Greenhow, D. E., and Marshall, B. E.: The hypotensive response to rapid intravenous administration of hypertonic solutions in man and in the rabbit. Anesthesiology, *50*:30, 1979.

42. Birndor, N.: DIC and renal failure. J. Lab. Invest., *24*:314, 1971.

FURTHER READING

Friedman, E. A., and Eliahou, H. E., (eds.): Proccedings, Conference on Acute Renal Failure. DHEW Publication No. (NIH) 74-608, 1973.

Levinsky, N. G., and Alexander, E. A.: Acute Renal Failure. *In* Brenner, B. M., and Rector, F. C. (eds.): The Kidney. pp. 806–837. Philadelphia, W. B. Saunders, 1976.

Levinsky, N. G., Alexander, E. A., and Venkatachalam, M. A.: Acute Renal Failure. *In* Brenner, B. M., and Rector, F. C. (eds.): The Kidney. ed 2. pp. 1181–1236. Philadelphia, W. B. Saunders, 1981.

Mazze, R. I.: Critical care of the patient with acute renal failure. Anesthesiology, *47*:138, 1977.

Schrier, R. W., and Conger, J. D.: Acute renal failure: Pathogenesis, diagnosis, and management. *In* Schrier, R. W. (ed.): Renal and Electrolyte Disorders. ed 2. pp. 375–408. Boston, Little, Brown and Co., 1980.

29 Polyuria

Jeffrey M. Baden, M.D., and Richard I. Mazze, M.D.

Polyuria is defined as daily urinary output greater than 2.5 L. in a 70-kg. man; the normal 24-hour urinary output ranges from 0.5 to 1.5 L. The number of physiological and pathological processes that may result in polyuria is large. They vary from a transitory excess intake of fluids to potentially fatal acute renal failure. In addition to conditions that may lead to polyuria but are not associated with surgery, surgical patients are also subject to conditions that occur only during anesthesia and operation.

RENAL CONCENTRATING-DILUTING MECHANISM

In order to diagnose and treat polyuria adequately, it is necessary to understand how urine is concentrated and diluted. More detailed descriptions of the concentrating-diluting mechanisms may be found in textbooks of renal physiology[1,2] and in Chapters 27 and 28. In brief, approximately 180 L. of glomerular filtrate are formed each day. Seventy to 80 per cent of this volume is reabsorbed iso-osmotically in the proximal tubule, and this segment of the nephron neither concentrates nor dilutes the filtrate (Fig. 29-1).[3] Thus, some 40 L. of isotonic fluid enters the descending limb of the loop of Henle each day. As filtrate passes through this segment, water diffuses from it into the hypertonic interstitium of the renal medulla, and salt passively diffuses from the interstitium into the descending limb. The so-called single effect of the medullary countercurrent system is provided by the ascending limb of the loop, which is impermeable to water but actively transports ions, probably chloride, into the medullary interstitium.[4] This results in progressive medullary hyperosmolality, concentrations reaching as high as 1200 mOsm. per kg., and hypotonicity of distal tubular fluid. Low medullary blood flow and countercurrent exchange of water, facilitated by the hairpin configuration of the vasa recta, help to maintain the high medullary osmolality. By the time the fluid reaches the distal tubule, the original 180 L. of glomerular filtrate has been reduced to about 25 L. It is at this point that antidiuretic hormone (ADH) acts.

ADH, an octapeptide, is formed in nerve cell bodies located mainly in the paraventricular and supraoptic nuclei. It migrates along the axons of these cells to perivascular nerve endings in the posterior lobe of the pituitary, where it is released into the blood. The primary stimulus for release of ADH is an increase in blood osmolality. Changes in osmolality of as little as 2 per cent can be detected by osmoreceptors in the pituitary gland and carotid body, ultimately leading to decreased urine production.[5] Volume depletion also is a potent stimulus for ADH release, whereas volume expansion inhibits the production of ADH; these effects may be mediated by left atrial stretch receptors. It is also thought that pain, anxiety, and administration of CNS depressant drugs, such as narcotics, lead to ADH release.

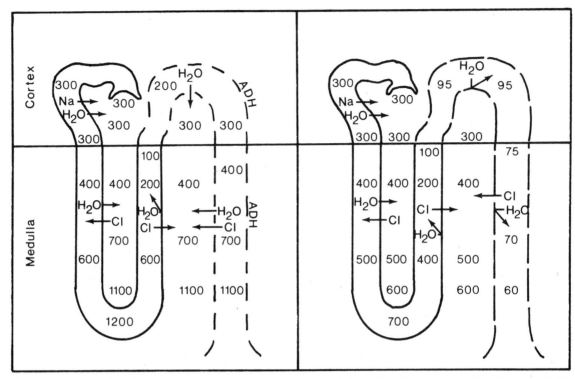

Fig. 29-1. A simplified version of the countercurrent system found within mammalian kidney. (*Left*) Alterations in tubular fluid and interstitial osmolality when ADH is present. (*Right*) The same system under circumstances in which there is no ADH. (Harrington, J. T., and Cohen, J. J.: Clinical disorders of urine concentration and dilution. Arch. Intern. Med., *131:* 810, 1973)

Ethanol administration inhibits ADH release and leads to polyuria. The major effect of ADH on the kidneys is to increase the permeability of both the distal tubule and epithelium of the collecting duct to water. This is most likely due to ADH stimulation of epithelial adenyl cyclase activity, leading to an increased production of 3'5'-adenosine monophosphate.[6] By altering epithelial permeability, ADH permits water to move passively down its concentration gradient, as shown in Figure 29-1 (*left*).

Thus, hypotonic distal tubular fluid loses water as it approaches osmotic equilibrium, initially with the isotonic cortical interstitium and, later, with the hypertonic renal medulla. Processes that interfere with the development or maintenance of the hypertonicity of the renal medulla, the production or release of ADH, or the ability of the kidney to respond to ADH will adversely affect the urine-concentrating mechanism. During diu-

resis, ADH is not present or levels are low, so that the epithelium of the distal convoluted tubules and collecting ducts is relatively impermeable to water This results in the formation of large volumes of dilute urine (Fig. 29-1, *right*).

CLINICAL PRESENTATION OF POLYURIA

Polyuria may first be noted by the patient who complains of passing more than the normal amount of urine. Alternatively, a nurse or physician may notice an increased urinary output. Prolonged and severe polyuria may result in dehydration and hypernatremia, which lead to neurological signs and symptoms, such as confusion, apathy, and coma. Under these circumstances, the symptom of increased urinary output cannot be elicited from the patient, and the diagnosis may be obscured. Similarly, during general anesthesia or if the patient is unconscious because of disease or trauma, it is more difficult to diagnose polyuria. In these instances, the only way to accurately assess the rate of urine formation is with an indwelling urethral catheter.

Pathological processes that result in an inability to concentrate urine may be grouped into two broad categories: those associated with no or low levels of ADH, and those in which ADH levels are normal.[7] Concentrating defects associated with no ADH or low levels of circulating ADH are called *central diabetes insipidus* (see the list below). Urine output is high, and osmolality typically varies from 50 to 200 mOsm. per kg. Central diabetes insipidus is most frequently acquired, secondary to trauma or disease of the pituitary-hypophyseal axis. Psychogenic polydipsia is the next most common cause of central diabetes insipidus. This condition is often difficult to distinguish from primary, idiopathic diabetes insipidus. In the latter case, water is imbibed because of dehydration secondary to persistent and uncontrollable polyuria. With time, there tends to be overcompensation, resulting in hyponatremia and serum hypo-osmolality. The compulsive water drinker is overhydrated from the start, manifesting hyponatremia, serum hypo-osmolality, and polyuria secondary to suppression of ADH formation. Deprivation of water for 24 hours or more, with frequent measurements of serum and urinary sodium and osmolality, will help to distinguish the two conditions. Patients with primary idiopathic diabetes insipidus cannot increase urinary osmolality to a great extent, in spite of hypernatremia and serum hyperosmolality, whereas patients with psychogenic polydipsia, ultimately, can concentrate their urine. It is not usually possible to eliminate the underlying cause of central diabetes insipidus, even when one can be found. Thus, hormonal replacement therapy often is required. Vasopressin tanate in oil, administered by injection, or vasopressin snuff or lysine vasopressin spray, by the inhalational route, are most commonly used.[11] In less severe cases, nonhormonal measures may suffice. Reducing the obligatory solute load by dietary restriction occasionally is of value. More success has been achieved by administration of thiazide diuretics, which act by contracting extracellular fluid volume and by reducing delivery of filtrate to the distal nephron.[12] Chlorpropamide also is effective in patients who have some residual ADH release from the posterior pituitary gland.[3]

Causes of Central Diabetes Insipidus (No ADH or Low Levels)

Acquired[8,9]
  Brain tumor
  Head trauma
  Post-neurosurgical
  Infectious disorders (e.g., encephalitis)
  Vascular disorders (e.g., postpartum pituitary necrosis)
  Systemic disorders (e.g., Hand-Schüller-Christian disease, sarcoidosis)
Psychogenic polydipsia (compulsive water drinking)[10]
Primary, idiopathic[8]
Familial[8]

The second major type of diabetes insipidus is called *nephrogenic* (see the list below).[13] Patients with this condition have an impaired renal tubular response to adequate levels of ADH. Nephrogenic diabetes insipidus following administration of methoxyflurane is the most clearly definable, anesthesia-related cause of polyuria. Since the origin of diabetes insipidus is usually apparent, whether it is central or nephrogenic, the discussion below does not distinguish between these two major categories. For additional information, Harrington and Cohen have published an excellent review on clinical disorders of urine concentration and dilution.[3]

POLYURIA IN THE PREOPERATIVE PERIOD

When investigating the cause of polyuria in surgical patients, it is useful to determine the onset of increased urinary output in relation to the time of the operation. Polyuria associated with the majority of the processes in the two lists above may be present prior to operation. In many patients, the etiology of polyuria can be readily determined from the history, physical examination, and a few simple laboratory investigations. For example, the syndrome of polyuria, urinary tract infection, weight loss, signs of peripheral vascular disease, neuropathy, and glycosuria are very likely associated with diabetes mellitus, whereas polyuria, headache, and failing vision suggest a hypothalamic tumor.[8,18] However, when chronic renal diseases, such as pyelonephritis[21] and nephrocalcinosis,[16] or systemic diseases, such as amyloidosis[34] and malnutrition,[31] result in polyuria, it is more difficult to be certain of the exact cause. In all cases of polyuria, a careful history of drug intake should be obtained to identify agents that may be directly nephrotoxic, such as lithium carbonate,[26] tetracycline,[25] and gentamicin.[24] Also, diuretic treatment may result in polyuria, either primarily as a therapeutic effect or secondarily as a toxic phenomenon, if postassium replacement has not been adequate.[15] Every effort should be made to determine the etiology and, if possible, to treat the causes of polyuria. Recognizing prior to operation that a surgical patient is polyuric is important in planning intraoperative and postoperative fluid therapy. Careful preoperative investigation also may prevent errors in management that may occur when polyuria that is present prior to operation is first discovered during or after operation.

Causes of Nephrogenic Diabetes Insipidus (Normal Levels of ADH)

Congenital, with or without hydronephrosis[13,14]
Acquired
    Hypokalemia (e.g., secondary to diuretic therapy)[15]
    Hypercalcemia, nephrocalcinosis[16,17]
    Osmotic diuresis (e.g., diabetes mellitus)[18]
    Non-oliguric acute renal failure[19,20]
    Recovery phase of oliguric acute renal failure,[19,20]
    Chronic pyelonephritis or hydronephrosis[21]
    Drug induced
        Methoxyflurane[22]
        Demeclocycline[23]
        Gentamicin[24]
        Tetracycline (outdated)[25]
        Lithium carbonate[26]
        Amphotericin B[27]
    After relief of urinary tract obstruction[28]
    Miscellaneous conditions
        Hypertension[29]
        Cirrhosis[30]
        Malnutrition[31]
        Anorexia nervosa[32]
        Sickle cell disease[33]
        Amyloidosis[34]

POLYURIA IN THE INTRAOPERATIVE PERIOD

Water and Diuretics

One of the most frequent causes of diuresis in surgical patients is the parenteral administration of excessive amounts of water during the preoperative period. Traumatized patients and patients having extensive operative procedures frequently require large volumes of intravenous fluids in order to maintain an adequate circulating blood volume. Fluid requirements in these individuals are difficult to quantitate, owing to the shift of large volumes of fluid from the intravascular compartment into an extravascular, interstitial compartment, the so-called "third space." The problem is further complicated if large quantities of crystalloids have been administered, since approximately three-fourths of the amount infused rapidly leaves the intravascular compartment and passes interstitially. Elimination of excess fluids in some cases begins during operation. If isotonic fluids have been administered, ADH secretion is reduced in response to expanded intravascular volume; if hypotonic fluids have been given, decreased serum osmolality is an additional stimulus to reduction of ADH secretion. Most frequently, however, renal excretion of sequestered water begins on the 2nd or 3rd postoperative day.

An additional cause of intraoperative polyuria is that due to osmotic diuresis secondary to hyperglycemia. The proximal tubules of the kidney usually reabsorb all filtered glucose, provided that a threshold limit, normally 180 to 200 mg. per dL. of arterial plasma, is not exceeded. During anesthesia and operation, this value may be lower, and glucose intolerance may be present. If the threshold for glucose is exceeded, the transport mechanism becomes saturated, the glucose appears in the urine, obligating the excretion of water. A source of excess glucose during operation may be parenterally administered fluids, since each liter of 5-per-cent dextrose contains 50 g. of glucose. Marked inoperative hyperglycemia usually can be prevented by restricting parenteral glucose intake during operation to 100 g.

Intraoperative polyuria may follow administration of diuretics. These agents may be administered during operation for the prevention and treatment of surgical renal failure, to reduce intraocular pressure, or to reduce brain size. Mannitol is the most extensively employed osmotic agent, although urea and glucose have been used in the past. The potent loop diuretics, furosemide and ethacrynic acid, also have been employed during operation. They are of undisputed value in the management of acute fluid overload and have been administered instead of or in addition to mannitol for the prevention and treatment of surgical renal failure.

Neurosurgical Trauma

Surgical interference with the supraopticohypophyseal axis may lead to an absolute or relative lack of circulating ADH.[8,9] In humans, in concentrations within the physiological range, the half-life of endogenous ADH is approximately 15 min.[35] However, after complete surgical ablation of the pituitary gland, polyuria does not occur for at least 12 hours postoperatively, if it occurs at all. Presumably, sufficient stores of ADH remain in cell bodies and can be released at the pituitary stalk or other sites, to prevent the immediate occurrence of polyuria. Nevertheless, urinary output should be carefully monitored whenever surgical procedures are carried out near the pituitary gland.

POLYURIA IN THE POSTOPERATIVE PERIOD

Most instances of polyuria in surgical patients first become manifest during the postoperative period. Although there are a number of causes of postoperative polyuria, the one most clearly related to anesthetic administration is the inorganic fluoride nephropathy characteristic of high-dose methoxyflurane anesthesia.

Methoxyflurane Nephrotoxicity

Crandell reported that 13 of 41 patients anesthetized with methoxyflurane for abdominal surgical procedures developed postoperative polyuria.[36] Inability to concentrate urine despite fluid deprivation and vasopressin administration suggested that polyuria was of renal origin. In most instances, normal urine-concentrating ability was restored in 10 to 20 days, although in three patients, abnormalities persisted for more than 1 year. Mazze extended Crandell's findings with a controlled, randomized, prospective clinical study, in which all patients anesthetized with methoxyflurane developed renal abnormalities.[22,37] Those most affected exhibited ADH-resistant polyuria, marked weight loss, hypernatremia, serum hyperosmolality, elevated blood urea nitrogen (BUN) and serum creatinine, increased serum uric acid, and decreased uric acid clearance. None of the control patients anesthetized with halothane developed renal abnormalities.

Subsequent studies in Fischer 344 rats[38,39] and in humans[40] demonstrated a direct relationship between methoxyflurane exposure, serum levels of the methoxyflurane metabolite, inorganic fluoride, and the degree of postoperative renal dysfunction. In humans, methoxyflurane exposures of 2 MAC hours or less resulted in peak serum inorganic fluoride concentrations below 40 μM and were not associated with nephrotoxicity. Exposures of 2.5 to 5 MAC hours resulted in peak serum inorganic fluoride levels of 50 to 80 μM and were associated with mild biochemical abnormalities and delayed return to maximum preoperative urine-concentrating ability. Longer methoxyflurane exposures resulted in fluoride levels greater than 100 μM and in signs and symptoms of marked renal dysfunction. Patients with methoxyflurane nephrotoxicity also have elevated serum and urinary oxalic acid levels, and oxalic acid crystals have been found in their renal biopsy specimens.[37,41] However, most evidence suggests that inorganic fluoride, rather than oxalic acid, is the primary nephrotoxic methoxyflurane metabolite.[39,40]

Also of interest in this nephropathy is the role of enzyme induction. Studies in Fischer 344 rats have shown that phenobarbital pretreatment increases methoxyflurane defluorination and the degree of nephrotoxicity associated with a given dose of anesthetic.[39] The significance of enzyme induction in the development of nephrotoxicity

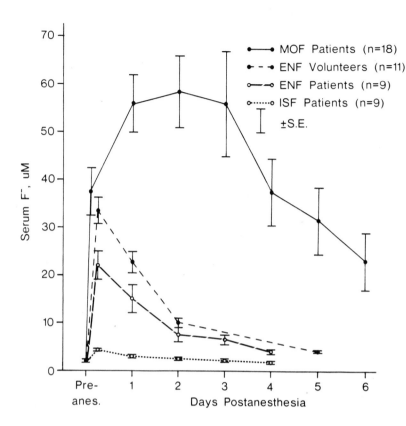

Fig. 29-2. Serum inorganic fluoride (F⁻) concentrations in patients and volunteers prior to and following enflurane (ENF) anesthesia and in patients prior to and following isoflurane (ISF) and methoxyflurane (MOF) anesthesia. There was a significant increase in serum F⁻ concentration immediately following enflurane anesthesia, reaching near peak values of 22.2±2.8 μM in patients and 33.6±2.8 μM in volunteers, 4 hours after anesthesia was terminated. Following methoxyflurane, mean peak serum F⁻ concentration was higher, 61±8 μM and declined more slowly than after enflurane. After isoflurane, mean peak serum F⁻ concentration was 4.4±0.4 μM.

in humans has not been established. An additional factor in the development of methoxyflurane nephropathy is the interaction of the anesthetic with nephrotoxic antibiotics. Treatment with both tetracycline[42] and gentamicin in humans[43] and animals[24] increases the severity of methoxyflurane-induced renal lesions.

It is unlikely that administration of other fluorinated anesthetics will result in nephrotoxicity. Enflurane is biochemically more stable than methoxyflurane and also not as soluble in fat; solubility in fat is directly related to how long an anesthetic is available for postoperative metabolism. In surgical patients exposed to an average of 2.9 MAC hours of enflurane, serum inorganic fluoride levels peaked at 22.2 μM[44]; in volunteers exposed to 9.7 MAC hours of enflurane, fluoride levels peaked at 33.6 μM (Fig. 29-2).[45] Polyuria was not seen in either group of subjects, although

the volunteers had a 26-per-cent decrease in maximum urinary osmolality in response to vasopressin administration compared to preanesthetic values. Polyuric nephrotoxicity, possibly related to enflurane metabolism to inorganic fluoride, has been reported in three surgical patients with poor preoperative renal function.[45] It is possible that damaged kidneys may be more susceptible to the nephrotoxic effects of inorganic fluoride and that higher inorganic fluoride levels may develop in patients with renal disease because of impaired fluoride excretion. Thus, enflurane should probably be avoided in patients with abnormal renal function. Isoflurane also is metabolized to inorganic fluoride, but to a lesser extent than its isomer, enflurane.[46] Serum inorganic fluoride levels have not exceeded 10 μM (Fig. 29-2), and polyuria has not been observed in humans or animals exposed to this anesthetic.[46,47]

Isoflurane administration should not result in polyuric nephrotoxicity, even in patients with preexisting renal abnormalities.

Polyuria Associated With Renal Failure

Depressed renal function usually returns to normal within a few hours after termination of operation. Occasionally, however, renal function does not rapidly recover, and the patient may develop acute renal failure.[48] A number of factors are responsible for this syndrome, including shock, hypotension, inadequate perioperative fluid replacement, mismatched blood transfusion, and heart failure. Except in patients to whom a large dose of methoxyflurane has been administered, the choice of anesthetic used is seldom a consideration. Although oliguria has been regarded as a cardinal sign of acute renal failure, some patients develop renal failure with normal or somewhat elevated urinary output.[19,20] This condition, known as non-oliguric acute renal failure, may be associated with marked biochemical abnormalities, as urinary solute content is relatively low, approximately 300 mOsm. per kg., and urinary volume is fixed. It is increasingly recognized as a more common form of acute renal failure, making up 50 per cent of all cases in several recent reports.[19,20] Patients with non-oliguric acute renal failure have a more benign clinical course than do patients with the oliguric variety: They spend less time in the hospital and have fewer episodes of sepsis, neurologic abnormalities, and gastrointestinal bleeding; they require less frequent dialysis; and, they survive more often (74% vs. 50% in oliguric renal failure).[20] Presumably, this is because more nephrons are spared, and patients retain some ability to execrete water, electrolytes, and metabolic products. It is important that the diagnosis of non-oliguric acute renal failure be made, otherwise serious errors in patient management may occur. Several deaths due to overhydration have occurred in patients whose urinary output was fixed in the normal range.[19] Additionally, electrolyte administration, particularly potassium, may be dangerous in patients with non-oliguric renal failure.

Polyuria frequently occurs as the first phase in the recovery process in patients with the oliguric form of acute renal failure. Daily urinary output doubles for several days, reaching as much as 3 to 6 L. before returning to normal. Approximately one-fourth of the mortality in patients with oliguric renal failure occurs during the polyuric phase, so management must be as careful as when urinary output is very low.[48]

REFERENCES

1. Pitts, R. F.: Physiology of the Kidney and Body Fluids. ed. 3. pp. 99–139. Chicago, Year Book Medical Publishers, 1974.
2. Marsh, D. J.: Osmotic concentration and dilution of the urine. *In* Rouiller, C., and Muller, A. F. (eds.): The Kidney: Morphology, Biochemistry, Physiology. vol. 3. pp. 71–127. New York, Academic Press, 1971.
3. Harrington, J. T., and Cohen, J. J.: Clinical disorders of urine concentration and dilution. Arch. Intern. Med., *131*:810, 1973.
4. Burg, M. B., and Green, N.: Function of the thick ascending limb of Henle's loop. Am. J. Physiol., *224*:659, 1973.
5. Verney, E. B.: Croonian lecture: The antidiuretic hormone and the factors which determine its release. Proc. R. Soc. London (Biol.), *135*:25, 1947.
6. Orloff, J., and Handler, J.: The role of adenosine 3'5'-phosphate in the action of antidiuretic hormone. Am. J. Med., *42*:757, 1967.
7. Randall, R. V., Clark, E. C., and Bahn, R. C.: Classification of the causes of diabetes insipidus. Proc. Mayo Clin., *34*:299, 1959.
8. Blotner, H.: Primary of idiopathic diabetes insipidus: a systemic disease. Metabolism, *7*:191, 1958.
9. Coggins, C. H., and Leaf, A.: Diabetes insipidus. Am. J. Med., *42*:807, 1967.
10. Barlow, E. D., and de Wardener, H. E.: Compulsive water drinking. Q. J. Med., *28*:235, 1959.
11. Miller, L., Fisch, L., and Kleeman, C. R.: Relative potency of arginine-8-vasopressin and lysine-8-vasopressin in humans. J. Lab. Clin. Med., *69*:270, 1967.
12. Earley, L. E., and Orloff, J.: The mechanism of antidiuresis associated with the administration of hydrochlorothiazide to patients with vasopressin resistant diabetes insipidus. J. Clin. Invest., *41*:1988, 1962.
13. Miller, M., and Moses, A. M.: Urinary antidiuretic hormone in polyuric disorders and in inappropriate ADH syndrome. Ann. Intern. Med., *77*:715, 1972.
14. Bode, H. H., and Crawford, J. D.: Nephrogenic diabetes insipidus in North America: the Hopewell hypothesis. N. Engl. J. Med., *280*:750, 1969.
15. Relman, A. S., and Schwartz, W. B.: The kidney in potassium depletion. Am. J. Med., *24*:764, 1958.
16. Epstein, F. H.: Calcium and the kidney. Am. J. Med., *45*:700, 1968.
17. Mayock, R. L., Bertrand, P., and Morrison, C. E.: Manifestations of sarcoidosis: analysis of 145 patients, with a

review of nine series selected from the literature. Am. J. Med., *35*:67, 1963.

18. Berliner, R. W.: Outline of renal physiology. *In* Strauss, M. B., and Welt, L. G., (eds.): Diseases of the Kidney. ed. 2. pp. 31–88. Boston, Little Brown, 1971.

19. Vertel, R. M., and Knochel, J. P.: Nonoliguric acute renal failure. J.A.M.A., *200*:598, 1967.

20. Anderson, R. J., Linas, S. L., Berns, A. S., et al.: Nonoliguric acute renal failure. N. Engl. J. Med., *296*:1134, 1977.

21. Kaye, D., and Rocha, H.: Urinary concentrating ability in early experimental pyelonephritis. J. Clin. Invest., *49*:1427, 1970.

22. Mazze, R. I., Trudell, J. R., and Cousins, M. J.: Methoxyflurane metabolism and renal dysfunction. Anesthesiology, *35*:247, 1971.

23. Roth, H., Becker, K. L., and Shalhoub, R. J.: Nephrotoxicity of demethylchlorotetracycline hydrochloride: a prospective study. Arch. Intern. Med., *120*:433, 1967.

24. Barr, G. A., Mazze, R. I., Cousins, M. J., et al.: An animal model for combined methoxyflurane and gentamicin nephrotoxicity. Br. J. Anaesth., *45*:306, 1973.

25. Frimpter, G. W., Timpanelli, A. E., Eisenmenger, W. J., et al.: Reversible "Fanconi syndrome" caused by degraded tetracycline. J.A.M.A., *184*:111, 1963.

26. Lee, R. V., Jampol, L. M., and Brown, W. V.: Nephrogenic diabetes insipidus and lithium intoxication: complications of lithium carbonate therapy. N. Engl. J. Med., *284*:93, 1971.

27. Douglas, J. B., and Healy, J. K.: Nephrotoxic effects of amphotericin B including renal tubular acidosis. Am. J. Med., *46*:154, 1969.

28. Witte, M. H., Short, F. A., and Hollander, W., Jr.: Massive polyuria and naturesis following relief of urinary tract obstruction. Am. J. Med., *37*:320, 1964.

29. Baldwin, D. S., Gombos, E. A., and Chasis, H.: Urinary concentrating mechanism in essential hypertension. Am. J. Med., *38*:864, 1965.

30. Jick, H., Kamm, D. E., and Snyder, J. G.: On the concentrating defect in cirrhosis of the liver. J. Clin. Invest., *43*:258, 1964.

31. Klahr, S., Tripathy, K., and Garcia, F. T.: On the nature of the renal concentrating defect in malnutrition. Am. J. Med., *43*:84, 1967.

32. Russell, G. F. M., and Bruce, J. T.: Impaired water diuresis in patients with anorexia nervosa. Am. J. Med., *40*:38, 1966.

33. Levitt, M. F., Hauser, A. D., and Levy, M. S.: The renal concentrating defect in sickle cell disease. Am. J. Med., *29*:611, 1960.

34. Carone, F. A., and Epstein, F. H.: Nephrogenic diabetes insipidus caused by amyloid disease. Am. J. Med., *29*:539, 1960.

35. Lauson, H. D.: Metabolism of antidiuretic hormones. Am. J. Med., *46*:713, 1967.

36. Crandell, W. B., Pappas, S. G., and Macdonald, A.: Nephrotoxicity associated with methoxyflurane anesthesia. Anesthesiology, *27*:591, 1966.

37. Mazze, R. I., Shue, G. L., and Jackson, S. H.: Renal dysfunction associated with methoxyflurane anesthesia: a randomized, prospective clinical evaluation. J.A.M.A., *216*:278, 1971.

38. Mazze, R. I., Cousins, M. J., and Kosek, J. C.: Dose-related methoxyflurane nephrotoxicity in rats: a biochemical and pathologic correlation. Anesthesiology, *36*:571, 1972.

39. Cousins, M. J., Mazze, R. I., and Kosek, J. C.: The etiology of methoxyflurane nephrotoxicity. J. Pharmacol. Exp. Ther., *190*:523, 1974.

40. Cousins, M. J., and Mazze, R. I.: Methoxyflurane nephrotoxicity: a study of dose response in man. J.A.M.A., *225*:1611, 1973.

41. Franscino, J. A., Vanamee, P., and Rosen, P. P.: Renal oxalosis and axotemia after methoxyflurane anesthesia. N. Engl. J. Med., *283*:676, 1970.

42. Kuzucu, E. Y.: Methoxyflurane, tetracycline, and renal failure. J.A.M.A., *211*:1162, 1970.

43. Mazze, R. I., and Cousins, M. J.: Combined nephrotoxicity of gentamicin and methoxyflurane anaesthesia in man. Br. J. Anaesth., *45*:394, 1973.

44. Cousins, M. J., Greenstein, L. R., Hitt, B. A., et al.: Metabolism and renal effects of enflurane in man. Anesthesiology, *44*:44, 1976.

45. Mazze, R. I., Calverley, R. K., and Smith, N. T.: Inorganic fluoride nephrotoxicity. Anesthesiology, *46*:265, 1977.

46. Hitt, B. A., Mazze, R. I., Cousins, M. J., et al.: Metabolism of isoflurane in Fischer 344 rats and man. Anesthesiology, *40*:62, 1974.

47. Mazze, R. I., Cousins, M. J., and Barr, G. A.: Renal effects and metabolism of isoflurane in man. Anesthesiology, *40*:536, 1974.

48. Mazze, R. I.: Critical care of the patient with acute renal failure. Anesthesiology, *47*:138, 1977.

FURTHER READING

Harrington, J. T., and Cohen, J. J.: Clinical disorders of urine concentration and dilution. Arch. Intern. Med., *131*:810, 1973.

Maffly, R. H.: Diabetes insipidus. *In* Andreloi, T. E., Grantham, J. J., and Rector F. C., Jr. (eds.): Disturbances in the Body Fluid Osmolality. pp. 285–307. Bethesda, American Physiological Society, 1977.

30 Urinary Retention

Jeffrey M. Baden, M.D., and Richard I. Mazze, M.D.

Acute urinary retention is a common complication following surgery and anesthesia. Several mechanisms are involved, including spasm of sphincters, bladder neck obstruction, and paralysis of the detrusor muscle. Additionally, narcotic and parasympatholytic drug administration may result in the inability to void. The serious consequences of unrecognized urinary retention make early diagnosis and correct treatment of this condition mandatory.

FUNCTIONAL ANATOMY OF THE BLADDER

The smooth muscle of the bladder is arranged in three layers. Only the outer layer, known as the detrusor muscle, is responsible for micturition; it is supplied by parasympathetic nerve fibers from the S2–4 spinal cord segments. (Fig. 30-1). Smooth muscle fibers from the detrusor muscle make up the internal sphincter, whereas the external urethral sphincter is made up of skeletal muscle. The latter is under conscious control and is supplied by somatic nerve fibers (S3–4) carried in the pudendal nerves. The bladder also has sympathetic nerve supply from the inferior mesenteric ganglion. Sympathetic stimulation inibits bladder contraction and increases the tone of the internal vesical sphincter. During micturition, however, no function has yet been attributed to these nerve fibers.

Micturition is an autonomic spinal reflex that is both facilitated and inhibited by higher centers. The urge to void occurs when intravesical pressure reaches 10 cm. H_2O; this is usually felt when bladder volume is approximately 150 ml. At a volume of 400 ml., there is a marked sense of fullness. The mechanism of micturition involves initial relaxation of the perineal muscles and external urethral sphincters, followed by contraction of the detrusor muscle. Proper function, therefore, requires an intact neuromuscular system and an unobstructed pathway for flow of urine.[1]

PATHOPHYSIOLOGY OF URINARY RETENTION

There are a number of reasons why postoperative urinary retention may occur. Operations in and around the pelvis and bladder, with subsequent trauma to the detrusor muscle and damage to the pelvic nerves, may inhibit bladder action. Edema around the bladder neck and reflex spasm of the sphincters due to pain or anxiety may contribute to postoperative retention. It is not surprising then, that operations on the genitourinary tract, rectum, and other pelvic structures lead to the highest incidence of postoperative urinary retention.[2,3]

Drugs used by the anesthesiologist may result in urinary retention. This is particularly true in

423

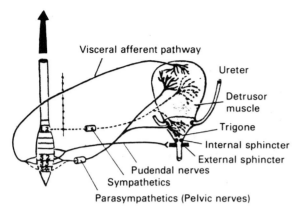

Fig. 30-1. The innervation of the urinary bladder. (Modified from Guyton, A. C.: Textbook of Medical Physiology. ed. 6. p. 472. Philadelphia, W. B. Saunders, 1981)

the presence of preexisting obstructive urinary tract disease, as may occur in the patient with prostatism. The belladona alkaloids, atropine and scopolamine, are used commonly as drying agents; additionally, atropine is administered in combination with neostigmine for reversal of paralysis produced by muscle relaxants. In addition, the use of the synthetic parasympatholytic glycopyrrolate can also result in urinary retention. Contraction of the urinary bladder due to parasympathetic nerve stimulation is only partly inhibited by these drugs. They do, however, lower intravesical pressure, increase bladder capacity, and reduce the frequency of bladder contractions by antagonizing parasympathetic control of this organ.[4]

It is not easy to assess the contribution of these drugs to postoperative urinary retention, but their potential for adversely affecting micturition should be considered, especially when administered to the patient with lower urinary tract obstructive disease.

Patients who remain heavily sedated at the end of an operation are subject to urinary retention, for they may be unaware of bladder distention. Overdistention leads to atony of the bladder wall, so that immediate recovery of function may not occur when the bladder is emptied.[5] Prolonged treatment, that is, indwelling urethral catheteri-

zation, may then be necessary. On the other hand, excessive postoperative pain may make urination impossible, so that perioperative administration of narcotics and sedatives must be accomplished with great skill.

Conduction anesthesia is commonly believed to cause a higher incidence of postoperative urinary retention than general anesthesia. The mechanism is presumed to be delayed recovery of autonomic and somatic nerve function, eventually leading to overdistention of the bladder and atony. However, that conduction anesthesia leads to more difficulty than general anesthesia has not been supported by experimental data. In the most comprehensive study to date, Scarborough analyzed data collected from 65,000 patients having either spinal or general anesthesia, and he concluded that there was no difference between the groups in the incidence of postoperative urinary retention.[6] As in other reports,[2,3,7] the site of operation appeared to be more important than the type of anesthesia in determining whether urinary retention would occur.

CLINICAL PRESENTATION OF URINARY RETENTION

The overall incidence of urinary retention is reported to be 1 to 3 per cent, and most cases occur after genitourinary, pelvic, and rectal operations or in the presence of prostatic hypertrophy.[7] Inability to void postoperatively, associated with an urgent desire to do so, is the usual clinical presentation. The diagnosis is made by palpating the often tender, distended bladder above the symphysis pubis. Generally, urinary retention may be present in any patient who has not voided in a reasonable period of time, during or after operation. The exact length of time is variable and depends upon the duration of the operative procedure and the amount of fluid administered. A careful assessment of any patient who is unable to void must be made if bladder atony and long-term catheterization are to be avoided. However, catheterization may finally be necessary, both to confirm the diagnosis and as part of the treatment.

DIFFERENTIAL DIAGNOSIS OF URINARY RETENTION

There are several reasons why a surgical patient may be unable to void. Administration of general anesthesia is associated with decreased urine formation, probably because of decreased renal blood flow and glomerular filtration rate. Inadequate fluid intake before, during, or after operation also may lead to oliguria and consequent delay in voiding. Patients with acute renal failure usually present with oliguria, although occasionally a patient may be anuric. Anuria is an important sign of total urinary tract obstruction, such as that due to bilateral ureteral calculi, surgical damage, or blood clots obstructing outflow.

TREATMENT OF URINARY RETENTION

Lesser degrees of urinary retention are best treated conservatively by encouraging the patient to urinate. Most patients are not used to voiding in the horizontal position and can be considerably benefited by sitting or standing; early ambulation also is helpful if circumstances permit. Audibly running water, hot or cold baths, or the suggestion that catheterization may be necessary are devices that have been successful in inducing patients to void. In general, good nursing care and encouragement give the best results.

When conservative measures fail, one may often increase the tone of the detrusor muscle sufficiently to promote micturition by using a parasympathomimetic agent (i.e., pilocarpine, up to 6–8 mg., p.o., or bethanechol, up to 20–50 mg., s.c.). These drugs are administered in small incremental doses (i.e., bethanechol, 5 mg., s.c., hourly) until a satisfactory response is obtained or symptoms of excessive cholinergic stimulation, such as biliary or intestinal colic, supervene. These drugs should not be used in cases of obstructive urinary retention (e.g., prostatism).

When prostatism is likely to be present or either the bladder or surrounding structures have been seriously traumatized, further damage should be avoided, and retention should be allevi-ated by the use of an indwelling catheter. In the case of a patient with vesical neck obstruction undergoing surgery other than prostatic, an indwelling urethral catheter should be inserted at the start of the operation and retained until the patient is active. A similar procedure should be followed if it can be predicted that surgery will lead to bladder dysfunction. In other circumstances, catheterization should be performed without delay, as soon as it becomes apparent that the patient is unable to void. Great care must be employed to insert the catheter in a sterile fashion and to avoid further trauma to already damaged tissues. Furthermore, it is important that correct management of the catheterized patient be maintained. First, the catheter must be kept patent by preventing kinkage and obstruction. Although controversial, irrigation of the bladder with either normal saline or a weak acidifying and antiseptic agent, such as mandelamine, may be necessary if catheterization is protracted and should be done aseptically, using a closed system. The urine should be kept acid to minimize bladder stone formation and infection, and routine bacterial cultures should be performed. Appropriate treatment with acidifying agents or antibiotics should be instituted when necessary. Catheters should be changed at regular intervals to prevent the deposit of urinary salts, which can serve as a nidus for infection and for formation of bladder stones. After removal of the catheter, it is most important that the patient be observed frequently to ensure that urinary retention does not recur.

PREVENTION OF URINARY RETENTION

Providing that sedatives and parasympatholytic drugs are used with caution, the type of anesthesia appears to have little effect on the occurrence or severity of postoperative urinary dysfunction. On the other hand, careful surgery, with avoidance of injury to the genitourinary tract, is the best form of prophylaxis. In any case, both the anesthesiologist and surgeon should be constantly alert for this potentially serious, but eminently treatable complication.

REFERENCES

1. Karu, M.: Nervous control of micturition. Physiol. Rev., *45*:425, 1965.
2. Bomze, E. J.: Bladder dysfunction following gynecological surgery. West J. Surg., *62*:325, 1954.
3. Egbert, L. D.: Spinal anesthesia for anorectal surgery. Int. Anesthesiol. Clin., *1*:811, 1963.
4. Weiner, N.: Atropine, scopolamine and related antimuscarinic drugs. *In* Gilman, A. G., Goodman, L. S., and Gilman, A. (eds.): The Pharmacological Basis of Therapeutics. ed. 6. pp. 120–137. New York, Macmillan, 1980.
5. Creevy, C. D.: The care of the urinary bladder after operation. Surgery, *7*:423, 1940.
6. Scarborough, R. A.: Spinal anesthesia from the surgeon's standpoint. J.A.M.A., *168*:1324, 1958.
7. Lund, P. C.: Principles and Practice of Spinal Anesthesia. pp. 631–632. Springfield, Charles C. Thomas, 1971.

Part Eight

The Gastrointestinal System

31 Postoperative Nausea and Vomiting

Eldon J. Swenson, M.D., and Fredrick K. Orkin, M.D.

Although nausea and vomiting are associated with significant morbidity in virtually any practice of anesthesia, they are discussed infrequently. This is true despite the fact that they constitute the single most memorable distress for many patients who have an otherwise uncomplicated anesthetic and surgical course. Even when other complications occur, nausea and vomiting may stand out as uniquely unpleasant.

Nausea is that vague sensation, difficult to describe or localize, which is often a prodrome to vomiting. *Vomiting* is a complex physiologic reflex involving coordinated activity of many skeletal muscles and of the autonomic nervous system, resulting in the forceful expulsion of gastric and even intestinal contents. This chapter will review the physical basis of nausea and vomiting, their incidence, treatment, and prevention.

APPLIED ANATOMY AND PHYSIOLOGY OF NAUSEA AND VOMITING

Neural Connections

Like other reflexes, nausea and vomiting have afferent pathways, a central integrator, and efferent pathways.[1,2] Much of our knowledge of the mechanism of nausea and vomiting derives from the work of Borison and Wang, who identified a vomiting center located bilaterally in the dorsol-ateral border of the lateral reticular formation in the medulla at the level of the olivary nuclei.[3] The vomiting center is particularly well situated in the midst of the nuclei and centers that regulate the visceral and somatic responses involved in vomiting. These regulatory structures include the spasmodic respiratory center, inspiratory and expiratory respiratory centers, vasomotor center, salivary nuclei, and bulbar facilitory and inhibitory systems.

This central integrator receives stimuli from various sites throughout the gastrointestinal tract via vagal and sympathetic afferents, higher cerebral centers, and a chemoreceptor trigger zone (CTZ) located on the floor of the fourth ventricle (Fig. 31-1). Additional stimuli include distention of the uterus, renal pelvis, or urinary bladder; rotation or unequal stimulation of the vestibular labyrinths (transmitted by way of the cerebellum and the CTZ); increased intracranial pressure; and pain.[2]

Efferent impulses leave the vomiting center by way of the fifth, seventh, ninth, tenth, and twelfth cranial nerves to the upper gastrointestinal tract and through the spinal nerves to the diaphragm and abdominal muscles.

The Act of Vomiting

Often as a prodrome to vomiting, the awake individual experiences nausea as a feeling of im-

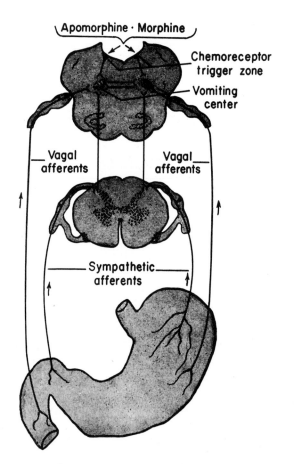

Fig. 31-1. The vomiting center and some of its afferent pathways. (From Guyton, A. C.: Textbook of Medical Physiology. edition 5. p. 899. Philadelphia, W. B. Saunders, 1976.)

minent desire to vomit. Accompanying vasomotor and autonomic disturbances include a feeling of faintness, weakness, anorexia, and emptiness, with simultaneous pallor, pupillary dilatation, diaphoresis, and tachycardia or, sometimes, bradycardia with hypotension. Salivation increases, breathing becomes deep, rapid, and irregular, and retching begins. The latter consists of simultaneous and poorly coordinated spasmodic contractions of the chest and abdominal muscles, with descent and sudden spasm of the diaphragm.[4] Contraction of abdominal musculature

forces gastric contents up into the esophagus; relaxation following each contraction allows refilling of the stomach from the esophagus.

Nausea gives rise to vomiting when retching becomes a coordinated and forceful expulsion of gastric contents through the mouth. Vomiting begins with a deep breath, followed immediately by the ascent of the hyoid bone and larynx; which raises the cricoesophageal sphincter. The glottis closes and remains shut until expulsion has occurred, thereby preventing pulmonary aspiration of vomitus. Similarly, the soft palate rises, closing the posterior nares. Then the diaphragm moves caudally as the abdominal muscles contract forcefully, squeezing the stomach and thereby raising intragastric pressure. The gastroesophageal sphincter and esophagus relax, with the expulsion of gastric contents up the esophagus.[4] The more forceful or prolonged the vomiting, the more likely that bile-stained duodenal contents or even material from lower intestinal levels are forced into the stomach and then expelled.

Regurgitation

Frequently confused with vomiting, *regurgitation* is a passive event. Loss of the sphincter-like activity of the lower esophagus and of the pharyngoesophageal musculature, loss of esophageal peristalsis, and reversal of normal pressure gradients in the upper gastrointestinal tract are factors that allow the passive transfer of gastric contents into the pharynx. All of these may occur in anesthetized patients. Indeed, "silent regurgitation" is a rather common occurrence in patients who receive "uneventful" anesthesia by mask but who experience pulmonary aspiration of small volumes of gastric contents (see Chap. 10).

ETIOLOGY OF NAUSEA AND VOMITING

The diverse afferent pathways to the vomiting center permit an equally diverse set of stimuli to cause nausea and vomiting (Fig. 31-2). Although a variety of etiologic classifications can be used (and are equally arbitrary), these stimuli will be discussed here according to the neural pathways insofar as they are known.[5]

Cortical Pathways

Emotional responses that are themselves manifestations of stress, fear, or depression may result in nausea and vomiting. Similar stimuli include sights (such as blood), odors, tastes, associations peculiar to the individual, and even neuroses and psychoses. Organic disturbances such as pain, severe hypotension, vascular headache (migraine), hypoxia, and increased intracranial pressure are also subserved by cortical pathways.

Visceral Afferent

Abdominal visceral stimuli subserved by vagal and sympathetic afferents include traction on viscera, intestinal obstruction, acute inflammation (such as appendicitis), acute inflammation of nonintestinal viscera accompanied by ileus (such as pancreatitis, cholecystitis), visceral pain,[6] functional gastrointestinal disorders (such as aerophagia), irritation of gastrointestinal mucosa (such as gastric acid, aminophylline, salicylate,

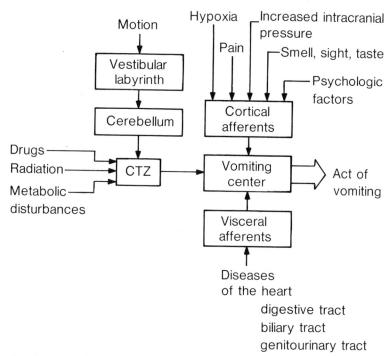

Fig. 31-2. A schematic view of some of the stimuli causing nausea and vomiting, organized by their afferent pathways.

-mycin antibiotics, endotoxin), and heart disease (acute myocardial infarction, congestive failure). A common factor in many of these situations is delayed gastric emptying with resultant gastric distention, which is not only a stimulus for vomiting, but also predisposes to regurgitation and aspiration (Chap. 10). Other causes of delayed gastric emptying include narcotic analgesic administration, intra-abdominal mass (such as gravid uterus), increased intracranial pressure, pain, and anxiety.

Vestibular Pathways

Motion, otitis media, and tumors and vascular changes of the labyrinth are stimuli subserved by the vestibular impulses that pass by way of the auditory nerve to the cerebellum and then the CTZ en route to the vomiting center. Opiates can sensitize the vestibular apparatus to motion. Motion sickness is also enhanced by visual, psychic, olfactory, and proprioceptive stimuli that are subserved by the cortical pathways.

Afferents from the CTZ

A variety of drugs, including apomorphine, morphine (and other narcotic analgesics), cardiac glycosides, amphetamines, ergot derivatives, and nitrogen mustard act directly on the CTZ to cause nausea and vomiting. Very likely, the nausea and vomiting associated with deficiency states (such as hypovitaminous, hypothyroidism, hypoadrenalism), electrolyte imbalance (ketoacidosis), ionizing radiation, and uremia is due to an effect on the CTZ and/or nearby hypothalamic and medullary centers.

INCIDENCE OF POSTOPERATIVE NAUSEA AND VOMITING

Postoperative sickness is a very common problem, with an incidence of 27–82 per cent reported in surveys performed during the past four decades.[7-27] Fortunately, with newer anesthetics and other improvements in surgical care, the overall incidence is now about 30 per cent.[1,8,11-13,24,27] What precludes an accurate prediction in a given patient is the multitude of predisposing factors whose relative importances and interrelations have not been evaluated systematically.

Predisposing Factors

Age. The highest incidence is present in children and adolescents; above age 20, the incidence of postoperative nausea and vomiting decreases.[11,13,14,17,19] Although some believe that the higher incidence reported in children is due to the deep level of ether anesthesia they received for procedures common in that age group (i.e., tonsillectomy),[11] the association is noted even in institutions in which light halothane anesthesia is used.[19]

Sex. Women are two to four times more prone to nausea and vomiting than men. Bellville notes that the incidence is particularly high for women in the third or fourth week of the menstrual cycle and suggests that a high gonadotropin level is responsible for this increased susceptibility.[1,14] Additional evidence that he cites for this explanation includes the nausea that follows orally administered estrogens, the nausea and high gonadotropin levels associated with hyperemesis gravidarum, and the fact that the incidence of nausea and vomiting remains high (as do gonadotropin levels) in postmenopausal and oophorectomized women but falls in women over age 70 (when gonadotropin levels fall).

Body Habitus. Obese patients have a higher incidence of nausea and vomiting,[14] possibly because their larger fat compartment serves as a reservoir for the slow and prolonged release of larger amounts of anesthetic. In effect, the body is exposed to the anesthetic for a longer period, a factor which is also associated with a higher incidence of nausea and vomiting.

Individual Predisposition. Patients with a history of motion sickness or prior postanesthetic vomiting are about three times more likely to have nausea and vomiting than patients without such a history.[19,28,29] Similarly, those with diseases associated with nausea and vomiting (i.e., renal failure, intestinal obstruction) also experience such symptoms more often postoperatively.[15]

Preanesthetic Medication. Patients receiving narcotic analgesics preoperatively are about three times more likely to have postoperative nausea and vomiting than those not receiving such drugs.[30-32] There is a close relationship between movement and sickness after morphine administration; the sickness may be delayed for hours after its administration,[33] and the effect can last as long as 18 hours.[34] Whether morphine is associated with more postoperative sickness than meperidine is controversial.[1,11,25,29,35] The administration of a parasympatholytic agent, such as atropine or scopolamine, with the narcotic diminishes the effect of the latter;[24] alone the parasympatholytics are associated with a lower incidence of nausea and vomiting. Similarly, barbiturates[10] (pentobarbital), antihistamines[8] (diphenhydramine), and especially, phenothiazines[10,29,35-37] (chlorpromazine, promethazine) and butyrophenones[16,27,38] (droperidol) can decrease the incidence of nausea and vomiting to as low as 5 to 10 per cent. Although the data are contradictory, metoclopramide—an interesting new drug that is efficacious in preventing regurgitation and thereby decreasing the risk of pulmonary aspiration (Chap. 10)—may also be an effective antiemetic.[5,39-42] Unfortunately, this drug is not available for clinical use in the United States.

The Anesthetic. There seems to be a lower incidence of nausea and vomiting when intravenous barbiturates rather than inhalation agents are used for induction.[24,43] Anesthesia with diethyl ether and especially cyclopropane is associated with a higher incidence of emesis[1,8,11-13,17,19,24,43,44] and halothane (and presumably enflurane) with a lower incidence than nitrous oxide.[17,19,43,45] The differences among agents are less pronounced after the first few hours following anesthesia.[19,24] Although the incidence of sickness following the administration of regional anesthesia is relatively unstudied, the same general stimuli that may cause sickness in patients anesthetized with inhalation or intravenous agents are operative. That is, anxiety, reflux esophagitis, traction reflex, hypotension, hypoxia, or hypocarbia may cause nausea and vomiting.

Duration of Anesthesia. The longer the anesthetic, the higher the incidence of postoperative nausea and vomiting,[11,13,14,46,47] which has been explained on a dose-response basis.[1]

Site of Operation. Intra-abdominal procedures are associated with the highest incidence of emetic symptoms;[8,19] head and neck, especially eye, procedures are also more likely to be followed by sickness.[11,13]

TREATMENT AND PREVENTION OF POSTOPERATIVE NAUSEA AND VOMITING

Although it is often difficult to decide which patients with postoperative nausea and vomiting should be treated, the prophylactic use of antiemetic drugs is unjustified. This is because only about 30 per cent are affected; in many of them the symptoms are mild and transient, the antiemetic drugs may not be effective, and the side effects of such drugs can be more harmful than the symptoms for which they are administered. Nevertheless, there are specific types of patients who benefit from therapy, including those with a history of postoperative sickness, those who have had intraocular surgery and who are at risk for loss of vitreous, and those whose retching and vomiting is particularly vigorous and therefore threatens esophageal laceration with hemorrhage (Mallory-Weiss syndrome) or mediastinitis.

General Measures

Patients who are likely to have delayed gastric emptying with gastric distention (see p. 152 and 160) benefit from gentle suction through a nasogastric tube.[10,11,13,14] Particular care should be used to avoid inflating the stomach during the administration of general anesthesia. Since pain can cause nausea and vomiting, relief of pain can be therapeutic.[6] The correction of hypotension, hypoxia, and hypercarbia can also relieve symptoms. Nausea and vomiting occurring after the administration of spinal and epidural anesthesia can be treated with atropine, 0.5–1.0 mg. intravenously, ephedrine, 10–25 mg. intravenously (if hypotension is present), oxygen by mask, judicious sedation, and skillful psychological support. Regardless of the type of anesthesia administered, the patient should be transported gently following anesthesia and frequent changes in position should be avoided.

Antiemetic Drugs

A variety of drugs in the minor and major tranquilizer and antihistamine classes have antiemetic activity. Generally these drugs are more effective when given prophylactically than therapeutically, with the phenothiazines being particularly useful for postoperative emesis.[48] For example, chlorpromazine administered preoperatively decreases postoperative sickness about 50 per cent,[11] whereas administered therapeutically it controls symptoms in about 30 per cent of patients.[10] The intramuscular administration of 1 mg. of the butyrophenone haloperidol controls symptoms in 80 per cent of patients within an hour and 100 per cent by an hour and a half.[26] The drawback of these drugs, however, is that they prolong emergence from general anesthesia, potentiate the respiratory depression produced by a variety of drugs, and can cause hypotension. In one institution, the prophylactic use of chlorpromazine, which proved to be an excellent sedative and antiemetic, had to be discontinued because many patients became hypotensive upon the induction of anesthesia.[49] In addition, both the phenothiazines and butyrophenones can cause extrapyramidal reactions, especially Parkinson-like symptoms; rarely, the phenothiazines cause blood dyscrasias and cholestatic jaundice. Even the new antiemetic benzquinamide, a benzoquinolizine derivative unrelated to the phenothiazines, which controls symptoms in up to 96 per cent of patients,[50] can cause arrhythmias during intravenous use, hypertension, and increased temperature and flushing. However, this drug is the only antiemetic that does not synergize with general anesthetics in causing respiratory depression and thereby prolongs emergency from anesthesia.[51]

REFERENCES

1. Bellville, J. W.: Postanesthetic nausea and vomiting. Anesthesiology, 22:773, 1961.
2. Brown, H. G.: The applied anatomy of vomiting. Br. J. Anaesth., 35:136, 1963.
3. Borison, H. L., and Wang, S. C.: Physiology and pharmacology of vomiting. Pharmacol. Rev., 5:193, 1953.
4. McCarthy, L. E., Borison, H. L., Spiegel, P. K., et al.: Vomiting: radiological and oscillographic correlates in the decerebrate cat. Pharmacol. Rev., 5:193, 1953.
5. Gibbs, D.: Diseases of the alimentary system. Nausea and vomiting. Br. Med. J., 2:1489, 1976.
6. Anderson, R. M.: Present status of cyclopropane. Canad. Anaesth. Soc. J., 23:366, 1976.
7. Waters, R. M.: Present status of cyclopropane. Br. Med. J., 2:1013, 1936.
8. Dent, S. J., Ramachandra, V., and Stephen, C. R.: Postoperative vomiting: incidence, analysis and therapeutic measures in 3,000 patients. Anesthesiology, 16:564, 1955.
9. Boulton, T. B.: Oral chlorpromazine hydrochloride: a clinical trial in thoracic surgery. Anaesthesia, 10:233, 1955.
10. Knapp, M. R., and Beecher, H. K.: Postanesthetic nausea, vomiting retching. J.A.M.A., 160:376, 1956.
11. Burtles, R., and Peckett, B. W.: Postoperative vomiting. Br. J. Anaesth., 29:114, 1957.
12. Bonica, J. J., Crepps, W., Monk, B., et al.: Postoperative nausea and vomiting. West. J. Surg. Obstet. Gynecol., 67:332, 1959.
13. Smessaert, A., Schehr, C. A., and Artusio, J. F.: Nausea and vomiting in the immediate postanesthetic period. J.A.M.A., 170:2072, 1959.
14. Bellville, J. W., Bross, I. D. J., and Howland, W. S.: Postoperative nausea and vomiting. IV: Factors related to postoperative nausea and vomiting. Anesthesiology, 21:186, 1960.
15. Dundee, J. W., Nicholl, R. M., and Moore, J.: Studies of drugs given before anaesthesia. III: A method for the studying of their effects on postoperative vomiting and nausea Br. J. Anaesth., 34:572, 1962.
16. Dyrberg, V.: Haloperidol (Serenase) in the prevention of postoperative nausea and vomiting. Acta Anaesthesiol. Scand., 6:37, 1962.
17. Coppolino, C. A., and Wallace, W.: Trimethobenzamide antiemetic in immediate postoperative period: double blind study in 2,000 cases. J.A.M.A., 180:326, 1962.
18. Dundee, J. W., Moore, J., and Clarke, R. S. J.: Studies of drugs given before anesthesia. V: Pethidine 100 mg. alone and with atropine or hyoscine before anaesthesia. Br. J. Anaesth., 36:703, 1964.
19. Purkis, I. E.: Factors that influence postoperative vomiting. Can. Anaesth. Soc. J., 11:335, 1964.
20. Heal, P. C.: Post-operative vomiting: methoxyflurance and halothane. Anaesthesia, 20:275, 1965.
21. Holmes, C. McK.: Postoperative vomiting after ether/air anaesthesia. Anaesthesia, 20:199, 1965.
22. Dundee, J. W.. Evaluation of the effect of halothane on postoperative vomiting. Br. J. Anaesth., 40:633, 1968.
23. Morrison, J. D., Hill, G. B., and Dundee, J. W.: Studies of drugs given before anaesthesia. XV: Evaluation of the method of study after 10,000 observations. Br. J. Anaesth., 40:890, 1968.
24. Gold, M. I.: Postoperative vomiting in the recovery room. Br. J. Anaesth., 41:143, 1969.
25. Dundee, J. W., Loan, W. B., and Morrison, J. D.: Studies of drugs given before anaesthesia. XIX: The opiates. Br. J. Anaesth., 42:54, 1970.
26. Barton, M. D., Libonati, M., and Cohen, P. J.: The use of

haloperidol for treatment of postoperative nausea and vomiting—a double-blind placebo-controlled trial. Anesthesiology, *42*:508, 1975.

27. Winning, T. J., Brock-Utne, J. G., and Downing, J. W.: Nausea and vomiting after anesthesia and minor surgery. Anesth. Analg., *56*:674, 1977.

28. Armer, A. L.: The control of postoperative nausea with the use of dimenhydrinate. J. Oral Surg., *10*:225, 1952.

29. Robbie, D. S.: Postanesthetic vomiting and antiemetic drugs. Anaesthesia, *14*:349, 1959.

30. Phillips, O. C., Nelson, A. J., Lyons, W. B., *et al.:* The effect of Trilafon on postanesthetic nausea, retching and vomiting: a controlled study. Anesth. Analg., *37*:341, 1958.

31. Phillpis, O. C., Nelson, A. C., Lyons, W. B., *et al.:* The effect of Trilafon on postanesthetic nausea, retching and vomiting: continued study. Anesth. Analg., *39*:38, 1960.

32. Riding, J. E.: Postoperative vomiting. Proc. R. Soc. Med., *53*:671, 1960.

33. Comroe, J. H., and Dripps, R. D.: Reactions to morphine in ambulatory and bed patients. Surg. Gynecol. Obstet., *89*:221, 1948.

34. Wangeman, C. P., and Hawk, M. H.: The effects of morphine, atropine and scopolamine on human subjects. Anesthesiology, *3*:24, 1942.

35. Feldman, S. A.: A comparative study of four premedications. Anaesthesia, *18*:169, 1963.

36. Adriani, J., Summers, F. W., and Antony, S. O.: Is the prophylactic use of antiemetics in surgical patients justified? J.A.M.A., *175*:661, 1961.

37. Bellville, J. W., Bross, I. D., and Howland, W. S.: Postoperative nausea and vomiting. V: Antiemetic efficacy of trimethobenzamide and perphenazine. Clin. Pharmacol. Ther., *1*:590, 1960.

38. Patton, C. M., Jr., Moon, M. R., Dannemiller, F. J.: The prophylactic antiemetic effect of droperidol. Anesth. Analg., *53*:361, 1974.

39. Lind, B., and Breivik, H.: Metoclopramide and perphenazine in the prevention of postoperative nausea and vomiting. Br. J. Anaesth., *42*:614, 1970.

40. Ellis, F. R., and Spence, A. A.: Clinical trials of metoclopramide (Maxolon) as an anti-emetic in anaesthesia. Anaesthesia, *25*:368, 1970.

41. Breivik, H., and Lind, B.: Anti-emetic and propulsive peristaltic properties of metoclopramide. Br. J. Anaesth., *43*:400, 1971.

42. Shah, Z. P., and Wilson, J.: An evaluation of metoclopramide (Maxolon) as an anti-emetic in minor gynaecological surgery. Br. J. Anaesth., *44*:865, 1972.

43. Riding, J. E., Dundee, J. W., Rajogopalan, M. S., *et al.:* Clinical studies of induction agents. VI.: Miscellaneous observations with G29.505. Br. J. Anaesth., *35*:480, 1963.

44. Moore, D. C., Bridenbaugh, L. D., VanAckeren, E. G., *et al.:* Control of postoperative vomiting with perphenazine (Trilafon): a double blind study. Anesthesiology, *19*:72, 1958.

45. Howat, D. D. C.: Antiemetic drugs in anaesthesia. Anaesthesia, *15*:289, 1960.

46. Smith, J. M.: Postoperative vomiting in relation to anaesthetic time. Br. Med. J., *2*:217, 1945.

47. Bodman, R. I., Morton, H. J., and Thomas, E. T.: Vomiting by out-patients after nitrous oxide anaesthesia. Br. Med. J.: *1*:327, 1960.

48. Drugs for relief of nausea and vomiting. Med. Lettr. Drugs Ther., *16*(11):46, 1974.

49. Dripps, R. D., Vandam, L. D., and Pierce, E. C.: The use of chlorpromazine in anesthesia and surgery. Arch. Surg., *142*:774, 1955.

50. Lutz, H., and Immich, H.: Antiemetic effect of benzquinamide in postoperative vomiting. Curr. Therp. Res., *14*:178, 1972.

51. Mull, T. D., and Smith, T. C.: Comparison of the ventilatory effects of two antiemetics benzquinamide and prochlorperazine. Anesthesiology, *40*:581, 1974.

FURTHER READING

Borison, H. L., and Wang, S. C.: Physiology and pharmacology of vomiting. Pharmacol. Rev., *5*:193, 1953.

Brown, H. G.: The applied anatomy of vomiting. Br. J. Anaesth., *35*:136, 1963.

Purkis, I. E.: Factors that influence postoperative vomiting. Can. Anaesth. Soc. J., *11*:335, 1964.

Roth, J. L. A.: Symptomatology other than pain and discomfort. In Bockus, H. L. (ed.): Gastroenterology. edition 8. Philadelphia, W. B. Saunders, 1974. pp. 71–102.

Seigel, L. J., and Longo, D. L.: The control of chemotherapy-induced emesis. Ann. Intern. Med., *95*:352, 1981.

32 Inhalation Anesthetics and Hepatic Injury

Burnell R. Brown, Jr., M.D., Ph.D., and Dwight C. Geha, M.D.

A well recognized feature of potent inhalation anesthetics is nonspecificity of action. From a pharmacologic viewpoint, anesthetics act at neither specific loci nor at receptors, nor are the effects of these drugs reversed by specific antagonists. Thus, a wide variety of physiologic and biochemical alterations, in addition to changes in consciousness, occur during the course of anesthesia. Obvious examples are reductions in myocardial contractility, blood pressure, and renal function. These changes, which, strictly defined, can be called pathologic, are accepted and tolerated simply because it can be fairly well predicted that they are ephemeral and will dissipate at the conclusion of the anesthetic period.

Specifically concerning the liver, a large number of transitory depressant actions, both physiologic and biochemical, are observed in the presence of clinical concentrations of anesthetics. A partial list includes inhibition of mitochondrial oxidation, urea synthesis, bilirubin formation, and drug biotransformation.[1,2] Temporary alterations in standard liver function tests (such as bromsulphalein (BSP) retention) may result, not unexpectedly when enzymatic processes are interrupted. However, these are fully reversible changes and, akin to unconsciousness and negative inotropic effects, are temporary and diminish in magnitude with decreasing concentrations of anesthetic. This chapter is concerned with immutable changes in the liver following general anesthesia, a relatively rare and unpredictable phenomenon.

INHALATION ANESTHETICS AND HEPATIC INJURY

Reports of jaundice and hepatic necrosis following the administration of inhalation anesthetics have appeared for more than 75 years. The early clinical and experimental work on the association of chloroform with fatal liver injury, which led to condemnation of the anesthetic by the Committee on Anesthesia of the American Medical Association in 1912, has been reviewed by Dykes.[3] Although "delayed chloroform poisoning" (alias hepatic necrosis) following chloroform was anecdotally recognized as a true entity, neither incidence nor absolute cause and effect relationship was proven following anesthesia in humans during the 7 decades of its popularity. In fact, Sykes stated the death rate with chloroform anesthesia was 1 in 3000, comparable to statistics of modern times, and the majority of these were due to cardiac, not hepatic complications.[4]

Because of the association of halogenated hydrocarbons and hepatic necrosis, the effects of halothane on liver function were extensively studied in the 1950s in animals and humans prior to release for widespread clinical use. Minor degrees of morphologic change, primarily fatty infiltration without necrosis, were observed in some animals following exposure to halothane.[5] The likelihood of hepatic necrosis in humans was considered to be no greater with halothane than with other inhalation anesthetics, but the only abnormality was a transient increase in BSP retention,[6,7] which is also observed with non-halogenated inhalation anesthetics. All currently employed halogenated anesthetics, at least anecdotally, have been associated with liver damage following surgery. Throughout this chapter, reference is frequently made to halothane. This particular halogenated anesthetic was selected because of its widespread use and because many toxicologists have studied it.

Early Reports of Halothane Hepatotoxicity

Shortly after the clinical introduction of halothane in 1958, isolated case reports appeared suggesting a link between halothane and postanesthetic hepatic necrosis.[8,9,10] In 1963, three series of cases of severe hepatic dysfunction following halothane anesthesia were reported.[11,12,13] Of the 15 patients studied, six died of massive hepatic necrosis, and six developed liver injury following a second halothane anesthetic.

These and other early case reports indicated that liver injury associated with halothane administration strongly resembled viral hepatitis. Clinical features included fever, anorexia, nausea, vomiting, malaise, lethargy, and pain in the right upper quadrant, which appeared prior to clinical jaundice. Physical findings included minimal to moderate liver enlargement, with tenderness. Laboratory findings were consistent with nonspecific hepatocellular dysfunction: elevations of serum bilirubin, transaminases, prothrombin time, and BSP retention. Pathologic findings at autopsy included massive hepatic necrosis with centrolobular and midzonal necrosis, which frequently extended to entire hepatic lobules. Vacuolar cytoplasmic degeneration was present in cells peripheral to the central necrosis. These observations were so nonspecific that they engendered (and still do engender) debate regarding whether such an entity as "halothane-related" jaundice or "halothane hepatotoxicity" exists.

Two interesting corollaries that would subsequently receive a great deal of attention emerged from these early clinical reports: the association of hepatic necrosis with the administration of a second halothane anesthetic; and Lindenbaum and Lieffer's observation of leukopenia and eosinophilia in several patients,[12] suggesting an allergic process. Thus, halothane "sensitization," by way of an immunologic process leading to liver damage on subsequent exposure, was hypothesized. This hypothesis received support by Tygstrup, who reported that a patient became jaundiced following a second and third halothane anesthetic.[14] Liver biopsies on both occasions did not confirm a specific histologic pattern, but rather revealed changes similar to viral hepatitis. Publication of these early reports stimulated investigation to determine the etiologic role of halothane in postanesthetic liver dysfunction and the incidence of this problem. Perhaps because of failure to reproduce this hepatic dysfunction in the laboratory, early efforts utilized epidemiologic methods, principally large-scale retrospective case analysis. Later, intense laboratory immunologic and biochemical studies were employed.

The National Halothane Study

Shortly after the first isolated case reports of massive hepatic necrosis following halothane anesthesia, the Committe on Anesthesia of the National Academy of Sciences—National Research Council appointed a group to study clinical aspects of halothane anesthesia, with special attention to the association of postanesthetic hepatic necrosis. Initially, a prospective, randomized clinical trial was planned. Following publication of several new case reports, however, the prospective study was abandoned in favor of a retrospective survey, with the hope that this would quickly clarify the issue and obviate extensive clinical trials.

The National Halothane Study surveyed 856,515 general anesthetic administrations in 34 hospitals during the period of 1959 to 1962. The study had two major goals. The first was to compare halothane with other general anesthetics regarding incidence of fatal hepatic necrosis within 6 weeks after surgery. The second was to compare halothane with other general anesthetics with regard to hospital mortality. There were 16,840 deaths, with 10,171 autopsies in the series. A panel of pathologists examined microscopically liver sections from cases of suspected hepatic necrosis and independently rated the extent of the necrosis.

Eighty-two of the autopsied cases had massive hepatic necrosis (1:10,000 anesthetic administrations). This was intermediate compared to the highest incidences of 1.7 in 10,000 with cyclopropane, 0.69 in 10,000 with nitrous oxide-barbiturate and 0.49 in 10,000 with ether. None of the 82 cases could be explained on the basis of usual clinical causes of hepatic necrosis. Seven received halothane, and four of these seven had received a previous halothane anesthetic within 6 weeks. The clinical course of these unexplained cases of massive hepatic necrosis included fever, followed in rapid progression by jaundice, confusion, and hepatic coma. Clinical signs appeared within 2 to 3 days following surgery. The course was rapid and similar to fulminant viral hepatitis. Histologic appearance was similar to viral or drug-induced hepatitis in six of the seven cases. Although the overall incidence of explained jaundice was higher with cyclopropane, there was a definite association of *unexplained* massive hepatic necrosis following exposure to halothane.

The conclusions of the National Halothane Study were that fatal postoperative hepatic necrosis following single or multiple administrations could not be excluded. It is interesting that halothane had a high record of safety, with an overall mortality of 1.87 per cent, compared to the average mortality of 1.93 per cent based on standardized patient populations, for the entire study. It is unfortunate that this large study was not conclusive. This study can be interpreted to verify or contradict the existence of "halothane hepatitis." Its retrospective nature and its volunteer bias were salient deficiencies. That is, prior to initiation of the National Halothane Study, four of the seven cases of unexplained fatal necrosis had been published, and two more were known to be a stimulus for the study.

The Problem Posed by Multiple Administrations of Halothane

Many of the early case reports indicated a higher incidence of unexplained jaundice following second administrations of halothane. Dykes and associates specifically looked for this relationship in a retrospective study of 47,000 general anesthetics.[15] Eight patients developed clinical and laboratory evidence of hepatic disease following halothane. Four of these eight had been anesthetized previously with halothane, without evidence of liver problems. Little reviewed the literature prior to 1968 and found 404 cases of liver dysfunction following halothane anesthesia.[16] Data concerning the number of administrations were available for 346 patients. Forty-nine per cent had two or more exposures. Klatskin reported 41 cases of "well-documented" halothane-associated hepatitis from the literature and another nine from personal records.[17] In 68 per cent, jaundice followed a second exposure to the anesthetic.

The Fulminant Hepatic Failure Surveillance Study was established to collect and review cases of liver failure to determine possible etiologic factors. Starting such a registry was one recommendation of the National Halothane Study. By 1970, 318 patients in all stages of hepatic coma had been reported.[18] Sixty-four of the 318 patients (20%) were assumed to have halothane-associated hepatic failure. Some of these patients, however, had blood transfusions, usually during operation. A history of multiple halothane exposures was present in 40 of the 64 cases (77%).

Two major criticisms have been made of the Fulminant Hepatic Failure Surveillance Study and, indeed, can be applied to all such series. First, significant and indeterminate bias is introduced when cases are reported with the presumptive diagnosis made by the reporting physician. In fact, McPeek stated, "In voluntary case reporting, persons report what they want. There is no control over bias nor even any good way of knowing what the bias is towards."[19] Second, the lack of a known sample group or patient population makes a determination of incidence impossible.

Sharpstone reported 11 cases of hepatic dysfunction following two or more halothane anesthetics, at two hospitals, over a 4-year period.[20] There were six deaths in this series from massive liver necrosis of the hepatocellular type, but many of these patients had other disorders that could have resulted in liver damage, such as blood transfusion and sepsis.[21] Moult and Sherlock reviewed the clinical and laboratory findings of 26 patients among those referred to their liver unit whose illness was attributed to halothane and in whom no other cause for liver disease could be found.[22] All had the onset of jaundice within 15 days of a halothane anesthetic, and none had perioperative hypotension or severe congestive failure prior to development of hepatic problems. Eight had received a blood transfusion within the previous month, however, before the onset of jaundice. Twenty-four of these 26 patients had multiple halothane anesthetics, including 18 who had halothane twice within 28 days. Two other findings of importance in this study were the lack of positive immunologic correlates, using lymphocyte transformation and antimitochondrial antibodies, and an inability to exclude viral hepatitis histologically. It is interesting that Sherlock, who previously had hypothesized that the so-called syndrome of halothane hepatitis was an immunologic phenomenon, suggested other etiologic factors following this report.

There are several other retrospective reviews of interest. Carney and Van Dyke reviewed nearly 600 cases, from the literature and from their own institution, of jaundice or hepatitis occurring within 4 weeks following exposure to halothane.[23] To reduce bias, they selected cases for analysis based on certain criteria, rather than upon the reporting author's diagnosis. Cases were eliminated when a cause other than halothane was demonstrated convincingly; when there was postoperative jaundice but no histologic or biochemical evidence of hepatocellular damage; when minimal abnormalities of liver function (serum glutamic-oxaloacetic transaminase (SGOT) less than 100 international units) were unaccompanied by clinical findings; when minimal focal hepatic necrosis was found incidentally in autopsies; when cases were reported in groups without individual details; when the patient was less than 13 years of age; and, when there were circumstances of occupational exposure. Using these criteria, a series of 234 cases was developed. Of these, 120 were from the National Halothane Study, 102 were published subsequent to that study, and 12 were from the investigators' own institution, collected over a 3-year period. It was possible to analyze the number of halothane exposures and the interval between them in all 234 cases. The incidence of postoperative liver dysfunction following repeated halothane exposure within a 3-month period was 50 per cent.

Mushin analyzed 67 cases of jaundice after halothane anesthesia that were reported at the Committee of Safety of Drugs of England and Wales between 1964 and 1970.[24] Of these, 68 per cent had two halothane anesthetics within a 4-week period. He then reviewed 74 patients who developed jaundice following a second halothane anesthetic and found that in 85 per cent halothane had been administered twice within 1 month. Mushin extrapolated a 10-year analysis of anesthetic practice in his own institution to the total surgical population in England and Wales for the years 1964 to 1967. Based upon this data, he estimated the incidence of jaundice following two halothane anesthetics within 1 month to be between 1 in 11,000 and 1 in 38,000. This study, however, has been criticized because, similar to the National Halothane Study, it is highly unlikely that a causal relationship existed between halothane and postanesthetic jaundice in each case that he reported.

An article that created considerable resurgence of interest in this problem was that of Trowell.[25] In a series of 39 patients with carcinoma of the cervix treated with radium and requiring repeated general anesthetics, it was found that the group anesthetized with halothane had a far greater elevation of serum glutamic-pyruvic transaminase (SGPT) levels than a control group whose primary anesthetic was nitrous oxide. None of the 21 patients in the group treated with nitrous oxide had SGPT levels rising above 100 units. It must be noted that none of the patients in this series developed overt liver disease; they merely showed SGPT elevations. However, in direct contrast to this, Allen and Downing studied 400 African women with multiple exposures to both halothane and enflurane anesthesia.[26] They found no changes in the concentrations of SGOT and SGPT, or serum LDH, alkaline phosphatase, or bilirubin. The differences in these studies have yet to be resolved. Obviously, the following question comes to mind: Is there a genetic predisposition among Caucasian females to development of this syndrome, or are there environmental or drug-related differences?

Factors Contributing to Hepatic Injury

A number of possible contributing factors have been associated with halothane-related liver injury. Among these are obesity, age, sex, previous allergic history, preexisting liver disease, and major surgery. Obesity was present in 56 per cent and 40 per cent of patients in two series.[24,27] Another report has stated that obesity and middle age are common findings and cause the most concern of the possible contributing factors that have been linked to halothane liver injury.[28] Carney and Van Dyke substantiated the finding that unexplained jaundice following the administration of halothane anesthesia was higher in the obese, middle-aged individual.[23] In fact, all but one of the 26 patients reported by Moult and Sherlock were over 40.[22] Thus, from an epidemiologic point of view, it appears that the middle-aged, obese woman is at highest risk for development of jaundice following the administration of halothane.

Early in its clinical use, halothane use was restricted in patients with concurrent liver disease or a past history of liver disease. The scientific evidence indicating that halothane administration may have an adverse effect upon patients with cirrhosis or patients who have had viral hepatitis is very tenuous, to say the least. The National Halothane Study did not find an increased incidence of massive hepatic necrosis following biliary tract surgery. A review of a large series of patients who had cirrhosis of the liver

and clinical and laboratory evidence of liver dysfunction and were also undergoing portocaval shunting procedures found no difference in mortality or in postoperative hepatic failure between halothane and non-halothane anesthetics.[29] At the present time the consensus is that preexisting liver disease such as hepatitis or cirrhosis does not enhance the susceptibility of the liver to injury by halothane.[30,31] It must be remembered that these results come from retrospective surveys, usually based on a report of a small personal series and often enlarged by cases collected from the literature. In only a relatively few of these cases were new serologic tests employed to exclude viral hepatitis. Unexplained postoperative fever does not contraindicate the use of halothane for subsequent anesthetics.[32]

PROPOSED ETIOLOGIES OF HALOGENATED ANESTHETIC HEPATITIS

Relationship of Halogenated Anesthetic Hepatitis to Viral Hepatitis

The inability to distinguish clinically and histologically viral hepatitis from halothane-associated hepatitis has generated considerable controversy.[21] It has been suggested that the stress of anesthesia and surgery unmasks incubating or subclinical viral hepatitis and results in a fulminant course of the disease that culminates in massive, fatal hepatic necrosis. Such a fulminant course has been described following laparatomy in patients with jaundice and suspected extrahepatic biliary obstruction, in whom viral hepatitis was eventually found to be the etiologic agent.[33] Indeed, many cases of hepatic necrosis routinely ascribed to halothane anesthesia are probably due to viral hepatitis. Although several investigators have reported histologic and electron microscopic features that differentiate viral and halothane-associated hepatitis, the consensus is that the two disease entities cannot be separated on a morphologic basis.[34] Sherlock has stated that, although there are some cases in which interesting differences have been shown, both by light and electron microscopy, between halothane and viral hepatitis, the detection depends on the experience of the pathologist, and there are absolutely no diagnostic characteristics that distinguish one form from the other.[22,35]

Infectious hepatitis characterized by a relatively short incubation period following fecal-oral transmission is categorized as hepatitis A. Serum hepatitis with a longer incubation period and transmitted by parenteral exposure to human blood or blood products is known as hepatitis B. It is now recognized, however, that the overlap of incubation periods, 31 to 53 days for hepatitis A and 41 to 69 days for hepatitis B, is too great to make such differentiation useful clinically.[36] Current hepatitis antigen testing methods in widespread use have yielded significant information concerning the prevalence of hepatitis B in its carrier state. Approximately 0.1 per cent of the general population has B antigen when tested. Endemic hepatitis among an urban adult population may be secondary to the hepatitis B virus, transmitted by a route other than parenteral.[37] Although incubation periods may be useful in differentiating viral from halothane-associated hepatitis, the incubation period may be less than 1 month in nearly 5 per cent of hepatitis cases.[25] The presence of hepatitis B antigen is of diagnostic value only if seroconversion can be documented. Demonstrating a lack of hepatitis B antigen is of little value, however, because the antigen may be present for only several days.[36] A recent report described 22 patients with hepatitis associated with transfusion in whom no serologic evidence of hepatitis A, hepatitis B, or cytomegalic virus could be found.[38] Currently, about 90 per cent of transfusion-associated hepatitis is caused by non-A, non-B hepatitis with an incubation period and clinical course that are similar to those of hepatitis B (see Chap. 55).[38a]

It is interesting to note that a death from massive hepatic necrosis following enflurane anesthesia was eventually found to be due to a type of herpes virus, although the initial diagnosis had implicated the anesthetic as the cause.[39] Thus, the distinction between viral hepatitis and the syndrome of halothane hepatitis is certainly not clear.

Sensitivity as a Mechanism of Halothane-Associated Hepatitis

Following the early case reports of death from massive liver necrosis associated with halothane anesthesia, investigators attempted to reproduce this syndrome in animals. They were universally unsuccessful in these studies, and it was postulated that "halothane hepatitis" was an allergic phenomenon specific only to humans. The supporting evidence for this theory included the higher incidence of liver necrosis following second administrations of the anesthetic, although many cases were reported in which only one anesthetic had been given. Several other features that suggested an immunologic or allergic basis for halothane-associated hepatitis included arthralgias, eosinophilia, and skin rashes. This theory of halothane-associated liver damage predominated throughout the 1960s.

It was reinforced by two clinical studies. In the first, that of Paronetto and Popper, lymphocytes from suspected "halothane hepatitis" patients were harvested and incubated with halothane in the presence of tritiated thymidine.[40] An increased incorporation of this nucleic acid, a test for allergy, was detected. The other evidence suggesting an allergic mechanism was that reported by Klatskin and Kimberg.[41] A subanesthetic concentration of halothane had been administered to an anesthesiologist who was known to have liver disease, possibly connected with occupational exposures. Shortly following this challenge, serum enzyme and other levels indicating abnormal liver function were elevated.

The difficulty with these studies is now apparent. The nonspecificity of the lymphocyte stimulation test has been documented[42,43]; in particular, lymphocyte stimulation has been noted following hepatitis B infection.[44] Moreover, an idiosyncratic reaction that follows administration of a drug does not indicate the mechanism but merely that a drug reaction has occurred. When alterations in liver function follow administration of a small dose of halothane, an allergic reaction is not necessarily the cause. Many other mechanisms may be operant. Animal studies have failed to substantiate an allergic basis with either halothane or its primary metabolite, trifluoroacetic acid.[45] Moreover, it is curious that the syndrome is almost unknown among infants and children, who constitute the largest group at risk for allergic diseases.

Nonetheless, given this theory of allergy, safe intervals between halothane exposures were postulated. Various investigators stated that halothane anesthesia should not be given for a period of 3 to 12 months.[46] These intervals were based upon theoretic considerations, however, rather than upon actual data. In fact, Bruce has stated that, given the absence of a reaction, the subsequent choices of anesthesia for the patient should be made by the anesthesiologist, based upon his experience and the requirements for surgery. He also noted that halothane may be the agent of choice in patients with chronic liver disease, for, if overall liver function is poor, then mechanisms that produce liver damage also probably function poorly.

Presently, then, the allergic theory is debatable at best. However, if an allergy to halothane should be proven to occur, then once there has been a "sensitization," the patient should not be given halothane anesthetics again, irrespective of the interval.

Biotransformation as a Mechanism of Anesthetic Hepatotoxicity

Hepatotoxicity of alkyl halides such as carbon tetrachloride and chloroform is attributed to interaction of highly reactive intermediates with liver cell macromolecules. The reactive intermediates are of an ephemeral nature and are produced by biotransformation of the parent molecules by the hepatic microsomal enzymes. Such bioactivation of relativity inert substances into toxic intermediates is well documented as a major mechanism of chemical toxicity.[47–51] Little interest in biotransformation as a cause of anesthetic hepatotoxicity was apparent until the demonstration that clinically employed halogenated inhalation anesthetics are biotransformed in animals[52] and man.[53,54]

It is now possible to produce two models of

centrolobular necrosis in animals, using clinical concentrations of halothane: Pretreatment of animals with a single dose of Arochlor 1254 (a mixture of polychlorinated biphenyls) is followed by 1-per-cent halothane anesthesia in oxygen for 1 hour; or, pretreatment with oral phenobarbital for 5 days is followed by 1 hour of 1-per-cent halothane in a reduced oxygen environment (F_{IO_2} = 0.14). Increases in SGOT, SGPT, and serum bilirubin occur concomitantly with liver injury. These models of hepatotoxicity assume that there is qualitative and quantitative alteration of halothane biotransformation, particularly by a reductive or non-oxygen-dependent route.*[55]

In a very elaborate study, Cohen and colleagues demonstrated urinary metabolites of halothane in humans; the investigators suspected these metabolites were reactive intermediates.[56] They included a defluorinated alkene derivative. Recently, Cohen and colleagues demonstrated low concentrations of trifluoromonochloroethane in air exhaled by humans following halothane anesthesia.[57] It was speculated previously that this compound was a reduction metabolite of halothane and it was demonstrated to have hepatotoxic potential.[58] The levels of this metabolite measured by Cohen (approximately 1 p.p.m.) following halothane anesthesia were too low to produce hepatic necrosis, and this probably explains why none of the patients in his series developed detectable liver injury.

Another important finding in animal studies related to halogenated anesthetic toxicity is the phenomenon of covalent binding. Covalent binding to liver proteins, lipids, and phospholipids indicates that a reactive substance has chemically combined with and become linked to important cell constituents. Studies have suggested that this binding inactivates these constituents, probably in a dose-related manner, leading to cell death and necrosis. Halothane and chloroform both form covalent bonds to liver macromolecules, but chloroform does this to a far greater extent than

---

*Personal communication, G. E. McLain, Jr., B. R. Brown, Jr., and I. G. Sipes.

halothane.[59–61] A most interesting finding is that the extent of this covalent binding of halothane metabolites is increased with low oxygen concentrations in vitro.[55,62,63] Hence, reductive or "low-oxygen-tension" biotransformation produces intermediates that form covalent bonds with important cell components and reach sufficient magnitude to produce gross necrosis of the liver.

The terminal enzyme of the microsomal, mixed-function oxidase system that is utilized for inhalation anesthetic metabolism, cytochrome P-450, is not a single enzyme, but is actually a family of related enzymes. Each component handles substrates differently, exists in different concentrations, and is inducible by different drugs or environmental contaminates. Thus, a speculative mechanism of hepatic necrosis by a halogenated anesthetic can be postulated as follows:

In certain adults, a variant of cytochrome P-450 ("low-oxygen-dependent") may be responsible for biotransformation of various halogenated alkyls to reactive intermediates. This variant may be activated genetically by the environment (presence of inducing drugs) and/or by diminutions in regional blood flow to the liver, which reduce electron flow from NADPH to "high-oxygen" cytochrome P-450. When blood flow to the liver is reduced, the "normal" variant of cytochrome P-450, responsible for oxidative biotransformation, is relatively inactivated, and the effects of "low-oxygen" cytochrome P-450 become more manifest. Biotransformation under these circumstances to reactive reductive intermediates would lead to the sequence of attack by these intermediates on liver macromolecules, with subsequent covalent binding, cellular structure alteration, functional death, and necrosis. It is well known that liver blood flow, particularly hepatic artery flow, generally falls with anesthesia and surgery.[64,65] Obese patients retain more anesthetic, metabolize more of it, and, hence, may be at greater risk. Drugs of low solubility in general are quantitatively biotransformed less than those of higher solubility. Newborn infants may be less susceptible than adults to toxic effects mediated by reactive intermediates, since their drug-metabolizing systems are not fully developed. For example, newborn rats are less susceptible to certain toxins than adult rats.[66]

Within a short period, repeated administrations of anesthetics may produce induction and/or buildup of covalent binding, such that liver function is eventually impaired. It is theoretically possible that the initial event is biotransformation to allergenic metabolite-protein complexes. However, it is quite unlikely that the parent molecule of the anesthetic is a "sensitizing" agent.[67] Biotransformation to quantities of reactive intermediates sufficient to produce manifest liver injury would thus depend upon many factors, such as genetics, environment, molecular configuration of the specific drug, liver blood flow, weight and age of the patient, and solubility of the anesthetic.

It must be emphasized that this mechanism is speculative and based on animal studies entirely. There are few clinical reports presently that confirm this hypothesis.[68]

CLINICAL IMPLICATIONS OF ANESTHETIC HEPATOTOXICITY

Does such an entity as halogenated anesthetic hepatotoxicity exist? The evidence is overwhelming that it does. The fact that centrolobular necrosis can be produced in animals certainly means that such an occurrence is at least a possibility in humans. There is also reason to believe that other conditions are frequently misdiagnosed as halogenated anesthetic hepatotoxicity. The authors are aware of many anecdotal situations in which "classic halothane hepatitis" was diagnosed by misinformed physicians. Patients with postoperative jaundice, in whom nitrous oxide or regional anesthesia was used, and who were incubating viral hepatitis, with abnormal preoperative liver function studies, ligated common bile ducts, and Weil's disease, have been so labelled in our experience. At present there is no confirmatory diagnostic test for this syndrome. Diagnosis is predicated on exclusion. Good medical practice dictates that exclusion should not be the first conclusion. This is a disservice to the patient and does not fulfill the diagnostic role of the physician.

The halogenated inhalation anesthetics are reasonably safe drugs. The rare unpredictable occurrence of a toxic reaction should not preclude their use. Were that the case, we would use the same logic and abandon many drugs, including antibiotics, oral contraceptives, phenylbutazone, and others associated with a much higher idiosyncratic death rate than the halogenated anesthetics. Epidemiologic evidence in humans and data from studies in animals predict that the middle-aged, obese individual is at highest risk. Repeated anesthetic administration poses an unanswered question. Some studies indicate that repeated anesthesia with halothane within a short period, particularly in the high-risk group, might be unwise; but the evidence is not definitive. There is no evidence to impose any time limit on repeated administration of the halogenated drugs. Although covalent binding could theoretically account for problems associated with frequent administrations, the environmental factors leading to this phenomenon (if it exists) have not been elucidated. Does the ill patient who requires second or multiple administrations undergo changes in microsomal enzymes induced by drugs, such as steroids, sedatives, and hypnotics, so that abnormal biotransformation is increased? Are alterations in splanchnic blood flow common in obese patients? These are unanswered questions.

In light of present knowledge, which unfortunately is scant, only the following general rules can be formulated as aids in clinical management: The neonate and infant are probably at very low risk, even if they are given repeated anesthetic administrations; the obese, middle-aged patient, particularly if he is taking various microsomal enzyme inducing drugs (e.g., barbiturates), may be at relatively high risk; unexplained postoperative jaundice following a halogenated anesthetic should preclude the use of that anesthetic for the duration of the patient's life; frequent, repeated anesthetic administration may not be ideal, particularly in high-risk patients.

Halogenated anesthetic hepatotoxicity is a perplexing, unresolved question. Until more data are available, good clinical judgment should be exercised.

REFERENCES

1. Biebuyck, J. F.: Anesthesia and hepatic metabolism: current concepts of carbohydrate homeostasis. Anesthesiology, *39*:188, 1973.
2. Brown, B. R., Jr.: The diphasic action of halothane on the oxidative metabolism of drugs by the liver: an in vitro study in the rat. Anesthesiology, *35*:241, 1971.
3. Dykes, M. H. M.: The early years: 1846–1912. Int. Anesthesiol. Clin., 8:175, 1970.
4. Sykes, W. S.: Essays on the First Hundred Years of Anesthesia. vol. II Edinburgh, Churchill Livingstone, 1961.
5. Jones, W. M., Margolis, G., and Stephen, C. R.: Hepatotoxicity of inhalation anesthetic drugs. Anesthesiology, *19*:715, 1958.
6. Little, D. M., Jr., and Barbour, C. M.: Hepatic function following Fluothane anesthesia. Anesthesiology, *19*:105, 1958.
7. Little, D. M., Jr., Barbour, C. M., and Given, J. B.: Effects of Fluothane, cyclopropane, and ether anesthesia on liver function. Surg. Gynecol. Obstet., *197*:712, 1958.
8. Burnap, T. K., Galla, S. J., Vandam, L. D.: Anesthetic, circulatory, and respiratory effects of Fluothane. Anesthesiology, *19*:307, 1958.
9. Virtue, R. W., and Payne, K. W.: Postoperative death after Fluothane. Anesthesiology, *19*:562, 1958.
10. Temple, R. L., Cote, R. A., and Gorens, S. W.: Massive hepatic necrosis following general anesthesia. Anesth. Analg., *41*:586, 1962.
11. Brody, G. L., and Sweet, R. B.: Halothane anesthesia as a possible cause of massive hepatic necrosis. Anesthesiology, *24*:29, 1963.
12. Lindenbaum, J., and Leiffer, E.: Hepatic necrosis associated with halothane anesthesia. N. Engl. J. Med., *268*:525, 1963.
13. Bunker, J. P., and Blumenfeld, C. M.: Liver necrosis after halothane anesthesia. N. Engl. J. Med., *268*:531, 1963.
14. Tygstrup, M.: Halothane hepatitis. Lancet, 2:466, 1963.
15. Dykes, M. H. M., Wolzer, S. G., Slater, E. M., et al.: Acute parenchymatous hepatic disease following general anesthesia. J.A.M.A., *193*:89, 1965.
16. Little, D. M.: Effect of halothane in hepatic function. *In* Greene, N. M. (ed.): Halothane. Philadelphia, F. A. Davis, 1968.
17. Klatskin, G.: Mechanisms of toxic and drug induced hepatic injury. *In* Fink, B. R. (Ed.): Toxicity of Anesthetics. pp. 159–175. Baltimore, Williams & Wilkins, 1968.
18. Trey, O.: Case records of the Massachusetts General Hospital, Case 10-1970. N. Engl. J. Med., *282*:558, 1970.
19. McPeek, B., and Gilbert, J. P.: Onset of postoperative jaundice related to anaesthetic history. Br. Med. J., 3:615, 1974.
20. Sharpstone, P., Medley, D. R. K, and Williams, S. R.: Halothane hepatitis—a preventable disease. Br. Med. J., 50:448, 1971.
21. Simpson, B. R., Strunin, L., and Walton, B.: The halothane dilemma: a case for the defense. Br. Med. J., *4*:96, 1971.

22. Moult, P. G. A., and Sherlock, S.: Halothane related hepatitis. Q. J. Med., *44*:99, 1975.
23. Carney, F. M. T., and Van Dyke, R. A.: Halothane hepatitis: a critical review. Anesth. Analg., *51*:135, 1972.
24. Mushin, W. W., Rosen, M., and Jones, E. B.: Post-halothane jaundice in relation to previous administration of halothane. Br. Med. J., *3*:18, 1971.
25. Trowell, J., Peto, R., Crampton-Smith, A., et al.: Controlled trial of repeated halothane anesthetics in patients with carcinoma of the uterine cervix treated with radium. Lancet, *1*:821, 1975.
26. Allen, P. J., and Downing, J. W.: A prospective study of hepatocellular function after repeated exposures to halothane or enflurane in women undergoing radium therapy for cervical cancer. Br. J. Anaesth., *49*:1035, 1977.
27. Peters, R. L., Edmondson, H. A., Reynolds, T. B., et al.: Hepatic necrosis associated with halothane anesthesia. Am. J. Med., *47*:748, 1969.
28. Bottiger, L. E., Dalen, E., and Hallen, B.: Halothane induced liver damage: an analysis of the material reported to the Swedish Adverse Reaction Committee, 1966–1973. Acta Anaesthesiol. Scand., *20*:40, 1976.
29. Jones, R. R., Dawson, B., Adson, M. A., et al.: Halothane and non-halogenated anesthetic agents in patients with cirrhosis of the liver: mortality and morbidity following porto-systemic venous anastomoses. Surg. Clin. North. Am., *45*:983, 1965.
30. La Mont, J. T., and Isselbacher, K. J.: Postoperative jaundice. N. Engl. J. Med., *288*:305, 1973.
31. Brown, B. R., Jr.: General anesthetics and hepatic toxicity. Ariz. Med., *34*:5, 1977.
32. Dykes, M. H. M.: Unexplained post-operative fever; its value as a sign of halothane sensitization. J.A.M.A., *216*:641, 1971.
33. Morley, T. J.: Halothane hepatitis. J.A.M.A., *225*:1659, 1973.
34. Summary of the National Halothane Study. J.A.M.A., *197*:775, 1966.
35. Sherlock, S.: Progress report: halothane hepatitis. Gut., *12*:324, 1971.
36. Blumberg, B. S., Sutnick, A. I., London, W. T., et al.: Australia antigen and hepatitis. N. Engl. J. Med., *283*:349, 1970.
37. Prince, A. N., Hargrove, R. L., Sznuness, W., et al.: Immunologic distinction between infectious and serum hepatitis. N. Engl. J. Med., *282*:987, 1970.
38. Feinstone, S. M., Kapikian, A. Z., Purcell, R. H., et al.: Transfusion associated hepatitis not due to viral hepatitis A or B. N. Engl. J. Med., *292*:767, 1975.
38a. Feinstone, S. M., and Purcell, R. H.: Non-A, non-B hepatitis. Annu. Rev. Med., *29*:359, 1978.
39. Douglas, H. J., Eger, E. I., II, Biava, C. G., et al.: Halothane hepatic necrosis associated with viral infection after enflurane anesthesia. N. Engl. J. Med., *296*:553, 1977.
40. Paronetto, F., and Popper, N.: Lymphocyte stimulation induced by halothane in patients with hepatitis following exposure to halothane. N. Engl. J. Med., *283*:277, 1970.
41. Klatskin, G., and Kimberg, D. V.: Recurrent hepatitis attributable to halothane sensitization in an anesthetist. N. Engl. J. Med., *280*:515, 1969.
42. Moult, P. G. A., Adjukiewicz, A. B., Gaylarde, P. M., et al.: Lymphocyte transformation in halothane-related hepatitis. Br. Med. J. *2*:69, 1975.

43. Walton, B., Dunmond, D. C., and Williams, C.: Lymphocyte transformation, absence of increased responses in alleged halothane jaundice. J.A.M.A., *225*:494, 1973.
44. Tong, M. J., Wallace, A. M., Peters, R. L., et al.: Lymphocyte stimulation of hepatitis B infections. N. Engl. J. Med., *293*:318, 1975.
45. McCracken, L. E.: Failure to induce halothane hepatic pathology in animals sensitized to halothane metabolites and subsequently challenged with halothane. Anesth. Analg., *55*:235, 1976.
46. Bruce, D. L.: What is the safe interval between halothane exposures. J.A.M.A., *221*:1140, 1972.
47. Butler, T. C.: Reduction of carbon tetrachloride in vivo and reduction of carbon tetrachloride and chloroform in vitro by tissue and tissue constituents. J. Pharmacol. Exp. Ther., *134*:311, 1961.
48. Slater, T. E.: Necrogenic action of carbon tetrachloride in the rat: a speculative mechanism based on activation. Nature, *209*:36, 1966.
49. Recknagel, R. O.: Carbon tetrachloride hepatotoxicity. Pharmacol. Rev., *19*:145, 1967.
50. Castro, J. A., Sasame, H., Sussman, H., et al.: Diverse effects of SKF 525-A and antioxidants on carbon tetrachloride-induced changes in liver microsomal P-450 content and ethylmorphine metabolism. Life Sci., *7*:129, 1968.
51. Scholler, K. L.: Modification of the effects of chloroform in the rat liver. Br. J. Anaesth., *42*:602, 1970.
52. Van Dyke, R. A., Chenoweth, M. B., Van Poznak, A.: Metabolism of volatile anesthetics I. Conversion in vivo of several anesthetics to $C^{14}O_2$ and chloride. Biochem. Pharmacol., *13*:1239, 1964.
53. Stier, A., Alter, H., Hessler, O., et al.: Urinary excretion of bromide in halothane anesthesia. Anesth. Analg., *43*:723, 1964.
54. Holaday, D. A., Rudofsky, S., and Treuhaft, P. S.: The metabolic degradation of methoxyflurane in man. Anesthesiology, *33*:579, 1970.
55. Sipes, I. G., and Brown, B. R., Jr.: An animal model of hepatotoxicity associated with halothane anesthesia. Anesthesiology, *45*:622, 1976.
56. Cohen, E. N., Trudell, G. R., Jr., Edwards, H. N., et al.: Urinary metabolites of halothane in man. Anesthesiology, *43*:392, 1975.
57. Cohen, E. N., and Trudell, G. R., Jr.: Anesthesiology [In Press].
58. Brown, B. R., Jr., Sipes, I. G., and Baker, R. R.: Halothane hepatotoxicity and the reduced derivative 1, 1, 1-trifluro-2 chlorethrane. Environ. Health Perspect., *21*:185, 1977.
59. Brown, B. R., Jr., Sipes, I. G., and Sagalyn, A.: Mechanisms of acute hepatic toxicity: chloroform, halothane, and glutathione. Anesthesiology, *41*:554, 1974.
60. Cohen, E. N.: The metabolism of halothane C^{14} in the mouse. Anesthesiology, *31*:560, 1969.
61. Van Dyke, R. A., and Wood, C. L.: In vitro studies on the irreversible binding of halothane metabolites to microsomes. Drug. Metab. Dispos., *3*:51, 1975.
62. Widger, L. A., Gandolfi, A. J., and Van Dyke, R. A.: Hypoxia and halothane metabolism in vivo: release of inorganic fluoride and halothane metabolite binding to cellular constituents. Anesthesiology, *44*:197, 1976.
63. Uehleke, H., Hillmer, K. H., and Tabarelli-Poplawski, S.: Metabolic activation of halothane and its covalent bind-

ing to liver endoplasmic proteins in vitro. Naunyn-Schmiedebergs Arch. Pharmakol., *279:*39, 1973.

64. Benumoff, J. L., Brookstein, J. J., Saidman, L. J., et al.: Diminished hepatic arterial flow during halothane administration. Anesthesiology, *45:*545, 1976.

65. Epstein, R. M., Deutsch, S., Cooperman, L. H., et al. Splanchnic circulation during halothane anesthesia and hypercapnia in normal man. Anesthesiology, *27:*654, 1966.

66. Gillette, J. R.: Stripp, B.: Pre- and post-natal enzyme capacity for drug metabolite production. Fed. Proc., *34:*172, 1975.

67. Williams, B. D., White, N., Amlot, P. L., et al.: Circulating immune complexes after repeated halothane anaesthesia. Br. Med. J., *2:*159, 1977.

68. Reynolds, E. S., Brown, B. R., Jr., and Vandam, L. D.: Massive hepatic necrosis after fluroxene anesthesia—a case of drug interaction? N. Engl. J. Med., *286:*530, 1972.

FURTHER READING

Brown, B. R., Jr. (ed.): Anesthesia and the Patient with Liver Disease. Philadelphia, F. A. Davis, 1981.

Strunin, L.: The Liver and Anaesthesia. London, W. B. Saunders, 1977.

33 Salivary Gland Enlargement

Lee H. Cooperman, M.D.

Salivary gland enlargement in association with general anesthesia is an unusual complication first described in 1968.[1] Since then, several additional reports have appeared, so a fuller description of the syndrome can be given.[2-6]

CLINICAL PRESENTATION OF SALIVARY GLAND ENLARGEMENT

Salivary gland enlargement is a benign, painless, although often puzzling and alarming enlargement of the salivary glands. Onset is variable, sometimes beginning shortly after induction of anesthesia (within 15 minutes), sometimes just before the termination of anesthesia, or, rarely, several hours after termination. Usually, all three glands are involved bilaterally. The severity of the disorder ranges from a barely noticeable swelling to a massive enlargement that actually impairs the airway. Salivary gland enlargement is usually transient, lasting several hours at most, although occasional patients have sialadenopathy for several days. Long-term sequelae have not been reported.

Several prospective studies suggest that salivary gland enlargement occurs in about 0.16 to 0.20 per cent of patients who undergo general anesthesia.

ETIOLOGY OF SALIVARY GLAND ENLARGEMENT

A number of causes of salivary gland enlargement are well known, including mumps, suppora- tive parotitis, lymphoma, leukemia, sarcoidosis, Sjögren's syndrome, and salivary duct stones. None of these, however, accounts for the salivary gland enlargement associated with general anesthesia. In fact, its exact cause is not known; but several factors are probably involved.

Enlargement often follows a period of coughing and straining with increased venous pressure and engorgement of the glands. Reflexes initiated by manipulation in the mouth (e.g., airway insertion, laryngoscopy, tracheal intubation) may stimulate parasympathetic hyperactivity and glandular hyperemia. Drugs, especially atropine and succinylcholine, may be inciting agents, although the exact mechanism is at best a matter of speculation. Perhaps they cause inspissation of secretions or marked changes in autonomic activity. Salivary gland enlargement is also seen in patients undergoing endoscopy by way of the oral route; several reports have appeared in the gastro-enterologic literature.[7,8] Because patients undergoing endoscopy do not receive general anesthesia, intraoral and pharyngeal stimulation may be the most important etiologic factors.

MANAGEMENT OF SALIVARY GLAND ENLARGEMENT

No special treatment is required; the adenopathy disappears in minutes, hours, or (rarely) days. There has been one report of salivary gland enlargement in association with malignant hyperthermia[9]; here, of course, prompt treatment for the metabolic derangement of hyperthermia is mandatory (see pp. 305–307).

REFERENCES

1. Attas, M., Sabawala, P.B., and Keats, A.S.: Acute transient sialadenopathy during induction of anesthesia. Anesthesiology, *29*:1050, 1968.
2. Bonchek, L.I.: Salivary gland enlargement during induction of anesthesia. J.A.M.A., *209*:1716, 1969.
3. Reilly, D.J.: Benign transient swelling of the parotid glands following general anesthesia: "Anesthesia mumps." Anesth. Analg., *49*:560, 1970.
4. Smith, G.L., Mainous, E.G., and Crowell, N.T.: Unilateral submandibular gland swelling after induction of general anesthesia: Report of case. J. Oral Surg., *30*:911, 1972.
5. Couper, J.L.: Benign transient enlargement of the parotid glands associated with anaesthesia. S. Afr. Med. J., *47*:316, 1973.
6. Matsuki, A., Wakayama, S., and Oyama, T.: Acute transient swelling of the salivary glands during and following endotracheal anaesthesia. Anaesthetist, *28*:125, 1975.
7. Gordon, M.J.: Transient submandibular swelling following esophagogastroduodenoscopy. Dig. Dis., *21*:507, 1976.
8. Shields, H.M., Soloway, R.D., Long, W.B., et al.: Bilateral recurrent parotid gland swelling after endoscopy. Gastroenterology, *73*:164, 1977.
9. Katz, D.: Recurrent malignant hyperpyrexia during anesthesia. Anesth. Analg., *49*:225, 1970.

34 Dental Complications

Jeffrey G. Garber, D.M.D., and Andrew Herlich, D.M.D.

The clinical practice of anesthesia involves working in and about the oral cavity. In spite of this working relationship with the mouth, most anesthesiologists profess little knowledge of its hard and soft structures. Yet, understanding and recognizing significant oral pathological changes and differences in prosthetic restorations may aid the clinician in avoiding dental complications when he is providing anesthetic care.

The patient's expectations of competent anesthetic care include reasonable protection from dental injury, which can be demonstrated by a growing body of case law. Protection from dental injury can be assured only when precautionary measures based on a rational understanding of potential hazards are undertaken. Since recognition is the first step toward prevention, and since most dental complications that occur during anesthetic care are usually a direct result of unrecognized potential problems, a major aim of this chapter is to develop a basic awareness of normal and abnormal oral structure.

DEVELOPMENT OF DENTITION

At birth, the oral cavity is usually devoid of teeth. The gum pads are relatively firm in comparision with other oral tissue but must be protected from trauma during airway manipulation. The oral structure of most significance to airway management is the tongue. The relative macroglossia of infants should be noted.

By the age of about 6 months, the primary (deciduous) dentition begins to erupt and is usually complete by 2 years of age (Table 34-1). When complete, the primary dentition consists of 20 teeth (10 maxillary, 10 mandibular). There are important differences in tooth morphology between the primary and permanent (adult, succedaneous) dentition. The primary teeth are smaller than their permanent analogues. Roots of primary teeth tend to be long and slender following initial development and are resorbed as eruption of the underlying adult teeth progresses. When the roots of these primary teeth have nearly been resorbed, they are held in place by only ligamentous and soft-tissue attachments. Hence, there is excessive mobility owing to the loss of alveolar support.

The eruption of the permanent dentition generally begins at age 6 and is usually complete by age 13 or 14, with the exception of the third molars (wisdom teeth; see Table 34-1). The third molars have an extremely variable sequence of eruption, if they erupt at all.[1-4] A mixed dentition consisting of primary and permanent teeth is present during this period of exfoliation and eruption (Table 34-1). When complete, the adult dentition consists of 32 teeth: 16 maxillary teeth and 16 mandibular teeth.

PEDIATRIC DENTAL COMPLICATIONS

During infancy, laryngoscopy may cause damage to the gum pads and soft oral mucosal linings.

Table 34-1   Chronology of the Human Dentition

TOOTH	ERUPTION	ROOT COMPLETED	EXFOLIATION
Primary Dentition			
Maxillary			
Central incisor	7½ mos.	1½ yrs.	7 yrs.
Lateral incisor	9 mos.	2 yrs.	8 yrs.
Cuspid	18 mos.	3¼ yrs.	11 yrs.
First molar	14 mos.	2½ yrs.	9 yrs.
Second molar	24 mos.	3 yrs.	11 yrs.
Mandibular			
Central incisor	6 mos.	1½ yrs.	6 yrs.
Lateral incisor	7 mos.	1½ yrs.	7 yrs.
Cuspid	16 mos.	3¼ yrs.	10 yrs.
First molar	12 mos.	2¼ yrs.	9 yrs.
Second molar	20 mos.	3 yrs.	10 yrs.
Permanent Dentition			
Maxillary			
Central incisor	7- 8 yrs.	10 yrs.	
Lateral incisor	8- 9 yrs.	11 yrs.	
Cuspid	11-12 yrs.	13-15 yrs.	
First bicuspid	10-11 yrs.	12-13 yrs.	
Second biscuspid	10-12 yrs.	12-14 yrs.	
First molar	6- 7 yrs.	9-10 yrs.	
Second molar	12-13 yrs.	14-16 yrs.	
Mandibular			
Central incisor	6- 7 yrs.	9 yrs.	
Lateral incisor	7- 8 yrs.	10 yrs.	
Cuspid	9-10 yrs.	12-14 yrs.	
First bicuspid	10-12 yrs.	12-13 yrs.	
Second biscuspid	11-12 yrs.	13-14 yrs.	
First molar	6- 7 yrs.	9-10 yrs.	
Second molar	11-13 yrs.	14-15 yrs.	

(Modified from Logan, W.H.G., and Kronfeld, R.: Development of the human jaws and surrounding structures from birth to the age of 15 years. D. Record, *20*:379, 1933, and Parfitt, G.J.: Variations in the age of shedding of deciduous teeth and eruption of permanent teeth. J.A.D.A., *20*:279, 1954)

Trauma to the gum pads owing to laryngoscopy or compression secondary to the presence of an orotracheal tube may lead to infection and injury of the unerupted tooth buds and result in maleruption or abnormal development.[5,6] Traumatic injury to the oral mucosa of neonates and infants is particularly likely because of the relatively large tongue, which affords a small working space to the anesthesiologist. Macroglossia frequently contributes also to the difficulty of maintaining the airway. When airway support is necessary, the use of a lubricant facilitates the placement of an oropharyngeal airway and may prevent needless trauma.[5]

Eruption of the primary dentition proceeds from about 6 months to 2 years of age. When children of this age undergo surgery, anesthesiologists must be prepared to care for these teeth. Premature loss may lead to malocclusion and abnormal development of the permanent teeth. When developmentally complete, the slender roots of the primary teeth are prone to fracture during laryngoscopy if undue pressures are placed upon them. Also, oropharyngeal airways frequently used as bite blocks during general anesthesia contact the teeth in the incisor region and exert inappropriate forces on these teeth (Fig. 34-1A). If additional force is exerted when the patient bites or clamps down on the airway, then the likelihood of fracture or displacement of these incisor teeth is increased greatly. If a bite block is needed to prevent the endotracheal tube from being compressed, then the use of a suitable mouth prop, placed in the posterior portion of the mouth and supported by the molar teeth, is preferred (Fig. 34-1B,C). The molar teeth are positioned in such a manner that evenly distributes the forces along their long axis and makes fracture less likely. Similarly, if a mouth gag is required for the surgical procedure (e.g., tonsillectomy), one should choose a broad-bladed gag that distributes pressure over a wide area.

Once development of the primary dentition is complete at age 2, a period follows in which the resorption of these teeth progresses as the underlying permanent successors erupt. This process continues until the last primary molar is exfoliated at about age 11. As the primary roots are resorbed, the teeth lose their alveolar support and loosen. This makes avulsion of these teeth considerably more likely during routine manipulation in the mouth.

Hence, preoperative visual examination of the teeth alone is not sufficient to assess their mobility, for their appearance will be the same as the other nonmobile teeth. Children should be asked which teeth are loose, and examination should follow to determine the extent of mobility. When it appears that teeth can be removed easily by fingertip pressure, then elective preoperative removal is indicated. If it is necessary to remove a loose primary tooth during a general anesthetic, this can be accomplished easily by grasping the tooth with a gauze pad and applying a quick twisting and snapping motion. Caution must be taken by placing a gauze pack in the back of the mouth, to prevent the tooth from being swallowed or aspirated.

It is important to remember that should a tooth be avulsed, it must be located and recovered. In almost all cases, the recovered primary tooth consists of only a crown, as the roots are normally resorbed.

With the many advances of pediatric dentistry and the early recognition and treatment of orthodontic problems, anesthesiologists encounter a

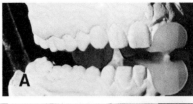
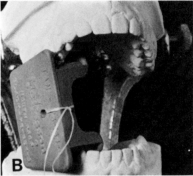
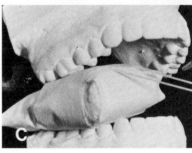

Fig. 34-1. Application of bite blocks. (*A*) An oropharyngeal airway placed in the midline subjects the incisors to forces that tend to displace or fracture them. Injury occurs because the incisors are aligned so that they normally slide over one another; now they must absorb forces normally absorbed by the premolars and molars. As a result, the upper incisors tend to move forward and the lower incisors tend to dislocate. In contrast, (*B*) a rubber or (*C*) an adhesive tape-covered gauze mouth prop placed posteriorly over the premolars and molars allows the distribution of force over sturdier, multi-rooted teeth that are aligned in the axis of the applied force.[5] Strings are attached to mouth props to facilitate their removal.

wide variety of oral appliances in daily practice. These appliances function to maintain spaces where premature loss of primary teeth has occurred, to correct malocclusions, and to break

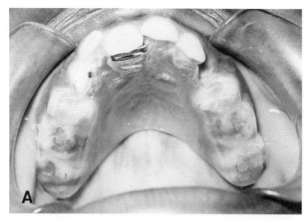

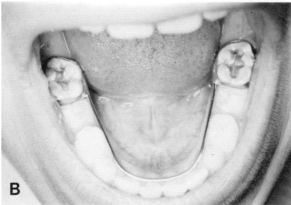

Fig. 34-2. Orthodontic retainers that may dislodge during airway manipulations and result in airway obstruction. (Courtesy of John Hunter, D.D.S.)

existing oral habits, such as thumb sucking and tongue thrust. Oral appliances may be fixed permanently in place, or they may be removable. Some may even interfere with space in the oral cavity and make placement of airway adjuncts difficult or impossible. In particular, appliances used for breaking tongue thrusting and thumb sucking often hang down from the hard palate and interfere with the free space above the tongue. Removable space maintainers, such as orthodontic retainers, if not recognized, may loosen during airway manipulation and become obstructive hazards (Fig. 34-2). Particular care must be taken to avoid damaging permanent appliances, for often these are quite costly. When necessary, dental consultation to ascertain the best methods

of protection is indicated. Anesthesiologists should protect the primary teeth as they would the permanent teeth. Damage or loss to these teeth may lead to severe occlusal and untoward developmental sequelae.

DENTAL COMPLICATIONS IN ADULTS

An adult's dentition, like a child's, presents potential hazards to unwary anesthesiologists. Teeth basically consist of enamel, a hard, heavily calcified outer layer; dentin, a softer, partially clacified organic matrix that underlies the enamel; and an innermost pulpal tissue, composed of vascular and neural elements.[2,3,7] Normal teeth have an exposed crown, supported by unexposed roots housed in the alveolus of the maxilla and mandible.

Functionally, the anterior teeth consisting of incisors and canines have single roots, as well as crowns that slice food. The maxillary and mandibular antagonists overlap slightly in the normal occlusion and have a slight forward inclination, which subjects them to the risk of being used as a fulcrum during laryngoscopy. The posterior teeth, the premolars and molars, are multirooted and function to grind food and support the occlusion. The multiple roots of the molar impart a significant lateral and vertical stability to the tooth in the arch. Because of the stability of the posterior dentition, a bite block should be placed in this area of the mouth, as opposed to the more usual anterior resting place (Fig. 34-1). The bite block acts as a wedge between the vertex of the angle formed by the maxilla and the mandible and provides maximum separation between the anterior teeth. However, a bite block placed between the incisors permits minimal opening of the mouth and subjects these teeth to greater chances of fracture or displacement. The oropharyngeal airway should be used as an airway and not as a bite block.[5,8] If an oropharyngeal airway is needed, a flexible plastic airway is preferred to a metal airway.

Fracture, Displacement, and Avulsion

Since the incisor teeth, positionally and structurally, are the most likely to fracture, some anesthesiologists utilize commercially produced, rubber or plastic tooth guards during laryngoscopy. However, the use of tooth guards is probably not necessary on a routine basis if proper technic is utilized during laryngoscopy. In addition, the tooth guard may give anesthesiologists a false sense of security, and fracture of the anterior teeth can still occur when excessive forces are applied.[9]

Rarely, a skilled anesthesiologist causes fracture, displacement, or avulsion of a permanent tooth. When this misfortune occurs, he should know the proper steps to take as well as the possible sequelae. Fractures of the teeth may involve the crown or root, may be displaced or nondisplaced, and may not require treatment. Root fractures may easily go unnoticed until oral radiographs reveal them, or they may be suspected when the patient complains of pain or if there is excessive mobility. There is little danger to the patient during the intraoperative period, unless the root fracture is associated with avulsion.

Coronal fractures may involve the outer enamel layer only or also the underlying dentinal layer and vital pulp tissue. If displacement of a portion of the crown occurs, location of the missing piece is imperative. Postoperatively, restorative dentistry can return fractured teeth to satisfactory esthetics and normal function. Fractures within the dentinal layer may cause the patient to experience pain and thermal sensitivity. Symptomatic relief of this discomfrot may be required until the tooth is restored. When the tooth is damaged to the point of exposing the vital pulp tissue, there is usually postoperative pain, and endodontic or oral surgical treatment is indicated.[10]

Total or partial avulsion of teeth is unfortunate and, with the rarest of exceptions, can be avoided by careful laryngoscopic technique and airway placement. Partially avulsed teeth usually can be pushed back into position at the time of the incident. Postoperatively, the tooth should be splinted to allow healing of the disrupted ligamentous attachment. The need for future endodontic treatment is likely. When total avulsion occurs, immediate retrieval is necessary. Frequently, the avulsed teeth are found in the mouth or nearby drapes. If it is impossible to locate the tooth, complete radiographs of the head, neck, chest, and abdomen may be required. The unconscious anesthetized patient can easily aspirate not only the avulsed tooth itself, but also restorative portions of the tooth: the crown, inlay, silver filling, or composite filling.

If an avulsed tooth is found, then reimplanting it in its socket should be considered. In order to preserve the delicate periodontal ligament attached to the tooth, it should be rinsed gently in cold physiologic saline prior to reimplantation. The reimplanted tooth should be shielded from further trauma and then splintered as soon as possible.[10,11]

Dental Disease That Predisposes Patients to Injury

Rampant caries refers to decay of gross proportions, affecting almost all of the existing teeth. Young adults and children are most likely to present with this advanced disease. Particularly characteristic is the circumferential location of much of the decay in the cervical area of the crown, that is, at the gumline. Decay in this area undermines the support of the crown and makes fracture more likely when forces are directed against it. Contributing factors for this aggressive carious process include salivary composition, diet, oral hygiene, and composition of oral flora. Xerostomia secondary to head and neck radiation, Mikulicz's disease, and Sjögren's syndrome make the finding of cervical caries more likely.[12,13] When this condition is noted by an anesthesiologist, additional care must be taken to prevent tooth fracture during laryngoscopy and airway insertion.

Periodontal disease, sometimes called *pyorrhea*, is probably the most widespread chronic disease in the world. It primarily affects adults over the age of 25; significant changes affecting anesthetic care occur after age 40. At present it is best defined as a multifactorial disease, resulting in an inflammatory destruction of the bony and ligamentous support of the teeth.[14] The overlying gingival tissues also undergo characteristic inflammatory changes. The resulting tooth mobility from loss of supporting structures may be

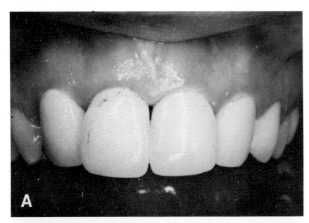

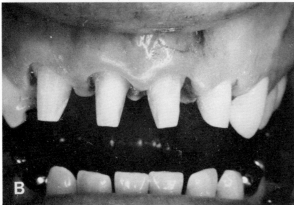

Fig. 34-3. (*A*) Underlying esthetically pleasing crowns are (*B*) structurally weak teeth. (Courtesy of John Hunter, D.D.S.)

minimal or in advanced states may cause spontaneous exfoliation or avulsion when the tooth is minimally traumatized. For this reason, it is imperative that anesthesiologists be aware of loose teeth preoperatively.

Peridontosis, an idiopathic degenerative destruction of alveolar bone that is now thought to be a very early and aggressive form of peridontal disease, is also of interest to anesthesiologists. It tends to affect patients between puberty and age 30 and is more common in blacks than whites. During this age span, one would not expect to find advanced tooth mobility. The most severely affected teeth are the incisors and first molars. The teeth appear extruded and loosened without significant gingival changes.[14]

Dentinogenesis imperfecta, also known as hereditary opalescent dentin, is a rare dominantly inherited disturbance that results in discolored, structurally weak teeth and affects both the primary and permanent dentition. The teeth have a peculiar opalescent brown color and are fractured or abraded easily. Associated with this condition, some patients have osteogenesis imperfecta with unusually brittle bones and, in many cases, blue sclerae. Any airway manipulation may damage these weak teeth.[4,13] Frequently these teeth are fitted with full coverage crowns soon after eruption.

Problems Related to Dental Prostheses

Prosthetic correction of dental disease states involves the splinting, replacement, and repair of mobile, missing, or broken teeth. These appliances may be fixed or removable, and they may involve individual teeth, groups of teeth, or complete arches. These prosthetic restorations may improve esthetics or function, or both. They are particularly prone to breakage and are likely to cause airway interference or obstruction.

Individual crowns or bridges (a series of crowns joined together) are subject to the greatest risk of fracture and avulsion. Crowns and bridges are made from porcelain, from procelain fused to metal (gold or nonprecious metal), from pure metal, from acrylic fused to metal, and from pure acrylic.[15] It is usually the porcelain and acrylic portions that are liable to fracture under pressure from undue forces. Porcelain crowns are particularly delicate and are usually found in the front of the mouth. Any tooth prepared for a crown has been greatly reduced structurally and is therefore at greater risk to fracture (Fig. 34-3).

All fixed restorations such as crowns and bridges require cement. Difficult or improper laryngoscopy may result in dislodgement of the prosthesis owing to breakage of the cement bond. If dislodgement of a crown or bridge occurs, retrieval of it and protection of the remaining tooth structure with an oil-soluble lubricant, such as petroleum jelly, are sufficient.

The removal prosthetic appliances likely to be encountered by anesthesiologists include the partial denture and full denture. A partial denture in most instances consists of a metal framework of chrome-colbalt upon which rests acrylic, in which porcelain or plastic teeth are embedded. The partial denture is held in place by metal arms or clasps that partially surround selected teeth.

Partial dentures tend to exert excessive forces upon the teeth to which they are clasped. This may cause advanced loss of bony support with resultant tooth mobility and risk of avulsion. It is helpful for anesthesiologists to have patients remove the partial denture during the preoperative visit and then to inspect the edentulous area and surrounding teeth for evidence of trauma, mobility, and loss of structural integrity (e.g., broken teeth).

Patients should be instructed to remove a partial denture before undergoing surgery, for dislodgment may occur at an inappropriate time and lead to airway obstruction.[16,17] Prostheses may also be swallowed and require surgical removal.[4]

As the name implies, *full dentures* replace a complete arch of teeth. For the most part, they are made from processed acrylic bases with either porcelain or plastic teeth.[18] Full dentures, like other prosthetic devices, are prone to fracture and may become an obstructive hazard because they are not permanently secured in the mouth. As with partial dentures, anesthesiologists should inspect the oral mucosa under the dentures for areas of trauma and describe these areas in the preoperative note. In most cases, patients are instructed to remove their dentures prior to surgery. However, sometimes tight-fitting dentures worn during surgery aid mask fit and airway management by supporting the facial skin and musculature. When laryngoscopy is attempted, the dentures should be removed and stored in a cup with water for return to the patient postoperatively.[5,8]

Since dental prostheses are quite costly and frequently affect the patient's psyche, it behooves the anesthesiologist during his preoperative visit to ask the simple question, "Do you have any caps, crowns, or bridges?" Knowing the answer to this may prevent much intra- and postoperative difficulty.

Problems Related to Skeletal Abnormalities

Complications involving the teeth and their prosthetic replacements are more likely to occur in patients in whom laryngoscopy and placement of artificial airways are technically more difficult. Certainly patients with known orofacial skeletal abnormalities must be assessed particularly carefully to minimize dental trauma, because difficult airway management and manipulation are likely to be encountered. Other skeletal changes that involve the occlusive function of the temporomandibular joint may greatly increase the difficulty of airway management and thereby increase the likelihood of dental complications.

Skeletal malposition of the mandible frequently increases the difficulty of orotracheal intubation.[19] Patients with excessively protruding (prognathic) or retruding (retrognathic) mandibles are difficult for the unsuspecting anesthesiologist to intubate. Arch shape, as well as position, should alert the clinician to possible pitfalls. The narrow, arched maxilla and mandible usually cause a technically more difficult laryngoscopy (see Chap. 8).

Although they are rare, occasional hyperplastic or hypertrophic anomalies of the coronoid process cause significant limitation of mandibular movement.[20,21] More commonly, temporomandibular joint abnormalities or dysfunction may decrease mandibular movement sufficiently to make airway maintenance difficult. Arthritic and traumatic changes of the temporomandibular joint are the most likely etiologies. Others include acute reversible traumatic arthritis and condylar head and neck fractures[3,22,23] (see Chap. 8).

Soft-Tissue Injury

Oral soft-tissue injury may also occur during anesthetic care.[9,24,25] Difficult laryngoscopy, especially with extended periods of cricoid pressure, can result in transient lingual nerve injury. Typically, numbness and loss of taste appear on the 1st postoperative day and disappear within 1 to 4 weeks.[24,25] Laceration or abrasion of the lips, palate, and cheeks, with possible ulceration and infection, may occur as the result of careless placement of the laryngoscope blade.

CLINICAL RECOMMENDATIONS FOR PREVENTION OF DENTAL COMPLICATIONS

The special importance attached to teeth in our highly civilized society and the ease with which they may be damaged during the administration of anesthesia give rise to several general suggestions.[26] It is particularly important for anesthesiologists to maintain a constant awareness of the problems that can occur in the mouth.

As part of the preoperative visit, the anesthesiologist should note which of his patient's teeth are loose, decayed, or heavily restored; whether other oral disease that weakens support of the teeth may be present; where prosthetic devices are located; and whether direct laryngoscopy and tracheal intubation are likely to be difficult as a result of some skeletal abnormality. In children the location of recently erupted teeth ought to be noted, too, because both primary and permanent teeth have only partially formed roots when they erupt. Abnormalities should be mentioned briefly in the preanesthetic note. When the risk of dental complications seems high, the anesthesiologist should inform the patient and should consider ways to minimize the risk. Steps taken to minimize risk may include greater care in direct laryngoscopy and orotracheal intubation, the use of a nasopharyngeal rather than an oropharyngeal airway or nasotracheal rather than orotracheal intubation, general anesthesia without intubation, and regional analgesia instead of general anesthesia. However, regardless of which anesthetic technique is used, unavoidable dental complications may occur as a result of actions necessary in an emergency and constitute a risk that the surgical patient must accept.

Should a dental complication occur, the anesthesiologist should seek dental consultation, as well as describe the injury on the patient's chart. Displaced teeth should be placed in chilled saline for later reimplanation. If lost teeth and prostheses cannot be found, appropriate radiographs must be obtained. Finally, the anesthesiologist should tell the patient and his family of any dental complication that may have occurred.[5,26-28]

REFERENCES

1. Finn, S. B. (ed.): Clinical Pedodontics. pp. 45–70. Philadelphia, W. B. Saunders, 1973.
2. Kraus, B. S., Jordan, R. G., and Abrams, L.: A Study of the Masticatory System: Dental Anatomy and Occlusion. pp. 245–262. Baltimore, Williams & Wilkins, 1969.
3. Sicher, H., and DuBrul, L.: Oral Anatomy. ed. 6. pp. 217–252, 504–512. St. Louis, C. V. Mosby, 1975.
4. Zegarelli, E. V., and Kutsler, A. W.: Diagnosis of Diseases of the Mouth and Jaws. ed. 2. pp. 503–507. Philadelphia, Lea and Febiger, 1978.
5. Dornette, W. H. L., and Hughes, B. H.: Care of the teeth during anesthesia. Anesth. Analg., 38:206, 1959.
6. Boice, J. B., Krous, H. F., and Foley, J. M.: Gingival and dental complications of orotracheal intubation. J.A.MA., 236:957, 1976.
7. Ingle, J. D., and Langeland, K. E.: Etiology and prevention of pulp inflammation, necrosis and dystrophy. *In* Ingle, J. D., and Beveridge, E. E. (eds.): Endodontics. ed. 2. pp. 313–340. Philadelphia, Lea and Febiger, 1976.
8. Dornette, W. H. L.: Care of the teeth during endoscopy and anesthesia. Clin. Anesth., 8:217, 1972.
9. Applebaum, E. L., and Bruce, D. L.: Tracheal Intubation. p. 81. Philadelphia, W. B. Saunders, 1976.
10. Hale, M. L.: Traumatic injuries of the teeth and alveolar processes. *In* Kruger, G. O. (ed.): The Textbook of Oral Surgery. ed. 4. pp. 307–313. St. Louis, C. V. Mosby, 1974.
11. Boyne, P. J.: Tissue transplantation. *In* Kruger, G. O. (ed.): The Textbook of Oral Surgery. ed. 4. pp. 263–283. St. Louis, C. V. Mosby, 1974.
12. Lorhan, P. H.: Anesthesia for the Aged. p. 39. Springfield, Charles C Thomas, 1971.
13. Shafer, W. C., Hine, M. K., and Levy, B. M.: A Textbook of Oral Pathology. ed. 3. pp. 366–432, 622–664. Philadelphia, W. B. Saunders, 1974.
14. Glickman, I.: Clinical Periodontology. ed. 4. pp. 421–426. Philadelphia, W. B. Saunders, 1972.
15. Johnston, J. F., Phillips, R. W., and Dykema, R. W.: Modern Practice of Crown and Bridge Prosthodontics. ed. 3. pp. 72–101, 356–373, 381–534. Philadelphia, W.B. Saunders, 1971.
16. Mehta, R. M., and Pathak, P. N.: A foreign body in the larynx. Br. J. Anaesth., 45:755, 1973.
17. Nash, P. J.: A foreign body in the larynx. Br. J. Anaesth., 48:371, 1976.
18. Hearthwell, C. M., Jr., and Rahn, A. O.: Syllabus of Complete Dentures. ed. 2. pp. 81–89. Philadelphia, Lea and Febiger, 1974.
19. White, A., and Kander, P. L.: Anatomic factors in difficult direct laryngoscopy. Br. J. Anaesth., 47:468, 1975.
20. Allison, M. L., Wallance, W. R., and Von Wyl, H.: Coronoid abnormalities causing limitation of mandibular movement. J. Oral Surg., 27:229, 1969.
21. Shurman, J.: Bilateral hypertrophy of the coronoid processes. Anesthesiology, 42:491, 1975.
22. Shira, R. B., and Alling, C. C.: Traumatic injuries involving the temporomandibular joint articulation. *In* Schwartz, L., and Chayes, C. M. (eds.): Facial Pain and Mandibular Dysfunction. pp. 129–139. Philadelphia, W. B. Saunders, 1968.

23. Guralnick, W., Kaban, L. B., and Merrill, R. G.: Temporomandibular joint afflictions. N. Engl. J. Med., *299*:123, 1978.

24. Jones, B. C.: Lingual nerve injury: a complication of intubation. Br. J. Anaesth., *43*:730, 1971.

25. Teichner, R. L.: Lingual nerve injury: a complication of orotracheal anaesthesia. Br. J. Anaesth., *43*:413, 1971.

26. Wright, R. B., and Manfield, F. F. V.: Damage to teeth during the administration of general anesthesia. Medical Protection Society bulletin, reprinted in ASA Newsletter, May 1974.

27. Dripps, R. D., Eckenhoff, J. E., and Vandam, L. D.: Introduction to Anesthesia: The Principles of Safe Practice. ed. 5. pp. 11–21. Philadelphia, W. B. Saunders, 1977.

28. Jackson, C., and Jackson, C. L.: Bronchoesophagology. pp. 13–34. Philadelphia, W. B. Saunders, 1950.

FURTHER READING

Applebaum, E. L., and Bruce, D. L.: Tracheal Intubation. Philadelphia, W. B. Saunders, 1976.

Finn, S. B. (ed.): Clinical Pedodontics. Philadelphia, W. B. Saunders, 1973.

Dornette, W. H. L.: Care of the teeth during endoscopy and anesthesia. Clin. Anesth., 8:213, 1972.

Shafer, W. C., Hine, M. K., and Levy, B. M.: A Textbook of Oral Pathology. ed. 3, Philadelphia, W. B. Saunders, 1974.

Part Nine

The Blood

35 Problems Posed by Transfusion

Ronald D. Miller, M.D.

When blood stored in either acid-citrate dextrose (ACD) solution or citrate-phosphate-dextrose (CPD) solution is infused, problems such as coagulation defects, adverse metabolic changes, or hepatitis may occur. This chapter describes the diagnosis and treatment of these problems.

ACD- VERSUS CPD-STORED BLOOD

Whole blood is stored in either ACD or CPD solution. Although most of the problems described here apply to both ACD- and CPD-stored blood, there are two major exceptions: Red blood cells and 2,3-diphosphoglycerate (2,3-DPG), an organic phosphate affecting the affinity of hemoglobin for oxygen, are better maintained in CPD solution. By definition, blood is deemed unsuitable for transfusion, and thus considered outdated, when the 24-hour post-transfusion survival of the transfused red cells is less than 70 per cent. Blood becomes outdated by this criterion when stored for 21 days in ACD solution and 28 days in CPD solution. Despite better survival of red blood cells, blood legally cannot be infused when it has been stored in CPD solution longer than 21 days. Intraerythrocytic 2,3-DPG levels decrease rapidly during the first 4 to 5 days of storage in ACD solution. A similar decrease in 2,3-DPG levels does not occur in CPD-stored blood until after about 2 weeks (Fig. 35-1). Although the phosphate present in CPD solution is helpful in maintaining ATP levels, the slightly higher pH of that solution accounts for the greater 2,3-DPG levels.[1] Other differences between ACD- and CPD-stored blood are the following: CPD solution has citrate and potassium levels that are 20 per cent lower; the pH of CPD-stored blood is approximately 0.1 to 0.3 units higher; ATP levels are better maintained in CPD-stored blood; although the volumes of microaggregates are about the same in blood stored in either solution, the particles are larger in CPD-stored blood.

Although not enormous, the advantages appear sufficient to indicate that blood should be stored in CPD rather than ACD solution. In spite of these advantages, coagulation, pulmonary and metabolic problems, and transfusion reactions occur when blood is stored in either solution.

2,3-DIPHOSPHOGLYCERATE AND THE OXYHEMOGLOBIN DISSOCIATION CURVE

In 1954, Valtis and Kennedy described a leftward shift of the oxyhemoglobin dissociation curve in vitro. The magnitude of this shift is related directly to the time blood has been stored.[2] After transfusion of ACD or CPD blood stored 7 days or longer, the dissociation curves of all patients also shift to the left. The magnitude of the leftward shift is related to volume and storage

461

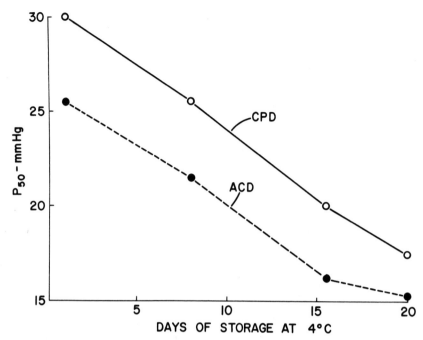

Fig. 35-1. Relationship between P_{50} (P_{O_2} at which hemoglobin is 50% saturated with oxygen) and days of storage of ACD- and CPD-stored blood. (Dawson, R. B., Jr., and Ellis, T. J.: Hemoglobin function of blood stored at 4°C in ACD and CPD with adenine and inosine. Transfusion, *10:* 113, 1970)

time of the infused blood. In some cases, the curve remains shifted to the left for as long as 24 hours after transfusion.

This observation was largely ignored until 1965. However, many investigators have suggested recently that because of the leftward shift in the dissociation curve, tissue hypoxia may develop from infusion of stored blood.

The Oxyhemoglobin Dissociation Curve

The oxyhemoglobin dissociation curve is obtained by plotting the partial pressure of oxygen (P_{O_2}) in blood against the per cent of hemoglobin saturated with oxygen (Fig. 35-2).

As hemoglobin becomes more saturated, its affinity for oxygen also increases. This is reflected in the sigmoid shape of the curve, which indicates that a decrease in $P_{A_{O_2}}$ makes considerably more oxygen available to the tissues than if the curve were straight. This allows greater efficiency of blood transport of oxygen to the tissues.

Shifts in the dissociation curve are quantitated by the P_{50}, which, by convention, is that partial pressure of oxygen at which hemoglobin is half saturated at 37°C and *p*H of 7.4. A low P_{50} indicates a left shift in the oxygen dissociation curve and an increased affinity of hemoglobin for oxygen. Thus, with the leftward shift of the curve, a lower than normal oxygen partial pressure will saturate hemoglobin in the lung, and the subsequent release of oxygen to the tissues will occur at a capillary oxygen partial pressure that is lower than normal. An increased affinity may be enough to insure that oxygen will not be released to the tissues, unless tissue P_{O_2} is in the hypoxic range. The theoretical and clinical evidence supporting the hypothesis, that tissues may become hypoxic during infusion of stored blood with a low P_{50}, is discussed below.

Theoretical Evidence That Stored Blood Interferes with Oxygen Delivery to Tissues

A close relationship between oxygen affinity of stored blood and intraerythrocytic 2,3-DPG has

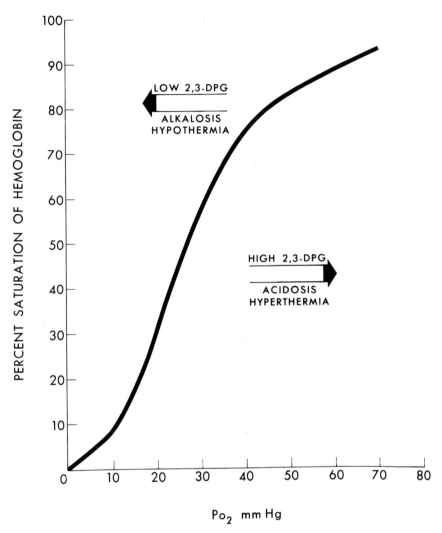

Fig. 35-2. Factors that shift position of the oxyhemoglobin dissociation curve.

been established.[3,4] The 2,3-DPG levels decrease with both CPD- and ACD-stored blood, although the decrease is less in CPD-stored blood (Fig. 39-1). For example, after storage for 7 days in ACD solution, the normal P_{50} and 2,3-DPG levels of 26.5 torr (3.5 kPa) and 4.8 μmol. per ml., respectively, are decreased to 18 torr (2.4 kPa) and 1.0 μmol. per ml. Alkalosis and hypothermia shift the curve leftward even more (Fig. 35-2).

Oftentimes, in studies of tissue oxygenation, mixed venous oxygen partial pressure (Pv_{O_2}) is measured, for it reflects the relationship between oxygen consumption and cardiac output. A low Pv_{O_2} suggests that the cardiac output cannot meet tissue oxygen demands. Studies in rats undergoing exchange transfusion with ACD-stored, 2,3-DPG-depleted blood suggest that impaired tissue oxygenation may occur. After infusion of ACD-stored blood, skin bubble oxygen partial pressure (a measure of Pa_{O_2}), central venous oxygen tension, and P_{50} decrease significantly and remain depressed for at least 9 hours.[5] These values decrease even more in acidotic rats.[6] Infusion with fresh blood instead of ACD-stored blood results in minimal changes in these measurements. These studies suggest that massive transfusion with ACD- or CPD-stored blood does interfere with delivery of oxygen to the tissues.

Clinical Evidence That Stored Blood Interferes With Oxygen Delivery to Tissues

The clinical evidence of the effects of storage is not consistent and reflects the difficulty of conducting a systematic study of seriously ill patients in varied clinical settings. Kopriva found that 2,3-DPG levels increased in severely injured battle casualties, each of whom had received 12 or more units of ACD-stored blood.[7] Furthermore, transfusion of fresh or stored blood did not influence 2,3-DPG levels. Yet, the more common finding is that P_{50} and 2,3-DPG levels do decrease following infusion of stored blood.[8] The resultant left shift in the oxyhemoglobin dissociation curve and the increased affinity for oxygen may increase cardiac output and work of the heart.* If a patient has marginal cardiac reserve and cannot increase cardiac output, tissue hypoxia may result.

Although the evidence is suggestive, it has not been shown that specific organ hypoxia results from infusion of blood with a low P_{50} or increased affinity for oxygen. In fact, Bowen and Fleming have shown that arteriovenous oxygen extraction by organs or tissues may not be altered by changes in oxyhemoglobin affinity, although affinity increases after transfusion of stored blood, particularly if compensatory flow occurs at the capillary level.[9] This compensatory flow may open capillaries; this permits increased blood flow to tissues and thereby increases cardiac output and reduces the capillary-tissue gradient to maintain the rate of tissue oxygen extraction.

Clinical Implications of the Effects of Stored Blood

Because of its low P_{50} and increased oxyhemoglobin affinity, assessment of specific organ function is necessary to substantiate the possible injurious effects of stored blood. Since such data are not yet available, conclusions are difficult to

*Personal communication, C. R. Valeri.

make. If the increased oxyhemoglobin affinity is important, it can be minimized by the following steps:

Steps to Minimize Increased Oxyhemoglobin Affinity of Stored Blood

Warm all blood.
Avoid excessive bicarbonate administration.
Use CPD- rather than ACD-stored blood.
Infuse blood that has been stored less than 5 to 7 days in patients whose cardiac output cannot be increased. (This may be difficult for most blood banks to accomplish.)
If available, use frozen blood,[10] which remains unchanged metabolically during frozen storage.

COAGULATION DEFECTS

The major causes of a hemorrhagic diathesis, which may include bleeding from venipuncture sites, excessive oozing of blood into the surgical field, hematuria, gingival bleeding, ecchymoses, or petechiae, are the following:

Major Causes of Hemorrhagic Diathesis

Dilutional thrombocytopenia
Low levels of factors V and VIII
Disseminated intravascular coagulation (DIC) and fibrinolysis
Hemolytic transfusion reaction

Blood transfusion-induced coagulopathies often present a vicious cycle. The bleeding is usually caused by blood that lacks certain coagulation factors. To replace a continuing blood loss, more ACD- or CPD-stored blood must be given; yet, this is the blood that initially caused coagulopathy. Thus, a bleeding tendency may be exacerbated by infusion of the required amount of stored blood; this establishes the vicious cycle, which must be interrupted by appropriate therapy.

Thrombocytopenia

In our experience, dilutional thrombocytopenia is the most important cause of a hemorrhagic diathesis from transfusion.[11] Although primarily quantitative, the platelet defect is also qualita-

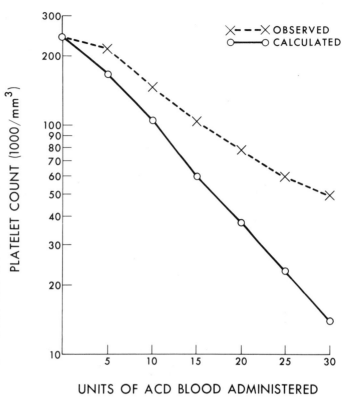

Fig. 35-3. Comparison between mean observed platelet counts in 21 patients receiving more than 15 units of ACD-stored blood and platelet count (predicted) in a person receiving platelet-free blood. The moderately close approximation of these two curves suggests that the thrombocytopenia is dilutional, resulting from infusion of platelet-free solutions (ACD blood stored for longer than 24 hours). (Miller, R. D., Robbins, T. O., and Tong, M. J.: Coagulation defects associated with massive blood transfusions. Ann. Surg., *174:* 794, 1971)

tive, and a storage temperature of 4°C accounts for most of the damage to platelets.[12] Taking into account viability and survival time, platelets retain only 60 per cent of their hemostatic function after 3 hours of storage. After 24 hours, only 12 per cent of the original platelet function is still present. When blood stored for more than 24 hours is infused, especially in patients who have lost large amounts of blood, the available platelet pool is diluted (Fig. 35-3). When the platelet count decreases below 65,000 per mm.[3], a bleeding problem is likely to develop.[11,12]

Utilization of the absolute platelet count alone can be criticized. For example, patients with leukemia may have platelet counts of less than 10,000 per mm.[3] and yet not bleed. However, these patients have *chronic* thrombocytopenias but no large surgical wounds. In patients without a chronic bleeding problem, spontaneous bleeding begins when the patelet count is less than about 65,000 per mm.[3]

Factors V and VIII

Although levels of factors V and VIII gradually decrease to 20 to 50 per cent of normal after 21 days of storage, these usually are not low enough to be the primary cause of a bleeding diathesis.[11,13] Therefore, the practice of giving fresh frozen plasma containing all the clotting factors except platelets, either prophylactically or therapeutically for bleeding from blood transfusion, is questionable. A possible exception may be patients with liver disease who are unable to produce these clotting factors.

DIC and Fibrinolysis

DIC and fibrinolysis have been reported to occur in patients given bank blood[14] and in patients undergoing certain operative procedures, such as removal of abruptio placenta,[15] prostatic surgery,[16] portocaval shunt, and neurosurgery resulting in brain injury.[17] Although the precise

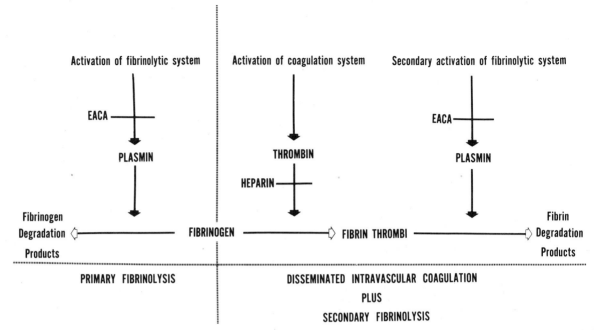

Fig. 35-4. Schematic representation of primary fibrinolysis and fibrinolysis secondary to disseminated intravascular coagulation. Although EACA inhibits primary fibrinolysis, it also inhibits secondary fibrinolysis, one of the main defenses against DIC. (Miller, R. D.: Complications of massive blood transfusion. Anesthesiology, *39:* 82, 1973)

causes are unknown, some hormone or toxic material releases tissue thromboplastin as a result. The thromboplastin, in turn, triggers the coagulation system, resulting in consumption and, therefore, decreased blood levels of factors I, II, V, and VIII and platelets. Thrombi and fibrin are deposited in the microcirculation of vital tissues, possibly interrupting their blood flow. In response to this hypercoagulable state, the fibrinolytic system is activated, lysing some of the excess fibrin. This is called *secondary fibrinolysis* (Fig. 35-4); primary fibrinolysis refers to activation of the fibrinolytic system without concomitant DIC. Heparin is used for treatment of DIC with secondary fibrinolysis, while epsilon-aminocaproic acid (EACA) is used to treat primary fibrinolysis.

Specific diagnosis of a bleeding problem, particularly in the operating room, is difficult. This is especially true if the bleeding problem occurs at times when the coagulation laboratory cannot perform diagnostic tests. The following tests are helpful: platelet count; partial thromboplastin time; plasma fibrinogen level; examination of a clot for lysis; and examination of plasma for free hemoglobin.[18,19]

If the platelet count is less than 100,000 per mm.[3], thrombocytopenia may be the cause of bleeding[11]; if the count is less than 50,000 per mm.[3], this diagnosis is confirmed. Treatment consists of administration of fresh blood stored for less than 6 hours or platelet concentrates. One unit of platelet concentrate will increase the platelet count approximately 10,000 per mm.[3] If the partial thromboplastin time is increased and all other coagulation tests are normal, the bleeding is probably a result of low levels of factors V and VIII.[11] Although this is unusual, it can be treated with fresh frozen plasma that contains all the coagulation factors except platelets.

Plasma fibrinogen levels are almost normal in bank blood. Therefore, hypofibrinogenemia (<150 mg./dl.) is unlikely to result from dilutional coagulopathy and, if present, strongly suggests fibrinolysis and/or DIC. Although the inhibition of plasmin by EACA administration is an effec-

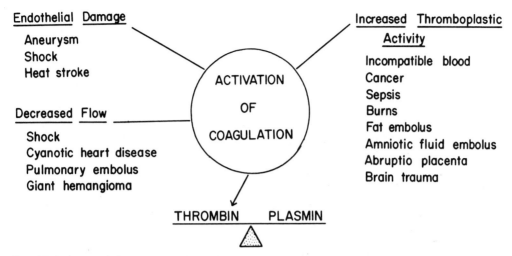

Fig. 35-5. Some of the many causes of activation of the coagulation mechanism leading to thrombin deposition and resultant disseminated intravascular coagulation.

tive treatment for primary fibrinolysis, it may enhance DIC by attenuating secondary fibrinolysis,[20] which represents one of the few defenses against extensive thrombosis in DIC. Since tests to distinguish primary from secondary fibrinolysis are not readily available, EACA should be given only after a patient is heparinized[21] and in conjunction with expert consultation. Although controversial, primary fibrinolysis either does not exist or is almost always secondary to DIC,[22] thus casting further doubt on the wisdom of EACA administration.

Although theoretically sound, the efficacy of heparin therapy for DIC is questionable, because DIC is not a distinct disease but rather a manifestation of a number of diseases (Fig. 35-5). If the precipitating cause of DIC (e.g., hypovolemic shock or sepsis) is eliminated, it will stop without heparin administration. But, if the precipitating cause is not eliminated, heparin administration will not improve survival.[23] Thus, the role of heparin therapy probably is limited to restoring the platelet count and fibrinogen level and attenuating bleeding while the precipitating cause is treated. (We usually start with 50 units/kg. of heparin intravenously.) Additional determinations of the platelet count and fibrinogen level in 2 to 4 hours may indicate a need for more heparin. When laboratory results indicate that platelet counts have begun to return to normal and the

intensity of the bleeding is decreased, heparin therapy may be discontinued. After the administration of heparin, the "consumed" factors, such as fibrinogen and platelets, may have to be replaced in the form of fresh blood, platelet concentrates, or fresh frozen plasma. Administration of these factors before heparin is administered results only in their consumption.

METABOLIC CHANGES

Acid-Base Balance

The *p*H of ACD and CPD solution is approximately 5.0 and 5.5, respectively. When either solution is added to a unit of freshly drawn blood, the *p*H of the blood immediately decreases to approximately 7.0 to 7.1. Owing to accumulation of lactic and pyruvic acids from erythrocyte metabolism and glycolysis, the *p*H of bank blood continues to decrease to about 6.6 after 21 days of storage. Much of the acidosis can be explained by the P_{CO_2} of 150 to 220 torr (20.0–29.3 kPa; see Table 35-1). The P_{CO_2} is high because the plastic blood container does not permit escape of carbon dioxide; however, with adequate pulmonary ventilation in the recipient, the high P_{CO_2} should be of little consequence.

Even when P_{CO_2} is returned to 40 torr (5.3 kPa), acidosis is still present in stored blood (Table 35-1), and some physicians recommend that alka-

Table 35-1. Comparison of Values in Normal and ACD-stored Whole Blood

	NORMAL RANGE	AFTER 14 DAYS OF STORAGE
pH	7.40	6.6–6.9
Pa_{CO_2}	40 torr (5.3kPa)	150–210 torr (20.0–27.9kPa)
Base deficit	Zero	9–15 mEq./L.
Factors V and VIII	100% of normal	20 to 50% of normal
Potassium	3.5–5.0 mEq./L. (3.5–5.0 mmol./L.)	18–26 mEq./L. (18–26 mmol./L.)
Temperature	37°C	4 to 6°C

linizing agents be given empirically. For example Howland and Schweizer recommend intravenous administration of sodium bicarbonate, 44.6 mEq. for every 5 units of bank blood infused, particularly in patients who have abnormal respiratory or renal compensatory mechanisms.[24] Recently, more controlled studies have indicated that empirical administration of sodium bicarbonate is not indicated. Furthermore, it may actually be unwise without concommitant analysis of arterial blood for P_{CO_2} and pH.[25,26] We found that the acid-base response to blood transfusion is quite variable (Fig. 35-6).[26] There is little logic in empirical administration of bicarbonate for prophylactic treatment of an unpredictable acid-base abnormality.

Bicarbonate therapy should be started when metabolic acidosis is diagnosed by analysis of arterial blood for Pa_{CO_2} and pH. We perform these measurements after administration of each 5 units of blood.[18,26] When a suitable artery is inaccessible during a particular operative procedure, peripheral venous blood can be utilized for these determinations. During anesthesia, the Pv_{O_2} of peripheral venous blood is usually greater than 60 torr (8.6 kPa); therefore, this blood is arterialized, Pa_{CO_2} and pH can be determined, and the amount of bicarbonate required can be calculated.[27] The total bicarbonate deficit is approximated as follows:

$$\text{(Body weight in kilograms) (0.4)} \times ([HCO_3']_{\text{desired}} - [HCO_3']_{\text{measured}})$$

Customarily, about half of the calculated deficit is administered, and the patient is reevaluated. If the patient's serum potassium concentration is low initially or a large bicarbonate deficit is corrected, one should monitor the serum potassi-

um level as well, because potassium enters the cell during correction of acidosis and hypokalemia may result.

Although treatment of metabolic acidosis with bicarbonate is important, is there any harm from excessive bicarbonate administration or its resultant metabolic alkalosis? Alkalosis augments a left shift of the oxyhemoglobin dissociation curve. Because of the citrate metabolism, exogenous bicarbonate, and administration of Ringer's lactated solution, metabolic alkalosis commonly occurs following infusion of several units of ACD- or CPD-stored blood. Also, excessive bicarbonate administration may result in a hyperosmolal state, causing intracellular dehydration. Administration of 0.5 to 1.0 mEq. per L. of sodium bicarbonate increases the plasma osmolality to 349 mOsm. per kg. in dogs experimentally and in humans during treatment of cardiac arrest.[28,29] Although plasma osmolality has not been measured when bicarbonate has been given empirically, the amount recommended is in the range described above. Thus, a hyperosmolal state seems possible. Bicarbonate administration should be reserved for patients in whom severe metabolic acidosis (base excess greater than −7mEq./L.) has been diagnosed.

Citrate Intoxication and Hyperkalemia

Citrate intoxication is not caused by the citrate ion per se, but by the binding of citrate to calcium. Thus, the signs of citrate intoxication are those of hypocalcemia: hypotension, narrow pulse pressure, elevated intraventricular end-diastolic pressure and central venous pressures, and a prolonged Q-T interval on the ECG.[30] Until recently, most investigators felt that citrate intoxication occurred only when at least one unit of blood was infused every 3 to 4 min. in a 70-kg. patient. With the advent of an electrode to measure ionized calcium, more precise information is now available. Although the data are incomplete, a serum ionized calcium concentration less than 0.6 mmol. per L may produce clotting difficulties, suggesting that cardiac arrest will occur before serum ionized calcium levels are low enough to cause a coagulopathy.[31] Therefore, the existence of a hypocalcemic coagulopathy without severe hypotension is unlikely.

Do serum ionized calcium levels decrease sufficiently during infusion of ACD- or CPD-stored blood to cause cardiac depression? Hinkle and Cooperman found that serum ionized calcium levels decrease during infusion of 500 ml. of ACD-stored blood.[32] However, within minutes after completion of the infusion, these levels rapidly rise toward normal. Furthermore, ionized calcium levels vary directly with Pa_{CO_2}. More recently, Denlinger found that infusion of 150 ml. per 70 kg. per min. of citrated blood depresses calcium levels a maximum of 0.6 mmol. per L. (Fig. 35-7),[33] although infusion of one-third of that amount has little effect. However, the serum ionized calcium level returns to normal immediately after cessation of the infusion. The rapid return of these levels to normal can be explained by the metabolism of citrate by the liver and mobilization of calcium from endogenous stores. Hypothermia, liver disease, and hyperventilation might increase the possibility that citrate intoxication can occur. Excluding these conditions, ionized calcium levels begin to decrease only when 1 unit of blood is infused every 10 min. Therefore, citrate intoxication is rare.

Serum potassium levels may be as high as 32 mEq. per L. (32 mmol./L.) in blood stored for 21 days. For consistent increases in serum potassium, bank blood must be given at a rate of 120 ml. per min.[34] This suggests that the potassium ion must leave the extravascular space either by diffusion into intravascular space or by way of the kidneys.

Because hyperkalemia and citrate intoxication are rare, routine administration of calcium is not justified. In fact, calcium may cause cardiac arrhythmias, particularly in patients anesthetized

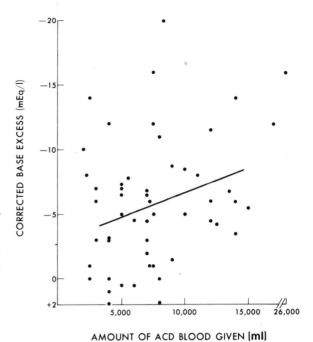

Fig. 35-6. Correlation between amount of ACD-stored blood administered and corrected base excess intraoperatively. (Miller, R. D., Tong, M. J., and Robbins, T. O.: Effects of massive transfusions of blood on acid-base balance. J.A.M.A., *216:* 1762, 1971. Copyright © 1971, American Medical Association)

with cyclopropane or halothane. Calcium administration should be based on diagnostic signs of hypocalcemia (prolonged Q-T interval) or hyperkalemia (peaked T wave).[18,19] Though reported to be irritating to veins, 10-per-cent calcium chloride provides three times more calcium than does an equal volume of 10-per-cent calcium gluconate, because the former has a molecular weight of 147, and the latter, of 448.

Hypothermia

Administration of bank blood that has been stored at 4°C can decrease the recipient's temperature. If the temperature decreases to less than 30°C, ventricular irritability and even cardiac arrest can occur. This can be prevented by warming blood before transfusion (see Chap. 19).[35] I believe that there are more subtle reasons for warming all blood, even in patients receiving only 1 or 2 units intraoperatively. Because of the cool temperature of the operating room, body tempera-

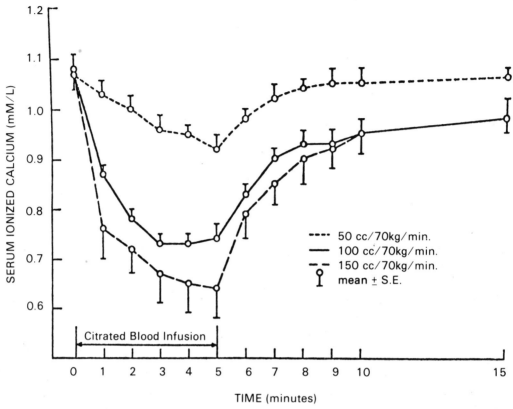

Fig. 35-7. Correlation between time during and after citrated whole blood infusion and serum ionized calcium. (Denlinger, J. K., Nahrwold, M. L., Lecky, J. H., et. al.: Hypocalcemia during rapid blood transfusion in anaesthetized man. Br. J. Anaesth., *48:* 995, 1976)

ture will often decrease, particularly in patients undergoing extensive abdominal surgery; administration of cold blood will augment this decrease in temperature (see Chap. 19).[36] A body temperature decrease as little as 0.5 to 1.0°C may induce shivering postoperatively, and this in turn may increase oxygen consumption as much as 400 per cent. To meet the demands of an elevated oxygen consumption, cardiac output must be increased. Is this too much stress for the patient with marginal cardiac reserve?[37] More studies are required to evaluate this concern.

Perhaps the safest and most common method for warming blood is to pass it through plastic coils immersed in a warm water (37–38°C) bath. Microwave warmers have many advantages,[18] but blood may overheat in them, resulting in severe hemolysis.[38,39] As a result, the following procedure is recommended before using the microwave

warmer: Once or twice each day, plastic blood bags containing saline should also be warmed to determine whether the warmer is functioning properly; temperature of the blood bag should be monitored by placing a probe in the folds of the exterior of the bag; and, only trained personnel should warm blood in this device.[39]

PULMONARY EFFECTS OF BLOOD TRANSFUSION

Pulmonary Hypersensitivity Reaction

Pulmonary edema, not secondary to circulatory overload, occasionally can occur after infusion of only 2 or 3 units of blood.[40] Presumably the edema is caused by recipient sensitivity to donor platelets or leukocytes. The presence of eosinophilia or urticaria helps confirm this diagnosis. Because this reaction is so rare, no one has had sufficient experience to determine which therapeutic manuvers are indicated. Some investigators have suggested that in addition to the usual treatment for pulmonary edema, steroids, antihistamines, and dextran may be helpful.[41]

Infusion of Unfiltered Debris ("Shock Lung")

In 1970, Moseley and Doty demonstrated that the amounts of clot and debris in bank blood increase with the length of storage.[42] Some of this particulate matter is not removed by the standard 170-μm. filter during routine transfusion, and it enters the recipient's circulation. Moseley and Doty suggest, therefore, that the accumulation of these microaggregates in the lungs results in vascular obstruction, which, in turn, results in respiratory insufficiency in patients with severe trauma and hemorrhage ("shock lung"). Several filters with pore sizes less than 40μm. (micropore filters) are now available to remove microaggregates before they enter the recipient. When giving massive transfusions of stored blood, the use of micropore filters should eliminate this potential contributor to the development of "shock lung."[43]

What is the evidence supporting this hypothesis and the need for micropore filters during massive transfusion of stored blood? First, what are the microaggregates and when do they develop in stored blood? The volume of microaggregates is about the same in blood stored in either ACD or CPD solution, although the particles are larger in CPD-stored blood.[44] Platelet aggregates form during the 2nd to 5th day of storage; but, the larger fibrin-white blood cell-platelet aggregates do not begin to accumulate until after 10 days of storage.[45] If the risk of pulmonary damage is primarily from the larger fibrin-white cell-platelet microaggregates, then micropore filters would not be needed unless the blood has been stored for 10 days or more. Also, screen filtration pressures (pressures developed when blood is forced through a screen with a pore size of 20–40 μm. at a defined flow) do not increase until blood has been stored for 5 to 9 days (Fig. 35-8).[46] These results indicate that *micropore filters are not necessary unless blood that has been stored for at least 5 and possibly 10 days is being infused.*

Are the micropore filters necessary at all? Most of the evidence supporting their use is based upon electron micrographs of debris on both the filters and pulmonary biopsy specimens.[47,48] When micropore filters are used, fewer structural changes are noted in the lung during hypotension.[48] Unfortunately, most of these studies were performed in animals. Other animal studies have shown increases in pulmonary vascular resistance after infusion of ACD-stored blood.[49] The assumption is that the microaggregates cause mechanical obstruction of the pulmonary vasculature. However, it is possible that the microaggregates release vasoactive materials that would increase pulmonary vascular resistance. The importance of the infused ACD-stored blood is difficult to ascertain, since these animals usually have had anesthesia, thoracotomy, artificial ventilation, and heparinization. In attempt to avoid these factors, Tobey studied the effect of hemorrhagic shock and massive blood transfusion in unanesthetized, spontaneously breathing baboons. He found no change in pulmonary gas exchange, including pulmonary artery pressure.[50] Also, electron microscopy did not reveal pulmonary microembolism from the transfused blood. More recent animal studies also suggest that microaggregates may not be significant in the development of the adult respiratory distress syndrome.[51]

Since animal studies are not convincing, do clinical observations support the need for micropore filters? With proper respiratory therapy, the incidence of respiratory failure ("shock lung") is very low in patients who have received large amounts of stored blood through a 170-μm. filter and who have no direct pulmonary injury.[52,53] Similar observations in dogs cast doubt on the contribution of the debris in stored blood to the development of "shock lung."[54] It is quite possible that the micropore filters are not needed during massive transfusion of stored blood and may even harm the cellular elements of stored blood.

Our main concern is whether patients who receive blood through the 170-μm. filter have poorer pulmonary function than those who receive blood through the micropore filters. Although Reul attempted to answer this question, his experimental design casts doubt on the conclu-

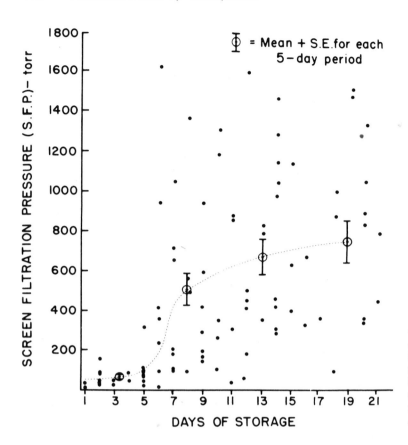

Fig. 35-8. Screen filtration pressures in ACD blood stored for 21 days. The pressures are an index of the amount of debris in blood. (Harp, J. R., Wyche, M. Q., Marshall, B. E., et al.: Some factors determining rate of microaggregate formation in stored blood. Anesthesiology, *40:* 398, 1974)

sions.[55,56] A large, well controlled study should be undertaken, preferably by a large trauma service or a service that performs extensive surgical procedures. Filters should be used randomly, and the pulmonary physiologic function of patients should be measured postoperatively or after injury; the anesthesiologist should not rely upon subjective observation of respiratory function. A common approach is to use the micropore filters for patients who receive more than 20 to 35 ml. per kg. of stored blood, even though there is no conclusive clinical evidence that the microaggregates are harmful.

TRANSFUSION REACTIONS

Minor Reaction to Blood Transfusion

Minor reactions to blood transfusions usually are not serious and are either febrile or allergic. A febrile reaction is characterized by chills, fever, and urticaria and probably is caused by antigens to which the recipient has leukocyte antibodies. Allergic reactions are very similar and are characterized by urticaria or, in more severe cases, by chills and fever as well. Although the cause of these reactions is rarely determined, they are more frequent in patients who have had a previous transfusion reaction or who have a history of allergies. Supportive therapy that includes antihistamines or aspirin may be needed. If the reaction begins with chills and fever with no urticaria, the plasma and urine should be examined for free hemoglobin to exclude a hemolytic transfusion reaction. Although chills and fever may signal bacterial contamination, this is rare with the use of plastic blood containers.

Hemolytic Reaction to Blood Transfusion

A hemolytic transfusion reaction is one of the most unfortunate complications in medicine. It is usually a result of incorrect laboratory work or mislabeling or misreading of labels on blood. In severe hemolytic reactions, there is a mortality rate of 40 to 60 per cent. Under general anesthesia, the signs may be hypotension, a bleeding diathesis, or hemoglobinura, which is the most common.

The primary sequelae of intravascular hemolysis are renal failure and DIC. Renal failure probably results from precipitation of hemoglobin as acid hematin in the distal tubules. The amount of the precipitate is related inversely to urine volume, flow rate, and *p*H. DIC commonly occurs because red cell stroma is disrupted, releasing erythrocytin, which activates the coagulation system. Because DIC may not occur immediately after the infusion of incompatible blood, blood for coagulation tests should be drawn to provide baseline values for future comparison.

Steps for the Treatment of Hemolytic Reaction

1. Stop the Transfusion!
2. Maintain a urine output of at least 75–100 ml./hour by the following:
   Generous administration of intravenous fluids
   Mannitol, 12.5–50 g., given slowly, intravenously
   If intravenous fluids and mannitol are insufficient, administer furosemide, 40 mg., intravenously.
3. Alkalinize the urine. Since bicarbonate is preferentially excreted in the urine, only 40–70 mEq. of sodium bicarbonate/70 kg. body weight is usually required to raise the urine *p*H to 8, whereupon repeated urine *p*H determinations indicate the need for additional bicarbonate.
4. Assay plasma and urinary hemoglobin concentrations.
5. Determine platelet count, partial thromboplastin time, and serum fibrinogen level.
6. Return unused blood to blood bank for re-cross match.
7. Prevent hypotension to insure adequate renal blood flow.

Recognizing the possibility of severe morbidity and even mortality, Seager utilized a different approach in treating a patient who had received 3000 ml. of incompatible blood.[57] He reasoned that the kidneys might be spared exposure to massive amounts of hemolyzed red blood cells by replacing all blood with compatible blood. This was performed using an extracorporeal circuit.

Normal urinary function returned rapidly, supporting further consideration of this method.

Hepatitis

In a recent prospective survey conducted in 14 medical centers, nearly 5000 patients received an average of 7.7 units of blood. A 2.8-per-cent incidence of symptomatic hepatitis and 0.1-percent fatality rate occurred, with much variability from center to center.[58] The incubation period ranged from 16 to 180 days following surgery, and 30 to 60 days was the most common. Although this study found that hepatitis was not attentuated by intramuscular injections of immune serum globulin containing low amounts of hepatitis B antibody,[58] Katz found that the addition of immune globulin to the bag of blood before transfusion is only partly effective.[59] However, interpretation of clinical studies of the efficacy of immune serum globulin should take into account the variable titer of hepatitis B antibody in the immune globulin.[60] Evaluation of such studies is complicated further because hepatic dysfunction following transfusion may also be the result of hepatitis A or non-A, non-B hepatitis[61] (see Chap. 55). Finally, the incidence of hepatitis in patients receiving multiple-donor plasma is about 9 per cent, and in patients receiving fibrinogen, between 10 and 50 per cent. Since hypofibrinogenemia is rare, but usually associated with DIC, the administration of fibrinogen is rarely, if ever, indicated.

CLINICAL RECOMMENDATIONS FOR TRANSFUSION

When administering whole blood, the following guidelines may be helpful:

To avoid coagulation problems, consider ordering fresh blood or having platelet concentrates available when 10 units have been given and more transfusions are anticipated. This will allow immediate treatment of a hemorrhagic diathesis from dilutional thrombocytopenia. Monitor platelet count and clot for lysis for at least every 5 to 10 units of CPD-stored blood administered. Also consider monitoring the partial thromboplastin time and plasma fibrinogen level after every 10 units of CPD-stored blood is administered.

To avoid infusion of unfilterable debris and low levels of 2,3-DPG, administer blood that is as fresh as possible and consider use of a micropore filter.

Warm all blood before transfusion.

Analyze arterial or arterialized venous blood for Pa_{O_2}, Pa_{CO_2}, and pH periodically (i.e., every 5 units of blood) to allow precise bicarbonate administration and to monitor oxygenation.

Monitor the ECG continuously to detect changes in calcium or potassium concentration in circulating blood.

REFERENCES

1. Dawson, R. B., Jr., Liken, M. F., and Crater, D. H.: Hemoglobin function in stored blood. Transfusion, *12*:46, 1972.
2. Valtis, D. J., and Kennedy, A. C.: Defective gas-transport function of stored red blood cells. Lancet, *1*:119, 1954.
3. Bunn, H. F., May, M. H., Kocholaty, W. F., et al.: Hemoglobin function in stored blood. J. Clin. Invest., *48*:311, 1969.
4. Benesch, R. E., and Benesch, R.: The reaction between diphosphoglycerate and hemoglobin. Fed. Proc., *29*:1101, 1970.
5. Guy, J. T., Bromberg, P. A., Meta, E. N., et al.: Oxygen delivery following transfusion of stored blood. I. Normal rats. J. Appl. Physiol., *37*:60, 1974.
6. Mondzelewski, J. P., Guy, J. T., Bromberg, P. A., et al.: Oxygen delivery following transfusion of stored blood. II. Acidotic rats. J. Appl. Physiol., *37*:64, 1974.
7. Kopriva, C. J., Ratliff, J. L., Fletcher, J. R., et al.: Biochemical and hematological changes associated with massive transfusion of ACD-stored blood in severely injured combat casualties. Ann. Surg., *176*:585, 1972.
8. McConn, R., and Derrick, J. B.: The respiratory function of blood: transfusion and blood storage. Anesthesiology, *36*:119, 1972.
9. Bowen, J. C., and Fleming, W. H.: Increased oxyhemoglobin affinity after transfusion of stored blood: evidence for circulatory compensation. Ann. Surg., *180*:760, 1974.
10. Valeri, C. R.: Blood components in the treatment of acute blood loss: use of freeze-preserved red cells, platelets, and plasma proteins. Anesth. Analg., *54*:1, 1975.
11. Miller, R. D., Robbin, T. O., and Tong, .M. J.: Coagulation defects associated with massive blood transfusions. Ann. Surg., *174*:794, 1971.
12. Lim, R. C., Jr., Olcott, C., IV, Robinson, A. J., et al.: Platelet response and coagulation changes following massive blood replacement. J. Trauma, *13*:577, 1973.
13. Simmons, R. L., Collins, J. A., and Heisterkamp, C. A.: Coagulation disorders in combat casualties. Ann. Surg., *169*:455, 1969.
14. Attar, S.: Alteration in coagulation and fibrinolytic mechanisms in acute trauma. J. Trauma, *9*:939, 1969.
15. Himansu, K. B.: Fibrinolytic and abruptio placenta. Br. J. Obstet. Gynaecol., *76*:481, 1969.

16. Friedman, N. J., Hoag, M. S., and Robinson, A. J.: Hemorrhagic syndrome following transurethral prostatic resection for benign adenoma. Arch. Intern. Med., *124*:341, 1969.
17. Goodnight, S. H., Kenoyer, G., Rapaport, S. I., et al.: Defibrination after brain-tissue destruction. N. Engl. J. Med., *290*:1043, 1974.
18. Miller, R. D.: Complications of massive blood transfusion. Anesthesiology, *39*:82, 1973.
19. Miller, R. D.: Transfusion therapy and associated problems. Refresher Courses in Anesthesiology, *1*:101, 1973.
20. Ratnoff, O. D.: Epsilon aminocaproic acid—dangerous weapon. N. Engl. J. Med., *280*:1124, 1969.
21. Robboy, S., Colman, R., and Minna, J.: Fibrinolysis vs. disseminated intravascular coagulation. N. Engl. J. Med., *281*:222, 1969.
22. Gans, H.: Is primary fibrinolysis a real entity? Surg. Gynecol. Obstet., *136*:975, 1973.
23. Priano, L. L., Wilson, R. D., and Traber, D. L.: Lack of significant protection afforded by heparin during endotoxic shock. Am. J. Physiol., *220*:901, 1971.
24. Howland, W. S., and Schweizer, O.: Physiologic compensation for storage lesion of bank blood. Anesth. Analg., *44*:8, 1965.
25. Collins, J. A., Simmons, R. L., James, P. M., et al.: The acid-base status of seriously wounded combat casualties: I. Resuscitation with stored blood. Ann. Surg., *173*:6, 1971.
26. Miller, R. D., Tong, M. J., and Robbins, T. O.: Effects of massive transfusions of blood on acid-base balance. J.A.M.A., *216*:1762, 1971.
27. France, C. J., Eger, E. I., II, and Bendixen, H. H.: The use of peripheral venous blood for pH and carbon dioxide tension determinations during general anesthesia. Anesthesiology, *40*:311, 1974.
28. Mattor, J. A., Weil, M. H., Shubin, H., et al.: Cardiac arrest in the critically ill. II. Hyperosmolal states following cardiac arrest. Am. J. Med., *56*:162, 1974.
29. Bishop, R. L., and Weisfeldt, M. L.: Sodium bicarbonate administration during cardiac arrest. J.A.M.A., *235*:507, 1976.
30. Bunker, J. P., Bendixen, H. H., and Murphy, J. A.: Hemodynamic effects of intravenously administered sodium citrate. N. Engl. J. Med., *266*:372, 1962.
31. Dixon, W. G.: Does transfusion citrate cause hemorrhage? Am. Surg., *24*:818, 1958.
32. Hinkle, J. E., and Cooperman, L. H.: Serum ionized calcium changes following citrated blood transfusion in anaesthetized man. Br. J. Anaesth., *43*:1108, 1971.
33. Denlinger, J. K., Nahrwold, M. L., Lecky, J. H., et al.: Hypocalcemia during rapid blood transfusion in anaesthetized man. Br. J. Anaesth., *48*:995, 1976.
34. Smith, N. T., and Corbascio, A. N.: The hemodynamic effects of potassium infusion in dogs. Anesthesiology, *26*:633, 1965.
35. Boyan, C. P.: Cold or warmed blood for massive transfusions. Ann. Surg., *160*:282, 1964.
36. Morris, R. H.: Influence of ambient temperature on patient temperature during intra-abdominal surgery. Ann. Surg., *173*:230, 1971.
37. Bay, J., Nunn, J. F., and Prys-Roberts, C.: Factors influencing arterial P_{O_2} during recovery from anaesthesia. Br. J. Anaesth., *40*:398, 1969.

38. Staples, P. J., and Griner, P. F.: Extracorporeal hemolysis of blood in a microwave blood warmer. N. Engl. J. Med., *285*:317, 1971.
39. Arens, J. F., and Leonard, G. L.: Danger of overwarming blood by microwave. J.A.M.A., *218*:1045, 1971.
40. Byrne, J. P., Jr., and Dixon, J. A.: Pulmonary edema following blood transfusion reaction. Arch. Surg., *102*:91, 1971.
41. Ward, H. N., Lipscomb, T. S., and Cawley, L. P.: Pulmonary hypersensitivity reaction after blood transfusion. Arch. Intern. Med., *122*:362, 1968.
42. Moseley, R. V., and Doty, D. B.: Changes in the filtration characteristics of stored blood. Ann. Surg., *171*:329, 1970.
43. Walker, A. K. Y.: Blood microfiltration. A review. Anaesthesia, *33*:35, 1978.
44. Gervin, A. S., Mason, K. G., and Wright, C. B.: Microaggregate volumes in stored human blood. Surg. Gynecol. Obstet., *139*:519, 1974.
45. Arrington, P., and McNamara, J. J.: Mechanism of microaggregate formation in stored blood. Ann. Surg., *179*:146, 1974.
46. Harp, J. R., Wyche, M. Q., Marshall, B. E., et al.: Some factors determining rate of microaggregate formation in stored blood. Anesthesiology, *40*:398, 1974.
47. Goldiner, P. L., Howland, W. S., and Ray, C., Jr.: Filter for prevention of microembolism during massive transfusions. Anesth. Analg., *51*:712, 1972.
48. Swank, R. L., Connell, R. S., and Webb, M. C.: Dacron wool filtration and hypotensive shock: an electron microscopical study. Ann. Surg., *179*:427, 1974.
49. Bennett, S. H., Geelhoed, G. W., Aaron, R. K., et al.: Pulmonary injury resulting from perfusion of stored bank blood in the baboon and dog. J. Surg. Res., *13*:295, 1972.
50. Tobey, R. E., Kopriva, C. J., Homer, L. D., et al.: Pulmonary gas exchange following hemorrhagic shock and massive blood transfusion in the baboon. Ann. Surg., *179*:316, 1974.
51. Giordano, J., Zinner, M., Hobson, R. W., et al.: The effect of microaggregates in stored blood on canine pulmonary vascular resistance. Surgery, *80*:617, 1976.
52. Horovitz, J. H., Carrico, C. J., and Shires, G. T.: Pulmonary response to major injury. Arch. Surg., *108*:349, 1974.
53. Proctor, J. H., Ballantine, T. V. N., and Broussard, N. D.: An analysis of pulmonary function following non-thoracic trauma, with recommendations for therapy. Ann. Surg., *172*:180, 1970.
54. Marshall, B. E., Soma, L. R., Harp, J. R., et al.: Pulmonary function after exchange transfusion of stored blood in dogs. Ann. Surg., *179*:46, 1974.
55. Reul, G. J., Greenberg, S. D., Lefrak, E. A., et al.: Prevention of post-traumatic pulmonary insufficiency. Arch. Surg., *106*:386, 1973.
56. Reul, G. J., Beall, A. C., and Greenberg, S. D.: Protection of pulmonary microvasculature by fine screen blood filtration. Chest, *66*:4, 1974.
57. Seager, O. A., Nesmith, M. A., Begelman, K. A., et al.: Acute hemodilution for incompatible blood reaction. J.A.M.A., *229*;790, 1974.
58. National Transfusion Hepatitis Study: Risk of post-transfusion hepatitis in the United States. J.A.M.A., *220*:692, 1972.
59. Katz, M., Rodriquez, J., and Ward, R.: Post-transfusion hepatitis: effect of modified gamma globulin added to blood in vitro. N. Engl. J. Med., *285*:925, 1971.
60. Maynard, J. E.: Passive immunization against hepatitis B: a review of recent studies and comments on current aspects of control. Am. J. Epidemiol., *107*:77, 1978.
61. Feinstone, S. M., and Purcell, R. H.: Non-A, non-B hepatitis. Annu. Rev. Med., *29*:359, 1978.

FURTHER READING

Miller, R. D.: Complications of massive blood transfusion. Anesthesiology, *39*:82, 1973.
Miller, R. D., and Brzica, S. M.: Blood, blood component, colloid, and autotransfusion therapy. *In* Miller, R. D. (ed.): Anesthesia. pp. 885–922. New York, Churchill Livingstone, 1981.

36 Difficulties in Sickle Cell States

Sharon B. Murphy, M.D.

Sickle cell disease is any disorder caused by sickling of erythrocytes and commonly includes homozygous hemoglobin SS disease, the simultaneous heterozygous states of SC disease and S-thalassemia, and hemoglobin S (HbS) in combination with the hereditary persistence of fetal hemoglobin. Sickle cell trait (hemoglobin genotype, AS) is not a disease and is exceedingly rarely associated with symptoms. Patients with sickle cell disease have an increased risk of morbidity and mortality with anesthesia and surgery. Whether or not this is true for patients with sickle cell trait is currently somewhat controversial. It is probable that an anesthetic that is unsafe for a person with sickle cell trait is also unsafe for a person without the trait. No strict guidelines for anesthetic management of patients with sickle cell disease may be dictated; each case must be considered individually in its clinical setting. Best results are likely to be achieved by prior recognition of the presence of a sickling disorder, preoperative preparation for elective surgery, careful monitoring, and strict avoidance of factors known to precipitate sickling, such as acidosis, hypoxia, hypotension, stasis, and hypothermia. Despite these precautions, patients with sickle cell disease still may experience unpredictable perioperative complications. Treatment of these disorders is not completely satisfactory.

This chapter examines difficulties encountered in the perioperative and anesthetic management of patients with sickle cell disease. Proper management is predicated on the incidence and clinical features that characterize the common sickle cell diseases and on an understanding of the pathophysiology of these disorders, which affects oxygen transport, circulatory rheology, and cardiopulmonary function. Complications that may arise are primarily due to vaso-occlusion from sickled erythrocytes. Recommendations for care include hydration, simple transfusion, preoperative elective hypertransfusion, and emergency partial exchange transfusion. Careful monitoring of the sickle cell patient should not cease upon recovery from the anesthetic, since the postoperative period may be characterized by fever, painful crisis, pulmonary problems, and jaundice. A team approach involving anesthesiologist, surgeon, and hematologist will provide the comprehensive care necessary for these patients.

CLINICAL FEATURES OF SICKLE CELL STATES

Incidence of Sickle Cell Disorders

Hemoglobin SS disease is the most serious sickling disorder. Its frequency in the U.S. black population at birth is roughly 1 in 625.[1] The other sickle cell diseases are HbS-β-thalassemia, HbS-C disease, and HbS-persistence of HbF (fetal hemoglobin). Their frequencies in blacks at birth are estimated to be, respectively, 1 in 1667, 1 in 833, and 1 in 25,000.[1] The actual prevalence of sickling disorders is less than their frequency at birth, but

Table 36-1. Summary of the Usual Findings in the Common Sickling Disorders

| | | | | BLOOD CELLS | | |
CONDITION	SYMPTOM-ATOLOGY	SPLENO-MEGALY	CIRCULATING Hb, g./dl.	SICKLED CELLS	TARGET CELLS	HbS PRESENT ON ELECTROPHORESIS
SS disease	++++	0	6–8	Many	Many	90–100% S, remainder F
S-thalassemia	++−+++	++	7–8	Few	Many	65–85% S, remainder A, A$_2$ & F
SC disease	+−++	++−+++	9–11	Few	Very many	40–60%, each S & C
S—hereditary persistence of Hb F	0−+	0	Normal	0	±	70–80% S, 20–30% F
S—trait	0	0	Normal	0	0	20–40% S, remainder normal A

this depends on the mortality of the disease, which makes it difficult to predict the exact frequency with age. The prevalence of sickle cell trait is 8 per cent among black Americans.[1]

Clinical Findings of Sickle Cell Disorders

Comparison of the clinical characteristics of the sickle cell disorders is given in Table 36-1. Hemoglobin SS disease is a severe disorder characterized by chronic hemolytic anemia and repeated episodes of vaso-occlusive crises, producing tissue infarction and organ dysfunction. Manifestations of the disease are protean and commonly include painful crises of the abdomen, back, and extremities; jaundice; renal insufficiency; bone deformities; leg ulcers; and neurologic manifestations such as hemiplegia and blindness. Congestive heart failure and severe infections, such as pneumonia and osteomyelitis, may occur.[2]

Symptomatology in hemoglobin SC disease and S-thalassemia is similar to that in SS disease but is generally less severe and less frequent. Hemoglobin SC disease is extremely variable in its severity, which ranges from an asymptomatic state to severe disability. S-thalassemia is likewise variable in severity but may be as severe as SS disease and difficult to distinguish both clinically and by laboratory results; family studies are usually necessary. HbS in association with hereditary persistence of HbF is quite rare, and affected patients usually have been asymptomatic.

People with sickle cell trait are asymptomatic, and studies of death rates have shown no increase in mortality.[3] Ordinarily there is no anemia, and the peripheral blood findings are normal; if anemia is found in a person with sickle cell trait, another cause might be sought. Except in unusual circumstances, sickle cell trait is a benign condition.[3a,4] Occasionally people with sickle cell trait exhibit hyposthenuria and hematuria. Nearly the whole spectrum of vaso-occlusive phenomena observed in patients with sickle cell disease has been reported in people with sickle cell trait. However, most of these reports are anecdotal, and the data, equivocal. Nevertheless, certain noxious effects are well recognized, such as splenic infarction associated with high-altitude flight in an unpressurized aircraft.[5] In what must be an exceedingly rare occurrence, apparently fatal extensive in vivo sickling may take place in sickle cell trait under conditions of extreme hypoxia, dehydration, or stasis.[6,7]

Diagnosis of Sickle Cell Disease

The diagnosis of sickle cell disease is not difficult and is generally evident after a complete history, physical examination, laboratory evaluation of the hemoglobin level and the peripheral blood smear, and a test for detection of sickle hemoglobin. For screening and detection, the tube solubility test for HbS has now generally replaced the less recent, 2-per-cent sodium metabisulfite test, which employed sealed, wet preparations of blood. The tube solubility (dithionite) test is based on the insolubility of reduced HbS in a solution of a strong phosphate buffer at slightly acid *p*H, which produces a turbid solution. The test can be performed with a drop of blood and takes only 5 minutes.[8] A commercial test kit is available (Sickledex, Ortho Diagnostics, Raritan, N.J.) Definitive diagnosis involves confirmatory hemoglobin electrophoresis. All black patients should be screened at least for the presence of HbS prior to anesthesia and surgery.

PATHOPHYSIOLOGY OF SICKLE CELL DISEASE

The pathogenesis of sickle cell disease is exceptionally well understood. The inherited substitution of an amino acid in the hemoglobin molecule permits stacking of hemoglobin molecules upon deoxygenation. This leads to the sickled distortion of the erythrocyte, which, in turn, accounts for the chronic hemolytic anemia and the vascular occlusion characteristic of the disease.

The Molecular Basis of Sickling

HbS is indicated as follows: $\alpha_2\beta_2^{6Glu \to Val}$; that is, a valine is substituted for glutamic acid in the sixth amino acid position from the aminoterminal end of the beta globin chains. This protein abnormality results in sickling upon deoxygenation of the hemoglobin molecule.

The physical mechanisms involved in formation of linear aggregates of deoxygenated molecules of HbS have been reviewed recently.[9] Briefly, deoxygenation produces an intramolecular rearrangement in such a way that the distance between two β-chain heme groups increases by 0.65 nm. This apparently allows certain surface regions of one deoxygenated molecule to line up in register with a neighboring molecule, so that weak intermolecular forces (hydrogen bonds, van der Waals forces, and electrostatic forces) produce

linear polymers that arrange themselves into helical bundles and produce filaments of sufficient rigidity to sickle the cell. These forces holding together deoxygenated molecules are relatively weak and easily reversed by temperature changes, hemoglobin concentration changes, and by the addition of ligands (oxygen or carbon monoxide).

The presence of types of hemoglobin other than S (A, C, or F) within the erythrocyte also clearly influences the tendency to form linear aggregates on deoxygenation. Either HbA or HbC can definitely copolymerize, but HbF is nearly completely excluded from the filaments. This exclusion accounts for the usually asymptomatic state of people simultaneously heterozygous for HbS and persistence of fetal hemoglobin, despite the presence of 70- to 80-per-cent HbS within their erythrocytes. In that condition, the HbF molecules are homogeneously distributed throughout the red cell population, and the amount of F per cell is apparently sufficient to prevent sickling. The presence of HbF also accounts for the mildness of sickle cell anemia in the first 6 months of life.

Oxygen Transport

Normal mechanisms of oxygen transport and the physiologic adaptations to anemia, including increased intraerythrocyte 2,3-diphosphoglycerate (2,3-DPG) content, have been well described.[10,11] Intact SS red cells have a higher concentration of 2,3-DPG than normal red cells, and the blood of patients with sickle cell anemia exhibits decreased affinity for oxygen compared to normal blood.[12] The oxygen-hemoglobin dissociation curve for SS blood is shifted far to the right. P_{50}, the partial pressure of oxygen at which hemoglobin is 50-per-cent saturated, is 49.7 torr (6.6 kPa) for whole SS blood, compared to the normal value of 30 to 32 torr (4.0–4.3 kPa) at *p*H of 7.13 and 37°C.[13] The increase in P_{50} of whole blood observed in sickle cell disease is not explained entirely by the increased 2,3-DPG, for P_{50} increases in sickle cell disease as the percentage of irreversibly sickled cells and the mean intracorpuscular hemoglobin concentration increase.[13] Hence, the reduced oxygen-carrying capacity of the blood in sickle cell disease due to the lowered hematocrit does not necessarily imply reduced oxygen delivery, because of this considerable shift to the right of the oxygen-hemoglobin dissociation curve.[14] Furthermore, in sickle cell anemia, there is a marked increase in the cardiac output, which, by itself, corrects the oxygen flux deficit. In sickle cell anemia, the mean cardiac index is 6.7 L. per m.[2] per min., and the calculated mean oxygen tension of venous blood is 44 torr (5.9 kPa).[15]

Rheology

Clinical symptomatology in sickle cell disease is related not to the anemia per se but rather to the altered rheologic properties of the blood caused by the presence of HbS.[16] An increase in blood viscosity, due to the decreased deformability of deoxygenated, reversibly sickled cells and oxygenated, irreversibly sickled cells, is the primary factor responsible for impedance to blood flow and capillary blockade. Harris showed that, as the oxygen saturation of the whole blood from sickle cell anemia patients is decreased, an increase in the viscosity is observed, which is directly related to the number and degree of sickled cells.[17] A similar effect was observed with blood from persons with sickle cell trait, but only at oxygen tensions below 15 torr (2.0 kPa).[17]

The clinical severity of various sickle cell disorders correlates with the rate of increase of viscosity during deoxygenation and is influenced by interaction with the types of hemoglobin other than S present within the red cell.[18] Increase in viscosity on deoxygenation is greatest for SS, followed in order by SC, SF, and AS. Acquisition of decreased red cell deformability upon deoxygenation takes a finite time. Harris and Messer note that red cells from patients with SS disease become less filterable within 0.12 seconds of deoxygenation, while no change takes place within 5 seconds for cells from persons with sickle cell trait.[19] This emphasizes the importance of transit time of erythrocytes in the hypoxic microcirculation.

A number of other known factors (and some presumably unknown) will also influence the viscosity of sickle cell blood. Admixture of nor-mal cells with sickle cells and, therefore, transfusion diminish the increase in viscosity observed on deoxygenation.[20] A fall in temperature has been shown to increase the viscosity of sickle cell blood[21] and confirms the well known clinical observation that exposure to cold may precipitate a crisis. Laasberg and Hedley-Whyte examined the effect of halothane on the viscosity of normal, AS, and SS blood. They found that, if deoxygenated sickle cell blood is equilibrated with halothane in clinical concentrations, with time the viscosity is increased, while that of normal blood is unaffected.[22] Drug effects on the vascular components determining flow, pressure, and vessel caliber in sickle cell disease are, no doubt, important but have not been investigated adequately.

The Vicious Cycle

An understanding of the altered rheologic properties of sickle cell whole blood and of the factors that precipitate sickling provides a ready appreciation of the so-called "vicious cycle" that is primarily responsible for the symptomatology of sickle cell disease.[23] During deoxygenation in the slow flow of the capillary microcirculation, sickled cells arise and produce an increase in blood viscosity. The increased viscosity further impedes the circulation, resulting in further deoxygenation and acidosis. Additional sickling occurs and eventually results in a static mass of sickled erythrocytes. These changes take place in patients with sickle cell disease within the usual physiologic ranges of oxygen tension. Similar changes can be induced in sickle cell trait, but only under exceptional nonphysiologic circumstances.

A schematic representation of the interrelated factors that may precipitate the vicious cycle and produce vaso-occlusion in sickle cell disease is shown in Figure 36-1. Strict avoidance of acidosis, hypoxia, hypotension, cooling, and circulatory stasis is necessary in management of the patient undergoing anesthesia and surgery.

Cardiopulmonary Dysfunction

Repeated vaso-occlusive insults over the course of a lifetime lead to compromised organ function in patients with sickle cell disease. In particular,

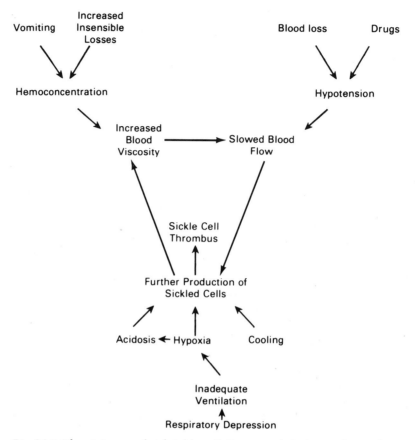

Fig. 36-1. The vicious cycle of sickle cell disease and the interrelationship of factors precipitating crisis in the patient undergoing anesthesia and surgery.

cardiopulmonary and renal function may be significantly deranged in such patients, and an appreciation of these derangements is necessary for optimal management.

Cardiovascular abnormalities, manifested clinically by cardiomegaly, a hyperdynamic circulation (full pulses, anterior parasternal lift, enlarged, laterally displaced apical impulse), murmurs, a third heart sound, and an accentuated second sound, are nearly always present in sickle cell disease.[24] The observed cardiovascular abnormalities are the result of long-term stresses on the system, including a chronically raised cardiac output, decreased arterial oxygen saturation due to ventilation–perfusion inequality and venoarterial shunting, and gradual thrombotic occlusion of the pulmonary vascular bed. No ECG features are specifically diagnostic, but evidence of both left and right ventricular hypertrophy is common.[24] As a rule, these cardiovascular abnormalities are observed only in the homozygous sickle state. They appear to be far less common in the heterozygous sickle hemoglobinopathies, and, of course, are not found in patients with sickle cell trait.

Pulmonary infection and vascular occlusion with infarction, often difficult to distinguish, are common in sickle cell disease and may cause acute and chronic alterations in pulmonary function.[25] Pulmonary function studies in SS patients exhibit abnormalities relevant to an understanding of their gas exchange.[25–27] Resting Pa_{O_2} generally ranges from 70 to 90 torr (9.3–12.0 kPa). $P_{(A-a)O_2}$ is increased compared to normal values and is frequently in excess of 20 torr (2.7 kPa), due to shunting through undefined pathways and to an abnormal degree of heterogeneity of ventilation–perfusion ratios in the lung. The mean membrane-diffusing capacity and pulmonary-diffusing capacity of patients with SS or SC disease are both below normal.[26]

Renal Dysfunction

Inability to concentrate the urine and consequent excretion of large daily volumes are consistent manifestations of sickle cell disease; this is also observed in sickle cell trait, but less consistently.[28,29] Hence, patients with sickle cell disease should not be left for long periods perioperatively without adequate intravenous fluid replacement. Further, while the volume and concentration of urine excreted by a normal patient usually provide a simple and reliable method of assessing the volume of intravenous fluid to be administered, these measures are much less reliable in the patient with sickle cell disease, in whom one should measure serum electrolytes and osmolarity to better assess hydration. In addition to hyposthenuria, these patients may develop renal papillary necrosis and the nephrotic syndrome.

ANESTHETIC COMPLICATIONS OF SICKLE CELL STATES

Complications of Sickle Cell Disease

Virtually every conceivable anesthetic and operative complication has been reported in patients with sickle cell disease, including splenic infarction,[30] atelectasis, pulmonary infarction and pneumonia,[31,32,33] unexpected death,[32,34] pulmonary embolization,[35] wound infection,[31] jaundice,[32] painful crisis,[32] renal failure,[36] and transient blindness.[37]

The true incidence of excess complications of anesthesia and surgery attributable to sickle cell disease is difficult to estimate. It is likely that the literature is heavily biased: Deaths and other complications are more likely to be reported than uncomplicated procedures. It appears certain, however, that morbidity and mortality are greater in patients with sickle cell disease than in normals. Searle collected 144 cases of sickle cell disease from the literature; these involved patients to whom general anesthesia had been administered.[38] There was a mortality rate of 7.6 per cent; of course, some of these patients were gravely ill, and death may have been unavoidable.

Estimates of the true incidence of morbidity are even more difficult to obtain than that of mortality. In an effort to document the frequency of complications and to analyze factors contributing to morbidity, a retrospective analysis of 69 surgical procedures, performed in 45 patients with sickle cell disease (36 SS, 9 SC patients) at Children's Hospital of Philadelphia and the Hospital of the University of Pennsylvania, from 1960 to 1972, was performed.* There were no deaths. In 59 procedures performed on patients with SS disease, complications occurred in 14 (24% morbidity rate); of 11 patients with SC disease, complications occurred in 4 (36%). The most common types of complications were postoperative fevers of unknown origin, painful crises, wound infections, and transfusion-related problems. Complications in each case were typically multiple and generally unpredictable. There was no clear relationship to the preoperative physical findings or laboratory data or to premedications employed. The general anesthetic agents employed included diethyl ether, cyclopropane, nitrous oxide, halothane, methoxyflurane, and ketamine, used singly and in combination. No one agent was associated with an increased frequency of complications. None of the patients with SC disease were managed with preoperative transfusion. Prophylactic transfusion was administered before 47 of the 58 procedures performed in SS patients but did not appreciably influence the complication rate. The combination of preoperative transfusion with intravenous hydration of to two to three times maintenance fluid requirements appeared to reduce but did not eliminate morbidity.

The following case history is typical:

---

*Personal communication, G. Packman, S. B. Murphy, and S. Chung.

Case 36-1. A 15-year-old black boy with SS disease was admitted to Children's Hospital of Philadelphia because of aseptic necrosis of the right hip, progressive after 8 weeks of conservative management. Despite troublesome transfusion therapy due to frequent febrile reactions and an anti-Kell antibody, the patient was prepared for surgery with multiple, packed cell transfusions to suppress formation of sickle cells and effectively to replace his circulating cells with normal ones. The patient had a preoperative Hb of 12.7 g. per dl. and a preoperative Hb electrophoresis showing 88-per-cent HbA and 11-per-cent HbS. He then underwent a subtrochanteric varus osteotomy of the right hip with a Phemister bone graft and adductor tenotomy under general endotracheal anesthesia with nitrous oxide, curare, and halothane after premedication with morphine, pentobarbital, and atropine. Surgery lasted 4 hours, 45 min., and the estimated blood loss was 2000 ml. Replacement consisted of 1000 ml. of packed red cells, 2700 ml. of intravenous fluid during surgery, with an addition 1500 ml. of packed cells over 5 days following surgery. Postoperatively, his course was complicated by fever, persistent tachycardia, and abdominal pain. Two months after surgery, the patient developed hyperbilirubinemia and a transient elevation of serum transaminases. A chronic tibial ulceration also developed, aggravated by spica casting.

Thus, despite careful management, numerous problems frequently arise in patients with sickle cell disease.

Complications of Sickle Cell Trait

Defining the risks of anesthesia in sickle cell trait is difficult. Because serious medical complications of sickle cell trait are so uncommon as to be "reportable," the literature is filled with numerous anecdotal reports. McGarry and Duncan reported deaths occurring in four children with sickle cell trait during or shortly after general anesthesia.[39] Schenk reported a fatal case of seizures, coma, superior longitudinal sinus thrombosis, and renal failure, which ensued 8 days following a tonsillectomy characterized by a difficult induction in a 12-year-old.[40] The importance of recognizing sickle cell trait in persons requiring open heart surgery is emphasized by the report of a fatality associated with multiple sickle thrombi and infarctions following cardiopulmonary bypass.[41]

These risks must be placed in perspective with regard to the incidence of sickle cell trait, which is common and affects millions of people, and of separation of cause from association, which is not always simple and straightforward. Provided that hypoxia, acidosis, and circulatory stasis are avoided, the actual excess risk (if there is one) of surgery and anesthesia in patients with sickle cell trait must be very slight. Searle reviewed 513 cases of sickle cell trait, involving patients who received anesthesia for procedures other than open heart surgery. He found that only four died. In three of the four, the deaths were not related to the anesthesia.[38] Atlas performed a matched-pair analysis of 56 black patients with sickle cell trait; they were matched for procedure, type of anesthesia, age, and sex, to black subjects with normal hemoglobin. No significant differences between the two groups in frequency, types of complications, or length of hospital stay were found. [42]

PREVENTION AND TREATMENT OF ANESTHETIC COMPLICATIONS OF SICKLE CELL STATES

Measures for the prevention and treatment of complications of sickle cell disease, arising as a result of surgery and anesthesia, should be considered together, because the rationale for their use is common to both, and because some measures may be preventive as well as therapeutic. Furthermore, the treatment of established complications is quite unsatisfactory and consists mainly of supportive measures. Therefore, emphasis should be placed on prevention.

No strict guidelines for the preoperative preparation or for the conduct of anesthesia may be formulated. Each case should be treated individually, with management dependent upon the condition of the patient, the type of surgical procedure, and the degree of emergency. Many techniques have been used successfully. Searle has stated aptly that the actual technique of general anesthesia employed is less important than the skill of the anesthetist using it.[38]

Management of the Patient with Sickle Cell Trait

The anesthetic and operative management of the patient with sickle cell trait should consist of such basic measures as preoxygenation prior to induction, scrupulous maintenance of adequate oxygenation during anesthesia, careful monitoring (including arterial blood gases), avoidance of acidosis and hypotension, and postanesthetic oxygen therapy. While such an anesthetic is desirable for all patients, it is obligatory for persons with sickle cell trait.

Management of the Patient with Sickle Cell Disease

The following remarks are directed toward management of sickle cell patients, particularly homozygous SS disease.

Preoperative Preparation. Recognition of the patient with sickle cell disease is the necessary first step in management (see p. 477). Elective procedures are best avoided but, if necessary, should be scheduled when the patient is in the best overall medical condition, free of symptoms of pain or infection. Premedication should not produce respiratory or circulatory depression.

Preoperative Transfusion. Transfusion with packed red cells prior to surgery is not without risks, such as acute transfusion reactions, hepatitis, and the probability of isosensitization. A number of investigators suggest that transfusion should not routinely be employed preoperatively and should be employed only for hemoglobin values less than 5 to 7 g. per dl.[30,32–35,43]

The efficacy of preoperative transfusion in reducing the morbidity and mortality of anesthesia and surgery in SS patients has never been shown clearly by a randomized controlled clinical trial. Nevertheless, the rationale for such an approach recommends itself, particularly when the nature of the operation or state of the patient makes the anesthetic particularly hazardous. The rationale for preoperative transfusion is reduction of the level of HbS by dilution or partial exchange with HbA blood. By their presence, normal red cells limit the maximum increase in viscosity resulting from conditions of lowered pH and decreased oxygen tension.[20] If surgery is elective, packed cell transfusions may be administered for 2 to 3 weeks prior to surgery. This raises the hemoglobin level to normal or slightly above and thereby suppresses endogenous erythropoiesis and allows time for short-lived sickle cells to be removed from the circulation.[44,45] If the surgery is an emergency, partial exchange transfusion may be carried out. Such a procedure simultaneously dilutes the sickle cells with normal cells and increases the blood oxygen-carrying capacity without increasing the blood volume and producing circulatory overload. One method for partial exchange for adults has been described as follows: (1) Remove 500 ml. of blood from the patient, using a plasmapheresis set; (2) infuse 300 ml. of isotonic sodium chloride solution through the female Luer connection; (3) remove 500 ml. of blood, using a transfer set to attach the blood container to the plasmapheresis set; stop this procedure if the patient becomes apprehensive or tachycardic; (4) infuse one unit of packed red blood cells, followed by four more units during the next 6 to 8 hours.[46] This method has the advantages of first reducing the patient's own red cell mass and then of not subsequently removing and discarding any transfused normal blood. Exchange transfusion has been used successfully in sickle cell disease for the treatment of symptomatic crisis,[46,47] for preoperative management,[48] and for management of the later stages of pregnancy and delivery.[49]

Other Measures to Prevent Sickling. Numerous measures, other than transfusion, have been suggested as a means of preventing sickling or of treating established crises. These include alkalinization,[30,32,43,50] hydration,[30] prophylactic folic acid,[30,32,34] magnesium sulfate,[30,32,50] heparinization,[30,32] and low-molecular-weight dextran.[51] The large number and variety of measures advocated provides eloquent testimony to the fact that none is completely satisfactory. There are almost no data to support any particular point of view, and generally favorable initial reports are most often followed by controlled trials demonstrating little or no efficacy.

Alkalinization is frequently recommended for management of the surgical patient[30,32,43,50] but is not thought to be necessary by others.[33,34] Suggested bicarbonate regimens have been either oral (1 g./kg./day in divided doses) or intravenous (3.3 mmol./kg./hour), with recommendations for use before, during, and after surgery. While it is true that prevention of acidosis or its prompt detection and correction are necessary, it has never been shown clearly that production of alkalosis will prevent vaso-occlusive crises. Good hydration, however, is essential.

There has been a flurry of recent interest in experimental agents to prevent sickling, such as urea or cyanate, though neither is currently approved for clinical use by the FDA. The theoretical promise of agents that interfere with aggregation of molecules of HbS is great but has not been demonstrated so far in practice.[46] The relative effectivenss of alkali, urea, and invert sugar administered intravenously for the treatment of painful crisis was compared in a controlled study, and no significant differences in responses were observed.[52]

Management of the Anesthetic. Among the wide variety of agents and techniques of anesthesia used in reported series of patients with sickle cell disease, none has been found to have a particularly deleterious effect. Hence, no particular anesthetic agent or technique is contraindicated. Wherever possible, local infiltration or nerve block is preferred to general anesthesia, however.

Careful positioning of the patient in an operating room that is not excessively cold is important. The use of tourniquets is best avoided, though several investigators have employed them with apparent safety. Monitoring of cardiopulmonary function, acid-base status, and renal function is essential. Arterial blood gas analysis should be carried out intraoperatively for major surgery.

Maintenance of adequate oxygenation is mandatory. Thus, administration of 100-per-cent oxygen prior to induction is recommended, while during the anesthetic itself, inspired oxygen should be adjusted so that a P_{O_2} of at least 80 to 100 torr (10.6–13.3 kPa) is achieved. Administration of 100-per-cent oxygen prior to extubation and supplemental oxygen postoperatively until full recovery has taken place are necessary. Generous intravenous hydration with replacement of blood loss ensures maintenance of an adequate circulating blood volume. Particular attention must be directed also to respiratory care, because atelectasis and pneumonia may occur more frequently in these patients,[33] and these complications may initiate the vicious cycle of sickling.[53]

REFERENCES

1. Motulsky, A. G.: Frequency of sickling disorders in U.S. blacks. N. Engl. J. Med., 288:31, 1973.
2. Karayalcin, G., Rosner, F., Chandra, P., et al.: Sickle cell anemia—clinical manifestations in 100 patients and review of literature. Am. J. Med. Sci., 51:51, 1976.
3. McCormick, W. F., and Kashgarian, M.: Age at death of patients with sickle cell trait. Am. J. Hum. Genet., 17:101, 1965.
3a. Sears, D. A.: The morbidity of sickle cell trait. Am. J. Med., 64:1021, 1978.
4. Ashcroft, M. T., and Desai, P.: Mortality and morbidity in Jamaican adults with sickle-cell trait and with normal haemoglobin followed up for twelve years. Lancet, 2:784, 1976.
5. Conn, H. O.: Sickle-cell trait and splenic infarction associated with high-altitude flying. N. Engl. J. Med., 251:417, 1954.
6. Oker, W. B., Bruno, M. S. Weinberg, S. B., et al.: Fatal intravascular sickling in a patient with sickle-cell trait. N. Engl. J. Med., 263:947, 1960.
7. Jones, S. R., Binder, R. A., and Donowho, E. M.: Sudden death in sickle-cell trait. N. Engl. J. Med., 282:323, 1970.
8. Diggs, L. W.: Screening tests for sickle cell disease. Postgrad. Med., 51:267, 1972.
9. Bertles, J. F.: Hemoglobin interaction and molecular basis of sickling. Arch. Intern. Med., 133:538, 1974.
10. Finch, C. A., and Lenfant, C.: Oxygen transport in man. N. Engl. J. Med., 286:407, 1972.
11. Torrance, J., Jacobs, S., Restrepo, A., et al.: Intraerythrocytic adaption to anemia. N. Engl. J. Med., 283:165, 1970.
12. Charache, S., Grisolia, S., Fiedler, A. J., et al.: Effect of 2,3-diphosphoglycerate on oxygen affinity of blood in sickle cell anemia. J. Clin. Invest., 49:806, 1970.
13. Seakins, M., Gibbs, W. N., and Milner, P. F.: Erythrocyte Hb-S concentration: an important factor in the low oxygen affinity of blood in sickle cell anemia. J. Clin. Invest., 52:422, 1973.
14. Milner, P.: Oxygen transport in sickle cell anemia. Arch. Intern. Med., 133:565, 1974.
15. Leight, L., Snider, T. H., Clifford, G. O., et al.: Hemodynamics studies in sickle cell anemia. Circulation, 10:653, 1954.
16. Klug, P., Lessin, L., and Radice, P.: Rheologic aspects of sickle cell disease. Arch. Intern. Med., 133:577, 1974.
17. Harris, J. W., Brewster, H. H., Ham, T. H., et al.: Studies

on the destruction of blood cells. X. The biophysics and biology of sickle cell disease. Arch. Intern. Med., *97*:145, 1956.

18. Charache, S., and Conley, C. L.: Rate of sickling of red cells during deoxygenation of blood from persons with various sickling disorders. Blood, *24*:25, 1964.

19. Messer, M. J., and Harris, J. W.: Filtration characteristics of sickle cells: rates of alteration of filterability after deoxygenation and reoxygenation, and correlations with sickling and unsickling. J. Lab. Clin. Med., *76*:537, 1970.

20. Anderson, R., Cassell, M., Mullinax, G. L., et al.: Effect of normal cells on viscosity of sickle-cell blood. Arch. Intern. Med., *111*:286, 1963.

21. Rubenstein, E.: Studies on the relationship of temperature to sickle cell anemia. Am. J. Med., *30*:95, 1961.

22. Laasberg, L. H., and Hedley-Whyte, J.: Viscosity of sickle disease and trait blood; changes with anesthesia. J. Appl. Physiol., *35*:837, 1973.

23. Harris, J. W., and Kellermeyer, R. W.: The Red Cell. rev. ed. pp. 168–202. Cambridge, Harvard University Press, 1970.

24. Lindsay, J., Jr., Meshel, J. C., and Patterson, R. H.: The cardiovascular manifestations of sickle cell disease. Arch. Intern. Med., *133*:643, 1974.

25. Bromberg, P. A.: Pulmonary aspects of sickle cell disease. Arch. Intern. Med., *133*:652, 1974.

26. Femi-Pearse, D., Gazioglu, K. M., and Yu, P. N.: Pulmonary function studies in sickle cell disease. J. Appl. Physiol., *28*:574, 1970.

27. Sproule, B. J., Holden, E. R., and Miller, W. F.: A study of cardiopulmonary alterations in patients with sickle cell disease and its variants. J. Clin. Invest., *37*:486, 1958.

28. Levitt, M. F., Hauser, A. D., and Levy, M. S.: The renal concentrating defect in sickle cell disease. Am. J. Med., *29*:611, 1960.

29. Schlitt, L., and Keitel, H.: Renal manifestations of sickle cell disease: A review. Am. J. Med. Sci., *239*:773, 1960.

30. Hilary-Howells, T., Huntsman, R. G., Boys, J. E., et al.: Anaesthesia and sickle cell haemoglobin. With a case report. Br. J. Anaesth., *44*:975, 1972.

31. Spiegelman, A., and Warden, M. J.: Surgery in patients with sickle cell disease. Arch. Surg., *104*:761, 1972.

32. Gilbertson, A. A.: Anaesthesia in West African patients with sickle-cell anaemia, haemoglobin SC disease, and sickle-cell trait. Br. J. Anaesth., *37*:614, 1965.

33. Holzmann, L., Finn, H., Lichtman, H. C., et al.: Anesthesia in patients with sickle cell disease: a review of 112 cases. Anesth. Analg., *48*:566, 1969.

34. Oduro, K. A., and Searle, J. F.: Anaesthesia in sickle-cell states: a plea for simplicity. Br. Med. J., *2*:596, 1972.

35. Oduntan, S. A., and Isaacs, W. A.: Anaesthesia in patients with abnormal haemoglobin syndromes: a preliminary report. Br. J. Anaesth., *43*:1159, 1971.

36. McPhillips, F. L., and Bickers, J. N.: Operations on patients with sickle cell anemia at Charity Hospital in New Orleans. Surg. Gynecol. Obstet., *135*:870, 1972.

37. Lewin, P., and Goodell, R. A.: Post-operative blindness with complete recovery in a patient with sickle-cell anemia. Br. Med. J., *2*:1373, 1962.

38. Searle, J. F.: Anaesthesia in sickle cell states. Anaesthesia, *28*:48, 1973.

39. McGarry, P., and Duncan, C.: Anesthetic risks in sickle cell trait. Pediatrics, *51*:507, 1973.

40. Schenk, E.: Sickle cell trait and superior longitudinal sinus thrombosis. Ann. Intern. Med., *60*:465, 1970.

41. Leachman, R. D., Miller, W. T., and Atias, I. M.: Sickle cell trait complicated by sickle cell thrombi after open-heart surgery. Am. Heart J., *74*:268, 1967.

42. Atlas, S. A.: The sickle cell trait and surgical complications. A matched-pair patient analysis. J.A.M.A., *229*:1078, 1974.

43. Browne, R. A.: Anaesthesia in patients with sickle-cell anaemia. Br. J. Anaesth., *37*:181, 1965.

44. Nadel, J. A., and Spivack, A. S.: Surgical management of sickle cell anemia: the use of packed red blood cell transfusions. Ann. Intern. Med., *48*:399, 1958.

45. Donegan, C. C., MacIhavaine, W. A., and Leavell, B. S.: Hematologic studies on patients with sickle cell anemia following multiple transfusions. Am. J. Med., *17*:29, 1954.

46. Charache, S.: The treatment of sickle cell anemia. Arch. Intern. Med., *133*:698, 1974.

47. Brody, J. I., Goldsmith, M. H., Park, S. K., et al.: Symptomatic crises of sickle cell anemia treated by limited exchange transfusion. Ann. Intern. Med., *72*:327, 1970.

48. Macleod, J.: Exchange transfusion in a 7-year-old girl with sickle cell anaemia as preparation for adenoidectomy. Proc. R. Soc. Med., *62*:1095, 1969.

49. Ricks, P.: Exchange transfusion in sickle cell anemia and pregnancy. Obstet. Gynecol., *25*:117, 1965.

50. Hugh-Jones, K., Lehmann, H., and McAlister, J. M.: Some experiences in managing sickle cell anaemia in children and young adults, using alkalis and magnesium. Br. Med. J., *2*:226, 1964.

51. Watson-Williams, E. J.: Sickle cell crisis treated with Rheomacrodex. Lancet, *1*:1053, 1963.

52. Cooperative urea trials group: clinical trials of therapy for sickle cell vaso-occulsive crises. J.A.M.A., *228*:1120, 1974.

53. Aldrete, J. A.: Hematologic disease. *In* Katz, J., and Kadis, L. B. (eds.): Anesthesia and Uncommon Diseases. pp. 244–250. Philadelphia, W. B. Saunders, 1973.

FURTHER READING

Conley, C. L.: Sickle-cell anemia—the first molecular disease. *In* Wintrobe, M. W. (ed.): Blood, Pure and Eloquent: A Story of Discovery, of People and Ideas. pp. 318–371. New York, McGraw-Hill Book Co., 1980.

Finch, C. A.: Pathophysiologic aspects of sickle cell anemia. Am. J. Med., *53*:1, 1972.

Flye, M. W., and Silver, D.: The role of surgery in sickle cell disease. Surg. Gynecol. Obstet., *137*:115, 1973.

Harris, J. W., and Kellermeyer, R. W.: The Red Cell. rev. ed. pp. 168–202. Cambridge, Harvard University Press, 1970.

Howells, T. H., Huntsman, R. G., Boys, J. E., et al.: Anaesthesia and sickle cell haemoglobin. Br. J. Anaesth., *44*:975, 1972.

Searle, J. F.: Anaesthesia in sickle cell states. Anaesthesia, *28*:48, 1973.

Tam, J. A., and Epstein, B. S.: Sickle cell disease and anesthesia. Anesth. Crit. Care Med., *1*(9):March 1978.

37 Immune Suppression

David L. Bruce, M.D.

There is literature, spanning over 70 years, that suggests that general anesthetic agents are immunosuppressant.[1-3] To date, no human data are available to support this contention conclusively. This subject deserves careful consideration in today's practice, since we encounter with increasing frequency patients whose immune defenses against infectious organisms and metastatic tumor cells are already weakened by sepsis, drugs, or nutritional deficits caused by an underlying infection and/or malignancy. When these patients require anesthesia, the informed anesthesiologist should be aware of evidence that suggests that anesthetic agents exert an additional depressant effect on these patients' defenses. In order to understand the role of anesthesia, the principal features of the immune response must first be reviewed. Necessarily, much of the following is speculative. Further studies are needed to assess the clinical relevance of anesthetic-induced immunosuppression.

THE IMMUNE RESPONSE

The word *immunity* is derived from the Latin word *immunitas*, meaning freedom from public service or, more generally, freedom from a burden. The body recognizes anything that is not "self" as a burden, such as bacteria, viruses, pollens, normal cells from another person, or its own malignant cells. Underlying the processes by which the body recognizes and then protects against foreign substances are both nonspecific and specific immune mechanisms that may act separately or jointly.

Nonspecific Immune Mechanisms

Nonspecific immune mechanisms tend to be genetically determined and as such do not require prior contact with foreign substances. Among numerous examples are the cilia of the respiratory epithelium that sweep foreign substances toward the pharynx, the bactericidal enzymes in saliva and tears, and the lytic action of fatty acids in sweat and sebaceous secretions.

Once a foreign particle such as an infecting organism has penetrated the barriers located at the interface of the body and the environment, the acute inflammatory response contains and then destroys the intruder. This nonspecific immune mechanism involves sequentially an increase in regional blood flow (to deliver plasma proteins and leukocytes to the site of injury), an increase in endothelial permeability (to permit the accumulation of phagocytic cells and bactericidal agents), an increase in venular sphincter tone (to promote stasis and hypoxia at the injury site), immune adherence between intruder and phagocytic cells, phagocytosis, and digestion of the intruder within the phagocytic cell.

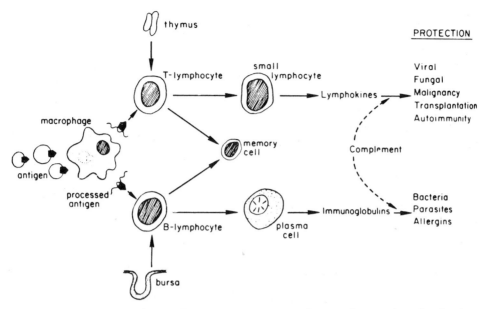

Fig. 37-1. Pathways of specific immunity. Macrophages phagocytize the foreign particles (antigen), process the antigenic information, and then pass on antigen-specific RNA to circulating lymphocytes. The transfer of antigenic information to B-lymphocytes results in a morphological alteration to form plasma cells that produce antigen-specific immunoglobulins (antibodies). Similar stimulation of T-lymphocytes results in their transformation to small circulating lymphocytes that produce chemical mediators (lymphokines) upon direct cellular interaction with the antigen. Either type of lymphocyte can form a memory cell capable of an accelerated response to that antigen in the future. The complement system can facilitate either humoral or cellular immunity. The usual protective roles of each type of immune cell are listed. (Duncan, F. G., and Cullen, B. F.: Anesthesia and immunology. Anesthesiology, *45:* 522, 1976)

Specific Immune Mechanisms

Immunity resulting from specific immune mechanisms is acquired. As a result of prior exposure to the particular intruder, specific proteins, called *antibodies,* are synthesized to react with these intruders and may be found in the body fluids (humoral antibodies) or bound to the surface of effector cells (cellular antibodies). There are several classes of antibodies and two principal types of lymphocytes involved in their production.

The thymus gland processes lymphocytes to become T cells. The other principal type of lymphocyte-derived cell is designated by the letter *B,* because these cells are produced in the bursa of Fabricius, an organ near the cloaca in birds. The "bursal" cells in man are produced most likely in the lymphoid tissue found throughout the gastrointestinal tract and in the spleen. The two lymphocyte types are grossly indistinguishable but may be differentiated by the ability of T cells to bind sheep erythrocytes, forming rosettes. The T-lymphocytes form effector cells whose functions include delayed hypersensitivity, transplant rejection, and tumor immunity. The B-lymphocytes give rise to plasma cells that synthesize circulating antibody. There is evidence of cooperation between T and B cells in many immune reactions, but the nature of this interaction is not clear.

In both the T cell and B cell activation pathways (Fig. 37-1), antigenic stimulation of sensitized cells results in their transformation into enlarged, blast forms, which then divide to produce a logarithmic curve of cell numbers. The humoral response involves differentiation of B cell progeny to plasma cells rich in endoplasmic reticulum, responsible for protein synthesis of antibodies, which are then released into circulation. In both cell-mediated and humoral pathways, "memory" cells are created. These cells do not progress further, forming a reserve of specifically sensitized cells that may be activated readily by reintroduction of antigen. This hastens the response to a second challenge, the basis of the "anamnestic" reaction.

The stimuli for specific reactions are antigens, which are further characterized as complete and incomplete. Complete antigens are macromolecules, usually proteins, that both elicit a response and react specifically with the products of that response. Incomplete antigens, designated *haptens*, are smaller molecules that combine with a carrier protein to form an antigen that can elicit a response that neither hapten nor carrier can cause by itself. There is considerable evidence that many antigens are phagocytized and "processed" by macrophages to render them suitable to stimulate appropriate lymphocytes.

Response to antigens involves the formation of antibodies. These are proteins that migrate electrophoretically as slow beta or gamma globulins. Collectively they are called *immunoglobulins (Ig)*. Each Ig molecule consists of two pairs of polypeptide chains, each joined by disulfide bonds. One pair, the light (L) chain pair, is common to all Ig. The other pair, the heavy (H) chain, has five varieties, so there are five classes of Ig: IgG, IgM, IgA, IgD, and IgE. Each class of immunoglobulin has specific functions. For example, IgG and IgM are involved in bacterial defense; IgG leaves the circulation to protect extravascular compartments, whereas the larger IgM antibody remains within the circulation. IgA is found in secretions such as saliva and protects the digestive and upper respiratory tracts.

Having described the eliciting antigen, the responding cells, and the immunoglobulin product, a final class of reacting products must be mentioned. Complement is a system of at least eleven distinct serum proteins organized into nine components, designated C1 to C9. Complement can be activated and bound by IgM and most IgG antibodies. Depending upon the antibody, a characteristic chain reaction follows this activation and leads to processes such as chemotaxis, phagocytosis, and cytolysis.

CELLULAR EFFECTS OF ANESTHETICS

General anesthetic agents inhibit a variety of processes involving intracellular contractility. These processes occur all along the pathway of the immune response, and any of them might be depressed by these drugs. Some of these processes are as follows:

Processes Involving Intracellular Contractility and Inhibited by Anesthetics

Phagocytosis of antigen by macrophages
Expulsion (exocytosis) of "processed" antigen
Uptake (pinocytosis) of processed antigen by lymphocytes
Blastic transformation of stimulated lymphocytes
Division of blast cells and clonal proliferation
Expulsion of synthesized antibodies

Phagocytosis and pinocytosis are special cases of the general category endocytosis, which includes active processes by which macromolecules are ingested by the cell. They differ chiefly in the size of particles engulfed; phagocytosis is macroscopic relative to pinocytosis. The return of material from cell to environment is called *exocytosis*. There are data that show inhibition of these cellular transport functions by anesthetics, although the experiments often were not designed to test immunologic functions directly.

The effects of ether, chloroform, and, more recently, halothane have been investigated in the ameba, a prototype of actively contractile cells.[4] These studies demonstrated reversible cessations of cytoplasmic streaming and phagocytosis when the cell is exposed to volatile anesthetic agents. In 1911 Graham showed that ether anesthesia reversibly depresses phagocytosis by neutrophils taken from patients during operation.[5] For 60 years afterward, similar studies in animals appeared sporadically in the European literature. Rekindled interest in this area is now evident and is discussed elsewhere.

Although the effect of anesthetics on endo- and exocytosis is still unclear, much has been learned recently about the effect of anesthesia on the blastic transformation of human lymphocytes in vitro following stimulation by phytohemagglutinin (PHA). PHA is a plant extract that nonspecifically induces T-lymphocytes to enlarge, synthesize protein, RNA, and DNA, and then to divide. This sequence is thought to mimic the specific reaction of sensitized cells to antigens. Halothane causes dose-dependent depression of human lymphocyte transformation in vitro[6,7]; inhibition in the presence of clinically significant anesthetic concentrations requires an exposure of more than 24 hours, however. A concentration of 2-per-cent halothane inhibits the nuclear enlargement[8] and protein and RNA synthesis[9] that normally follow addition of PHA to the lymphocyte cultures. Lymphocyte function is normal in patients following brief operations[10] and in volunteers after prolonged anesthesia with halothane or enflurane without surgery.[11] Diminished lymphocyte transformation does occur with nitrous oxide anesthesia in volunteers,[12] but not in vitro[13] and the depressed lymphocyte reactivity correlates inversely with the cortisol response to light anesthesia.[12] This suggests that impaired lymphocyte function results from the neurohumoral responses, such as increases in adrenocorticosteroid and catecholamine levels, accompanying surgical stress.[14,15]

Once the antigen has caused blastic transformation, the immune response involves repeated cell division to produce a logarithmic increase in progeny from that one cell. The family of cells so derived is known as a clone. Cell division is thus at the heart of the matter of immunity, and it has been known since Claude Bernard's studies that anesthetics do inhibit cell division.[16]

Thus, there is a suggestion that the administration of general anesthetics *may* result in immune suppression. The alterations owing to surgery and its attendant stress probably overshadow any changes caused by anesthetics, since a clinical confirmation of the effect of anesthesia has not been demonstrated. An anesthetic effect on immunity should affect the response to infection, transplants, tumors, and anaphylaxis.

CLINICAL SIGNIFICANCE OF ANESTHETIC-INDUCED IMMUNE SUPPRESSION

Infections

Resistance to infection involves many modes of defense. For example, an infective agent may elicit a high titer of circulating antibodies in a host that is adequately equipped with complement and phagocytic cells, but these elements must be delivered to the site of infection by an adequate blood supply and tissue perfusion or they will be of no benefit. The discussion that follows assumes that blood supply, nutrition, and other nonspecific factors are adequate and will focus on the specific immune response itself; however, it should not be forgotten that anesthetics may alter many of these nonspecific factors, too.

Alexander and Good estimate that the critical number of bacteria in an inoculum necessary to cause a clinical infection is 10^6 organisms in normal human tissue, 10^2 when specific antibody is absent, and only 10^0 when phagocytic cells are absent.[17] The predominant antibody to gram-negative bacteria is IgM. To other bacteria, as well as to some viruses, it is IgG. The reactions of these antibodies with bacterial antigens activate the complement system, producing several important effects, including the following: chemotaxis, in which phagocytes are drawn to the site of infection; immune adherence, whereby bacterial surfaces are "opsonized" by direct coating with antibody, facilitated by complement, and causing the organisms to be more easily attached to phagocytic cell membranes; phagocytosis of the bacteria; and activation of intracellular digestion of these phagocytized organisms.

Infections with many viruses, fungi, and bacteria of relatively low virulence, such as mycobacteria, are combated by cell-mediated immune mechanisms. The antibody on T cell walls combines with surface antigens, activating the lymphocytes to synthesize and release lymphotoxin, which enzymatically disrupts the foreign cell membrane. These reactions occur in vitro, where there is no complement. Patients with severely compromised cellular immunity, such as those with disseminated tuberculosis, advanced malignancy, or immunosuppression by drug therapy, are inordinately susceptible to usually trivial infections such as rubeola, chicken pox, and cytomegalovirus disease.

In 1903 Snel showed that anesthesia with ether or chloroform increases guinea pig mortality from anthrax.[18] The immune response to this disease is probably primarily cellular, but studies soon followed that employed infectious agents to which the response is humoral. In 1904 Rubin reported that these same anesthetic agents increase the virulence of streptococcal and pneumococcal infections in rabbits.[19] A number of other studies followed, and anesthesia was generally regarded in those days as detrimental to the patient's resistance to infection. The interest in these experiments seems to have lessened around 1925, and for many years thereafter, little mention was made of this subject in surgical texts. More recently, Kosciolek reported that neutrophils removed from rabbits and men anesthetized with halothane or ether were defective in their capacity to phagocytize staphylococci.[20] Although the patients had the stress of surgery superimposed on anesthesia, the rabbits did not, and the results from the two species are similar.

The rabbits also had a circulating lymphopenia, as did the rats studied by Bruce and Koepke.[21] Although those rats were exposed to halothane for days, the lymphopenia was seen early. In addition, the neutrophil compartments were shifted, suggesting a "damming up" of dividing myeloid cells. If this were to occur in patients, one would expect the peripheral neutrophils not to reflect any change until several days postoperatively.[22] Neutrophil function was found to be deficient in mice infected with salmonella, with a reduction from 24.6 to 2.7 bacteria ingested per peritoneal neutrophil.[23] More recently, Cullen[1,24] and others[2,3] have concluded that the effect of anesthesia on phagocytosis is of only minor importance compared to the impairment associated with surgical trauma, and they have suggested that these earlier findings may have been caused by nonspecific "stress" responses. Thus, the evidence that anesthetics affect the numbers and functions of phagocytes is inconclusive and controversial.

Since these experiments involve processes in which immunity is of the humoral type, there has been interest in the effect of anesthesia on antibody production. The only studies of this function have been reported by Wingard, Humphrey, and Lang, who described depression of splenic antibody-producing cells in rats and mice anesthetized with halothane for 2 to 4 hours.[25,26] In general, the reduction in these antibody-producing cells correlates with the duration of exposure to anesthetic, and recovery may require 72 hours. Yet, only insignificant changes in immunoglobulin levels have been found in patients having routine surgery.[27–29] Nevertheless, both cellular and humoral components of immunity may be depressed in the postoperative period when wound infections or pneumonia can develop. Since viral hepatitis is kept in check by a predominantly humoral immune response, postoperative liver dysfunction might occasionally be related to compromised immunity.

The capacity of complement to interact with antibodies in the presence of anesthetics has not been studied directly. One of the many processes affected by complement is chemotaxis. In studies of peritoneal neutrophil response to both bacterial endotoxin and live salmonella, there was a marked reduction in numbers of neutrophils mobilized into this site in mice anesthetized with halothane.[23] This may have involved complement but also could have been caused by changes in the fine structure of the neutrophils or even by reduced splanchnic blood flow. The latter is unlikely, however, since Evans blue dye appeared at a normal rate in peritoneal cavities of mice anesthetized under identical conditions. Although death occurred earlier in mice receiving halothane following the intraperitoneal injection of bacteria, the ultimate mortality of the anesthetized animals was similar to that of the control group. Recently, using a fecal peritonitis model that is more sensitive to the effects of anesthesia, Duncan, Cullen, and Pearsall have shown that mortality in mice receiving halothane is 81 per cent compared to 44 per cent in a control group.[30] Because halothane did not affect the size of a *Candida albicans* skin lesion in another series of animals, they felt that the anesthetic probably has little effect on the mobilization and deposition of phagocytic cells at the site of infection. Heat-sterilization of the fecal material removes the lethality of halothane, suggesting that death in this model results from active infection rather than endotoxin. They postulated that the halothane-increased mortality is caused by decreased plasma opsonization with substances like complement and antibodies and/or impaired reticuloendothelial phagocytosis.

Even less is known about the effect of anesthetics on those infections combated by cell-mediated immunity. The only study of anesthetic effect on such an infection was that reported by Snel, in which anesthesia was associated with an increased mortality from anthrax in mice. In view of the tendency of anesthetic agents to modify neurohumoral responses to surgery,[12,14,15] depth of anesthesia may be important in the clinical response to infections combated by cell-mediated immunity.

The following sequence of events can occur during operation: Pathogenic bacteria contaminate the wound; neutrophils are inhibited both from reaching these extravascular sites of contamination and, once there, from ingesting the organisms normally; the bacteria-proliferate, being relatively resistant to anesthetic inhibition of their rate of cell division and also exposed only to a low tension of the agent at that site; some of the bacteria that do reach regional lymph nodes are not phagocytized normally by the macrophages in the nodal cortex; the underlying B-lymphocytes in germinal centers of the nodes do not undergo blastic transformation in response to the antigenic material that is "processed" by those macrophages; and, there is a resultant lag in the production of plasma cells synthesizing circulating antibody to the bacterial antigens. Consequently, by the 2nd or 3rd postoperative day, the bacteria have had a "head start"; their growth exceeds the rate of antibody production, and the number of neutrophils in circulation is less than if there had not been a block of division of precursors to maturing marrow myeloid compartments during anesthesia. Adding to this picture the effect of elevated corticosteroids and catecholamines in response to the surgical stress, causing diminished vascular reactivity and lymphopenia, and considering also the foreign bodies of the suture material, which afford relatively inaccessible environments for bacteria to multiply, the stage is set for infection.

If this hypothetical sequence is accurate, even in part, it is remarkable that serious infections do not occur more often. Although definitive prospective studies are required to determine the role of anesthesia in postoperative infections, prolonged anesthesia and surgery are associated with a higher incidence of wound infections.[31,32] Undoubtedly, numerous factors are responsible for postoperative infections (e.g., advanced age, severe obesity, malnutrition, diabetes),[33-37] but the relative importance of each is unknown. It is possible that the surgeon may have to reevaluate the importance of minimizing anesthesia time.

Transplants and Tumors

The immune response is highly specific, so much so that substitution of one amino acid in a long polypeptide chain of a protein is recognized as different by antibody-forming cells. It is no wonder, then, that cells from a person of different genetic constitution elicit an immune response. For the same reason, malignant cells arising from the host's own tissues have undergone enough change to be recognized as different and they, too, are antigenic. Moreover, malignancy is often associated with progressive immune deficiency and/or immunosuppressive therapy.[38-41]

Because anesthesia under some circumstances may depress the T cells responsible for cellular immunity,[12] anesthesia can affect adversely the defenses against cancer and favor the successful "take" of transplanted tissue. However, the experimental evidence for this expectation is contradictory. Although some studies suggest that anesthesia enhances the development of metastases,[42,43] others do not.[44-46] Halothane and nitrous oxide[47] and thiopental[48,49] inhibit tumor cell killing mediated by sensitized leukocytes in vitro, with the degree of inhibition depending upon the duration of exposure to the anesthetic, or anesthetics.

If future studies show that anesthetic agents do favor the spread of tumor cells and inhibit the rejection of transplanted tissue, the significance of these findings would be different in each case, depending on the duration of anesthesia and, perhaps, other factors. Yet, even a few hours of anesthetic-induced immunosuppression might allow these cells to get a "head start" in a manner analogous to that hypothesized for a bacterial nidus. This subject should be investigated further before discounting the possibility that the growth of some tumors, in some patients, is aided by general anesthesia.

Anaphylaxis

Allergic reactions may occur in the anesthetized patient, and the most serious type is anaphylaxis. In a review of anaphylaxis detected in a series of 11,526 monitored medical inpatients, blood and its derivatives were the chief offending agents.[50] The anaphylactic reaction consists of an acute, severe set of symptoms that follow the combination of administered antigen with tissue mast cells sensitized with antibody to that antigen. The antibody class is IgE, which, when combined with antigen, causes the mast cells to degranulate by a process of exocytosis. The released "granules" are packets of pharmacologically active substances that cause smooth muscle to contract. In man, these substances are chiefly histamine and slow reacting substances of anaphylaxis (SRS-A). Histamine acts quickly to contract smooth muscle and is blocked by antihistamines, whereas SRS-A acts more slowly to cause such contraction and is antagonized by atropine. In man, the end organ most affected is bronchial smooth muscle, which contracts to produce severe bronchospasm.

Cyclic AMP (3',5'-adenosine monophosphate) is involved both in the mast cell degranulation and in the smooth muscle contraction. Agents that elevate intracellular cAMP inhibit both these processes and thus help abort the anaphylactic reaction. Such an elevation can result from increased synthesis of cAMP, caused by beta-adrenergic agonists, and from decreased degradation of the cAMP by phosphodiesterase, an enzyme inhibited by methylxanthines. This explains the rationale of the treatment of acute bronchial asthma with epinephrine and aminophylline.

Animal studies of the influence of anesthesia on anaphylaxis have been inconsistent and contradictory.[51] Problems are posed by species differences, route of administration of antigen, respiratory depression attendant to anesthesia, and imprecise methods of anesthetic administration. All of these make interpretation of the data difficult. Although early work suggested that ether offers some protection,[52] the effect is limited to inhaled antigen and is not shared by other anesthetics.[53] In the light of the more recent findings concerning mechanisms of mediator release and cAMP, this action of ether may be secondary to catecholamine release, rather than a result of a primary effect of the anesthetic molecule itself. Ether and halothane are known to relax bronchospastic muscle.[54] Whether this action is caused by an anesthetic effect on cAMP of that tissue is unknown at present. Workers in anesthesiology are just beginning to study cAMP and cyclic nucleotides as mediators for anesthetic action.[55] For the present, then, one must assume that anesthetics do not affect the release of mediators by antigens or their interactions with target organs, although the clinical manifestations (e.g., bronchospasm) may be modified.

CLINICAL RECOMMENDATIONS FOR ANESTHETIC MANAGEMENT

In a compendium of complications of anesthesia, immune suppression is possibly the most speculative. Little is known about anesthetic effect on immunity, despite an interest that began with modern surgery, when patients were given deep anesthesia by open drop methods and were subject to postoperative pneumonia. Little was known of respiratory physiology, and neither ventilators nor antibiotics were available. Later, anesthesiology became more sophisticated, ventilation was better maintained, and muscle relaxants and antibiotics became available. Postoperative pneumonia occurred less often, and when it did happen, it was more easily treated.

Why, then, is there an apparent resurgence of interest in researching this subject? It is probably a measure of maturity within the specialty of anesthesiology. We have passed the point at which the administration of anesthesia was considered an art, devoid of more monitoring than the intuition of the anesthesiologist. Today we provide safe anesthesia for patients who, in the past, would have been rejected as unfit for surgery. Operations have become longer, more complicated, and more traumatic. Today anesthesiologists consider the total impact of anesthetic agents and techniques on the recovery of these patients. Effects on immunity fall within this category of concern.

Given our present knowledge of the effects of anesthetics on the immune system, no firm recommendations can be made regarding the choice of anesthetic agents and techniques. We have some laboratory evidence to support the avoidance of elective surgery in infected patients, as well as prolonged surgery and anesthesia. However, we need more information about the relative immunosuppressive potencies of our agents and techniques, and how they interact with variables such as the patient's age, drug therapy, nutritional status, and surgical procedure in altering the immune system.

REFERENCES

1. Duncan, P. G., and Cullen, B. F.: Anesthesia and immunology. Anesthesiology, 45:522, 1976.
2. Moudgil, G. C., and Wade, A. G.: Anaesthesia and immunocompetence. Br. J. Anaesth., 48:31, 1976.
3. Walton, B.: Anaesthesia, surgery and immunology. Anaesthesia, 33:322, 1978.
4. Bruce, D., and Christiansen, R.: Morphologic changes in the giant amoeba *Chaos Chaos* induced by halothane and ether. Exp. Cell Res., 40:544, 1965.
5. Graham, E. A.: The influence of ether and ether anesthesia in bacteriolysis, agglutination, and phagocytosis. J. Infect. Dis., 8:147, 1911.
6. Bruce, D. L.: Halothane inhibition of phytohemagglutinin-induced transformation of lymphocytes. Anesthesiology, 36:201, 1972.
7. Cullen, B. F., Sample, W. F., and Chretien, P. B.: The effect of halothane on phytohemagglutinin-induced transformation of human lymphocytes *in vitro*. Anesthesiology, 36:206, 1972.
8. Bruce, D. L.: Halothane effect on nuclear volume of PHA treated human lymphocytes. Reticuloendothel. Soc., 15:497, 1974.
9. Bruce, D. L.: Halothane inhibition of RNA and protein synthesis of PHA treated human lymphocytes. Anesthesiology, 42:11, 1974.
10. Cullen, B. F., and Van Belle, G.: Lymphocyte transformation and changes in leukocyte count: effect of anesthesia and operation. Anesthesiology, 43:563, 1975.
11. Duncan, P. G., Cullen, B. F., Calverly, R., et al.: Failure of enflurane and halothane anesthesia to inhibit lymphocyte transformation in volunteers. Anesthesiology, 45:661, 1976.
12. Lecky, J. H.: Anesthesia and the immune system. Surg. Clin. North Am., 55:795, 1975.
13. Bruce, D. L.: Failure of nitrous oxide to inhibit transformation of lymphocytes by phytohemagglutinin. Anesthesiology, 44:155, 1976.
14. Bancewicz, J., Gray, A. C., and Lindop, C.: The immunosuppressive effect of surgery—a possible mechanism. Br. J. Surg., 60:314, 1973.
15. Wilmore, D. W., Long, J. M., Mason, A. D., et al.: Stress in surgical patients as a neurophysiologic reflex response. Surg. Gynecol. Obstet., 142:257, 1976.
16. Sturrock, J. E., and Nunn, J. F.: Mitosis in mammalian cells during exposure to anesthetics. Anesthesiology, 43:21, 1975.
17. Alexander, J. W., and Good, R. A.: Immunobiology for Surgeons. Philadelphia, W. B., Saunders, 1970.
18. Snel, J. J.: Immunitat und narkose. Berlin Klin. Wschr., 40:212, 1903.
19. Rubin, G.: The influence of alcohol, ether and chloroform on natural immunity in its relation to leukocytosis and phagocytosis. J. Infect. Dis., 1:425, 1904.
20. Kosciolek, E.: Fagocytarna aktywnosc leukocytow krwi i whysieku otrzewnowego wogolnym znieczuleniu fluotanowyn. Roczn. Pom. Akad. Med. Swierca., 13:149, 1967.
21. Bruce, D. L., and Koepke, J. A.: Changes in granulopoiesis in the rat associated with prolonged halothane anesthesia. Anesthesiology, 27:811, 1966.
22. Bruce, D. L., and Koepke, J. A.: Clinical implications of the effect of halothane on depressed rat bone marrow. Anesthesiology, 34:573, 1971.
23. Bruce, D. L.: Effect of halothane anesthesia on experimental salmonella peritonitis in mice. J. Surg. Res., 7:180, 1967.
24. Cullen, B. F.: The effect of halothane and nitrous oxide on phagocytosis and human leukocyte metabolism. Anesth. Analg., 53:531, 1974.
25. Wingard, D. W., Lang, R., and Humphrey, L. J.: Effect of anesthesia on immunity. J. Surg. Res., 7:430, 1967.
26. Wingard, D. W., and Humphrey, L. J.: Depression of antibody production by halothane: a dose response. Anesthesiology, 30:353, 1969.
27. Cohen, P. J.: Response of human immunoglobulins to halothane anesthesia and surgery. Fed. Proc., 31:534, 1972.
28. Slade, M. S., Simmons, R. L., Yunis, E., et al.: Immunodepression after major surgery in normal patients. Surgery, 78:363, 1975.

29. Fuller, J. M., and Keyser, J. W.: Serum immunoglobulins after surgical operation. Clin. Chem., *21*:667, 1975.

30. Duncan, P. G., Cullen, B. F., and Pearsall, N. N.: Anesthesia and the modification of response to infection in mice. Anesth. Analg., *55*:776, 1976.

31. National Academy of Sciences-National Research Council Ad Hoc Committee of the Committee on Trauma: Postoperative wound infections: the influence of ultraviolet irradiation of the operating room and of various other factors. Ann. Surg., *160*[Suppl. 2]:1, 1964.

32. Jepsen, O. B., Larsen, S. O., and Thomsen, V. F.: Postoperative wound sepsis in general surgery. II. An assessment of factors influencing the frequency of wound sepsis. Acta Chir. Scandinav., *396* [Suppl.]:80, 1969.

33. Cruse, P. J. E., and Foord, R.: A five-year prospective study of 23,649 surgical wounds. Arch. Surg., *107*:206, 1973.

34. MacLean, L. D., Meakin, J. L., Taguchi, K., et al.: Host resistance in sepsis and trauma. Ann. Surg., *182*:207, 1975.

35. Miller, W. E., and Counts, G. W.: Orthopedic infections: a prospective study of 378 clean procedures. South Med. J., *68*:386, 1975.

36. Stevens, D. B.: Postoperative orthopaedic infections. J. Bone Joint Surg., *46*:96, 1964.

37. Stone, H. H., and Hesser, T. R.: Incisional and peritoneal infection after emergency celiotomy. Ann. Surg., *177*:669, 1973.

38. Failkow, P. J.: Immunologic oncogenesis. Blood, *30*:388, 1967.

39. Penn, L., Hammond, W., Brettschneider, L., et al.: Malignant lymphomas in transplantation patients. Transplant. Proc., *1*:106, 1969.

40. Miller, D. G.: The immunologic capability of patients with lymphoma. Cancer Res., *28*:1441, 1968.

41. Southam, C. M.: The immunologic status of patients with nonlymphomatous cancer. Cancer Res., *28*:1433, 1968.

42. Agostino, D., and Cliffton, E. E.: Anesthetic effect on pulmonary metastases in rats. Arch. Surg., *88*:735, 1964.

43. Gaylord, H. R., and Simpson, B. T.: The effect of certain anesthetics and loss of blood upon the growth of transplanted mouse cancer. J. Cancer Res., *1*:379, 1916.

44. Cullen, B. F., and Sundsmo, J. F.: Failure of halothane anesthesia to alter growth of sarcoma in mice. Anesthesiology, *41*:580, 1974.

45. Fisher, B., and Fisher, E. R.: Experimental studies of factors influencing hepatic metastases. III. Effect of surgical trauma with special reference to liver injury. Ann. Surg., *150*:731, 1959.

46. Van Den Brenk, H. A. S., and Shapington, C.: Effect of phenobarbital on growth of metastasizing allogeneic sarcoma in the rat. Experientia, *28*:686, 1972.

47. Cullen, B. F., Duncan, P. G., and Ray-Keil, L.: Inhibition of cell-mediated cytotoxicity by halothane and nitrous oxide. Anesthesiology, *44*:386, 1976.

48. Duncan, P. G., Cullen, B. F., and Ray-Keil, L.: Thiopental inhibition of tumor immunity. Anesthesiology, *46*:97, 1977.

49. Lundy, J., Lovett, E. J. II, and Conran, P.: Pulmonary metastases, a potential biologic consequence of anesthetic-induced immunosuppression by thiopental. Surgery, *82*:254, 1977.

50. Jick, H., and Shapiro, S.: Drug-induced anaphylaxis. A cooperative study. J.A.M.A., *224*:613, 1973.

51. Bruce, D. L., and Wingard, D. W.: Anesthesia and the immune response. Anesthesiology, *34*:271, 1971.

52. Carron, H.: Anaphylaxis and anesthesia. Anesthesiology, *8*:625, 1947.

53. Parrish, W. E., Hall, L. W., and Coombs, R. R. A.: The effects of anesthesia on anaphylaxis in guinea pigs. Immunology, *6*:462, 1963.

54. Fletcher, S. W., Flacke, W., and Alper, M. H.: The actions of general anesthetic agents on tracheal smooth muscle. Anesthesiology, *29*:517, 1968.

55. Wiklund, R. A.: Cyclic nucleotides. Anesthesiology, *41*:490, 1974.

FURTHER READING

Duncan, P. G., and Cullen, B. F.: Anesthesia and immunology. Anesthesiology, *45*:522, 1976.

Norman, J., and Whitwam, J. G. (eds.): Symposium on immunology in anaesthesia and intensive care. Br. J. Anaesth., *51*:1, 1979.

Mathieu, A., and Kahan, B. D. (eds.): Immunologic Aspects of Anesthetic and Surgical Practice. New York, Grune & Stratton, 1975.

Moudgil, G. C., and Wade, A. G.: Anaesthesia and immunocompetence. Br. J. Anaesth., *48*:31, 1976.

Samter, M. (ed.): Immunological Diseases. ed. 3. Boston, Little, Brown & Co., 1979.

Walton, B.: Anaesthesia, surgery and immunology. Anaesthesia, *33*:322, 1978.

38 Acquired Methemoglobinemia and Sulfhemoglobinemia

Fredrick K. Orkin, M.D.

The sudden appearance of cyanosis usually suggests such cardiorespiratory catastrophes as airway obstruction, pneumothorax, cardiac dysrhythmia, and cardiac arrest, among others discussed in Parts 4 and 5 of this book. Typically, cyanosis is a manifestation of hypoxia. Rarely, however, cyanosis results because the hemoglobin structure has been altered, for example, to form methemoglobin or sulfhemoglobin, which impairs oxygen transport. This chapter is a discussion of how alterations in hemoglobin structure are produced by drugs administered either during or in proximity to anesthesia.

THE PHYSICAL BASIS OF METHEMOGLOBINEMIA AND SULFHEMOGLOBINEMIA

The respiratory molecule hemoglobin consists of four subunits, each with an iron-containing porphyrin heme united with a globin polypeptide chain (Fig. 38-1). The iron contained in heme is in the reduced, or ferrous, state. Each iron atom binds to the four pyrrole rings that comprise heme; a fifth bond of the iron attaches to a histidine residue of globin, leaving a sixth valence bond to combine reversibly with one molecule of oxygen.

The binding of oxygen to hemoglobin is a complex, sequential, *cooperative* process. As oxygen binds to each heme, the affinity of the re-

maining hemes for oxygen increases. Hence, the oxyhemoglobin dissociation curve at first rises slowly, then more steeply, finally, once an oxygen molecule has combined with each of the four hemes, it flattens again (see Fig. 35-2). To account for heme–heme interactions that occur while the four hemes in hemoglobin are not touching, Perutz has proposed that hemoglobin shifts back and forth between two alternative structures.[1] In

Fig. 38-1. The structure of the iron-containing porphyrin heme (ferroprotoporphyrin) consists of an iron atom in the ferrous state bound to four pyrrole rings joined in a plane by methene bridges. For the sale of clarity, the carbon atoms of the pyrrole ring are represented as the corners of the pentagons, with the hydrogen atoms omitted. On one side of this plane the iron binds with a globin polypeptide chain and on the other, oxygen. Four heme-polypeptide subunits comprise hemoglobin, with each heme nestled at the surface of the molecule.

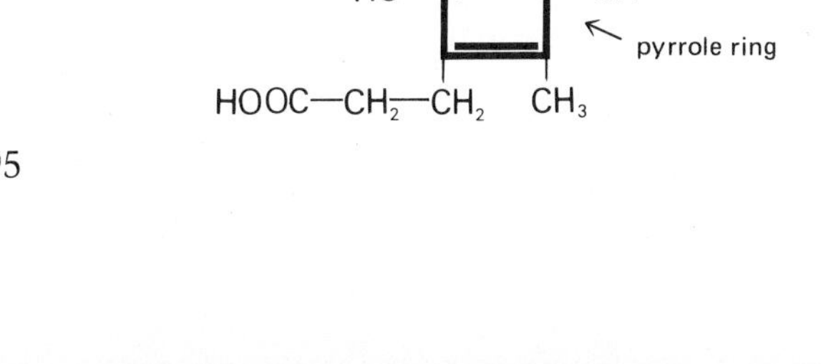

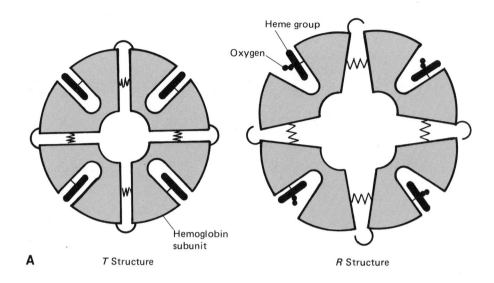

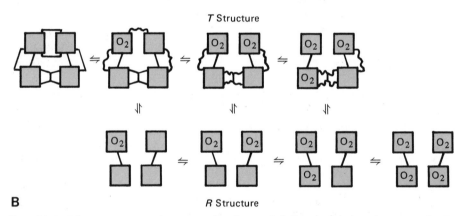

Fig. 38-2. The transport of oxygen by hemoglobin is postulated to involve a transition between two structures. A. In the *T* structure the subunits are clamped tightly by salt bridges against springs, narrowing the heme pockets; in the *R* structure the salt bridges have ruptured, allowing the heme pockets to open wide enough to admit oxygen easily. B. The transition from the *T* structure to the *R* structure involves the progressive rupture of salt bridges as oxygen is bound. Simultaneous weakening of salt bridges (wavy lines) occurs elsewhere in the molecule (allosteric effect), enhancing the likelihood of further oxygen binding. (Perutz, M. F.: Hemoglobin structure and respiratory transport. Sci. Am. *239:*92, December 1978.)

the *T* (tense) structure, the heme pockets in the hemoglobin subunits are so narrow that oxygen cannot enter, whereas in the *R* (relaxed) structure the heme pockets are wide enough to permit oxygen to bind easily with heme (Fig. 38-2A). The

binding of oxygen to heme in the lungs is associated with breakage of the salt bridges that link the subunits tightly in the *T* structure (Fig. 38-2B). Breakage of the salt bridges, in turn, causes conformational changes in hemoglobin that increase the affinity of heme elsewhere in the molecule for oxygen (allosteric effect). Loss of oxygen molecules in the capillary allows the salt bridges to reestablish, with resultant narrowing of the heme pockets and return to the *T* structure. According to this theory, any alteration in hemoglobin structure that prevents the transition between the *R* and *T* structures would impair oxygen transport by hemoglobin.

METHEMOGLOBINEMIA

Under normal circumstances, a very small fraction of hemoglobin in living erythrocytes undergoes oxidation. As a result, some of the heme iron is in the ferric state, forming methemoglobin ($HbFe^{3+}$) that exists in equilibrium with hemoglobin ($HbFe^{2+}$):

$$HbFe^{2+} + H_2O \rightleftharpoons 2HbFe^{3+} - OH$$

In the oxidized state, the sixth valence bond combines with a hydroxyl group (in the alkaline form, as in Fig. 38-2) or a water molecule (in the acid form) and can no longer combine with oxygen.[2] In terms of Perutz's model, methemoglobin is stabilized in the *R* structure and cannot shift between the *T* and *R* structures.[1]

Methemoglobinemia exists when more than 1 per cent of hemoglobin is methemoglobin. This small but relatively constant concentration of methemoglobin reflects the difference between the rate of which methemoglobin is being formed spontaneously and the rate at which it is being reduced to hemoglobin.

Four intraerythrocytic mechanisms reduce methemoglobin to hemoglobin (Fig. 38-3). Quantitatively, the most important reducing mechanism involves reduced nicotinamide adenine dinucleotide (NADH), which is generated during the oxidation of glucose. A NADH-dependent methemoglobin reductase reduces cytochrome b_5, using NADH as a hydrogen donor, and the reduced cytochrome b_5 then reduces methemoglobin.[3] A second enzymatic reducing mechanism involves reduced nicotinamide adenine dinucleotide phosphate (NADPH), which is generated in the hexose monophosphate shunt during the conversion of glucose-6-phosphate to 6-phosphoglucose in the presence of glucose-6-phosphate dehydrogenase.[4] If NADPH is present, a NADPH-dependent methemoglobin reductase reduces methemoglobin; however, this mechanism functions only when a cofactor or an artificial electron carrier, such as methylene blue, is present. In fact, administering methylene blue causes methemoglobin reduction to occur at a rate much greater than the rate during normal red cell metabolism[5,6] (Fig. 38-4). Nonenzymatic reduction of small amounts of methemoglobin also occurs following the administration of glutathione[7] and ascorbic acid.[8]

SULFHEMOGLOBINEMIA

Unlike methemoglobin, sulfhemoglobin has not been characterized structurally. Moreover, sulfhemoglobin is formed under normal conditions. Exposure to any of the chemical agents that may cause methemoglobin to form may also cause formation of sulfhemoglobin, (see "Etiology"), but once formed, sulfhemoglobin cannot be converted back to hemoglobin. Instead, sulfhemoglobin is removed from the circulation only when the red blood cells reach the end of their life span.

ETIOLOGY OF METHEMOGLOBINEMIA AND SULFHEMOGLOBINEMIA

Methemoglobinemia may be either inherited or acquired; except for a single report of a possibly congenital case, sulfhemoglobinemia has been known to occur only in acquired form. The inherited forms are rarely, if ever, encountered in anesthetic practice, so they will be discussed briefly.

INHERITED METHEMOGLOBINEMIA

Hereditary deficiency of NADH-methemoglobin reductase is a rare disorder; only a few hundred cases have been reported. It may be caused by actual deficiency of the enzyme or by synthesis of an abnormal enzyme, resulting in reduced activity. About half the hemoglobin of people homozygous for the disorder is in the form of methemoglobin. Although they are cyanotic from birth, these patients are otherwise well, and treatment with methylene blue or ascorbic acid is

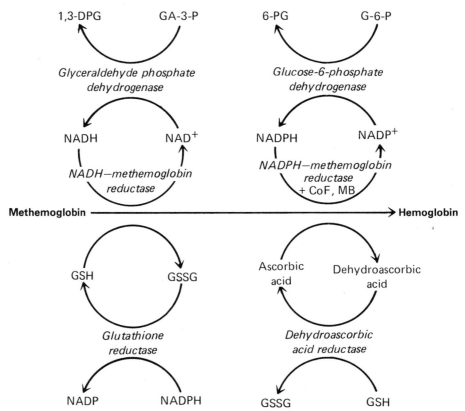

Fig. 38-3. A schematic view of the metabolic mechanisms for the reduction of methemoglobin to hemoglobin in the red blood cell and the regeneration of the reducing agents. Abbreviations: 1,3-DPG = 1,3-diphosphoglucose; GA-3-P = glyceraldehyde-3-phosphate; 6-PG = 6-phosphoglucose; G-6-P = glucose-6-phosphate; NADH = reduced nicotinamide adenine dinucleotide; NADPH = reduced nicotinamide adenine dinucleotide phosphate; CoF = cofactor; MC = methylene blue; GSSG = oxidized glutathione; GSH = reduced glutathione.

undertaken for cosmetic reasons only. Patients who are heterozygous for the disorder are generally not cyanotic, but they are highly susceptible to drugs and chemicals that produce the acquired form of methemoglobinemia (see section on acquired forms). Only in exceedingly rare instances does this disorder account for cyanosis during anesthesia.[9]

Hemoglobin M disease is as equally rare a cause of hereditary methemoglobinemia as hereditary NADH-methemoglobin reductase deficiency. There are five variants of the disorder. In each, an amino-acid substitution occurs in the globin polypeptide chain close to heme, which coexists with hemoglobin A. Once it has been formed by spontaneous oxidation, methemoglobin M becomes an unsuitable substrate for enzymatic reduction because of the abnormal structure. No homozygous cases have been described, presumably because such a disorder would be incompatible with life. In individuals with the heterozygous disorder, as much as one-third of the hemoglobin is in the form of methemoglobin, the specific amount depending upon the quantities of hemoglobin M and hemoglobin A present. Methylene blue and ascorbic acid are ineffective in treating the cyanosis. There have been no reports of this disorder in association with anesthesia.

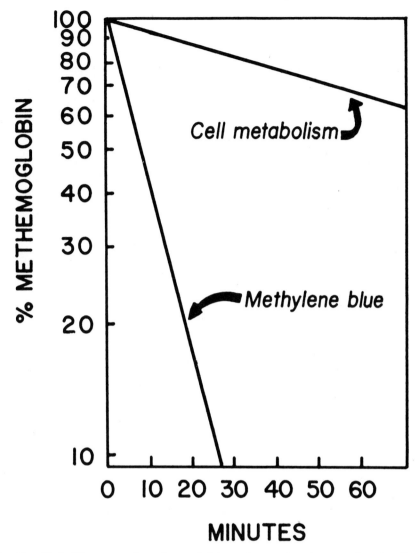

Fig. 38-4. The rate of methemoglobin reduction with normal red cell metabolism and with the addition of methylene blue. The ordinate represents the percentage of the initial concentration of methemoglobin, between 2 and 5 g. per dl. in the patients studied (Modified from Finch, C. A.: Methemoglobinemia and sulfhemoglobinemia. N. Engl. J. Med., *239*:470, 1948).

ACQUIRED METHEMOGLOBINEMIA AND SULFHEMOGLOBINEMIA

Acquired or toxic methemoglobinemia is far more common than the hereditary forms. It is caused by a variety of drugs and chemicals that cause the rate of hemoglobin oxidation to exceed the reductive capacity of the erythrocyte. Except for nitrates and nitrites, the same oxidants that cause methemoglobinemia may cause sulfhemoglobinemia. Industrial exposure to chemicals capable of oxidizing hemoglobin (e.g., chlorates, nitrobenzenes, quinones)[10] has decreased as a result of improved occupational health standards,[11,12] but methemoglobinemia may still occur because oxidants are present in many therapeutic agents to which patients may be exposed during or near anesthesia. In general, no widely used drug produces methemoglobinemia or sulfhemoglobinemia if clinical dosage is used. Most of the case reports involve uncommonly used drugs given in excessive dosage or more rarely, drugs given to patients having NADH-methemoglobin reductase deficiency. The oxidant in most cases is a metabolite rather than the drug itself.

Analgesic-Antipyretic Agents

Phenacetin and **acetaminophen,** as well as less commonly used *p*-aminophenol derivatives (e.g., acetanilide, *p*-aminosalicylic acid), cause dose-related methemoglobinemia,[12] although generally only when taken in excess. Phenacetin abuse is especially prevalent in Great Britain, where one report associated the drug with nine of ten cases of methemoglobinemia occurring in surgical patients in one hospital during a three-year period.[13] Recently, the drug has been implicated in cases of methemoglobinemia[14] and sulfhemoglobinemia[15] occurring during anesthesia in the United States. Although therapeutic doses of phenacetin generally do not cause methemoglobin production sufficient to cause cyanosis, some patients have a heightened sensitivity because they metabolize a greater proportion of the drug to an oxidizing metabolite.[16] Newborns are particularly sensitive to these drugs because the hepatic glucuronide conjugation enzymes that detoxify *p*-aminophenol are immature at birth.[17] Moreover, newborns are sensitive to a variety of oxidants because their NADH-methemoglobin reductase is immature.[18]

Antimicrobials and Antiseptics

Methemoglobinemia following administration of the antimalarials chloroquine and dapsone, other sulfonamide derivatives, and the urinary tract antiseptic phenazopyridine, as well as less commonly used drugs, has been reported.[12]

Vasodilators

Amyl nitrite and **nitroglycerin** are potent oxidants; glyceryl trinitrate is converted to a nitrite by intestinal bacteria and may also cause methemoglobinemia if used continually. Nitrates and nitrites used as meat preservatives have also been implicated.[11] Methemoglobinemia has also developed in a person with NADH-methemoglobin reductase deficiency who sniffed butyl nitrite as an aphrodisiac,[19] and in others following accidental overdosage[19a] and customary clinical dosage[19b] of nitroglycerin.

Sodium nitroprusside as a cause of methemoglobinemia in a patient with an acute myocardial infarction was reported by Bower and Peterson.[20] Others have shown that production of methemoglobin is an intermediate state in the production of cyanmethemoglobin and cyanide that occurs after administration of nitroprusside[21]; however, the clinical importance of these findings is uncertain.

Local Anesthetics

Prilocaine, a toluidine derivative, is an anesthetic drug infamous for its ability to produce methemoglobin.[22-37] Introduced in the early 1960s as a rational alternative to other local anesthetics (its advantages being longer clinical duration and less CNS toxicity), prilocaine in fact never achieved wide popularity owing to this property. As with other drugs that may cause methemoglobinemia, a metabolite of prilocaine, probably *o*-toluidine, is the oxidant, not prilocaine as such.[24,25] Cyanosis occasionally appears after administration of dosages as low as 400 mg. following major nerve blocks or epidural anesthesia[22,25,27-29]; however, it usually occurs following administration of considerably larger doses (e.g., 600–1600 mg.), such as might be administered during prolonged continuous epidural anesthesia.[22,25,26-30] Although the likelihood that cyanosis will appear is dose-related,[25] the correlation between dosage and methemoglobin production is sufficiently poor to suggest that other pharmacokinetic considerations, such as the injection site, the patient's metabolism rate, and vasoconstrictor use, are critical factors. Cyanosis appears 90 minutes to 6 hours after administration, depending on the type of block used and the presence of vasoconstrictor; it usually disappears within 24 hours if not treated. None of the published reports describe tachycardia, hypertension, or clinical symptoms of hypoxia accompanying the cyanosis. Concern about using prilocaine during a prolonged epidural block for obstetrical labor is justified, however, because the drug affects the fetus to the same extent as the mother,[31–33] and, as already mentioned, the drug-metabolizing system[17] and the NADH-methemoglobin reductase[17] of a fetus and immature.

Benzocaine, a *p*-aminobenzoic acid derivative, has been implicated in cases of cyanosis occurring in infants following topical[38] and rectal[39–41] use, and in a case where an older child became cyanotic after tracheal intubation with a tube whose lubricant contained benzocaine.[42] A benzocaine-containing topical anesthetic spray (Cetacaine) caused rapid onset of methemoglobinemia in three critically ill adults, at least two of whom had received an excessive dose; a three-second spray deposits sufficient benzocaine to produce methemoglobinemia.[43,43a]

Lidocaine, which bears a structural similarity to prilocaine, is listed among agents causing methemoglobinemia in two standard reference works[44,45] on the basis of three case reports: One case involved an obstetrical patient who had received a total of 1.8 g. of lidocaine during a period of about 8 hours and who appeared cyanotic 9 hours after delivery.[46] Methemoglobinemia was confirmed spectrophotmetrically, and the cyanosis disappeared after administration of methylene blue. This patient had also received phenacetin after the delivery, however, making it impossible to ascribe the methemoglobinemia solely to lidocaine; in addition, methemoglobinemia sufficient to cause cyanosis does not occur following clinical doses of lidocaine.[28,36] Furthermore, the response to methylene blue required "a few hours" rather than several minutes, suggesting that the patient may have had glucose-6-phosphate deficiency (see Fig. 43-3).[47] The other case involved a young man who had full-mouth dental extractions with local anesthesia (300 mg. lidocaine).[48] Following the procedure he received codeine and remained hospitalized overnight; 4 hours after returning home the next morning, he suddenly became dizzy and lost consciousness. He was readmitted to the hospital, where he was observed to be cyanotic. The cyanosis disappeared after methylene blue administration, but, again,

more slowly than expected. The acute problem occurred almost 24 hours after the nerve blocks, at a time when lidocaine would have been almost entirely cleared from the body. Perhaps the patient also received an analgesic containing phenacetin—"APC," for example, or even another unmentioned drug rather than just codeine. A third patient developed methemoglobinemia after the administration of an unknown volume of 4 per cent liodcaine to the posterior pharynx, twice in an hour, less than a day after experiencing methemoglobinemia with benzocaine.[43a] Although no predisposing hematologic defect could be found, one must question whether the normal reductive mechanisms had returned to normal after the first episode of cyanosis. In short, there is insufficient evidence with which to implicate lidocaine as a cause of methemoglobinemia.

Surface-Acting Agents

Mafenide acetate, a sulfonamide derivative used as a topical agent in the treatment of burns, caused severe methemoglobinemia in two children who had suffered burns over about half their body surface.[49] The agent is absorbed rapidly through the burn surface and reaches a peak plasma concentration within a few hours. The two children came from communities in which intermarriage was common, raising the possibility of an inherited metabolic defect (e.g., NADH-methemoglobin reductase deficiency) that would have made them more sensitive to the oxidant.

Silver nitrate therapy for burns has also been implicated in a few cases of methemoglobinemia.[50–52] Bacterial infection probably converts the nitrate to nitrite, which is the oxidant.

Aniline dyes used for laundry marking of diapers have been associated with nursery epidemics of methemoglobinemia.[53]

CLINICAL SIGNIFICANCE OF METHEMOGLOBINEMIA AND SULFHEMOGLOBINEMIA

Whereas 5 mg. per dl. of reduced hemoglobin must be present before cyanosis is evident, cyanosis of equal severity can be caused by as little as 1.5 mg. of methemoglobin or 0.5 mg. of sulfhemoglobin per dl. The cyanosis reflects diminished oxygen-carrying capacity of the blood and greater affinity of the remaining hemoglobin for oxygen (i.e., the oxyhemoglobin dissociation curve shifts to the left, with decreased release of oxygen to the tissues at low partial pressures of oxygen.[54] The clinical signs and symptoms, in turn, reflect not only the amount of methemoglobin and/or sulfhemoglobin present but also the ability of the patient's cardiorespiratory system to compensate. For example, 600 mg. of prilocaine, the maximum recommended dose for a single administration, causes a loss of about 5 per cent of the blood's oxygen-carrying capacity, a deficit that is offset easily by an increase in cardiac output. Even the deficits imposed by much larger prilocaine dosages (e.g., 20% after 1200–1600 mg.) pose little challenge, for cardiac output in a healthy adult can increase about 300 per cent during exercise. Difficulty arises, however, with greater loss of oxygen-carrying capacity, especially in persons with limited cardiac reserve. At levels above 20 per cent—which are not uncommon following the ingestion of nitrates and nitrites—weakness, fatigue, headache, dizziness, and tachycardia appear. At levels above 50 per cent, methemoglobinemic stupor appears; levels over 60 to 70 per cent cause coma and death.

DIAGNOSIS OF ACQUIRED METHEMOGLOBINEMIA AND SULFHEMOGLOBINEMIA

Generally, cyanosis unresponsive to oxygen therapy suggests a diagnosis of acquired methemoglobinemia or sulfhemoglobinemia, particularly when there is no evidence of cardiorespiratory disease. The venous blood of patients with these disorders has been described as chocolate brown, reddish brown, or mauve brown. The color persists after the blood sample has been mixed with air, whereas reduced hemoglobin (e.g., from a patient with a large right-to-left shunt) turns bright red. Usually, a spectrophotometric oximeter (e.g., IL 182 CO-Oximeter) will indicate the hemoglobin saturation as being relatively low for a given Pa_{O_2}, but the measured saturation corresponds to the color of the blood and the degree of the patient's cyanosis. More-

over, because the computer's program assumes that only oxyhemoglobin, deoxyhemoglobin, and carboxyhemoglobin are present in the sample,[43] such devices calculate a falsely low value for hemoglobin and a negative value for carboxyhemoglobin. For definitive diagnosis, spectrophotometry is used. Methemoglobin absorbs maximally at 502 and 632 nm., whereas sulfhemoglobin has its peak absorption at 620 nm. Finally, adding a few drops of a 10-per-cent cyanide solution to a brown sample of blood produces a bright red pigment (cyanmethemoglobin) and removes the peaks from the methemoglobin spectrum.

TREATMENT OF ACQUIRED METHEMOGLOBINEMIA AND SULFHEMOGLOBINEMIA

Therapy is generally undertaken for cosmetic reasons, not because of medical necessity. Intravenous administration of methylene blue (1 mg./kg.) promptly relieves cyanosis due to methemoglobinemia (Fig. 38-4). The dose should be given over a period of 5 minutes to avoid symptoms of toxicity, such as restlessness, apprehension, tremor, and precordial pain, which also occur following very large doses (500 mg. or more).[55] Methylene blue should not be given to patients with glucose-6-phosphate deficiency lest acute hemolysis result.[47] There is no specific therapy for sulfhemoglobinemia; the administration of offending agent should be discontinued.

REFERENCES

1. Perutz, M. F.: Stereochemistry of cooperative effects in haemoglobin (haem-haem interaction and the problem of allostery). Nature, 228:726, 1970.
2. Jaffe, E. R., and Heller, P.: Methemoglobinemia in man. Prog. Hematol., 4:48, 1964.
3. Hultquish, D. E., and Passon, P. G.: Catalysis of methaemeoglobin reduction by erthyrocyte cytochrome B5 and cytochrome B5 reductase. Nature (New Biol.), 229:252, 1971.
4. Gibson, Q. H.: The reduction of methaemoglobin in red blood cells and studies on the cause of idiopathic methaemoglobinaemia. Biochem. J., 42:13, 1948.
5. Wendel, W. B.: Control of methemoglobinemia with methylene blue. J. Clin. Invest., 18:179, 1939.
6. Bodansky, O., and Gutmann, H.: Treatment of methemogolbinemia. J. Pharmacol. Exp. Therp. 89:46, 1947.

7. Morrison, D. B., and Williams, E. F.: Methemoglobin reduction by glutathionone or cysteine. Science, *87*:15, 1938.

8. Gibson, Q. H.: Reduction of methaemoglobin by ascorbic acid. Biochem. J., *37*:615, 1943.

9. Gabel, R. A., and Bunn, H. F.: Hereditary methemoglobinemia as a cause of cyanosis during anesthesia. Anesthesiology, *40*:516, 1974.

10. Hooper, R. R., Husted, S. R., and Smith, E. L.: Hydroquinone poisoning aboard a navy ship. Morbidity Mortality Weekly Report, *27*:237, 1978.

11. Bodansky, O.: Methemoglobinemia and methemoglobin-producing compounds. Pharmacol. Rev., *3*:144, 1951.

12. Smith, R. P., and Olson, M. V.: Drug-induced methemoglobinemia. Semin. Hematol., *10*:253, 1973.

13. Joseph, D.: Methaemoglobinaemia and anaesthesia. Br. J. Anaesth., *34*:309, 1962.

14. Easley, J. E., and Condon, B. F.: Phenacetin-induced methemoglobinemia and renal failure. Anesthesiology, *41*:99, 1974.

15. Schmitter, C. R., Jr.: Sulfhemoglobinemia and methemoglobinemia—uncommon causes of cyanosis. Anesthesiology, *43*:586, 1975.

16. Shahidi, N. T., and Hemaidan, A.: Acetophenetidin-induced methemoglobinemia and its relation to the excretion of diazotizable amines. J. Lab. Clin. Med., *74*:581, 1969.

17. Vest, M. F., and Streiff, R. R.: Studies on glucoronide formation in newborn infants and older children. Am. J. Dis. Child., *98*:688, 1959.

18. Ross, J. D.: Deficient activity of DPNH-dependent methemoglobin diaphorase in cord blood erythrocytes. Blood, *21*:51, 1963.

19. Horne, M. K., Waterman, R. R., Simon, L. M., et al.: Methemoglobinemia from sniffing butyl nitrite. Ann. Intern. Med., *91*:417, 1979.

19a. Marshall, J. B., and Ecklund, R. E.: Methemoglobinemia from overdose of nitroglycern, J.A.M.A., *24244*:330, 1980.

19b. Fibuch, E. E., Cecil, W. T., and Reed, W. A.: Methemoglobinemia associated with organic nitrate therapy. Anesth. Analg. *58*:521, 1979.

20. Bower, P. J., and Peterson, J. N.: Methemoglobinemia after sodium nitroprusside therapy. N. Engl. J. Med., *293*:865, 1975.

21. Smith, R., and Kruszyna, H.: Nitroprusside produces cyanide poisoning via a reaction with hemoglobin. J. Pharm. Exp. Therp., *191*:557, 1975.

22. Daly, D. J., Davenport, J., and Newland, M. C.: Methaemoglobinaemia following the use of prilocaine ("Citanest"). Br. J. Anaesth., *36*:737, 1964.

23. Sadove, M. S., Rosenberg, R., Heller, F. N., et al.: Citanest. a new local anesthetic agent. Anesth. Analg. *43*:527, 1964.

24. Onji, Y., and Tyuma, I.: Methemoglobin formation by a local anesthetic and some related compounds. Acta Anaesth. Scand. [Suppl.], XVI:151, 1965.

25. Crawford, O. B., Hollis, R. W., and Covino, B. G.: Clinical tolerance and effectiveness of propitocaine, a new local anesthetic agent. J. New Drugs, *5*:162, 1965.

26. Lund, P. C., and Cwik, J. C.: Citanest, a clinical and laboratory study. Part 2. Anesth. Analg., *44*:712, 1965.

27. Hjelm, M., and Holmdahl, M. H.: Clinical chemistry of prilocaine and clinical evaluation of methaemoglobinaemia induced by this agent. Acta Anaesth. Scand. [Suppl.], XVI:161, 1965.

28. Hjelm, M., and Holmdahl, M.H.: Biochemical effects of aromatic amines. II. Cyanosis, methaemoglobinaemia and heinz-body formation induced by a local anaesthetic agent (prilocaine). Acta Anaesth. Scand., *9*:99, 1965.

29. Sadove, M. S., Jobgen, E. A., Heller, F. N., et al.: Methemoglobinemia—an effect of a new local anesthetic, L-67 (prilocaine). Acta Anaesth. Scand. [Suppl.] XVI:175, 1965.

29a. Lund, P.C., and Cwik, J.C.: Propitocaine (Citanest) and methemoglobinemia. Anesthesiology, *26*:569, 1965.

30. Scott, D. B.: Toxicity and clinical use of prilocaine. Proc. Roy. Soc. Med., *58*:420, 1965.

31. Poppers, P. J., Vosburgh, G. J., and Finster, M.: Methemoglobinemia following epidural analgesia during labor. A case report and literature review. Am. J. Obstet. Gynecol., *95*:630, 1966.

32. Climie, C. R., McLean, S., Starmer, G. A., et al.: Methaemologbinaemia in mother and foetus following continuous epidural analgesia with prilocaine. Clinical and experimental data. Br. J. Anaesth., *39*:155, 1967.

33. Marx, G. F.: Fetal arrhythmia during caudal block with prilocaine. Anesthesiology, *28*:222, 1967.

34. Mazze, R. I.: Methemoglobin concentrations following intravenous regional anesthesia. Anesth. Analg., *47*:122, 1968.

35. Harris, W. H., Cole, D. W., Mital, M., et al.: Methemoglobin formation and oxygen transport following intravenous regional anesthesia using prilocaine. Anesthesiology, *29*:65, 1968.

36. Bridenbaugh, P. O., Bridenbaugh, L. D., and Moore, D. C.: Methemoglobinemia and infant response to lidocaine and prilocaine in continuous caudal anesthesia: A double-blind study. Anesth. Analg. *48*:824, 1969.

37. Arens, J. F., and Carrera, A. E.: Methemoglobin levels following peridural anesthesia with prilocaine for vaginal deliveries. Anesth. Analg., *49*:219, 1970.

38. Haggerty, R. J.: Blue baby due to methemoglobinemia. N. Engl. J. Med., *267*:1303, 1962.

39. Peterson, H. DeC.: Acquired methemoglobinemia in an infant due to benzocaine suppository. N. Engl. J. Med., *263*:454, 1960.

40. Hughes, J. R.: Infantile methemoglobinemia due to benzocaine suppository. J. Pediatr., *66*:797, 1965.

41. Bloch, A.: More on infantile methemoglobinemia due to benzocaine suppository. J. Pediatr., *67*:509, 1965.

42. Steinberg, J. B., and Zepemick, R. G.: Methemoglobinemia during anesthesia. J. Pediatr., *67*:885, 1962.

43. Douglas, W. W., and Fairbanks, V. F.: Methemoglobinemia induced by topical anesthetic spray (Cetacaine). Chest, *71*:587, 1977.

43a. O'Donohue, W. J., Jr., Moss, L. M., and Angelillo, V. A.: Acute methemoglobinemia induced by topical benzocaine and lidocaine. Arch. Intern. Med., *140*:1508, 1980.

44. Beutler, E.: Methemoglobinemia and sulfhemoglobinemia. In Williams, W. J., Beutler, E., Erslev, A. J., et al. (eds.): *Hematology*, Ed. 2, pp. 491–494. New York, McGraw-Hill, 1977.

45. Cartwright, G. E.: Methemoglobinemia and sulfhemoglobinemia. In Thorn, G. E., Adams, R. D., Braunwald, E. et al. (eds.): *Principles of Internal Medicine*, Ed. 8, pp. 1710–1713. New York, McGraw-Hill, 1977.

46. Burne, D., and Doughty, A.: Methaemoglobinaemia following lignocaine. Lancet, 2:971, 1964.
47. Rosen, P. J., Johnson, C., McGehee, W. G., et al.: Failure of methylene blue treatment in toxic methemoglobinemia. Association with glucose-6-phosphate deficiency. Ann. Intern. Med., 75:83, 1971.
48. Deas, T. C.: Severe methemoglobinemia following dental extractions under lidocaine anesthesia. Anesthesiology, 17:204, 1956.
49. Ohlgisser, M., Adler, M., Ben-Dov, D., et al.: Methaemoglobinaemia induced by mafenide acetate in children. A report of two cases. Br. J. Anaesth. 50:299, 1978.
50. Ternberg, J. L., and Luce, E.: Methemoglobinemia: A complication of the silver nitrate treatment of burns. Surgery, 63:328, 1968.
51. Cushing, A. H., and Smith, S.: Methemoglobinemia with silver nitrate therapy of burns. Report of a case. Pediatrics, 74:613, 1969.
52. Strauch, B., Buch, W., Grey, W., et al.: Successful treatment of methemoglobinemia secondary to silver nitrate therapy. N. Engl. J. Med., 281:257, 1969.
53. Graubarth, J., Bloom, C. J., Coleman, F. C., et al.: Dye poisoning in the nursery: A review of seventeen cases. J. A. M. A., 128:1155, 1945.
54. Darling, R. C., and Roughton, F. J. W.: Effect of methemoglobin on equilibrium between oxygen and hemoglobin. Am. J. Physiol., 137:56, 1942.
55. Finch, C. A.: Methemoglobinemia and sulfhemoglobinemia. N. Engl. J. Med., 239:470, 1948.

FURTHER READING

Beutler, E.: Energy metabolism and maintenance of erythrocytes. In Williams, W. J., Beutler, E., Erslev, A. J., et al. (eds.): *Hematology*, ed. 2, pp. 177–190. New York, McGraw-Hill, 1977.
Finch, C. A.: Methemoglobinemia and sulfhemoglobinemia. N. Engl. J. Med., 239:470, 1948.
Perutz, M. F.: Hemoglobin structure and respiratory transport. Sci. Am., 239:92, December 1978.
Smith, R. P., Olson, M. V.: Drug-induced methemoglobinemia. Semin. Hematol., 10(3):253, 1973.

39 Exacerbation of Inducible Porphyria

Fredrick K. Orkin, M.D.

More than 25 years ago, anesthesiologists were exhorted never to use thiopental or other barbiturates in the anesthetic management of patients known or suspected to have porphyria[1,2] The "dire" effects of barbiturate anesthesia in these patients included an acute and bizarre neurologic syndrome consisting of abdominal pain, nausea and vomiting (among other autonomic dysfunctions), mental disturbances, and peripheral neuropathy, often leading to respiratory paralysis, with death occurring in as many as two thirds of those affected. Apart from an appreciation of an inheritable predisposition to this complication, there was no understanding of its underlying pathogenesis and, hence, no effective therapy until recently.

Porphyria is now recognized as a clinically heterogeneous group of diseases, acquired as well as inherited. In these disorders, there are underlying disturbances in the biosynthesis of heme, the prosthetic group in essential respiratory pigments such as hemoglobin and the cytochromes. Each of the porphyrias has a characteristic pattern of overproduction and accumulation of porphyrin precursors and porphyrins, tetrapyrrole pigments which are intermediates in the heme biosynthetic pathway.

Acute clinical episodes of three porphyrias—*acute intermittent porphyria*, *variegate porphyria*, and *hereditary coproporphyria*—may be precipitated by barbiturates and other drugs that, under experimental conditions, can induce porphyrin biosynthesis. Hence, these diseases may be termed *inducible*.[3] This chapter reviews the physical basis, symptomatology, treatment, and prevention of life threatening, though rare, acute episodes of these inducible porphyrias that are of particular interest to the anesthesiologist.

CLASSIFICATION OF THE PORPHYRIAS

But for an acquired form, the porphyrias represent classic examples of disorders resulting from inborn errors of metabolism, first described by Garrod.[4] Hence, the porphyrias are as much metabolic disorders as hematologic diseases. Because a mutant *somatic* gene is responsible for the metabolic derangement in each type, the porphyrias must be considered *cellular* diseases. Indeed, in a given form of porphyria, the accumulation of characteristic porphyrins and porphyrin precursors is generally found in all tissues studied. This is not surprising because all mammalian cells can synthesize the porphyrin required for essential heme containing enzymes, such as cytochromes, catalase, and peroxidase. Although a classification according to defined enzymatic defects at specific sites in heme biosynthesis is near, the current classification schemes are based upon the major site where the metabolic error appears.[5]

Classification of the Porphyrias
Erythropoetic porphyrias
   Cogenital erythropoietic porphyria
   Erythropoietic coproporphyria
Erythrohepatic porphyria
   Protoporphyria
Hepatic porphyrias
   Acute intermittent porphyria
   Variegate porphyria
   Hereditary coproporphyria
   Porphyria cutanea tarda
   Cutaneous porphyrias

Functionally, the porphyrias may also be classified on the basis of symptomatology. Acute intermittent porphyria, variegate porphyria, and hereditary coproporphyria are the only forms that have an acute neurologic syndrome induced by drugs and, thus are of principal interest to the anesthesiologist. Some patients with variegate porphyria and hereditary coproporphyria also have eruptions in areas exposed to sunlight.

Photosensitivity with dermatologic manifestations, however, rather than a neurologic syndrome, is characteristic of the *non*inducible porphyrias.[6,7] There have been only 7 dozens cases of congential erythropoietic porphyria (Gunther's disease) which expresses itself early in childhood and is associated with mutilating skin lesions, facial hirsutism, hemolytic anemia, port-wine-colored urine, and early death. Erythropoietic croporphyria is a milder disorder which has been described in only one family. *Protoporphyria* begins early in life with skin rashes after exposure to sunlight and progresses to hepatic disease, with liver failure in some patients. *Porphyria cutanea tarda* is probably the most common form of porphyria and is characterized by chronic skin lesions in areas exposed to sunlight and by hepatic siderosis. Finally, there are several *cutaneous porphyrias*, resembling porphyria cutanea tarda, associated with lupus erythematosus, chronic alcoholism, hepatic tumors, hemolytic anemias, and hexachlorobenzene poisoning.

In addition to the major site of metabolic expression and sympotomatology, the porphyrias may be differentiated on the basis of the mode of inheritance and laboratory abnormalities (Table 39-1).

THE PHYSICAL BASIS OF INDUCIBLE PORPHYRIAS

HEME BIOSYNTHESIS

Figure 39-1 presents a schematic view of the heme biosynthetic pathway. Within the mitochondrion, succinate (from the metabolism of acetate in the Krebs' tricarboxylic acid cycle) is converted to succinyl-coenzyme-A which condenses with glycine in the presence of the enzyme δ-aminolevulinic acid synthetase (ALA-S) to form a five-carbon chain, δ-aminolevulinic acid (ALA). The next several steps occur in the cytosol: the condensation of two chains to form the porphyrin precursor, porphobilinogen (PBG), and deamination and further condensation by uroporphyrinogen I synthetase (porphobilinogen deaminase) and uroporphyrinogen III cosynthetase (porphobilinogen isomerase) to form uroporphyrinogen III which is converted to coproporphyrinogen III by uroporphyrinogen decarboxylase. Upon reentering the mitochondrion, further oxidation and decarboxylation of coproporphyrinogen III by coproporphyrinogen oxidase results in the formation of protoporphyrinogen IX. The latter is converted to protoporphyrin IX by protoporphyrinogen oxidase, prior to the insertion of ferrous iron by ferrochelatase to form heme which, upon combining with four globin subunits (see Chap. 38), in turn, forms hemoglobin.

REGULATION OF HEME BIOSYNTHESIS

Many of the steps in heme biosynthesis are favored thermodynamically, and the degradation of heme (to bile pigments) proceeds along a different pathway. As a result, heme biosynthesis is unidirectional and irreversible. Control mechanisms for such pathways are usually located at the first enzymatic step uniquely involved in the synthesis of the end product.[8] In heme biosynthesis, this step is the formation of ALA. That ALA-S is the rate-limiting enzyme is suggested by its much lower activity than that of enzymes later in the pathway, that succinyl-coenzyme-A and glycine are present in abundance, and that distal heme precursors are present in only trace quantities.[9]

Table 39-1. Clinical and laboratory features of the porphyrias.

CHARACTERISTICS	ERYTHROPOIETIC PORPHYRIA (CONGENITAL ERYTHROPOIETIC PORPHYRIA)	ERYTHROHEPATIC PORPHYRIA (PROTOPORPHYRIA)	HEPATIC PORPHYRIAS ACUTE INTERMITTENT PORPHYRIA (latent)	(acute)	VARIEGATE PORPHYRIA (latent)	(acute)	HEREDITARY COPROPORPHYRIA (latent)	(acute)	PORPHYRIA TARDA
Inheritance	Autosomal recessive	Autosomal dominant	Autosomal dominant		Autosomal dominant		Autosomal dominant		Autosomal dominant
Symptomatology									
Photosensitivity cutaneous lesions	yes	yes	no	no	no	yes/no	no	no/yes	yes
Neurologic syndrome	no	no	no	yes	no	yes	no	yes	no
Laboratory Findings									
Red Blood Cells									
Uroporphyrin	↑↑↑	↑	N	N	N	N	N	N	N
Coproporphyrin	↑↑	↑	N	N	N	N	N	N	N
Protoporphyrin	N or ↑	↑↑↑	N	N	N	N	N	N	N
Urine									
Color*	Red*	N*	N*	Red*	N*	N or red*	N*	N or red*	Red*
ALA	N	N	↑	↑↑↑	N	↑↑	↑	↑↑	N
PBG	N	N	↑↑	↑↑↑	N	↑↑	N or ↑	↑↑	N
Uroporphyrin	↑↑↑	N	↑↑	↑↑	N	↑↑↑	N	↑↑↑	↑↑
Coproporphyrin	↑↑	N	↑	↑	N	↑↑	N or ↑	↑↑	↑
Feces									
Coproporphyrin	↑	N	N	↑	↑↑↑	↑↑	↑↑	↑↑↑	N
Protoporphyrin	N or ↑	N or ↑	N	↑	↑↑↑	↑↑	N	↑	N

*Freshly voided. On standing, the urine may become deep brownish red or black.

N, normal; ↑, increased; ↑↑↑, greatly increased; ALA, δ-aminolevulinic acid; PBG, porphobilinogen

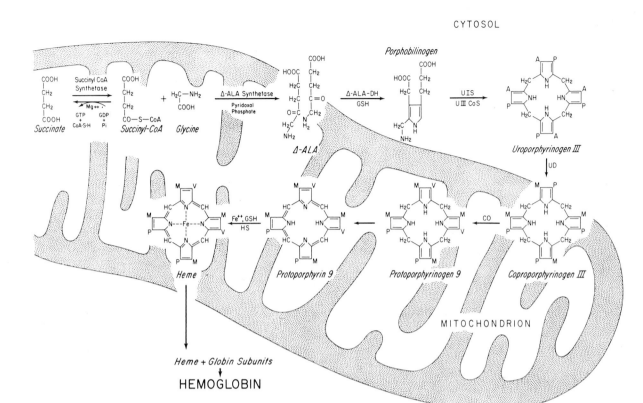

Fig. 39-1. The biosynthesis of heme. The following abbreviations are used: CoA, coenzyme A; GTP, guanosine triphosphate; GDP, guanosine diphosphate; Pi, inorganic phosphorous; GSH, glutathione; δ-ALA-DH, δ-aminolevulinate dehydrase; UIS, uroporphyrinogen I synthetase; UIII CoS, uroporphyrinogen III cosynthetase; UD, uroporphyrinogen decarboxylase; CO, coproporphyrinogen oxidase; and, HS, heme synthetase. (Bunn H. F.: Pallor and anemia. In Isselbacher, K. J., Adams, R. D., Braunwald, E., et al. (eds.): Harrison's Textbook of Internal Medicine. ed. 9. p. 265. New York, McGraw-Hill, 1980.)

FEEDBACK REPRESSION OF ALA-S

Under normal circumstances, heme biosynthesis is regulated to supply the heme required for the various hemoproteins efficiently. This is accomplished, as shown in Figure 39-2, by the negative-feedback regulation of the end product, heme, upon ALA-S.[10,11] Inhibition of ALA-S *activity*, as a result of conformational changes consequent to physical binding with heme, is a possible control mechanisn;[12] however, such feedback inhibition has been demonstrated only with purified enzyme preparations. The principal mode of ALA-S regulation appears to be repression of enzyme *synthesis*.

Although the precise mechanism of this end-product inhibition is unclear, the data are consistent with the general regulatory model of protein synthesis proposed by Jacob and Monod.[13] Applied to heme biosynthesis (Fig. 39-3), that model proposes that heme combines with a protein, termed an aporepressor, whose synthesis is directed by a regulator gene.[14] The combination of heme, acting as a corepressor, and the aporepressor is termed a repressor. The latter acts upon the operator gene which represses the transcription of the structural gene responsible for synthesizing the messenger RNA which, in turn, controls the synthesis of ALA-S on the ribosomes in the cytosol. Hence, the availability of excess heme serves to decrease the availability of ALA-S at the rate-limiting step, diminishing the synthesis of heme itself.

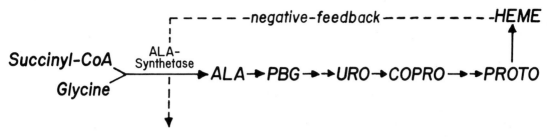

Fig. 39-2. In heme biosynthesis, heme exerts negative-feedback regulation upon δ-aminolevulinic acid synthetase (ALA-S). The other abbreviations are PBG, porphobilinogen; URO, uroporphyrinogen; COPRO, coproporphyrinogen; and PROTO, protoporphyrin.

Fig. 39-3. Regulatory mechanisms for heme biosynthesis. Heme, acting as a corepressor, combines with a repressor substance whose synthesis is directed by a regulator gene. The resultant repressor influences an operator gene to "turn off" the structural gene directing the synthesis of the messenger RNA (mRNA) for the synthesis of δ-aminolevulinic acid synthetase (ALA-S) on the ribosomes. Decreased availability of mRNA and, in turn, ALA-S at the rate-limiting step results in diminished synthesis of heme precursors. Heme may also combine with ALA-S, changing the conformation of the enzyme and thereby inhibiting its activity. Less repressor is present when there is increased demand for heme, and the repressor may be inactivated when heme is displaced from its binding site by certain drugs, resulting in increased mRNA and ALA-S synthesis and permiting increased heme production.

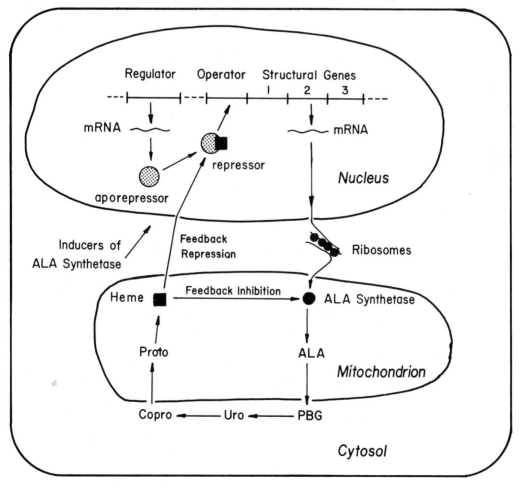

INDUCTION OF ALA-S

In accordance with this scheme for the regulation of heme biosynthesis, an increased heme utilization *de*represses the operator gene, and more ALA-S is synthesized, providing more heme precursors to satisfy the demand for heme (see Fig. 39-3). Under normal circumstances, most of the hepatic heme synthesized is used for the synthesis of cytochrome P_{450}, a group of microsomal enzymes which function as the terminal oxidase in drug metabolism.[6] The administration of many diverse lipophilic chemicals and drugs induces increased synthesis of cytochrome P_{450} and, in turn ALA-S.[9] Although barbiturates are well-known inducers of drug-metabolizing enzymes, other inducing agents are insecticides, endogenous and exogenous steroids, and a variety of therapeutic agents, principally antibiotics and nonbarbiturate hypnotics. Not unexpectedly, porphyria produced in the laboratory by chemicals that impair the regulatory mechanism and permit excessive ALA-S synthesis is termed *chemical* or *experimental porphyria*.[9,15,16]

MODIFICATION OF ALA-S INDUCTION

A variety of exogenous and endogenous factors, some having clinical relevance, can modify the induction of ALA-S synthesis.[17] Increased intake of carbohydrate or protein can block induction; the mechanism of this *glucose effect* is unknown.[15,18] On the other hand, fasting enhances ALA-S induction, probably through increased breakdown of heme.[6,19] Chelated iron in the form of ferric citrate or iron dextran also results in loss of heme and marked increase in ALA-S induction as a secondary, expected event.[6] A diverse group of steroids, including metabolites of gonadal and adrenocortical hormones[20] and intermediates in bile acid degradation,[21] can induce ALA-S, as well. In adrenalectomized animals, hydrocortisone exhibits a "permissive" effect on ALA-S induction.[22]

METABOLIC DEFECTS IN INDUCIBLE PORPHYRIAS

Given the regulatory interdependence between the availability of heme and the synthesis of ALA-S (see Fig. 39-2), it is apparent that any partial block in a biosynthetic step between ALA and heme should result in increased ALA-S synthesis and an accumulation of heme precursor immediately proximal to the defect. In fact, in each of the inducible porphyrias there is a seemingly inappropriate increased ALA-S activity and a specific pattern of heme precursor accumulation and excretion (Table 39-1, Fig. 39-4). In no case, however, is the enzymatic defect a complete blockage, for the absence of heme synthesis is incompatible with life.

ACUTE INTERMITTENT PORPHYRIA

In this disorder there is deficient uroporphyrinogen I synthetase, resulting in the accumulation of ALA and PBG in the urine.[23,24] The pathogenic gene is located on autosome 11.[25]

VARIEGATE PORPHYRIA

The excretion pattern suggests that the enzyme defect is between protoporphyrinogen and heme, and one study notes that the defect is a deficiency of ferrochelatase in this disease.[26] As a result, the excretion products consist in ALA and PBG in the urine, and a variety of porphyrin compounds in the feces.

HEREDITARY COPROPORPHYRIA

The defect here is probably a deficiency of coproporphyrinogen oxidase.[27–29] Thus, ALA, PBG, and a variety of porphyrins are also excreted, as in variegate prophyria.

PATHOGENESIS OF THE SYMPTOMATOLOGY

Whereas much is known about the biochemistry of heme biosynthesis and of porphyria, relatively little is understood about the relationships between the enzymatic defects and the symptomatology, particularly the neurologic syndrome. However, a superficial differentiation of symptomatology is possible on biochemical grounds:[30] acute attacks of all of the inducible porphyrias are associated with a neurologic syndrome and the excretion of ALA and PBG; photosensitivity occurs in variegate porphyria and hereditary coproporphyria, both of which are associated with the

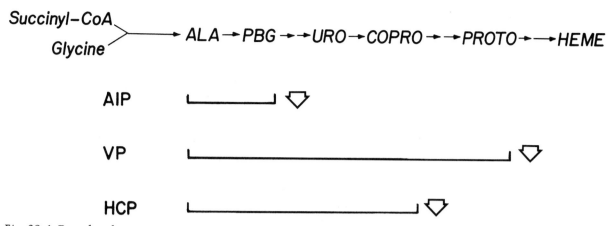

Fig. 39-4. Postulated primary enzyme deficiencies (outlined arrow) and urinary excretion patterns (in brackets) during acute attacks of the inducible porphyrias. The following abbreviations are used: ALA, δ-aminolevulinic acid; PBG, porphobilinogen; URO, uroporphyrinogen; COPRO, coproporphyrinogen; PROTO, protoporphyrinogen; AIP, acute intermittent porphyria; VP, variegate porphyria; and HCP, hereditary coproporphyria.

additional accumulation of porphyrins, but not in acute intermittent porphyria which is not associated with porphyrin excess.

PHOTOSENSITIVITY

Porphyrins fluoresce intensely in the ultraviolet light region corresponding to a wavelength of about 400 nm. Ultraviolet radiation in this band happens to evoke maximal cutaneous photosensitivity under experimental conditions.[6] Although the mechanism of the dermatologic lesion is understood incompletely, it is known that porphyrins capable of causing photosensitization are stored in lysosomes.[31] Absorption of light in the 400 nm band, in the presence of oxygen, may cause leakage of hydrolytic enzymes also stored in the lysosomes, with resultant disruption of the cell and the release of substances that give rise to the characteristic erythema, blistering, and, later, scarring.

NEUROLOGIC SYNDROME

It is tantalizing to postulate that the ALA and PBG that accumulate in the blood during acute attacks are neurotoxic. These compounds can cause presynaptic inhibition of neurotransmitter release, inhibition of ATPase in brain, inhibition of monosynaptic reflexes in the spinal cord, and decrease in resting membrane potential of muscle.[32] However, neither compound penetrates the blood–brain barrier sufficiently to achieve concentrations in nervous tissue approximating those required for such effects. Moreover, rising blood levels of these compounds may not be associated with neurologic deterioration.[33] More plausible is the presence of a concomitant defect in *neural* heme biosynthesis, resulting in demyelination, with secondary axonal degeneration.[32] Interestingly, asymptomatic persons who exhibit the biochemical defect, but who have never experienced an acute attack, demonstrate a peripheral neuropathy electromyographically.[34] Thus, it is likely that the latent genetic defect present in neural cells, as in other somatic cells, is activated during acute episodes.

CLINICAL CORRELATES OF INDUCIBLE PORPHYRIAS

PREVALENCE OF INDUCIBLE PORPHYRIAS

The inducible porphyrias are transmitted genetically as autosomal dominant traits, with variable individual expressivity and with marked geographic and ethnic variability in prevalence. Because of the variable expressivity—with some patients suffering frequent acute episodes of porphyria and other individuals with the same enzymatic defect never experiencing an attack—one cannot identify all affected persons without costly screening procedures. As a result, there is little precision in estimates of the prevalences of inducible porphyrias. In turn, there are no accurate estimates of the incidence of acute episodes.

ACUTE INTERMITTENT PORPHYRIA

The most common type of inducible porphyria, this disorder accounts for three quarters of the cases encountered in unselected populations in the United States. In a study of hospital admissions in metropolitan Seattle during the period 1952–1962, when porphyria was beginning to attract widespread clinical interest, the hospital records of 66 patients with porphyrias of undetermined types were identified.[35] These patients accounted for one in 7088 admissions, generally for other medical problems. Although these patients were obviously highly selected, as well as incompletely characterized, this study represents the only such survey conducted in this country. This disease is most common in Sweden—especially in Lapland where its prevalence has been estimated to be greater than 1:1000[36]—hence, it has been termed the Swedish type of porphyria. Lower prevalence has been noted in other countries: Northern Ireland, 1:5,000; Ireland, 1:80,000; and Western Australia, 3:100,000.[35,37] In all of these series, the prevalence in women is higher than that in men, suggesting a hormonal role in the etiology of the acute episodes.[37]

VARIEGATE PORPHYRIA

Accounting for perhaps one fifth of inducible porphyria cases in the United States, this disorder is most prevalent in South Africa; hence it is often termed the South African type. The prevalence is as great as 3:1000 among the whites in South Africa where the disorder was introduced by one of the original colonists from Holland in 1688.[37] The prevalence is considerably lower elsewhere.

HEREDITARY COPROPORPHYRIA.

This disorder accounts for the remaining five percent of inducible porphyria cases seen in this country. Because of its rarity and the fact that at least one half of affected patients are asymptomatic, there are no estimates of prevalence.

ETIOLOGY OF ACUTE EPISODES

Largely accounting for the variable expressivity of the genetically determined tendency toward acute episodes of neurologic dysfunction is an interaction of the defective biochemistry with several factors. These superimposed triggering factors include drugs, endogenous and exogenous steroids, infection, and starvation.[37]

DRUGS

Historically, barbiturates were among the earliest described triggering agents; but, over time, other therapeutic chemicals have been added to the growing list of drugs to be avoided in susceptible persons (Table 39-2).

Until recently, the anecdotal case report was the basis for adding a drug to the list of harmful drugs. With understanding of the defective biochemistry, it has become possible to "screen" potentially porphyrinogenic drugs pospectively in intact animals and in cell systems.[16,44–46] Drugs capable of inducing ALA-S, the rate-controlling enzyme in porphyrin metabolism, are suspect of being porphyrinogenic. Such screening procedures quantitate the accumulation of excess porphyrins and porphyrin precursors associated with the induction of ALA-S.[15,16,53,55] That is, drugs capable of inducing ALA-S are suspect of being porphyrinogenic. In addition, iron, lead, and other heavy metals can depress the activity of many of the enzymes in the heme biosynthetic pathway.[6]

Yet, the sensitivities and specificities of the different screening procedures vary, and drugs that induce ALA-S synthesis in an experimental system are not necessarily porphyrinogenic in man.[37] Moreover, an acute attack may not necessarily follow the administration of a known triggering agent to a susceptible person[6,37,40] or may occur after a variable and unpredictable time. The dose of the porphyrinogenic agent may have been too small in some cases to produce an identifiable attack, whereas in others an erroneous diagnosis of an *inducible* porphyria may account for the absence of an attack. Finally, susceptibility is

Table 39-2. Drugs and other stimuli implicated in precipitating acute attacks of porphyria.

Sedatives
  Barbiturates[6,39,40,45]
  Nonbarbiturate hypnotics[40,41,45]
    Chlordiazepoxide[47]
    Glutethimide
    Isopropylmeprobamate
    Meprobamate
    Methyprylon
Analgesics
  Pentazocine[45]*
  Pyrazolone-derivative antipyretics[40]
    Amidopyrine
    Antipyrine
    Isopropylantipyrine
    Dipyrone
Inhalation anesthetics[45]
  Enflurane*
  Methoxyflurane*
Local anesthetics[45]
  Lidocaine*
Anticonvulsants[48]
  Phenytoin[39,41]
  Mephenyltoin[15]*
  Methsuximide[41]
  Phensuximide[15]*
  Primidone
Antibiotics
  Chloramphenicol[15]*
  Griseofulvin[6,40,42,43]
  Sulfonamides[6,39,43]
Steroids[37]
  Althesin[45]*
  Hydroxydione
  Estrogens[50,51]
  Progesterone[51,52]
  Metapyrone[53]*
Hypoglycemic sulfonylureas[37]
  Chlorpropamide
  Tolbutamide[54]
Toxins
  Arsenic[6]
  Ethanol[40]
  Hexachlorobenzene[6]
  Lead[6,44]
Miscellaneous drugs
  Amphetamine
  Dichlorophenazone[40]
  Ergot preparations[40]
  Ferric chloride[6]
  Imipramine[41]
  Nikethimide[53]*

*Induces δ-aminolevulinic acid synthetase synthesis *in vitro* or produces porphyria in experimental systems *in vivo* but has not been unequivocally implicated in precipitating acute porphyria in man.

influenced by other superimposed factors, such as diet and hormonal status.

Compounding attempts to characterize drugs which are porphyrinogenic is the presence of more than one drug, as well as other factors, in the clinical setting. However, high lipid solubility is a characteristic of these drugs which facilitates their passage across membranes and contact with microsomal enzymes in the cytosol.[37] Apart from ancedotal case reports and literature reviews,[1,2,56–69] there has been only one systematic study[45] of the ability of anesthetic drugs to induce ALA-S *in vitro*.

Ultra-Short-Acting Barbiturates

Infamous among barbiturates, thiopental, the most commonly used induction agent, was highlighted in early case reports of acute porphyris.[1,2,58,61] Thiopental is especially hazardous because it is administered intravenously in large dosages and often given to patients already experiencing symptoms; that is, their abdominal pain may simulate an acute appendicitis or other urgent abdominal disorder requiring surgery.[37] More recently, there have been reports of the absence of an acute attack after thiopental administration in some patients who were found later to have an inducible porphyria.[35,39,65–67] The survey conducted among Seattle hospitals noted that acute attacks were uncommon after barbiturate (usually thiopental) administration, with only three attacks occurring following 36 thiopental inductions.[35] This survey, however, did not document the diagnosis of "porphyria" sufficiently to be certain that all patients had an inducible porphyria. The diagnoses seem firmly established in other reports[39,65–67] which demonstrate that, even in a given patient,[39,65] an acute attack does not necessarily follow a thiopental induction. Of particular interest is the absence of an attack when the disease was in the latent phase at the time of the induction and the worsening of symptoms in most of those anesthetized during an acute attack.[67]

Methohexital also induces the synthesis of ALA-S,[45] although this drug has not been associated with acute attacks in man, probably because it is used so infrequently.

Etomidate

Although there are no reports of acute porphyria associated with etomidate, this imidazole derivative also induces ALA-S synthesis *in vitro*.[45]

Ketamine

This potential alternate induction agent has been used in a susceptible patient on two occasions without acute porphyria occurring in the postoperative period.[68] However, as with other drugs, extrapolations from experiences with a single patient or small series can be misleading, given the unpredictability of the attacks. Ketamine does not induce ALA-S synthesis in rat liver when given in a dosage of 20 mg./kg., twice the maximum recommended dosage for a single administration in man;[45] however, in the more sensitive chick embryo liver model, slightly higher dosages are porphyrinogenic.[69] Further clinical experience is needed to determine whether, for example, prolonged ketamine anesthesia with higher dosages might be porphyrinogenic.

Inhalational Anesthetics

Enflurane and methoxyflurane induce ALA-S synthesis *in vitro*,[45] although they have not been implicated in causing clinical attacks. Curiously, halothane, which is metabolized to a greater degree than enflurane, was not found to be porphyrinogenic. Given the ability of all inhalation agents, with the exception of cyclopropane, to stimulate microsomal enzymes nonspecifically,[70] it is surprising that only two of these drugs have been found to be potentially porphyrinogenic. However, the multiplicity of drugs used pre- and intraoperatively, as well as the almost universal use of barbiturate induction agents, mitigates against implicating inhalation anesthetics in acute attacks.

Local Anesthetics

Lidocaine is porphyrinogenic, yet procaine *decreases* ALA-S synthesis in the rat liver model.[45] Whereas lidocaine is highly lipid soluble and metabolized by microsomal enzymes, procaine has been reported to induce remission in acute porphyria.[71]

Analgesics

Capable of inducing ALA-S synthesis *in vitro*,[45] pentazocine has an allyl group in its chemical structure which sterically hinders hydrolysis and which has been found in other porphyrinogenic drugs.[72]

Anticholinesterases

Neostigmine and other anticholinesterases have been assumed to be porphyrinogenic because certain insecticides (*e.g.*, chlordane, lindane) have anticholinesterase activity and can cause demyelinization. However, axonal degeneration rather than demyelinization occurs during acute porphyria; moreover, anticholinesterase agents have been used during attacks without aggravating the symptoms. Hence, there does not seem to be a rational basis to consider anticholinesterases porphyrinogenic.

STEROIDS

Considerable circumstantial evidence implicates female sex hormones as triggering agents: onset of biochemical and clinical manifestations after puberty, a predominance of women affected, attacks just before menstruation in many women, activation of the disease during pregnancy, precipitation of attacks by exogenous estrogens and oral contraceptives, and weak porphyrinogenicity of estradiol, estrone, progesterone, and testosterone in the chick embryo liver model.[37] Yet, in some patients, estrogens and oral contraceptives can prevent attacks. In particular, exogenous and endogenous steroids having a 5ß-H configuration which is found in many steroid metabolites are porphyrinogenic.

Althesin

This mixture of two steroids, alphaxalone and alphadolone, induces ALA-S synthesis *in vitro*.[45]

INFECTION

Bacterial and viral infections appear to trigger acute porphyria. Whether the underlying mechanism relates to increased 5ß-H steroid production (*i.e.*, increased catabolism) or decreased food intake (*i.e.*, starvation) is unknown.[37]

Table 39-3. Clinical features noted in acute attacks of porphyria.

FEATURES	MARKOWITZ[76] 69 PATIENTS 1954	WALDENSTROM[36] 233 PATIENTS 1957	GOLDBERG[77] 50 PATIENTS 1959	EALES[78] 80 PATIENTS 1962	STEIN & TSCHUDY[39] 46 PATIENTS 1970
Disorder	AIP	AIP	AIP	VP	AIP
Females	61%	60%	62%	70%	76%
Abdominal pain	95	85	94	90	95
Vomiting	52	59	78	80	43
Mental changes	80*	55	56	55	40
Constipation	46	48	74	80	48
Paralysis	72	42	68	53	32
Hypertension	49	40	56	55	40
Fever	36	37	14	38	9
Tachycardia	51	28	64	83	80
Cranial nerve involvement	51	?	29	9	?
Seizures	?	10	18	12	20
Sensory loss	24	9	38	15	26
Amaurosis	?	4	3	3	6
Diarrhea	11	9	12	8	5
Azotemia	67	9	6	69	32
Proteinuria	?	9	14	8	0
Leukocytosis	48	7	24	20	11
ECG abnormalities	47	?	44	23	37

*Includes seizures
AIP, acute intermittent porphyria; VP, variegate porphyria

STARVATION

This was identified as a triggering agent during studies of experimental models.[73] Conversely, a diet rich in carbohydrate results in decreased porphyrin and porphyrin precursor excretion.[37,74,75] This "glucose effect" constitutes the basis for part of the therapy of acute attacks.

CLINICAL PRESENTATION OF ACUTE EPISODES

As diverse as the triggering factors are the features that comprise the acute attack. Although there is often marked variability in symptomatology from patient to patient, usually a particular disease pattern recurs in a given patient. Taken collectively, however, the clinical features noted in one series of patients resemble those in others remarkably well (Table 39-3).

Underlying the symptomatology, but not well understood, is a polyneuropathy consisting of axonal degeneration. Although predominantly a motor neuropathy, almost any part of the nervous system can be involved, accounting for the diverse and bizarre presentations. Simulating so many other disorders, acute porphyria has been termed "the little imitator."[79] Compounding the diagnostic difficulties is the fact that symptomatology may not closely follow exposure to triggering agents. Although pain may be experienced within hours of exposure, other neurologic symptoms may appear a month later. As a result, the precipitating agent may pass unrecognized. This may explain, in part, how some patients appear to have tolerated thiopental, for example, "without complications."

Some features of the acute attack are particularly relevant to anesthesiology practice.

AUTONOMIC INSTABILITY

Autonomic neuropathy results in diffuse instability of the autonomic nervous system. Imbalance in the innervation of the gut, with resultant spasm and relaxation, probably accounts for the severe abdominal pain that is almost universally

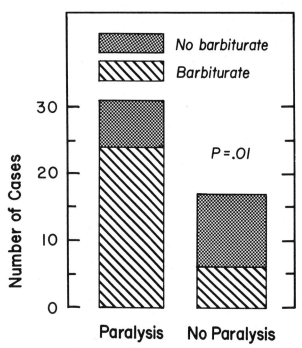

Fig. 39-5. Barbiturate administration is overrepresented among patients experiencing paralysis or paresis. (Data from Goldberg, A.: Acute intermittent porphyria: A study of 50 cases. Quart. J. Med., 28:183, 1959.)

experienced. Because the pain simulates that due to acute abdominal disorders and fever and leukocytosis may be present, the patient is likely to be subjected to unnecessary laparotomy. Autonomic instability also manifests itself as tachycardia, labile hypertension, and postural hypotension. There may also be incontinence or urinary retention.

Paralysis

Generally following the abdominal pain by days to months, peripheral neuropathy is manifested often by pain felt in the back and extremities. Sometimes flaccid paralysis appears within days; if there is concomitant involvement of bulbar cranial nerves, there may be aphonia, dysphagia, and respiratory paralysis. In particular, paralysis or paresis may be more common among patients who have received barbiturates[77] (Fig. 39-5). Unlike the Guillain-Barré syndrome, the paralysis generally progresses caudad, with the upper extremities more severely affected than the lower ones.[80]

Mental Changes

Often, these patients suffer from insomnia and restless, predisposing them to exposure to barbiturates. The resultant mental changes are highly variable from one patient to another, ranging from a mild, acute confusional state to acute psychosis. In fact, "mad" King George III, against whom the American colonists fought for their independence, probably had acute intermittent porphyria.[81]

Fluid and Electrolyte Imbalances

With vomiting and diarrhea, there is excessive fluid and electrolyte loss from the gastrointestinal tract. This results in sodium loss and hypovolemia. In most patients, however, there is free water retention, failure of normal renal sodium conservation, and resultant hyponatremia owing to the inappropriate release of antidiuretic hormone.[82–84] Concomitantly there is often a metabolic encephalopathy, heralded by seizures that may linger beyond restoration of fluid and electrolyte balance. There may also be hypomagnesemia of a sufficient degree to produce tetany.[82,83] A syndrome of neurogenic hyperventilation, leading to marked alkalosis and secondary coma, has also been described.[85]

DIAGNOSIS OF INDUCIBLE PORPHYRIAS

The detection of latent forms of inducible porphyria is extraordinarily difficult, for routine laboratory studies do not screen patients for these disorders. Generally, the diagnosis is suggested by episodes of bizarre symptomatology, perhaps related to an identifiable triggering agent. Once suggested, the diagnosis is established principally by chemical analysis of urine and possibly blood and feces, too (see Table 39-1). Exposure to potential triggering agents should cease and therapy (see next section) should be instituted promptly while waiting for the laboratory to confirm the clinical diagnosis.

ACUTE INTERMITTENT PORPHYRIA

The diagnosis of acute intermittent porphyria is established by documenting an increase in urinary ALA or PBG, as one would expect from the biochemical defect. Generally, only PBG is assayed because the analysis for ALA is very difficult; the levels of urine and stool porphyrins are normal.

There are several ways to determine whether the level of PBG is elevated. Urine containing very high levels turns black upon standing, particularly if acidified. The presence of lower levels of urinary PBG can be determined with the Watson–Schwartz[86] or the simpler and more specific Hoesch[87] test, both of which are generally positive (urine turns red upon addition of reagents) at PBG concentrations greater than 10 mg./24 hr.[88] Chromatography can also be used.

Unfortunately, during the latent phase between attacks and even during some attacks, the levels of ALA and PBG may be near normal (*e.g.*, 3–9 mg./24 hr.). A definitive diagnosis can be made by demonstrating a deficiency of uroporphyrinogen I synthetase in red blood cells.[89] This test is also useful for screening relatives for this disorder.

VARIEGATE PORPHYRIA AND HEREDITARY COPROPORPHYRIA

During acute attacks, levels of urinary ALA and PBG are elevated as in acute intermittent porphyria, although not as much. However, during the latent phase, urinary ALA, PBG, and porphyrins are normal. Fecal levels of coproporphyrin and protoporphyrin remain elevated, even during the latent phase; the former is higher in hereditary coproporphyria, whereas the latter is higher in variegate porphyria.

TREATMENT OF ACUTE EPISODES OF INDUCIBLE PORPHYRIAS

GENERAL MEASURES

Treatment is largely supportive, with correction of fluid and electrolyte imbalances, especially dehydration, hyponatremia, and hypomagnesemia. If hyponatremia coexists with normovolemia, the underlying syndrome of inappropriate secretion of antidiuretic hormone is treated with fluid restriction.

Excessive tachycardia and hypertension, as well as possibly anxiety and abdominal discomfort, can be treated safely with ß-adrenergic blocking drugs (*e.g.*, propranolol).[90] Pain can be treated with commonly used narcotics (*e.g.*, meperidine, morphine); however, there is justifiable concern about the potential for narcotic addiction in these patients. Curiously, chlorpromazine, in doses of 25 to 100 mg, orally or parenterally, is often effective as an analgesic.[91] Seizures may be treated with diazepam or clonazepam[92] as safe alternatives to barbiturates, hydantoins, and succinimides. All nonessential drugs should be discountinued. Of course, potential triggering agents (see Table 39-2), if present, should be withdrawn and assiduously avoided. Ventilatory support should be instituted for impending as well as frank respiratory failure.

SPECIFIC MEASURES

PYRIDOXINE

Some patients with porphyric neuropathy are deficient in vitamin B_6, a neurologically active substance that is a cofactor for ALA-S activity, among other essential steps in intermediary metabolism.[93] Given its low toxicity, it should be administered, even though its efficacy has yet to be established.

GLUCOSE

The intravenous infusion of glucose, 10 to 20 g./hr., to approach 500 g./day, takes advantage of the "glucose effect," in which this simple carbohydrate blocks the induction of ALA-S.[37,74,75] Unfortunately, for unknown reasons, the clinical response is often variable and, once the infusion is stopped, rebound increases in ALA-S activity and porphyrin precursor excretion occur.

HEMATIN

Should neurologic symptoms appear or any symptomatology progress despite the use of glucose infusion and supportive care, an intravenous infusion of hematin, 4 mg./kg. every 12 hr., should be started. Hematin is the heme extracted from red cells and acts like heme in repressing ALA-S synthesis.[94] Like glucose and heme, hematin lowers porphyrin and porphyrin precursor excretion, producing a remission within 48 hr.[95-98] Upon discontinuing the hematin infusion, levels of ALA and PBG may rise, but clinical illness does not necessarily coincide.[33] Although hematin infusion is reliable and effective therapy, it can cause acute renal failure and its discontinuation results in rebound increase in porphyrin and prophyrin precursor excretion.

PREVENTION OF ACUTE EPISODES OF INDUCIBLE PORPHYRIAS

GENERAL CONSIDERATIONS

The most important element in prevention is educating susceptible persons about their disease and particularly about the need for strict avoidance of triggering agents, such as certain drugs (see Table 39-2) and deliberate fasting. This, in turn, requires that susceptible persons be identified by screening relatives of those known to have an inducible porphyria. All those found to be at risk should wear wrist bands or similar identification and take as few medications as possible.

ANESTHETIC MANAGEMENT

Part of the preoperative evaluation should be a thorough neurological assessment to document existing deficits, particularly those affecting respiratory and other bulbar functions. Existing fluid and electrolyte imbalances should be corrected.

Because the use of regional anesthetic techniques introduces confounding considerations should an attack occur or become more severe, general anesthesia is generally chosen. However, apart from the strict avoidance of drugs listed in Table 39-2, there are no proscriptions in the choice of anesthetic technique and agents. Given the large number of drugs which hospitalized patients often receive and the diversity of potentially porphyrinogenic drugs, as few drugs as possible should be administered. For those patients with variegate porphyria or hereditary coproprophyria with dermal lesions, special care should be exercised during positioning and transporting.

REFERENCES

1. Dean, G.: Porphyria. Br. Med. J., 2:1291, 1953.
2. Dundee, J. W., and Riding, J. E.: Barbiturate narcosis in porphyria. Anaesthesia, 10:55, 1955.
3. Watson, C. J., Pierach, C. A., Bossenmaier, I., et al.: Postulated deficiency of hepatic heme and repair by hematin infusions in the "inducible" hepatic porphyrias. Proc. Natl. Acad. Sci. U.S.A., 74:2118, 1977.
4. Garrod, A. E.: Inborn Errors of Metabolism. ed. 2. London, Frowde, Hodder, and Stoughton, 1923.
5. Meyer, U. A.: Hepatic porphyrias: New findings on the nature of metabolic defects. Prog. Liver Dis., 5:280, 1976.
6. Meyer, U. A., and Schmid, R.: The porphyrias. In Stanbury, J. B., Wyngaarden, J. B., and Frederickson, D. S. (eds.): The Metabolic Basis of Inherited Disease. ed. 4. pp. 1166–1220. New York, McGraw-Hill, 1978.
7. Elder, G. H., Gray, C. H., and Nicholson, D. C.: The porphyrias: A review, J. Clin. Path., 25:1013, 1972.
8. Kaplan, B. H.: Synthesis of heme. In Williams, W. J., Beutler, E., Erslev, A. J., et al.: Hematology. ed. 2. pp. 149–157. New York, McGraw-Hill, 1977.
9. Granick, S., and Urata, G.: Increase in activity of δ-aminolevulinic acid synthetase in liver mitochondria induced by feeding of 3'5-dicarbethoxy-1, 4-dihydrocollidine. J. Biol. Chem., 238:821, 1963.
10. Burnham, B. F., and Lascelles, J.: Control of porphyrin biosynthesis through a negative-feedback mechanism. Studies with preparations of δ-aminolaevulinate synthetase and δ-aminolaevulate dehydrase from *Rhodopseudomonas* spheroids. Biochem. J., 87:462, 1963.
11. Granick, S., and Sassa, S.: δ-aminolaevulinic acid synthetase and the control of heme and chlorophyll synthesis. In Vogel, H. J. (ed.): Metabolic Regulation. p. 77. New York, Academic Press, 1971.
12. Monod, J., Changeux, J. B., and Jacob, F.: Allosteric proteins and cellular control systems. J. Mol. Biol., 6:306, 1963.
13. Jacob, F., and Monod, J.: Genetic regulatory mechanisms in the synthesis of proteins. J. Mol. Biol., 3:318, 1961.
14. Granick, S., and Levere, R. D.: Heme synthesis in erythroid cells. Prog. Hematol., 4:1, 1964.
15. Granick, S.: The induction in vitro of the synthesis of δ-aminolevulinic acid synthetase in chemical porphyria: A response to certain drugs, sex hormones and foreign chemicals. J. Biol. Chem., 241:1359, 1966.
16. Tschudy, D. P., and Bonkowski, H. L.: Experimental porphyria. Fed. Proc., 31:147, 1966.
17. DeMatteis, F.: Drug interactions in experimental hepatic porphyria. Enzyme, 16:266, 1973.
18. Tschudy, D. P., Welland, F. H., Collins, A., et al.: The effect of carbohydrate feeding on the induction of aminolevulinic acid synthetase. Metabolism, 13:396, 1964.
19. Rose, J. A., Hellman, E. S., and Tschudy, D. P.: Effect of diet on the induction of experimental porphyria. Metabolism, 10:514, 1961.
20. Granick, S., and Kappas, A.: Steroid control of porphyrin and heme biosynthesis: A new biological function of steroid hormone metabolites. Proc. Natl. Acad. Sci. U.S.A., 57:1463, 1967.
21. Javitt, N. B., Rifkind, A., and Kappas, A.: Porphyrin-heme pathway: Regulation by intermediates in bile acid synthesis. Science, 182:841, 1973.
22. Marver, H. S., Collins, A., and Tschudy, D. P.: The permissive effect of hydrocortisone on the induction of ALA-S. Biochem. J., 99:31C, 1966.

23. Strand, J. L., Felsher, B. F., Redeker, A. G., et al.: Heme biosynthesis in intermittent acute porphyria: Decreased hepatic conversion of porphobilinogen and increased δ-aminolevulinic acid synthetase activity. Proc. Natl. Acad. Sci. U.S.A., 67:1315, 1970.

24. Meyer, U. A., Strand, L. J., Doss, M., et al.: Intermittent acute porphyria: Demonstration of a genetic defect in porphobilinogen metabolism. N. Engl. J. Med., 286:1277, 1972.

25. McKusick, V. A.: The anatomy of the human genome. Am. J. Med., 69:267, 1980.

26. Becker, D. M., Viljoen, J. D., Katz, J., et al.: Reduced ferrochelatase activity: A defect common to variegate porphyria and protoporphyria. Br. J. Haematol., 36:171, 1977.

27. Elder, G. H., Evans, J. D., Thomas, N., et al.: The primary enzyme defect in hereditary coproporphyria. Lancet, 2:1217, 1976.

28. Brodie, M. J., Thompson, G. G., Moore, M. R., et al.: Hereditary coproporphyria: Demonstration of the abnormalities in haem biosynthesis in peripheral blood. Q. J. Med., 46:229, 1977.

29. Nordmann, Y., Grandchamp, B., Phung, N., et al.: Coproporphyrinogen-oxidase deficiency in hereditary coproporphyria. Lancet, 1:140, 1977.

30. Brodie, M. J., Moore, M. R., and Goldberg, A.: Enzyme abnormalities in the porphyrias. Lancet, 2:699, 1977.

31. Allison, A. C., Magnus, I. A., and Young, M. R.: Role of lysosomes and of cell membranes on photosensitization. Nature, 209:974, 1966.

32. Shanley, B. C., Percy, V. A., and Neethling, A. C.: Pathogenesis of neural manifestations in acute porphyria. S. Afr. Med. J., 51:458, 1977.

33. Watson, C. J.: Hematin and porphyria. N. Engl. J. Med., 293:605, 1975.

34. Mustajoki, P., and Seppalainen, A. M.: Neuropathy in latent hereditary hepatic porphyria. Br. Med. J., 2:310, 1975.

35. Ward, R. J.: Porphyria and its relation to anesthesia. Anesthesiology, 26:212, 1965.

36. Waldenstrom, J.: The prophyrias as inborn errors of metabolism. Am. J. Med., 22:758, 1957.

37. Tschudy, D. P., Valsamis, M., and Madnussen, C. R.: Acute intermittent porphyria: clinical and selected research aspects. Ann. Intern. Med., 83:851, 1975.

38. Dean, G., and Barnes, H. D.: Porphyria: A South African screening experiment. Br. Med. J., 1:298, 1958.

39. Stein, J. A., and Tschudy, D. P.: Acute intermittent porphyria: A clinical and biochemical study of 46 patients. Medicine, 49:1, 1970.

40. Eales, L.: Acute porphyria: The precipitating and aggravating factors. S. Afr. J. Lab. Clin. Med., 17:120, 1971.

41. Cowger, M. L., and Labbe, R. F.: Contraindications of biological oxidation inhibitors in the treatment of porphyria. Lancet, 1:88, 1965.

42. Redeker, A. G., Sterling, R. E., and Bronow, R. S.: Effect of griseofulvin in acute intermittent porphyria. J. A. M. A., 188:466, 1964.

43. Berman, A., and Franklin, R. L.: Precipitation of acute intermittent porphyria by griseofulvin therapy. J. A. M. A., 192:1005, 1965.

44. Maxwell, J. D., and Meyer, U. A.: Drug sensitivity in hereditary hepatic porphyria. In Porphyrins in Human Disease: 1st Int. Porphyrin Meeting, Freiburg, 1975. pp. 1–9. Basel, Karger, 1976.

45. Parikh, R. K., and Moore, M. R.: Effect of certain anaesthetic agents on the activity of rat hepatic δ-aminolaevulinate synthetase. Br. J. Anaesth., 50:1099, 1978.

46. Eales, L.: Porphyria and the dangerous life-threatening drugs. S. Afr. Med. J., 56:914, 1979.

47. Goldberg, A., Rimington, C., and Lockhead, A. C.: Hereditary coproporphyria. Lancet, 1:632, 1967.

48. Birchfield, R. I., and Cowger, M. L.: Acute intermittent porphyria with seizures. Anticonvulsant medication-induced metabolic changes. Am. J. Dis. Child., 112:561, 1966.

49. Davidson, R.: Acute porphyria in an epileptic. Br. J. Clin. Pract., 17:33, 1963.

50. Welland, F. H., Hellman, E. S., Collins, A., et al.: Factors affecting the excretion of porphyrin precursors by patients with acute intermittent porphyria. II. The effect of ethynyl estradiol. Metabolism, 13:251, 1964.

51. Wetterberg, L.: Oral contraceptives and acute intermittent porphyria. Lancet, 2:1178, 1964.

52. Levit, E. J., Nodine, J. H., and Perloff, W. H.: Progesterone-induced porphyria. Am. J. Med., 22:831, 1957.

53. DeMatteis, F.: Disturbances of liver porphyrin metabolism caused by drugs. Pharmacol. Rev., 19:523, 1967.

54. Schlesinger, F. G., and Gastel, C.: Possible aggravation of abdominal symptoms by tolbutamide in a patient with diabetes and hepatic porphyria. Acta Med. Scand., 169:433, 1961.

55. DeMatteis, F.: Drugs and porphyria. S. Afr. J. Lab. Clin. Med., 17:126, 1971.

56. Dundee, J. W., and Riding, J. E.: Barbiturate narcosis in porphyria. Anaesthesia, 10:55, 1955.

57. Norris, W., and Macnab, G. W.: Anaesthesia in porphyria. Br. J. Anaesth., 32:505, 1960.

58. Dundee, J. W., McCleery, W. N. C., and McLoughlin, G.: The hazard of thiopental anesthesia in porphyria. Anesth. Analg., 41:567, 1962.

59. Lepinskie, F. F.: Porphyria as a problem in anaesthesia. Canad. Anaesth. Soc. J.: 10:286, 1963.

60. Murphy, P. C.: Acute intermittent porphyria: The anaesthetic problem and its background. Br. J. Anaesth., 36:801, 1964.

61. Eales, L.: Porphyria and thiopentone. Anesthesiology, 27:703, 1966.

62. Mees, D. E., Jr., and Frederickson, E. L: Anesthesia and the porphyrias. South. Med. J., 68:29, 1975.

63. Sumner, E.: Porphyria in relation to surgery and anaesthesia. Ann. Roy. Coll. Surg. Eng., 56:81, 1975.

64. Silvay, G., and Miller, R.: Porphyrias. Anesthesiol. Rev., 6(5):51, 1979.

65. Slavin, S. A., and Christoforides, C.: Thiopental administration in acute intermittent porphyria without adverse effect. Anesthesiology, 44:77, 1976.

66. Mustajoki, P., and Koskelo, P.: Hereditary hepatic porphyrias in Finland. Acta Med. Scand., 200:171, 1976.

67. Mustajoki, P., and Heinonen, J.: General anesthesia in "inducible" porphyrias. Anesthesiology, 53:12. 1980.

68. Rizk, S. F., Jacobson, J. H., II, and Silvay, G.: Ketamine as an induction agent for acute intermittent porphyria. Anesthesiology, 46:305, 1977.

69. Kostrzewska, E., Gregor, A., and Lipinska, D.: Ketamine in acute intermittent porphyria—dangerous or safe? Anesthesiology, 49:376, 1978.

70. Linde, H. W., and Berman, M. L.: Nonspecific stimulation of drug-metabolizing enzymes by inhalation anesthetic agents. Anesth. Analg., 50:656, 1971.

71. Grubschmidt, H. A.: A case of acute porphyria remissions

induced with procaine intravenously. Calf. Med., 77:243, 1950.

72. Racz, W. J., and Moffat, J. A.: Drug metabolism in cell cultures. I. Importance of steric factors for activity in porphyrin inducing drugs. Biochem. Pharmacol., 23:215, 1974.

73. Rose, J. A., Hellman, E. S., and Tschudy, D. P.: Effect of diet on the induction of experimental porphyria. Metabolism, 10:514, 1961.

74. Welland, F. H., Hellman, E. S., Collins, A., et al.: Factors affecting the excretion of porphyrin precursors by patients with acute intermittent porphyria. I. The effect of diet. Metabolism, 13:232, 1964.

75. Perlroth, M. G., Tschudy, D. P., Ratner, A., et al.: The effect of diet in variegate (South African genetic) porphyria. Metabolism, 17:571, 1968.

76. Markowitz, M.: Acute intermittent porphyria: A report of five cases and a review of the literature. Ann. Intern. Med., 41:1170, 1954.

77. Goldberg, A.: Acute intermittent porphyria: A study of 50 cases. Quart. J. Med., 28:183, 1959.

78. Eales, L., and Linder, G. C.: Porphyria—the acute attack—an analysis of 80 cases. S. Afr. Med. J., 36:284, 1962.

79. Waldenstrom, J.: Neurological symptoms caused by so-called acute porphyria. Acta Psychiatr. Scand., 14:375, 1939.

80. Sergay, S. M.: Management of neurologic exacerbations of hepatic porphyria. Med. Clin. N. Am., 63(2):453, 1979.

81. Macalpine, I., and Hunter, R.: Porphyria and King George III. Sci. Am., 221:38, July 1969.

82. Hellman, E. S., Tschudy, D. P., and Bartter, F. C.: Abnormal electrolyte and water metabolism in acute intermittent porphyria: The transient inappropriate secretion of antidiuretic hormone. Am. J. Med., 32:734, 1962.

83. Nielsen, B., and Thorn, N. A.: Transient excess urinary excretion of antidiuretic material in acute intermittent porphyria with hyponatremia and hypomagnesemia. Am. J. Med., 38:345, 1965.

84. Lipshutz, D. E., and Reiter, J. M.: Acute intermittent porphyria with inappropriately elevated ADH secretion. J. A. M. A., 230:716, 1974.

85. Baker, N. H., and Messert, B.: Acute intermittent porphyria with central neurogenic hyperventilation. Neurology, 17:559, 1967.

86. Watson, C. J., Taddeini, L., and Bossenmaier, I.: Present status of the Erhlich aldehyde reaction for urinary porphobilinogen. J. A. M. A., 190:501, 1964.

87. Lamon, J., With, T. K., and Redeker, A. G.: The Hoesch test: Beside screening for urinary porphobilinogen in patients with suspected porphyria. Clin. Chem., 20:1438, 1974.

88. Lamon, J. M., Frykholm, B. C., and Tschudy, D. P.: Screening tests in acute porphyria. Arch. Neurol., 34:709, 1977.

89. Magnussen, C. R., Levine, J. B., Doherty, J. M., et al.: A red cell enzyme method for the diagnosis of acute intermittent porphyria. Blood, 44:857, 1974.

90. Atsmon, A., Blum, I., and Fischl, J.: Treatment of acute attack of porphyria variegata with propranolol. S. Afr. Med. J., 46:311, 1972.

91. Monaco, R. N., Leeper, R. D., Robbins, J. J., et al.: Intermittent acute porphyria treated with chlorpromazine. N. Engl. J. Med., 256:309, 1957.

92. Larson, A. W., Wasserstrom, W. R., Felsher, B. R., et al.: Posttraumatic epilepsy and acute intermittent porphyria: Effects of phenytoin, carbamazepine, and clonazepam. Neurology, 28:824, 1978.

93. Elder, T. D., and Mengel, C. E.: Effect of pyridoxine deficiency on porphyrin precursor excretion in acute intermittent porphyria. Am. J. Med., 41:369, 1966.

94. Waxman, A. D., Collins, A., and Tschudy, D. P.: Oscillations of hepatic δ-aminolevulinic acid synthesis produced in vivo by heme. Biochem. Biophys. Res. Commun., 24:675, 1966.

95. Bonkowsky, H. L., Tschudy, D. P., Collins, A., et al.: Repression of the overproduction of porphyrin precursors in acute intermittent porphyria by intravenous infusions of hematin. Proc. Nat. Acad. Sci. USA, 68:2725, 1971.

96. Peterson, A., Bossenmaier, I., Cardinal, R., et al.: Hematin treatment of acute porphyria: Early remission of an almost fatal relapse. J. A. M. A., 235:520, 1976.

97. Lamon, J. M., Frykholm, B. C., Bennett, M., et al.: Prevention of acute porphyric attacks by intravenous haematin. Lancet, 2:492, 1978.

98. McColl, K. E. L., Thompson, G. T., Moore, M. R., et al.: Haematin therapy and leucocyte δ-aminolaevulinic-acid-synthase activity in prolonged attack of acute porphyria. Lancet, 1:133, 1979.

FURTHER READING

Elder, G. H., Gray, C. H., and Nicholson, D. C.: The porphyrias: A review. J. Clin. Path., 25:1013, 1972.

London, I. M.: Iron and heme: Crucial carriers and catalysts. In Wintrobe, M. M. (ed.): Blood, Pure and Eloquent. pp. 170–208. New York, McGraw-Hill, 1980.

Meyer, U. A., and Schmid, R.: The porphyrias. In Stanbury, J. B., Wyngaarden, J. B., and Frederickson, D. S. (eds.): The Metabolic Basis of Inherited Disease. ed. 4. pp. 1166–1220. New York, McGraw-Hill, 1978.

Mustajoki, P., and Heinonen, J.: General anesthesia in "inducible" porphyrias. Anesthesiology, 53:15, 1980.

Tschudy, D. P., Valsamis, M., and Magnussen, C. R.: Acute intermittent porphyria: Clinical and selected research aspects. Ann. Intern. Med., 83:851, 1975.

Part Ten

Obstetrics, Gynecology, and Neonatology

40 Teratogenicity

Bradley E. Smith, M.D.

During the past 15 years, increasing attention has been paid to the toxicities of our drugs to the fetus. The origin of this interest was the thalidomide tragedy in Europe.[1] Even though the drug laws then in force prevented a similar disaster from occurring in the United States, our medical practice has probably never been so profoundly altered by any single event. The resulting revisions of our drug laws now regulate almost every aspect of drug therapy in this country.

INCIDENCE OF TERATOGENIC EFFECTS OF ANESTHETICS

Reports alleging potential teratogenic effects of anesthetics (or at least the state of surgical anesthesia) appeared even before thalidomide was introduced.[2] In fact, it is estimated that as many as 2 per cent of all pregnant women receive an anesthetic for a surgical procedure.[3,4] Reproductive malfunction, including abortion, premature delivery, and perinatal mortality, also is much higher in women undergoing surgery during pregnancy. The perinatal mortality rate is estimated to be between 5 and 35 per cent. Pertinent studies, necessarily limited to relatively few pregnancies, have demonstrated only questionable evidence of an increased incidence of fetal malformation. Because of the great number of stress factors involved in any one of these exposures and the limited numbers of humans that have been studied, inferences concerning causal relationships should be drawn very cautiously from the incidental reports available.[3]

PROBLEMS OF STUDYING TERATOGENICITY

There are several problems posed by studying drug toxicity to reproductive function. Research in this area is probably more difficult to control than in any other area of human biology. For example, the "normal" incidence of human reproductive malfunction is not totally clear. Additionally, the incidence of human congenital anomalies is much greater than generally appreciated. Some reports suggest that the incidence is only 1 to 2 per cent; however, careful studies suggest that the true incidence is probably 7 per cent. In fact, it is estimated that congenital anomalies cause 29 per cent of neonatal deaths and 17 per cent of fetal deaths in the United States[5,6]. Many current studies have referred to erroneously low "established rates of congenital anomalies," in lieu of obtaining proper "control" data, in an attempt to demonstrate increased rates of malformation "caused" by suspected drugs. As a result, these studies have only confused the situation further.

Besides the uncertainty regarding the incidence of teratogenicity, the definition of the term *teratology* or *congenital anomaly* is vague. Moreover, the potential variety of toxic effects of drugs or other agents taken by the mother is so great as to stagger the imagination. Under experimental conditions in animals, a drug that is toxic to reproduction is more likely to cause abortion or resorption than to produce a defect in a live-born animal.[7] Similarly, specific teratogenic drugs have been shown to cause sterility by affecting sperm, by inhibiting impregnation of the ovum, or by preventing implantation of the fertilized egg.

This spectrum of effects of toxicity includes fetal death, expulsion of the developing fetus, lethal or nonlethal anatomic defects, and functional abnormalities. There is also a potential for causing congenital defects that are not apparent at birth and that may appear later during growth or only under certain types of stress. We can even conjecture that genetic damage may occur but not be manifested until reproduction is attempted or, indeed, only in subsequent generations.[5] Therefore, it is far more reliable to declare a drug teratogenic, using as evidence its dramatic effects, than it is to say that a drug is free of reproductive toxicity.[8]

Even after 15 years of widespread scrutiny, very few drugs have been proven to be teratogenic in humans.[9] These include thalidomide, diethylstilbestrol, diazepam, certain cancer chemotherapeutic agents, and vitamin A. These specific teratogens were identified because either a unique anatomic or functional defect is produced in relatively high incidence, or specific observations have been made in large groups of patients.

For many other alleged human teratogens, anecdotal reporting, statistical bias, or lack of "control" data makes the allegation questionable. One current example is the presumed human reproductive toxicity of chronic exposure to trace concentrations of anesthetic agents.[10] (see chap. 56).

There is the distinct possibility that some agents now thought to be "safe" may be toxic but produce effects that have not yet been identified. Like the recent investigation of diazepam, these may await only the design and application of specific, subtle tests before being demonstrated to be human teratogens. Although surgical anesthesia has not been proven clearly to be teratogenic to humans, it might well be a member of this category.

Contrasting with the very short list of proven teratogens in humans is the seemingly endless list of pharmacologic agents known to be teratogenic to animals. Anesthetics are not exceptions. Nearly every inhalation anesthetic now available can be shown to be potentially teratogenic to some species under specific conditions.[11]

There are several reasons why animal data obtained from teratogenicity research are particularly difficult to interpret or to extrapolate to humans. A great deal of the early research on teratogenicity has been episodic, uncontrolled, or has failed to consider some very important variables.[5]

For example, until recently dose equivalency has been poorly controlled. Most drugs that are toxic to some degree are embryocidal at some dosage range. Frequently, the dosage concentration necessary for a "litter LD_{50}" is well below half the maternal LD_{50}. Usually the teratogenic range is at or below the lowest range of maternal toxicity. The dosage range that produces the greatest number of anomalous fetal survivors usually is in the litter LD_{50} range. However, this range is very narrow, and usually there are no observable toxic effects on embryos at a dosage range of one half the litter LD_{50} and below. Research in which the exposure exceeds or does not approach this range may give a totally erroneous impression of the safety of the test substance. Of course, there are rare exceptions. For example, it appears that methoxyflurane may produce anomalies in nearly half of the litter at a litter LD_{10}.[12]

Another problem is that drugs given at one stage of gestation may produce totally different anomalies than those produced at other stages. For example, high oxygen tension on day 3 of incubation in the chick results in a very high incidence of wing and leg anomalies. However, the same oxygen exposure on day 5 of incubation results in a low incidence of limb defects but a very high incidence of anophthalmia and other eye defects. These differences probably relate to difference in tissue metabolic rates at different stages of development. Similarly, in the C57 black mouse there is very little danger to the embryo after repeated exposure to surgical anesthetic concentrations at days 6 through 11. However, anesthetic exposure on days 12 and 13 results in a sudden, tremendous increase in the incidence of congenital anomalies.[12] If research had not examined the effect of this agent at all stages of development methodically, this prominent effect would have been overlooked.

Differences in susceptibility to a given teratogen are influenced not only by the species, but even by different strains of the same species. Cortisone, which causes a 100-per-cent incidence of cleft palate in A-Jax mice, is associated with only about a 12-per-cent incidence with the same dose in C57 black mice. Other differences in species responses may be caused by diversity in drug detoxification pathways. For example, in one strain of mice, 5-fluorouracil is destroyed by hepatic enzymes, thereby affording protection against the teratogenicity demonstrated in another strain of mice lacking this enzyme system.[11]

The bone teratogenicity of methoxyflurane illustrates an indirect pathway: A product of the breakdown of the administered drug is the toxicant, and not the administered drug itself.[13] This particular mouse strain has the ability to release significant amounts of fluoride from the methoxyflurane molecule. Fluoride becomes peculiarly toxic at the 12th and 13th days because the ossification centers first become active at about the 11th day. The free fluoride combines with the calcium in these centers, especially in the vertebrae and ribs.[12]

MECHANISMS OF TERATOGENICITY

How do teratogens cause defects? One of the most obvious mechanisms is damage to genetic materials. Many potent teratogens, such as a number of anti-cancer drugs, do have the ability to damage DNA or messenger RNA. The antibiotic actinomycin D forms a stable complex with DNA, thereby preventing the formation of messenger RNA and ultimately leading to a complete breakdown of protein synthesis within the cell.[5] Diethyl ether, while not inhibiting RNA synthesis, may inhibit transport of messenger RNA, ultimately leading to a similar effect.[14] Many agents exhibit competitive metabolic blockade of essential nucleic acid substrates. For example, methotrexate and azaserine inhibit the synthesis of purines and pyrimidines, leading to a block of DNA production and, therefore, teratogenicity. It is intriguing to recall that in the laboratory anesthetics can be shown to have effects on DNA also; one may postulate that, perhaps, some of the teratogenic effects noted in animals might be brought about by this mechanism.[15]

Higher oxides of nitrogen are also known to be mutagenic by causing DNA damage. As contaminants in commercial nitrous oxide, they have been implicated but not proven to be sources of teratogensis.[5] Also, nitrogen mustard forms a stable complex between two adjacent guanine molecules in DNA, thereby leading to DNA damage and subsequent mutations. Since, under some circumstances, some chlorinated anesthetics release minute quantities of similar toxic substances, this possibility is potentially of interest in relation to the teratogenicity of inhalation anesthetics. Extensive studies in lower animal forms have demonstrated that anesthetic agents damage chromosomes. However, studies have failed so far to verify that this damage occurs in humans.[16]

Another mechanism by which drugs cause malformations is metabolic alteration. Anesthetics have profound effects on normal energy metabolism and, in particular, depress oxidation in the electron transfer chain and oxidative phosphorylation.[17] In general, energy requirements are high during gestation. In addition, both general energy use and requirements for specific substrate metabolism increase greatly and abruptly in specific organs and structures as they enter their respective periods of rapid development and change.

Experimentally, it appears that during rapid development of an organ system, its tissues may be more sensitive to the decreased availability of energy or specific substrates resulting from exposure to certain teratogens. Thus, cellular death or abnormal development may result in these organs. This leads ultimately to development of an anatomic or functional defect, but the total development of the embryo is relatively unaffected.[11] For example, antimycin, a cytochrome C antagonist, causes widespread death of myoblasts in the chick embryo when administered at a specific time in development. However, if it is administered earlier or later, there is no effect. Therefore, it can be assumed that the myoblasts have a high requirement for the substrate acted upon by cytochrome C (succinate) or have a deficiency of cytochrome C relative to its metabolic needs at that time.

Anesthetic agents (some of which appear to depress this same pathway), administered at the same time, might easily have the same type of effect as antimycin. Indeed, this mechanism of damage and cell death is reminiscent of the anomalies induced by exposure of chick embryos to diethyl ether. On the days following exposure, there is immediate death of eye cells leading to necrosis and resorption of these tissues. However, the rest of the embryo continues its normal path of development.[18]

Another possible teratogenic mechanism is the known antimitotic effect of anesthetics, even in low concentrations. For example, nitrous oxide is a well known metaphase blocker in cell culture.[19] Definite antimitotic effects occur in developing embryos exposed to nitrous oxide, cyclopropane, and halothane.[20]

Besides these postulated direct teratogenic effects of anesthetics, there is the potential insult of various complications of surgical anesthesia. Anesthesia, even when not complicated by airway obstruction or grossly observable hypoventilation, may lead to hypoxia resulting from subtle effects such as right-to-left shunt, owing to atelectasis, or shifts in the oxygen-hemoglobin dissociation curve, caused by metabolic acidosis. Although hypoxia is incontrovertibly teratogenic, the effect is demonstrated more easily in lower forms than in mammals.[5] Protective mechanisms utilized by the mammalian embryo include its favorable oxygen-hemoglobin dissociation curve, greater hemoglobin concentration, and ability to dilate the capillaries of the placenta and to increase its own cardiac output in response to maternal hypoxia. Human fetuses, for example, appear to survive hypoxic insult such as maternal cyanotic heart disease and prolonged artificial circulation during cardiac surgery.[12]

In the human, teratogenicity from prolonged exposure to elevated oxygen tension has not been demonstrated. However, high oxygen tension in other species is potentially teratogenic and is directly related to the degree of elevation of oxygen tension and duration of the exposure.[11]

Hypercapnia increases the incidence of still-born fetuses and cardiac anomalies in rats. In addition, there is a synergism of hypercapnia with anesthetic teratogens such as methoxyflurane.[21] Both hypercapnia and hypoxia alter the permeability of biologic membranes to some drugs. Therefore, these states might allow a greater concentration of teratogenic drugs to accumulate in the fetus. Maternal responses to asphyxia or hypotension, as well as to the many adjuvant drugs used in anesthesia, are possible teratogens, too. Catecholamines, both exogenous and those released during such stress, cause a marked decrease in uterine blood flow (see Chaps. 4 and 41) and have a teratogenic effect in mammals.[5]

Although the effects of respiratory alkalosis owing to hyperventilation are still controversial, there is certainly sufficient evidence to question whether the alkalosis produced during a long anesthetic might harm the fetus. A prolonged decrease in placental blood flow and inhibition of normal placental transfer of metabolites and nutrients might be the cause.

Since almost all anesthetic and hypnotic drugs are highly lipid-soluble, they pass from mother to fetus easily. But some anesthetics, such as trichloroethylene and methoxyflurane, achieve a higher concentration in fetal than in maternal blood during prolonged exposure. This increases their potential for causing defects.[5]

Some potential teratogens administered to the mother may accumulate to very high levels in the fetus, because the fetus has immature ability to degrade and excrete these drugs. Fetal hepatic glucuronyltransferase has very low activity, for example, leading to difficulty with conjugation and excretion of bilirubin, sulfobromophthalein, lidocaine, mepivacaine, and meprobamate. Fetal liver microsomal enzymes also degrade barbiturates and other drugs slowly. In addition, renal clearance of some drugs (e.g., penicillin) is markedly depressed. These defects not only lead to unexpectedly high blood levels but may also prolong the exposure of the fetus to these toxic drugs, heightening the potential teratogenic effect.

ANESTHETIC TERATOGENICITY

Inhalation Agents

There have been extensive reports demonstrating the teratogenic capabilities of almost all inhalation anesthetic drugs in laboratory animals. Incubation with 80-per-cent nitrous oxide greatly decreases the rate of hatching of chick eggs and results in a significant number of neurologic defects in the few surviving chicks.[22] Exposure for only 6 hours at that concentration leads to a significantly elevated rate of embryo death. A mild degree of hypoxia, in itself insufficient to affect the developing embryo, combined with nitrous oxide greatly increases this toxicity, indicating a synergism.[23] Inhalation of 50-per-cent nitrous oxide for 24 to 48 hours produces a high incidence of intrauterine death and resorption, multiple skeletal deformities, and a significant decrease in embryo size in rats.[24]

Diethyl ether in clinical concentrations results in an elevated death rate of chick embryos and produces anomalies in 21 per cent of the survivors. In contrast, the incidence of death and anomalies in unexposed embryos is less than 1 per cent. The concentration of ether in the blood of exposed embryos is less than that achieved in humans during surgical ether anesthesia.[18]

Cyclopropane causes death and an increased incidence of abnormality in surviving chick embryos in a dose-related fashion. These anomalies include stunted growth, anophthalmia, and brain malformations.[25]

Similarly, exposure of C57 black mice on day 12 or 13 of gestation to methoxyflurane, under conditions that produce no maternal deaths, results in an exceedingly high incidence of bone anomalies. Despite this teratogenic activity, rates of embryo death and resorption are relatively low.[12]

The teratogenicity of halothane in chick embryos is directly related to concentration and duration of exposure.[23] Bone and developmental anomalies appear in rat fetuses when the mother is exposed to low concentrations of halothane for

12 to 48 hours.[26] A 3-hour halothane exposure on day 13, 14, or 15 in the Swiss mouse results in a highly significant increase in cleft palate and limb anomalies in the surviving fetuses.[27] The incidence of anomalies among the surviving fetuses is 46 per cent when pregnant mice are exposed to 1.5-per-cent halothane for only 3 hours on day 13 of gestation, but there is no lethality in the mothers. Similar defects are not found in unexposed fetuses. Blood halothane concentration is in the same range as that during clinical anesthesia in humans.[27] A 2-hour halothane anesthetic during early gestation in rats is followed by learning deficits in the adult offspring[28]; whether this "behavioral teratogenicity" is the result of the anesthetic agent or some other unstudied variable in the experiment must still be studied.

Adjuvants

The potential teratogenicity of barbiturates is disputed. However, in one very well controlled investigation, no anomalies were detected in offspring of Rhesus monkeys given large doses of pentobarbital during middle and late gestation. The weight of these conflicting reports suggests that barbiturates are not teratogenic in mammals.[11] Meprobamate appears to be associated with the impairment of learning ability after treatment of pregnant rats. Even though glutethemide is clinically very similar to thalidomide, it did not induce malformations either in animals or in humans when it was carefully studied during the first trimester.[5]

Although not studied as extensively, narcotics also appear to be relatively free of teratogenic potential. Despite some disagreement, observation of babies born to addicted mothers seems to verify this conclusion.[5]

The ethylamine structure in antihistaminics and antiemetics is highly suggestive of teratogenicity. However, extensive studies in rats have failed to demonstrate teratogenicity even when four times the human dose of dimenhydrinate was used. Cyclizine appears to be teratogenic in animals, but this has not been verified in humans. Similarly, meclizine, chlorpromazine, and prochlorperazine are teratogenic in animals, but there is no proof that they are teratogenic in humans. In fact, trifluperazine, promethazine, and imipramine do not seem to be teratogenic in humans.[5,29]

TERATOGENICITY OF TRACE ANESTHETIC CONCENTRATIONS

Anesthetists, surgeons, and nursing personnel are exposed to detectable concentrations of anesthetic gases that are vented or "spilled" from anesthetic equipment into the operating room.[30–36] Concern that these "trace concentrations" may be toxic to reproductive function or mental performance, or cause carcinogenesis in operating room personnel and anesthetists has been voiced strongly.[37] The problems addressed are complex and multifaceted. Although only reproductive aspects are reviewed here, other aspects are discussed in Chapter 56.

The National Institute for Occupational Safety and Health is considering recommending regulations that would require that operating room environments contain no more than 25 parts per million (p.p.m.) nitrous oxide and 0.5 p.p.m. of halogenated anesthetics used with nitrous oxide, or 2.0 p.p.m. used alone.[38] However, the validity of these target levels has not been substantiated. The implied stringent restriction of allowable level is in sharp contrast to levels presently accepted by several governments in regulating industrial workers', exposure to anesthetics. These regulations permit exposure to 1/25 of the concentration of the "threshold" limit of the drug's biologic activity. Specifically, 1/12 of the anesthetic concentration of certain anesthetics has been accepted as a safe limit.[39]

Therefore, if shown to be valid, the current suggestion that anesthetics are toxic in concentrations from 1/1000 to 1/100 of the anesthetic levels would reduce the allowed limits for suspect chemicals far below the previously established occupational safety standards.

Owing to the relatively small volume of anesthetic mixtures that are spilled into the operating room air and the very high ventilation rate of modern operating rooms (approximately 700 cubic ft./min.), the concentration of these gases breathed by operating personnel is very low. For example, with methoxyflurane the concentration inhaled by the anesthetist ranges from 0.001 to 0.01 per cent near the anesthesia machine.[40] The minimum effective anesthetic concentration of the same agent is from 160 to 1,600 times greater. In the case of halothane, the inhaled atmosphere near the anesthesia machine varies from 0.001 to 0.04 per cent[10,33,41]; again, the minimum effective anesthetic concentration is hundreds of times greater. The greatest concentration of nitrous oxide usually breathed under normal circumstances by the anesthetist is from 0.03 to 0.97 per cent,[30,32,33] 100 to 1000 times less than the minimum concentration necessary to produce anesthesia. Blood concentration of these anesthetics in anesthetists and operating room personnel can also be detected by extremely sensitive devices. These concentrations generally approximate one-tenth the inhaled anesthetic concentration and persist at even lower levels for several hours.[10,31,40]

Animal Studies of Teratogenicity of Trace Anesthetic Concentrations

Animal investigations of the alleged reproductive toxicity of trace concentrations of the anesthetics have been generally unsatisfactory, inconsistent, or negative in their findings. These studies usually investigated very small numbers of pregnant animals, utilized concentrations of anesthetics far greater than those in the actual operating room environment, or presented multiple internal inconsistences in handling of data.[32,41] For example, in one study rats were exposed to 1-per-cent nitrous oxide 24 hours per day from days 8 through 13 of pregnancy. This concentration and duration are greater than usually breathed by the anesthetist. In another portion of the same report resorption rates in ten pregnant rats exposed to 0.01-per-cent nitrous oxide for 8 hours per day from day 10 to 13 were reported to be 2.5 times greater than rates in other females, in which inhalation of the same concentration was continued from days 8 through 19 of gestation, thereby implying diminished toxicity from a greater exposure![32]

Another report indicated that 8 to 10 p.p.m. of halothane inhaled by 30 pregnant rats, 5 hours per day, 5 days per week during mating and gestation resulted in no effect on fertility or birth indices of the resulting 280 fetuses.[41] However, when exposure to the same concentration was continued during and after birth and during the lactation-suckling period, significant perinatal mortality occurred but was reported as reproductive toxicity of the anesthetic! Since nursing mothers rarely bring their infants to the operating room each day, that study involved a stress greater than the clinical situation.

More recently, Bruce has been unable to demonstrate reproductive toxicity in mice after chronic inhalation of trace concentrations of halothane.[42] Similarly, other studies have failed to demonstrate reproductive toxicity resulting from chronic expousre to trace concentrations of methoxyflurane[43] or halothane[44] in Sprague-Dawley rats. In studies of graded exposure, reproductive toxicity does not appear until the exposure to halothane,[45,46] nitrous oxide,[46] or methoxyflurane[46] is at least 40 times that found in unscavenged operating rooms. Spermatogenic cell injury manifested by reduced production of mature spermatozoa occurs in rats exposed to 20-per-cent nitrous oxide for several weeks.[47] Whether this effect occurs following the much lower concentrations noted in the operating room is unknown. The "behavioral teratogenicity," consisting of learning deficits in adult offspring of rats receiving halothane early in gestation,[28] also occurs with chronic exposure to trace (10 p.p.m.) concentrations of halothane.[48,49]

Clinical Studies of Teratogenicity of Trace Anesthetic Concentrations

Reports dealing with alleged reproductive toxicity in operating room personnel have many features in common. All were retrospective and carried out by mailed questionnaires. All but one included relatively small numbers of women actually exposed to the operating theater environment. Generally, either no controls have been used,[34] or the control group of women has been selected in a method possibly subject to bias.[30,36] In some cases the studied anesthetists were significantly older than the "control" women.[10] In another report, the reproductive performance of the same anesthetists, at an older age, was compared with their own reproductive performance at a younger age. This is an extremely significant bias, because reproductive malfunction increases rapidly during the age span considered in this study.

A closely related, prominent bias was involved in a British study of 563 female anesthetists.[35] There was no significant difference between the children born to the two groups with respect to sex ratio, stillbirth, neonatal death, or congenital abnormality. The study clearly states that "no such association (. . . with the known teratogenicity of the volatile anesthetic agents in other species. . .) can be derived from our survey. . . " However, the report also compared the incidence of spontaneous abortion during regular employment and during periods of unemployment, while "resting" at home, in the same anesthetists; there was indeed a greater incidence of reproductive malfunction in working anesthetists. However, no control was offered, and this suggested that any other type of regular employment, as opposed to "resting" at home, might increase reproductive malfunction to the same degree. Even more significantly, this study states that offspring of anesthetists working during pregnancy do not have a significantly different rate of congenital abnormalities (6.5%) than those of nonanesthetist controls (4.9%). Although they experience a frequency of spontaneous abortion that is greater than the control group, this incidence is not different from anesthetists who did not work during pregnancy.

There are many possible explanations for the higher incidence of spontaneous abortion in working anesthetists: for example, increased physical activity, disturbed sleep, and the emotional stresses of the operating room. The last explanation suggests that qualities necessary to become a successful anesthetist may coincide with those of the well known "abortion-prone personality." This personality type and the prominent influence of emotion and stress on successful reproductive function in humans have been discussed extensively.[50]

The United States national study presents some evidence that supports this suspicion.[35] Female anesthesiologists who had no exposure to anesthetics during the first trimester or during the entire year before pregnancy had a rate of spontaneous abortion of 15.7 per cent. The abortion rate among these unexposed anesthesiologists was nearly twice that of female pediatricians and was almost identical to the rate found in exposed female anesthesiologists (17.1%).

Although attention was not drawn to the fact, the data presented in the United States national study demonstrated that female anesthesiologists at work actually had a lower incidence of infants with birth defects than an employed group of nonanesthetist general duty nurses. The same report claimed that the female anesthesiologists have a higher abortion rate than do "controls." However, the study correctly noted that the "control" group of female pediatricians display a "remarkably low," abnormally favorable rate of spontaneous abortions. Had employed members of the American Nursing Association been chosen as the "controls," rather than the female pediatricians, there would have been no statistically significant difference between the abortion rates.

Additional objections have been raised regarding inconsistencies in the experimental design and statistical analysis utilized in this report.[51–53] Further, there was no "dose response effect" apparent in the alleged reproductive toxicity among the groups. The anesthetist is exposed to a greater "dose" than the operating room nurse; therefore, she should experience a greater incidence of toxicity. This was not demonstrated.

Finally, it is likely that biased reporting contributed to the higher rages of spontaneous abortion and fetal malformation in operating room personnel.[52] For example, the questionnaire used in the national study was entitled, "Effects of Waste Anesthetics on Health."[36] That title probably encouraged people with operating room exposure to report past events more fully than those without this exposure. That the response rates of the operating room personnel were much higher than those of the unexposed groups suggests that the reports were biased. Moreover, given the emotional sequelae of the birth of a deformed infant or even spontaneous abortion, there may also have been a strong bias toward response.

Avoiding such ascertainment bias by using an existing health registry, a recent study among Swedish operating room nurses found no increased incidence of threatened abortion or congenital malformations.[54]

There are many other uncontrolled factors in most of the human studies. These include differences in the use of contraceptives between study and control periods, the observed greater frequency of irregular menstrual periods and dysmenorrhea among anesthetists, and the implications of these findings for successful reproduction. Only scant comment has been made concerning the reproductive implications of frequent irradiation in the operating room or of the well established greater exposure to all types of viral infections (particularly hepatitis) among operating room personnel.

CLINICAL RECOMMENDATIONS FOR PREVENTION OF ANESTHETIC TERATOGENICITY

There is extensive evidence that inhalation anesthetic agents are toxic to reproductive function when inhaled in concentrations sufficient to establish surgical anesthesia in pregnant laboratory animals. Although there is no actual evidence that the human fetus is similarly affected, it seems prudent and reasonable to exercise some caution in anesthetizing pregnant patients.

Therefore, totally elective surgery for a pregnant patient should probably be deferred until after termination of the pregnancy. There is good reason to question the prevailing view that, even if a drug has teratogenic potential, the threat disappears after the first trimester of pregnancy.

If, on the other hand, the patient requires surgery during pregnancy, anesthetic techniques that utilize the least toxic drugs in the lowest possible concentration, for the shortest possible time, should be chosen. For example, spinal anesthesia is preferable when it is as applicable as general anesthesia (avoiding hypotension, of course).

If general anesthesia is necessary, on the basis of evidence from laboratory animals, the use of barbiturates, narcotics, and muscle relaxants seems to be the least toxic to the reproductive system than all other current methods of general anesthesia. The use of minimal concentrations of nitrous oxide may be permissible, but only because it appears to be the least toxic of the inhalation anesthetics.

Imposing pronouncements have been made concerning the alleged danger to operating room personnel of inhalation of the minute concentrations of anesthetic gases in their environment. Close inspection of these reports and their data suggests that convincing evidence of a real danger has not been presented yet. While it is apparent that anesthetists at work in the operating room experience a greater incidence of reproductive malfunction than other women, this statistic may result from inherent differences in the anesthetist population, to the stress of this type of employment, or to other teratogens encountered in the environment, and not to the anesthetic agents.

However, since relatively efficient and inexpensive devices are available to reduce markedly even this small exposure to suspected toxicants, it seems entirely reasonable to support the use of these devices. The adoption of regulations limiting the exposure of operating room personnel to these trace amounts of anesthetics would have extensive (and possibly totally unjustified) legal and economic ramifications and effects on recruitment; therefore, the adoption of these regulations should be postponed until more convincing evidence of reproductive toxicity is found.

REFERENCES

1. Taussig, R. B.: A study of the German outbreak of phocomelia. J.A.M.A., *180*:1106, 1962.
2. Ingalls, T. H., and Philbrook, F. R.: Monstrosities induced by hypoxia. N. Engl. J. Med., *245*:558, 1958.
3. Smith, B. E.: Fetal prognosis after anesthesia during gestation. Anesth. Analg., *42*:521, 1963.
4. Shnider, S. M., and Webster, G. M.: Maternal and fetal hazards of surgery during pregnancy. Am. J. Obstet. Gynecol., *92*:891, 1965.
5. Smith, B. E.: Teratogenic capabilities of surgical anaesthesia. *In* Woolam, D. H. M. (ed.): Advances in Teratology. vol. 3. pp. 127–180. Cambridge, Logos Press, 1968.
6. Mellin, G. W.: The fetal life study. *In* Chipman, S. S. (ed.): Methodology and Needs in Perinatal Studies. pp. 88–117. Springfield, Charles C Thomas, 1966.
7. Runner, M. N.: Comparative pharmacology in relation to teratogenesis. Fed. Proc., *26*:1131, 1967.
8. Neel, J. V.: Some genetic aspects of congenital defects. *In* Fishbein, M. (ed.): First International Congress of Congenital Malformations. pp. 130–142. Philadelphia, J. B. Lippincott, 1962.
9. Wilson, J. G.: Present status of drugs as teratogens in man. Teratology, *7*:3, 1973.
10. Cohen, E. N., Bellville, J. W., and Brown, B. W., Jr.: Anesthesia, pregnancy, and miscarriage: a study of operating room nurses and anesthetists. Anesthesiology, *35*:343, 1971.
11. Smith, B. E.: Teratogenicity of inhalation anesthetics. *In* Progress in Anesthesiology. pp. 589–593. London, Excerpta Medica, 1970.
12. Smith, B. E.: Teratology in anesthesia. Clin. Obstet. Gynecol., *17*:145, 1974.
13. Fiserova-Bergerova, V.: Changes of fluoride content in bone: an index of drug defluorination *in vivo*. Anesthesiology, *38*:345, 1973.
14. Korfsmeier, K. H., and Schoof, J.: The action of diethyl ether in RNA metabolism. Autoradiographic studies on human fibroblast cultures. Pflugers Arch. Ges. Physiol., *293*:357, 1967.
15. Green, C. D.: The effect of nitrous oxide on ribonucleic and deoxyribonucleic acid content of rat bone marrow. *In* Fink, B. R. (ed.): Toxicity of Anesthetics. pp. 114–122. Baltimore, Williams and Wilkins, 1968.
16. Usubiaga, L. E., and Smith, B. E.: Studies of the effects of halothane on chromosomes in human leukocyte cultures. *In* Advances in Anaesthesiology and Resuscitation. pp. 1019–1024. Prague, Czechoslovak Medical Press, 1972.
17. Cohen, P. J., and Marshall, B. E.: Effects of halothane on respiratory control and oxygen consumption of rat liver mitochondria. *In* Fink, B. R. (ed.): Toxicity of Anesthetics. pp. 24–36. Baltimore, Williams and Wilkins. 1968.
18. Smith, B. E., Gaub, M. L., Usubiaga, L., et al.: Teratogenic effects of diethyl ether. *In* Fink, B. R. (ed.): Toxicity of Anesthetics. pp. 269–278. Baltimore, Williams and Wilkins, 1968.
19. Rao, P. N.: Mitotic synchrony in mammalian cells treated with nitrous oxide at high pressure. Science, *160*:774, 1968.
20. Snegireff, S. L., Cox, J. R., and Eastwood, D. W.: The effect of nitrous oxide, cyclopropane or halothane on neural tube mitotic index, weight, mortality, and gross anomaly rate in the developing chick embryo. *In* Fink, B. R. (ed.): Toxicity of Anesthetics. pp. 279–293. Baltimore, Williams and Wilkins, 1968.
21. Smith, B. E., Gaub, M. L., and Moya, F.: Investigations into the teratogenic effects of anesthetic agents. The fluorinated agents. Anesthesiology, *26*:260, 1965.
22. Rector, G. H. M., and Eastwood, D. W.: The effects of nitrous oxide and oxygen on the incubating chick. Anesthesiology, *25*:109, 1964.
23. Smith, B. E., Gaub, M. L., and Moya, F.: Teratogenic effects of anesthetic agents: nitrous oxide. Anesth. Analg., *44*:726, 1965.
24. Fink, B. R., Shepard, T. H., and Blandau, R. J.: Teratogenic activity of nitrous oxide. Nature, *214*:146, 1967.
25. Andersen, N. B.: The teratogenicity of cyclopropane in the chicken. Anesthesiology, *20*:113, 1968.
26. Basford, A. B., and Fink, B. R.: The teratogenicity of halothane in the rat. Anesthesiology, *29*:1167, 1968.

27. Smith, B. E., Usubiaga, L. E., and Lehrer, S. B.: Cleft palate induced by halothane anesthesia in C-57 mice. Teratology, 4:242, 1971.
28. Smith, R. F., Bowman, R. E., and Katz, J.: Behavioral effects of exposure to halothane during early development in the rat: sensitive period during pregnancy. Anesthesiology, 49:319, 1978.
29. Yerushalmy, J., and Milkovich, L.: The evaluation of the teratogenic effect of meclizine in man. Am. J. Obstet. Gynecol., 93:533, 1965.
30. Askrog, V., and Harvald, B.: Teratogen effekt of inhalations-anesthetika. Nord. Med., 83:498, 1970.
31. Corbett, T. H.: Anesthetics as a cause of abortion. Fertil. Steril. 23:866, 1972.
32. Corbett, T. H., and Endres, J. L.: Chronic exposure to nitrous oxide: a possible occupational hazard to operating room personnel (abstr). pp. 249–250. American Society of Anesthesiologists, Annual Meeting, 1972.
33. Whitcher, C. E., Cohen, E. N., and Trudell, J. R.: Chronic exposure to anesthetic gases in the operating room. Anesthesiology, 35:348, 1971.
34. Vaisman, A. I.: Working conditions in surgery and their effect on the health of anesthesiologists. Eksp. Khir. Anesteziol., 3:44, 1967.
35. Knill-Jones, R. P., Moir, D. D., Rodrigues, L. V., et al.: Anaesthetic practice and pregnancy. Lancet, 1:1326, 1972.
36. Cohen, E. N., Brown, B. W., Jr., Bruce, D. L., et al.: Occupational disease among operating room personnel: a national study. Anesthesiology, 41:321, 1974.
37. Greene, N. M.: Traces of anesthetics. Anesthesiology, 41:317, 1974.
38. National Institute for Occupational Safety and Health (NIOSH): Criteria for a Recommended Occupational Exposure to Waste Anesthetic Gases and Vapors. DHEW Pub. No. (NIOSH) 77-140.
39. McGowen, J. C.: Effects of anaesthetics and related substances on the division of living cells. Lancet, 2:279, 1972.
40. Corbett, T. H., and Ball, G. L.: Chronic exposure to methoxyflurane: a possible occupational hazard to anesthesiologists. Anesthesiology, 34:532, 1971.
41. Katz, J., and Clayton, W.: Fetal mortality in rats chronically exposed to low concentrations of halothane (abstr). pp. 57–58. American Society of Anesthesiologists, Annual Meeting, 1973.
42. Bruce, D. L.: Murine fertility unaffected by traces of halothane. Anesthesiology, 38:473, 1973.
43. Corbett, T. H., Cornell, R. G., Page, A., et al.: Occupational disease among operating room personnel. Anesthesiology, 41:321, 1974.
44. Lansdown, A. B. G., Pope, W. D. B., Halsey, M. J., et al.: Analysis of fetal development in rats following maternal exposure to subanesthetic concentrations of halothane. Teratology, 13:299, 1976.
45. Wharton, R. S., Mazze, R. I., Baden, J. M., et al.: Fertility, reproduction and postnatal survival in mice chronically exposed to halothane. Anesthesiology, 48:167, 1978.
46. Pope, W. D. B., Halsey, M. J., Lansdown, A. B. G., et al.: Fetotoxicity in rats following chronic exposure to halothane, nitrous oxide, or methoxyflurane. Anesthesiology, 48:11, 1978.
47. Kripke, B. J., Kelman, A. D., Shah, N. K., et al.: Testicular reaction to prolonged exposure to nitrous oxide. Anesthesiology, 44:104, 1976.
48. Quimby, K. L., Aschkenaze, L. J., Bowman, R. E., et al.: Enduring learning deficits and cerebral synaptic malformation from exposure of 10 parts of halothane per million. Science, 185:625, 1974.
49. Quimby, K. L., Katz, J., and Bowman, R. E.: Behavioral consequences in rats from chronic exposure to 10 ppm halothane during early development. Anesth. Analg., 54:628, 1975.
50. Mann, E. T.: Psychiatric investigation of habitual abortion. Obstet. Gynecol., 7:589, 1956.
51. Walts, L. F., Forsythe, H. B., and Moore, J. G. M.: Critique: occupational disease among operating room personnel. Anesthesiology, 42:608, 1975.
52. Vessey, M. P.: Epidemiological studies of the occupational hazards of anaesthesia—a review. Anaesthesia, 33:430, 1978.
53. Ferstandig, L. L.: Trace concentrations of anesthetic gases: a critical review of their disease potential. Anesth. Analg., 57:328, 1978.
54. Ericson, A., and Källén, B.: Survey of infants born in 1973 or 1975 to Swedish women working in operating rooms during their pregnancies. Anesth. Analg., 58: 302, 1979.

FURTHER READING

Ferstandig, L. L.: Trace concentrations of anesthetic gases: a critical review of their disease potential. Anesth. Analg., 57:328, 1978.
Johnson, E. M.: Screening for teratogenic hazards. Ann. Rev. Toxicol., 21:417, 1981.
Pedersen, H., and Finster, M.: Anesthetic risk in the pregnant surgical patient. Anesthesiology, 51:439, 1979.
Smith, B. E.: Teratology in anesthesia. Clin. Obstet. Gynecol., 17:145, 1974.
Wilson, J. G.: Present status of drugs as teratogens in man. Teratology, 7:3, 1973.
Vessey, M. P.: Epidemiological studies of the occupational hazards of anaesthesia—a review. Anaesthesia, 33:430, 1978.

41 Aorto-caval Compression

Otto C. Phillips, M.D.

Mauriceau called pregnancy a disease of 9 months' duration.[1] There has been objection to this concept, since the pregnant state is considered a natural and anticipated condition in women. Nonetheless, physiological changes that would be considered signs or symptoms of disease in the normal, non-pregnant female do occur during pregnancy. Some of these are adaptations to the physiological demands of pregnancy (increased minute ventilation and cardiac output), while others (increased blood volume and fibrinogen) are in anticipation of problems and needs that might arise. Some changes demand compensatory adaptations that sometimes are not totally successful. This is true of the increasing size of the uterus and its contents.

The average weight of the normal non-gravid uterus is 45 to 80 g. At term, the uterus itself weighs about 1100 g., and the total weight, with contents (fetus, placenta, amniotic fluid), is about 6000 g., approximately a hundred-fold increase. This substantial intra-abdominal mass impinges on and influences other structures and their function, not the least of which are the inferior vena cava and the abdominal aorta. Blood flow through these vessels is compromised.

HISTORICAL BACKGROUND OF AORTOCAVAL COMPRESSION

In 1943 McLennan described the discrepancy between upper and lower extremity venous pressures during pregnancy and the puerperium.[2] He noted that the mean antecubital venous pressure in antepartum patients was 7.7 cm. H_2O (0.75 kPa), and in postpartum patients, 8.0 cm. H_2O (0.78 kPa); these values differed little from pressures in non-pregnant subjects. In contrast, femoral venous pressure rose from 9.1 cm. H_2O (0.89 kPa) during the first trimester to 24 cm. H_2O (2.35 kPa) at term (Fig. 41-1) and fell rapidly after delivery to non-pregnant levels. Also, the femoral venous pressure showed a marked decline after removal of the fetus during cesarean section. McLennan pointed out the similarity in response of these patients to those with large pelvic tumors.

In 1951 McRoberts discussed "postural shock" in pregnancy; he noted hypotension in the supine position in patients who had no serious underlying disease.[3] In 1953, Howard, Goodson, and Mengert noted that hypotension in the supine position was relieved during uterine contractions or when the patient assumed a lateral position (Fig. 41-2). The same phenomenon occurred when the vena cava of a pregnant dog near term was occluded with a ligature; when the ligature was released, the pressure returned quickly to normal (Fig. 41-3). The aorta was not affected, because it has thicker walls and a higher pressure than the vena cava. Pregnant animals do not normally assume the supine position; this unnatural position is assumed by humans only for the convenience of the obstetrician with his forceps.

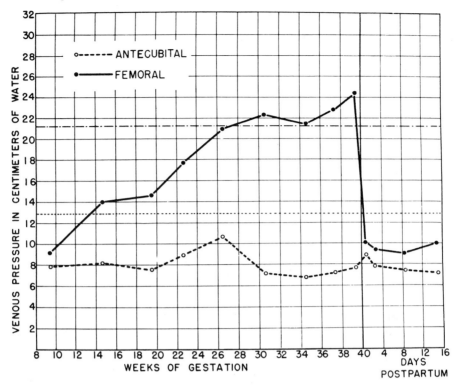

Fig. 41-1. Femoral and antecubital venous pressure. (McLennan, C. E.: Antecubital and femoral venous pressure in normal and toxemic pregnancy. Am. J. Obstet. Gynecol., *45*:568, 1943)

Fig. 41-2. Supine hypotensive syndrome: measurements of blood pressure and pulse during labor. (Howard, B. K., Goodson, J. H., and Mengert, W. F.: Supine hypotensive syndrome in late pregnancy. Obstet. Gynecol., *1*:371, 1953)

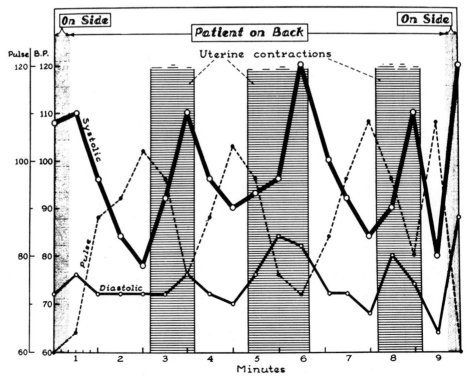

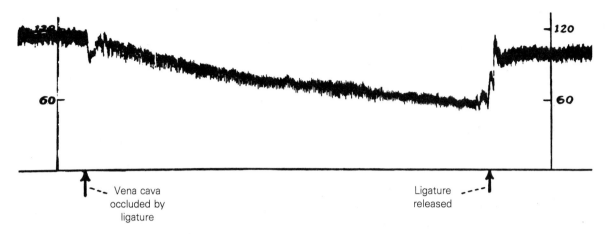

Fig. 41-3. Vena cava occlusion in a pregnant dog. (Howard, B. K., Goodson, J. H., and Mengert, W. F.: Supine hypotensive syndrome in late pregnancy. Obstet. Gynecol., *1*:371, 1953)

Kerr,[4,5] in 1964 and 1965 and Scott[6] in 1968 demonstrated that occlusion of the vena cava is the rule rather than the exception in the supine position at term, and that the main channel for venous return is through collateral vessels emptying into the azygous vein. Narrowing of the vena cava occurs even in the lateral position, but cardiac output is 25 per cent less in the supine as compared to the lateral position. One of the variables in the response to supine hypotension, therefore, is the extent to which collateral circulation has developed. More recently, Bieniarz has demonstrated pressure on and displacement of the aorta through use of pelvic arteriograms.[7]

Thus, the gravid uterus compresses both the inferior vena cava and the abdominal aorta. Pressure on the vena cava impedes venous return to the heart and leads to diminished cardiac output and arterial hypotension. Pressure and obstruction of the aorta lead to diminished perfusion of the uterus, and symptoms of this deficiency are observed in 30 per cent of fetuses.

INCIDENCE OF AORTOCAVAL COMPRESSION

Reports vary on the percentage of patients showing symptoms of aortocaval compression. Cappe and Surks noted an incidence of less than 1 per cent in 2,000 patients undergoing cesarean section.[8] Quilligan and Tyler reported an incidence of 3 per cent in 196 patients.[9] Howard noted an incidence of 11.2 per cent in 160 third-trimester patients,[10] while Holmes reported that 70 per cent of 500 patients studied in the last lunar month of pregnancy had supine hypotensive symptoms.[11] In only 8 per cent of the latter series, however, was the response to the supine position severe. A number of factors may influence the frequency and severity of the syndrome; an understanding and recognition of its mechanism is important.

TREATMENT OF AORTOCAVAL COMPRESSION

Treatment of the supine aortocaval syndrome begins with recognition of problems that can be anticipated and averted by identifying susceptible patients. Comparison of blood pressure in the supine and lateral positions during the last trimester of pregnancy would be a valuable adjunct to customary prenatal observations. In addition, patients themselves can usually recognize a problem. Those affected may feel weak or have difficulty breathing in the supine position, and they learn that symptoms are relieved when they turn on the side or sit up. A note should be placed on the chart identifying these patients, so that they are not placed in a supine position while in labor.

Correction of hypotension depends upon an

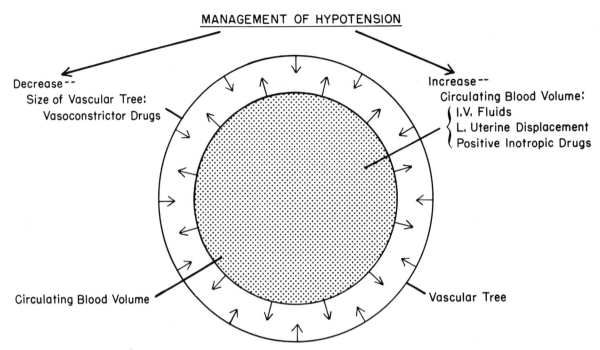

Fig. 41-4. Management of hypotension is based on correction of the discrepancy between the size of the vascular tree and circulating blood volume.

understanding of all the factors involved in maintaining blood pressure and their relationships. *Arterial blood pressure* is defined as pressure exerted by the blood on the arterial walls. This pressure can be increased by expanding the effective circulating blood volume or by decreasing the size of the arterial tree (Fig. 41-4). The opposite of these actions will lead to a drop in pressure. Each of these effects can be accomplished in several ways, and a decrease in one factor can be compensated for by an increase in another. Intelligent management of a physiological or clinical problem, however, consists of replacing the missing "ingredient." Neglect of this concept may lead to use of unsound and indirect compensatory measures that may place an undue and unnecessary burden on the cardiovascular system of the patient.

Hypotension from uterine pressure on the vena cava is due to inadequate venous return, diminished cardiac output, and decreased effective circulating blood volume. Many patients can compensate for this problem with increased sympathetic activity and cardiac output. Conversely,

the problem can be accentuated by blood loss, contraction of the blood volume, and, through vigorous positive pressure breathing, diminished cardiac output. Sympathetic blockade with spinal or epidural anesthesia, by expanding the vascular tree, can lead to serious problems if other hypotensive factors have not been corrected. Vena caval compression, therefore, does not occur by itself; it must be looked upon as just one of a number of factors that influence blood pressure, either favorably or unfavorably. A disturbing drop in pressure from vena caval compression can become a serious problem if other hypotensive influences are already present or are superimposed.

The answer to the problem comes directly from these physiologic considerations. The uterus must be displaced away from the vena cava. Howard and associates demonstrated the effect of this maneuver very well.[10] Kennedy reported that left uterine displacement is effective in restoring blood pressure to normal in 93.4 per cent of the patients who develop hypotension following spinal anesthesia for vaginal delivery.[12] Ueland showed that a change from the supine to the lateral position increases cardiac output 21.7 per cent.[13] In the same manner, uterine contractions in the supine position increase cardiac output by 15.3 per cent; the effect is less notable in the lateral position. Ueland also confirmed the observations of other investigators, that a decline in blood pressure almost always follows spinal anesthesia for cesarean section[14]; the degree of hypotension is not directly related to the dose of agent or to the height of the block. This hypotension is completely reversed by turning the patient on her side. In addition, delivery is followed by a 52-percent increase in cardiac output.

Time sequences in the development of this entity are important. It may take 5 to 10 minutes in the supine position for vena caval compression and pooling to reach the point at which cardiac output is impaired and hypotension develops. One or two normal readings of blood pressure might assure attendants that all is well and lead to complacency. Ten minutes later, hypotension may develop; inadequate cerebral blood flow in an unobserved patient may follow and possibly result in permanent brain damage. The obstetrical patient in the supine position should be observed at all times. If she has received a major conduction anesthetic, such as spinal or epidural, constant and repeated monitoring of blood pressure is even more imperative.

There are several measures that may be taken to relieve uterine pressure on the vena cava. Movement of the uterus by hand is probably the best of these. The hand is sensitive, its shape and direction of pressure are adaptable, and there is practically always a hand around during labor and delivery. Many delivery tables can be tilted to the left; after manually displacing the uterus, it will frequently remain in a position away from the vena cava. If the table cannot be tilted, pads or folded sheets can be placed under the right hip of the patient. Mechanical braces that can be attached to the table are now available. Occasionally there is movement of the uterus or patient that these devices cannot detect and to which they cannot adapt; therefore, use of the hand still has some advantages.

Unphysiologic correction of symptoms alone can lead to problems. It is possible to correct hypotension associated with vena caval compression by constricting the arterial tree with potent sympathomimetics. This approach demonstrates ignorance of the fundamental problem. Upon release of pressure on the vena cava following delivery, circulating blood volume will be increased while the vascular tree remains constricted. Blood pressure can rise dramatically, leading to an abnormal burden on both the vessels and the heart. This type of mismanagement has led to congestive heart failure and to cerebrovascular accidents. Concommitmant use of a vasoconstricting oxytocic, such as ergonovine, will magnify the hypertensive epidsode.

REFERENCES

1. DeLee, J.: Principles and Practice of Obstetrics. ed. 7. p. xiii. Philadelphia, W. B. Saunders, 1938.
2. McLennan, C. E.: Antecubital and femoral venous pressure in normal and toxemic pregnancy. Am. J. Obstet. Gynecol., *45*:568, 1943.
3. McRoberts, W. A.: Postural shock in pregnancy. Am. J. Obstet. Gynecol., *62*:627, 1951.
4. Kerr, M. G., Scott, D. B., and Samuel, E.: Studies of the inferior vena cava in late pregnancy. Br. Med. J., *1*:532, 1964.
5. Kerr, M. G.: The mechanical effects of the gravid uterus in late pregnancy. J. Obstet. Gynaecol. Br. Commonw., *72*:513, 1965.
6. Scott, D. B.: Inferior vena caval occlusion in late pregnancy and its importance in anaesthesia. Br. J. Anaesth., *40*:120, 1968.
7. Bieniarz, J., Crottogini, J. J., Curuchet, E., et al.: Aortocaval compression by the uterus in late human pregnancy. Am. J. Obstet. Gynecol., *100*:203, 1968.
8. Cappe, B. E., and Surks, S. N.: Inferior vena cava syndrome in late pregnancy. Am. J. Obstet. Gynecol., *79*:162, 1960.
9. Quilligan, F. J., and Tyler, C.: Postural effects on the cardiovascular status in pregnancy: a comparison of the lateral and supine postures. Am. J. Obstet. Gynecol., *79*:162, 1960.
10. Howard, B. K., Goodson, J. H., and Mengert, W. F.: Supine hypotensive syndrome in late pregnancy. Obstet. Gynecol., *1*:371, 1953.
11. Holmes, F.: The supine hypotensive syndrome, its importance to the anaesthetist. Anaesthesia, *15*:298, 1960.
12. Kennedy, R. L., Friedman, D. L., Katchka, D. M., et al.: Hypotension during obstetrical anesthesia. Anesthesiology, *20*:153, 1959.
13. Ueland, K., and Hansen, J. M.: Maternal cardiovascular dynamics II: posture and uterine contractions. Am. J. Obstet. Gynecol., *103*:1, 1969.
14. Ueland, K., Gills, R. E., and Hansen, J. M.: Maternal cardiovascular dynamics I: cesarean section under subarachnoid block anesthesia. Am. J. Obstet. Gynecol., *100*:42, 1968.

42 Uterine Atony

Otto C. Phillips, M.D.

Hemorrhage is consistently one of the leading causes of obstetrical mortality[1,2] and may occur during either the antepartum or postpartum period. Uterine atony, in turn, is the basis for 90 per cent of postpartum hemorrhage. Atony is therefore a significant factor in obstetrical mortality, and case reports on this problem still appear.[3]

ETIOLOGY OF UTERINE ATONY

Postpartum uterine atony may be associated with the use of anesthetic drugs, or it may result from trauma. Following the introduction of chloroform in obstetrics by Simpson, it became evident that this agent can cause profound relaxation of the uterus; chloroform therefore became the agent of choice when intrauterine manipulations were desired. With the introduction of a technique to study uterine contractility by recording intra-amniotic fluid pressures, objective measurements of the influence of numerous anesthetic agents and techniques have been made.

Vasicka and Kretchmer demonstrated that diethyl ether almost completely abolishes uterine contractions at surgical planes of anesthesia and that this effect is not counteracted by simultaneous intravenous infusion of an oxytocic drug.[4] Similar effects are observed with halothane, although the time sequences are shorter. Also notable is the residual, marked influence of these agents on uterine tone even after the patient is awake. More recently, Munson and Embro have demonstrated that halothane, enflurane, and iso-flurane are equipotent in producing dose-dependent depression of uterine contractility.[5]

These studies have been supported by clinical observation. Albert and associates reported that 75 per cent of patients receiving halothane for 30 minutes or more have an atonic uterus postpartum[6]; excessive bleeding is a problem in some instances. Similarly, McKay noted an undesirable degree of uterine relaxation in half the vaginal deliveries in his series.[7]

At first it was believed that halothane exerted its influence on the uterus only at term and not early in pregnancy. Cullen, Margolis, and Eger, however, noted that blood loss is more than 11 times greater (283 vs. 25 ml.) when halothane is used for elective therapeutic abortion in contrast to paracervical block.[8] The differential is nine-fold with fluroxene versus paracervical block. Similar results have been reported with isoflurane.[9] Thus, halothane and other volatile agents should be used cautiously in obstetrics. Their application should be reserved for patients with prepartum uterine tetany and for patients in whom uterine relaxation is required for the obstetrician to accomplish delivery. Again, it must emphasized that the relaxant effect of volatile anesthetic agents dissipates slowly after anesthesia is discontinued; and, that while under their influence, the uterus remains unresponsive to oxytocic drugs.

Changing obstetrical practice has resulted in fewer requests by the obstetrician for uterine relaxation. Cesarean section has become the conservative approach of choice, as opposed to a difficult and traumatic operative vaginal delivery. Also, obstetricians have learned to accomplish operative vaginal deliveries without the flaccid uterus some of their forebearers deemed imperative.

Confusion has resulted from the lack of discrimination between the terms *anesthesia* and *analgesia.* Smith and Moya have demonstrated that most anesthetic agents, when used in low concentrations, can be valuable analgesic agents without the problems that accompany anesthetic concentrations.[10] Other investigators, on the other hand, have referred to the safety of halothane as an *anesthetic* agent, while using it in *analgesic* concentrations. Stoelting, for instance, in studying halothane in obstetric anesthesia, states that it is an excellent drug with little effect on uterine relaxation, when the concentration is kept low.[11] However, concentrations reported were 0.6 to 0.8 per cent, just above the 0.5-per-cent level used by Smith and Moya for analgesia.

Thus, the volatile anesthetic agents, used as such, depress uterine tone and contractility and will frequently lead to disturbing and even dangerous increases in postpartum bleeding. This influence on uterine musculature begins early in pregnancy and persists until term. This effect is not evident if the agents are used only in analgesic concentrations.

DIFFERENTIAL DIAGNOSIS OF UTERINE ATONY

In addition to uterine atony, there are several other causes of postpartum hemorrhage: anatomic defects, retained secundae, and coagulation defects. These must all be considered, and the proper diagnosis must be made before appropriate treatment can be instituted. Delay in identifying the cause of bleeding delays the institution of proper therapy.

Anatomic Defects

Thornton reported cervical lacerations in 4.7 per cent and vaginal lacerations in 4.1 per cent of spontaneous deliveries.[12] A three-fold incidence of vaginal or cervical tears occurs in instrumented

or forceps deliveries in contrast to spontaneous deliveries. Defects extending into the broad ligament or through the body of the uterus may result in more extensive bleeding.

Vaginal and cervical lacerations should be suspected and sought whenever bleeding continues after delivery. Hemorrhage into the broad ligament is often subserosal and not apparent, while rents in the body of the uterus may lead to extensive bleeding into the peritoneal cavity. If instability of the circulation cannot be explained, bleeding and hypovolemia from an anatomic defect should be suspected and promptly investigated. Signs of either overt or occult bleeding usually occur early in the postpartum period, almost always while the patient is still on the delivery table.

Uterine trauma is a common denominator in many cases of uterine atony and anatomic defects and may be associated with prolonged labor, tumultuous labor (oxytocic stimulation), a large baby, multiple pregnancy, hydramnios, high parity, and operative delivery. All of these place demands on the uterus beyond those of a normal, uncomplicated, nonoperative delivery. As a result, the uterus may become flaccid, engendering excessive bleeding.

Retained Secundae

Postpartum bleeding will occur unless there is an intact uterus firmly contracted on an empty uterine cavity. Large vessels that develop in the uterine wall during pregnancy are compressed by the contracting musculature after the uterus is evacuated. There is retention of placental fragments or membranes in about 4 per cent of postpartum patients,[13] possibly leading to inadequate contraction of the uterus and continued bleeding until removed. This has led some obstetricians to explore the uterine cavity manually promptly after each delivery. Retained secundae, clots, or an atonic uterus can then be detected early, and proper management can be instituted.

Coagulation Defects

A coagulation defect or fibrinolytic disorder leading to excessive bleeding almost always follows some other clinical problem. Toxemia, placenta previa, septic abortion, intrauterine fetal death, amniotic fluid embolism, and, in particular, excessive bleeding from any cause should arouse a high index of suspicion of coagulation defects. Obstetrical hemorrhage may be compared to a prairie fire; the longer it continues, the bigger and more complex the problem. Lack of prompt attention to many obstetrical problems invites the development of disseminated intravascular coagulation and a chain of aberrations in the complex coagulation mechanisms.

TREATMENT OF UTERINE ATONY

Since uterine atony is always a possibility, attendants of the obstetrical patient should be familiar with the fundamental causes and their treatment. Therapy involves three considerations: prevention, detection, and management.

Prevention of Uterine Atony

Prevention of uterine atony is based upon avoiding the factors that cause or contribute to the problem. Trauma may be an integral part of an obstetrical problem or may be related to the efforts of the accoucheur. In either case, adverse effects on uterine contractility should be anticipated. Either alone or as adjunct factors, volatile inhalation anesthetic agents should be avoided if possible. When their use is indicated, extended effect on the uterus should be considered, and the risk must be balanced against the benefit. Also, following delivery, the uterus is firmer, and there is less need for treatment if an oxytocic is given.[14]

Detection of Uterine Atony

Brisk or bright red bleeding in the presence of a firm, contracted uterus suggests a laceration. Slow, continuous oozing is more characteristic of retained secundae or an atonic uterus. Since obstetrical hemorrhage may occur unexpectedly and often suddenly, all parturients should have vital signs monitored closely.

Management of Uterine Atony

All obstetrical patients should have secure intravenous routes, and blood should be typed prior to the time of delivery. For those patients particularly at risk for postpartum bleeding, blood should be crossmatched upon admission. If a bleeding problem occurs, preparations should be made for transfusion of whole blood and/or blood components to maintain adequate blood volume. The obstetrician should search for residual fragments of placenta or membranes in the uterine cavity and lacerations. After delivery of the placenta, the fundus should be palpated to make sure that it is firm and well contracted. If not, it should be massaged gently with the finger tips. Bimanual pressure compresses the uterine veins in addition to stimulating the uterus. This can be accomplished by compressing the posterior aspect of the uterus through the abdominal wall, against the anterior surface, with the fist in the vaginal cavity.

Packing the uterine cavity is no longer an accepted procedure, because intrauterine contents deter firm and continuous contraction of the uterus and may increase rather than diminish uterine bleeding. Fribourg has proposed intrauterine lavage with very warm water.[15] He has reviewed reports of this approach and noted good results in his own practice. Finally, if there is no response to therapy, hysterectomy should be performed. Too much time cannot be lost before making this decision, since prolonged periods of bleeding make the patient susceptible to a superimposed coagulation defect.

REFERENCES

1. Phillips, O. C., Davis, G. H., Frazier, T. M., et al.: The role of anesthesia in obstetric mortality. Anesth. Analg., *40*:557, 1961.
2. Phillips, O. C., Hulka, J. F., and Christy, W. C.: Obstetric hemorrhage: 28-year review of death at the Magee-Womens Hospital. Anesth. Analg., *43*:453, 1965.
3. Jewett, J. F.: Multiparous uterine atony. N. Engl. J. Med., *286*:778, 1972.
4. Vasicka, A., and Kretchmer, H. E.: Effect of conduction and inhalation anesthesia on uterine contractions. Am. J. Obstet. Gynecol., *82*:600, 1961.
5. Munson, E. S., and Embro, W. J.: Enflurane, isoflurane, and halothane on isolated human uterine muscle. Anesthesiology, *46*:11, 1977.
6. Albert, C. A., Anderson, G., Wallace, W., et al.: Fluothane for obstetric anesthesia. Obstet. Gynecol., *13*:282, 1959.

7. McKay, I. M.: Clinical evaluation of Fluothane with special reference to a controlled percentage of vaporizer. Can. Anaesth. Soc. J., *4*:235, 1957.

8. Cullen, B. F., Margolis, A. J., and Eger, E. I., II: The effects of anesthesia and pulmonary ventilation on blood loss during elective therapeutic abortion. Anesthesiology, *32*:108, 1970.

9. Dolan, W. M., Eger, E. I., II, and Margolis, A. J.: Forane increases bleeding in therapeutic suction abortion. Anesthesiology, *36*:96, 1972.

10. Smith, B. E., and Moya, F.: Inhalational analgesia with methoxyflurane for vaginal delivery. South Med. J., *61*:386, 1968.

11. Stoelting, V. K.: Fluothane in obstetric anesthesia. Anesth. Analg., *43*:243, 1964.

12. Thornton, W. N.: Discussion of Newton, M.: Postpartum hemorrhage. Am. J. Obstet. Gynecol., *94*:711, 1966.

13. Briscoe, C.: Discussion of Newton, M.: Postpartum hemorrhage. Am. J. Obstet. Gynecol., *94*:711, 1966.

14. Newton, M.: Postpartum hemorrhage. Am. J. Obstet. Gynecol., *94*:711, 1966.

15. Fribourg, S. R., Rothman, I. A., and Rovinsky, J. J.: Intrauterine lavage for control of uterine atony. Obstet. Gynecol., *41*:876, 1973.

43 Fetal Depression

Jay S. DeVore, M.D.

Providing pain relief for childbirth has been an accepted part of medical practice since the 19th century, when Queen Victoria removed the stigma attached to it by receiving chloroform for the birth of her eighth child. For most of the intervening time, however, little attention has been paid to the effects of anesthetic techniques on the fetus and newborn. While risks to the mother from anesthesia have been recognized for some time, it is only rather recently that critical attention has been paid to the newborn. Recent techniques have been aimed at minimizing fetal depression, yet a significant number of newborns show measurable residual effects of anesthesia.

FETAL PHYSIOLOGY

In order to understand the causes, treatment, and prevention of anesthetic-induced fetal depression, a brief discussion of fetal physiology is necessary.

Placental Transport

All drugs used in anesthesia, with the exception of the neuromuscular blocking agents, cross the placenta in clinically significant amounts.[1] Succinylcholine, curare, and related drugs do cross the placenta, but unless a massive overdose is given, there is no measurable effect on the fetus. The following factors affect placental transport: lipid solubility—the more lipid soluble a molecule is, the more readily it will cross the placenta; degree of ionization—unionized forms cross the placenta more readily than do ionized forms; concentration gradient—the amount of drug that crosses the placenta to the fetal circulation is directly proportional to its concentration in the maternal circulation; and molecular weight— drugs with molecular weights of less than 300 cross the placenta readily, while those of greater than 1000 cross only with great difficulty, if at all. The latter are particularly significant, for drugs bound to maternal proteins are less likely to cross the placenta.[1]

Fetal Circulation

The fetal circulation is also an important consideration in determining the response to anesthesia. The fetus receives its oxygen through the placenta by way of the uterine artery and excretes carbon dioxide through the placenta by way of the uterine vein. Obviously, any drug or phenomenon that decreases uterine flow will interfere with fetal respiratory function, and any drug or phenomenon that decreases maternal P_{O_2} will interfere with fetal oxygenation. There are also certain peculiarities of the fetal circulation that influence anesthetic effect. Especially important is the large percentage of blood that enters the fetus by way of the umbilical vein, which passes through the liver prior to entering the central circulation; in addition, the liver acts as a biologic filter, taking up a significant proportion of the drug before it reaches the fetal heart and brain.

CAUSES OF FETAL DEPRESSION

Anesthetic-related fetal depression can be divided into three etiological categories: depression caused by drugs; by maternal hypotension; and by maternal hypoxia.

Drug-Induced Fetal Depression

Inhalation anesthetic agents such as nitrous oxide, cyclopropane, halothane, methoxyflurane, and enflurane all cross the placenta.[1] The degree of fetal depression is related to the total dose of anesthetic; that is, both inspired concentration and time must be considered. Subanesthetic concentrations (e.g., 50% nitrous oxide, 0.25% methoxyflurane, 0.5% halothane, or 0.5% enflurane) will not depress the fetus even if given for long periods.[2-4] As the concentration is increased, the time required for depression decreases, so that when anesthetic concentrations, such as 70-percent nitrous oxide, are given, depression ensues in 7 to 10 min. Of course, general anesthetic-induced depression of the fetus can be reversed by assisting respiration with a mask, which hastens pulmonary clearance of the anesthetic agent.

Narcotics can cause respiratory and, to a lesser extent, cardiovascular depression of the fetus and newborn. In general, small doses like 50 mg. of meperidine, 50 µg. of fentanyl, or 20 mg. of alphaprodine have only slight effects on the fetus. These effects can be further decreased by avoiding administration of narcotics within 1 hour of delivery. It must be remembered, however, that the duration of the respiratory depression on the fetus and newborn is markedly longer than the analgesic effect of the narcotics.[5]

Barbiturates, for the most part, have little place in obstetric anesthesia. They are not analgesic and cause fetal depression that is not readily reversible, particularly since the fetal liver is not fully capable of metabolizing these drugs. The ultra-short-acting barbituates such as thiopental seem to be somewhat safer. An induction dose of 4 mg. per kg. of thiopental does not significantly affect the fetus.[6,7] This is caused partly by the great uptake of drug by the fetal liver.

Tranquilizing agents have a wide use in obstetrics because they are able to relieve that component of discomfort of labor that is caused by anxiety, and they potentiate the analgesic action of the narcotics. Tranquilizers have rather minimal depressant effects on the fetus, particularly if doses are kept within a reasonable range. Doses of 50 to 75 mg. of hydroxyzine, 10 mg. of propiomazine, or 25 mg. of promethazine have little effect on the fetus. Diazepam, while generally considered a very safe agent, causes an inordinate amount of depression in the fetus, leading to skeletal and smooth muscle hypotonia, hypothermia, and urinary and fecal retention.[8] Additionally, the vehicle in which the drug is dissolved competes with bilirubin for albumin binding sites, so that jaundice occurs more often.[9]

Ketamine, while an excellent analgesic, seems to have only a limited use in obstetrics. Early studies using ketamine anesthesia for cesarean section and vaginal delivery in doses greater than 1 mg. per kg. showed marked depression of the newborn, and skeletal muscle rigidity made resuscitation quite difficult.[10] More recent studies using subanesthetic doses, such as 0.25 mg. per kg., have shown no appreciable effect on the fetus.[11,12] Women given this dose are not really anesthetized and may continue to vocalize and move; however, they do not seem to remember the procedure.

Regional anesthesia is generally considered to be the safest method of providing pain relief for the mother. However, local anesthetics are not without depressant effects. The drug can reach the fetus either by the maternal circulation or by direct injection. The newborn, thus, demonstrates the systemic effects of cardiovascular and CNS depression (see chap. 4).

Local anesthetics are weak bases, with dissociation constants in the range of 7.9 to 9.0. Therefore, they are largely unionized at body *p*H. This means that transport across the placenta is quite free. Lipid solubility of local anesthetics is variable, but all of them are reasonably lipid soluble; and, they are relatively small molecules. Therefore, the primary factors influencing placental transport are the concentration of the local anesthetic in maternal blood and the degree to which the agent is bound to maternal protein (and, thus, incapable of crossing the placenta).

The concentration of the local anesthetic in the maternal (and, in turn, fetal) blood depends upon several factors that include the route of injection, dose of the agent, rate of metabolism, and frequency of injection. When the drug is given by the epidural route, the maternal blood level peaks at about 10 min., and the fetal level, 10 min. later. The rate of metabolism is determined largely by the structure of the local anesthetic. Those with an ester structure, such as procaine and chloroprocaine, are hydrolyzed rapidly in the serum by maternal pseudocholinesterase, and only rarely is a very high blood level reached in the mother; hence, fetal toxicity from these drugs is unusual. The agents with an amide structure, however, are metabolized slowly by the hepatic microsomal enzyme system, and repeated injections by any route result in a progressively increasing maternal (and, thus, fetal) level. Great care must be taken to avoid exceeding the toxic dose of local anesthetic on a cumulative basis.

A very high degree of protein binding is an important characteristic of the recently developed agents, bupivacaine and etidocaine, and as a result, they cross the placenta to a much lesser degree than do lidocaine and mepivacaine. Once the local anesthetic has crossed the placenta, however, the relationship between fetal and maternal blood levels is dependent upon the fetal pH. At normal pH, about one-third of the local anesthetic is present in the unionized form, which penetrates the placenta readily, and the fetal–maternal ratio of blood levels is between 0.2 and 0.5. Because the dissociation constant of the agent is reasonably close to blood pH, acid-base imbalance between mother and fetus can result in clinically important changes in the ratio of unionized to ionized forms of the agent. For example, if the fetal pH is considerably lower than the maternal pH, as in asphyxia, the dissociation of the agent in the fetus shifts such that there is "trapping" of the ionized form, with an inordinately high fetal blood level (Fig. 43-1).

Administration by the pudendal route produces a high blood level of local anesthetics in the mother; however, fetal toxicity is rarely a problem in this case, because delivery is generally accomplished prior to the peak blood level. Paracervical block is associated with a high incidence of fetal depression.[13] The local anesthetic is absorbed by the rich vascular plexus around the uterus and by the uterine circulation. Mepivacaine and bupivacaine, both highly lipid soluble, have been particularly incriminated in this technique.

Of course, the highest maternal blood levels result from intravascular injection of local anesthetic. Obviously, intravascular injection never occurs intentionally, but it is always possible when injections are made in highly vascular areas. When an inadvertent intravascular injection occurs, resulting high maternal blood levels of local anesthetics lead to high fetal levels also.

Direct intoxication of the fetus with local anesthetics is also possible under certain circumstances. In paracervical block, the fetal head is quite close to the site of injection. It is possible to accidentally deposit the local anesthetic in the fetal scalp, with resultant massive intoxication, unless the needle placement is extremely meticulous and care is taken to insert the needle only a few millimeters. One of the greatest catastrophes in obstetric anesthesia can occur during caudal anesthesia, particularly when it is given shortly prior to delivery, when the fetal head has moved well down into the maternal pelvis.[14] Under these circumstances, owing to distortion of the mother's anatomy, it is possible to insert the needle through the mother's rectum into the fetal head, where a large dose of local anesthetic is then deposited. Case reports have indicated that some permanent damage is almost a certainty. The performance of a rectal examination prior to the injection of any local anesthetic in the caudal canal should prevent this disaster.

Even apparently vigorous babies may have some subtle neurobehavioral changes after delivery under regional anesthesia.[15] These changes, primarily relating to muscle tone and responsiveness, are transient, lasting only a few hours, and seem to be more common with mepivacaine and lidocaine than with the other local anesthetics.[16] The clinical significance of these changes has yet to be determined.

Maternal Hypotension

Anesthesia can depress the fetus indirectly by effects on the mother. Major conduction anesthesia, such as lumbar epidural, caudal, or spinal,

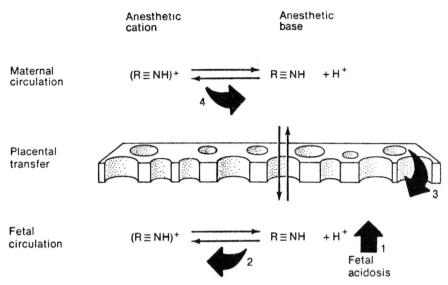

Anesthetic cation   Anesthetic base

Maternal circulation $(R \equiv NH)^+$ ⇌ $R \equiv NH$ + H^+ 4

Placental transfer

Fetal circulation $(R \equiv NH)^+$ ⇌ $R \equiv NH$ + H^+ 2   1   Fetal acidosis   3

Fig. 43-1. Fetal acidosis increases the transfer of local anesthetics across the placenta. The dissociation equilibrium local anesthetic in the fetus is driven to the left, and this reduces the amount of anesthetic base available. As the dissociation equilibrium in the maternal circulation shifts to the right, more anesthetic base is transferred to the fetus. (Albright, G. A.: Anesthesia in Obstetrics: Maternal, Fetal, and Neonatal Aspects. p. 116. Menlo Park, Addison-Wesley, 1978)

may produce maternal hypotension owing to the sympathetic block. If the maternal blood pressure drops below the critical level needed to perfuse the placenta, fetal asphyxia will ensue. The maternal systolic pressure is the primary determinant of placental perfusion, and fetal depression is likely to occur if this pressure is allowed to decrease more than 25 per cent or is allowed to remain below 100 torr.[17] Persistent maternal hypotension results in hypoxia and metabolic acidosis in the fetus. If severe or protracted enough, this results in permanent damage, even though the degree of hypotension may not be dangerous to the mother (see chap. 4).

Maternal Hypoxia

Fetal oxygenation is also dependent upon the oxygen content of the blood delivered from the maternal umbilical artery. If the mother is allowed to become hypoxic from respiratory depression or inadvertent delivery of an inadequate concentration of oxygen, the fetus, too, eventually becomes hypoxic. Even though fetal hemoglobin does have a greater affinity for oxygen than adult hemoglobin, the fetus still requires a P_{O_2} above approximately 25 torr for adequate cellular functioning.

EVALUATION OF FETAL DEPRESSION

When a newborn is depressed, it is important to determine whether the depression is caused by a drug or condition like asphyxia and trauma.

Several methods can be used to evaluate fetal depression. A proper history is extremely useful. If depressant drugs have been administered, particularly 1 to 2 hours prior to delivery, anesthetic-related depression must be considered. This is especially true if general anesthesia has been used for delivery. If there have been signs of asphyxia during labor, such as late decelerations in fetal heart rate, or if the mother is diabetic or toxemic, asphyxia is the most likely diagnosis. Finally, if the delivery is operative, such as a mid- or high forceps, trauma with a concussion-like syndrome must be considered.

Table 43-1. Apgar Scoring Method

Sign	Score		
	0	1	2
Heart rate	Absent	< 100/min.	> 100/min.
Respiratory effort	Absent	Weak cry; hypoventilation	Good; strong cry
Muscle tone	Limp	Some flexion of extremities	Active motion; extremities well flexed
Reflex irritability	No response	Grimace	Cry
Color	Blue; pale	Body pink; extremities blue	Completely pink

(Based on Apgar, V.: A proposal for a new method of evaluation of the newborn infant. Anesth. Analg., *32*: 260, 1953)

For nearly 25 years the Apgar score[18] has been a standard method for evaluation of the newborn (Table 43-1). One minute after delivery, the five signs are evaluated, and each is given the appropriate score. A total score of 10 indicates the infant is in the best possible condition. Typically, the anesthetic-depressed newborn has a good heart rate but loses one point in each of the other categories. Additionally, these newborns respond to stimulation by breathing more vigorously but, if left unstimulated, will again become hypotonic with depressed respirations. The asphyxiated newborn is much more likely to have bradycardia and much less likely to respond to simple stimulation.

While the Apgar score is a very valuable tool for immediate evaluation of the newborn, it does have its limitations, for it is only a very gross estimation of vigor. The acid-base status is a much more precise measure of the newborn's condition.[19] Again, this is useful also in differentiating depression owing to drugs from that owing to other causes. Specifically, the drug-depressed newborn has normal umbilical cord blood gases at birth but deteriorates thereafter, and he lags behind his unmedicated counterpart for as long as 24 hours in recovery to a normal acid-base status. Asphyxiated newborns, on the other hand, have grossly abnormal blood gases, with low P_{O_2}, high P_{CO_2}, and low pH. Depression from umbilical cord compression can generally be differentiated from that owing to uteroplacental insufficiency. In the former, levels of umbilical artery blood gases are far more abnormal than those from the umbilical vein, whereas in placental insufficiency, the P_{CO_2} may be relatively normal compared to P_{O_2}.

Drug-induced fetal and neonatal depression can be evaluated directly, by assaying the drug in neonatal blood, or indirectly, by determining maternal blood levels, which can be used to estimate the fetal levels. The technical difficulty of determining narcotic levels has limited precise estimation of the toxic level of narcotics in the fetus. This is further complicated by the fact that metabolites of narcotics, particularly meperidine, may be more depressant than the narcotics themselves.[20] Toxic levels of local anesthetics, on the other hand, have been elucidated. The fetus begins to show toxicity at a blood level of approximately 3 μg. per ml. of lidocaine[21] and approximately 1 μg. per ml. of bupivacaine. The rapid metabolism of chloroprocaine by plasma cholinesterase makes a determination of blood levels extremely difficult and estimation of toxicity quite problematical.

Recently, simple mortality statistics and Apgar scores have been supplemented by sophisticated neurobehavioral testing.[15,16] The latter are designed to assess motor organization and responsiveness to external stimuli and extend observations of the newborn well beyond the 5 min. of the Apgar score. Using these techniques, it has been shown that for as long as 8 hours after birth, there are detectable differences in newborns of mothers receiving epidural anesthesia with mepivacaine or lidocaine.[15] Such changes are not apparent in newborns of mothers receiving epidural anesthesia with bupivacaine.[16] It should be pointed out that newborns evaluated under this method are vigorous and seemingly normal. Similar observations have been made with newborns of mothers who have received narcotics[22] or general anesthesia. In these cases, extremely subtle changes have been observed for far longer periods.

TREATMENT OF FETAL DEPRESSION

Treatment of fetal depression is based on the most recent evaluation of the Apgar score. Newborns with mild to moderate depression from general anesthetics and with Apgar scores of 5 or 6 need simply to be supported like any anesthetized patient. For the most part, adequate suctioning, stimulation, and occasionally positive pressure ventilation with a mask are all that is necessary to support these newborns until the general anesthetic is excreted through the lungs. When newborns are depressed from narcotics, stimulation and ventilatory support are still adequate to prevent any damage, but the slow metabolism of narcotics by the fetus necessitates more direct therapy. Depression in a newborn whose mother has received narcotics probably is partially the result of narcotic administration. These infants should receive 5 μg. per kg. of naloxone intramuscularly. Failure of naloxone to improve the newborn's condition within 2 or 3 min. is *prima facie* evidence that narcotics are not important in the depression, and other causes should be sought. There is apparently no danger in this technique, since naloxone itself does not produce depression. It should be remembered that the duration of action of naloxone is shorter than that of most narcotics, and these newborns may require a second dose again, later in the nursery.

Depression owing to barbituates or tranquilizers is far more difficult to treat. There is no effective antidote for these drugs, so infants depressed from these agents require supportive treatment until the effect of the drug is dissipated.

If the depression is mild, simple observation, suctioning of the airway, and stimulation may be all that is necessary. Severe depression may have to be treated by mechanical ventilation. If hypotension is associated with the depression, transfusion with plasma is usually the preferred treatment, although cardiotonic agents may be necessary.

The depression induced by local anesthetics is usually manifested by hypotonia, respiratory depression, and frequently bradycardia. Again, in mild depression, stimulation, suctioning, and supplemental oxygen should be adequate. If depression is severe, ventilatory support will be required and, quite possibly, external cardiac massage and, occasionally, cardiotonic agents. If there has been massive overdose with local anesthetics (e.g., from inadvertent direct fetal injection), attempts should be made to remove the drug from the fetus because metabolism will be quite slow. The most effective and direct method is exchange transfusion with fresh whole blood. If this is not feasible owing to either lack of whole blood or technical problems with the exchange transfusion, a significant amount of local anesthetic can be removed by gastric lavage. Since the gastric pH is considerably lower than the systemic pH, the ion trapping effect similar to that in the asphyxiated fetus will develop, and high concentrations of local anesthetics will be concentrated in the stomach.[23] Repeated lavage with saline removes large quantities of local anesthetic. If convulsions occur, anticonvulsive medication such as phenobarbital should be administered. Of course, ventilatory support is mandatory in these cases, and the airway should be protected with an endotracheal tube during lavage.

When severe depression (e.g., Apgar score less than 4) is present from any cause, resuscitation will be facilitated by placement of an umbilical vein catheter. This catheter permits analysis of blood pH, as well as drug therapy: sodium bicarbonate, 2 mEq. per kg., immediately to counter the metabolic and respiratory acidosis, with subsequent doses dictated by serial blood pH analysis; 10 per cent dextrose in water, 100 ml. per kg. per 24 h., to provide metabolic substrate and plasma volume expansion; epinephrine, 0.1 mg.

per kg., to stimulate the heart and peripheral circulations; and, naloxone, 0.01 mg. per kg., to reverse narcotic-induced depression.

PREVENTION OF FETAL DEPRESSION

It is apparent that most of the neonatal complications of obstetrical anesthesia are preventable. A few simple precautions in the use of anesthetic agents can minimize these problems. The primary principle involves use of the least amount of anesthesia necessary to provide satisfactory conditions. If general anesthesia is used, the concentrations of the agent should be kept to a minimum, and the duration of anesthesia should be only that which is absolutely necessary. For instance, in cesarean section, the patient should be prepared and draped, and the surgeons should be ready to operate prior to the induction of anesthesia. If vaginal delivery is anticipated, the patient should be placed in stirrups and the fetal head should be on the perineum prior to the institution of general anesthesia. With parenteral agents, such as narcotics or tranquilizers, the smallest possible dose of short-acting agents and care in the timing of administration are important.

When regional anesthesia is elected, similar considerations are in order. Again, the lowest possible concentration and dose of local anesthetic are used. Precise needle placement and careful aspiration before any injection are important to avoid inadvertent intravascular injection. A rectal examination should be performed prior to injection of drug in a caudal technique; and continuous fetal heart rate monitoring should be performed with paracervical block. With epidural anesthesia, the anesthesiologist must monitor blood pressure frequently and assure adequate hydration of the patient. If the blood pressure falls, it should be treated promptly by displacing the uterus from the vena cava and, if necessary, by administering intravenous ephedrine, 5 to 15 mg. (see Chaps. 4, 5, and 41).

If all of the above are considered, pain relief for childbirth can be provided safely. It must always be kept in mind, however, that millions of women have delivered children without pain relief. While it is certainly desirable that the mother be comfortable and happy, it may not be always appropriate to administer anesthetics if the fetus must pay the price. Certainly, no anesthesia is preferable to improperly administered anesthesia.

REFERENCES

1. Albright, G. A.: Anesthesia in Obstetrics: Maternal, Fetal, and Neonatal Aspects. pp. 58–64. Menlo Park, Addison-Wesley, 1978.
2. Finster, M., and Poppers, P. J.: Cesarean section. *In* Bonica, J. J. (ed.): Principles and Practice of Obstetric Analgesia and Anesthesia. pp. 1338–1365. Philadelphia, F. A. Davis, 1967.
3. Moir, D. D.: Anaesthesia for cesarean section: an evaluation of a method using low concentrations of halothane and 50 percent oxygen. Br. J. Anaesth., *42*:136, 1970.
4. Galbert, M. W., and Gardner, A. E.: Use of halothane in a balanced technic for cesarean section. Anesth. Analg., *51*:701, 1972.
5. Stechler, G.: Newborn attention as affected by medication during labor. Science, *144*:315, 1964.
6. Finster, M., and Poppers, P. J.: Safety of thiopental used for the induction of general anesthesia in elective cesarean section. Anesthesiology, *29*:190, 1968.
7. Dawes, G. S.: The distribution and actions of drugs on the foetus in utero. Br. J. Anaesth., *45*:766, 1973.
8. Flowers, C. E., Rudolph, A. J., and Desmond, M. M.: Diazepam (Valium) as an adjunct in obstetric analgesia. Obstet. Gynecol., *36*:68, 1969.
9. Schiff, D., Chan, G., and Stern, L.: Fixed drug combinations and the displacement of bilirubin from albumin. Pediatrics, *48*:139, 1971.
10. Little, B., Chang, T., Chucot, L., et al.: Study of ketamine as an obstetric anesthetic agent. Am. J. Obstet. Gynecol., *113*:247, 1972.
11. Akamatsu, T. J., Bonica, J. J., Rehmet, R., et al.: Experiences with the use of ketamine for parturition: 1. Primary anesthetic for vaginal delivery. Anesth. Analg., *52*:284, 1974.
12. Janeczko, G. F., El-Etr, A. A., and Younes, S.: Low-dose ketamine anesthesia for obstetrical delivery. Anesth. Analg., *53*:828, 1974.
13. Asling, J. H., Shnider, S. M., Margolis, A. J., et al.: Paracervical block anesthesia in obstetrics. Am. J. Obstet. Gynecol., *107*:626, 1970.
14. Finster, M., Poppers, P. J., Sinclair, J. C., et al.: Accidental intoxication of the fetus with local anesthetic drug during caudal anesthesia. Am. J. Obstet. Gynecol., *92*:922, 1965.
15. Scanlon, J. W., Brown, W. U., Weiss, J. B., et al.: Neurobehavioral responses of newborn infants after maternal epidural anesthesia. Anesthesiology, *40*:121, 1974.
16. Scanlon, J. W., Ostheimer, G. W., Lurie, A. O., et al.: Neurobehavioral responses and drug concentrations in newborns after maternal epidural anesthesia with bupivacaine. Anesthesiology, *45*:400, 1976.
17. Moya, F., and Smith, B. E.: Maternal hypotension and the newborn. Proc. 3rd World Congr. Anaesth., *2*:28, 1964.

18. Apgar, V.: A proposal for a new method of evaluation of the newborn infant. Anesth. Analg., *32*:260, 1953.

19. Saling, E.: Technical and theoretical problems in electronic monitoring of the fetal heart. Int. J. Gynecol. Obstet., *10*:211, 1972.

20. Morrison, J. C., Whybrew, M. S., Rosser, S. I., et al.: Metabolites of meperidine in the fetal and maternal serum. Am. J. Obstet. Gynecol., *126*:997, 1976.

21. Shnider, S. M., and Way, E. L.: Plasma levels of lidocaine (Xylocaine) in mother and newborn following obstetrical conduction anesthesia. Anesthesiology, *29*:958, 1968.

22. Brackbill, Y., Kane, J., Manniello, R. L., et al.: Obstetric meperidine usage and assessment of neonatal status. Anesthesiology, *40*:116, 1974.

23. Brown, W. U., Bell, G. C., and Alper, M. H.: Acidosis, local anesthetics and the newborn. Obstet. Gynecol., *48*:27, 1976.

FURTHER READING

Albright, G. A.: Anesthesia in Obstetrics: Maternal, Fetal, and Neonatal Aspects. Menlo Park, Addison-Wesley, 1978.

Gregory, G. A.: Resuscitation of the newborn. Anesthesiology, *43*:225, 1975.

Pedersen, H., and Finster, M.: Anesthetic risk in the pregnant surgical patient. Anesthesiology, *51*:439, 1979.

Shnider, S. M., and Levinson, G.: Anesthesia for Obstetrics. Baltimore, Williams & Wilkins, 1979.

44 Hypoventilation and Apnea in the Newborn

Lawrence S. Berman, M. D., and Russell C. Raphaely, M. D.

HYPOVENTILATION

Hypoventilation frequently occurs postoperatively in the neonate. Whenever possible, the cause of the hypoventilation should be identified so that the most appropriate treatment can be administered. However, a more general therapy should be used immediately if hypoxemia and acidemia accompany the hypoventilation.

PATHOPHYSIOLOGY OF HYPOVENTILATION

Hypoventilation is present when Pa_{CO_2} is above 40 torr (5.3 kPa). Carbon dioxide reacts with water to form H_2CO_3 which dissociates into H^+ and HCO_3^- in the plasma and red cells. When H^+ production exceeds the buffering capacity of plasma and red cells, *p*H decreases and respiratory acidemia exists.

Equally serious is the hypoxemia that can accompany hypoventilation and apnea. In the newborn, when there is open communication between the pulmonary and systemic circulations, the direction of blood flow through the ductus arteriosus and foramen ovale depends on the balance between the pressures of the two circuits. Normally, it is from left to right. But, the pulmonary vasculature of the newborn is extremely sensitive to *p*H and Pa_{O_2}. When acidemia and hypoxemia are present, pulmonary artery pressure increases and causes right-to-left shunting, with subsequent hypoxemia.

CAUSES, DIAGNOSIS, AND THERAPY OF HYPOVENTILATION

Upper Airway Obstruction

The hypoventilation in the newborn may be caused by an obstructed airway. Secretions are the most common cause of obstruction and can occur at any point from the nares to the alveoli. Hence, initial therapy for hypoventilation is to rectify the obstructed airway by removing all secretions.

Choanal stenosis and atresia can also cause upper airway obstruction, since the neonate must breathe through his nose. To diagnose the latter, pass a suction catheter through the nares into the nasopharynx. If the catheter does not pass, an oral airway should be inserted immediately, and the patient should be fed through an orogastric tube. If choanal atresia is bilateral, it should be corrected surgically during the neonatal period.

A congenital anomaly frequently associated with upper airway obstruction is the Pierre Robin syndrome, which is characterized by micrognathia in association with cleft palate and glossoptosis. In newborns with this condition, airway obstruction is more likely to occur when the infant is supine, because it is then that the tongue drops into the pharynx; placing the infant prone may alleviate the airway obstruction. However, in cases of acute obstruction, an artificial airway may be necessary. Surgery to keep the tongue forward will maintain airway patency until the infant outgrows the defect. (See Chap. 8 for a more complete discussion of congenital defects that predispose to upper airway obstruction.)

A variety of congenital anomalies of the trachea (e.g., laryngeal web, vocal cord paralysis, vascular ring, and neoplasm) may also cause hypoventilation. In addition, there may be defects in the tracheal cartilage that support the neonatal tracheal lumen. Small, absent, or malformed tracheal cartilage permit tracheal weakening (tracheomalacia) and collapse, resulting in a functional tracheal stenosis and obstruction. Normal contraction of the lumen during expiration is exaggerated because the trachea is not adequately supported. The lumen may also be small during inspiration. The patient may wheeze or have stridor, dyspnea, tachypnea, or cyanosis. The diagnosis is made by bronchoscopy, fluoroscopy, or tracheogram. Secondary cartilage damage from external compression, such as a vascular ring or neoplasm, must be considered. Since cartilage continues to develop and eventually supports the airway, treatment should be conservative. Artificial support with an endotracheal tube or tracheostomy is rarely required but, when necessary, is usually prolonged.

Another possible source of upper airway obstruction is an external mass, such as a congenital goiter, neoplasm, or lingual thyroid.

Lower Airway Obstruction

Congenital diaphragmatic hernia with translocation of the abdominal contents into the thorax causes severe hypoventilation in the neonate. This lesion most commonly occurs on the left side of the diaphragm. The majority of patients have symptoms in the first 72 hours of life. Important physical signs, such as absent breath sounds, a scaphoid abdomen, and characteristic radiographic findings will lead to the correct diagnosis. Immediate surgical intervention is needed.

The small airways are blocked after aspiration of meconium. More common in large, full-term infants, this obstruction is best treated by suctioning the trachea immediately after delivery, if the amniotic fluid is noted to be stained with meconium. These patients may progress to severe respiratory failure and require mechanical ventilation. End-expiratory pressure has been found beneficial in the therapy of meconium aspiration.

Respiratory Distress Syndrome

The most common cause of neonatal hypoventilation is the respiratory distress syndrome (RDS). It accounts for approximately 25,000 deaths per year in the United States. Primarily a disease of premature infants, RDS may also occur in full-term infants, particularly those delivered by cesarean section or those of diabetic mothers in whom fetal surfactant production or activity is decreased. Patients with RDS grunt on expiration and have tachypnea. A chest radiograph typically shows a diffuse, fine granularity throughout. Oxygen, distending airway pressure, and ventilatory support can all be used to resuscitate and treat these patients.

CNS Depression

In contrast to the patient with airway obstruction, other neonates may have slow, shallow respiration and make less effort to breathe. This condition of drug-induced hypoventilation is caused by barbiturates, narcotics, or inhalation anesthetic agents administered to the mother during labor and delivery or to the neonate during surgery. An infant with residual barbiturate or inhalation anesthetic is treated with ventilatory support until redistribution, excretion, and metabolism reduce the effect of the drug. Naloxone hydrochloride, a short-acting narcotic antagonist that is not a respiratory depressant, effectively reverses narcotic-induced hypoventilation. Recent evidence suggests that this antagonist may inhibit the metabolism or even prolong the respiratory depressant effect of the narcotic. If this drug is the only therapy given, the patient must be observed particularly closely for several hours after its administration, because the respiratory depression produced by the narcotic outlasts the effect of the naloxone. Therefore, it is particularly important that in the hours immediately after delivery, a note should be made of all drugs given to the mother during labor.

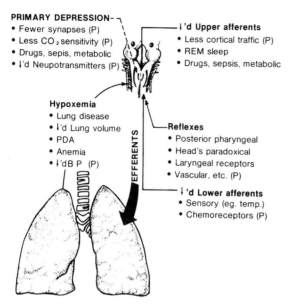

Fig. 44-1. Proposed pathogenetic pathways for neonatal apnea. (Kattwinkel, J.: Neonatal apnea: pathogenesis and therapy. J. Pediatr., *90*:342, 1977)

Residual Neuromuscular Blockade

Residual effects of neuromuscular blocking agents can also cause hypoventilation in the neonate postoperatively. Though conflicting data exist;[1—3] studies using twitch depression or electromyography[4,5] show the average dose of d-tubocurarine required for surgery, based on weight, affect neonates no more than the older child and adult. However, there is greater individual variation in sensitivity with neonates than with older patients; there is up to a fourfold difference in the range of effective doses for individual neonates. Therefore, administering a standard dose for infants under 10 days of age may, for a particular neonate, be twice the amount of drug necessary needed. The result of this miscalculation is a degree of neuromuscular blockade that may be difficult to antagonize after surgery. Similarly, smaller doses of pancuronium have been found to cause apnea more commonly in newborns than in older infants.

If infants and older patients have a similar degree of muscular weakness, the infants have a greater degree of respiratory impairment than do the older patients. Although the reason for this is not clear, there are several possible explanations. The closing volume of airways of the small child is very high.[6] Hence, a diminished tidal volume can close the airways even more. Respiratory muscles of the infant may be more sensitive to muscle relaxants than adults, but conclusive evidence is lacking. Whatever the cause, it is clear that low dosages of nondepolarizing muscle relaxants can cause hypoventilation in neonates. *All nondepolarizing muscle relaxants administered to the infant should be antagonized with an anticholinesterase agent (e.g., neostigmine).*

APNEA

The breathing of premature newborns may be regularly interrupted by periods of apnea lasting 3 seconds or more. This is a normal ventilatory pattern and occurs in 30 to 45 per cent of premature infants.[8] *Neonatal apnea* is the absence of breathing for 20 seconds or longer, or an apneic period associated with cyanosis or bradycardia.

Neonatal apnea results from a variety of causes (Fig. 44-1). In response to hypoxemia, newborns increase their ventilation and then may experience periodic breathing, respiratory depression, and apnea.[9] Hence, any disorder that results in hypoxemia can also cause apnea. Lung disease associated with decreased lung volume, a patent ductus arteriosus with a right-to-left shunt, anemia, and hypotension can all cause a degree of hypoxemia sufficient to result in apnea.

Abnormal or hyperactive cardiorespiratory reflexes can also cause neonatal apnea. Stimulation of the posterior pharynx during suctioning,[10] lung inflation,[11] and chemical stimuli[12] can cause apnea, bradycardia, or both.

Activity of the medullary respiratory center depends on a variety of afferent inputs from the respiratory tract. When input is decreased, respiratory drive decreases.[13] Chemoreceptors function as early as 28 weeks of gestation.[14,15] Respiratory frequency and amplitude of neonates vary with different sleep states, which are regulated by the cerebral cortex. For instance, there may be a decrease in respiratory center activity and elimination of lung inflation reflexes during rapid eye movement (REM) sleep.[17,18] Also, neonatal apnea occurs during abnormal neurological states, such as seizures, and abnormal metabolic states, such as hypoglycemia.

In some infants, the number of synapses in the respiratory center may be decreased.[19] But, the relatively greater respiratory afferent activity traveling over a smaller number of pathways may lessen the incidence of apnea by increasing total respiratory afferent activity. The carbon dioxide response curve of infants resembles that of the adult when corrected for weight, but other data suggest that the carbon dioxide response curve changes as the central nervous system matures.[20]

TREATMENT OF APNEA

Many techniques have been proposed to treat apnea of premature infants. The technique should be approriate to the cause of the apnea, for each cause, there is an optimal technique. Possible causes are shown in Figure 44-1.

When hypoxemia is the cause of apnea, increasing the concentration of inspired oxygen, applying end-expiratory pressure, or providing mechanical ventilation can overcome the apnea. However, the administration of oxygen is not without its risk to the neonate. Retrolental fibroplasia is a danger to eyes not fully developed. When administering supplemental oxygen to infants, the arterial blood gases should be monitored closely (see Chap. 23). Low level continuous positive-pressure airway pressure (CPAP) can reverse hypoxemia and decrease the incidence of apnea. Congestive heart failure or a patent ductus arteriosus should be treated. Transfusion improves oxygen delivery in the anemic patient.

Reflexes known to trigger apnea should be avoided. Thus, nasopharyngeal suction catheters and nipple feedings should be avoided if possible, as well as hyperinflation during manual ventilation. The trigeminal area of the face is sensitive to cold, and very warm stimuli which may precipitate apnea.[22] The face should be kept in as neutral a thermal environment as possible. However, thermal[23,24] and cutaneous stimulation[21] to other parts of the body have been used to stimulate afferents of the patient with deficient afferent activity.

Apnea associated with sepsis, metabolic disorders, or an overdose of narcotics should be treated by correcting the primary cause. Aminophylline has been proposed to treat apnea in the premature infant.[25] While the mechanism of action is not clear, elevation of cyclic AMP activity has been suggested.[26] A loading dose of 5.5 mg. per kg. orally, followed by 1.1 mg. orally every 8 hours, has been recommended.[27]

MONITORING FOR HYPOVENTILATION AND APNEA

Detection of alveolar hypoventilation or apnea requires monitoring by both instruments and medical staff. Infrared devices or mass spectrometers that analyze exhaled gas permit continuous assessment of the adequacy of ventilation; the measurement of P_{CO_2} of exhaled gas correlates with Pa_{CO_2}.

Thermography and impedance pneumography are techniques readily adaptable for apnea detection in neonates. These devices can be equipped with auditory and visual alarms to warn personnel when periods of breathlessness occur. Additionally, cardiotachometry is useful to detect bradycardia. A transcutaneous oxygen monitoring system can also be equipped with alarms, both visual and auditory, which signal when responses are not within the range set on the instrument.

APPROACH TO APNEA AND HYPOVENTILATION IN THE POSTOPERATIVE PERIOD

Postoperatively, apnea and hypoventilation can be diagnosed by laboratory evidence of carbon dioxide retention. Once the diagnosis is made, causes, such as respiratory distress syndrome, hypoglycemia, hypocalcemia, sepsis, anemia, hypothermia, drug effects, and starvation should be either excluded or treated, if present.

Therapy should be started and may take the form of intermittent stimulation or more chronic stimulation devices such as water beds. Nasal

CPAP may effectively stimulate breathing and decrease hypoxemia.

In particular, adequate oxygenation and hemoglobin levels should be maintained. Supplemental oxygen may be required to maintain a Pa_{O_2} level of 50 to 80 torr. Aminophylline therapy should be considered, particularly for the premature infant.[27] If these means fail to reverse hypoventilation or apnea in the neonate, mechanical ventilation should be instituted.

REFERENCES

1. Stead, A. L.: The responses of the newborn infant to muscle relaxants. Br. J. Anaesth., *27*:124, 1955.
2. Lim, H. S., Davenport, H. T., and Robson, J. G.: The response of infants and children to muscle relaxants. Anesthesiology, *25*:161, 1964.
3. Churchill-Davidson, H. C., and Wise, R. P.: The response of the newborn infant to muscle relaxants. Can. Anaesth. Soc. J., *11*:1, 1964.
4. Long, G., and Bachman, L.: Neuromuscular blockade by *d*-tubocurarine in children. Anesthesiology, *23*:723, 1967.
5. Walts, L. F., and Dillon, J. B.: The response of newborns to succinylcholine and *d*-tubocurarine. Anesthesiology, *31*:35, 1969.
6. Mansell, A., Bryan, C., and Levinson, H.: Airway closure in children. J. Appl. Physiol., *33*:711, 1972.
7. Bennett, E. J., Ramamurthy, S., Dalal, F. Y., *et al.:* Pancuronium and the neonate. Br. J. Anaesth., *47*:75, 1975.
8. Chernick, V., Heldrick, F., and Avery, M. E.: Periodic breathing of premature infants. J. Pediatr., *64*:330, 1964.
9. Cross, K. W., and Oppe, T. E.: The effect of inhalation of high and low concentrations of oxygen on the respiration of the premature infant. J. Physiol., *117*:38, 1952.
10. Cardero, L. and Hon, E.: Neonatal bradycardia following nasopharyngeal stimulation. J. Pediatr., *78*:441, 1971.
11. Cross, K. W., Klaus, M., Tooley, W. H., *et al.:* The response of the newborn baby to inflation of the lungs. J. Physiol., *151*:551, 1960.
12. Downing, S. E., and Lee, J. C.: Laryngeal chemosensitivity: a possible mechanism for sudden infant death. Pediatrics, *55*:640, 1975.
13. Burns, B. D.: The central control of respiratory movements. Br. Med. Bull., *19*:7, 1963.
14. Rigatto, H., and Brady, J. P.: Periodic breathing and apnea in preterm infants. I. Evidence of hypoventilation possibly due to central respiratory depression. Pediatrics, *50*:202, 1972.
15. Kraus, A. N., Tori, C. A., Brown, J., *et al.:* Oxygen chemoreceptors in low birthweight infants. Pediatr. Res., *7*:569, 1973.
16. Finer, N., Abroms, I., and Taeusch, H.: Influence of sleep state on the control of ventilation. Pediatr. Res., *9*:365, 1965.
17. Gabriel, M., Albani, M., and Schulte, F. J.: Apneic spells and sleep states in preterm infants. Pediatrics, *57*:142, 1976.
18. Finer, N. N. Abroms, I. F., and Taeusch, H. W.: Ventilation and sleep states in newborn infants. J. Pediatr., *89*:100, 1976.
19. Parmelee, A. H., Stern, E., and Harris, M. A.: Maturation of respiration in prematures and young infants. Neuropaediatrie, *3*:351, 1972.
20. Avery, M. E., and Fletcher, B.: The Lung and Its Disorders in the Newborn Infant. Philadelphia, W. B. Saunders Company, 1974.
21. Kattwinkel, J., Nearman, H. S., Fanaroff, A. A., *et al.:* Apnea of prematurity. J. Pediatr., *86*:588, 1975.
22. Mestyan, I., Jarai, G. B., and Fekete, M.: Surface temperature versus deep body temperature and the metabolic response to cold of hypothermic premature infants. Biol. Neonate, *7*:230, 1964.
23. Perlstein, H., Edward, K., and Sutherland, J.: Apnea in premature infants and incubator air temperature changes. N. Engl. J. Med., *282*:461, 1970.
24. Daily, W. J. R., Klause, J. H., and Meyer, H. B. P.: Apnea in premature infants: Monitoring incidence, heart rate changes and effect of environmental temperature. Pediatrics, *43*:510, 1969.
25. Bednarek, F. J., and Roloff, D. W.: Treatment of apnea of prematurity with aminophylline. Pediatrics, *55*:595, 1975.
26. Uauy, R., Shapiro, D. L., Smith, B., *et al.:* Treatment of severe apnea in prematures with orally administered theophylline. Pediatrics, *55*:595, 1975.
27. Kattwinkel, J.: Neonatal apnea: Pathogenesis and therapy. J. Pediatr., *90*:342, 1977.

Part Eleven

Special Techniques

45

Complications Associated with the Use of Muscle Relaxants

Ronald L. Katz, M.D., and Leah E. Katz, C.R.N.A., Ed. D.

There are a number of reviews that deal with complications of muscle relaxants.[1-6] The reader is referred to these, since some related topics are discussed only briefly here. For example, prolonged respiratory depression may be regarded as a complication of the pharmacology of the relaxant or a failure of the person who administers the relaxant to appreciate the pharmacology of the drug. Since this subject has been covered extensively and the factors that prolong the action of relaxants have been recently reviewed well,[6] prolonged respiratory depression is not covered here. However, the anesthesiologist should keep in mind the factors that may modify the action of relaxants and thereby produce prolonged effects: blood flow, liver disease, protein binding, renal failure, acid-base balance, temperature and electrolyte abnormalities, acetylcholinesterase inhibitors, pseudocholinesterase inhibitors, local anesthetics, lithium, antibiotics, antiarrhythmic agents, and inhalation anesthetics. All of these may exert pharmacologic effects on the muscle relaxants or physiologic effects on the neuromuscular junction that may significantly modify the action of relaxants.

HYPERKALEMIA FOLLOWING SUCCINYLCHOLINE ADMINISTRATION

The Use of Succinylcholine in Burn Patients

It has been known since 1958 that the use of succinylcholine in burn patients may be associated with cardiac arrhythmia and arrest,[7] although the mechanism was not known. In 1961 Allen speculated that ionic shifts produced by succinylcholine might account for the ventricular fibrillation.[8] He suggested that potassium is the only ion that can be mobilized from its depots and translocated rapidly enough to produce arrhythmias and fibrillation. However, it was not until 1967 that Tolmie and colleagues demonstrated that, indeed, hyperkalemia is the mechanism responsible for cardiac arrest.[9] They described a patient who had undergone 10 uneventful anesthetics in a 26-day period following massive burns and soft-tissue destruction. At his 11th operation, which occurred on the 31st day following injury, he received 60 mg. of succinylcholine and suffered a cardiac arrest, from which he was successfully resuscitated. On the 36th day following injury, he again received succinylcholine and developed ventricular fibrillation; the ECG suggested hyperkalemia. Following successful resuscitation, the patient was anesthetized again and received succinylcholine on the 40th day, as well as on several other occasions. Although ventricular fibrillation did not recur, his ECG showed evidence of hyperkalemia following succinylcholine, with a maximum rise in serum potassium of 8 mmol. per L.

The Use of Succinylcholine in Patients With Trauma

Around the time when Tolmie's report was published, there were reports that succinylcholine could produce hyperkalemia under other circumstances. In 1968, Mazze and Dunbar[10] and others,[11-13] 1 year later, reported hyperkalemia in patients with massive trauma who had received succinylcholine. In 1969, Roth and Wüthrich reported an increase in serum potassium level in tetanus patients given succinylcholine.[14]

The Use of Succinylcholine in Patients With Neurological Disease

Cooperman reported hyperkalemia after succinylcholine administration in patients with paraplegia following spinal cord trauma, hemiparesis, multiple sclerosis, muscular dystrophy, and cerebrovascular accidents.[15,16] Others reported succinylcholine-induced hyperkalemia in patients with paraplegia due to spinal cord injury[17,18] and tetanus.[14] Subsequently, the Guillain-Barré syndrome, with diffuse anterior horn cell involvement,[19] peripheral nerve injuries,[20] Duchenne type of muscular dystrophy,[21] encephalitis,[22] and CNS injuries were implicated.[23] Some studies (see below) have demonstrated that disuse atrophy produced by experimental skeletal fixation may increase the likelihood of potassium release following succinylcholine. In short, any central nervous system lesion may under certain circumstances result in marked hyperkalemia following succinylcholine.

The Use of Succinylcholine in Patients With Renal Disease

Roth and Wüthrich described two hyperkalemic patients with severe renal disease who suffered cardiac arrest following succinylcholine.[14] As a result, they suggested that the use of depolarizing muscle relaxants in such patients is dangerous. This view was supported by Powell, who reported a similar incident.[24] However, the response of patients with renal failure to succinylcholine is controversial; the majority of studies suggest that the use of succinylcholine in these patients is not associated with hyperkalemia. These studies suggest, in general, that the succinylcholine-induced increases in serum potassium are no greater in uremic patients than in normal patients.[25,26,27] The increase in potassium

levels produced by succinylcholine in the normal patient is approximately 0.5 mmol. per L., depending upon the induction and anesthetic agents used.[2,28,29] However, a second or third dose of succinylcholine may produce a greater rise in potassium than is normally seen after a first dose in patients with chronic renal failure.[24,25,30] For example, Walton and Farman reported a uremic patient whose serum potassium remained at 4.5 mmol. per L. following 50 mg. of succinylcholine; after a second dose of 25 mg., the potassium rose to 7.3 mmol. per L., for a total rise of 2.8 mmol. per L.[30] Yet, in 11 patients with renal failure undergoing renal transplantation, three doses of succinylcholine did not produce increases in potassium greater than 0.6 mmol. per L.[31] A complicating factor in interpreting these studies is that polyneuropathy, a common feature of uremia, may explain the development of hyperkalemia that had been attributed to chronic renal failure.

Although the results of these studies differ somewhat, in a given patient, under appropriate conditions, a second or third dose may result in potassium increases of more than the usual 0.5 mmol. per L. Therefore, repeated doses of succinylcholine are not contraindicated in patients with chronic renal failure, but the ECG should be monitored, and if evidence of hyperkalemia is observed, samples should be withdrawn for analysis of potassium. Though rare, if severe ECG changes occur, treatment with intravenous administration of calcium chloride and sodium bicarbonate should be started.

The Time Factor

One of the puzzling observations concerning succinylcholine-induced hyperkalemia is the following: Burn patients who were anesthetized without difficulty on several occasions following their burn developed arrhythmia and arrest on a subsequent occasion for no apparent reason. In the case reported by Tolmie, the patient had undergone ten successful anesthetics without difficulty[9]; it was only during the subsequent procedures that cardiac arrest occurred. This can now be explained by a time factor that is involved in the hyperkalemic response. Schaner and colleagues observed elevations in serum potassium of at least 6 mmol. per L. in 16 of 52 patients.[32] They found that the period of time that the patient was susceptible to succinylcholine-induced hyperkalemia was from the 20th to the 60th day following burn. The period of risk with other disorders is not identical. For example, Mazze reported that in trauma patients, the period of danger extended from 3 weeks until the lesion was covered by skin.[18] Cooperman reported that the susceptible period following spinal cord injury was usually less than 6 months but could be longer when the neurological disease was progressive.[16] Tobey, who studied lower motor neuron injuries, found a similar duration.[20]

The time course, mechanism, and site of potassium release following succinylcholine has been studied by several groups. The maximum increase in serum potassium in burn patients occurs 2 to 4 min. after succinylcholine injection, with a gradual slow decline over the next 10 to 15 min.; however, normal values are seldom reached within this time, and there is a marked variation in the rise of potassium following 1 mg. per kg. of succinylcholine. Between the 10th and 50th day, the increase can be as high as 5 mmol. per L., or the increase may be insignificant. After more than 14 days, the maximum increase in serum potassium correlates with the burn index (burn index = the per cent of full thickness of burn area + the per cent of partial thickness of burn area).[33] Several studies in a variety of species, including humans, have shown that following succinylcholine administration, there is a higher potassium concentration in the blood draining a denervated limb than in the control limb.[12,20,34,35,36] Hyperkalemia is not observed in animals in which only the skin is burned; but it is observed when the skin is burned and muscle destruction occurs. Thus, potassium efflux occurs in both normal and injured muscle, but the greatest amount of potassium is lost from the latter.

Mechanism of Succinylcholine-Induced Hyperkalemia

The normally innervated muscle cell undergoes depolarization only when acetylcholine is applied to the end-plate. However, following denervation, supersensitivity develops after approximately 2 weeks. At this time, the entire muscle membrane becomes sensitive to acetylcholine and acts as if it were an end-plate. Thus, depolarization occurs along the entire length of the fiber. The movement of sodium and potassium that normally occurs when acetylcholine is applied to the end-plate now occurs over the entire length. It is this increased area of permeability to sodium and potassium following denervation that accounts for the marked increase in serum potassium following succinylcholine. Support for this comes from the demonstration that the denervated muscle membrane responds to succinylcholine in a fashion similar to acetylcholine.[36] Potassium efflux from denervated muscle following succinylcholine is 20 times greater than that in normal muscle.[37] Walts pointed out that although this explains the hyperkalemic response of denervated muscle, it does not explain the hyperkalemic response in traumatized patients without muscle injury.[5] He referred to the work of Katz and Miledi, who reported that hypersensitivity of muscle to acetylcholine can occur following injury and does not require denervation.[38] Furthermore, damage to nerve or muscle is not necessary to produce a hyperkalemic response to succinylcholine or an increase in acetylcholine sensitivity. Immobilization of an extremity, producing disuse atrophy, can result in hypersensitivity to acetylcholine.[39] After succinylcholine administration, the greatest potassium flux occurs in denervated muscle, followed by paraplegic muscle; the least flux occurs in immobilized muscle.[35,37,40]

Thus, succinylcholine-induced hyperkalemia is related to increased chemosensitivity of the membrane, owing to the development of receptor sites in extrajunctional areas. Although succinylcholine induces a small release of potassium in normal muscle, it produces a potentially lethal efflux in the presence of increased sensitivity. This potassium-releasing action of succinylcholine begins about 5 to 15 days after injury and persists for 2 to 3 months in patients who have sustained burns or trauma, and perhaps 3 to 6 months in patients with upper motor neuron lesions.

Prevention of Succinylcholine-Induced Hyperkalemia

It is well established that nondepolarizing agents diminish or block the response to a variety of the unwanted effects of succinylcholine. *d*-Tubocurarine (6 mg.) given prior to succinylcholine may markedly decrease the potassium elevation after succinylcholine.[12,13] However, the curare does not predictably abolish the succinylcholine-induced hyperkalemia in all patients.[16] Birch reported that curare essentially abolished the potassium rise after succinylcholine.[12] However, Gronert criticized this report by indicating that the curare was given before a *second* injection of succinylcholine.[40] Gronert showed that if curare preceded a *first* injection of succinylcholine, it did not abolish the rise in potassium. Since nondepolarizing agents do not necessarily abolish the increase in potassium following succinycholine in all patients, it would seem prudent to avoid succinylcholine in patients at risk, rather than expose the patient to pharmacological roulette. Nondepolarizing relaxants do not increase plasma potassium.[41]

DECREASED PSEUDOCHOLINESTERASE ACTIVITY IN BURN PATIENTS

Burn patients may have deficiencies in pseudocholinesterase activity, and the magnitude and rate of fall correlates with the severity of burn injury.[42] The lowest levels are often reached 5 to 6 days after the injury, when pseudocholinesterase activity may be depressed by more than 80 per cent. In patients with mild burns, pseudocholinesterase activity returns to normal in 6 to 14 days, but in others with severe burns, pseudocholinesterase is often depressed for months. In addition to the severity of the burn, other factors determine the level of pseudocholinesterase activity, including the presence of local or systemic infections and recent surgery. In patients who received blood transfusions, there is a marked increase in pseudocholinesterase activity. There is a good correlation between burn index (see p. 559) and the lowest level of pseudocholinesterase, and between burn index and time of recovery of pseudocholinesterase activity to normal. The possible mechanisms for the prolonged depression of pseudocholinesterase activity include the following: increased pseudocholinesterase catabolism; the presence of inhibiting substances in the plasma; and depression of hepatic synthesis and/or release of the enzyme. The most likely cause of prolonged depression is the last.

MYOGLOBINURIA FOLLOWING SUCCINYLCHOLINE ADMINISTRATION

Bennike and Jarnum reported postoperative myoglobinuria in a patient who experienced vigorous fasciculations following succinylcholine.[43] On the 1st postoperative day, the patient voided dark red urine that contained myoglobin, and he subsequently developed acute renal failure. The investigators suggested that since acute attacks of myoglobinuria may be precipitated by some type of exercise, possibly the vigorous fasciculations produced by succinylcholine might have caused the myoglobinuria. Following this study, there were several case reports, usually in children, of myoglobinuria following anesthesia, in which succinylcholine was implicated. Jensen described postoperative myoglobinuria in a 15-year-old girl who received halothane and, interestingly, was given 3 mg. of curare prior to 100 mg. of succinylcholine.[44] She did not relax and was given additional succinylcholine. Postoperatively, she developed myoglobinuria but recovered rapidly. Other investigators have described similar patients.[45,46]

Because of these case reports of myoglobinuria, Tammisto and associates undertook a number of studies.[47–50] They measured levels of creatinine phosphokinase (CPK), using it as a sign of muscle injury, and they reported that succinylcholine can regularly cause myoglobinuria. Myoglobinuria and CPK elevation do not occur in patients who receive a single dose of succinylcholine during halothane anesthesia, nor in those who receive multiple doses of succinylcholine during nitrous oxide, nor in those who receive halothane plus succinylcholine by continuous infusion. However, in patients who receive halothane plus repeated doses of succinylcholine, there is a marked increase in CPK. In cases in which CPK elevations are marked, myoglobinuria is also observed.

Reviewing their data, it is apparent that the patients who received halothane and succinylcholine can be divided into two groups, depending upon whether thiopental was used. In the patients who did not receive thiopental, the level of CPK was markedly elevated, while in those who did receive thiopental, there was only a small increase in CPK. Finally, they reported an inhibitory effect of *d*-tubocurarine on the increase of serum CPK activity produced by intermittent succinylcholine administration during halothane anesthesia.

Ryan studied the frequency of myoglobinemia in 58 children and 30 adults.[51] Forty children and all adults received succinylcholine, 1 mg. per kg., intravenously, while 12 children received the same dose intramuscularly. Measurements were also made in six children who received halothane but no succinylcholine. In 16 of the 40 children (40%), myoglobinemia developed. However, of the 30 adult patients, only one developed myoglobinemia. In the six children who did not receive succinylcholine, and in the 12 children who received the relaxant intramuscularly, myoglobinemia was not noted. The frequency of myoglobinemia was greatest in the children in whom halothane was the primary agent. Thus, in this study, as in that of Tammisto, halothane appears to be related to the release of myoglobin. To determine whether the intravenous barbiturate commonly used for induction in adults, but not children, might prevent the myoglobinemia and thus account for the different results in children and adults, Ryan studied seven children in whom anesthesia was induced with thiopental. This did not lessen the frequency of myoglobinemia.

In a report describing five cases of malignant hyperpyrexia, Ryan and Papper noted two patients who failed to relax with the initial dose of succinylcholine and who subsequently developed myoglobinuria.[52] There have been reports of several families in whom one member developed myoglobinuria following succinylcholine and halothane, whereas another member who received these agents developed malignant hyperpyrexia. It may be that these are different expressions of related muscle diseases.

Thus, myoglobinuria, myoglobinemia, or a rise in CPK may occur in patients who receive multiple doses of succinylcholine, especially with concomitant halothane. (Studies of other potent agents may reveal a similar problem.) Moreover, myoglobinuria or myoglobinemia is more likely to occur in children than in adults. One possible explanation for the release of myoglobin is that muscle in children may behave as if it were chronically denervated. Perhaps an abnormal efflux of muscle protein leading to myoglobinemia follows succinylcholine administration and results from breaks in membrane of the muscle. This hypothesis was tested by Hegab, who studied normal and chronically denervated rat skeletal muscle with and without succinylcholine.[53] Sarcolemma breaks did not appear in the 28 days following denervation, nor were they seen following succinylcholine challenge. Thus, the sarcolemma remains intact in denervated muscles, and succinylcholine does not induce membrane breaks in either normal or denervated muscle.

INCREASED INTRAOCULAR PRESSURE FOLLOWING SUCCINYLCHOLINE ADMINISTRATION

Early Studies of the Effect of Succinylcholine on Intraocular Pressure

Hofmann and Lembeck reported in 1952 that succinylcholine and decamethonium produced contraction of the extraocular muscles.[54] In 1953 Hofmann and Holzer reported that succinylcholine increased intraocular pressure as much as 18 torr in unanesthetized volunteers.[55] An increase in intraocular pressure in patients under general anesthesia was also noted, but the magnitude was somewhat less. These workers astutely observed that coincident with the rise in intraocular pressure, the eyes became divergent and remained fixed. As intraocular pressure decreased, movement of the eyes returned. Therefore, they suggested that the increase in intraocular pressure is produced by contraction of the extraocular muscles, an effect of succinylcholine that they had noted earlier.[54] In 1955 Lincoff reported that following succinylcholine the extraocular muscles contracted and the intraocular pressure of cats increased.[56] Only a slight increase in intraocular pressure was observed when all of the extraocular muscles were cut. He concluded that the contraction of the extraocular muscles produced by succinylcholine compresses the globe and increases intraocular pressure. He also reported that in patients receiving succinylcholine (0.3 mg/kg), intraocular pressure increased an average of 7.9 torr, with a maximum increase of 39 torr.

In 1957, Dillion[57,58] and Lincoff[59] reported cases of vitreous expulsion in humans, attributable to the increase in intraocular pressure produced by succinylcholine. Succinylcholine contracted the extraocular muscles of cats and humans,[57,58] and this effect was blocked by curare[57,59,60] and is markedly reduced by sectioning all six extraocular muscles.[61] These studies corroborated the conclusions of Lincoff: The contraction of the extraocular muscles produced by succinylcholine is responsible for the increased intraocular pressure. With repeated injections of succinylcholine, however, tachyphylaxis occurs.[61] Similarly, with continuous infusion of succinylcholine, the pressure returns to normal. Craythorne demonstrated in 1960 that succinylcholine increases intraocular pressure in children and that patients with glaucoma do not experience a greater rise in intraocular pressure than those without glaucoma.[62]

Although these studies suggest a relationship between the increased intraocular pressure and extraocular muscles, other studies have questioned this correlation. Some patients who receive succinylcholine do not develop a rise in intraocular pressure, and the pretreatment with curare may not prevent the phenomenon.[63,64] At least one investigator suggested that an intrabulbar cause, such as a direct vasodilatory effect of succinylcholine, is responsible for the pressure rise.[65] Thus, in the early 1960s, the mechanism and magnitude of intraocular pressure rise produced by succinylcholine were in doubt.

Mechanism of Increase in Intraocular Pressure

As a result of this disagreement, Katz and Eakins began a series of studies in the early 1960s to determine whether succinylcholine does increase intraocular pressure and, if so, by what mechanism.[66–70] They found that extraocular muscles in vivo respond to succinylcholine with an increase in tension. In subsequent studies, they stimulated the third cranial nerve and recorded the twitch response of the extraocular muscles.

With small doses of succinylcholine, there is no change in twitch height, but the previously observed increase in muscle tension is again seen. As increasing doses of succinylcholine were given, the tension of muscle increased further, but the twitch response began to diminish. It was possible to find a dose of succinylcholine that abolished the twitch response of the extraocular muscles but simultaneously produced a marked increase in tension, equal to or even greater than the maximum force generated by nerve stimulation. These results suggest that there are two kinds of neuromuscular systems in the extraocular muscles: twitch and tonic (Table 45-1). The response of the tonic system to succinylcholine is an increase in tension; in contrast, the twitch system is inhibited. Cutting all of the extraocular muscles markedly decreases but does not abolish the increased intraocular pressure produced by succinylcholine. Katz and Eakins also studied the response of the nictitating membrane to succinylcholine. The nictitating membrane was used as an index of orbital smooth muscle response. They found that succinylcholine contracted the nictitating membrane and orbital smooth muscle; therefore, they concluded that the rise in intraocular pressure produced by succinylcholine, while in large measure a result of the contraction and increase in tension of the extraocular muscles, was also, in part, caused by orbital smooth muscle contraction. Curare blocked the contraction of the extraocular muscles, nictitating membrane, and orbital smooth muscle, and it prevented the rise in intraocular pressure.

Thus, succinylcholine increases intraocular pressure in cats and humans. While this increase results predominantly from the contraction of the extraocular muscles, the contraction of orbital smooth muscle that surrounds the eye is also contributory. Another possible contributing factor is arterial hypertension, which is sometimes associated with succinylcholine administration. Every 10-torr rise in arterial pressure produces a 1-torr rise in intraocular pressure.

Prevention of Succinylcholine-Induced Increase in Intraocular Pressure

The use of a small dose of curare prior to succinylcholine is discussed on page 564. A dose

Table 45-1. The Two Nerve-Muscle Fiber Systems of Mammalian Extraocular Muscle

	TWITCH (Fibrillenstruktur)	TONIC (Feldenstruktur)
Fibrils	Small, regular, well-defined	Large, irregular, poorly defined
Nerve endings	Single, large nerve endings derived from large-diameter motor fiber	Numerous, small grape-like endings derived from small-diameter eflerent nerves
Stimulation of motor nerve	Fast twitch contraction Propagated muscle action potential Contraction produced by single shocks	Slow graded muscle contraction Non-propagated muscle action potential of long duration Tetanic rate of stimulation required for excitation
Function	Rapid eye movements	Control of overall tension of eye muscle (i.e., tone of muscle)

of 3 to 6 mg. may be given to prevent the expected rise in intraocular pressure, but a recent study suggests that nondepolarizing neuromuscular blocking drugs may not prevent this effect of succinylcholine.[71] Among several aspects that make that study difficult to evaluate, however, is the unusual intramuscular administration of the curare or gallamine, which may account for the lack of efficacy.

Since this dose of curare diminishes the muscle relaxant effect of succinylcholine, an increase in the dose of succinylcholine of approximately 50 per cent is required to produce an equivalent effect (1.5 mg./kg. produces effects similar to 1 mg./kg.) This is important, because if curare is given prior to an inadequate dose of succinylcholine, such that the patient coughs on the endotracheal tube, the rise in intraocular pressure can be much greater than that which would have been produced by succinylcholine alone.

Hexafluorenium, if given 5 min. before succinylcholine, is also capable of blocking the response. However, hexafluorenium is rarely used today. Acetazolamide has also been reported to prevent the rise in intraocular pressure if given 2 minutes prior to succinylcholine.[72] This effect, however, has not yet been confirmed.

In the clinical situation, although hexafluorenium and curare usually prevent the rise in intraocular pressure, the technique chosen to prevent this rise in situations in which it is potentially dangerous (*e.g.*, the open eye) should depend upon the familiarity of the anesthesiologist with curare and hexafluorenium.

INCREASED INTRAGASTRIC PRESSURE FOLLOWING SUCCINYLCHOLINE ADMINISTRATION

It is common practice to manage the patient with a "full stomach" by rapid induction of anesthesia with thiopental and succinylcholine, followed by tracheal intubation. It has been suggested that the fasciculations produced by succinylcholine may raise the intragastric pressure sufficiently to overcome the opening pressure of the gastroesophageal junction and thereby produce regurgitation of gastric contents. Of ten adult patients who had balloon catheters in their stomachs, four had marked fasciculations following succinylcholine, and intragastric pressure was elevated in three of the four.[73] Similarly, three of 25 patients had elevations in intragastric pressure greater than 19 cm. H_2O above a resting level of 4 to 16 cm. H_2O.[74] Intragastric pressure can rise as much as 40 to 85 cm. H_2O above a resting level of 0 to 17 (mean = 7) cm. H_2O.[75,76,77]

Miller and Way noted that there is a correlation between the intensity of fasciculations and the increase in intragastric pressure.[77] Although the increase in intragastric pressure may be caused by the skeletal muscle fasciculations, it is also possible that the acetylcholine-like effect of succinylcholine (which is essentially two acetylcholine molecules joined together) may also play some role in increasing intragastric pressure.

Is the increase in intragastric pressure following succinylcholine sufficient to cause incompetence of the cardioesophageal junction? Regurgitation can occur when intragastric pressure rises to 28 cm. H_2O.[78] The gastric opening pressure depends upon the angle of entry of the esophagus into the stomach. In six of 15 patients, the opening pressure was less than 28 cm. H_2O, while the average opening pressure of the stomach in normal position was 36 cm. H_2O.[79] Pressing or clamping the fundus of the stomach lowered the opening pressure, but a bulging fundus raised it. The esophageal angle of entry into the stomach is critical in determining the opening pressure. Any alteration in this normally oblique angle may change the intragastric pressure required to produce incompetence at the cardioesophageal junction. A change of this angle may occur in pregnancy, obesity, and in the presence of bowel obstruction, hiatal hernia, or ascites. Under these circumstances, the cardioesophageal junction may become incompetent at pressures less than 15 cm. H_2O. Therefore, there are two major variables affecting competence of the cardioesophageal junction: presence of circumstances affecting the angle of entry of the esophagus into the stomach; and the variable increase in intragastric pressure produced by succinylcholine.

There are several ways to prevent the increase in intragastric pressure sometimes produced by succinylcholine. Curare (4–6 mg.) injected prior to succinylcholine, prevents this increase.[76] Miller and Way noted that the injection of curare (3 mg.) or gallamine (20 mg.) is also efficacious.[77] They also reported that pre-injection of lidocaine (6 mg./kg.) is effective as well, although this study was abandoned because of hypotension in some patients.

An alternate approach to preventing regurgitation after succinylcholine is to increase the opening pressure of the stomach. Intravenous atropine (0.6 mg.) raises gastric opening pressure to about 54 cm. H_2O.[80] Since succinylcholine rarely raises intragastric pressure to this level, this is one approach to handling this problem. Moreover, in the study of Miller and Way, pa-

tients premedicated with atropine had lesser increases in intragastric pressure, but this was not statistically different from that in un-premedicated patients.[77] Thus, although atropine does not appear to significantly modify the change produced by succinylcholine, it does increase the gastric opening pressure to a level greater than that usually produced by succinylcholine. An alternate way of diminishing the likelihood of regurgitation and aspiration is Sellick's maneuver, pressure on the cricoid cartilage sufficient to compress the esophagus against the vertebral body.[81] If carried out properly, this maneuver is effective in preventing gastric regurgitation during rapid induction with thiopental and succinylcholine followed by intubation. Patients with a full stomach may also be managed by awake intubation (see Chap. 10).

It appears that the effect of succinylcholine on intragastric pressure in infants and children differs from that in adults. In most children studied, there was a fall in intragastric pressure following succinylcholine, but in five of the older children, there was a slight rise, with a maximum of 4 cm. H_2O.[82] The investigators related the lack of a rise in intragastric pressure to the lack of strong muscle fasciculations.

COMPLICATIONS OF RELAXANTS IN PREGNANCY

An unusual response to muscle relaxants may occur in parturients who receive magnesium sulfate for treatment of toxemia. Morris and Giesecke found that in these patients, less succinylcholine is required.[83] In normal patients, 7.4 mg. per kg. per hour is required during uncomplicated caesarean section; in contrast, in the parturients who have received magnesium sulfate, 4.7 mg. per kg. per hour is required. In patients in whom the response to muscle relaxants is not monitored with a peripheral nerve stimulator and the "usual" dose of succinylcholine is given, prolonged apnea following succinylcholine may occur in patients who have received magnesium sulfate. Studies in animals demonstrate an additive neuromuscular effect of magnesium sulfate and succinylcholine, which thus explains the prolonged apnea following the administration of both drugs.[84]

An interaction between magnesium and curare also occurs. Several case reports describe patients undergoing caesarean section who have had prolonged response to curare when their magnesium levels were about 7 mEq. per L. (3.5 mmol./L.).[85,86] Following recovery, the magnesium levels were noted to be normal: 2 mEq. per L. (1.0 mmol./L.). One patient had received magnesium sulfate prior to caesarean section and had adequately recovered from curare. However, 1 hour postoperatively, the patient was given an additional dose of 10 g. of magnesium sulfate. The patient began to have respiratory difficulty, 10 min. later, when her serum magnesium level was 8.4 mg. per L. (4.2 mmol./L.) Ghoneim and Long established dose-response curves for curare, decamethonium, and succinylcholine, using the rat phrenic-diaphragm preparation, with and without the presence of magnesium sulfate.[86] In each case, the combination of the muscle relaxant and magnesium sulfate shifted the dose-response curve to the left. Magnesium produces the following: a decrease in the amount of acetylcholine liberated at the neuromuscular junction; a decrease in sensitivity of the end-plate to the depolarizing action of acetylcholine; and a decrease in excitability of the muscle membrane.[87] Probably, the decreased liberation of acetylcholine from the motor nerve terminal is the most important action of magnesium, since transmission can be restored by the administration of calcium, which increases the release of acetylcholine but does not alter the reduced end-plate sensitivity or the increased threshold of the muscle membrane.

There are also case reports of prolonged apnea following the administration of succinylcholine in pregnant patients who have not received magnesium.[88–91] Shnider attributed the apnea in his patient to a low level of pseudocholinesterase.[88] The decreased enzyme level occurs in the first trimester of pregnancy and then remains constant until after the early postpartum period. According to Hazel and Monier,[92] the decrease is approximately 20 to 30 per cent, while Robertson found serum levels of pseudocholinesterase below normal in 35 per cent of pregnant women and in 7.5 percent of nonpregnant women.[89]

An unusual case of hypoventilation in both the newborn and mother followed caesarean section, in which a total dose of 140 mg. of succinylcholine had been administered.[93] In the mother, the neuromuscular block lasted for 5.5 hours, while in the infant, ventilatory support was necessary for 10 min. In both, pseudocholinesterase activity was markedly diminished. It should be remembered that Kvisselgard and Moya found no demonstrable amounts of the drug in umbilical vein blood when the maternal dose was less than 300 mg.[94]; however, their patients had normal pseudocholinesterase activity.

Arthrogryposis following the treatment of maternal tetanus with muscle relaxants has been reported.[95] The patient developed tetanus during the 10th to 12th week of pregnancy and required curarization. A total of 1281 mg. had been given intramuscularly and intravenously over a 10-day period. Upon delivery, the infant was noted to have arthrogryposis multiplex congenita. According to Drachman and Banker, this may be seen in a number of pathological processes that immobilize the fetal limbs at some period during or shortly after the formation of the joints.[96] It is possible to produce arthrogryposis in chick embryos by intravenous curarization.[97]

HISTAMINE RELEASE CAUSED BY MUSCLE RELAXANTS

Histamine Release Following Succinylcholine Administration

Histamine release by succinylcholine has been suggested by occasional reports of bronchospasm associated with its use.[98–103] Additional manifestations include generalized skin rash, facial edema, and hypotension.[102,104–107] The case reported by Katz and Mulligan is typical: A 53-year-old woman received succinylcholine (80 mg.). Approximately 1 min. later, there were inspiratory and expiratory wheezes, a prolonged expiratory phase, and difficulty in ventilation requiring a peak inspiratory pressure greater than usual. Subsequently, the patient received a challenge dose of succinylcholine (10 mg.). Within 1 min.

wheezes and ventilatory difficulties recurred, lasting 12 min. An intradermal skin wheal was positive. Bronchospasm has also occurred when hexafluorenium was used with succinylcholine.[101]

Histamine Release Following *d*-Tubocurarine Administration

Although rare following succinylcholine, histamine release following intravenous curare is common. As early as 1936, occasional bronchospasm was associated with the use of curare.[108] Swelling of the eyelids, edema of the face and neck, giant hives over most of the body, and pharyngeal and epiglottic edema have all occurred after the injection of curare.[109] Histamine concentrations in the patient's blood may be more than twice that of pre-injection level.[109,110–112] Intracutaneous and intra-arterial injection of curare may produce wheals, flares, edema, and itching.[113–115] In the dog, a histamine-releasing agent causes similar bronchoconstriction, which may be blocked by pretreatment with an antihistamine.[116] The dose of curare injected is an important determinant of the magnitude of side effects caused by histamine release: Small doses of curare, (e.g., 0.1–0.2 mg./kg.) rarely are associated with clinical histamine release;[115] however, when large amounts (e.g., 0.6–0.7 mg./kg.) are injected rapidly, hypotension, erythema, and bronchospasm occur not uncommonly. Edema of the face, pharynx, and epiglottis is much less common, even after these large doses of curare. Many of these early studies used a curare preparation that we now know to be impure. It is difficult to tell whether the results observed by early workers were due to the curare per se or to the impurities. Nevertheless, it is clear that curare itself can release histamine and produce elevated plasma histamine levels in man. Several investigative groups have demonstrated a rise in plasma histamine in some of the patients they studied.[111,112,117] However, some patients who demonstrate clinical signs of histamine release do not show an increase in plasma histamine levels. It has been speculated that the plasma histamine concentrations are low, because of the marked uptake of histamine by the effector end organ.

In studies of airway resistance, marked increases occur in a small minority of patients given curare. For example, Landmesser reported a decrease in compliance in one of nine patients given curare,[118] while Westgate reported an increase in airway resistance in three of 23 patients.[119] However, more recent studies have found no significant or consistent changes in respiratory resistance. [120] Thus, bronchospasm and increased airway resistance occur only occasionally following the administration of curare.

Histamine Release Following Administration of Other Relaxants

Decamethonium, pancuronium, diallyl nortoxiferine, and gallamine have been reported to release histamine, but to a much lesser extent than curare.[121–124] Although implicated in one case,[122] various studies have found no increase in plasma histamine following use of pancuronium.[125,126]

CHANGES IN HEART RATE AND RHYTHM

Cardiovascular Effects of Succinylcholine

Shortly after its introduction into clinical practice, bradycardia following the injection of succinylcholine was reported in both adults[127] and children.[128] Besides bradycardia, sinus arrest and supraventricular and ventricular arrhythmias occur following repeated intravenous injection of succinylcholine in patients of all ages anesthetized with nitrous oxide, trichloroethylene, ether, halothane, and cyclopropane.[129–134] However, it is important to distinguish between bradycardia in children from that in adults. Bradycardia in children is often noted following the first dose of succinylcholine, whereas bradycardia in adults is rarely observed until after the second dose, when it occurs in more than 80 per cent of patients given doses at 5-min. intervals.[132,135]

In humans, several investigative groups[130,136,137] reported that atropine protects against cardiac slowing and arrhythmias after succinylcholine, though this has not been confirmed by others.[134,138,139] These conflicting results may be explained by different modes of administration of atropine. Intravenous atropine blocks succinylcholine-induced bradycardia; however, when given intramuscularly for premedication, atropine does not block the cardiac slowing.[134] When the interval between two doses of succinylcholine is less than 3 min. or greater than 30 min., arrhythmias are not seen; with an interval of 5 min., arrhythmias are consistently observed.

Craythorne[130] and Williams[134] suggested that the succinylcholine-induced bradycardia and arrhythmias in adults are caused by stimulation of the sympathetic and parasympathetic nervous system. That trimethaphan can suppress the circulatory responses to succinylcholine suggests that these responses are mediated by sympathetic and parasympathetic efferent nerves, rather than by a direct effect of succinylcholine on the heart or on vascular smooth muscle. The general anesthetic agents are also important. With thiopental or diethyl ether, the change in pulse rate produced by the first or subsequent doses of succinylcholine is variable. With halothane or cyclopropane, the first injection produces tachycardia, and the second commonly results in cardiac slowing. In one study, succinylcholine did not produce arrhythmias in five patients in whom anesthesia was induced with thiopental and maintained with halothane, but it did produce arrhythmias in five patients in whom anesthesia was induced and maintained with halothane. Furthermore, three of the patients in the latter group, after an injection of thiopental, no longer developed cardiac arrhythmias with repeated injections of succinylcholine.[133] Perhaps the rarity of cardiac arrhythmias after succinylcholine is related to the common use of thiopental for induction.

Patients who receive hexafluorenium also do not develop arrhythmias after succinylcholine; similarly, patients given acetylcholine do not develop arrhythmias after second doses of acetylcholine, but four of five patients given succinylcholine after acetylcholine developed bradycardia or asystole.[133] These results suggest that choline, which is produced by the hydrolysis of succinyldicholine to succinylmonocholine and choline, sensitizes the patient to subsequent doses of succinylcholine. Following sensitization by choline, the arrhythmias are produced by the entire succinylcholine molecule.

In more than one-third of patients given small amounts of succinylcholine injected directly into the common carotid artery and, thus, presumably, into the pressoreceptors of the carotid sinus, an immediate bradycardia occurred.[135] Therefore, it has been postulated that succinylcholine is able to stimulate peripheral sensory receptors, such as carotid sinus baroreceptors, and produce reflex bradycardia. Other investigators have demonstrated a stimulant action of acetylcholine on pressoreceptors and on other sensory receptors.[140–142]

There have been a number of studies of attempts to prevent the bradycardia produced by succinylcholine. Investigations involving atropine are discussed on page 566; the ability of hexafluorenium to prevent bradycardia following a second dose of succinylcholine is discussed above. Small doses of nondepolarizing agents also block bradycardia: curare, 5 mg.,[135,143,144] alcuronium, 3.5 mg.,[143,144] c-toxiferine, 0.4 mg.,[143] and pancuronium, 2 mg.[143]

Ventricular arrhythmias associated with succinylcholine have also been observed in cats, dogs, and monkeys. Galindo and Davis studied the effects of succinylcholine on the excitability of the heart, expressed in terms of the strength and duration of electrical current required to produce extrasystoles at various intervals of the cardiac cycle.[145] They observed in monkeys anesthetized with halothane that succinylcholine lowered the cardiac excitability threshold and produced severe ventricular arrhythmias. These were explained in terms of the following: changes in cell membrane permeability for potassium, with the loss of potassium from the cell, a decrease in resting membrane potential, and an increase in serum potassium; sympathetic postganglionic stimulation; and a direct effect on the myocardium. It was reported by Katz that succinylcholine produced cardiac arrhythmias in 45 per cent of decerebrate cats inhaling 1-per-cent halopropane.[4] Alpha-adrenergic blockade does not consistently prevent the arrhythmias produced by succinylcholine, but beta-adrenergic blockade does. Ganglionic blockers are also able to prevent these arrhythmias. Probably part of the effect in cats is caused by the release of acetylcholine and catecholamines owing to a ganglionic-stimulating action of succinylcholine.

Dowdy and Fabian found in digitalized cats,

dogs, and humans, that injection of succinylcholine could produce ventricular arrhythmias, some of which could be abolished by curare.[131] Subsequent studies by Perez,[146] List,[147] and this author did not confirm these results.

Cardiovascular Effects of Gallamine

Tachycardia and hypertension following the injection of gallamine have long been known[148] and are due to vagal blockade.[149] The injection of gallamine during cyclopropane anesthesia can produce ventricular arrhythmias in addition to tachycardia and hypertension.[150] Brown and Crout suggested that the tachycardia produced by gallamine might not be attributable solely to a vagal-blocking action of the drug, but that it might be due to the release of catecholamines from cardiac adrenergic nerves.[151,152] This was based on the demonstration that gallamine increased myocardial contractile force in ventricle of cats and that this could be blocked by propranolol. Furthermore, in guinea pigs pretreated with reserpine (which depleted catecholamines), the increase in myocardial contractile force produced by gallamine was inhibited.

More recently, there have been a number of studies of the cardiovascular effects of gallamine in humans. Heart rate, systolic pressure, and cardiac output increase, and peripheral vascular resistance decreases following gallamine in patients anesthetized with nitrous oxide and halothane.[153] Similar effects are noted during nitrous oxide and trichloroethylene anesthesia.[154] Eisele and colleagues found that the onset and extent of the increase in heart rate parallels the degree of neuromuscular block of the hand muscles after gallamine, though the increase outlasts the duration of neuromuscular block.[155] In one set of studies, they showed a progressive increase in heart rate after 20-mg. increments of gallamine, until a total of 60 mg. had been given. The average increase in heart rate at this point was approximately 90 per cent of the maximum increase obtained, which occurred with a cumulative dose of 100 mg. Additional gallamine did not increase the heart rate further. However, 2 mg. of atropine does produce a further increase in heart rate, thus indicating that gallamine dose not produce complete vagolysis. No changes in heart rate or blood pressure occurred when gallamine was given after 2 mg. of atropine. This suggests that inhibition of the cardiac vagus, although different from that caused by atropine, is the only cardiac effect of gallamine. In addition, the increase in heart rate and contractile force reported by Brown and Crout[151,152] is probably a phenomenon that occurs in guinea pigs and cats, but not in humans. Others have not demonstrated an increase in myocardial contractile force following gallamine in humans.[156,157] Thus, it would seem that the catecholamine release by gallamine that occurs in some species does not occur in humans.

An unusual study compared the effects of gallamine to curare in two groups of patients undergoing hysterectomy.[158] Although the two groups were not matched, a difference between the two relaxants in their effect on blood loss during hysterectomy was noted. The most likely cause is the higher heart rate, probably associated with a higher cardiac output, in the group that received gallamine.

Cardiovascular Effects of Pancuronium

Pancuronium was introduced partly because physicians believed that it would produce fewer cardiovascular effects than curare. The early studies showed little or no changes in heart rate or blood pressure.[159–161] However, subsequent studies found that there are increases in mean arterial pressure, heart rate, and cardiac output following pancuronium, and all of these can be prevented by the prior administration of atropine.[162–164] These differences in cardiovascular responses may be reconciled in the following fashion: In patients who receive a belladonna premedication and are anesthetized with moderate to deep levels of anesthesia, pancuronium produces little or no cardiovascular change. However, in lightly anesthetized patients not premedicated with belladonna drugs, pancuronium does increase heart rate, blood pressure, and cardiac output. The increase in heart rate produced by pancuronium is unrelated to the concentration of halothane or the doses of pancuronium.[165] Furthermore, there is no significant increase in pulse rate following pancuronium in patients who receive atropine (0.5–0.6 mg.). The maximum increase in heart rate occurs in patients who have the lowest heart rates immediately prior to injection of pancuronium. Recently, it was reported that in dogs pancuronium acts on postganglionic nerve endings and causes the release of norepinephrine; this was said to account for the tachycardia and hypertension sometimes seen with large doses of pancuronium.[166] These potentially adverse cardiovascular effects can be avoided by combining pancuronium, in smaller dosage, with either metocurarine or *d*-tubocurarine. Such combinations also demonstrate synergism in the neuromuscular blockade produced by the components, often used in remarkably small doses.[166a]

Cardiovascular Effects of *d*-Tubocurarine

The cardiovascular effects of curare are markedly different from those of gallamine or pancuronium. Shortly after its introduction into clinical practice, many physicians reported hypotension following injection of curare.[167,168] The fall in pressure is greater during halothane than during nitrous oxide anesthesia and increases with higher concentrations of halothane.[169,170] Although systolic pressure and total peripheral resistance are decreased commonly, effects on heart rate, stroke volume, and cardiac output are variable.[171–173] Despite the hypotension, there is no change in myocardial contractile force.[174]

There are a number of studies of the mechanism by which hypotension is produced by curare. It has been known since at least 1890 that curare has a ganglionic-blocking action and is capable of releasing histamine. To what degree hypotension can be attributed to each of these is still debatable. Curare produces only minor changes in blood pressure in dogs depleted of histamine.[175] However, in humans, pretreatment with antihistamines prevents hypotension in only 50 per cent of cases.[176] It is likely that hypotension following curare in humans is caused by a combination of histamine release and ganglionic blockade.

Dowdy reported a decrease in myocardial contractile force of the rabbit atrium perfused with curare.[177] However, more recent studies have shown that curare without preservative and antibacterial agent does not have a cardiac depressant effect.[178,179] Still other studies in humans found that, although the preservatives do not produce hypotension, curare can.[180] Therefore, hypotension associated with curare in humans, but not animals, is caused by curare itself and not by the preservative. The hypotension associated with curare, like the cardiovascular stimulation that accompanies pancuronium, can be avoided by combining small doses of curare and pancuronium.[166a]

MYOTONIC RESPONSE TO SUCCINYLCHOLINE

Myotonia is an inability to relax a muscle normally after a contraction and is attributable to repetitive discharge of the motor end-plate. The disorder is most commonly seen in the adductor of the thumb, and this is manifested by an inability of the patient to release his hand after shaking hands.

Generalized myotonia has been reported in patients with myotonia dystrophica and myotonia congenita following the injection of succinylcholine. Myotonia dystrophica is a hereditary disease usually beginning in middle or late life, characterized by myotonia, muscle wasting, cataract, testicular atrophy, and frontal baldness. Myotonia congenita is a familial disorder in which lifelong myotonia is present. The myotonia is often severe after excitement or anxiety. This disease is much more benign than myotonia dystrophica.

Patients with myotonia may develop generalized tonic contractions of all skeletal muscles following succinylcholine.[181–184] Ventilation, as well as tracheal intubation, may be difficult or impossible. This response is produced by all depolarizing agents.[185]

Not all myotonic patients respond to succinylcholine in this manner. There have been several reports of patients with myotonia who have responded to succinylcholine in a normal fashion or in whom only some of the muscles showed a myotonic response.[181,186–189]

If the anesthesiologist is presented with a

myotonic patient, it would be reasonable for him to avoid succinylcholine administration. If succinylcholine is necessary, a nondepolarizing agent should be available, in case a myotonic response occurs. Both the author and Baraka are aware of cases in which curare aborted the myotonic response to succinylcholine.[184]

NEOSTIGMINE AND LARGE BOWEL ANASTOMOSIS LEAKAGE

Bell and Lewis reported that neostigmine had an adverse effect on the integrity of iliorectal anastomoses.[190] They observed a high incidence of anastamotic leakage following intraoperative neostigmine, compared with a similar group of patients in whom cyclopropane anesthesia was administered and neostigmine was not used. They therefore suggested that neostigmine caused disruption of the intestinal anastomosis, possibly because of mechanical forces that pulled the suture material through the bowel wall or because of temporary ischemia of the bowel in the anastomotic areas. Subsequent studies in animals and in humans have failed to confirm these results.[191,192]

MUSCLE PAINS FOLLOWING SUCCINYLCHOLINE ADMINISTRATION

Shortly after succinylcholine was introduced into clinical practice, muscle pain was reported in association with its clinical use. Bourne stated in 1952 that the fasciculations caused by succinylcholine produced complaints of muscle stiffness postoperatively.[193] Subsequently, there have been numerous reports of muscle pain and stiffness following succinylcholine.[194–207] The pain and stiffness usually occur 12 to 24 hours after the patient has received succinylcholine,[196–200] but symptoms may appear as early as 3 hours postoperatively or as late as the 4th postoperative day.[201,202] The pain usually lasts 1 to 2 days but may occasionally persist for 5 to 6 days.[199,203] The sites most commonly involved are the neck and shoulders, chest, abdomen, and back. The jaw and limbs are sometimes also affected.[199–206] Pa-

tients frequently say that the pain and stiffness are similar to that observed following strenuous exercise of untrained muscles.[200,202,204,207] Before the relationship between succinylcholine and muscle pain was appreciated, these patients sometimes presented diagnostic problems and were thought to have pleurisy, meningitis, or poliomyelitis.[204,208] Even today, the muscle pain is sometimes mistakenly attributed to the hardness of the operating table or the uncomfortable position of the patient during operation. While both of these undoubtedly contribute to postoperative muscle pain, it is clear in many cases that the pain is caused mainly by succinylcholine.

Incidence of Muscle Pains Following Succinylcholine Administration

The frequency with which muscle pain has been reported varies from 0.7 to 89 per cent.[198,199,201,207,209–213] The differences in frequency depend upon the patient population studied. The incidence of muscle pain is higher in women than in men.[194,197–200,204] It varies with age: The highest incidence occurs in the 20- to 50-year-old age-group.[196,201,202,204,210,211] It was originally believed that muscle pains did not occur in children; however, Bush and Roth reported an incidence of 3 per cent in children 5 to 9 years of age and of 23 per cent in children 10 to 14 years of age.[196] The most important factors are the nature of the operative procedure and the time postoperatively when the patient is up and about. Patients undergoing minor operative procedures who are up and about in the immediate postoperative period have the highest incidence of muscle pains, compared to patients undergoing major operative procedures who stay in bed postoperatively.[199,200,202,206] Perhaps the best demonstration of this phenomenon can be seen in the study of Churchill-Davidson.[206] He reported muscle pain in 66 per cent of outpatients who received succinylcholine, but in only 14 per cent of inpatients who underwent similar procedures but were confined to the hospital for 48 hours.

The reported frequency of muscle pains is affected significantly by the time at which the patient is questioned and by whom the patient is questioned. In one study, 35 per cent of dental patients discharged from the hospital on the 1st postoperative day complained of pain on the day of discharge.[203] However, the frequency of complaints on the 5th postoperative day was 72 per cent. Thus, if one were studying outpatient anesthesia, patients would report little or no muscle pain when discharged on the operative day. However, a subsequent interview at the 3rd or 5th postoperative day would reveal a higher incidence of pain. The frequency of reports of muscle pain is also affected by the interviewer. For example, fewer patients complain about muscle pain to their physician than to the ward nurses.[210] This may be caused by a reluctance of the patient to complain to a physician to whom he feels indebted. Finally, a lower incidence of pain occurs in the well exercised patient compared to the less physically fit.[214]

Mechanism of Succinylcholine-Induced Muscle Pain

Although there are numerous reports on the subject of muscle pain, the mechanism by which succinylcholine produces pain and stiffness is not understood. Although the pain was thought originally to be related in some way to muscle fasciculations,[193] most investigators have been unable to correlate the incidence and magnitude of visible muscle fasciculations to the incidence and severity of pain. This lack of correlation, however, may be due to poor relationship between visible fasciculations and EMG-recorded fasciculations. However, Collier found a relationship with the frequency of motor unit function following succinylcholine.[215] There was a statistically significant association between postoperative symptoms and high-frequency discharge rates. In 39 of 42 patients with discharge frequencies greater than 50 Hz, typical succinylcholine-induced pains occurred. All of the patients in the study who developed symptoms (55%) displayed frequencies in the range of 48 to 72 Hz. Within this range, however, neither the severity nor the nature of the symptoms were directly related to the actual frequency. The occurrence of the symptoms is an "all or none" response that occurs above a certain threshold frequency. Collier suggested that the muscle pain is caused by

activation of muscle spindles, and this theory accounts for the finding that pain and stiffness are usually experienced in the back of the neck and lower chest: The highest counts of spindle density per gram of muscle are obtained in the small muscles of the neck, as well as in the lower intercostal muscles. Furthermore, muscle spindles have been found in virtually all striated muscles, and this could account for the generalized distribution of symptoms in some patients with severe pains. Collier further suggested that damage to the muscle spindles might account for the post-exertional pain and stiffness commonly seen after unaccustomed exercise, which is similar to the pain seen following succinylcholine. This theory is an interesting one but requires additional studies before it can be accepted as the main mechanism of muscle pain and stiffness.

Other mechanisms that have been suggested include mechanical damage to the muscle cell, the release of large amounts of lactic acid, release of potassium, and an effect produced by one of the breakdown products of succinylcholine, possibly succinylmonocholine.[2,4,212,213]

Another possibility recently suggested by Waters and Mapleson is unsynchronized contraction.[216] When a nerve is stimulated, there is a simultaneous uniform contraction of all muscle fibers. However, when the muscle is stimulated by succinylcholine, the fibers will eventually contract if the concentration of succinylcholine reaches an adequate level. If the concentration required for one fiber to contract is slightly different from that for another fiber, then an unsynchronized contraction may occur, the fascia may become deformed, and a shearing force may be applied to the connective tissue.

Shearing force produces damage, and pain follows later. On the basis of unsynchronized contraction, certain predictions can be made: With increasing doses, the degree of pain will increase, but if the dose becomes sufficiently large, there should be a decrease in the frequency of pain. The prior injection of a nondepolarizer should prevent the muscle pains, since many of the fibers are already paralyzed. Thus, the muscle twitching would be confined only to unblocked fibers, and, therefore, there would be less pain. If multiple doses are given, each dose will subject a portion of muscle fibers to the risk of damage. Therefore, the number of muscle fibers damaged will increase with the number of doses. Waters and Mapleson tested these hypotheses. In studying doses of 12.5 to 200 mg. of succinylcholine, they found an initial increase in frequency of pain as dosage increased, followed by a decrease as the dosage increased further. They also found that the prior injection of a nondepolarizer (gallamine, 20 mg.) decreased the incidence of pain. It was also observed that the degree of pain was higher with multiple doses than with a single dose. These workers concluded that succinylcholine-induced muscle pain is the result of damage produced in muscle by the unsynchronized contraction of adjacent muscle fibers just before the onset of paralysis.

Prevention of Succinylcholine-Induced Muscle Pains

There have been numerous attempts to prevent the muscle pain and stiffness, which in some patients may be extremely troublesome. Although several investigators reported that the slow injection of succinylcholine did not decrease the incidence of muscle pain, Lamoreaux and Urbach reported that a slow intravenous drip of 0.2-per-cent succinylcholine produced a 14-per-cent incidence of muscle pain, compared with a 40-per-cent incidence after the rapid intravenous injection of 50 mg. of succinylcholine.[207] The use of succinylcholine bromide rather than chloride did not decrease the incidence of muscle pains nor did chlorpromazine, atropine, and neostigmine.[203,211]

Morris and Dunn found that the prior intravenous injection of procaine (100–200 mg.) decreased the incidence of muscle pain from 72 to 44 per cent.[203] Usabiaga showed that the prior administration of lidocaine (6 mg./kg.) significantly reduced postoperative muscle pain in frequency, intensity, and duration.[217] It is, of course, obvious that 6 mg. per kg. is a rather large single dose of lidocaine to inject intravenously. It has recently been reported that a smaller dose of lidocaine, 3 to 4 mg. per kg., given intravenously, will decrease the incidence of muscle pain.[218] In

the control group who received thiopental (150–300 mg.), followed by succinylcholine (30–50 mg.), the incidence of pain was 52 per cent and was greatest in the 21- to 30-year-old age-group and lowest in children under 10. No pain was reported in the control group of patients over 50 years old. The group given lidocaine had an incidence of muscle pain of 14 per cent and experienced small but significant changes in blood pressure and pulse rate after lidocaine was administered.

Many studies have demonstrated that succinylcholine-induced muscle pain may be prevented by the prior injection of a nondepolarizing neuromuscular blocking agent: Gallamine (20–40 mg.) and curare (3–5 mg.) decrease the incidence in large groups of patients by at least half when given several minutes before succinylcholine.[203,207,211,213] However, if the nondepolarizing drug is given just before succinylcholine, it has no preventive effect.[200] One drawback of the prior injection of a nondepolarizer is that a larger dose of succinylcholine is necessary to produce the desired effect.[219] Approximately 50 per cent more succinylcholine is required when a dose of 3 to 5 mg. of curare or comparable doses of other nondepolarizers are injected prior to succinylcholine.[220]

Another approach to the prevention of succinylcholine muscle pains is the injection of hexafluorenium, which extends the action of succinylcholine by inhibition of pseudocholinesterase.[221]

Hexafluorenium may prevent pain by way of its weak nondepolarizing action or by inhibition of succinylcholine breakdown, so that the small dose of succinylcholine administered becomes, in effect, a large dose that does not produce muscle pain (Waters-Mapleson hypothesis).[216] Another drug that extends succinylcholine action, tetrahydroaminocrine (tacrine), has been reported by some but not all investigators to decrease the incidence of muscle pain.[222]

Whether thiopental prevents succinylcholine-induced muscle pain is controversial.[201,210,223] Craig reported a decrease in frequency of pain from 55 to 14 per cent.[202] It should be pointed out, however, that the dose of succinylcholine used in his study was 25 mg., and the dose of thiopental used was 4.7 mg. per kg. If the interval between thiopental and succinylcholine administration was 5 min., the incidence was reduced only from 55 to 41 per cent; but, if succinylcholine was given immediately after thiopental, the incidence of muscle pain was reduced to 14 per cent.

Another report stated that succinylcholine-induced muscle pains could be prevented by vitamin C,[224] which has been shown to alleviate pain and stiffness after strenuous exercise of untrained muscles.[225] Vitamin C is known to be essential for the proper formation of collagen and intracellular material, possibly helping to stabilize the muscle cell wall. A series of 240 patients undergoing endoscopy was studied. These patients were ambulatory 2 to 3 hours after anesthesia and therefore should have had a high incidence of muscle pain. Patients in the treated group received vitamin C, 1 g. per day, during the perioperative period. The patients remained in the hospital for 2 to 3 hours after the procedure and then went home. The patients were recalled to the hospital and interviewed on the 3rd postoperative day. In the control group, the incidence of muscle pain was 37 per cent; in the group given vitamin C, the incidence was 12 per cent. Before vitamin C can be recommended for routine use, however, additional clinical studies will be necessary, particularly since it has been recently reported that vitamin C did not prevent muscle pain produced by succinylcholine.[226] Diazepam (0.05 mg./kg.) was recently reported to decrease the incidence of succinylcholine muscle pain from 60 to 15 per cent.[227]

Significance of Muscle Pains Following Succinylcholine Administration

The significance of muscle pains following succinylcholine is often questioned. Are there adverse effects more serious than the discomfort caused by muscle stiffness and pain? Shibuya and colleagues suggests that this is so.[228] The muscle pain and stiffness in some patients prevents breathing deeply. They therefore studied the ventilatory effects of succinylcholine-induced muscle pain in three groups of patients: One group did not receive succinylcholine, one received 40 to 50 mg. of succinylcholine, and one

received 40 mg. of gallamine prior to succinylcholine. The only significant differences noted in ventilation were in the maximum voluntary ventilation (MVV) and the breathing reserve ratio (BRR), which were reduced in the group that received only succinylcholine. The other two groups did not report muscle pain. These differences in ventilation seemed related to the extent and distribution of painful muscles. The investigators suggested that such an inability to breathe deeply postoperatively following succinylcholine might contribute to morbidity and mortality, particularly in aged or debilitated patients.

To put the problem of muscle pain and its prevention in perspective, the following must be appreciated: The greatest incidence occurs in young patients undergoing brief procedures who are up and about in the immediate postoperative period. These patients are at great risk and, thus, the use of techniques designed to minimize the amount of muscle pain is indicated. Among the choices available are a small dose of nondepolarizer prior to succinylcholine, the prior injection of hexafluorenium or tetrahydroaminocrine, prior injection of lidocaine, and the injection of thiopental immediately before succinylcholine. It is, of course, possible to use combinations of these techniques. The choice will depend upon the training and experience of the practitioner. Although the use of preventive measures is clearly worthwhile in some patients, their routine use in all patients must be decried. There seems little point in taking preventive measures in aged patients undergoing major surgery who will not be up and about in the immediate postoperative period, since the incidence of muscle pain in these patients is low and similar to that observed in patients in whom preventive drugs and techniques are used. Therefore, the routine use of preventive drugs in all patients receiving succinylcholine does not seem logical.

OVERVIEW

The nature of a review of complications of relaxants is such that the reader may obtain a distorted view of these agents. Despite the many complications discussed, it is important to remember that the muscle relaxants are extremely safe drugs. They have a very wide margin of safety, perhaps greater than that for any other class of drugs. Relaxants have transformed the practice of medicine and made it possible to undertake operations that were once thought impossible.

REFERENCES

1. Foldes, F. F.: Muscle Relaxants in Anesthesiology. Springfield, Charles C Thomas, 1957.
2. Paton, W. D. M.: The effects of muscle relaxants other than muscular relaxation. Anesthesiology, 20:453, 1959.
3. Foldes, F. F.: Factors which alter the effects of muscle relaxants. Anesthesiology, 20:464, 1959.
4. Katz, R. L., and Katz, G. J.: Complications associated with the use of muscle relaxants. Clin. Anesth., 4:121, 1966.
5. Walts, L. F.: Complications of muscle relaxants. In Katz, R. L. (ed.): Muscle Relaxants. p. 209. Amsterdam, Excerpta Medica, 1975.
6. Miller, R. D.: Factors affecting the action of muscle relaxants. In Katz, R. L. (ed.): Muscle Relaxants. p. 163. Amsterdam, Excerpta Medica, 1975.
7. Moncrief, J. A.: Complications of burns. Ann. Surg., 147:443, 1958.
8. Allen, C. M., Cullen, W. G., and Gillies, D. M. M.: Ventricular fibrillation in a burned boy. Can. Med. Assoc. J., 84:432, 1961.
9. Tolmie, J. D., Joyce, T. H., and Mitchell, G. D.: Succinylcholine danger in the burned patient. Anesthesiology, 28:467, 1967.
10. Mazze, R. I., and Dunbar, R. W.: Intralingual succinylcholine administration in children: an alternative to intravenous and intramuscular routes? Anesth. Analg., 47:605, 1968.
11. Weintraub, H. D., Heisterkamp, D. V., and Cooperman, L. H.: Changes in plasma potassium concentration after depolarizing blockers in anesthetized man. Br. J. Anaesth., 41:1048, 1969.
12. Birch, A. A., Jr., Mitchell, G. D., Playford, G. A., et al.: Changes in serum potassium response to succinylcholine following trauma. J.A.M.A., 210:490, 1969.
13. Mazze, R. L., Escrue, H. M., and Houston, J. B.: Hyperkalemia and cardiovascular collapse following administration of succinylcholine to the traumatized patient. Anesthesiology, 31:540, 1969.
14. Roth, F., and Wüthrich, H.: The clinical importance of hyperkalemia following suxamethonium administration. Br. J. Anaesth., 41:311, 1969.
15. Cooperman, L. H., Strobel, G. E., Jr., and Kennell, E. M.: Massive hyperkalemia after administration of succinylcholine. Anesthesiology, 32:161, 1970.
16. Cooperman, L. H.: Succinylcholine-induced hyperkalemia in neuromuscular disease. J.A.M.A., 213:1867, 1970.
17. Stone, W. A., Beach, T. P., and Hamelberg, W.: Succinylcholine-danger in the spinal-cord-injured patient. Anesthesiology, 32:168, 1970.
18. Tobey, R. E.: Paraplegia, succinylcholine and cardiac arrest. Anesthesiology, 32:359, 1970.
19. Beach, T. P., Stone, W. A., and Hamelberg, W.: Circulatory collapse following succinylcholine: report of a patient with diffuse lower motor neuron disease. Anesth. Anagl., 50:431, 1971.
20. Tobey, R. E., Jacobsen, P. M., Kahle, C. T., et al.: The serum potassium response to muscle relaxants in neural injury. Anesthesiology, 37:332, 1972.
21. Genever, E. E.: Suxamethonium-induced cardiac arrest in unsuspected pseudohypertrophic muscular dystrophy. Br. J. Anaesth., 43:984, 1971.
22. Cowgill, D. B., Mostello, L. A., and Shapiro, H. M.: Encephalitis and a hyperkalemic response to succinylcholine. Anesthesiology, 40:409, 1974.
23. Smith, R. B., and Grenvik, A.: Cardiac arrest following succinylcholine in patients with central nervous system injuries. Anesthesiology, 33:558, 1970.
24. Powell, J. N.: Suxamethonium-induced hyperkalaemia in a uraemic patient. Br. J. Anaesth., 42:806, 1970.
25. Koide, M., and Waud, B. E.: Serum potassium concentrations after succinylcholine in patients with renal failure. Anesthesiology, 36:142, 1972.
26. Miller, R. D., Way, W. L., Hamilton, W. K., et al.: Succinylcholine-induced hyperkalemia in patients with renal failure? Anesthesiology, 36:138, 1972.
27. Walton, J. D., and Farman, J. V.: Suxamethonium, potassium and renal failure. Anaesthesia, 28:626, 1973.
28. Stovner, J., Endresen, R., and Bjelke, E.: Suxamethonium hyperkalaemia with different induction agents. Acta Anaesth. Scand., 16:46, 1972.
29. Dhanaraj, V. J., Narayanamurthy, J., Sitadevi, C., et al.: A study of the changes in serum potassium concentration with suxamethonium using different anaesthetic agents. Br. J. Anaesth., 47:516, 1975.
30. Walton, J. D., and Farman, J. V.: Suxamethonium hyperkalaemia in uraemic neuropathy. Anaesthesia, 28:666, 1973.
31. Powell, D. R., and Miller, R.: The effect of repeated doses of succinylcholine on serum potassium in patients with renal failure. Anesth. Analg., 54:746, 1975.
32. Schaner, P. J., Brown, R. L., Kirksey, T. D., et al.: Succinylcholine-induced hyperkalemia in burned patients—I. Anesth. Analg., 48:764, 1969.
33. Viby-Mogensen, J., Hanel, H. K., Hansen, E., et al.: Serum cholinesterase activity in burned patients. II: Anaesthesia, suxamethonium and hyperkalaemia. Acta Anaesth. Scand., 19:169, 1975.
34. Stone, W. A., Beach, T. P., and Hamelberg, W.: Succinylcholine-induced hyperkalemia in dogs with transected sciatic nerves or spinal cords. Anesthesiology, 32:515, 1970.
35. Gronert, G. A., and Theye, R. A.: Serum potassium changes after succinylcholine in swine with thermal trauma or sciatic nerve section. Can. Anaesth. Soc. J., 18:558, 1971.
36. Kendig, J. J., Bunker, J. P., and Endow, S.: Succinylcholine-induced hyperkalemia: effects of succinylcholine on resting potentials and electrolyte distribution in normal and denervated muscle. Anesthesiology, 36:132, 1972.
37. Gronert, G. A., Lambert, E. H., and Theye, R. A.: The responses of denervated skeletal muscle to succinylcholine. Anesthesiology, 39:13, 1973.
38. Katz, B., and Miledi, R.: The development of acetylcholine sensitivity in nerve-free segments of skeletal muscle. J. Physiol. (Lond.), 170:389, 1964.

39. Solandt, D. Y., Partridge, R. C., and Hunter, J.: The effect of skeletal fixation on skeletal muscle. J. Neurophysiol., 6:17, 1943.

40. Gronert, G. A., and Theye, R. A.: Pathophysiology of hyperkalemia induced by succinylcholine. Anesthesiology, 43:89, 1975.

41. Bali, I. M., Coppel, D. L., and Dundee, J. W.: The effect of nondepolarizing muscles relaxants on plasma potassium. Br. J. Anaesth., 47:505, 1975.

42. Viby-Mogensen, J., Hanel, H. K., Hansen, E., et al.: Serum cholinesterase activity in burned patients. I: Biochemical findings. Acta Anaesth. Scand., 19:159, 1975.

43. Bennike, K. A., and Jarnum, S.: Myoglobinuria with acute renal failure possibly induced by suxamethonium: a case report. Br. J. Anaesth., 36:730, 1964.

44. Jensen, K., Bennike, K. A., Hanel, H. K., et al.: Myoglobinuria following anaesthesia including suxamethonium. Br. J. Anaesth., 40:329, 1968.

45. McLaren, C. A. B.: Myoglobinuria following the use of suxamethonium chloride: a case report. Br. J. Anaesth., 40:901, 1968.

46. Auerback, V. H., DiGeorge, A. M., Mayer, B. W., et al: Rhabdomyolysis and hyperpyrexia in children after administration of succinylcholine. *In* Gordon, R. A., Britt, B. A., and Kalow, W. (ed.): International Symposium on Malignant Hyperthermia. p. 30. Springfield, Charles C Thomas, 1971.

47. Tammisto, T., and Airaksinen, M. M.: Suxamethonium-induced myoglobinuria. Br. J. Anaesth., 37:464, 1965.

48. Tammisto, T., and Airaksinen, M.: Increase of creatine kinase activity in serum as sign of muscular injury caused by intermittently administered suxamethonium during halothane anaesthesia. Br. J. Anaesth., 38:510, 1966.

49. Airaksinen, M. M., and Tammisto, T.: Myoglobinuria after intermittent administration of succinylcholine during halothane anesthesia. Clin. Pharmacol. Ther., 7:583, 1966.

50. Tammisto, T., Leikkonen, P., and Airaksinen, M.; The inhibitory effect of d-tubocurarine on the increase of serum-creatine-kinase activity produced by intermittent suxamethonium administration during halothane anaesthesia. Acta Anaesthesiol. Scand., 11:333, 1964.

51. Ryan, J. F., Kagen, L. J., and Hyman, A. I.: Myoglobinemia after a single dose of succinylcholine. N. Engl. J. Med., 285:824, 1971.

52. Ryan, J. F., and Papper, E. M.: Malignant fever during and following anesthesia. Anesthesiology, 32:196, 1970.

53. Hegab, E., Schiff, H. I., Smith, D. J., et al.: An electron microscopic study of normal and chronically denervated rat skeletal muscle following succinylcholine challenge. Anesth. Analg., 53:650, 1974.

54. Hofmann, H., and Lembeck, F.: The response of the external ocular muscles to curare, decamethonium and succinylcholine. Arch. Exp. Path. Pharmakol., 216:552, 1952.

55. Hofmann, H., and Holzer, H.: Die Wirkung von muskelrelxantien auf den intraokularen Druck. Klin. Mbl. Augenheik, 123:1, 1953.

56. Lincoff, H. A., Ellis, C. H., .DeVoe, A. G., et al.: The effect of succinylcholine on intraocular pressure. Am. J. Ophthalmol., 40:501, 1955.

57. Dillon, J. B., Sabawala, P., Taylor, D. B., et al.: Action of succinylcholine on extraocular muscles and intraocular pressure. Anesthesiology, 18:44, 1957.

58. Dillon, J. B., Sabawala, P., Taylor, D. B., et al.: Depolarizing neuromuscular blocking agents and intraocular pressure in vivo. Anesthesiology, 18:439, 1957.

59. Lincoff, H. A., Breinn, G. M., and DeVoe, A. G.: The effect of succinylcholine on the extraocular muscles. Am. J. Ophthalmol., 43:440, 1957.

60. Macri, F. J., and Grimes, P. A.: The effects of succinylcholine on the extraocular striate muscles and on the intraocular pressure. Am. J. Ophthalmol., 44:221, 1957.

61. Schwartz, H., and deRoetth, A.: Effect of succinylcholine on intraocular pressure in human beings. Anesthesiology, 19:112, 1958.

62. Craythorne, N. W. B., Rottenstein, H. S., and Dripps, R. D.: The effect of succinylcholine on intraocular pressure in adults, infants, children during general anesthesia. Anesthesiology, 21:59, 1960.

63. Lewallen, W. M., Jr., and Hicks, B. L.: The use of succinylcholine in ocular surgery. Am. J. Ophthalmol., 49:773, 1960.

64. Wretline, A., and Wahlin, A.: The effect of succinylcholine on the orbital musculature of the cat. Acta Anaesth. Scand., 3:101, 1959.

65. Sobel, A. M.: Hexafluorenium, succinylcholine and intraocular tension. Anesth. Analg. 41:399, 1962.

66. Katz, R. L., and Eakins, K. E.: A comparison of the effects of neuromuscular blocking agents and cholinesterase inhibitors on the tibialis anterior and superior rectus muscles of the cat. J. Pharmacol. Exp. Ther., 152:304, 1966.

67. Eakins, K. E., and Katz, R. L.: The action of succinylcholine on the tension of extraocular muscles. Br. J. Pharmacol., 26:205, 1966.

68. Katz, R. L., and Eakins, K. E.: Mode of action of succinylcholine on intraocular pressure. J. Pharmacol. Exp. Ther., 162:1, 1968.

69. Katz, R. L., and Eakins, K. E.: A comparison on the effects of neuromuscular blocking agents and cholinesterase inhibitors on the tibialis anterior and superior rectus muscles of the cat. J. Pharmacol. Exp. Ther., 152:304, 1966.

70. Katz, R. L., Eakins, K. E., and Lord, C. O.: The effects of hexafluorenium in preventing the increase in intraocular pressure produced by succinylcholine. Anesthesiology, 29:70, 1968.

71. Meyers, E. F., Krupin, T., Johnson, M., et al.: Failure of nondepolarizing neuromuscular blockers to inhibit succinylcholine-induced increased intraocular pressure, a controlled study. Anesthesiology, 48:149, 1978.

72. Carballo, A. S.: Succinylcholine and acetazolamide (diamox) in anaesthesia for ocular surgery. Can. Anaesth. Soc. J., 12:486, 1965.

73. Andersen, N.: Changes in intragastric pressure following the administration of suxamethonium: preliminary report. Br. J. Anaesth., 34:363, 1962.

74. Roe, R. B.: The effect of suxamethonium on intragastric pressure. Anaesthesia, 17:179, 1962.

75. La Cour, D.: Rise in intragastric pressure caused by suxamethonium fasciculations. Acta Anaesth. Scand., 13:255, 1969.

76. La Cour, D.: Prevention of rise in intragastric pressure due to suxamethonium fasciculations by prior dose of d-tubocurarine. Acta Anaesth. Scand., 14:5, 1970.

77. Miller, R. D., and Way, W. L.: Inhibition of suc-

cinylcholine-induced increased intragastric pressure by nondepolarizing muscle relaxants and lidocaine. Anesthesiology, *34*:185, 1971.

78. Marchand, P.: The gastro-oesophageal 'sphincter' and the mechanism of regurgitation. Br. J. Surg., *42*:504, 1955.

79. Greenan, J.: The cardio-oesophageal junction. Br. J. Anaesth., *33*:432, 1961.

80. Clark, C. G., and Riddoch, M. E.: Observations on the human cardia at operation. Br. J. Anaesth., *34*:875, 1962.

81. Sellick, B. A.: Cricoid pressure to control regurgitation of stomach contents during induction of anaesthesia. Lancet, *2*:404, 1961.

82. Salem, M. R., Wong, A. Y., and Lin, Y. H.: The effect of suxamethonium on the intragastric pressure in infants and children. Br. J. Anaesth., *44*:166, 1972.

83. Morris, R., and Giesecke, A. H., Jr.: Potentiation of muscle relaxants by magnesium sulfate therapy in toxemia of pregnancy. South. Med. J., *61*:25, 1968.

84. Giesecke, A. H., Jr., Morris, R. E., Dalton, M. D., et al.: Of magnesium, muscle relaxants, toxemic parturients, and cats. Anesth. Analg., *47*:689, 1968.

85. De Silva, A. J. C.: Magnesium intoxication: an uncommon cause of prolonged curarization. Br. J. Anaesth., *45*:1228, 1973.

86. Ghoneim, M. M., and Long, J. P.: The interaction between magnesium and other neuromuscular blocking agents. Anesthesiology, *32*:23, 1970.

87. Del Castillo, J., and Engbaek, L.: The nature of neuromuscular block produced by magnesium. J. Physiol. (Lond.), *124*:370, 1954.

88. Shnider, S. M.: Serum cholinesterase activity during pregnancy, labor and the puerperium. Anesthesiology, *26*:335, 1965.

89. Robertson, G. S.: Serum cholinesterase deficiency II: Pregnancy. Br. J. Anaesth., *38*:361, 1966.

90. MacDonald, A. G., and Graham, I. H.: Suxamethonium aponea in a pregnant patient. Br. J. Anaesth., *40*:711, 1968.

91. Wildsmith, J. A. W.: Serum pseudocholinesterase, pregnancy and suxamethonium. Anaesthesia, *27*:90, 1972.

92. Hazel, B., and Monier, D.: Human serum cholinesterase: variations during pregnancy and postpartum. Can. Anaesth. Soc. J., *18*:272, 1971.

93. Owens, W. D., and Zeitlin, G. L.: Hypoventilation in a newborn following administration of succinylcholine to the mother: a case report. Anesth. Analg., *54*:38, 1975.

94. Kvisselgaard, N., and Moya, F.: Investigation of placental thresholds to succinylcholine. Anesthesiology, *22*:7, 1961.

95. Jago, R. H.: Arthrogryposis following treatment of maternal tetanus with muscle relaxants. Arch. Dis. Child., *45*:277, 1970.

96. Drachman, D. B., and Banker, D. Q: Arthrogryposis multiplex congenita. Arch. Neurol., *5*:77, 1961.

97. Drachman, D. B., and Coulombre, A. J.: Experimental clubfoot and arthrogryposis multiplex congenita. Lancet, *2*:523, 1962.

98. Fellini, A. A., Bernstein, R. L., and Zauder, H. L.: Bronchospasm due to suxamethonium. Br. J. Anaesth., *35*:657, 1963.

99. Smith, N. L.: Histamine release by suxamethonium. Anaesthesia, *12*:293, 1957.

100. Selvin, B., and Howland, W. S.: Bronchospasm associated with the use of a combination of succinylcholine and Mylaxen to produce muscle relaxation. Anesth. Analg., *38*:332, 1959.

101. Mostert, J. W., and Kundig, H.: Experimental study of arrhythmias and bronchospasm associated with the use of hexafluorenium. Br. J. Anaesth., *36*:83, 1964.

102. Kepes, E. R., and Haimovici, H.: Allergic reaction to succinylcholine. J.A.M.A., *171*:548, 1959.

103. Mandappa, J. M., Chandrasekhara, P. M., and Nelvigi, R. G.: Anaphylaxis to suxamethonium. Br. J. Anaesth., *47*:523, 1975.

104. Jerums, G., Whittingham, S., and Wilson, P.: Anaphylaxis to suxamethonium. Br. J. Anaesth., *39*:73, 1967.

105. Eustace, B. R.: Case report: suxamethonium induced bronchospasm. Anaesthesia, *22*:638, 1967.

106. Bele-Binda, N., and Valeri, F.: A case of bronchospasm induced by succinylcholine. Can. Anaesth. Soc. J., *18*:116, 1971.

107. Katz, A. M., and Mulligan, P. G.: Bronchospasm induced by suxamethonium. Br. J. Anaesth., *44*:1097, 1972.

108. West, R.: Intravenous curarine in the treatment of tetanus. Lancet, *1*:12, 1936.

109. Westgate, H. D., Schultz, E. A., and Van Bergen, F. H.: Urticaria and angioneurotic edema following d-tubocurarine administration. Anesthesiology, *22*:286, 1961.

110. Alam, M., Anrep, G. V., Barsoum, G. S., et al.: Liberation of histamine from the skeletal muscle by curare. J. Physiol. (Lond.), *95*:148, 1939.

111. Gerecke, W. B., Imasato, Y., and Keats, A. S.: Histamine release by drugs used in association with anesthesia in man. p. 127. Abstract of Scientific Papers, ASA Meeting, 1969.

112. Miyashita, K.: The release of histamine in the blood following the administration of pancuronium bromide in man. Jap. J. Anesth., *20*:947, 1971.

113. Comroe, J. H., and Dripps, R. D.: The histamine-like action of curare and tubocurarine injected intracutaneously and intra-arterially in man. Anesthesiology, *7*:260, 1946.

114. Grob, D., Lilienthal, J. L., Jr., and Harvey, A. M.: On certain vascular effects of curare in man. "Histamine" reaction. Bull. Johns Hopkins Hosp., *80*:299, 1947.

115. Mongar, J. L., and Whelan, R. F.: Histamine release by adrenaline and d-tubocurarine in the human subject. J. Physiol. (Lond.), *120*:146, 1953.

116. Landmesser, C. M.: A study of the bronchoconstrictor and hypotension actions of curarizing drugs. Anesthesiology, *8*:506, 1947.

117. Westgate, H. D., and Van Bergen, F. H.: Changes in histamine blood levels following d-tubocurarine administration. Can. Anaesth. Soc. J., *9*: 497, 1962.

118. Landmesser, C. M., Converse, J. G., and Harmel, M. H.: Quantitative evaluation of the bronchoconstrictor action of curare in the anesthetized patient: a preliminary report. Anesthesiology, *13*:275, 1952.

119. Westgate, H. D., Gordon, J. R., and Van Bergen, F. H.: Changes in airway resistance following intravenously administered d-tubocurarine. Anesthesiology, *23*:65, 1962.

120. Gerbershagen, H. U., and Bergman, N. A.: The effect of d-tubocurarine on respiratory resistance in anesthetized man. Anesthesiology, *28*:981, 1967.

121. Sniper, W.: The estimation and comparison of histamine release by muscle relaxants in man. Br. J. Anaesth., *24*:232, 1952.

122. Buckland, R. W., and Avery, A. F.: Histamine release following pancuronium: a case report. Br. J. Anaesth., 45:518, 1973.

123. Mushin, W. W., Wien, R., Mason, D. F. J., et al.: Curare-like actions of tri (Diethylaminoethoxy)-benzene triethyliodide. Lancet, 1:726, 1949.

124. Stovner, J., and Lund, I.: Alloferin, et nytt muskelrelaxans i anesthesien. Nord. Med., 72:1505, 1964.

125. Buckett, W. R., Marjoribanks, C. E. B., Marwick, F. A., et al.: The pharmacology of pancuronium bromide (org. NA97), a new potent steroidal neuromuscular blocking agent. British Journal of Pharmaceutical Chemotherapy, 32:671, 1968.

126. Dobkin, A. B., Arnadia, H. Y., and Levy, A. A.: Effect of pancuronium bromide on plasma histamine levels in man. Anesth. Analg., 52:772, 1973.

127. Phillips, H. S.: Physiologic changes noted with the use of succinylcholine chloride, as a muscle relaxant during endotracheal intubation. Anesth. Analg., 33:165, 1954.

128. Leigh, M. D., McCoy, D. D., Belton, M. K., et al.: Bradycardia following intravenous administration of succinylcholine chloride to infants and children. Anesthesiology, 18:698, 1957.

129. Barreto, R. S.: Effect of intravenously administered succinylcholine upon cardiac rate and rhythm. Anesthesiology, 21:401, 1960.

130. Craythorne, N. W. B., Turndorf, H., and Dripps, R. D.: Changes in pulse rate and rhythm associated with the use of succinylcholine in anesthetized children. Anesthesiology, 21:465, 1960.

131. Dowdy, E. G., and Fabian, L. W.: Ventricular arrhythmias induced by succinylcholine in digitalized patients. Anesth. Analg., 42:501, 1963.

132. Lupprian, K. G., and Churchill-Davidson, H. C.: Effect of suxamethonium on cardiac rhythm. Br. Med. J., 2:1774, 1960.

133. Schoenstadt, D. A., and Whitcher, C. E.: Observations on the mechanism of succinyldicholine-induced cardiac arrhythmias. Anesthesiology, 24:358, 1963.

134. Williams, C. H., Deutsch, S., Linde, H. W., et al.: Effects of intravenously administered succinylcholine on cardiac rate, rhythm and arterial blood pressure in anesthetized man. Anesthesiology, 22:947, 1961.

135. Mathias, J. A., and Evans-Prosser, C.: An investigation into the site of action of suxamethonium on cardiac rhythm. p. 1153. Proceedings of IVth World Congress of Anaesthesiologists, London, 1968.

136. Bullough, J.: Intermittent suxamethonium injections. Br. Med. J., 1:786, 1959.

137. Foster, B.: Suxamethonium and cardiac rhythm. Br. Med. J., 1:129, 1961.

138. Verner, I., and Comty, C.: Intermittent suxamethonium injections. Br. Med. J., 1:1239, 1959.

139. Stoelting, R. K., and Peterson, C.: Heart-rate slowing and junctional rhythm following intravenous succinylcholine with and without intramuscular atropine preanesthetic medicine. Anesth. Analg., 54:705, 1975.

140. Daly, M. B.: Acetylcholine and transmission at chemoreceptors. Pharmacol. Rev., 6:79, 1954.

141. Douglas, W. W., and Gray, J. A. B.: The excitant action of acetylcholine and other substances on cutaneous sensory pathways and its prevention by hexamethonium and d-tubocurarine. J. Physiol. (Lond.), 119:118, 1953.

142. Diamond, J.: Observations on the excitation by acetylcholine and by pressure of sensory receptors in the cat's carotid sinus. J. Physiol. (Lond.), 130:513, 1955.

143. Mathias, J. A., Evans-Prosser, C. D. G., and Churchill-Davidson, H. C.: The role of the non-depolarizing drugs in the prevention of suxamethonium bradycardia. Br. J. Anaesth., 42:609, 1970.

144. Karhunen, U., Heinonen, J., and Tammisto, T.: The effect of tubocurarine on suxamethonium-induced rate and rhythm. Acta Anaesth. Scand., 16:3, 1972.

145. Galindo, A. H., and Davis, T. B.: Succinylcholine and cardiac excitability. Anesthesiology, 23:32, 1962.

146. Perez, H. R.: Cardiac arrhythmia after succinylcholine. Anesth. Analg., 49:33, 1970.

147. List, W. F. M.: Succinylcholine induced cardiac arrhythmias. Anesth. Analg., 50:361, 1971.

148. Bovet, D., Depiette, F., Courvoisier, S., et al.: Recherches sur les poisons curarisants de synthese. Arch. Int. Pharmacodyn., 80:172, 1949.

149. Riker, W. F., Jr., and Wescoe, W. C.: The pharmacology of Flaxedil, with observations on certain analogs. Ann. N.Y. Acad. Sci., 54:373, 1951.

150. Walts, L. F., and Prescott, F. S.: The effects of gallamine on cardiac rhythm during general anesthesia. Anesth. Analg., 44:265, 1965.

151. Brown, B. R., and Crout, J. R.: The sympathomimetic effect of gallamine on the heart. Anesthesiology, 29:179, 1968.

152. Brown, B. R., Jr., and Crout, J. R.: The sympathomimetic effect of gallamine on the heart. J. Pharmacol. Exp. Ther., 172:266, 1970.

153. Smith, N. T., and Whitcher, C. E.: Hemodynamic effects of gallamine and tubocurarine administered during halothane anesthesia. J.A.M.A., 199:114, 1967.

154. Kennedy, B. R., and Farman, J. V.: Cardiovascular effects of gallamine triethiodide in man. Br. J. Anaesth., 40:773, 1968.

155. Eisele, J. H., Marta, J. A., and Davis, H. S.: Quantitative aspects of the chronotropic and neuromuscular effects of gallamine in anesthetized man. Anesthesiology, 35:630, 1971.

156. Longnecker, D. E., Stoelting, R. K., and Morrow, A. G.: Cardiac and peripheral vascular effects of gallamine in man. Anesth. Analg., 52:931, 1973.

157. Reitan, J. A., Fraser, A. I., and Eisele, J. H.: Lack of cardiac inotropic effects of gallamine in anesthetized man. Anesth. Analg., 52:974, 1973.

158. Casale, F. F., and Farman, J. V.: Blood loss during hysterectomy associated with the use of tubocurarine or gallamine. Br. J. Anaesth., 42:65, 1970.

159. Baird, W. L. M., and Reid, A. M.: The neuromuscular blocking properties of a new steroid compound, pancuronium bromide. Br. J. Anaesth., 39:775, 1967.

160. McDowell, S. A., and Clarke, R. S. J.: A clinical comparison of pancuronium with d-tubocurarine. Anaesthesia, 24:581, 1969.

161. McIntyre, J. W. R., and Gain, E. A.: Initial experience during the clinical use of pancuronium bromide. Anesth. Analg., 50:813, 1971.

162. Kelman, G. R., and Kennedy, B. R.: Cardiovascular effects of pancuronium in man. Br. J. Anaesth., 43:335, 1971.

163. Stoelting, R. K.: The hemodynamic effects of pancuronium and d-tubocurarine in anesthetized patients. Anesthesiology, 36:612, 1972.

164. Coleman, A. J., Downing, J. W., Leary, W. P., et al.: The

immediate cardiovascular effects of pancuronium, alcuronium and tubocurarine in man. Anaesthesia, 27:415, 1972.

165. Miller, R. D., Eger, E. I., Stevens, W. C., et al.: Pancuronium-induced tachycardia in relation to alveolar halothane, dose of pancuronium, and prior atropine. Anesthesiology, 42:352, 1975.

166. Domenech, J. S., Garcia, R. C., Sasiaen, J. M. R., et al.: Pancuronium bromide: an indirect sympathomimetic agent. Br. J. Anaesth., 48:1143, 1976.

166a. Lebowitz, P. W., Ramsey, F. M., Savarese, J. J., et al: Potentiation of neuromuscular blockade in man produced by combinations of pancuronium and metocurine of pancuronium and d-tubocurarine. Anesth. Analg., 59:604, 1980.

167. Cullen, S. C.: The use of curare for the improvement of abdominal muscle relaxation during inhalation anesthesia. Surgery, 14:261, 1943.

168. Whitacre, R. J., and Fisher, A. J.: Clinical observations on the use of curare in anesthesia. Anesthesiology, 6:124, 1945.

169. Stoelting, R. K., and Longnecker, D. E.: Influence of end-tidal halothane concentration on d-tubocurarine hypotension. Anesth. Analg., 51:364, 1972.

170. Munger, W. L., Miller, R. D., and Stevens, W. C.: The dependence of d-tubocurarine-induced hypotension on alveolar concentration of halothane, dose of d-tubocurarine, and nitrous oxide. Anesthesiology, 40:442, 1974.

171. Smith, N. T., Whitcher, C. E.: Hemodynamic effects of gallamine and tubocurarine administered during halothane anesthesia. J.A.M.A., 199:144, 1967.

172. Stoelting, R. K.: The hemodynamic effects of pancuronium and d-tubocurarine in anesthetized patients. Anesthesiology 36:612, 1972.

173. Coleman, A. J., Downing, J. W., Leary, W. P., et al.: The immediate cardiovascular effects of pancuronium, alcuronium and tubocurarine in man. Anaesthesia 27:415, 1972.

174. Longnecker, D. E., Stoelting, R. K., and Morrow, A. G.: Cardiac and peripheral vascular effects of d-tubocurarine in man. Anesth. Analg., 49:660, 1970.

175. Lee, D. C., and Johnson, D. L.: Effects of d-tubocurarine and anesthesia upon cardiac output in histamine depleted dogs. Fed. Proc., 29:2804, 1970.

176. Stoelting, R. K., and Longnecker, D. E.: Effect of promethazine on hypotension following d-tubocurarine use in anesthetized patients. Anesth. Analg., 51:509, 1972.

177. Dowdy, E. G., Dugger, P. N., and Fabian, L. W.: Neuromuscular blocking agents on isolated digitalized mammalian hearts. Anesth. Analg., 44:608, 1965.

178. Dowdy, E. G., Holland, W. C., Yamanaka, I., et al.: Cardioactive properties of d-tubocurarine with and without preservatives. Anesthesiology, 34:256, 1971.

179. Carrier, O., Jr., and Murphy, J. C.: The effects of d-tubocurarine and its commercial vehicles on cardiac function. Anesthesiology, 33:627, 1970.

180. Stoelting, R. K.: Blood-pressure responses to d-tubocurarine and its preservatives in anesthetized patients. Anesthesiology, 35:315, 1971.

181. Kaufman, L.: Anaesthesia in dystrophia myotonica. Proc. R. Soc. Med., 53:183, 1960.

182. Paterson, I. S.: Generalized myotonia following suxamethonium. Br. J. Anaesth., 34:340, 1962.

183. Thiel, R. E.: The myotonic response to suxamethonium. Br. J. Anaesth., 39:815, 1967.

184. Baraka, A., Haddad, C., Afifi, A., et al.: Control of succinylcholine-induced myotonia by d-tubocurarine. Anesthesiology, 33:669, 1970.

185. Örndahl, G.: Myotonic human musculature: stimulation with depolarizing agents. II. A clinicopharmacological study. Acta Med. Scand., 172:753, 1962.

186. Bourke, T. D., and Zuck, D.: Thiopentone in dystrophia myotonica. Br. J. Anaesth., 29:35, 1957.

187. Haley, F. C.: Anaesthesia in dystrophia myotonia. Can. Anaesth. Soc. J., 9:270, 1962.

188. Cobham, I. G., and Davis, H. S.: Anesthesia for muscle dystrophy patients. Anesth. Analg., 43:22, 1964.

189. Talmage, E. A., and McKechnie, F. B.: Anesthetic management of patient with myotonia dystrophica. Anesthesiology, 20:717, 1959.

190. Bell, C. M., and Lewis, C. B.: Effects of neostigmine on integrity of ileorectal anastomoses. Br. Med. J., 3:587, 1968.

191. Wilkins, J. L., Hardcastle, J. D., Mann, C. V., et al.: Effects of neostigmine and atropine on motor activity of ileum, colon, and rectum of anaesthetized subjects. Br. Med. J., 1:793, 1970.

192. Cofer, T. W., Jr., Ray, J. E., and Gathright, J. B., Jr.: Does neostigmine cause disruption of large-intestinal anastomoses?: A negative answer. Dis. Colon. Rectum, 17:235, 1974.

193. Bourne, J. G., Collier, H. O. J., and Somers, G. F.: Succinylcholine. Lancet, 1:1225, 1952.

194. Currie, T. T.: Subcostal pain following controlled respiration. Br. Med. J., 1:1032, 1953.

195. Sanger, C.: Subcostal pain following controlled respiration. Br. Med. J., 1:1162, 1953.

196. Bush, G. H., and Roth, F.: Muscle pains after suxamethonium chloride in children. Br. J. Anaesth., 33:151, 1961.

197. Enderby, G. E. H.: Low incidence of muscle pain after suxethonium bromide (Brevidil E). Br. J. Anaesth., 31:530, 1959.

198. Hegarty, P.: Postoperative muscle pains. Br. J. Anaesth., 28:209, 1956.

199. Parbrook, G. D., and Pierce, G. F. M.: Comparison of postoperative pain and stiffness after the use of suxamethonium and suxethonium compounds. Br. Med. J., 2:579, 1960.

200. White, D. C.: Observations on the prevention of muscle pain after suxamethonium. Br. J. Anaesth., 34:332, 1962.

201. Burtles, R., and Tunstall, M. E.: Suxamethonium chloride and muscle pains. Br. J. Anaesth., 33:24, 1961.

202. Craig, H. J. L.: The protective effect of thiopentone against muscular pain and stiffness which follows the use of suxamethonium chloride. Br. J. Anaesth., 36:312, 1965.

203. Morris, D. D. B., and Dunn, C. H.: Suxamethonium chloride administration and postoperative muscle pain. Br. Med. J., 1:383, 1957.

204. Leatherdale, R. A. L., Mayhew, R. A. J., and Hayton-Williams, D. S.: Incidence of muscle pain after short-acting relaxants. Br. Med. J., 1:904, 1959.

205. Bryson, T. H. L., and Ormston, T. O. G.: Muscle pains following the use of suxamethonium in caesarean section. Br. J. Anaesth., 34:476, 1962.

206. Churchill-Davidson, H. C.: Suxamethonium (succinyl-

choline) chloride and muscle pains. Br. Med. J., *1*:74, 1954.

207. Lamoreaux, L. F., and Urbach, K. F.: Incidence and prevention of muscle pain following the administration of succinylcholine. Anesthesiology, *21*:394, 1960.

208. Price, J. M.: Suxamethonium and muscular pain. Br. Med. J., *1*:273, 1954.

209. Edmonds-Seal, J., and Eve, N. H.: Minor sequelae of anaesthesia: a pilot study. Br. J. Anaesth., *34*:44, 1962.

210. Burtles, R.: Muscle pains after suxamethonium and suxethonium. Br. J. Anaesth., *33*:147, 1961.

211. Foster, C. A.: Muscle pains that follow administration of suxamethonium. Br. Med. J., *2*:24, 1960.

212. Bennike, K., and Nielson, E.: Muscle pain following suxamethonium. Danish Med. Bull., *11*:122, 1964.

213. Mayrhofer, O.: Die wirksamkeit con d-Tubocurarin zur verhutung der muskelschmerzen nach succinylcholin. Der Anaesthetist, *8*:1313, 1959.

214. Newman, P. T. F., and Loudon, J. M.: Muscle pain following administration of suxamethonium: the aetiological role of muscular fitness. Br. J. Anaesth., *38*:533, 1966.

215. Collier, C.: Suxamethonium pains and fasciculations. Proc. R. Soc. Med., *68*:105, 1975.

216. Waters, D. J., and Mapleson, W. W.: Suxamethonium pains: hypothesis and observations. Anaesthesia, *26*:127, 1971.

217. Usubiaga, J. E., Wikinski, J. A., Usubiaga, L. E., et al.: Intravenous lidocaine in the prevention of postoperative muscle pain caused by succinylcholine administration. Anesth. Analg., *46*:225, 1967.

218. Haldia, D. A., Chatterji, S., and Kackar, S. N.: Intravenous lignocaine for prevention of muscle pain after succinylcholine. Anesth. Analg., *52*:849, 1973.

219. Walts, L. F., and Dillon, J. B.: Clinical studies of the interaction between d-tubocurarine and succinylcholine. Anesthesiology, *31*:39, 1969.

220. Cullen, D. J.: The effect of pretreatment with nondepolarizing muscle relaxants on the neuromuscular blocking action of succinylcholine. Anesthesiology, *35*:572, 1971.

221. Foldes, F. F., Monte, A. P., Brunn, H. M., Jr., et al.: Studies with muscle relaxants in unanesthetized subjects. Anesthesiology, *22*:230, 1961.

222. Buley, R., Morgan, M., and Page, P.: Influence of tetrahydroaminacrine on muscle pains after suxamethonium. S. Afr. Med. J., *49*:85, 1975.

223. Ruddell, J. S.: Muscle pain after short acting relaxants. Br. Med. J., *1*:1623, 1959.

224. Gupte, S. R., and Savant, N. S.: Post suxamethonium pains and vitamin C. Anaesthesia, *26*:436, 1971.

225. Syed, I. H.: Muscle stiffness and Vitamin C. Br. Med. J., *2*:304, 1966.

226. Wood, J. B., Altwood, E. C., Wood, B. M., et al.: Vitamin C and postsuxamethonium pains. Anaesthesia, *32*:21, 1977.

227. Fahmy, N. R., and Malek, N. S.: Adverse effects of succinylcholine administration: their modification by diazepam. p. 177. Abstracts of Scientific Papers, 1976 ASA meeting.

228. Shibuya, J., Cuevo, N., Quarnstrom, F. C., et al.: Ventilatory disturbances resulting from muscle pain following the administration of succinylcholine chloride. Med. Ann. D. C., *37*:457, 1968.

FURTHER READING

Walts, L. F.: Complications of muscle relaxants. *In* Katz, R. L. (ed.): Muscle Relaxants. pp. 209–244. Amsterdam, Excerpta Medica, 1975.

46 Complications of Hyperbaric Oxygenation

Christopher W. Dueker, M.D.

The treatment of various disorders with increased atmospheric pressure has a complex history. In the 1920s, the popularity of compressed air therapy reached a peak, with the construction of entire hospitals designed for compression. These facilities mercifully became scrap iron, and hyperbaric therapy became less popular, except for its valuable employment in the treatment of decompression sickness and traumatic cerebral air embolism.

Early hyperbaric treatment used air. Even at five times normal pressure, the oxygen thus supplied did not exceed that available by administering pure oxygen at normal atmospheric pressure. In the 1950s, a revival of hyperbaric therapy began with the use of oxygen rather than air. It was widely recommended for use in radiation therapy, cardiac surgery, and many disease states.

Hyperbaric oxygen is obviously quite different from compressed air and is a valuable contribution to our armamentarium. Unfortunately, many of the claims made of hyperbaric oxygen therapy did not prove to be valid. Today, the popularity of hyperbaric oxygenation is again more restricted. Hyperbaric therapy is of great value in decompression sickness, arterial air embolism, carbon monoxide poisoning, and clostridial gas gangrene. Intensive investigation is concentrated on expanding its range of usefulness and minimizing the hazards associated with high-pressure environments.

Anesthesiologists may be involved in the care of surgical patients receiving general anesthesia in hyperbaric chambers. More frequently, they provide respiratory support to critically ill patients being treated with hyperbaric oxygenation.

Even an elementary familiarity with hyperbaric therapy requires some knowledge of the environment in which such therapy is provided. Chambers range in size from one-person tanks to those large enough for surgery. Regardless of size, they are closed spaces with limited access. Rapid transfer of personnel is not possible, because of the need for compression or decompression.

Increased gas pressure, which forms the basis of hyperbaric therapy, introduces several problems that dictate procedures for compression and decompression. Direct effects of pressure increase the risk of fire, cause barotrauma, and alter performance of anesthetic equipment. Indirect effects of pressure lead to decompression sickness, inert gas narcosis, and oxygen poisoning. These effects interact to limit the tolerance of patients and therapists to hyperbaric exposure.

Pressure within a chamber can be expressed in several, somewhat confusing ways. At sea level, a pressure gauge reads zero, but the atmosphere actually exerts a force of 760 torr (101.1 kPa) or 14.7 p.s.i. This pressure is called *one atmosphere absolute (ATA)*. Doubling the pressure creates two atmospheres absolute or one atmosphere gauge. Because of similarities to diving, the magnitude of pressurization is frequently stated as equivalent feet of salt water. Descent through each 33 ft. of salt water adds 14.7 p.s.i. to total pressure. Pressure expressed in feet of sea water can then be converted to atmospheres by dividing by 33 ft. This gives gauge atmospheres; to get absolute atmospheres, 1 must be added to this. It is the absolute pressure that is important; hence, pressures expressed herein will be in atmospheres absolute (ATA), unless otherwise noted.

FIRES AND EXPLOSIONS

Fire is a catastrophic risk in all operations performed in a hyperbaric chamber. At best, fire is dangerous in any small, closed space in which immediate evacuation is not possible. Further, during therapy, not every person in the chamber has the freedom from other duties necessary to help fight a fire. Finally, an oxygen-enriched environment supports combustion vigorously.

A fire ignites more easily (e.g., there is a lower temperature of ignition) and then burns more rapidly in an oxygen-enriched environment. Chambers are therefore dangerous in two ways: They may contain a higher percentage of oxygen, and the increased total pressure raises the partial pressure of a given oxygen percentage. Both percentage and partial pressure are important in determining fire hazard.

In general, a given partial pressure of oxygen mixed with an inert gas is more dangerous at lower rather than higher total pressures. That is, 2 ATA of pure oxygen burns more rapidly than air at 10 ATA, which would also contain 2 atm. of oxygen. The inert gas dampens combustion.

Gases with higher thermal conductivity cause greater elevation of the threshold for ignition. More heat is necessary to ignite flammable material in helium and oxygen than in nitrogen and oxygen.

Fire prevention requires stringent efforts to eliminate sources of ignition and fuel. Unless the gases are inherently flammable, sparking appears to be a minor risk. However, electrical arcs and local sources of heat are more difficult to eliminate.

Unfortunately, the very presence of a human provides fuel. The risk is minimized by using treated flameproof clothing, mattresses, blankets, and paint. However, materials that do not burn at sea level may burn under increased pressure.

The careful regulation of oxygen concentration in the chamber represents the best hope for fire protection. Oxygen concentrations below 5 per cent do not support combustion, regardless of total pressure.[1] This concentration is useful at depths in excess of 4 ATA. Even at only 2 ATA, an oxygen concentration of 10 per cent sustains life normally and markedly reduces combustibility, while the patient receives a higher concentration.

During most therapy, only the patient breathes oxygen, while the chamber is filled with air. Exhalation from the patient, however, usually raises the chamber oxygen level to 25 per cent. This small increment increases the burning rate by 25 per cent. Therefore, the patient's exhalations should be vented outside the chamber.

Anesthetic flammability under hyperbaric conditions has not been evaluated thoroughly. Theoretically, potent flammable agents might not be dangerous, since they would be used in very low concentrations because of the elevated total pressure. However, the introduction of halogenated agents has obviated the use of flammable agents. Halothane is probably the most widely used inhalation anesthetic for hyperbaric anesthesia. Halothane in concentrations up to 49 torr (6.5% surface equivalent) does not burn in oxygen with a total pressure of 4 ATA,[2] whereas higher partial pressures of halothane will burn at this pressure. Yet, halothane concentrations that are safe in oxygen alone may burn briskly in oxygen and nitrous oxide, which readily supplies its oxygen atom.

Rapid flame propagation frequently makes fire fighting in a hyperbaric chamber hopeless. In 1965, a chamber fire was caused by overheating of a motor in an atmosphere of 27-per-cent oxygen, 36.5-per-cent nitrogen, and 36.5-per-cent helium at 60 ft. Both occupants were killed almost immediately. The fire reached a temperature that raised the chamber pressure to 9 ATA within 1 min.[3] The most efficient extinguishing system is an automatic deluge system, operated through infrared emission or ultraviolet radiation detectors, which distinguish between flame and background levels.

BAROTRAUMA

The solid and liquid tissues of the body freely transmit increased pressure in all directions. Thus, these tissues are not affected by pressure changes. In rapid deep diving, there may be joint pain, but this does not occur in the low-pressure ranges utilized in therapy. However, gas-filled spaces are frequently affected by pressure. Damage caused by pressure is called *barotrauma* or, descriptively, "squeeze." Barotrauma may develop during either compression or decompression.

Barotrauma During Compression

By far, the most common site of barotrauma during compression is the middle ear. Pressure rises linearly with depth, but the greatest relative changes are in the shallow depths. Pain typically begins in the first 10 ft. of the descent. During compression, the tympanic membrane bows inward and the mucosa of the middle ear becomes engorged. Opening of the eustachian tube permits high-pressure air to enter the middle ear and equalize pressure, thus preventing tympanic membrane damage or mucosal transudation. Opening of the eustachian tube during compression usually requires a conscious act such as yawning, chewing, swallowing, moving the jaws, or performing a Valsalva's maneuver. Because of this, many facilities perform myringotomies on unconscious patients[4]; yet, other facilities have not found this to be necessary.*

Damage ranges from simple tympanic injection to actual rupture. The pain is so severe that few persons willingly proceed to the stage of rupture. Of course, perforation eliminates pain by providing a pathway for equalization. In a survey of submarine school candidates, 36 per cent suffered clinical otic barotrauma following compression to 4 ATA.[5]

Slow compression with careful attention to

---

*Personal communication, R. M. Smith.

"clearing the ears" makes hyperbaric exposures tolerable for most patients. The most common mistake is failure to begin equalization early in the descent. Persons with allergic, infectious, or mechanical obstruction of the eustachian tubes should not be subjected to compression. Submarine candidates with upper respiratory infections had a 61-per-cent incidence of barotrauma.[5] Systemic or topical decongestants may be useful.

Much more rarely, barotrauma may affect the inner ear. The stapes can be dislodged from the oval window, causing hearing loss. Recently, rupture of the round window, with subsequent vestibular disturbances, has been reported in divers.[6] These problems may accompany an intact tympanic membrane.

The sinuses are also frequently affected by compression. When the ostia are obstructed, mucosal congestion and hemorrhage result. The signs of sinus squeeze are pain and epistaxis. Unfortunately, there is no convenient way to equalize a blocked sinus, although decongestants may help. Similarly, repaired teeth sometimes have air spaces that can be "squeezed." However, much of the pain attributed to the teeth is probable due to sinus barotrauma.

Persons in a hyperbaric chamber do not have to worry about lung barotrauma during descent, for the free breathing of pressurized gas eliminates this problem. Barotrauma may occur, however, in breath-hold diving, since air at high pressure is not available to counteract the inward thoracic pressure.

Barotrauma During Decompression

During decompression, otic barotrauma is uncommon but will occur if air in the expanding middle ear cannot be vented through the eustachian tube. Under this condition, the tympanic membrane bulges outward. Generally, the eustachian tube opens spontaneously to release air at positive pressure.

Similarly, decompression may cause sinus and dental barotrauma. Gas in the gastrointestinal tract expands on ascent. In healthy persons who are free of bowel obstruction and have normal bowel volumes of gas, this is not a serious problem.

One of the most serious of all hyperbaric complications, lung barotrauma, occurs during ascent. During decompression, the lungs begin to distend as ambient pressure decreases. With normal exhalation, distention is immediately relieved as the gas escapes, and transthoracic pressure is equalized. Even a brief failure in exhalation can cause overdistention and rupture of the lungs. Divers using compressed air have died after ascending from depths as shallow as 10 ft. while breath holding.[7] Without exhalation, lung volume doubles during decompression from 33 ft.

Overdistention of the lungs may tear alveoli and release air into the interstitial tissue of the lung. Continued ascent after rupture results in expansion of this extra-alveolar air. Typically, the air passes along vascular sheaths to the mediastinum, resulting in pneumomediastinum. Having reached the hilum, air may dissect between the pleural layers to cause pneumothorax. Direct rupture into the pleural space is less common.[8] Air dissection up into the neck results in subcutaneous emphysema.

The ultimate disaster results from direct escape of alveolar air into the pulmonary blood vessels. Air carried directly to the left heart forms arterial emboli. In the upright position, the victim generally suffers embolization to cerebral vessels, though coronary arteries may also be affected. The body has a low tolerance for arterial embolization (see Chap. 18).

Typically, air embolism becomes apparent with the development of unconsciousness immediately upon surfacing. The other manifestations of lung barotrauma usually have a slower onset.

Victims of air embolism must be recompressed immediately, for any delay markedly reduces the chances for survival. Most commonly, recompression is carried to 6 ATA, and slow decompression is begun upon evidence of initial recovery. At best, air embolization is frequently fatal. Pneumothorax, pneumomediastinum, and subcutaneous emphysema usually do not require recompression.

Most cases of air embolism occur during submarine escape training or in scuba divers trying to make "free ascents" (surfacing while exhaling continuously due to real or simulated failure of the breathing apparatus). Lung barotrauma resulting from ascent should be very rare in hyperbaric chambers, since ascents are not rapid. Of course, a sudden failure in pressurization subjects all occupants to the hazards of lung rupture.

Lung rupture can also occur in persons who exhale normally. Localized areas of trapped air may expand dangerously. Broncholiths, mucus plugs, or weakened airway walls may permit inspiration while impeding exhalation. Also, bullae may rupture more easily than areas of normal lung tissue. All candidates for treatment in hyperbaric chambers should be evaluated carefully to exclude those with lung abnormalities. Patients with active respiratory infections should not be subjected to hyperbaric conditions.

Pressure changes can affect the equipment used for hyperbaric therapy. Intravenous fluids should be administered from bags or air-space vented bottles, so that the air space over the fluid cannot expand on decompression and force fluid and then air into veins. An air-filled tracheal tube cuff will shrink on descent and expand on ascent. Cuffs should be emptied before ascent or filled with liquid. Anesthetic flowmeters are affected by pressure, too (see p. 588).

DECOMPRESSION SICKNESS

During general anesthesia, uptake of the anesthetic causes blood and tissue anesthetic concentrations to gradually approach the inspired concentration. Many factors, including cardiac output, ventilation, inspired concentration, blood and tissue solubilities, and regional blood flow, affect the rate of uptake. The nitrogen found in air undergoes a similar process during compressed air exposure. As total gas pressure rises, the partial pressure of nitrogen correspondingly increases. Because of its low solubility (compared to anesthetics), nitrogen equilibrates rapidly. The total amount of anesthetic in a patient depends on the concentration administered and the duration of exposure. Similarly, in high-pressure air breathing, total nitrogen uptake depends on dose (which depends directly on exposure pressure or depth) and duration of exposure.

Upon stopping anesthetic inhalation, the blood carries anesthetic in solution to the lungs for excretion. Upon surfacing from a dive, nitrogen pressure begins to return to the lower, ambient partial pressure. Unlike suddenly stopping anesthesia, however, a sudden release in pressure can overwhelm the pathway for inert gas elimination. Instead of reaching the lungs in solution, the nitrogen may form bubbles within tissues and blood vessels. Through a variety of mechanisms, these bubbles cause the derangement known as *decompression sickness.* Decompression sickness has many manifestations, including skin rash, pruritus, fatigue, musculoskeletal pain, central and peripheral nervous system symptoms, respiratory distress, and shock.

Bubble formation is a complex subject and is still incompletely understood. Tissues can hold gas at partial pressures above the ambient pressure. However, above a threshold (varying from tissue to tissue and dependent on factors such as agitation), bubbles will form.

Bubbles have been considered the etiologic agent in decompression sickness, because they can cause ischemia by obstructing blood flow and by producing direct tissue damage when present extravascularly. In 1938, Edgar End described red blood cell aggregation in decompression sickness and postulated that this, rather than bubbles alone, impaired blood flow.[9] Only recently have End's findings been confirmed and appreciated. Current investigation has identified several other abnormalities. Although bubbles definitely do cause mechanical disruption and remain the basic problem in decompression sickness, the interface between gas bubble and blood is also very important. Protein denaturation can occur at these interfaces and may account for the observed erythrocyte and platelet clumping and the activation of coagulation factors.[11] In severe decompression sickness, platelet counts are markedly depressed. Plasma loss occurs in decompression sickness and aggravates the sluggish blood flow. Lipid emboli have also been implicated. Recently, evidence has been presented that spinal cord involvement results from obstruction of the epidural vertebral venous plexus, rather than from generalized gaseous embolization.[10]

Individual factors are important as well. Old, obese divers in poor physical condition appear more susceptible. There is evidently some actual adaptation to hyperbaric work. Signs of decompression sickness vary somewhat between divers and caisson workers. No thorough evaluation has been made of decompression sickness occurring in hyperbaric therapy facilities.

Musculoskeletal pain, usually in a large joint, is the most common presenting complaint. The popular term, "the bends," applies only to this manifestation of decompression sickness. In 60 to 95 per cent of stricken divers, it is the only symptom.[11] Typically, the deep, boring pain is not accompanied by local heat, tenderness, swelling, or discoloration.

CNS involvement is not uncommon. It most frequently involves the spinal cord but may include cerebral centers. Usually spinal cord derangement begins with paresthesias in the legs and progresses to weakness, paralysis, and autonomic loss.

Respiratory involvement, called "the chokes," develops more rarely. Perhaps bubbles in the pulmonary circulation cause the dyspnea and chest pain.

Recently, increased attention has been directed to the presence of aseptic bone necrosis in experienced divers. The incidence varies widely; one series reported a 50-per-cent incidence.[12] This avascular necrosis may be juxta-articular. Eventually it may cause symptoms, or it may affect the bone shaft, which generally is asymptomatic. Often, afflicted divers have never had any other manifestation of decompression sickness.

Prevention of decompression sickness depends on limiting the dose of inert gas and providing time for its orderly elimination. Since some overpressure is tolerable, decompression tables have been formulated to permit diving followed by immediate but gradual ascent (normally at a rate of 60 ft./min.). As depth of the dive increases, the duration of the dive must naturally decrease to limit the total amount of nitrogen absorbed. In theory, a 2-atm. exposure of any length can be followed by immediate ascent. However, very long dives to this depth may be followed by decompression sickness.[10]

When dives exceed the safe limits for direct ascent, gradual decompression must be employed. The U.S. Navy uses staged decompression: An initial ascent is followed by a pause to eliminate gas before making another ascent. The British often use a slower continuous ascent. Because gas elimination, like uptake, is exponential, the pauses can be brief in the deep depths but should lengthen as the excretion rate slows. Similarly, in continuous ascent, the rate can be faster initially but then must be slowed.

Even under the best of conditions, decompression sickness sometimes occurs despite proper adherence to decompression standards. Furthermore, ultrasonic bubble detectors demonstrate bubbling in the absence of clinical signs.[13] These "silent bubbles" are of undefined significance but may be responsible for chronic changes, such as aseptic necrosis.

Basic treatment of decompression sickness requires recompression followed by gradual decompression. Because of the high incidence of failure of treatment based on old tables, treatment based on schedules that utilize oxygen breathing has been introduced. Recompression to 60 ft. is followed by alternating oxygen and air breathing (to reduce the risk of oxygen toxicity), with subsequent decompression to 30 ft., and at this stage oxygen-air cycles are continued. Recompression reduces bubble size, and oxygen breathing provides a steep gradient for elimination of nitrogen.

Success depends on prompt treatment of well evaluated patients. Fifty to 85 per cent of decompression sickness develops within 1 hour after surfacing.[11] However, delays of over 24 hours are possible. Any person with symptoms compatible with decompression sickness deserves a trial of recompression therapy if he has had a hyperbaric exposure within 24 to 36 hours. The choice of treatment tables depends on the symptoms; serious cases receive longer therapy. Careful evaluation is essential, as severe joint pain may obscure early CNS signs. Delays in instituting treatment lessen the chance for complete recovery.

Many therapists supplement recompression therapy. Hemoconcentration is sometimes treated with plasma. Low-molecular-weight dextran may relieve erythrocyte and platelet clumping; steroids are employed frequently in cases involving the CNS.

Decompression sickness should be uncommon in modern hyperbaric therapy. Since the patient breathes oxygen rather than inert gases, he is not at risk. The low pressures employed to avoid oxygen toxicity in the patient engenders prolonged air exposure for the therapists. Because of inert gas accumulation, therapists should ideally be compressed for only one session each day. Many centers use oxygen during the last 30 ft. of decompression to further speed nitrogen elimination by the attendants. If an attendant develops decompression sickness, prompt treatment can be provided readily. Since decompression sickness may have a long latent period, all persons exposed to pressure should remain near a chamber for several hours and should carry obvious identification of their pressure exposure.

In hyperbaric surgery, the anesthetic gas may cause decompression sickness. This is not a problem with the potent agents, because the dose used is low. However, nitrous oxide can readily cause decompression sickness, since large amounts are taken up. Nitrous oxide breathed after an air dive increases symptoms in mice, presumably by enlarging small air bubbles.[14] Dogs that have breathed large doses of nitrous oxide (e.g., 80% at 3 ATA or 55% at 5 ATA) have a high incidence of fatal decompression sickness.[15] However, those exposed to 55% at up to 4 ATA have no fatalities or macroscopic bubbles.

The risk of decompression sickness, plus the limitation on oxygen concentration, has led some investigators to conclude that nitrous oxide is inappropriate in hyperbaric therapy. Faulconer has provided adequate anesthesia with 50-per-cent nitrous oxide at 2 ATA,[16] which agrees well with an independent determination of MAC. Since anesthesia depends on partial pressure and not on concentration of anesthetic, surgery at 3 ATA can be performed with about 33-per-cent nitrous oxide. This dose probably does not represent a serious risk of decompression sickness, especially if the nitrous oxide is discontinued before decompression, thus providing maximum washout.

OXYGEN TOXICITY

The toxic effects of oxygen pose the most significant limitation to the use of hyperbaric oxygen therapy. Illnesses such as respiratory failure might respond to hyperbaric oxygen, but the therapy itself damages the lungs. Besides the lungs, oxygen toxicity affects the CNS and eyes (see Chap. 23). It almost certainly is toxic to other organs such as the liver, kidney, and heart, though the data are limited. Oxygen affects single cells and all known forms of life. Oxygen toxicity is dose-dependent. The dose depends on the partial pressure of oxygen inspired and the length of exposure; an increase in either hastens the onset of toxicity.

Pulmonary oxygen toxicity is clinically significant in the management of critically ill patients. Hyperbaric oxygen speeds the development of lung damage. Healthy volunteers breathing oxygen at 2 ATA have severe chest pain and dyspnea after 8 to 10 hours.[18] Vital capacity begins to decline significantly within 4 hours of initiation of oxygen breathing; symptoms and changes in vital capacity persist hours after the exposure.

Visual abnormalities are associated with excessive oxygen in infants but are not a clinical problem in adults. However, in a 2-ATA exposure, five of 13 subjects had visual symptoms.[18] Only one (a man with a prior history of retrobulbar neuritis) had major signs: unilateral constriction of visual fields, scotoma, and decreased visual activity that necessitated termination of oxygen exposure.

At pressures exceeding 2 ATA, CNS toxicity limits tolerable oxygen exposure. Minor symptoms include nausea, muscle twitching (particularly facial), and numbness. Tonic clonic seizures follow unless oxygen exposure is promptly terminated. Unfortunately, seizures may occur without warning or so rapidly that halting administration of oxygen does not prevent them. No definite threshold can be established for oxygen toxicity to the CNS. Convulsions have been reported at only 2 ATA, though most persons can tolerate 2 hours of oxygen at 3 ATA while at rest.[19,20] Because of the risk of oxygen toxicity, hyperbaric therapy is almost always limited to 3 ATA.

Rather than seeking a threshold, it may be more reasonable to think in terms of latent periods before oxygen poisoning becomes manifest. In general, as pressure rises, the latent period decreases.

Latency is also affected by other factors. Carbon dioxide accumulation hastens seizures, though moderately high carbon dioxide levels may actually suppress oxygen convulsions.[21] The mechanism for the enhanced toxicity may be related to the increased cerebral blood flow associated with elevated carbon dioxide levels. Very high carbon dioxide partial pressure is itself convulsive, but such levels are not associated with hyperbaric therapy. Exercise markedly decreases latency. Whether this is a primary factor or related to carbon dioxide retention is unknown. Interestingly, wet chamber exposures seem to be tolerated less well than dry ones. This is true even for comparable levels of pressure.

The mechanism of oxygen toxicity remains undefined, despite extensive investigation. Its universality suggests interference with very basic metabolic pathways, and several enzyme systems have been implicated. Perhaps the syndrome results from interacting mechanisms rather than a single one.[22,23]

Treatment of CNS toxicity is simple: Remove the source of oxygen. Patients breathing oxygen should be switched to air. The chamber should not be decompressed during a seizure, for apnea or airway obstruction may lead to lung rupture. If the exposure is terminated and the seizure managed properly, residual effects do not accompany oxygen seizures. Apnea during the seizure is not a problem, since the patient is well oxygenated. Presumably, prolonging oxygen exposure causes permanent damage.

Prevention of toxicity requires limitations to exposure. Since the goal of hyperbaric therapy is to provide large amounts of oxygen, treatment schedules push the dose to toxic levels. Drugs may obtund the overt signs of poisoning, but in doing so they mask toxicity. Dogs given halothane or barbiturates have delayed or no seizures but may have residual changes of severe poisoning.[24]

The most promising preventive is the use of intermittent oxygen breathing. In animals and humans, oxygen tolerance has been extended by the interposition of brief periods of air breathing between periods of oxygen inhalation.[25] Apparently, these intermissions provide time for partial recovery from oxygen toxicity. An initial evaluation of the effect of intermittent oxygen exposure in man utilized a schedule of 20 min. of oxygen followed by 5 min. of air in volunteers at 2 ATA.[26] Changes in vital capacity were markedly delayed by this regimen. Longer periods of air breathing might further reduce oxygen toxicity, but at the expense of reducing the duration of oxygen administration.

NITROGEN NARCOSIS

Another constraint in hyperbaric therapy is the narcotic effect of high-pressure nitrogen. This, unlike oxygen toxicity, affects the attendants in the chamber rather than the patient who is protected by breathing only oxygen.

Almost all inert gases can be narcotic. However, narcosis has not been demonstrated with helium, though other CNS effects are noted at very high pressures.[27] Probably inert gas narcosis results from the same mechanism, or mechanisms, as general inhalation anesthesia. The narcotic potency of the inert gases correlates well with their lipid solubility. In mice, the narcotic potency of nitrous oxide is 28 times that of nitrogen.[28] The oil–gas partition coefficient of nitrous oxide is 20 times that of nitrogen (1.4 vs. 0.067). Using lipid solubility as a determinant of potency, air at 2.4 ATA (nitrogen at 1400 torr) should have the potency of 10-per-cent nitrous oxide inhaled at sea level,[29] which produces a mild euphoria. Air at sea level contains enough nitrogen to impair human performance slightly compared to a helium-oxygen mixture.[30]

Clinically it is difficult to demonstrate nitrogen narcosis in most people at pressures less than 4 ATA. However, performance tests show impairment at pressures as low as 3 ATA.[31] The choice of an appropriate test and the wide range of individual variability makes measurement difficult. Generally, mood change, usually euphoria, is the first symptom. Decrements occur in conceptual reasoning (most affected), reaction time, and mechanical dexterity (least affected). Performance continues to deteriorate with increasing air pressure until consciousness may be lost at depths below about 330 ft. (11 ATA). Presumably, surgical anesthesia is obtained at about 20 ATA of nitrogen (25 ATA of air), though air at this pressure would cause severe oxygen toxicity.

Some investigators believe there may be adaptation to narcosis, for experienced divers can often work at depths that incapacitate novices. More likely, these divers learn to work despite narcosis by narrowing their impaired attention to the task at hand. Narcosis makes simple tasks complex.

Carbon dioxide retention intensifies inert gas narcosis. This can be a problem in diving suits but should not be an issue in well ventilated hyperbaric chambers.

Nitrogen narcosis limits air diving to depths of 125 ft.; excursions to 200 ft. should be undertaken only in emergencies. Many scuba divers have died in their attempt to establish a diving record. Modern deep diving employs helium as a complete or partial substitute for nitrogen.

Even with the restricted pressures used for therapy, nitrogen narcosis may occasionally be a problem, for effects can be demonstrated at 3 ATA. Therapy at 4 ATA would be expected to introduce observable problems of narcosis. As a result, all chamber operations are supervised by observers at sea level, whose decisions override those of the attendants in the chamber.

ANESTHETIC OVERDOSE

Administration of inhalation anesthetics on the basis of the percentage given at sea level can be fatal in a hyperbaric chamber. Doses must be expressed as partial pressure and not percentage concentration. That is, 1 MAC of halothane (0.76%) is really 0.76 per cent of 760 torr, or 6 torr. At 2 ATA, this halothane pressure of 6 torr is still equivalent to 1 MAC but constitutes only 0.4 per cent of the total gas pressure. However, if the sea level concentration of halothane (0.76%) were continued at 2 ATA, the patient would receive 2 MAC and, thus, an overdose.

With gaseous anesthetics, the main concern is

reducing inspired percentage as total pressure increases. Vaporization of volatile anesthetics does not depend on total ambient pressure. At 20°C, the partial pressure of halothane is 243 torr, regardless of total pressure. Calibrated vaporizers (e.g., Fluotec), once set at sea level, compensate automatically for changes in ambient pressure. As total pressure rises, the pressure of emited halothane stays constant and represents a smaller fraction of the effluent. However, the constant partial pressure maintains an unchanged anesthetic potency. Severinghaus found that changes in gas turbulence lead to small variations in anesthetic output.[29] McDowell found that the accuracy of this type of vaporizer is better above 2 per cent than in the lower ranges.[32]

Vaporizers of the Copper Kettle type emit volatile anesthetics in accordance with the ratio of partial pressure of anesthetic to that of oxygen. As ambient pressure increases, the fraction represented by the anesthetic must decrease, since its pressure relative to total pressure decreases. For halothane at 2 ATA, each 100 ml. of oxygen takes up 20 ml. of halothane. If dilutent gas flows are unchanged, the percentage of halothane administered decreases. However, partial pressure of halothane is not changed.

Rotameter flow depends on gas density, which increases directly with pressure. The following equation predicts the effect of hyperbaric conditions:[32]

$$F_1 = F_0 \times \frac{\rho_0}{\rho_1}$$

where F_1 = true flow
F_0 = rotameter flow reading
ρ_0 = density at normal pressure
ρ_1 = density of gas at chamber pressure

Since doubling the pressure doubles the gas density, at 2 ATA true flow should be 71 per cent of indicated flow. Subsequent experiments support this approximation. However, each hyperbaric facility should calibrate its flowmeters at various pressures.

Removal of anesthetic gaseous waste ("scavenging") from the chamber is important to prevent anesthetic exposure of attendants, who are already at risk to the narcotic properties of nitrogen.

REFERENCES

1. Schmidt, T. C., Dorr, V. A., Hamilton, R. W., Jr.: Chamber Safety (Technical Memorandum UCRI-721). Tarrytown (N.Y.), Ocean Systems, Inc., 1973.
2. Gottlieb, S. F., Fegan, F. J., and Tieslink, J.: Flammability of halothane, methoxyflurane and fluroxene under hyperbaric oxygen conditions. Anesthesiology, *27*:195, 1966.
3. Harter, J. V.: Fire at high pressure. *In* Lambertsen, C. J. (ed.): Proceedings of the Third Symposium on Underwater Physiology. pp. 55–80. Baltimore, Williams & Wilkins, 1967.
4. Jacobson, J. H., II, and Peirce, E. C., II: Hyperbaric oxygenation. *In* Norman, J. C. (ed.): Cardiac Surgery. ed. 2. pp. 211–226. New York, Appleton-Century-Crofts, 1972.
5. Alfandre, H. J.: Aerotitis media in submarine recruits. U.S. Navy Submarine Medical Center Research Report, March 1966.
6. Edmonds, C., and Thomas, R. L.: Medical aspects of diving—Part 3. Med. J. Aust., *2*:1300, 1972.
7. Cooperman, E. M., Hogg, J., and Thurlbeck, W. M.: Mechanism of death in shallow-water scuba diving. Can. Med. Assoc. J., *99*:1128, 1968.
8. Schaefer, K. E., and McNulty, W. P.: Mechanism in development of interstitial emphysema and air embolism on decompression from depth. J. Appl. Physiol., *13*:15, 1958.
9. End, E.: The use of new equipment and helium gas in a world record dive. J. Industr. Hyg., *20*:511, 1938.
10. Elliott, D. H., Hallenbeck, J. M., and Bove, A. A.: Acute decompression sickness. Lancet, *2*:1193, 1974.
11. Rivera, J. C.: Decompression sickness among divers: an analysis of 935 cases. Milit. Med., *129*:314, 1964.
12. Edmonds, C., and Thomas, R. L.: Medical aspects of diving—Part 4. Med. J. Aust., *2*:1367, 1972.
13. Evans, A., Barnard, E. E. P., and Walder, D. N.: Detection of gas bubbles in man at decompression. Aerosp. Med., *53*:1095, 1972.
14. Van Liew, H. E.: Dissolved gas washout and bubble absorption in routine decompression. *In* Lambertsen, C. J. (ed.): Underwater Physiology. pp. 145–150. New York, Academic Press, 1971.
15. McIver, R. G., Fife, W. P., and Ikels, K. G.: Experimental decompression sickness from hyperbaric nitrous oxide anesthesia. U.S.A.F. School of Aerospace Medicine, June 1965.
16. Faulconer, A., Pender, J. W., and Bickford, R. G.: The influence of partial pressure of N_2O on the depth of anesthesia and the EEG in man. Anesthesiology, *10*:601, 1949.
17. Winter, P. M., Hornbein, T. F., Smith, G., et al.: Hyperbaric nitrous oxide anesthesia in man: determination of anesthetic potency (MAC) and cardiorespiratory effects (abstr.). pp. 103–104. American Society of Anesthesiologists, Annual Meeting, 1972.
18. Clark, J. M., and Lambertsen, C. J.: Rate of development of pulmonary O_2 toxicity in man during O_2 breathing at 2.0 ATA. J. Appl. Physiol., *30*:739, 1971.

19. Donald, K. W.: Oxygen poisoning in man. I and II. Br. Med. J., *1*:667 and 712, 1947.
20. Yarbrough, W. W., Briton, E. S., and Behnke, A. R.: Symptoms of oxygen poisoning and limits of tolerance at rest and at work. Experimental Diving Unit Project X-337 (sub no. 62), 1947.
21. Lambertsen, C. J.: Effects of oxygen at high partial pressure. *In* Fenn, W. O., and Rahn, H. (eds.): Handbook of Physiology. section 3. vol. II. pp. 1027–1046. Washington (D.C.), American Physiological Society, 1965.
22. Clark, J. M., and Lambertsen, C. J.: Pulmonary oxygen toxicity: a review. Pharmacol. Rev., *23*:37, 1971.
23. Haugaard, N.: The scope of oxygen poisoning. *In* Lambertsen, C. J. (ed.): Underwater Physiology. pp. 1–8. New York, Academic Press, 1971.
24. Harp, J. R., Gutsche, B. B., and Stephen, C. R.: Effect of anesthesia on central nervous system toxicity of hyperbaric oxygen. Anesthesiology, *27*:608, 1966.
25. Clark, J. M.: The toxicity of oxygen. Am. Rev. Resp. Dis., *110*:40, 1974.
26. Hendricks, P. L., Hall, D. A., Hunter, W. L., Jr., et al.: Extension of pulmonary oxygen tolerance in man at 2 ATA by intermittent oxygen exposure. J. Appl. Physiol., *42*:593, 1977.
27. Brauer, R. W., and Way, R. O.: Relative narcotic potencies of hydrogen, helium, nitrogen, and their mixtures. J. Appl. Physiol., *29*:23, 1970.
28. Brauer, R. W., Goldman, S. M., Beaver, R. W., et al.: Nitrogen, hydrogen, and nitrous oxide antagonism of high pressure neurological syndrome in mice. Undersea Biomed. Res., *1*:59, 1974.
29. Severinghaus, J. W.: Anesthesia and related drug effects. In Greenbaum, L., and Seeley, S. (eds.): Fundamentals of Hyperbaric Medicine (Publication 1298). pp. 115–127. Washington (D.C.), National Academy of Sciences, 1966.
30. Winter, P. M., Bruce, D. L., Bach, M. J., et al.: The anesthetic effect of air at atmospheric pressure. Anesthesiology, *42*:658, 1975.
31. Kiesling, R. J., and Maay, C. H.: Performance impairment as a function of nitrogen narcosis. U.S. Navy Experimental Diving Unit Research Report 3-60, 1960.
32. McDowall, D. G.: Anaesthesia in a pressure chamber. Anaesthesia, *19*:321, 1964.

FURTHER READING

Bennett, P. B., and Elliot, D. H.: Physiology and Medicine of Diving and Compressed Air Work. ed. 2. Baltimore, Williams & Wilkins, 1975.

Davis, J. C., and Hunt, T. K. (eds.): Hyperbaric Oxygen Therapy. Bethesda, Undersea Medical Society, Inc., 1977.

Dueker, C. W.: Medical aspects of sport diving. Cranbury, A. S. Barnes & Co., 1970.

Greenbaum, L., and Seeley, S. (eds.): Fundamentals of Hyperbaric Medicine (Publication 1298). Washington (D.C.), National Academy of Sciences, 1966.

47 Complications of Extracorporeal Circulation

Fredrick K. Orkin, M.D.

The development of cardiac surgery, considered perhaps the most important clinical advance in cardiovascular and pulmonary medicine since 1945, itself required the development and application of extracorporeal circulation to keep the patient alive while his heart is repaired.[1]

Traumatic cardiac wounds were repaired as early as 1897, and correction of some congenital and rheumatic heart defects was undertaken during the second quarter of the 20th century. Yet, until the development of a method to enable the circulation to bypass the heart and lungs, cardiac surgery was extremely limited. The only procedures attempted were those that could be performed under direct vision within the seven or eight minutes of circulatory interruption permitted by hypothermia. Not until Gibbon closed a large atrial septal defect in 1953, using a pump-oxygenator to bypass completely the patient's heart and lungs, did cardiac surgery begin to blossom.[2] That first successful application of extracorporeal circulation was itself dependent upon the confluence of developments such as the use of heparin in 1934, which is needed to prevent coagulation in the pump; the use of protamine in 1937 to neutralize heparin at the end of the artificial perfusion; the synthesis of plastics for pump tubing; and blood-banking procedures for the typing and preservation of blood, among many other requirements.[3]

Concomitant with this clinical achievement has been the emergence of a wide spectrum of complications which will be surveyed in this chapter.

TYPES OF EXTRACORPOREAL CIRCULATION

Extracorporeal circulation involves the diversion of venous blood through an external device that returns the blood to the arterial side of the circulation. In its most advanced form, the device consists of a pump to provide the motive force, an oxygenator to remove the carbon dioxide and add oxygen, tubing, a heat exchanger to promote hypothermia and rewarming, filters to trap bubbles and debris, and pressure transducers and thermistors to monitor its function.

Cardiopulmonary bypass, the principal application of extracorporeal circulation, diverts all or part of the blood returning to the right atrium away from the heart and lungs. *Total bypass* is used for procedures requiring exposure of the right side of the heart and main pulmonary artery, whereas *partial bypass* is used for operations on the left side of the heart, coronary arteries, and aorta. Details of bypass techniques and equipment, as well as adjuncts such as hemodilution, anticoagulation, and hypothermia, are beyond the scope of this chapter and are covered well elsewhere.[4-6] Problems related to induced hypothermia are discussed in Chapter 49.

THE SPECTRUM OF COMPLICATIONS FOLLOWING EXTRACORPOREAL CIRCULATION

The complications that occur following the use of extracorporeal circulation may be related to the patient's preexisting disease, the surgical procedure, and the anesthetic management, as well as the extracorporeal circulation itself. Despite such an arbitrary classification, the role of these other associated factors, singly or in combination, must not be forgotten when one is confronted with a given complication following the use of extracorporeal circulation.

COMPLICATIONS RELATED TO PREEXISTING DISEASE

Apart from its use in cardiac surgery, extracorporeal circulation has been used infrequently, if not rarely, in a variety of uncommon circumstances. These include the use of a pump for perfusion of an isolated organ or extremity with an antineoplastic agent; a pump-oxygenator for the treatment of malignant hyperthermia,[7] profound hypothermia, or severe acute respiratory failure;[8] partial cardiopulmonary bypass during liver transplantation;[9] and a left ventricular assist device for refractory cardiogenic shock following cardiac surgery.[10] Of course, each of these underlying clinical circumstances has its own set of potential complications.

In the first decade of cardiopulmonary bypass, when the technique and surgical procedures were being learned, complications occurred frequently, averaging one for each patient.[11–13] Complications were more frequent and serious among patients with valvular heart disease than among those with congenital heart defects because of more advanced cardiac disease and age, as well as longer duration of surgery, bypass, and anesthesia. During the past decade, myocardial revascularization has emerged and eclipsed other types of cardiac surgery in the United States (Fig. 47-1). Also, more recently, there has been a trend toward primary correction rather than palliative procedures in the treatment of infants under 1 year of age with congenital heart disease. Usually the complications have been (and continue to be) those medical problems to which these patients are especially susceptible. Only a few of the more salient complications related to preexisting disease will be mentioned here.

CARDIAC DYSRHYTHMIAS

So commonplace are dysrhythmias that precipitating factors should be sought and treated, when time permits, before pharmacologic agents are used symptomatically (see Chap. 14).

Etiology

Among the diverse precipitating factors that are present during the administration of anesthesia are laryngoscopy, tracheal intubation, and surgical incision, especially during a light level of anesthesia; hypoxemia; hypercarbia; hypovolemia; hypotension; hypertension; aortic cross-clamping; hypokalemia; and reflex stimulation of the autonomic nervous system, such as that accompanying traction on ribs, mesentery, pleura, heart, or great vessels. Other precipitating factors that are particularly common in these patients after cardiopulmonary bypass are atelectasis with or without hypoxemia, hypercarbia, hypokalemia with or without digitalis intoxication, other electrolyte disorders, pericarditis, pulmonary infection or embolism, and myocardial infarction. Estimates of the incidence of these dysrhythmias in current practice are not available. However, the type of dysrhythmia generally corresponds to the underlying cardiac disease: atrial fibrillation or flutter occurs commonly in patients with valvular disease, whereas ventricular tachycardia or fibrillation occurs most often in those with coronary artery disease; heart block is noted most often after procedures involving the interventricular septum (for example, septal defect repair, valve replacement).[14]

Treatment

Although many dysrhythmias disappear once the precipitating factor is identified and treated, others may require drug therapy (see p. 222) either

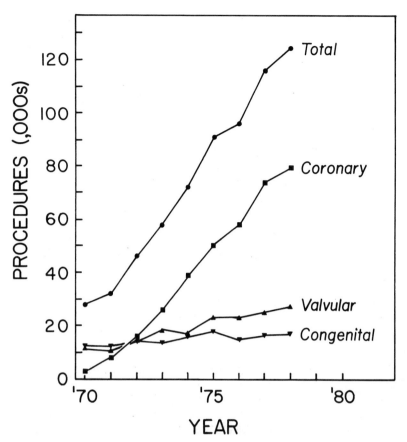

Fig. 47-1. The rapid growth of aggregate cardiac surgery using cardiopulmonary bypass in the United States, with its major categories (coronary revascularization procedures, surgery of heart valves, and repair of congenital heart defects), 1970 through 1977. (Drawn from data tabulated by Feldstein, P. J., and Viets, H. P.: Forecasting health manpower requirements: The case of thoracic surgeons. Ann. Thorac. Surg., 28:413, 1979.)

because no etiology can be found or the disturbance threatens perfusion to vital organs. Some patients will benefit from myocardial stimulation *via* atrial and ventricular epicardial electrodes placed during surgery; this topic is beyond the scope of this chapter but is covered well elsewhere.[15] These dysrhythmias are discussed further in Chapter 14.

MYOCARDIAL INFARCTION

Etiology

Although expected to be an increasingly common complication in current practice of predominantly myocardial revascularization, the incidence of postoperative myocardial infarction seems to have remained relatively stable, presumably because of concomitant improvements in cardiac surgical care. For example, in one report of

99 patients having either coronary artery bypass grafts or valve replacements, in whom the diagnosis of myocardial infarction was aggressively sought postoperatively, there was a 17 per cent incidence of this complication overall.[16] The incidence of infarction was greater among those having bypass grafts, but the difference was not statistically significant; instead, the duration of cardiopulmonary bypass and the extent of coronary artery disease correlated better with postoperative infarction, as has been noted by others (see p. 259). Although serum SGOT, LDH, and CPK enzyme levels were higher among those suffering postoperative infarction, enzyme elevations occurred among those not suffering infarction as a result of the tissue injury associated with surgery; this, too, has been noted following other types of surgery.[17–20] Curiously, chest pain was not commented upon in that report; however, characteris-

tic chest pain is absent in at least half of the cases of postoperative infarction following cardiopulmonary bypass, and other manifestations of infarction are often atypical.[21]

Prevention

Although controversy surrounds individual approaches, lowering the incidence of perioperative infarction in patients undergoing cardiopulmonary bypass requires an appreciation of the delicate balance between myocardial oxygen supply and demand.[22,23] Myocardial oxygen supply is dependent upon coronary blood flow and oxygen delivery which itself is dependent upon hemoglobin concentration and the degree of oxygen saturation; whereas myocardial oxygen demand is determined by arterial blood pressure (afterload), ventricular volume (perload), heart rate, and myocardial contractility. That clinical situations such as hypotension, hypoxemia, and anemia can reduce myocardial oxygen supply has been known for some time. Only relatively recently, however, has it been recognized that hypertension (increased afterload) increases myocardial oxygen demand. Ensuring a balance between myocardial oxygen supply and demand requires, in turn, an appreciation of cardiac hemodynamics.[24] Typically, preload, afterload, and heart rate are manipulated separately, and the optimal combination is obtained through trial and error with close cardiopulmonary monitoring. Shortly after bypass, for example, hypertension can occur which is so severe that it threatens subendocardial ischemia due to increased cardiac work, as well as pulmonary edema due to acute left ventricular failure; bleeding with resultant pericardial tamponade (see the following) is also a particularly common outcome. The underlying peripheral vasoconstriction is commonly treated with vasodilating agents, with a resultant decrease in cardiac work and, thus, myocardial oxygen demand.

ACUTE RESPIRATORY INSUFFICIENCY

Etiology

Preexisting cardiorespiratory disease also predisposes to pulmonary dysfunction following cardiopulmonary bypass.[25-27] Pulmonary function is frequently impaired in those requiring cardiac surgery,[27] since left ventricular failure results in increased pulmonary venous pressure and extravascular lung water, decreased compliance, and ventilation–perfusion mismatch.[28] Also, chronically congested, edematous lungs are prone to atelectasis and infection. The ability to sustain an adequate pulmonary ventilation and clear tracheobronchial secretions may be hampered by residual effects of preanesthetic medication, general anesthetics, neuromuscular blocking agents, and postoperative analgesics, as well as by the surgical trauma and incisional pain. Increased work of the respiratory muscles and further impairment of gas exchange result from atelectasis associated with pleural effusion or pneumothorax, pulmonary infection and emboli, low levels of pulmonary surfactant, and intrapulmonary hemorrhage due to clotting disorders which may occur during cardiopulmonary bypass.[28-31] (Aspects of respiratory dysfunction associated with "pump lung," a form of adult respiratory distress syndrome, are discussed on p. 601 among the problems related more directly to the use of extracorporeal circulation.) As a result of these various factors, some degree of hypoxemia and possibly hypercarbia is common following cardiac surgery.[32,33]

Unfortunately, the earliest *clinical* signs of respiratory decompensation—tachypnea, tachycardia, gasping, expiratory grunting, use of accessory muscles of respiration, flaring of the alae nasae, diminished breath sounds, and agitation—are relatively late, nonspecific *physiologic* manifestations. Without treatment, cyanosis, bradycardia, and hypotension supervene.

Treatment

The mainstay in the treatment of respiratory insufficiency after cardiac surgery has been tracheal intubation and controlled mechanical ventilation with humidified air sufficiently oxygen-enriched to maintain the patient's PaO_2 in the range 80 to 100 torr (10.6–13.3 kPa).[34-39] Physiologic measurements—particularly arterial blood gas values, tidal volume, and minute ventilation—are essential in assessing and modifying therapy. In addition, a pulmonary artery catheter permits sampling mixed venous blood from which may be calculated the degree of physiologic shunt and arteriovenous oxygen content difference (see p. 597).

Positive end-expiratory pressure (PEEP) may improve oxygenation and allow the use of lower inspired oxygen concentrations. However, high levels of PEEP can aggravate the pulmonary damage already present by causing increased transudation of fluid through injured capillary beds.[40,41] Also, the use of PEEP may not affect survival, which is related more to the severity of the hypoxemia prior to the institution of PEEP.[42]

As oxygenation improves, weaning from controlled ventilation may be undertaken if minimal criteria are met: inspiratory force of at least -20 to -30 cm H_2O (-2 to -3 kPa), alveolar–arterial oxygen gradient of less than 300 to 500 torr (40.0–46.7 kPa), deadspace-to-tidal volume ratio of less than 0.6, cardiovascular stability (absence of serious dysrhythmias, low cardiac index, hypotension, high dose of vasopressor), and adequate gag and cough reflexes.[43] Intermittent mandatory ventilation may facilitate the transition from controlled ventilation to spontaneous respiration by allowing the patient to assume his respiratory function gradually as the number of ventilator breaths per minute is decreased.[44] Prior to extubation, the patient should be alert, able to cough and gag adequately, and to breathe spontaneously through a T-piece (Briggs) adapter for at least an hour without tachycardia, tachypnea, or increase in $PaCO_2$.

Recently, the *routine* use of mechanical ventilation has been questioned[45] and early extubation advocated for those patients who are able to satisfy specified criteria for tracheal extubation.[46–48]

Prevention

An important element in the prevention of respiratory dysfunction is the identification of those patients particularly likely to experience such difficulty postoperatively. The use of full pulmonary function testing probably adds little to the sensitivity of careful clinical evaluation, including arterial blood gas studies.[50] Among those most susceptible to respiratory difficulty are patients having chronic lung disease and a history of many years' cigarette smoking, especially those with hypercapnia. These patients should be urged strongly to discontinue smoking at least 2 weeks prior to surgery and should receive postural drainage with percussion, bronchodilator therapy, and, depending upon the nature of the underlying pulmonary disease, antibiotics or steroids. General goals include reducing tracheobronchial secretions and bronchospasm.[51]

COMPLICATIONS RELATED TO THE SURGICAL PROCEDURE

The problems related to the actual surgical procedure are so diverse that only a sampling is presented here.

PROBLEMS RELATED TO SURGICAL ERROR

Surgical error includes errors in both preoperative diagnosis and surgical technique. Imprecision in diagnosis was responsible for the death of the first patient to undergo cardiopulmonary bypass[52] and contributed to morbidity during the technique's early years of development. With the great advances in diagnostic technology, as well as increasing experience, it is rare that a major error in diagnosis is made now. Yet, an *associated* lesion having lesser hemodynamic importance can be overlooked preoperatively and thereby either may not be treated or may surprise the surgeon intraoperatively, complicating the planned procedure. Among lesions notorious for eluding preoperative diagnosis in the past are patent ductus arteriosus, persistent left superior vena cava, and anomalous coronary artery circulation.[12] Clearly, accuracy in diagnosis is essential to successful cardiac surgery.

Errors in surgical technique have also decreased with increased clinical experience. Some of the more common technical errors include permitting peripheral embolization of calcium or tissue debris from a rheumatic valve with resultant necrosis in the organ involved, an excessively long ventricular incision with secondary impaired myocardial contractility, injury to a coronary artery with myocardial infarction, damage to the thoracic duct leading to chylothorax, injury to cardiac tissue produced by undue retraction and leading to dysrhythmias and excessive bleeding, and an excessively tight closure of the pericardium leading to diminished cardiac output.[12]

PERICARDIAL TAMPONADE

Etiology

Even when the pericardium is not closed completely, pericardial tamponade occurs in up to 15 per cent of patients following cardiac surgery, especially after procedures involving the aortic valve.[53,54] Although tamponade may occur days or weeks later, it usually occurs within hours of the procedure. Excessive bleeding, often in association with the removal of epicardial pacing wires or coagulation defects resulting from cardiopulmonary bypass (see p. 606), results in an acute cardiac compression syndrome. There are progressive increases in atrial and central venous pressures, and decreases in cardiac output and systolic and pulse pressures. The peripheral circulation constricts, and output falls.

Differential Diagnosis

Initially, the symptoms are quite nonspecific, including restlessness, dyspnea, tachypnea, and even anterior chest pain. Associated signs are also nonspecific. Pulsus paradoxus of at least 10 torr (1.3 kPa), very characteristic of pericardial tamponade,[55,56] may be absent if mechanical ventilation is in use[57] or may be present but due instead to other conditions, such as pneumothorax, bronchospasm, or myocardial failure. Other differential diagnoses to be considered when confronted by elevated atrial and venous pressures, with falling systemic pressures and cardiac output, include the low output syndrome (see p. 601), dissecting aneurysm of the aorta, the postperfusion lung syndrome (see p. 601), hemorrhage elsewhere in the chest or abdomen, and myocardial infarction. The most challenging and important differential diagnosis is that between conges-tive heart failure and pericardial tamponade. Patients with heart failure following cardiopulmonary bypass generally have less bleeding and respond less well to blood volume replacement than those with tamponade,[53] whose right atrial, pulmonary diastolic, and right atrial pressures usually approach each other.

Treatment

Prompt evacuation of pericardial blood and clots is therapeutic. Although circulatory function improves as soon as the chest is opened in the intensive care unit, even before a limited decompression is performed,[58] thorough exploration is generally required to secure hemostasis, especially when postoperative bleeding from chest tubes exceeds 300 ml./hr. for more than 2 hours.

COMPLICATIONS RELATED TO ANESTHETIC MANAGEMENT

In addition to many of the complications described in other chapters, several problems related to anesthetic management are particularly likely to occur in patients undergoing cardiopulmonary bypass.

HUMAN ERROR

Given the generally more severely ill patients having cardiac surgery, longer duration of these procedures, more complex anesthetic and adjunctive techniques, and greater use of monitoring, opportunities for human error abound. Human error includes inadvertent changes in administered gas flows, administration of the wrong drug as a result of confusing syringes, and failure to detect breathing circuit disconnection.[59] Human error, manifested as the mislabelling of blood specimens and misidentification of patients, is also responsible for the majority of hemolytic transfusion reactions.[60-62] A common feature of such events is a lapse of vigilance that itself may be fostered by poor communication among anesthesia personnel caring for a given patient, haste, fatigue, and distraction, among other factors.[59] In addition, personnel may also fall prey to the temptation to fixate upon the esoteric to the exclusion of the more mundane events.[63]

DIFFICULTIES RELATED TO MONITORING

The more intensive monitoring of vital organ function, required for safe management of the anesthetic in these patients, itself engenders complications.

Electrocardiogram

Thermal burns can occur at the site of ECG electrodes when a simultaneously used electrosurgical unit has defective grounding or a related problem.[64] Also, defective grounding in a variety of electrical equipment can cause electrocution in a patient who has a central venous catheter that conducts microampere currents directly to the myocardium;[65] electrical burns and electrocution and discussed more fully in Chapter 53. The ECG display is probably more susceptible to misinterpretation than other monitoring data owing to a variety of electrical and mechanical artifacts. Nonstandard electrode placement makes the intraoperative ECG reliable for the identification of only cardiac rate and rhythm. Although localization may not be possible, myocardial ischemia can often be detected only if lead V_5 is monitored.[66]

Direct Arterial Pressure

The need for constant blood pressure measurement and periodic sampling for laboratory studies has rendered arterial cannulation (and venous cannulations discussed later) commonplace during cardiac surgery. Although femoral and brachial arteries are larger and, thus, easier to cannulate, percutaneous radial artery cannulation is performed more often because there are fewer attendant problems.[67] Complications of arterial cannulation and, to a lesser degree, arterial puncture include pain at the site, trauma to the artery (e.g., dissection of the intima, and aneurysm[68] and pseudoaneurysm[69,70] formation) and neighboring structures (e.g., nerve[71,72]), hematoma formation, thrombosis,[73–76] distal ischemia and gangrene,[77,78]

local infection and bacteremia,[76,79] and embolization of air or debris.[74,77,80–82]

Etiology. Predisposing factors include preexisting arterial disease, prolonged cannulation,[73] hypotension, anticoagulation, use of vasopressors, and impaired host defenses, all of which are likely to be present at least at some time during bypass and the early postoperative period. Additionally, only recently have pressure transducers[83,84] and stopcocks[85] been identified as sources of nosocomial infection that is *not* prevented by disposable transducer domes.[86,87]

Prevention. Prevention requires that anesthesiology personnel sterilize and maintain meticulously the cannulation site and transducer, avoid using a radial artery whose Allen test[88] indicates poor collateral ulnar flow, avoid marked dorsiflexion that can compress the median nerve (and occlude the collateral flow through the transpalmar arch and thereby yield a falsely abnormal Allen test,[89] use nontapered catheters of small gauge relative to the vessel lumen diameter and of the least thrombogenic material (e.g., Teflon rather than polypropylene),[74,76,90–93] use a continuous heparin flush (e.g., heparin, 2 units/ml. at 3 ml./hr.[73,76,91] rather than intermittent, large volume flushing (which can result in cerebral embolization,[80] label potential injection sites along the flushing infusion to avoid inadvertent injection of drugs (which generally produce a severe arteritis with resultant distal gangrene of the extremity,[94–96] and, as expected, remove the catheter at the earliest time,[73] with syringe aspiration applied to remove thrombi.[97] A small wrist circumference (e.g., less than 18 cm in an adult) is predictive of subsequent vascular occlusion,[98] although recanalization is likely to occur in most cases.[73]

Central Venous Pressure

Etiology. The many problems that may result from central venous catheterization are divisible into those related to the presence of the indwelling catheter and those due to the insertion of the catheter. Among the complications associated with the presence of the catheter are air embolism (especially following disconnection of the infusion, see Chap. 18), catheter embolism (following shearing of the catheter at the insertion site), phlebitis, venous thrombosis, local bacterial and fungal infection, and septicemia.[99] The complications associated with catheter insertion include perforation of the heart, with hemopericardium or hydropericardium and resultant pericardial tamponade (p. 595).[100-102] Other injuries consequent to needle and catheter trauma are highly dependent upon the site of insertion and the experience of the personnel involved. For example, misinsertion of a subclavian catheter can result in subcutaneous emphysema, pneumothorax (see Chap. 12), subclavian or innominate artery puncture or laceration, hemothorax, hemomediastinum, brachial plexus or phrenic nerve injury, cerebral infarction, and puncture of the trachea (possibly with perforation of the cuff of the tracheal tube), thymus, or thyroid gland.[103,104] These complications are infrequent, if not rare, with internal jugular vein cannulation performed cephalad to the point where the external jugular vein crosses the lateral border of the sternocleidomastoid muscle.[105-109] However, inadvertent puncture of the common carotid artery is a particular hazard which can lead to life-threatening hemorrhage and airway encroachment if the punctured artery is then mistakenly dilated for insertion of a large-bore catheter.[110,111]

Prevention. Most of these complications can be prevented by meticulous attention to the various details of central venous catheterization: asepsis in skin preparation and catheterization site and infusion maintenance,[112,113] positioning of the patient so that the site is below heart level, use of a short-beveled needle with attention to surface landmarks specified for the particular site, confirmation of proper placement by demonstrating free flow and easy aspiration, strict avoidance of an intracardiac placement of the catheter tip and use of the catheter for infusion of large volumes, and removal of the catheter at the earliest practical time. The appropriate vein can be identified and entered with minimal trauma by using the Seldinger technique:[114] a relatively small-gauge needle (*e.g.*, 18 gauge) is used to identify and enter

the vessel, a flexible guide wire is passed into the lumen of the vessel and the needle removed, a tapered dilator-sheath is inserted over the wire into the vessel, the wire is removed, and the sheath serves as the catheter. The safety of the procedure is enhanced further by attaching the small-bore, exploratory needle to a transducer to exclude the possibility that an artery has been entered.

Pulmonary Artery Pressures

Apart form the complications encountered in performing a central venous cannulation just cited, a variety of problems, very infrequent though often life-threatening, have been associated with the placement or use of the flow-directed, balloon-tipped, pulmonary artery catheter: atrial and ventricular dysrhythmias,[115] intracardiac knotting,[116,117] infection,[118-120] air embolism,[121] complete heart block,[122] tricuspid valve chordae rupture,[123] thrombosis,[124-126] thrombocytopenia,[127] segmental pulmonary ischemia and infarction,[124,128] and pulmonary artery hemorrhage, often with exsanguination.[128-134]

Etiology. The hemorrhagic problems result from perforation of a pulmonary artery branch by the inflation balloon near the tip of the catheter or the relatively firm tip itself, which is more likely in the presence of hypothermia (which stiffens the catheter), pulmonary hypertension, and anticoagulation.[134]

Treatment. If blood issues from the tracheal tube following placement or during use of this type of catheter in the intensive care unit, the catheter should be withdrawn a few centimeters and a chest x-ray film should be examined promptly for distention of a pulmonary segment or rupture of the pleura. If either is present or should bleeding continue, surgical exploration, with possible segmental pulmonary resection, is indicated. During cardiac surgery, airway bleeding typically appears shortly after inflation of the balloon for a wedge pressure, just before discontinuation of the bypass. Prompt termination of the bypass, neutralization of the heparin anticoagulation with protamine, and exploration of the

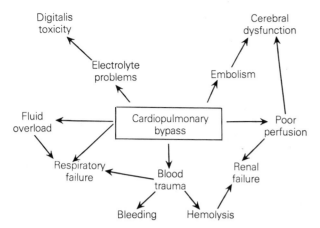

Fig. 47-2. The interrelationships among some of the complications related directly to the use of cardiopulmonary bypass in cardiac surgery. (Courtesy of Dr. R. T. Geer, University of Pennsylvania.)

lung and pleura may be life-saving. Other modalities include withdrawing the catheter a few centimeters, administering positive end-expiratory pressure to tamponade the bleeding site, and placing a double-lumen tracheal tube to isolate (and identify) the bleeding lung.

Prevention. Prevention begins with critical assessment of the need for such a catheter and, in particular, the necessity of obtaining true wedge pressures, as opposed to noting merely the pulmonary diastolic pressures. Once inserted, excessive manipulation of the catheter, as well as the heart and lungs, should be avoided. However, even then, migration of the catheter distally, especially as it warms to body temperature, is to be expected. Great care should be exercised to avoid overinflation of the balloon; the catheter should never be flushed during inflation of the balloon.

COMPLICATIONS RELATED TO EXTRACORPOREAL CIRCULATION

Problems related directly to cardiopulmonary bypass, by far the most common application of extracorporeal circulation, are diverse and often serious, if not life-threatening. Only some of the more common complications are discussed here, principally according to the organ system involved.[135] These complications rarely present individually, however. Rather, they are highly interrelated (Fig. 47–2). Impairment or failure of one organ system usually results in problems in other systems, with greatly increased morbidity and mortality. For example, renal failure severe enough to require dialysis may be associated with a mortality of 70% or more; the addition of sepsis or pulmonary insufficiency generally results in a fatal illness.

VASCULAR INJURY

Blood oxygenated by the heart–lung machine returns to the patient through a cannula placed in either the femoral artery or the ascending aorta. Cannulation can result in several types of serious vascular complications. Fortunately, these problems are generally preventable or can be treated without irreversible end-organ changes if recognized early.[136]

RETROGRADE AORTIC DISSECTION

Injury to the femoral artery during cannulation, coexistent vascular disease, or excessively high perfusion rates can cause intimal tears in as many as 3 per cent of femoral cannulations.[137,138] A sudden drop in systemic pressure occurs, followed by a bluish enlargement of the ascending aorta. Other signs include excessive pressure in the arterial return, a collapsed ascending aorta, and, somewhat later, oliguria or anuria. Failure to discontinue cardiopulmonary bypass promptly usually results in fatal aortic dissection; stenosis with distal ischemia and neuropathy,[139] traumatic aneurysm, and late hemorrhage occur less commonly. Once the problem is recognized, the cannula can be placed in the other femoral artery, some other location in the aorta, or even the same femoral artery if the true lumen can be identified, depending upon the extent of the dissection.[140–142] Prevention requires that the cannula be inserted gently, with the bevelled opening directed away from the wall of the vessel, pulsatile flow be observed prior to starting perfusion, and the perfusion be increased slowly. Largely to avoid this complication, cannulation is undertaken more commonly in the ascending aorta, unless aortic arch surgery is planned.

FEMORAL ARTERY OCCLUSION

Although this rare problem can occur as a result of surgical trauma to the vessel (*e.g.*, use of an excessively large-bore cannula), femoral artery occlusion occurs more often in patients having peripheral vascular disease with intermittent claudication. Treatment usually includes a femoral bypass graft. Prevention involves not only avoiding cannulation of diseased vessels but also not tying the anchoring tape tightly around the vessel and thereby occluding the vasa vasorum.[136]

ASCENDING AORTIC DISRUPTION

This rare, but usually fatal complication can present weeks to years following aortic cannulation. Typically, a nonmycotic false aneurysm has developed at the cannulation site following a major wound infection (*e.g.*, *S. aureus* infection of the sternotomy wound).[143] Yet, less commonly, poor quality tissue or faulty closure of the aortotomy site is implicated.

CEREBRAL HYPERPERFUSION

Anatomic variation or inadvertent common carotid cannulation results in a substantial portion of or the entire arterial return being directed cephalad.[144-147] Mean arterial pressure is lower than expected and does not respond to vasopressors; there may also be unilateral otorrhea, rhinorrhea, facial edema, petechiae, and conjunctival edema. Of greater concern is the increased mean cerebral perfusion that elevates intracranial pressure, leading to cerebral edema and capillary disruption. Without prompt recognition ·of the cerebral hyperfusion and the institution of aggressive treatment of the increased intracranial pressure (see Chap. 20), this complication is generally fatal.

CORONARY OBSTRUCTION

Selective coronary perfusion is used for aortic valve procedures. Cannulation of the coronary ostia can injure the media of the vessels, with subsequent intimal proliferation. Additionally, prolonged cannulation-related occlusion of the vasa vasorum can lead to necrosis and secondary scarring. The third mechanism of injury is the pressure exerted upon the vessel wall by the perfusion itself. The resultant coronary narrowing presents clinically as coronary insufficiency, with episodes of angina and the development of ventricular dysrhythmias.[136] Treatment includes coronary revascularization[148] and possibly angioplasty.

SYSTEMIC EMBOLISM

Nonspecific, often subtle impairment of most organ systems is common following cardiopulmonary bypass and probably related, at least in part, to diffuse defects in the microcirculation consequent to systemic embolism. Perhaps truer than with other complications, prevention here is easier (and associated with a better clinical outcome) than treatment which usually consists of supportive and symptomatic care; for, rarely is the embolized material sufficiently large or localized to be removed surgically.

ETIOLOGY

Emboli can be either gas (*e.g.*, oxygen, air) or particulate matter.

Gas Embolism

The incidence of gas embolism is dependent upon the type of oxygenator blood and oxygen flow rates, and the design of the bypass circuit. Membrane oxygenators are associated with a considerably lower risk of gas embolism than bubble oxygenators, unless the membrane is punctured. As the blood and oxygen flows are increased above 3 liter/min. and 6 liter/min., respectively, the concentration of microemboli in the effluent of the bubble oxygenator can rise 200-fold.[149] Bubbles can also form at sharp angulations and sudden changes in the lumen of the apparatus tubing, as well as when high negative pressure or rapid warming is applied. In addition, air accumulates in the heart and, to a lesser extent, in the great vessels during the surgical procedure. Large volumes of air can be pumped through the arterial return if the venous return to the oxygenator becomes occluded, with rapid emptying of the venous reservoir.

Particulate Matter Embolism

A variety of endogenous and exogenous debris collects in the pump-oxygenator and returns to the patient to embolize widely throughout the microcirculation. This material includes vegetations and calcium fragments from diseased valves, endocardial thrombi and clots, fat globules, formed blood elements aggregated or destroyed by the pump rollers or the natural aging of bank blood, and proteins denatured by the pump.

Treatment. Largely supportive and symptomatic therapy for the diverse manifestations of embolism is directed to the particular organs affected, as described in the remaining parts of this chapter.

Prevention. Attempts should be made to remove trapped air before bypass is discontinued—by lifting the heart to expel air, needle aspiration of air from the most superior site of the aorta, and gentle ventilation of the lungs to force air out of the pulmonary veins—yet, some gas undoubtedly remains. Since the source of much, if not all of the embolized air is the left cardiotomy, flooding the operative field with carbon dioxide has been suggested because this gas is tolerated intravascularly better than air, more soluble in blood, and more rapidly removed. However, this measure does not appear to be very effective, possibly because the gas diffuses rapidly away from the field; moreover, there is a danger of respiratory acidosis.[150] The more general problem of particulate matter microembolism is prevented by maintaining a high level of anticoagulation throughout the perfusion period, minimizing the amount of bank blood infused by using hemodilution, using a membrane rather than a bubble oxygenator, irrigating debris from the operative field before using cardiotomy suction, limiting the use of cardiotomy suction, limiting perfusion time, and, most important, using micropore filters (*e.g.*, pore size less than 40 μ) in the bypass circuit.[151–154]

CEREBRAL INJURY

Up to 60 per cent of patients exhibit some type of cerebral dysfunction following cardiopulmonary bypass.[155] The spectrum of disturbances noted is remarkably diverse, including subtle behavioral and personality changes, immediate memory loss, acute toxic psychosis, visual and other spotty deficits, paraplegia, hemiplegia, coma, and convulsions.[155–159] Fortunately, the majority of these disturbances are short-lived and clear spontaneously without residual deficits, the most severe and persisting problems occurring among those who die from yet other complications.

ETIOLOGY

Given imprecise methods for assessing cerebral function and inadequate understanding of how cerebral function can be deranged, compounded by the diverse symptomatology and still other variables related to the patient and his surgical procedure, there is little more than an empirical, if not circumstantial basis for relating cerebral complications to specific etiologic factors. Very likely, the symptomatology is related to the site and extent of cerebral injury, with the injury itself being a nonspecific, transient or persisting loss of cerebral perfusion. Two major etiologies have been implicated: microembolization of gas or particulate matter from the heart, oxygenator, or stored blood; and, inadequate cerebral perfusion resulting from low perfusion pressure, prolonged duration of bypass, or cerebrovascular disease.[155,160] The use of a membrane rather than bubble oxygenator,[161] micropore filters in the bypass circuit,[151,153,162–166] and maintenance of high perfusion flows and pressures during bypass[164,165] are associated with a reduced incidence of cerebral injury. The incidence of cerebral injury is enhanced by a variety of related variables such as advanced age,[158,160] cerebrovascular disease,[160,167] prolonged bypass,[160,164,166] and valvular procedures.[160,164,170]

DIFFERENTIAL DIAGNOSIS

The diverse clinical presentations of cerebral injury following cardiopulmonary bypass should suggest an equally diverse set of differential diagnoses. Intraoperative cerebral injury not uncommonly results in a prolonged emergence from anesthesia; the differential diagnosis of prolonged emergence and failure to regain consciousness is discussed in Chapter 26. Generally, the more severe the injury (*e.g.*, hemiparesis), the easier the diagnosis becomes. Diagnostic difficulty, however, is encountered with symptomatology at the other end of the spectrum. For example, agitation and confusion may be related to hypoxia, sleep deprivation, emotional stress in an unfamiliar setting, and an adverse drug reaction, among other etiologies (see Chap. 25). Even mental lucidity after a prolonged emergence does not guarantee an uneventful course, for some patients lapse into coma days later; this is reminiscent of the delayed neurologic deterioration described in persons resuscitated after exposure to an anoxic environment.[171]

TREATMENT

Therapy is largely supportive and symptomatic. Once hypoxia has been excluded, the agitated or confused patient may be treated with haloperidol, 2 mg. intravenously, two or three times daily. For the more severe injuries, the therapy is directed towards reducing the accompanying cerebral edema and secondary increased intracranial pressure, while maintaining adequate arterial oxygenation and cerebral perfusion (see Chap. 20).

PREVENTION

In accordance with current knowledge of etiology, prevention requires that cardiopulmonary bypass be conducted with a membrane oxygenator, with meticulous attention paid to avoiding embolization of gas or particulate matter (p. 600), maintenance of an adequate perfusion flow rate (*e.g.*, 2.5 liter/min) and mean arterial blood pressure (*e.g.*, 60 torr), and use of micropore filters. Nonessential drugs should be discontinued as soon as possible to minimize their contribution to depression and agitation. Also, as soon as practical, patients should be moved from the unfamiliar intensive care setting to their private rooms where they can be with family and friends. Additionally, consideration should be given to the use of a cerebral function monitor intraoperatively.[165] Simpler, more reliable, and less costly than a conventional EEG, this device permits earlier diagnosis and, thus, enables immediate

therapy; by detecting cerebral dysfunction earlier, this monitor should also assist in the prevention of further injury. Unfortunately, this device provides no information about the site or extent of injury.

LOW OUTPUT SYNDROME

The low output syndrome represents a potentially end-stage, multisystem failure that results from prolonged circulatory insufficiency.[172,173] Prominent features of the syndrome are hypotension, intense vasoconstriction, low cardiac output and mixed venous oxygen saturation, acidosis, oliguria, respiratory insufficiency, and mental obtundation. Without prompt therapy, the syndrome is generally fatal within hours.

ETIOLOGY

An exacerbation of congestive heart failure is the most common cause of the syndrome. Other etiologies include overdistention of the heart, inadequate intraoperative myocardial preservation, electrolyte imbalance, dysrhythmias, incomplete correction of the surgical defect, malfunction of or leak about an implanted valve, and pericardial tamponade.

TREATMENT

To reduce cardiac work and improve the circulation, vasodilatation is induced with a nitroprusside infusion. As the vascular space increases, volume replacement is begun, using the central venous pressure as a guide and remembering that the particular pressure required is dependent upon the given patient. If hypotension persists, administration of a peripherally dilating inotropic agent (*e.g.*, dopamine, 5–20 µg./kg./min.) is started. Of course, while the circulation is being supported, treatable causes should be sought.

POSTPERFUSION LUNG

Postperfusion lung is a form of acute respiratory insufficiency that generally begins within hours of cardiopulmonary bypass. Initially believed to be a unique clinical entity, the syndrome is now recognized to be merely another example of the adult respiratory distress syndrome that has been described following trauma, shock, sepsis, multiple blood transfusions, pulmonary aspiration, and fat embolism.[174-177] The syndrome begins insidiously and, without prompt therapy, progresses rapidly with a potentially fatal course that includes rales, wheezes, inspiratory retraction, severe tachypnea, marked cyanosis, cardiac failure (which it resembles), peripheral constriction, and multiple organ failure. Fortunately, owing to preventive measures (see following), the incidence of this syndrome has decreased in the past decade. Because the more general aspects of postoperative respiratory insufficiency have been mentioned already (p. 593), this section briefly examines only those aspects particularly associated with cardiopulmonary bypass.

ETIOLOGY

As with most of the other problems associated with bypass, the incidence of this complication has been related directly to the duration of bypass; not unexpectedly, both particulate matter microemboli and aspects of the actual perfusion have been implicated in the etiology. Platelet aggregates,[178] polymorphonuclear leukocytes,[179] and mast cells have been found trapped in the pulmonary capillaries in man and experimental animals after bypass. Although the number of such emboli is small, the platelets have been noted to be disaggregating, the leukocytes disintegrating and releasing lysosomal granules,[180] and the mast cells degranulating and releasing vasoactive substances. There is resultant swelling of the pulmonary capillary endothelial cells; damage also occurs among the alveolar epithelial calls. Initially there is capillary and bronchiolar constriction, followed by loss of vascular tone, increased capillary permeability, and capillary hemorrhage. Finally, there are patchy accumulations of both interstitial and alveolar edema, with the amounts related directly to the duration of bypass and the extent of pulmonary pathology *prior* to bypass. (Significantly, some degree of preexisting pulmonary disease, such as chronic pulmonary congestion or chronic pulmonary hypertension,

with associated damage to the pulmonary capillary bed, seems to be required for the development of this syndrome.[25-27,179]) Edema formation is enhanced further by the reductions in both pulmonary capillary hydrostatic pressure and plasma colloid pressure that occur during bypass. These pathophysiologic processes are enhanced further as the bypass flow rate increases. For, at low flow rates, the lungs are relatively protected because generally less than 1 per cent of the bypass flow reaches the atelectatic lungs, presumably through the thebesian circulation. At higher flow rates, however, there is increased blood flow through bronchial arteries, exposing the lungs to more microemboli and risking pulmonary venous congestion.

DIAGNOSIS

The presence of postperfusion lung is suggested clinically by tachypnea, dyspnea, decreased pulmonary compliance, and severely impaired oxygenation despite oxygen administration. Not unexpectedly, the alveolar-arterial oxygen gradient and the dead space-to-tidal volume ratio are both increased. The chest x-ray reveals a diffuse pulmonary opacification.

TREATMENT

In addition to respiratory support, the rudiments of which are described on page 593, fluid management is an important part of therapy. These patients tend to retain fluid extracellularly during bypass and intravascularly later as the compartmentalized fluid returns to the circulation, often leading to a dilutional hyponatremia (see p. 605); mechanical ventilation is also associated with water retention.[181] Fluid management generally includes rigid fluid restriction (*e.g.*, replacement of urinary loss plus an estimate for insensible losses), diuretic therapy, and the administration of salt-poor albumin, guided by left atrial or pulmonary artery pressure. Since pulmonary and cardiac function are interdependent, improving cardiac performance is also essential. Steroids (*e.g.*, methylprednisolone, 30 mg./kg.) have been recommended for their ability to stabilize membranes and theoretically minimize release of proteolytic enzymes;[182] however, their efficacy has yet to be established.

PREVENTION

Postperfusion lung is now uncommon, probably owing to improved pulmonary preparation of patients with preexisting cardiorespiratory disease (p. 594), measures to avoid microemboli in the perfusion (p. 600), and fluid management. The use of hemodilution rather than whole blood during bypass also serves to decrease the amount of debris perfused. Advocated prophylactically,[182] steroid administration is controversial. Although PEEP is am important part of therapy, it does not appear to have prophylactic value.[183]

RENAL FAILURE

Acute renal failure of some degree occurs in up to 30% of patients following cardiopulmonary bypass, with death in more than two thirds of those requiring dialysis.[184–188] Death is usually not due to the renal failure but rather to sepsis, cardiac failure, or pulmonary insufficiency. Oliguric renal failure is discussed in greater detail in Chapter 28.

ETIOLOGY

Receiving one fifth of the cardiac output, the kidneys are very sensitive to changes in blood pressure and organ blood flow consequent to extracorporeal circulation.[189,190] Among the predisposing causes of acute renal failure are factors related to preexisting renal disease and advanced age; surgical trauma, such as occult dissecting aortic aneurysm and renal emboli; and details of the cardiopulmonary bypass itself. Particularly relevant aspects of the bypass are its duration, as well as the duration of aortic cross-clamping, and the presence of postoperative acidosis (pH below 2.5), excessive hemolysis (plasma hemoglobin concentration greater than 200 mg./dl.), low urine flow rate (below 40 ml./hr.), perioperative hypotension (particularly bypass perfusion rates lower than 2.5 liter/min.), prolonged nonpulsatile perfusion (e.g., greater than 2.5 hr.), and exposure to nephrotoxic drugs (e.g., aminoglycosides, tetracyclines, methoxyflurane, iodinated contrast media).

DIFFERENTIAL DIAGNOSIS

Acute renal failure is heralded by anuria or, more likely, oliguria. Oliguria, a urinary output of less than 400 ml/24 hr, is not synonymous with renal failure, however. In fact, oliguria following cardiopulmonary bypass is usually due to inadequate intravenous fluid administration as replacement for sequestered "third space" fluid and the postoperative blood loss which can reach 1 liter in the first 24 hr. The differential diagnosis also includes other physiologic factors (e.g., increased antidiuretic hormone or aldosterone), other fluid losses (e.g., drainage, sweating, prior diuresis), cardiac tamponade (p. 595), low cardiac output syndrome (p. 601), congestive heart failure, hypotension, obstruction of the urinary tract (e.g., renal tubular obstruction by free hemoglobin released from red cells damaged during bypass), and acute renal failure. The latter may be due to prerenal causes that result in decreased renal blood flow and glomerular filtration rate (e.g., reduced effective plasma volume as in hypovolemia and heart failure) or intrinsic causes, such as renal ischemia with resultant acute tubular necrosis.

DIAGNOSIS

Generally, the differential diagnosis narrows considerably upon review of the patient's clinical course. An important distinction is whether the renal failure is due to prerenal or intrinsic causes —that is, has there been adequate intravenous fluid replacement or are the kidneys unable to excrete their customary salt and water load? Monitoring the left atrial pressure with a catheter inserted at surgery or measuring the wedge pressure with a pulmonary artery catheter can determine whether the patient requires further fluid administration. Finding a urinary sodium concentration of less than 10 mEq/liter (10 mmol./liter) in a random sample is also suggestive of a prerenal cause; that urine sample may also have a high specific gravity (*i.e.*, 1.018–1.030) and osmolarity. Fluid administration results in an increased urine flow. However, patients with intrinsic renal failure, such as acute tubular necrosis, exhibit poor urinary concentrating ability (*i.e.*, specific gravity of 1.010–1.015), have a much higher urinary sodium concentration (greater than 25 mEq. or mmol./liter), and do not respond to expansion of their vascular volume.

TREATMENT

Once a diagnosis of intrinsic renal failure is established, fluid, potassium, and protein intake must be reduced in accordance with the degree of oliguria. Typically, intravenous fluid is restricted to 500 ml. plus an estimate for insensible loss. Although mannitol can augment urine flow by increasing cortical blood flow, excessive use of osmotic diuretics can result in hyperosmolarity, hyponatremia, and pulmonary edema;[189] in addition, producing a large volume of dilute urine has yet to be shown to alter the course of the renal failure. Potentially nephrotoxic drugs should be discontinued or administered in smaller dosages.

Specific therapy is needed for the hyperkalemia that may develop in oliguric renal failure. Serum potassium level is determined at least daily and monitored also with the ECG. Characteristic tall, symmetrically spiked T waves appear when the serum potassium concentration rises above 6.5 mEq./liter (6.5 mmol./liter); above a potassium level of 8 mEq./liter atrial activity is absent and QRS prolongation occurs. The magnitude of the potassium elevation guides the therapy.[191] With a serum potassium level of 6.5 to 8.0 mEq./liter, therapy consists of eliminating the cause of the renal failure, where possible (*e.g.*, obstruction, hypotension), and neutralizing the accompanying acidosis with an alkali infusion (*e.g.*, sodium bicarbonate, 80 to 132 mEq., in 1 liter D_5W administered over several hours). Potassium levels above 8 mEq./liter require more aggressive therapy: calcium gluconate 10%, 10 to 30 ml., is infused over several minutes to lessen cardiac toxicity, and a glucose (*e.g.*, $D_{10}W$ 200–500 ml. in

30 min., another 500–1000 ml. over several hours) or glucose-insulin (*e.g.*, glucose 50%, 50 ml., and regular insulin, 50 units, as a bolus) is given to move potassium into cells. Potassium may be removed from the body by sodium polystyrene sulfonate, a cation exchange resin, administered as a retention enema. ·

With severe oliguria or anuria, peritoneal or hemodialysis is generally required by the time the serum creatinine has reached 5 mg./dl. (440 μmol./liter). Survival may be improved by instituting dialysis early.[192] Dialysis in these patients, however, is associated with a greater risk of dysrhythmias and hypotension; greater care in managing fluid balance, judicious use of vasopressor infusions (to avoid hypotension), and use of a dialysate with a higher than usual concentration of potassium (to avoid rapid changes in potassium level) may be needed.

PREVENTION

Preoperatively, BUN and creatinine levels should be determined to identify those patients with impaired renal function, generally those having BUN levels above 25 mg./dl. (8.9 mmol./liter), with creatinine levels above 1.5 mg/dl (133 μmol/liter. Particular care should be directed to avoiding exposure of these patients to potentially nephrotoxic drugs, excessive fluid loading, and hypotension. More than others, patients with preexisting renal disease will benefit from expeditious surgery, with a short duration of bypass and scrupulous attention to details such as adequate perfusion (*e.g.*, at least 2.5 liter/min., with an arterial pressure above 60 torr), avoidance of emboli, and maintenance of normal blood gas and electrolyte values. Once deterioration in renal function begins, prompt therapy may avert further problems.

ELECTROLYTE PROBLEMS

Because fluid and electrolyte disturbances are discussed in Chapter 27, only aspects of those problems particularly relevant to cardiopulmonary bypass are mentioned here. In general, most clinically important problems can be avoided by continual determination of electrolyte values and assessments of fluid losses and replacement, with prompt institution of changes in fluid administration.

HYPOKALEMIA

Common following cardiopulmonary bypass, hypokalemia can precipitate ventricular dysrhythmias, particularly in patients receiving digitalis.[193-196] Lowering the threshold for dysrhythmias is particularly important for the successful discontinuation of bypass. Although some of the potassium loss is due to overly vigorous preoperative diuretic therapy, most of the loss occurs during bypass owing variously to the use of prime solutions deficient in potassium, hemodilution with forced diuresis, activation of the renin–angiotensin–aldosterone system, and inadequate potassium replacement. So great are the losses that 100 mEq. or more of potassium chloride may be needed merely to maintain the potassium level. Postoperatively, the loss may be compounded by overly zealous use of diuretics without adequate potassium replacement, respiratory or metabolic alkalosis, and an increased insulin level that moves potassium into cells. Treatment, as well as prevention, requires frequent potassium determinations, with prompt and adequate replacement of losses as they are noted. Intraoperatively, bolus doses of less than 8 mEq. of potassium chloride may be given without vasoconstrictor effect.[197] Later, potassium infusions at rates up to 1 mEq./kg./hr. may be used with ECG monitoring for the tall, peaked T waves associated with *hyper*kalemia.

HYPERKALEMIA

In addition to renal failure (see p. 603), metabolic acidosis, hemoglobinuria secondary to blood trauma, accumulation of blood in the thorax, multiple transfusions, and large doses of potassium-containing medications (*e.g.*, potassium penicillin, 10 million units) can also raise the serum potassium level, although generally not to the same level as in renal failure. Therapy is the same as that discussed for hyperkalemia occurring with renal failure (see p. 604).

HYPONATREMIA

Mild hyponatremia (e.g., serum sodium level of 130 mEq. or mmol./liter) usually occurs following cardiopulmonary bypass as a result of overhydration with salt-poor fluids. Also, pain, emotional and surgical stress, administration of inhalation anesthetics and narcotics, and potitive-pressure ventilation can result in increased secretion of antidiuretic hormone (ADH) and the retention of free water.[198,199] Often there are no clinically recognizable signs or symptons. Restricting fluid intake to 300 to 500 ml./day, plus an estimate for insensible losses, results in spontaneous diuresis and correction of the hyponatremia. However, sufficient potassium may be lost to produce hypokalemia that threatens dysrhythmias, especially in the patient receiving digitalis. More severe hyponatremia, such as in water intoxication in which the sodium level may be as low as 110 mEq/liter, is accompanied by restlessness, confusion, disorientation, muscle twitching, and, with the lowest sodium levels, stupor, coma, and convulsions. In life-threatening circumstances, hypertonic saline may also be administered (see p. 394).

HYPOPHOSPHATEMIA

The administration of large doses of glucose can result in severe hypophosphatemia, associated with which is a reduced concentration of 2,3-diphosphoglyceric acid (2,3–DPG) in the red cell and secondary reduced oxygen delivery to the tissues.[200] Additional consequences of hypophosphatemia are reduced adenosine triphosphate (ATP) levels in the red cell leading to increased red cell hemolysis and in the leukocytes leading to impaired phagocytosis. First noted in patients receiving intravenous hyperalimentation,[200,201] this problem has been found recently following cardiopulmonary bypass in patients given a glucose–insulin–potassium infusion to improve cardiac performance and to decrease the incidence of dysrhythmias.[202] The clinical significance of the hypophosphatemia in cardiac surgery patients, however, may be small. In the only study of this problem, all patients experienced severe hypophosphatemia but the duration was just 12 hr; there was no change in red cell ATP and only small decreases in 2,3-DPG, and the decrease in the calculated P_{50} was just 1.2 torr (0.16 kPa).[110]

POSTPERFUSION BLEEDING

Bleeding in the late perfusion and early postoperative period is common, occurring in one quarter of patients and requiring exploration in many cases.[203]

ETIOLOGY

Although perhaps a more diverse set of etologies underlie this complication of cardiopulmonary bypass than others, it should not be forgotten that most postperfusion bleeding is due to inadequate hemostasis. Other causes include destruction of platelets by the pump rollers, destruction of leukocytes with the release of a fibrinolytic activator, destruction of all three formed elements with the development of disseminated intravascular coagulation and secondary fibrinolysis, dilution of platelets and coagulation factors (especially V and VIII), and a transfusion reaction leading to disseminated intravascular coagulation with secondary fibrinolysis. Although a variety of clotting defects has been described, there has been little success in accounting for the disparate results among the various studies.[204] The use of a membrane rather than bubble oxygenator does seem to impair hemostasis less, presumably because of less damage to blood elements.[205] Inadequate neutralization of heparin undoubtedly adds to bleeding problems, but "heparin rebound" is less common than believed.[206] Similarly, although protamine in excess has anticoagulant activity, that effect is not clinically important.[207] Finally, there are nonsurgical causes, such as a mild bleeding tendency (e.g., some forms of hemophilia, von Willebrand's disease, and platelet abnormalities), low vitamin K levels (as in liver dysfunction, chronic congestive heart failure), and drugs (e.g., aspirin, other nonsteroidal anti-inflammatory agents). Worthy of particular note is the bleeding tendency of patients with cyanotic congenital heart disease, who often demonstrate prolonged prothrombin time, increased partial thromboplastin time, and a modest decrease in platelet count.

DIAGNOSIS

Instead of drawing a battery of coagulation studies indiscriminately, one can make simple but important observations that can guide further evaluation and consultation. An important early distinction is whether the bleeding is localized (and, thus, related to the surgery) or generalizes (suggesting a diffuse coagulation defect). Freshly drawn blood should be observed for clotting and possible subsequent clot lysis. Specific studies can be obtained, although the bleeding problem usually will have been treated by the time that the test results become available.

TREATMENT

If exploration fails to reveal a localized site of bleeding, the problem is treated empirically with fresh frozen plasma, fresh whole blood, and platelets. Calcium is often administered, particularly if large volumes of bank blood have been given with in a short time; similarly, if the patient had taken warfarin anticoagulants preoperatively, one can give vitamin K, although the effect is not apparent for hours.

PREVENTION

The preoperative history should include a thorough medication history and also an inquiry about bleeding tendencies. Preoperative testing should include a prothrombin time, partial thromboplastin time, platelet count, and thrombin time. Neutralization of heparin should be undertaken with a heparin–protamine titration which is repeated within the early postoperative hours. But, above all, meticulous surgical technique must be used, with thorough exploration of the chest for bleeding prior to the closure.

POSTPERFUSION SYNDROME

One to three months following cardiopulmonary bypass, an occasional patient develops a syndrome consisting of fever, hepatosplenomegaly, and lymphocytosis, with a rare patient also exhibiting a skin rash and lymphadenopathy.[208,209] Self-limited and benign, the syndrome usually resolves within a few weeks. Although the etiologic agent is now known to be cytomegalovirus,[210,211] presumably transmitted by transfused blood or reactivation of a preexisting latent infection, the differential diagnosis is both diverse and difficult: subacute bacterial endocarditis, infectious mononucleosis, toxoplasmosis, drug fever, and serum hepatitis. The diagnosis is confirmed later when the results of specific serologic tests (*e.g.*, cytomegalovirus complement-fixing antibody, hepatitis B surface antigen) become available. Treatment is symptomatic, except in those experiencing hemolytic anemia, in whom a short course of prednisone may be given.

REFERENCES

1. Comroe, J. H., Jr., and Dripps, R. D.: Scientific basis for the support of biomedical research. Science, *192*:105, 1976.
2. Gibbon, J. H., Jr.: Application of a mechanical heart and lung apparatus to cardiac surgery. Minn. Med., *33*:52, 1953.
3. Comroe, J. H., Jr., and Dripps, R. D.: Ben Franklin and open heart surgery. Circ. Res., *35*:661, 1974.
4. Finlayson, D. C., and Kaplan, J. A.: Cardiopulmonary bypass. In Kaplan, J. A. (ed.): Cardiac Anesthesia. pp. 393–440. New York, Grune and Stratton, 1979.
5. Branthwaite, M. A.: Extracorporeal circulation and associated techniques. In Branthwaite, M. A. (ed.): Anaesthesia for Cardiac Surgery and Allied Procedures. ed 2. pp. 148–170. Oxford, Blackwell Scientific Publications, 1980.
6. Ionescu, M. I. (ed.): Current Techniques in Extracorporeal Circulation. ed. 2. London, Butterworth, 1981.
7. Ryan, J. F., Donlon, J. V., Malt, R. A., et al.: Cardiopulmonary bypass in the treatment of malignant hyperthermia. N. Engl. J. Med., *290*:1121, 1974.
8. Zapol, W. M., Snider, M. T., Hill, J. D., et al.: Extracorporeal membrane oxygenator in severe acute respiratory failure. A randomized prospective study. J.A.M.A., *242*:2193, 1979.
9. Calne, R. Y., Smith, D. P., McMaster, P., et al.: Use of partial cardiopulmonary bypass during the anhepatic phase of orthotopic liver grafting. Lancet, 2:612, 1979.
10. Berger, R. L., McCormick, J. R., Stetz, J. D., et al.:

11. Williams, J. F., Jr., Morrow, A. G., and Braunwald, E.: The incidence and management of "medical" complications following cardiac operations. Circulation, *32*:608, 1965.
12. Rosky, L. P., and Rodman, T.: Medical aspects of open-heart surgery. N. Engl. J. Med., *274*:833 and 886, 1966.
13. Gooch, A. S., Maranhao, V., Alblaza, S., at al.: Medical complications following open-heart surgery. Arch. Intern. Med., *120*:672, 1967.
14. Cordell, A. R.: Cardiac dysrhythmias associated with extracorporeal circulation. In Cordell, A. R., and Ellison, R. G. (eds.): Complications of Intrathoracic Surgery. pp. 53–59. Boston, Little, Brown & Company, 1979.
15. Waldo, A. L., and MacLean, W. A. H.: Diagnosis and Treatment of Cardiac Arrhythmias Following Open Heart Surgery: Emphasis on the Use of Atrial and Ventricular Epicardial Wire Electrodes. Mount Kisco (N.Y.), Futura, 1980.
16. Ghani, M. F., Parker, B. M., and Smith, J. R.: Recognition of myocardial infarction after cardiac surgery and its relation to cardiopulmonary bypass. Am. Heart J., *88*:18, 1974.
17. Killen, D. A.,: Serum enzyme elevations, a diagnostic test for acute myocardial infarction during the early postoperative period. Arch. Surg., *96*:200, 1968.
18. Hobson, R. W., Conant, C., Mahoney, W. D., et al.: Serum creatine phosphokinase. Analysis of postoperative changes. Am. J. Surg., *124*:625, 1972.
19. Alderman, E. L., Mattloff, H. J., Shumway, N. E., et al.: Evaluation of enzyme testing for the detection of myocardial infarction following direct coronary surgery. Circulation, *48*:135, 1973.
20. Dixon, S. H., Jr., Limbird, L. E., Roe, C. R., et al.: Recognition of postoperative acute myocardial infarction: application of isoenzyme techniques. Circulation, *47–48*(suppl.):III–137, 1973.
21. Driscoll, A., Hobika, J. H., Etsten, B. E., et al.: Postoperative myocardial infarction. N. Engl. J. Med., *264*:633, 1961.
22. Sonnenblick, E. H., and Skelton, L. L.: Oxygen consumption of the heart: Physiological principles and clinical implications. Mod. Concepts Cardiovasc. Dis., *40*:9, 1971.
23. Moroko, P. R., Kjekshus, J. E., Sobel, B. E., et al.: Factors influencing infarct size following experimental coronary artery occlusions. Circulation, *43*:67, 1971.
24. Gorlin, R.: Practical cardiac hemodynamics. N. Engl. J. Med., *296*:203, 1977.
25. Ellison, L. T., Duke, J. F., III, and Ellison, R. G.: Pulmonary compliance following open heart surgery and its relationship to ventilation and gas exchange. Circulation, *35*(suppl.):I-217, 1967.
26. Tilney, N. L., and Hester, W. J.: Physiologic and histologic changes in the lungs of patients dying after prolonged cardiopulmonary bypass. Ann. Surg., *166*:759, 1967.
27. Weintraub, H. D., Sullivan, S. F., Malm, J. R., et al.: Lung function and blood-gas exchange, before and after cardiac surgery. J. Appl. Physiol., *20*:483, 1965.
28. Kirklin, J. W.: Pulmonary dysfunction after open heart surgery. Med. Clin. North Am., *48*:1063, 1964.

Successful use of a paracorporeal left ventricular assist device in man. J.A.M.A., *243*:46, 1980.

29. Parker, D. J., Karp, R. B., Kirklin, J. W., et al.: Lung water and alveolar and capillary volumes after intracardiac surgery. Circulation, *45*(suppl.):I–139, 1972.

30. Thung, N., Herzog, P., Christlieb, I. I., et al.: Cost of respiratory effort in postoperative cardiac patients. Circulation, *28*:552, 1963.

31. Peters, R. M., Wellons, H. A., Jr., and Htwe, T. W.: Total compliance and work of breathing after thoracotomy. J. Thorac. Cardiovasc. Surg., *57*:348, 1968.

32. Fordham, R. M. M.: Hypoxaemia after aortic valve surgery under cardiopulmonary bypass. Thorax, *20*:505, 1965.

33. McClenahan, J. B., Young, W. E., and Sykes, M. K.: Respiratory changes after open-heart surgery. Thorax, *20*:545, 1965.

34. Bjork, V. O., and Engstrom, C. G.: The treatment of ventilatory insufficiency by tracheostomy and artificial ventilation. J. Thorac. Cardiovasc. Surg., *34*:228, 1957.

35. Spencer, F. C., Benson, D. W., Liu, W. C., et al.: Use of a mechanical respirator in the management of respiratory insufficiency following trauma or operation for cardiac or pulmonary disease. J. Thorac. Cardiovasc. Surg., *38*:758, 1959.

36. Dammann, J. E., Jr., Thung, N., Christlieb, H., et al.: The management of the severely ill patient after open heart surgery. J. Thorac. Cardiovasc. Surg., *45*:80, 1963.

37. Macrae, W. R., and Masson, A. H. B.: Assisted ventilation in the postbypass period. Br. J. Anaesth., *36*:711, 1964.

38. Zeitlin, G. L.: Artificial respiration after cardiac surgery. Anaesthesia, *20*:145, 1965.

39. Lefemine, A. A., and Harken, D. E.: Postoperative care following open-heart operations: Routine use of controlled ventilation. J. Thorac. Cardiovasc. Surg., *52*:207, 1966.

40. Toung, T., Saharia, P., Permutt, S., et al.: Aspiration pneumonia: Beneficial and harmful effects of positive end-expiratory pressure. Surgery, *82*:279, 1977.

41. Kudsk, K. A., Pflug, B., and Lowery, B. D.: Value of positive end-expiratory pressure in aspiration pneumonia. J. Surg. Res., *24*:321, 1978.

42. Springer, R. R., and Stevens, P. M.: The influence of PEEP on survival of patients in respiratory failure: A restrospective analysis. Am. J. Med., *66*:196, 1979.

43. Feeley, T. W., and Hedley-Whyte, J.: Weaning from controlled ventilation and supplemental oxygen. N. Engl. J. Med., *292*:903, 1975.

44. Downs, J. B., Klein, E. F., Jr., Desautels, D., et al.: Intermittent mandatory ventilation: A new approach to weaning patients from mechanical ventilators. Chest, *64*:331, 1973.

45. Midell, A. I., Skinner, D. B., DeBoer, A., et al.: A review of pulmonary problems following valve replacements in 100 consecutive patients. Ann. Thorac. Surg., *18*:219, 1974.

46. Prakash, O., Johnson, B., Meij, S., et al.: Criteria for early extubation after intracardiac surgery in adults. Anesth. Analg., *56*:703, 1977.

47. Klineberg, P. L., Geer, R. T., Hirsh, R. A., et al.: Early extubation after coronary artery bypass graft surgery. Crit. Care Med., *5*:272, 1977.

48. Quasha, A. L., Loeber, N., Feeley, T. W., et al.: Postoperative respiratory care: A controlled trial of early and late extubation following coronary-artery bypass grafting. Anesthesiology, *52*:135, 1980.

49. Barash, P. G., Lescovich, R., Katz, J. D., et al.: Early extubation following pediatric cardiothoracic operation: A viable alternative. Ann. Thorac. Surg., *29*:228, 1980.

50. Cain, H. D., Stevens, P. M., and Adaniya, R.: Preoperative pulmonary function and complications after cardiovascular surgery. Chest, *76*:130, 1979.

51. Ellison, R. G.: Respiratory complications of extracorporeal circulation. In Cordell, A. R., and Ellison, R. G. (eds.): Complications of Intrathoracic Surgery. pp. 60–71. Boston, Little, Brown & Company, 1979.

52. Dennis, C., Spreng, D. S., Jr., Nelson, G. E., et al.: Development of a pump-oxygenator to replace the heart and lungs: An apparatus applicable to human patients, and application to one case. Ann. Surg., *134*:709, 1951.

53. Nelson, R. M., Jenson, C. B., and Smoot, W. M., III: Pericardial tamponade following open-heart surgery. J. Thorac. Cardiovasc. Surg., *58*:510, 1969.

54. Cunningham, J. N., Jr., Spencer, F. C., Zeff, R., et al.: Influence of primary closure of the pericardium after open-heart surgery on the frequency of tamponade, postcardiotomy syndrome, and pulmonary complications. J. Thorac. Cardiovasc. Surg., *70*:119, 1975.

55. Shabetai, R., Fowler, N. O., and Guntheroth, W. G.: The hemodynamics of cardiac tamponade and constrictive pericarditis. Am. J. Cardiol., *26*:480, 1970.

56. Reddy, P. S., Curtiss, E. I., O'Toole, J. D., et al.: Cardiac tamponade: Hemodynamic observations in man. Circulation, *58*:265, 1978.

57. Weeks, K. R., Chatterjee, K., Block, S., et al.: Bedside hemodynamic monitoring: Its value in the diagnosis of tamponade complicating cardiac surgery. J. Thorac. Cardiovasc. Surg., *71*:250, 1976.

58. Thomas, T. V.: Emergency evacuation of acute pericardial tamponade. Ann. Thorac. Surg., *10*:566, 1970.

59. Cooper, J. B., Newbower, R. S., Long, C. D., et al.: Preventable anesthesia mishaps: A study of human factors. Anesthesiology, *49*:399, 1978.

60. Pineda, A. A., Brzica, S. M., Jr., and Taswell, H. F.: Hemolytic transfusion reaction: Recent experience in a large blood bank. Mayo Clin. Proc., *53*:378, 1978.

61. Myhre, B. A.: Fatalities from blood transfusion. J.A.M.A., *244*:1333, 1980.

62. Honig, C. L., and Bove, J. R.: Transfusion-associated fatalities: Review of Bureau of Biologics Reports 1976–1978. Transfusion, *20*:653, 1980.

63. Utting, J. E., Gray, T. C., and Shelley, F. C.: Human misadventure in anaesthesia. Can. Anaesth. Soc. J., *26*:472, 1979.

64. Becker, C. M., Malhotra, I. V., and Hedley-Whyte, J.: The distribution of radiofrequency current and burns. Anesthesiology, *38*:106, 1973.

65. Leeming, M. N.: Protection of the "electrically susceptible patient": A discussion of systems and methods. Anesthesiology, *38*:370, 1973.

66. Kaplan, J. A., and King, S. B., III: The precordial electrocardiographic lead (V$_5$) in patients who have coronary-artery disease. Anesthesiology, *45*:570, 1976.

67. Mortensen, J. D.: Clinical sequelae from arterial needle puncture, cannulation and incision. Circulation, *35*:1118, 1967.

68. Mathieu, A., Dalton, B., Fischer, J. E., et al.: Expanding

aneurysm of the radial artery after frequent puncture. Anesthesiology, *38*:401, 1973.

69. Russell, R. C., Steichen, J. B., and Zook, E. G.: Radial-arteries pseudoaneurysms—their diagnosis, treatment and prevention. Orthopaedic Rev., *8*:49, 1979.

70. Wolf, S., and Mangano, D. T.: Pseudoaneurysm, a late complication of radial-artery catheterization. Anesthesiology, *52*:80, 1980.

71. Macon, W. L., and Futrell, J. W.: Median-nerve neuropathy after percutaneous puncture of the brachial artery in patient receiving anticoagulants. N. Engl. J. Med., *228*:1396, 1973.

72. Marshall, G., Edelstein, G., and Hirshman, C. A.: Median nerve compression following radial artery puncture. Anesth. Analg., *59*:953, 1980.

73. Bedford, R. F., and Wollman, H.: Complications of percutaneous radial-artery cannulation: An objective prospective study in man. Anesthesiology, *38*:228, 1973.

74. Downs, J. B., Rackstein, A. D., Klein, E. F., Jr., et al.: Hazards of radial-artery catheterization. Anesthesiology, *38*:283, 1973.

75. Gardner, R. M., Schwartz, R., Wong, H. C., et al.: Percutaneous indwelling radial-artery catheters for monitoring cardiovascular function. Prospective study of the risk of thrombosis and infection. N. Engl. J. Med., *290*:1227, 1974.

76. Mandel, M. A., and Dauchot, P. J.: Radial artery cannulation in 1,000 patients: Precautions and complications. J. Hand Surg., *2*:482, 1977.

77. Bartlett, R. M., and Munster, H. W.: Improved technique for prolonged arterial cannulation. N. Engl. J. Med., *279*:92, 1968.

78. Mangano, D. T., and Hickey, R. F.: Ischemic injury following uncomplicated radial artery catheterization. Anesth. Analg., *58*:55, 1979.

79. Stamm, W. E., Colella, J. J., Anderson, R. L., et al.: Indwelling arterial catheters as a source of nosocomial bacteremia. An outbreak caused by flavobacterium species. N. Engl. J. Med., *292*:1099, 1975.

80. Lowenstein, E., Little, J. W., III, and Hing, H. L.: Prevention of cerebral embolization from flushing radial artery cannulas. N. Engl. J. Med., *285*:1414, 1971.

81. Michaelson, E. D., and Walsh, R. E.: Osler's node: A complication of prolonged arterial cannulation. N. Engl. J. Med., *283*:472, 1970.

82. Matthews, J. I., and Gibbons, R. B.: Embolization complicating radial artery puncture. Ann. Intern. Med., *75*:87, 1971.

83. Walton, J. R., Shapiro, B. A., Harrison, R. A., et al.: Serratia bacteremia from mean arterial pressure monitors. Anesthesiology, *43*:113, 1975.

84. Weinstein, R. A., Stamm, W. E., Kramer, L., et al.: Pressure monitoring devices overlooked source of nosocomial infection. J.A.M.A., *236*:936, 1976.

85. Dryden, G. E., and Brickler, J.: Stopcock contamination. Anesth. Analg., *58*:141, 1979.

86. Maki, D. G., and Band, J. D.: Septicemia from disposable pressure-monitoring chamber domes. "Beware of Greeks bearing gifts." Chest, *74*:486, 1978.

87. Buxton, A. E., Anderson, R. L., Klimek, J., et al.: Failure of disposable domes to prevent septicemia acquired from contaminated pressure transducers. Chest, *74*:508, 1978.

88. Allen, E. V.: Thromboangiitis obliterans: Methods of diagnosis of chronic occlusive arterial lesions distal to the wrist with illustrative cases. Am. J. Med. Sci., *178*:237, 1929.

89. Greenhow, D. E.: Incorrect performance of Allen's test—Ulnar artery flow erroneously presumed inadequate. Anesthesiology, *37*:356, 1972.

90. Bedford, R. F.: Percutaneous radial-artery cannulation—Increased safety using Teflon catheters. Anesthesiology, *42*:219. 1975.

91. Downs, J. B., Chapman, R. L., and Hawkins, I. F.: Prolonged radial artery catheterization: Evaluation of heparinized catheters and continuous irrigation. Arch. Surg., *108*:671, 1974.

92. Bedford, R. F.: Radial arterial function following percutaneous cannulation with 18- and 20-gauge catheters. Anesthesiology, *47*:37, 1977.

93. Davis, F. M.: Radial artery cannulation: Influence of catheter size and material on arterial occlusion. Anaesth. Intensive Care, *6*:49, 1978.

94. Stone, H. H., and Donnelly, C. C.: The accidental intra-arterial injection of thiopental. Anesthesiology, *22*:996, 1961.

95. Schanzer, H., Gribetz, I., and Jacobson, J. H., II: Accidental intra-arterial injection of penicillin G. A preventable catastrophe. J.A.M.A., *242*:1289, 1979.

96. Mazumder, J. K., Metcalf, I. R., and Holland, A. J. C.: Inadvertent intra-arterial injection of thiopentone. Can. Anaesth. Soc. J., *27*:395, 1980.

97. Bedford, R. F.: Removal of radial-artery thrombi following percutaneous cannulation for monitoring. Anesthesiology, *46*:430, 1977.

98. Bedford, R. F.: Wrist circumference predicts the risk of radial-arterial occlusion after cannulation. Anesthesiology, *48*:37, 1978.

99. Walters, M. B., Stanger, H. A. D., and Rotem, C. E.: Complications with percutaneous central venous catheters. J.A.M.A., *220*:1455, 1972.

100. Fitts, C. T., Barnett, L. T., Webb, C. M., et al.: Perforating wounds of the heart caused by central venous catheters. J. Trauma, *10*:764, 1970.

101. Dane, T. E. B., and King, E. G.: Fatal cardiac tamponade and other mechanical complications of central venous catheters. Br. J. Surg., *62*:6, 1975.

102. Defalque, R. J., and Cambell, C.: Cardiac tamponade from central venous catheters. Anesthesiology, *50*:249, 1979.

103. Defalque, R. J.: Subclavian venipuncture: A review. Anesth. Analg., *47*:677, 1968.

104. Schechter, D. C., and Acinapura, A. J.: Subclavian vein catheterization. Parts I and II. NY State J. Med., *79*:346 and 732, 1979.

105. English, I. C. W., Frew, R. M., Pigott, J. F. G., et al.: Percutaneous cannulation of the internal jugular vein. Anaesthesia, *24*:521, 1969.

106. Jernigan, W. R., Gardner, W. C., Mahr, M. M., et al.: Use of the internal jugular vein for placement of central venous catheter. Surg. Gynecol. Obstet., *130*:522, 1970.

107. Daily, P. O., Griepp, R. B., and Shumway, N. E.: Percutaneous internal jugular vein cannulation. Arch. Surg., *101*:534, 1970.

108. McConnell, R. Y., and Fox, R. T.: Experience with percutaneous internal-innominate vein catheterization. Calf. Med., *117*:1, 1972.

109. Defalque, R. J.: Percutaneous catheterization of the internal jugular vein. Anesth. Analg., 53:116, 1974.
110. McEnany, M. T., and Austen, W. G.: Life-threatening hemorrhage from inadvertent cervical arteriotomy. Ann. Thorac. Surg., 24:233, 1977.
111. McDaniel, M. M., and Grossman, M.: Aortic dissection complicating percutaneous jugular-vein catheterization. Anesthesiology, 49: 1978.
112. Maki, D. G., Goldmann, D. A., and Rhame, F. S.: Infection control in intravenous therapy. Ann. Intern. Med., 79:867, 1973.
113. Maki, D. G.: Nosocomial bacterimia: An epidemiologic overview. Am. J. Med., 70:719, 1981.
114. Seldinger, S. I.: Catheter replacement of the needle in percutaneous arteriography. Acta. Radio., 39:368, 1953.
115. Voukydis, P. C., and Cohen, S. I.: Catheter-induced arrhythmias. Am. Heart J., 88:588, 1974.
116. Lipp, H., O'Donoghue, K., and Resnekov, L.: Intracardiac knotting of a flow-directed balloon catheter. N. Engl. J. Med., 284:220, 1970.
117. Meister, S. G., Furr, C. M., Engel, T. R., et al.: Knotting of a flow-directed catheter about a cardiac structure. Cathet. Cardiovasc. Diagn., 3:171, 1971.
118. Cerra, F., Milch, R., and Lajos, T. Z.: Pulmonary artery catheterization in critically ill patients. Ann. Surg., 177:37, 1973.
119. Pracher, H., Dittel, M., Jobst, C., et al.: Bacterial contamination of pulmonary artery catheters. Intensive Care Med., 4:79, 1978.
120. Michel, L., Marsh, H. M., McMichan, J. C., et al.: Infection of pulmonary artery catheters in critically ill patients. J.A.M.A., 245:1032, 1981.
121. Conahan, T. J., III: Air embolization during percutaneous Swan-Ganz catheter placement. Anesthesiology, 50:360, 1979.
122. Abernathy, W. S.: Complete heart block caused by the Swan-Ganz catheter. Chest, 65:349, 1974.
123. Smith, W. R., Glauser, F. L.: and Jemison, P.: Rupture chordae of the tricuspid valve. The consequence of flow-directed Swan-Ganz catheterization. Chest, 70:790, 1976.
124. Foote, G. A., Schabel, S. I., and Hodges, M.: Pulmonary complications of the flow-directed balloon-tipped catheter. N. Engl. J. Med., 290:927, 1974.
125. Yorra, F. H., Oblath, R., Jaffe, H., et al.: Massive thrombosis associated with use of the Swan-Ganz catheter. Chest, 65:682, 1974.
126. Swan, H. J. C., Ganz, W., Forrester, J., et al.: Catheterization of the heart in man with the use of a flow-directed balloon-tipped catheter. N. Engl. J. Med., 283:447, 1970.
127. Kim, Y. L., Richman, K. A., and Marshall, B. E.: Thrombocytopenia associated with Swan-Ganz catheterization in patients. Anesthesiology, 53:261, 1980.
128. Meltzer, R., Kint, P. P., and Simoons, M.: Hemoptysis after flushing Swan-Ganz catheters in the wedge position. N. Engl. J. Med., 304:1980.
129. Pape, L. A., Haffajee, C. I., Markis, J. E., et al.: Fatal pulmonary hemorrhage after use of the flow-directed balloon-tipped catheters. Ann. Intern. Med., 90:344, 1979.
130. Chun, G. M. H., and Ellestad, M. H.: Perforation of the pulmonary artery by a Swan-Ganz catheter. N. Engl. J. Med., 284:1041, 1971.
131. Ohn, K. C., Cottrell, J. E., and Turndorf, H.: Hemoptysis from a pulmonary-artery catheter. Anesthesiology, 51:485, 1979.
132. Krantz, E. M., and Viljoen, J. F.: Hemoptysis following insertion of a Swan-Ganz catheter. Br. J. Anaesth., 51:457, 1979.
133. McDaniel, D. D., Stone, J. G., Faltas, A. N., et al.: Catheter-induced pulmonary artery hemorrhage: Diagnosis and management in cardiac operations, J. Thorac. Cardiovasc. Surg., 82:1, 1981.
134. Barash, P. G., Nardi, D., Hammond, G., et al.: Catheter-induced pulmonary artery perforation: Mechanisms, management, and modifications. J. Thorac. Cardiovasc. Surg., 82:5, 1981.
135. Branthwaite, M. A.: Complications of open heart surgery. In Branthwaite, M. A. (ed.): Anaesthesia for Cardiac Surgery and Allied Procedures. ed 2. pp. 198–209. Oxford, Blackwell Scientific Publications, 1980.
136. Najafi, H.: Vascular complications of extracorporeal circulation. In Cordell, A. R., and Ellison, R. G. (eds.): Complications of Intrathoracic Surgery. pp 78–83. Boston, Little, Brown & Company, 1979.
137. Jones, J. W., Vetto, R. R., Winterscheid, L. C., et al.: Arterial complications incident to cannulation in open-heart surgery with special reference to the femoral artery. Ann. Surg., 152:969, 1960.
138. Elliot, D. P., and Roe, B. B.: Aortic dissection during cardiopulmonary bypass. J. Thorac. Cardiovasc. Surg., 50:357, 1965.
139. Carey, J. S., Skow, J. R., and Scott, C.: Retrograde aortic dissection during cardiopulmonary bypass: "Nonoperative" management. Ann. Thorac. Surg., 24:44, 1977.
140. Serry, C., Najafi, H., Dye, W. S., et al.: Superiority of aortic over femoral cannulation for cardiopulmonary bypass, with special attention to lower extremity neuropathy. J. Thorac. Cardiovasc. Surg., 19:277, 1978.
141. Vatayanon, S., Kahn, D. R., and Sloan, H.: Retrograde aortic dissection during cardiopulmonary bypass. Report of a case with successful management. Ann. Thorac. Surg., 4:451, 1967.
142. Benedict, J. S., Buhl, T. L., and Henney, R. P.: Acute aortic dissection during cardiopulmonary bypass. Successful treatment of three patients. Arch. Surg., 108:810, 1974.
143. Soorae, A. S., Cleland, J., and O'Kane, H.: Delayed non-mycotic false aneurysm of ascending aortic cannulation site. Thorax, 32:743, 1977.
144. Kulkarni, M. G.: A complication of aortic cannulation. J. Thorac. Cardiovasc. Surg., 9:207, 1968.
145. Magner, J. B.: Complications of aortic cannulation for open-heart surgery. Thorax, 26:172, 1971.
146. Krous, H. F., Mansfield, P. B., and Sauvage, L. R.: Carotid hyperperfusion during open heart surgery. J. Thorac. Cardiovasc. Surg., 66:118, 1973.
147. Ross, W. T., Jr., Lake, C. L., and Wellons, H. A.: Cardiopulmonary bypass complicated by inadvertent carotid cannulation. Anesthesiology, 54:85, 1981.
148. Chawla, S. K., Najafi, H., Javid, H., et al.: Coronary obstruction secondary to direct cannulation. Ann. Thorac. Surg., 23:135, 1977.
149. Kessler, J., and Patterson, R. H., Jr.: Production of microemboli by various oxygenators. Ann. Thorac. Surg., 9:221, 1970.

150. Burbank, A., Ferguson, T. B., and Burford, T. H.: Carbon dioxide flooding of the chest in open-heart surgery. A potential hazard. J. Thorac. Cardiovasc. Surg., *50*:691, 1965.

151. Osborn, J. J., Swank, R. L., Hill, J. D., et al.: Clinical use of a Dacron wool filter during perfusion for open-heart surgery. J. Thorac. Cardiovasc. Surg., *60*:575, 1970.

152. Lawrence, G. H., McKay, H. A., and Sherensky, R. T.: Effective measures in the prevention of intra-operative air-embolus. J. Thorac. Cardiovasc. Surg., *62*:731, 1971.

153. Hill, J. D.: Blood filtration during extracorporeal circulation. Ann. Thorac. Surg., *15*:313, 1973.

154. Solis, R. T., Noon, G. P., Beall, A. C., Jr., et al.: Particulate microembolism during cardiac operation. Ann. Thorac. Surg., *17*:332, 1974.

155. Lee, W. H., Jr., and Brady, M. P.: Central nervous system complications of extracorporeal circulation. In Cordell, A. R., and Ellison, R. G. (eds.): Complications of Intrathoracic Surgery. ed 2. pp. 72–77. Boston, Little, Brown & Company, 1979.

156. Gilman, S.: Cerebral disorders after open-heart operations. N. Eng. J. Med., *272*:489, 1965.

157. Tufo, H. M., Ostfeld, A. M., and Shekelle, R.: Central nervous system dysfunction following open-heart surgery. J.A.M.A., *212*:1333, 1970.

158. Heller, S. S., Frank, K. A., Malm, J. R., et al.: Psychiatric complications of open-heart surgery. N. Engl. J. Med., *283*:1015, 1970.

159. Branthwaite, M. A.: Neurologic damage related to open heart surgery: Clinical survey. Thorax, *27*:748, 1972.

160. Kolkka, R., and Hilberman, M.: Neurologic dysfunction following cardiac operation with low-flow, low-pressure cardiopulmonary bypass. J. Thorac. Cardiovasc. Surg., *79*:432, 1980.

161. Carlson, R. G., Lande, A. J., Landis, B., et al.: The Lande-Edwards membrane oxygenator during heart surgery. Oxygen transfer, microemboli counts, and Bender-Gestalt visual motor test scores. J. Thorac. Cardiovasc. Surg., *66*:894, 1973.

162. Arrants, J. E., Gadsden, R. H., Huggins, M. B., et al.: Effects of extracorporeal circulation upon blood lipids. Ann. Thorac. Surg., *15*:230, 1973.

163. Page, U. S., Bigelow, J. C., Carta, C. R., et al.: Emboli (debris) produced by bubble oxygenators. Removal by filtration. Ann. Thorac. Surg., *18*:164, 1974.

164. Aberg, T., and Kihlgren, M.: Effect of open heart surgery on intellectual function. Scand. J. Thorac. Cardiovasc. Surg., 8 [Suppl. 15]:1, 1974.

165. Branthwaite, M. A.: Prevention of neurological damage during open-heart surgery. Thorax, *30*:258, 1975.

166. Clark, R. E., Margraf, H. W., and Beauchamp, R. A.: Fat and solid filtration in clinical perfusions. Surgery, *77*:216, 1975.

167. Lee, W. H., Jr., Brady, M. P., Rowe, J. M., et al.: Effects of extracorporeal circulation upon behavior, personality, and brain function. Part II. Hemodynamic, metabolic, and psychometric correlations. Ann. Surg., *173*:1013, 1971.

168. Hill, J. D., Aquilar, M. J., Baranco, A., et al.: Neuropatheological manifestations of cardiac surgery. Ann. Thorac. Surg., *7*:409, 1969.

169. Javid, H., Tufo, H. M., Najafi, H., et al.: Neurological abnormalities following open-heart surgery. J. Thorac. Cardiovasc. Surg., *58*:502, 1969.

170. Rabiner, C. J., Willner, A. E., and Fishman, J.: Psychiatric complications following coronary bypass surgery. J. Nerv. Ment. Dis., *160*:342, 1975.

171. Plum, F., Posner, J. B., and Hain, R. F.: Delayed neurological deterioration after anoxia. Arch. Intern. Med., *110*:56, 1962.

172. Dietzman, R. H., Erseck, R. A., Lillehei, C. W., et al.: Low output syndrome. J. Thorac. Cardiovasc. Surg., *57*:138, 1969.

173. Ankeney, J. L.: Cardiac complications of extracorporeal circulation (low cardiac output syndrome). In Cordell, A. R., Ellison, R. G. (eds.): Complications of Intrathoracic Surgery. ed 2. pp. 43–52. Boston, Little, Brown & Company, 1979.

174. Ashbaugh, D. G., Bigelow, D. B., Petty, T. L., et al.: Acute respiratory distress in adults. Lancet, 2:319, 1967.

175. Ellison, R. G.: Respiratory complications of extracorporeal circulation. In Cordell, A. R., and Ellison, R. G. (eds.): Complications of Intrathoracic Surgery. ed 2. pp. 60–71. Boston, Little, Brown & Company, 1979.

176. Edmunds, L. H., Jr., and Alexander, J. A.: Effects of cardiopulmonary bypass on the lungs. In Fishman, A. P. (ed.): Pulmonary Diseases and Disorders. pp. 1728–1738. New York, McGraw-Hill Book Company, 1980.

177. Byrick, R. J., and Noble, W. H.: Postperfusion lung syndrome. J. Thorac. Cardiovasc. Surg., *76*:685, 1978.

178. Dutton, R. C., Edmunds, L. H., Jr., Hutchinson, J. C., et al.: Platelet aggregate emboli produced in patients during cardiopulmonary bypass with membrane and bubble oxygenators and blood filters. J. Thorac. Cardiovasc. Surg., *67*:258, 1974.

179. Ratliff, N. B., Young, W. G., Jr., Hackel, D. B., et al.: Pulmonary injury secondary to extracorporeal circulation. J. Thorac. Cardiovasc. Surg., *65*:425, 1973.

180. Chenoweth, D. E., Cooper, S. W., Hugli, T. E., et al.: Complement activation during cardiopulmonary bypass. Evidence for generation of C3a and C5a anaphylatoxins. N. Engl. J. Med., *304*:497, 1981.

181. Sladen, A., Laver, M. B., and Pontoppidan, H.: Pulmonary complication and water retention in prolonged mechanical ventilation. N. Engl. J. Med., *279*:448, 1968.

182. Wilson, J. W.: Treatment or prevention of pulmonary cellular damage with pharmacologic doses of corticosteroids. Surg. Gynecol. Obstet., *134*:675, 1972.

183. Stanley, T. H., Liu, W.-S., and Gentry, S.: Effects of ventilatory techniques during cardiopulmonary bypass on post-bypass and postoperative pulmonary compliance and shunt. Anesthesiology, *46*:391, 1977.

184. Porter, G. A., Kloster, F. E., Herr, R. J., et al.: Renal complications associated with valve replacement surgery. J. Thorac. Cardiovasc. Surg., *53*:145, 1967.

185. Abel, R. M., Wick, J., Beck, C. H., et al.: Renal dysfunction following open-heart operations. Arch. Surg., *108*:175, 1974.

186. Casali, R., Simmons, R. L., Najarian, J. S., et al.: Acute renal insufficiency complicating major cardiovascular surgery. Ann. Surg., *181*:370, 1975.

187. Abel, R. M., Buckley, M. J., Austen, W. J., et al.: Etiology, incidence, and prognosis of renal failure following cardiac operations. J. Thorac. Cardiovasc. Surg., *71*:323, 1976.

188. Bhat, J. G., Gluck, M. C., Lowenstein, J., et al.: Renal

failure after open heart surgery. Ann. Intern. Med., *84*:677, 1976.

189. Yeh, T. J., Brackney, E. L., Hall, D. P., et al.: Renal complications of open-heart surgery: Predisposing factors, prevention and management. J. Thorac. Cardiovasc. Surg., *47*:79, 1964.

190. Cordell, A. R.: Renal complications of extracorporeal circulation. In Cordell, A. R., and Ellison, R. G. (eds.): Complications of Intrathoracic Surgery. pp. 35–42. Boston, Little, Brown & Company, 1979.

191. Levinsky, N. G.: Management of emergencies. VI. Hyperkalemia. N. Engl. J. Med., *274*:1076, 1966.

192. Gailiunas, P., Jr., Chawla, R., Lazarus, J. M., et al.: Acute renal failure following cardiac operations. J. Thorac. Cardiovasc. Surg., *79*:241, 1980.

193. Lockey, E., Longmore, D. B., Ross, D. N., et al.: Potassium and open-heart surgery. Lancet, *1*:671, 1966.

194. Marcial, M. B., Vedoya, R. C., Zerbini, E. J., et al.: Potassium in cardiac surgery with extracorporeal perfusion. Am. J. Cardiol., *23*:400, 1969.

195. Dieter, R. A., Neville, W. E., and Pifarre, R.: Hypokalemia following hemodilution cardiopulmonary bypass. Ann. Surg., *171*:17, 1970.

196. Dieter, R. A., Neville, W. E., and Pifarre, R.: Serum electrolyte changes after cardiopulmonary bypass with Ringer's lactate solution used for hemodilution. J. Thorac. Cardiovac. Surg., *59*:168, 1970.

197. Schwartz, A. J., Conahan, T. J., III, Jobes, D. R., et al.: Peripheral vascular response to potassium administration during cardiopulmonary bypass. J. Thorac. Cardiovac. Surg., *79*:237, 1980.

198. Soliman, M. G., and Brindle, G. F.: Plasma levels of anti-diuretic hormone during and after heart surgery with extra corporeal circulation. Can. Anaesth. Soc. J., *21*:195, 1974.

199. Philbin, D. M., and Coggins, C. H.: Plasma antidiuretic hormone levels in cardiac surgical patients during morphine and halothane anesthesia. Anesthesiology, *49*:95, 1978.

200. Travis, S. F., Sugarman, H. J., Ruberg, R. L., et al.: Alterations of red-cell glycolytic intermediates and oxygen transport as a consequence of hypothosphatemia in patients receiving intravenous hyperalimentation. N. Engl. J. Med., *285*:763, 1971.

201. Dudrick, S. J., MacFadyen, B. V., Van Buren, C. T., et al.: Parenteral hyperalimentation: Metabolic problems and solution. Ann. Surg., *176*:259, 1972.

202. Swaminathan, R., Morgan, D. B., Ionescu, M., et al.: Hypoposphatemia and its consequences for patients following open heart surgery. Anaesthesia, *33*:601, 1978.

203. Cordell, A. R.: Hematological complications of extracorporeal circulation. In Cordell, A. R., and Ellison, R. G. (eds.): Complications of Intrathoracic Surgery. pp. 27–34. Boston, Little, Brown & Company, 1979.

204. Kalter, R. D., Saul, C. M., Wetstein, L., et al.: Cardiopulmonary bypass: Associated hemostatic abnormalities. J. Thorac. Cardiovasc. Surg., *77*:427, 1979.

205. deJong, J. C. F., ten Duis, H. J., Smit Sibinga, C. T., et al.: Hematologic aspects of cardiotomy suction in cardiac operations. J. Thorac. Cardiovasc. Surg., *79*:227, 1980.

206. Ellison, N., Beatty, C. P., Blake, D. R., et al.: Heparin rebound: Studies in patients and volunteers. J. Thorac. Cardiovasc. Surg., *67*:723, 1974.

207. Ellison, N., Ominsky, A. J., and Wollman, H.: Is protamine a clinically important anticoagulant? A negative answer. Anesthesiology, *35*:621, 1971.

208. Kreel, I. L., Zaroff, L. I., Canter, J. W., et al.: A syndrome following total body perfusion. Surg. Gynecol. Obstet., *111*:317, 1960.

209. Wheeler, E. O., Turner, J. D., and Scannell, J. G.: Fever, splenomegaly, and atypical lymphocytes: A syndrome observed after cardiac surgery using a pump oxygenator. N. Engl. J. Med., *266*:454, 1967.

210. Lang, D. J., Scolnick, E. M., and Willerson, J. T.: Association of cytomegalovirus infection with the postperfusion syndrome. N. Engl. J. Med., *278*:147, 1968.

211. Kantor, G. L., and Johnson, B. L.: Cytomegalovirus infection associated with cardiopulmonary bypass. Arch. Intern. Med., *125*:488, 1970.

FURTHER READING

Branthwaite, M. A.: Complications of open heart surgery. In Branthwaite, M. A.: Anaesthesia for Cardiac Surgery and Allied Procedures. edition 2. pp. 198–209. Oxford, Blackwell Scientific Publications, 1980.

Cordell, A. R., and Ellison, R. G. (eds.): Complications of Intrathoracic Surgery. Boston, Little, Brown & Company, 1979.

Edmunds, L. H., Jr., and Alexander, J. A.: Effect of cardiopulmonary bypass on the lungs. In Fishman, A. P., (ed.): Pulmonary Diseases and Disorders. pp. 1728–1738. New York, McGraw-Hill Book Company, 1980.

Finlayson, D. C., and Kaplan, J. A.: Cardiopulmonary bypass. In Kaplan, J. A. (ed.): Cardiac Anesthesia. pp. 393–440. New York, Grune and Stratton, 1979.

48 Complications of Deliberate Hypotension

McIver W. Edwards, Jr., M.D.

Many physicians have criticized the deliberate induction of hypotension during surgical operations as a dangerous and unjustified "physiological trespass" with risks out of proportion to any possible benefits. Nevertheless, it continues to be a popular procedure, and it is worthwhile to review the complications of deliberate hypotension: their incidence, recognition, and avoidance.

It is often claimed that deliberate hypotension reduces surgical blood loss. Several studies of scoliosis surgery,[1] hip replacement,[2–5] portocaval shunting, craniotomy, and rhinoplasty[6] support this. Other purported benefits are decrease in operating time, better operating conditions, and less hematoma and fibrosis. A significant decrease in operating time has been shown for total hip replacement,[4,5] but not for portocaval shunting.

INCIDENCE OF COMPLICATIONS OF DELIBERATE HYPOTENSION

The risks of deliberate hypotension prior to 1953 were assessed by a questionnaire circulated by Hampton and Little.[7,7a] The overall mortality was 96 in 27,930 cases, an incidence of 0.34 per cent; in 0.24 per cent, death was thought to be related to anesthesia or hypotension. On the other hand, a selected series has experienced a much lower death rate. Enderby reported nine deaths in 9,107 cases (0.99%) before 1961; from his data, it appears that the deaths due to anesthe-

sia and hypotension were only 0.055 per cent.[8] There are no other series of comparable size. Five reports of prostatectomy in older patients resulted in a total of 76 in-hospital deaths in 1,411 patients rendered hypotensive (5.4%). The mortality rates in each report ranged from 3.6 to 10 per cent, compared with 4.2 to 10.7 per cent in unmatched controls; these results are inconclusive but suggest that there is no difference in mortality rates between hypotensive and normotensive prostatectomy.[9–13]

Nonfatal complications are, of course, more common. Hampton and Little reported 908 major and minor complications, an incidence of 3.3 per cent. The more common nonfatal complications are reactionary hemorrhage, delayed awakening, blurred vision, oliguria, anuria, and persistent hypotension. A significant practical point is that there were *no* major complications in patients whose systolic pressure was kept above 80 torr.[7] Most of the complications are related to inadequate perfusion of major organs, and risks are probably increased by vascular disease, preexisting hypertension, hypocapnia, very low arterial pressure (mean below 70 torr), anemia, hypovolemia, and careless monitoring.[14]

EFFECT OF HYPOTENSION ON THE NERVOUS SYSTEM

The symptoms of nervous system damage may range from yawning and fainting, to loss of intellect, convulsions, paralysis, and death. There are fairly specific brain lesions, which Adams has classified as ischemic, oligemic, or hypoxic.[15] Lesions of increasing severity are thought to first involve the neurons in a diffuse but selective manner, leading to some dysfunction; this is followed by damage to the neuroglia resulting in infarction; the most severe lesions cause necrosis of blood vessels, with subsequent hemorrhagic infarction if flow returns to normal levels. The histological changes are often very difficult to recognize if death occurs less than 24 to 48 hours after the insult.

There is no good prospective study of cerebral complications in a controlled series. Many authors have reported isolated cases of CNS damage.[10,12,16–18] In Hampton and Little's survey, the combined incidence of major and minor CNS complications was 1.3 per cent; cerebral thrombosis occurred in 0.014 per cent, and retinal arterial thrombosis, in 0.01 per cent.[7]

Mental function has been presumed to be a sensitive indicator of cerebral function, which should decrease following an ischemic episode. Two studies failed to show any differences between patients made hypotensive and patients kept normotensive. In one of these studies, aged patients undergoing retropubic prostatectomy were given a battery of psychometric tests before and after operation. Half were subjected to hypotension with an average decrease in mean pressure of 56 per cent, and half were not. All patients showed decreased intellectual function the 5th day after operation; 6 weeks later, all performed better than in the preoperative tests. There was no significant difference between the 13 controls and the 14 hypotensive patients.[19] A similar study of young, healthy patients also showed no difference.[20]

The EEG has been proposed as a means of monitoring cerebral function during hypotension, but to be useful it must detect changes while they are still reversible. How well does the EEG meet this criterion? In a study using monkeys, profound hypotension caused slowing and decreased amplitude of the EEG. The changes reverted to normal when blood pressure returned to normal. However, 2 to 2.5 hours later, some animals

began to deteriorate and died; death could not be predicted on the basis of the EEG changes during hypotension.[21] In dogs, hemorrhagic hypotension reduced the cerebral blood flow (CBF) to less than 20 per cent of control values without changing the electrocorticogram; there were few survivors.[22] In humans, careful studies of perfusion pressure and regional cerebral blood flow (rCBF) have shown that EEG changes are usually produced when regional cerebral blood flow falls below 18 ml. per min. per 100 g. The changes occur usually within 20 to 40 seconds and disappear when pressure returns to normal. However, there is no strict correlation between regional cerebral blood flow and EEG changes.[23–26] One should probably not rely on EEG changes as indicators of reversible cerebral ischemia.

Halothane may afford some protection to the brain in hypotension. Cerebral metabolic rate (CMR_{O_2}) is sometimes decreased by halothane.[27] This reduced demand for oxygen may allow the patient to better tolerate hypotension. In dogs made hypotensive with halothane, cerebral lactate increases less than in those made hypotensive with trimethaphan or hemorrhage.[28] Deep, halothane-induced hypotension in rats also produces little increase in cerebral lactate and pyruvate. Hypocapnia seems to be harmful; a Pa_{CO_2} of 20 torr (2.66 kPa) during hypotension causes a further increase in cerebral lactate, presumably by reducing cerebral blood flow. Hypercapnia does not afford any protection greater than that of normocapnia.[29] In man, hypocapnia produces a fall in cerebral blood flow and an increase in lactate production, but an insignificant decrease in CMR_{O_2}.[30] The combination of halothane, head-up tilt, and ganglionic block can produce hypotension without significantly lowering the jugular $P\bar{v}_{O_2}$. However, the addition of either positive airway pressure or hypocapnia produces cerebral hypoxia in some subjects.[31]

Sodium nitroprusside appears to dilate at least some cerebral vessels. It causes a decrease in systemic blood pressure without causing any fall in cerebral blood flow; in some local areas, cerebral blood flow increases.[32,33] One action of sodium nitroprusside is of special concern: It apparently decreases or abolishes autoregulation of cerebral blood flow for a longer time than it exerts its systemic hypotensive effect. After its discontinuation, intracranial pressure may rise significantly in animals with mass intracranial epidural lesions.[34]

Preexisting hypertension or carotid occlusive disease increases the risk from induced hypotension. In patients with occlusive disease, Boysen and colleagues found that regional cerebral blood flow was proportional to "stump pressure" distal to the occlusion. The stump pressure is, in turn, proportional to systemic arterial pressure, although quite different constants of proportionality were obtained in different patients, indicating great differences in the resistance of collateral vessels. The difference between mean systemic and stump pressure ranged from 5 to 80 torr. Boysen and colleagues investigated patients only during normotension and hypertension, but presumably these same patients made hypotensive would suffer further decreases in stump pressure, regional cerebral blood flow, and brain function.[26]

Hypertension is probably the most common disease that decreases the tolerance of the brain to hypotension. Hypertensive patients tend to have persistently high cerebral vascular resistance. When systemic pressure is lowered, regional cerebral blood flow falls to a critical level at a higher systemic pressure in hypertensive patients than in normal controls. For example, awake patients whose control blood pressures were 80 torr showed evidence of cerebral ischemia only when the mean arterial pressure was lowered to 29 torr. Mildly hypertensive patients with mean arterial pressure of 113 torr tolerated hypotension to 47 torr, while severe hypertensives with mean arterial pressure of 180 torr showed signs of cerebral ischemia at mean arterial pressure of 90 torr.[35] Other investigators have obtained similar results.[36]

Hypotension can cause minor to severe brain damage, but the reported incidence of cerebral complications is not high. Unfortunately, the EEG is not a reliable indicator of reversible ischemia. Normotensive patients probably tolerate a mean pressure as low as 30 torr, but hypertensives may be intolerant of low pressure even as high as 90 torr.

EFFECT OF HYPOTENSION ON THE HEART

The heart is probably less likely to be damaged by hypotension than the brain for two reasons: Hypotension reduces the work load of the heart and its oxygen requirements, and ECG monitoring can be a very sensitive indicator of reversible ischemia. In Hampton and Little's series, there was a 0.27-per-cent incidence of cardiac arrest, "coronary thrombosis," or "cardiovascular collapse," and a 0.079-per-cent incidence of fatality.[7] Enderby reported only one "cardiac collapse" in 9,107 hypotensive anesthetic administrations (0.01%), and this occurred 20 hours postoperatively.[8]

There is some evidence that hypocapnia should be avoided for myocardial as well as cerebral protection. During halothane-induced hypotension in dogs, myocardial oxygen consumption decreases in proportion to the decrease in blood flow, but this balance is disturbed by hypocapnia, which causes a further decrease in coronary flow without further decrease in oxygen consumption. Reduction of mean arterial pressure to 55 per cent of control values is accompanied by reduction of myocardial blood flow to 47 per cent and oxygen consumption to 55 per cent of control values. Then, hypocapnia of 26 torr (3.46 kPa) causes a further reduction of blood flow to 38 per cent of control values, without any decrease in oxygen consumption.[37]

Moderate hypotension caused by spinal anesthesia may also have little harmful effect on myocardial oxygenation. In one study, spinal anesthesia to the level of T4 caused a fall in mean arterial pressure from 120 to 62 torr, with a fall in coronary blood flow from 153 to 73 ml. per 100 g per min.[38] In only one of six subjects did coronary sinus oxygen content fall; there was a statistically insignificant decrease in myocardial oxygen extraction. The patients were, however, extremely sensitive to blood volume: A loss of 70 ml. of blood was reported to result in "vascular collapse" and myocardial ischemia.

Hypotension induced by sodium nitroprusside may result in an actual increase in coronary blood flow during moderate hypotension, but at more profound levels of hypotension, the flow decreases.[39] Flow in superior mesenteric and femoral arteries follows a similar course.[40] Hypotension-induced reflex tachycardia results in further decreases in coronary blood flow due to decreased diastolic filling time. Resultant increases in oxygen demand, with concomitant decreases in oxygen supply, pose a particular threat to patients with coronary artery disease.[40a]

A variety of ECG changes can occur during induced hypotension. All appear to be reversible. Rollason and Hough reported "major" changes, consisting of decreased P wave voltage, S-T segment elevation or depression, and T wave alterations, in about half the cases they studied. Other "minor" changes in the QRS and Q-T intervals, and P-Q and S-T segments brought the total incidence of transient changes to almost 80 per cent. Most of the "major" changes appear to result from rapid induction of hypotension, rather than from the depth of hypotension or the agent used.[41,42]

EFFECT OF HYPOTENSION ON THE LUNGS

There are no specific complications of hypotensive anesthesia that involve the lungs. However, when the head-up position is used, physiologic dead space will increase. Eckenhoff and colleagues showed that dead space calculated by the Bohr equation increased an average of 60 ml. during hypotension with head-up position.[43,44] The ratio of dead space to tidal volume V_D/V_T, increased from 0.32 to 0.45; one value of 0.92 was reported. Dead space also increased in patients who were placed in a head-up position without instituting hypotension. The likely explanation of this effect is that a fall in pulmonary artery pressure occurs, leading to poor perfusion of the lung apices and a larger *Zone 1*, the area of the lung that is ventilated but poorly perfused. The practical consequence is that it is necessary to ventilate these patients with higher minute volumes when they are put in the head-up position. Because of this effect and other dangers of hypocapnia, arterial blood gas tensions should be measured during most hypotensive anesthetics.

Arterial oxygenation may be affected by in-duced hypotension. Ganglionic blockade by pentolinium causes decreased pulmonary as well as systemic vascular resistance in halothane-anesthetized patients and may be accompanied by decreased intrapulmonary shunting $(\dot{Q}_s/\dot{Q}_t)$.[45] On the other hand, sodium nitroprusside infusion may impair arterial oxygenation: This may be due to lowered $P\bar{v}_{O_2}$ or impaired hypoxic vasoconstriction, as studied in an isolated lung preparation.[46] Two recent studies have demonstrated that nitroprusside infusion lowers Pa_{O_2} by reversing hypoxic pulmonary vasoconstriction in atelectatic portions of the lung.[46a,46b] However, in intact men and dogs, nitroprusside produces either a minimal increase or no significant change in pulmonary shunting.[47,48]

EFFECT OF HYPOTENSION ON THE SPLANCHNIC ORGANS

There have been no reports of ischemia of the liver or the bowel during induced hypotension, but nor have there been systematic studies of the problem. Most anesthetic agents decrease splanchnic blood flow even more than they reduce oxygen consumption.[49] Mild hypotension induced by nitroprusside increases superior mesenteric artery flow in chloralose-anesthetized dogs; more severe hypotension decreases it.[40] A similar effect occurs when nitroprusside is given to halothane-anesthetized dogs.[50] The clearance of indocyanine green dye from plasma can be used as an index of hepatic function: When hypotension is induced by nitroprusside or epidural blockade in dogs anesthetized with halothane, there is no change in the clearance, suggesting that there is no change in hepatic excretory function or hepatic blood flow.[51]

EFFECT OF HYPOTENSION ON THE KIDNEY

Anuria or oliguria occurred in 116 patients in the survey of Hampton and Little[7]; the total incidence was 0.42 per cent, and the fatalities were 0.032 per cent. Other investigators have reported reduced urine output without renal damage[52] or large numbers of cases with no renal problems.[8,53,54] Significantly, none of the patients whose systolic pressures were maintained above 80 torr developed anuria.[7]

Most anesthetics, except perhaps neuroleptanesthetics, cause a temporary decrease in renal function, with diminished filtration rates and electrolyte excretion. The changes can usually be explained by systemic hypotension, catecholamine release, or the release of antidiuretic hormone. Prolonged systemic hypotension may lead to oliguria, anuria, and renal failure.

Anesthetics may have a protective effect in certain circumstances. The renal vasoconstriction accompanying hemorrhagic hypotension leads to renal damage; in rats, some protection is afforded by barbiturates and possibly by halothane, but not by enflurane, droperidol, or ether.[55] Halothane has a similar protective effect in dogs.[56]

Hypotension produced by halothane and trimethaphan causes a decreased glomerular filtration rate and filtration fraction during mannitol-induced diuresis but a less consistent decline in effective renal plasma flow.[57] Hypotension with 2-per-cent halothane causes diminished renal blood flow, but apparently no intrarenal shunting; the ratio of renal blood flow to cardiac output remains constant.[58] Hypotension with nitroprusside and halothane results in a greater relative drop in renal blood flow than in iliac, celiac, or mesenteric blood flow; this probably means that these other vascular beds are further dilated by nitroprusside, while the renal vascular bed is limited in its capacity to so respond.[50]

Obviously, the renal effects of different hypotensive techniques should be studied more extensively. Many practitioners measure the urine output and give diuretics to maintain "adequate output" during the period of hypotension. There is no evidence that this is beneficial.

COMPLICATIONS OF DELIBERATE HYPOTENSION DUE TO SPECIFIC AGENTS

It is convenient to classify hypotensive agents as *short-acting*, comprising trimethaphan, nitroglycerin, and sodium nitroprusside, or *long-acting*, comprising all of the other hypotensive agents. The great advantages of short-acting agents are that their actions are easily controlled and that they do not produce postoperative hypotension. On the other hand, they require constant intraoperative regulation of infusion rate. The long-acting agents require less attention to pressure monitoring, fluid replacement, and anesthetic depth. They may prove to be less troublesome in an operation requiring a long duration of hypotension, but their effects extend into the postoperative period.

Trimethaphan

Trimethaphan is inactivated by serum cholinesterase, and its action may be prolonged in patients with deficient or blocked cholinesterase. In addition to ganglionic blockade, it produces histamine release and bronchoconstriction. Large doses can cause neuromuscular block, producing respiratory muscle weakness,[59] which is not reversed by neostigmine. Neostigmine may, in fact, retard the breakdown of trimethaphan, because it inhibits plasma cholinesterase. Eye signs that are valuable in assessing neurologic status may be obscured for hours.

NITROGLYCERIN

Acting more on capacitance than resistance vessels, nitroglycerin tends to reduce preload and, thus, cardiac output. As a result, the patient's sensitivity to the drug may be more dependent upon his blood volume adequacy than is the case with other vasodilators. Nitroglycerin prolongs neuromuscular blockade produced by pancuronium but not that resulting from other relaxants.

Sodium Nitroprusside

The most immediate danger from the infusion of sodium nitroprusside (SNP) is overdose and profound hypotension.[60] This complication can best be avoided by judicious administration. Long-term toxicity has been reported in one uremic patient: Hypothyroidism was caused by the metabolic product thiocyanate, which inhibits thyroid function.[61] This type of toxicity is unlikely to be important in anesthetic practice. A

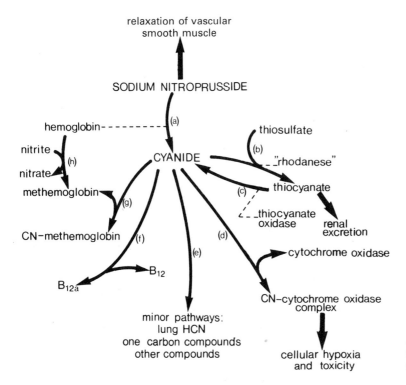

Fig. 48-1. Breakdown, toxicity, and detoxification of sodium nitroprusside and cyanide in the body.

third danger, raising some very interesting problems, is cyanide poisoning from the cyanide released by breakdown of sodium nitroprusside, a complication which has received much attention since reports of isolated cases in 1974.

Figure 48-1 summarizes the known pathways of breakdown of sodium nitroprusside in the body. The molecule of sodium nitroprusside, $Na_2Fe(CN)_5NO \cdot 2H_2O$ (molecular weight = 297.8) contains 44 per cent cyanide by weight and is degraded to cyanide by a reaction occurring in the presence of hemoglobin (reaction a); this reaction is complete within a few minutes in hemoglobin solutions but has a half-time of about 20 minutes with intact human erythrocytes in vitro.[62] There may be differences between species in red cell permeability to sodium nitroprusside that affect the rate of the reaction.[63]

The toxicity of cyanide results from the inhibitions of cellular respiration which occurs when cyanide combines with cytochrome oxidase (reaction d). Anaerobic metabolism increases and leads to metabolic acidosis, which allows the observant

practitioner to detect this cellular toxicity. Detoxification of cyanide occurs by reaction with thiosulfate to form thiocyanate; this irreversible reaction is catalyzed by the enzyme "rhodanese," found in liver and other tissues (reaction b). Thiocyanate is excreted in the urine. In large concentrations, it inhibits gastric acid secretion and thyroid function,[64] but this is unlikely to be an important problem. Thiocyanate is degraded slowly back to cyanide by thiocyanate oxidase (reaction c). It is uncertain whether nitroprusside must be broken down to cyanide before it can form thiocyanate. An abnormality of rhodanese or a deficiency of thiosulfate may limit the rate of detoxification, which explains the rationale for treating cyanide toxicity with thiosulfate.

Cyanide is readily bound to methemoglobin (reaction g). The recommended therapy for cyanide posioning is administration of nitrite, which oxidizes the Fe^{++} of hemoglobin to the Fe^{+++} of methemoglobin (reaction h) and shifts the equilibrium of reaction g toward the relatively stable and nontoxic cyanmethemoglobin. Another effective method is to give hydroxocobalmin, vitamin B_{12a}, which combines with cyanide (reaction f) to form the nontoxic B_{12}.[65] However, the dosage form and current availability of B_{12a} make this an impractical method at present. Other pathways exist for the excretion or detoxification of cyanide (reaction e), but they are not thought to be of practical importance. Sodium nitroprusside can cause the formation of cyanmethemoglobin in human erythrocytes in vitro, but methemoglobin concentrations are not elevated in patients receiving sodium nitroprusside infusions.[66]

Just what is the evidence that links nitroprusside and cyanide toxicity? First, we are certain that sodium nitroprusside is broken down to cyanide and that cyanide is toxic. The signs of suspected sodium nitroprusside toxicity resemble cyanide poisoning, and the concentration of cyanide in the blood is similar in both types of poisoning. In rats and mice, sodium nitroprusside is about four times as toxic per mole as is cyanide; this finding is consistent with liberation of the five cyanide radicals from sodium nitroprusside, particularly if one radical combines with each mole of hemoglobin in reactions h and g of Figure 48-1. Lethal blood concentrations of cyanide (90 μM) are found in rats and mice dying from administration of sodium nitroprusside.[63] Guinea pigs can be poisoned by sodium nitroprusside; B_{12a} prevents this toxicity. When baboons were made hypotensive with sodium nitroprusside, half failed to recover and died with a severe and increasing metabolic acidosis. Cerebral oxygen uptake was markedly reduced before death, although cerebral blood flow was the same as in the survivors. Animals that did not recover had demonstrated resistance or tachyphylaxis to the hypotensive effect of sodium nitroprusside and had required six times as much (7.3 mg./kg.) as the survivors.[67]

Numerous cases of probable human poisoning with sodium nitroprusside have been reported. They resemble cyanide poisoning with severe metabolic acidosis, often progressing to cardiac arrhythmias, cardiac arrest, and death.[68–73] In the one fatal case in which it was analyzed, blood cyanide concentration was 1.9×10^{-4} M (0.5 mg./100 ml.).[68] Fatal cyanide poisoning in hu-

mans has been associated with postmortem blood cyanide concentrations as low as 1.1×10^{-4} M and 1.5×10^{-4} M.[74,75] It is difficult to discuss further the toxic concentrations: Few analyses have been done, and many published values are given as plasma concentrations, which are about 1 to 2 per cent of the whole blood concentration.[76]

It is safe to say, however, that the usual doses of sodium nitroprusside are capable of yielding toxic amounts of cyanide. There is evidence that an absorbed dose of as little as 24 mg. of cyanide may be fatal to humans.[74] One ampule of 50 mg. of sodium nitroprusside contains 22 mg. (835 μmol.) of cyanide; thus, the recommended maximum doses for sodium nitroprusside of 1 to 3 mg. per kg. are capable of yielding harmful amounts of cyanide. In the fatal cases of sodium nitroprusside intoxication, adults received over 400 mg. and children over 300 mg. Yet, many other patients have received large doses without reported toxicity. Therefore, there must be great variations in tolerance between individuals, perhaps because of differing rates of breakdown of sodium nitroprusside or detoxification of cyanide.

To date, probably the most complete report of a death from sodium nitroprusside is that of Davies.[68] A boy of 14, anesthetized with halothane, required 400 mg. (10 mg./kg.) of sodium nitroprusside in 80 min. to control his blood pressure. Metabolic acidosis developed near the end of the infusion, with arterial blood pH, 7.27, P_{CO_2} 19 torr (2.53 kPa), and base excess, -12 mEq./L. He was treated with sodium bicarbonate, but 30 minutes later blood pressure and pulse rate fell, and he died. Blood cyanide concentration was 1.9×10^{-4}M; no thiocyanate was detectable by the method used. It is unknown whether this death was caused by an "absolute" overdose of sodium nitroprusside (if there is indeed such a thing) or whether something unusual in this patient's metabolism enhanced its toxicity. Some possibilities include accelerated release of cyanide from sodium nitroprusside, inability to detoxify cyanide due to rhodanese abnormality, and lack of thiosulfate as a substrate for detoxification. In a companion paper, the same investigators report the use of sodium thiosulfate to treat apparent cyanide toxicity in two patients; in one of these, plasma cyanide concentration was measured and was found to decrease after sodium thiosulfate (150 mg./kg.) had been given. They suggest that a small bodily reserve of thiosulfate may limit the rate of cyanide detoxification.[73]

Sodium nitroprusside may be contraindicated in patients with conditions that affect cyanide metabolism: impaired liver function, low plasma concentration of B_{12}, chronic cyanide intoxication, tobacco amblyopia, or Leber's optic atrophy.[77-79] In clinical concentrations, sodium nitroprusside is a potent inhibitor of platelet aggregation,[80] but no increased bleeding has been reported. Pretreatment with sodium nitroprusside enhances the response to clonidine, a fact which should be remembered in the treatment of hypertensive emergencies.[81]

Dosage of Sodium Nitroprusside

What are some practical solutions to the problem of nitroprusside dosage?

Limit the Dose of the Drug. Educated guesses of the maximum allowable dose have ranged from 1.5 to 3 mg. per kg.,[76] but even 1 mg. per kg. may be too high. Lawson found a high correlation between the effective dose for hip surgery and the ratio of age to weight, resulting in the following empirical relationship:[82]

$$\text{dose rate } (\mu g./min.) = 748.76 \times e^{(-2.63A/W)}$$

where A is the age in years and W the weight in kilograms. This was derived from data from patients of ages 14 to 79 and weighing about 20 to 90 kg. It predicts doses of 10 mg. per hour for a 40-yr-old, 70-kg patient, and 25 mg. per hour for a 20-yr-old, 90-kg. patient. Whether such a predictive approach will be useful remains to be seen. It may allow one to quantitate resistance or tachyphylaxis by stating how much an individual patient's drug requirement exceeds the predicted dose.

Measure Acid-Base Status Hourly. If metabolic acidosis begins to develop, nitroprusside should be stopped and sodium bicarbonate and specific antidotes given.

Be Prepared to Give the Specific Antidotes for Cyanide Poisoning.[83-85] Chronic nitroprusside administration should not exceed 0.5 mg./kg./h.[86] All should be given intravenously:

SODIUM NITRITE: 10 ml. of a 3-per-cent solution for adults; 0.2 ml. per kg. for children.

SODIUM THIOSULFATE: 150 mg. per kg. body weight, as a 25-per-cent solution.

HYDROXOCOBALMIN (B_{12a}): 5 mol. per mol. of sodium nitroprusside, or 1 g. per 50 mg. of sodium nitroprusside.

Consider prophylactic administration of sodium thiosulfate or hydroxocobalmin. It may be desirable to give these antidotes along with sodium nitroprusside.[73,78,83]

Consider simultaneous administration of propranolol. Nitroprusside requirement can be diminished by giving propranolol in a dose sufficient to slow heart rate during deliberate hypotension.[87] The underlying mechanism may be propranolol suppression of nitroprusside-induced renin release.[88,89] Not unexpectedly, adding or increasing the concentration of a potent inhalation anesthetic will also decrease nitroprusside requirement.

These are not entirely satisfactory guidelines, because of the anecdotal nature of most reports of sodium nitroprusside toxicity in humans, but they are, nevertheless, based on sound theoretical grounds and some experiments in animals. The overall experience with sodium nitroprusside suggests that it is a most useful drug. The number of cases of toxicity is probably small in relation to the number of times the drug has been used; but, it must be used only by a physician who is alert to the possible complications.

REFERENCES

1. McNeil, T. W., DeWald, R. L., Kuo, K. N., et al.: Controlled hypotensive anesthesia in scoliosis surgery. J. Bone Joint Surg., *56A*:1167, 1974.
2. Mallory, T. H.: Hypotensive anesthesia in total hip replacement. J.A.M.A., *224*:248, 1973.
3. Davis, N. J., Jennings, J. J., and Harris, W. H.: Induced hypotensive anesthesia for total hip replacement. Clin. Orthop., *101*:93, 1974.
4. Amaranath, L., Cascorbi, H. F., Singh-Amaranath, A. V., et al.: Relation of anesthesia to total hip replacement and control of operative blood loss. Anesth. Analg., *54*:641, 1975.
5. Thompson, G. E., Miller, R. D., Stevens, W. C., et al.: Hypotensive anesthesia for total hip arthroplasty: a study of blood loss and organ function (brain, heart, liver, and kidney). Anesthesiology, *48*:91, 1978.
6. Eckenhoff, J. E., and Rich, J. C.: Clinical experience with deliberate hypotension. Anesth. Analg., *45*:21, 1966.

7a. Hampton, L. J., and Little, D. M., Jr.: Complications associated with the use of "controlled hypotension" in anesthesia. Arch. Surg., *67*:549, 1953.

7. Little, D. M.: Induced hypotension during anesthesia and surgery. Anesthesiology, *16*:320, 1955.

8. Enderby, G.E.H.: A report on mortality and morbidity following 9,107 hypotensive anaesthetics. Br. J. Anaesth., *33*:109, 1961.

9. Bodman, R. I.: Dangers of hypotensive anaesthesia. Proc. R. Soc. Med., *57*:1184, 1964.

10. Way, G. L., and Clarke, H. L.: An anaesthetic technique for prostatectomy. Lancet, *2*:888, 1959.

11. Baker, A. H.: Prostatectomy without catheter. Proc. R. Soc. Med., *57*:1179, 1964.

12. Boreham, P.: Retropubic prostatectomy with hypotensive anaesthesia. Proc. R. Soc. Med., *57*:1181, 1964.

13. Rollason, W. N., and Hough, J. M.: A study of hypotensive anaesthesia in the elderly. Br. J. Anaesth., *32*:276, 1960.

14. Lindop, M. J.: Complications and morbidity of controlled hypotension. Br. J. Anaesth., *47*:799, 1975.

15. Adams, J. H.: Hypoxic brain damage. Br. J. Anaesth., *47*:121, 1975.

16. Brierly, J. B., and Cooper, J. E.: Cerebral complications of hypotensive anaesthesia in a healthy adult. J. Neurol. Neurosurg. Psychiat., *25*:24, 1962.

17. Siegel, P., Moraca, P. P., and Green, J. R.: Sodium nitroprusside in the surgical treatment of cerebral aneurysms and arteriovenous malformations. Br. J. Anaesth., *43*:790, 1971.

18. Hugosson, R., and Högström, S.: Factors disposing to morbidity in surgery of intracranial aneurysms with special regard to deep controlled hypotension. J. Neurosurg., *38*:561, 1973.

19. Rollason, W. N., Robertson, G. S., and Cordiner, C. M.: A comparison of mental function in relation to hypotensive and normotensive anaesthesia in the elderly. Br. J. Anaesth., *43*:561, 1971.

20. Eckenhoff, J. E., Compton, J. R., Larson, A., et al.: Assessment of cerebral effects of deliberate hypotension by psychological measurements. Lancet, *2*:711, 1964.

21. Gamache, F. W., Dold, G. M., and Myers, R. E.: Changes in cortical impedance and EEG activity induced by profound hypotension. Am. J. Physiol., *228*:1914, 1975.

22. Yashon, D., Locke, G. E., and Bingham, W. G., Jr.: Cerebral function during profound oligemic hypotension in the dog. J. Neurosurg., *34*:494, 1971.

23. Boysen, G., Engell, H. C., Pistolese, G. R., et al.: On the critical lower level of cerebral blood flow in man with particular reference to carotid surgery. Circulation, *49*:1023, 1974.

24. Boysen, G.: Cerebral hemodynamics in carotid surgery. Acta Neurol. Scand., *49*[Suppl. 52], 1973.

25. Sundt, T. M., Sharbrough, F. W., Trautmann, J. C., et al.: Monitoring techniques for carotid endarterectomy. Clin. Neurosurg., *22*:199, 1975.

26. Boysen, G., Engell, H. C., and Henricksen, H.: The effect of induced hypertension on internal carotid artery pressure and regional cerebral blood flow during temporary carotid clamping for endarterectomy. Neurology, *22*:1133, 1972.

27. Smith, A. L.: Effect of anesthetics and oxygen deprivation on brain blood flow and metabolism. Surg. Clin. North Am., *55*:819, 1975.

28. Yashon, D., Stone, W., Magness, A., et al.: Evidence of preservation of aerobic cerebral metabolism during halothane-induced hypotension. J. Neurosurg., *39*:712, 1973.

29. Nilsson, L., and Siesjö, B. K.: The effect of deep halothane hypotension upon labile phosphates and upon extra- and intracellular lactate and pyruvate concentrations in the rat brain. Acta Physiol. Scand., *81*:508, 1971.

30. Alexander, S. C., Smith, T. C., Strobel, G. E., et al.: Cerebral carbohydrate metabolism of man during respiratory and metabolic alkalosis. J. Appl. Physiol., *24*:66, 1968.

31. Eckenhoff, J. E., Enderby, G. E. H., Larson, A., et al.: Human cerebral circulation during deliberate hypotension and head-up tilt. J. Appl. Physiol., *18*:1130, 1963.

32. Griffiths, D. P. G., Cummins, B. H., Greenbaum, R., et al.: Cerebral blood flow and metabolism during hypotension induced with sodium nitroprusside. Br. J. Anaesth., *46*:671, 1974.

33. Ivankovich, D., Miletich, D. J., Albrecht, R. F., et al.: Sodium nitroprusside and cerebral blood flow in the anesthetized and unanesthetized goat. Anesthesiology, *44*:21, 1976.

34. Keykhah, M. M., Shapiro, H. M., Van Horn, K., et al.: Intracranial pressure response to nitroprusside during intracranial hypertension. Abstracts of Scientific Papers. 1976 Annual Meeting, American Society of Anesthesiologists, p. 243.

35. Finnerty, F. A., Witkin, L., and Fazekas, F. J.: Cerebral hemodynamics during cerebral ischemia induced by acute hypotension. J. Clin. Invest., *33*:1227, 1954.

36. Strandgaard, S.: Autoregulation of cerebral blood flow in hypertensive patients. Circulation, *53*:720, 1976.

37. Vance, J. P., Smith, G., Thorburn, J., et al.: The combined effect of halothane-induced hypotension and hypocapnia on canine myocardial blood-flow and oxygen consumption. Br. J. Anaesth., *47*:825, 1975.

38. Hackel, D. B., Sancetta, S. M., and Kleinerman, J.: Effect of hypotension due to spinal anesthesia on coronary blood flow and myocardial metabolism in man. Circulation, *13*:92, 1956.

39. Tountas, C. J., Georgopoulos, A. J., and Kyriakou, K. V.: The effect of sodium nitroprusside on coronary circulation. Bull. Soc. Int. Chir., *23*:267, 1964.

40. Ross, G., and Cole, P. V.: Cardiovascular action of sodium nitroprusside in dogs. Anaesthesia, *28*:400, 1973.

40a. Loeb, H. S., Sandje, A., Croke, R. P., et al.: Effects of pharmacologically-induced hypertension on myocardial ischemia and coronary hemodynamics in patients with fixed coronary obstruction. Circulation, *57*:41, 1978.

41. Rollason, W. N., Dundas, C. R., and Milne, R. G.: ECG and EEG changes during hypotensive anaesthesia. Proc. III Congr. Mund. Anaesth., *1*:106, 1964.

42. Rollason, W. N., and Hough, J. M.: Some electrocardiographic studies during hypotensive anaesthesia. Br. J. Anaesth., *31*:66, 1959.

43. Askrog, V. F., Pender, J. W., and Eckenhoff, J. E.: Changes in physiological dead space during deliberate hypotension. Anesthesiology, *25*:744, 1964.

44. Eckenhoff, J. E., Enderby, G. E. H., Larson, A., et al.: Pulmonary gas exchange during deliberate hypotension. Br. J. Anaesth., *35*:750, 1963.

45. Fahmy, N. R., Selwyn, A. S., Patel, D., et al.: Pulmonary vasomotor tone during general anesthesia and deliberate hypotension in man. Anesthesiology, *45*:3, 1976.

46. Arkin, D. B., and Wahrenbrock, E. A.: Hypoxemia following nitroprusside administration: Effect of cardiac output

and pulmonary autoregulation. Abstracts of Scientific Papers, 1975 Annual Meeting, American Society of Anesthesiologists, p. 161.

46a. Mookherjee, S., Keighley, J. F. H., Warner, R. A., et al.: Hemodynamic, ventilatory and blood gas changes during infusion of sodium nitroferricyanide (nitroprusside). Studies in patients with congestive heart failure. Chest, 72,:273, 1977.

46b. Colley, P. S., and Cheney, F. W.: Sodium nitroprusside increases $\dot{Q}_s/\dot{Q}_t$ in dogs with regional atelectasis. Anesthesiology, 47:338, 1977.

47. Parson, N. L., and Sullivan, S. F.: Effect of sodium nitroprusside hypotension on pulmonary blood/gas distribution. Abstracts of Scientific Papers. 1975 Annual Meeting, American Society of Anesthesiologists, p. 75.

48. Stone, J. G., Khambatta, H. J., and Matteo, R. S.: Pulmonary shunting during anesthesia with deliberate hypotension. Anesthesiology, 45:508, 1976.

49. Price, H. L., and Pauca, A. L.: Effects of anesthesia on the peripheral circulation. Clin. Anesth., 7(3):74, 1969.

50. Bagshaw, R. J., Cox, R. H., and Campbell, K. B.: Sodium nitroprusside and regional arterial haemodynamics in the dog. Br. J. Anaesth., 49:735, 1977.

51. Salam, A. R. A., Drummond, G. B., Bauld, H. W., et al.: Clearance of indocyanine green as an index of liver function during cyclopropane anaesthesia and induced hypotension. Br. J. Anaesth., 48:231, 1976.

52. Warner, W. A., Shumrick, D. A., and Caffrey, J. A.: Clinical investigation of prolonged induced hypotension in head and neck injury. Br. J. Anaesth., 42:39, 1970.

53. Cousins, M. J., and Mazze, R. I.: Anaesthesia, surgery and renal function. Anaesth. Intens. Care, 1:355, 1973.

54. Deutsch, S.: Effects of anesthetics on the kidney. Surg. Clin. North Am., 55:775, 1975.

55. Hillebrand, A., van der Meer, C., and Ariëns, A. T.: The effect of anesthetics on the occurrence of kidney lesions caused by hypotension. Eur. J. Pharmacol., 14:217, 1971.

56. MacDonald, A. G.: The effect of halothane on renal cortical blood flow in normotensive and hypotensive dogs. Br. J. Anaesth., 41:644, 1969.

57. Pannacciuli, E., Quarto DePalo, F. M., Trazzi, R., et al.: Renal function changes in controlled hypotension. Minerva Anestesiol., 36:625, 1970.

58. Engelman, R. M., Guy, H. H., Smith, S. J., et al: The effect of hypotensive anesthesia on renal hemodynamics. J. Surg. Res., 18:293, 1975.

59. Dale, R. C., and Schroeder, E. T.: Respiratory paralysis during treatment of hypertension with trimethaphan camsylate. Arch. Intern. Med., 136:816, 1976.

59a. Glisson, S. N., El-Etr, A. A., and Lim, R.: Prolongation of pancuronium-induced neuromuscular blockade by intravenous infusion of nitroglycerin. Anesthesiology, 51:47, 1979.

59b. Glisson, S. N., Sanchez, M. M., El-Etr, A. A., et al.: Nitroglycerin and the neuromuscular blockade produced by gallamine, succinylcholine, *d*-tubocurarine and pancuronium. Anesth. Analg., 59:117, 1980.

60. Tinker, J. H., and Michenfelder, J. D.: Sodium nitroprusside: pharmacology, toxicology and therapeutics. Anesthesiology, 45:340, 1972.

61. Nourok, D. S., Glasscock, R. J., Solomon, D. H., et al.: Hypothyroidism following prolonged sodium nitroprusside therapy. Am. J. Med. Sci., 248:129, 1964.

62. Vesey, C. J., Cole, P., and Simpson, P.: Changes in cyanide concentrations induced by sodium nitroprusside (SNP). Br. J. Anaesth., 48:268, 1976.

63. Smith, R. P., and Kruszyna, H.: Nitroprusside produces cyanide poisoning via a reaction with hemoglobin. J. Pharmacol. Exp. Ther., 191:557, 1974.

64. Davenport, H. W.: The inhibition of carbonic anhydrase and of gastric acid secretion by thiocyanate. Am. J. Physiol., 129:505, 1940.

65. Posner, M. A., Tobey, R. E., and McElroy, H.: Hydroxocobalmin therapy of cyanide intoxication in guinea pigs. Anesthesiology, 44:157, 1976.

66. Smith, R. P., and Carleton, R. A.: Nitroprusside and methemoglobinemia. N. Engl. J. Med., 294:502, 1976.

67. McDowall, D. G., Keaney, N. P., Turner, J. M., et al.: The toxicity of sodium nitroprusside. Br. J. Anaesth., 46:327, 1974.

68. Davies, D. W., Kadar, D., Stewart, D. J., et al.: A sudden death associated with the use of sodium nitroprusside for induction of hypotension during anaesthesia. Can. Anaesth. Soc. J., 22:547, 1975.

69. Merrifield, A. J., and Blundell, M. D.: Toxicity of sodium nitroprusside. Br. J. Anaesth., 46:324, 1974.

70. Jack, R. D.: Toxicity of sodium nitroprusside. Br. J. Anaesth., 46:952, 1974.

71. MacRae, W. R., and Owen, M.: Severe metabolic acidosis following hypotension induced with sodium nitroprusside. Br. J. Anaesth., 46:795, 1975.

72. Perschan, R. A., Modell, J. H., Bright, R. W., et al.: Suspected sodium nitroprusside-induced cyanide intoxication. Anesth. Analg., 56:533, 1977.

73. Davies, D. W., Greiss, L., Kadar, D., et al.: Sodium nitroprusside in children: observations on metabolism during normal and abnormal responses. Can. Anaesth. Soc. J., 22:553, 1975.

74. Gettler, A. O., and Baine, J. O.: Toxicity of cyanide. Am. J. Med. Sci., 195:182, 1938.

75. Ansell, M., and Lewis, F. A. S.: A review of cyanide concentrations found in human organs. J. Forensic Med., 17:148, 1970.

76. Vesey, C. J., Cole, P., and Simpson, P.: Sodium nitroprusside in anaesthesia. Br. Med. J., 3:229, 1975.

77. Vesey, C. J., Cole, P V., Linnell, J. C., et al.: Some metabolic effects of sodium nitroprusside in man. Br. Med. J., 2:140, 1974.

78. Vesey, C. J., and Cole, P. V.: Nitroprusside and cyanide. Br. J. Anaesth., 47:1115, 1975.

79. Wilson, J.: Leber's hereditary optic atrophy: a possible defect of cyanide metabolism. Clin. Sci., 29:505, 1965.

80. Saxon, A., and Kattlove, H. E.: Platelet inhibition by sodium nitroprusside, a smooth muscle inhibitor. Blood, 47:957, 1976.

81. Cohen, I. M., Mottet, M. M., Francis, G. S., et al.: Danger in nitroprusside therapy. Ann. Intern. Med., 85:205, 1976.

82. Lawson, N. W., Thompson, D. S., Nelson, C. L., et al.: Sodium nitroprusside-induced hypotension for supine total hip replacement. Anesth. Analg., 55:654, 1976.

83. Posner, M. A., Rodkey, F. L., and Tobey, R. E.: Nitroprusside-induced cyanide poisoning: antidotal effect of hydroxocobalamin. Anesthesiology, 44:330, 1976.

84. Lutier, F., Dusoleil, P., and DeMontgros, J.: Action de l'hydroxocobalmine à dose massive dans l'intoxication aigüe au cyanure. Arch. Mal. Prof., 32:683, 1972.

85. Done, A. K.: Clinical pharmacology of systemic antidotes. Clin. Pharmacol. Ther., *2*:750, 1961.

86. Michenfelder, J. D., and Tinker, J. H.: Cyanide toxicity and thiosulfate protection during chronic administration of sodium nitroprusside in the dog: Correlation with a human case. Anesthesiology, *47*:441, 1977.

87. Bedford, R. F., Berry, F. A., and Longnecker, D. E.: Impact of propranolol on hemodynamic responses and blood cyanide levels during nitroprusside infusion: A prospective study in anesthetized man. Anesth. Analg., *58*:466, 1979.

88. Khambatta, H. J., Stone, J. G., and Khan, E.: Propranolol abates nitroprusside-induced renin release. Anesthesiology, *51*:S74, 1979.

89. Marshall, W. K., Bedford, R. F., Arnold, W. P., et al.: Effects of propranolol on the cardiovascular and renin-angiotensin systems during hypotension produced by sodium nitroprusside in humans. Anesthesiology, *55*:277, 1981.

FURTHER READING

Adams, A. P.: Techniques of vascular control for deliberate hypotension during anesthesia. Br. J. Anaesth., *47*:777, 1975.

Cottrell, J. E., Casthely, P., Brodie, J. D., et al.: Prevention of nitroprusside-induced cyanide toxicity with hydroxocobalmin. N. Engl. J. Med., *298*:809, 1978.

Larson, A. G.: Deliberate hypotension. Anesthesiology, *25*:682, 1964.

Lindop, M. J.: Complications and morbidity of controlled hypotension. Br. J. Anaesth., *47*:799, 1975.

Tinker, J. H., and Michenfelder, J. D.: Sodium nitroprusside: pharmacology, toxicology and therapeutics. Anesthesiology, *45*:340, 1976.

49 Physiologic Disturbances Associated with Induced Hypothermia

Fredrick K. Orkin, M.D.

Induced hypothermia is by no means a new technique in anesthesia. Indeed, the use of hypothermia during surgery predates anesthesia, at least as we know it, by thousands of years. Hippocrates was among the first to note the analgesic property of cold, and refrigeration anesthesia, as it came to be called, was commonly used before the modern era of anesthesia, the most celebrated instances being the painless amputations performed by Napoleon's surgeon-general, Baron Larrey.[1]

Much more in keeping with our current use of hypothermia to decrease metabolism, however, are the early attempts by the eighteenth century English physiologist John Hunter to freeze fish in a state of suspended animation.[1] Forty years ago, Smith and Fay reported limited success in slowing the growth of cancer when cold was applied locally.[2] More recently, induced hypothermia has enjoyed sporadic use in carotid artery and intracranial surgery to decrease cerebral metabolism during periods of hypoperfusion.[3,4] Our principal current use of induced hypothermia in cardiac surgery results largely from the demonstration by Bigelow that hypothermia enables complete occlusion of blood flow to the heart and, thus, intracardiac surgery in a bloodless field.[5,6]

This chapter surveys the problems associated with induced hypothermia, placing special emphasis upon the altered physiology that underlies the problems. It will be apparent that the culprit is not the cold itself but rather the resultant altered physiology when inadequately monitored and controlled.

HYPOTHERMIA AND ITS CLINICAL PRESENTATIONS

THE THREE ZONES OF HYPOTHERMIA

Hypothermia is the clinical state of having a subnormal body temperature. In clinical circumstances, "core" (rectal, esophageal, or tympanic) temperature is measured, and "hypothermia" is generally regarded as being less than 35°C. Values down to about 32°C describe mild hypothermia, or a safe zone of hypothermia in which heat conservation and production mechanisms, such as peripheral vasoconstriction and shivering, are usually present. (Chapter 19 reviews the normal thermoregulatory mechanisms.) Between about 32°C and 24°C, there is a transitional zone characterized by progressive depression of tissue metabolism, development of maximal vasoconstriction, and cessation of shivering. Below 24°C, there is the danger zone of hypothermia in which the human behaves as a poikilothermic organism, assuming the temperature of his surroundings.[7]

ACCIDENTAL HYPOTHERMIA

Used without qualification, the term hypothermia conjures up images of the elderly person brought to the emergency room severely hypothermic afer prolonged exposure to the cold. Such cases of accidental hypothermia have become much more common in recent years as winter has become less mild and inflation has placed the cost of both heating and food almost beyond the reach of small, fixed incomes. Although particularly common among the elderly, accidental hypothermia is also seen in neonates, immobile and unconscious persons, and others who become physically exhausted in a cold environment. Not unexpectedly, associated conditions include endocrine deficiency states (*e.g.*, myxedema, hypoglycemia, Addison's disease, pituitary insufficiency), malnutrition, uremia, severe infection, cerebrovascular or other intracranial disease, myocardial infarction, cirrhosis, pancreatitis, and drug and ethanol ingestion.

Accidental hypothermia is frequently unrecognized, at least in part, because conventional clinical thermometers do not record temperatures low enough. Unchecked, hypothermia often leads to fatal, multiple-system failure that can include pneumonia, intractable ventricular dysrhythmias, congestive heart failure, pancreatitis, and cerebrovascular accidents.[8,9] Survival requires that accidental hypothermia be recognized as a medical emergency and managed with prompt institution of aggressive therapy to raise body temperature rapidly, establish and maintain an airway, assure oxygenation and blood volume expansion, and close monitoring for and treatment of dysrhythmias and acid–base and electrolyte disorders (*e.g.*, hypokalemia, acidosis).[8–11]

UNINTENTIONAL HYPOTHERMIA

A far less catastrophic, but rather common form of hypothermia is the unintentional hypothermia that results during anesthesia in a cold operating room. Preanesthetic sedation, anesthetics, and anesthetic adjuvants predispose the patient to suffer hypothermia by depressing the thermoregulatory center and voluntary muscular activity, increasing cutaneous vasodilatation, reducing peripheral thermal receptor sensitivity, and preventing shivering. In addition, hypothermia alters aspects of the pharmacology of inhalation anesthetics and adjuvant drugs. For example, muscle sensitivity to nondepolarizing neuromuscular blocking agents diminishes as body temperature decreases.[12] Upon rewarming, the clinical effect of the residual relaxant is increased ("recurarization"), disposing the patient to muscle weakness when it is least expected.

Of greater concern, however, is the shivering that occurs upon emergence from anesthesia, as the thermoregulatory system regains its integrity and attempts to return the body temperature to normal. The resultant greatly augmented oxygen utilization stresses the respiratory and circulatory systems at a time when they may not be able to meet the demand fully. Hypoxemia and secondary problems, such as cardiac dysrhythmias, can appear with little warning. Particularly at risk for unintentional hypothermia and postoperative shivering are infants and small children, who lose heat more readily because of their greater ratio of body-surface area to volume. This presentation of hypothermia is discussed more fully in Chapter 19.

INDUCED HYPOTHERMIA

In contrast to other presentations of hypothermia, induced hypothermia is a controlled and remarkably safe physiologic state. Uneventful recovery generally follows hypothermia induced to levels at which survial in accidental hypothermia is uncommon. This suggests not only that cold is not innately harmful but also that what determines morbidity is the manner in which hypothermia is managed.[10] Although hypothermia has been induced in a variety of ways,[13,14] today it is usually produced as an adjunct to extracorporeal circulation in cardiac surgery. Once induced, however, hypothermia must be managed with keen awareness of the resultant altered physiology to avoid complications.

THE ALTERED CLINICAL PHYSIOLOGY OF INDUCED HYPOTHERMIA

Hypothermia produces physiologic disturbances in most tissues and organ systems. Unfortunately, it is often difficult to predict how a given

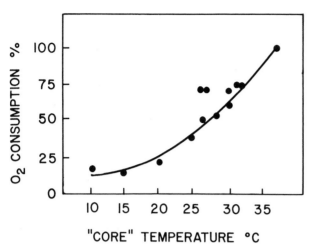

Fig. 49-1. The relationship between core temperature and whole-body oxygen consumption (compared to control values at 37 C), based upon values taken from various studies. (Data from Dills, D. B., and Forbes, W. H.: Respiratory and metabolic effects of hypothermia. Am. J. Physiol., *132*:685, 1941; Spurr, G. B., Hutt, B.K., and Horwath, S. M.: Reponses of dogs to hypothermia. Am. J. Physiol., *179*:139, 1954; Lougheed, W. H., Sweet, W. H., White, J. C., et al.: Use of hypothermia in surgical treatment of cerebral vascular lesions: Preliminary report. J. Neurosurg., *12*:240, 1955; Severinghaus, J. W., Stupfel, M., and Bradley, A. F.: Alveolar dead space and arterial to end-tidal carbon dioxide differences during hypothermia in dog and man. J. Appl. Physiol., *10*:349, 1957; Rosomoff, H. L.: Pathophysiology of the central nervous system during hypothermia. Acta Neurochirurgica, Suppl. *XIII*:11, 1964; Blair, E.: Physiologic and metabolic effects of hypothermia in man. *In* Muschia, X. J., and Saunders, J. F. (eds.): Depressed Metabolism. Proceedings of the First International Conference on Depressed Metabolism, Washington, D. C., August 22–23, 1968. New York, American Elsevier, 1969.)

patient will respond to induced hypothermia for a variety of reasons: thermoregulation is probably subject to greater individual variation than other bodily functions; some observations made in other species are not directly applicable to humans; observations in humans have been modified necessarily by the concomitant administration of general anesthetics and other drugs, as well as the given patient's state of health; and still other observations were made in the uncon-

trolled setting of accidental hypothermia. Nonetheless, some generalizations can be made.

To facilitate discussion, the more salient disturbances are discussed here largely by bodily systems, although the disturbances are usually interrelated. In particular, it should be noted that, by themselves, the disturbances resulting from well-conducted induced hypothermia are generally remarkably benign and limited to the period of hypothermia.

METABOLISM

Underlying the usefulness of induced hypothermia is the accompanying generalized depression of metabolism. Metabolic rate is quantitated most easily by measuring oxygen consumption. Whole-body oxygen consumption bears a direct linear relationship to core temperature, decreasing approximately 50 per cent for each 10°C change (Fig. 49-1). However, large temperature gradients develop between superficial and deep tissues, and, more importantly, tissues also vary innately in their oxygen requirements. In the most metabolically active tissues there is a threefold decrease in oxygen consumption for each 10°C drop in temperature; such tissues are said to have a Q_{10} of 3. In contrast, most physical processes, such as the diffusion of metabolic substrate, have a Q_{10} close to 1.[10] Thus, as temperature decreases, there is a disproportionately greater decrease in the use of metabolic substrate. Herein lies the metabolic benefit of hypothermia.

The beneficial effect of hypothermia may be offset, however, or, more likely, negated by shivering which occurs involuntarily as a centrally mediated, nonautonomic response to decreased core temperature. The intense muscular activity that occurs during shivering increases heat production and thereby tends to restore euthermia (pp. 632). Initially there is an increase in muscle tone that, in turn, increases basal heat production 50 per cent to 100 per cent. This is followed by the visible and more familiar vigorous muscular activity that results in a 50 per cent to 600 per cent increase in whole-body oxygen consumption.[21-23]

CENTRAL NERVOUS SYSTEM FUNCTION

CENTRAL NERVOUS SYSTEM

Cerebral blood flow decreases in direct proportion to the decrease in body temperature, at a rate of 6.7 per cent for each degree Celsius.[24] Hence, at 30°C, cerebral blood flow is about half normal, and at 25°C, about one fifth of its normothermic value. Concomitantly, mean systemic blood pressure falls by only about 5 per cent for each degree of temperature decrease, indicating that cerebrovascular resistance increases.[25-27] In the absence of shivering,[28] however, cerebral oxygen consumption falls at the same rate as that for cerebral blood flow.[24,26,27,29] As a result, arteriovenous oxygen difference is unchanged,[26,27] and, if cerebral perfusion is uninterrupted, cerebral hypoxia does not occur.[26,27] Associated with decreases in cerebral metabolism and blood flow are decreases in brain volume, cerebral venous pressure, and cerebrospinal-fluid volume.[30]

Coincident with the depression of cerebral metabolism is depression of all aspects of central nervous system function.[10] Subtle changes in consciousness accompany mild hypothermia, although the EEG appears normal, perhaps with slightly decreased frequency or amplitude of the waves. Consciousness is lost when body temperature drops below 28°C, at which point there is progressive electrical slowing, with the appearance of theta and then delta activity before electrical activity ceases in the temperature range of 15°C to 20°C.[31] The autonomic nervous system and the respiratory and cardiovascular centers also exhibit progressive depression with hypothermia. However, reflexes (*e.g.*, gag, pupillary light, and deep tendon reflexes) are generally intact until 25°C. Typically monosynaptic responses, such as muscle stretch, become polysynaptic or less pure during hypothermia, activating neighboring pathways.

PERIPHERAL NERVOUS SYSTEM

Not unexpectedly, hypothermia is associated with generalized depression in conduction of the nervous impulse, the magnitude of which is directly related to the fall in temperature. Thus, there is decreased excitability and rate of conduction in peripheral nerves[32,33] (and spinal pathways), as well as impaired neuromuscular transmission.[34] The larger, myelinated fibers are blocked first, whereas the small, unmyelinated sympathetic fibers are affected only during deep hypothermia. Also, as body temperature decreases, muscle tone becomes more prominent, with rigidity apparent at about 26°C. Spontaneous myoclonus, facial spasms, and other examples of muscle excitability may be noted below 30°C.

CARDIOVASCULAR FUNCTION

THE HEART

Heart rate increases transiently in response to the early sympathetic stimulation that accompanies hypothermia, especially if shivering is present.[35] Below 32° to 34°C, cooling results in a proportional decrease in heart rate[36-38] that ends in cardiac arrest at profound depths of hypothermia (*e.g.*, 10°C to 15°C). Probably caused by the direct effect of cold upon the sino-atrial tissue, this bradycardia is not affected by atropine or vagotomy.

In the absence of anesthetic-induced cardiac depression, stroke volume is preserved down through the transitional zone of hypothermia[39] and then usually increases.[40] Given the relatively stable stroke volume, the cardiac output necessarily mirrors the heart rate, rising initially and then falling proportionally with body temperature and, thus, tissue metabolism.[6,39,41] Some investigators[42,43] have reported that coronary blood flow falls progressively but in proportion to the decrease in cardiac work (and, hence, oxygen utilization)[44]; whereas, others[45] have noted an increase in coronary blood flow as body temperature falls. In either case, the coronary blood flow is adequate for the metabolic needs of the cooled heart, so myocardial ischemia is unlikely. However, below about 18°C, blood viscosity is so high that coronary blood flow is markedly diminished.[46,47]

The most important cardiovascular effects of

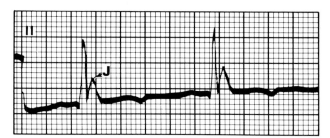

Fig. 49-2. The characteristic J or Osborn wave of hypothermia is noted during the terminal deflection of the QRS complex and may be mistaken for a T wave with a narrow QT interval.

hypothermia are those affecting myocardial conduction and irritability. During mild hypothermia, an inapparent skeletal-muscle tremor (due to thermal muscle tone) may completely obscure the P waves in the ECG. In addition to bradycardia, there is prolongation of the P–R interval, QRS complex, and Q–T interval as a result of retarded depolarization and repolarization.[48–51] The most characteristic ECG change below 31°C, consistently present below 25°C, is the J wave (Osborn wave,[52] or camel-hump sign), a slow deflection apparent in all leads and arising during the terminal deflection of and in the same direction as the QRS complex (Fig. 49-2). Initially thought to represent a "current of injury,"[53,54] the J wave is no longer regarded as a presage of ventricular fibrillation.[55] Neither is the J wave pathognomonic of hypothermia, for it has been noted in other circumstances, such as cerebral injuries.[56] During deep hypothermia, the ST segment is often elevated or depressed and the T wave biphasic and then deeply inverted,[36] as if to suggest myocardial ischemia.[57,58]

Also, as cooling progresses, sino-atrial tissue tends to be inhibited and lower areas assume pacemaker activity. When body temperature has decreased to 27° to 30°C, electrical evidence of myocardial irritability appears, although in a highly variable fashion. Irritability may appear first as an atrial ectopic focus or wandering atrial pacemaker but insidiously changes to atrial fibrillation, usually with a slow ventricular response; but, sometimes, there is an abrupt increase in heart rate that interrupts the typical bradycardia

of hypothermia. Although a first-degree heart block may be present, higher degrees of block are observed generally only in those with organic heart disease. As body temperature drops, other ectopic rhythms, such as atrial flutter, atrioventricular junctional rhythm, premature ventricular contractions, and ventricular fibrillation, may also appear. Ventricular fibrillation can develop without any forewarning during this part of the transitional zone of hypothermia.

PERIPHERAL CIRCULATION

The initial peripheral circulatory response to hypothermia is increased peripheral resistance due to cutaneous vasoconstriction.[48,59,60] The latter results, in turn, from the direct effect of cold on arterial walls[61] and reflex sympathetic stimulation initiated by cold receptors in the skin. Below 34°C, cutaneous vessels dilate owing to the direct effect of the cold,[62] but deeper vessels progressively constrict down to about 25°C, at which generalized vasodilatation begins.

Consequent to the vasoconstriction, blood volume shifts to the deep capacitance vessels, particularly those in the liver and lungs, stimulating volume receptors and thereby probably contributing to "cold diuresis" (see p. 630).[7] Also, water moves extravascularly to the tissues,[63] and the hematocrit rises secondarily.[64] Hemoconcentration raises the blood viscosity and thereby increases peripheral resistance further.

Blood pressure rises initially during the transient period of peripheral vasoconstriction and then falls as body temperature drops and cardiac depression develops.[35,60] Clinically important hypotension, however, generally appears only below about 25°C.[65]

Unfortunately, hypothermia is detrimental when continued for more than 24 hr., as it might be for cerebral resuscitation following cardiac arrest, head trauma, or near drowning.[66,67] With time, the favorable reductions in both cardiac output and whole-body oxygen consumption are themselves diminished to less than 10 per cent and 30 per cent of control values, respectively; both remain depressed upon rewarming. There is probably diffuse nonperfusion of capillary beds during prolonged hypothermia, with resultant trapping of acid metabolites in the unperfused tissues. Upon rewarming, vascular beds open and the accumulated metabolites enter the circulation and depress the cardiovascular system. Experimental animals[66,67] and humans[2] generally die of shock and severe metabolic acidosis following prolonged hypothermia.

RESPIRATORY FUNCTION

THE LUNG

As with cardiac function, the initial respiratory response to hypothermia is stimulation,[7,50,54,68] followed by depression in proportion to the fall in body temperature and rate of metabolism.[69-72] Generally, the respiratory rate and pulmonary minute ventilation decrease in tandem, as does the $PaCO_2$. More important, however, is the decreased ventilatory responsiveness to both increased carbon dioxide[71,72] and decreased oxygen[71] inhalation, even when anesthetic depth is constant relative to the body temperature. If controlled ventilation is not instituted, spontaneous respiration ceases when the body temperature has reached about 24°C.

In addition to disturbances in respiratory control there are changes in respiratory mechanics, albeit much less important in the clinical setting, that accompany hypothermia. These include increases in both anatomic and physiologic dead space, apparently the result of bronchodilatation.[73]

THE BLOOD

Respiratory function is also influenced by the complex ways in which gas transport is affected by temperature.

The oxyhemoglobin dissociation curve shifts to the left in hypothermia (Fig. 35-2); thus, the partial pressure of oxygen in the tissues must fall to a lower-than-normal value before the hemoglobin gives up its oxygen. Although tissues can manage with remarkably little oxygen, oxygen-starved tissues could resort, theoretically, to anaerobic metabolism. That would result in acidosis that, in turn, would shift the curve toward the

right again. A more realistic mechanism for offsetting the shift in the dissociation curve is the increased solubility of oxygen in blood (and other body fluids) during hypothermia. For example, compared to normal body temperature, the dissolved oxygen is 19 per cent greater at 30°C and 33 per cent greater at 25°C. As large as these increases are, dissolved oxygen alone is insufficient to meet tissue oxygen requirements until the body temperature has dropped to about 16°C.[74] Actually, there is no evidence that hypoxemia occurs during hypothermia, provided that tissue perfusion remains adequate.

Carbon dioxide is also more soluble in blood and other body fluids during hypothermia; in fact, the increase in carbon dioxide dissolved in plasma is the same as that noted for oxygen. However, because dissolved carbon dioxide comprises only about 5 per cent of the total carbon dioxide carried in blood under normal circumstances, the increased solubility has only a limited effect upon carbon-dioxide transport during hypothermia. Quantitatively more important is an increase in the plasma concentration of the bicarbonate ion that, under normal circumstances, accounts for 95 per cent of carbon-dioxide transport. The plasma-bicarbonate concentration rises because the ionization of carbonic acid (formed when carbon dioxide hydrates in body fluids) to bicarbonate is favored even more as body temperature decreases and the activity of blood buffers increases, allowing them to accept more hydrogen ions. These changes in carbon-dioxide carriage, coupled with the decreased production of carbon dioxide during depressed metabolism, result in a lower $PaCO_2$ for any given pulmonary minute ventilation than at normal temperature. Respiratory alkalosis, in turn, is associated with a leftward shift of the oxyhemoglobin dissociation curve.

RENAL FUNCTION

Renal function is also depressed reversibly during hypothermia, owing to both decreased systemic blood pressure (secondary to the cardiovascular depression) and the direct effect of the cold. Typically, as renal blood flow progressively falls, renal vascular resistance rises (causing renal blood flow to decrease further) and glomerular filtration decreases.[75–78] However, because tubular reabsorption of water is also depressed, urine flow is only mildly decreased, if at all.[79] Serum sodium and potassium levels generally remain normal, but enough impairment of sodium and water reabsorption occurs that relatively large volumes of dilute urine are excreted ("cold diuresis") down to at least 20°C. With deep hypothermia, sufficiently large shifts of fluid may occur to result in hypovolemia during cooling and oliguria during rewarming. Renal excretion of acid is also impaired, but acid–base disturbances are uncommon during induced hypothermia down to 27°C. In the absence of severe hypotension or myxedema, or very uncommon disorders such as cryoglobulinemia or cold agglutinin disease that result in acute renal failure in a cold environment,[80] these changes are transient. Recovery of renal blood flow and filtration rate is about three-quarters complete within 2 hr. of rewarming and normal by the following day.[79]

ALIMENTARY FUNCTION

THE GUT

Hypothermia causes a reversible depression of smooth muscle motility throughout the alimentary tract.[10] Thus, there is reduction in peristalsis in the esophagus, stomach, and intestines. Common manifestations include acute gastric dilation (often with abdominal distension), paralytic ileus, and colonic dilation. Gastric secretion and free-acid production are both markedly depressed, as is the absorption of drugs from the intestine.

THE LIVER

Splanchnic blood flow decreases directly in proportion to the decrease in temperature[81] but perhaps more than the fall in cardiac output.[82] Although the liver continues to utilize oxygen and avoid cellular hypoxia down to at least 25°C, it is less able to use the available glucose. This is due, in large part, to the inhibition of the release of insulin from the pancreas and of the peripheral uptake of glucose.[83] As a result, blood glucose rises and remains elevated but without the development of ketoacidosis.

A particularly important aspect of the liver's altered physiology is the generalized depression of drug metabolism. During induced hypothermia and general anesthesia, the liver's ability to conjugate steroids, excrete sodium sulfobromophthalein (Bromsulphalein), and detoxify and excrete drug is impaired.[10]

COAGULATION

Although clinical experience suggests that hypothermia is associated with a bleeding tendency, substantive studies of coagulation are scant and controversial. Some authors have noted evidence of impaired coagulation only when the temperature is below 26°C[84] or when the cooling technic is improper or a surgical procedure is performed in addition to hypothermia.[85] Others have reported that clotting time increases as body temperature decreases.[86–88] The longer the period of hypothermia, the greater the prolongation of the clotting time, perhaps related to the progressive thrombocytopenia.[89,90] Other clotting defects, such as fibrinolysis,[91] have been noted sporadically and are probably related to the surgical procedure rather than the hypothermia.

MANAGEMENT OF DISTURBANCES ASSOCIATED WITH INDUCED HYPOTHERMIA

GENERAL CONSIDERATIONS

Despite a large literature on the altered physiology associated with hypothermia, little has been written, particularly during the last 15 years, on the clinical management of the disturbances associated with induced hypothermia. In large part, this is because induced hypothermia is used almost exclusively as an adjunct to cardiopulmonary bypass, whose cardiopulmonary support effectively treats many of the most serious disturbances associated with hypothermia and whose complications are generally overshadowing (see Chap. 47). Nonetheless, some recommendations can be made.

TEMPERATURE MONITORING

As noted in the discussion of metabolism (p. 626), large temperature gradients develop among the tissues as hypothermia progresses. These gradients are accentuated during rapid cooling and warming.[92] However, even in the absence of rapid changes in body temperature, the gradients produced are sufficiently large to result in continued fall in body temperature after cooling has been discontinued. This inadvertent, usually unpredictable downward drift in body temperature is termed after-drop. Monitoring several representative body temperatures allows a more adequate assessment of the progress of hypothermia (and warming) and, in particular, the magnitude of the temperature gradients. As a result, after-drop should occur less frequently, and the resultant physiologic disturbances should be less severe.

Among those sites most commonly monitored are the rectum, esophagus, tympanic membrane, and nasopharynx. The highest temperature during normothermia is usually recorded in the rectum, which is generally regarded as representing core temperature. About half a degree lower than rectal, esophageal temperature reflects the temperature of the central blood volume, unless the probe is located high in the esophagus where it can be influenced by the cooler anesthetic gases passing through the trachea.[93] Rather close to esophageal temperature, tympanic membrane temperature reflects that of the nearby internal carotid artery which supplies the thermoregulatory centers in the hypothalamus.[94,95] Although tympanic membrane thermometry is simple and convenient and provides reliable information, the probe can damage the tympanic membrane, as well as cause aural bleeding.[96] Nasopharyngeal temperature reflects that of the brain, but only if the probe makes contact with the oral mucosa.[97] Owing to changes in cutaneous blood flow, skin temperature varies so much that monitoring it generally has limited usefulness during induced hypothermia.

A variety of thermistor and thermocouple thermometers are available commercially for use in clinical settings.

ARTERIAL BLOOD GAS ANALYSIS

Frequent assessment of arterial blood gases is also essential to variously diagnose, treat, or prevent cardiorespiratory problems that are particularly likely during hypothermia. For example, in addition to customary uses such as assessing adequacy of oxygenation, some have used blood gases for the early detection and therapy of developing acidosis in an attempt to minimize episodes of ventricular fibrillation.[98] In current practice, however, provided that tissue perfusion remains adequate, acidosis is uncommon because ventilation is controlled.

A much more likely problem is respiratory alkalosis which develops if ventilation is not decreased proportionately to match the diminished carbon dioxide load available for pulmonary excretion as metabolism slows and carbon dioxide becomes more soluble in body tissues and fluids. Respiratory alkalosis is especially undesirable because its physiologic concomitants counter the beneficial effects of hypothermia: cerebrovascular contriction with secondary cerebral hypoperfusion; increased ventricular irritability with ventricular dysrhythmias; and the leftward shift of the oxyhemoglobin dissociation curve with generalized diminished tissue oxygen delivery. Serial blood-gas analysis enables early detection and treatment of such acid–base disturbances as they are developing.

Unfortunately, the assessment of acid–base disturbances during hypothermia is complicated by the temperature dependence of the blood-gas values themselves. Although normal blood-gas values are well-known for the human at a body temperature of 37°C, "normal" values have not been established for the hypothermic human. Analysis is performed in an electrode system at 37°C, and nomograms are often used to correct the measured values to the patient's lower temperature.[99,100] The question then arises, what should be the ideal values, particularly of pH and P_aCO_2 when reported "temperature corrected" to the patient's actual body temperature or "uncorrected" at the measuring electrode's temperature? Recently, a theoretical basis has been advanced for using uncorrected values because the higher pH and lower P_aCO_2 that would be reported if corrected to the patient's temperature maintains constancy of ionic charges on active proteins, thereby preserving optimal enzyme function at the lower temperature.[101] At 37°C, however, the more familiar pH of 7.40 and P_{CO_2} of 40 torr are "normal" regardless of whether the patient is normothermic, hypothermic, or hyperthermic. Uncorrected values are not only simpler to use, they also offer ease of interpretation when serial measurements are made at different patient temperatures.[102]

INTRAVENOUS FLUID MANAGEMENT

As during normothermic conditions, intravenous-fluid management must relate to the patient's state of hydration, electrolyte balance, and ongoing fluid losses. Hypothermia poses two additional considerations: Owing to depressing of liver metabolism, glucose-containing infusions and excessive amounts of acid-citrate-dextrose blood should be avoided during the period of hypothermia, lest hyperglycemia result; however, mild hyperglycemia should not be treated because hypoglycemia is likely upon rewarming when the liver resumes normal metabolic function. Fluid input and estimates of overall fluid loss should be monitored particularly closely if the period of hypothermia is more than a few hours because of the possibility of cold diuresis and posthypotermia oliguria. During prolonged hypothermia, serial measurements of urine and serum electrolytes are also needed to plan optimal fluid management. Potassium supplementation is often required during the diuretic phase.

MANAGEMENT OF SPECIFIC PROBLEMS

SHIVERING

As noted during the discussions of the metabolic (p. 626) and cerebral (p. 627) effects of hypothermia, shivering is a protective reflex which during induced hypothermia is not only counterproductive, but potentially threatening to the well-being of the organism. This is because the increased oxygen requirement imposed by shivering places

undue and, very likely, excessive demands on the cardiorespiratory systems.[21-23] Should respiratory obstruction occur during emergence from hypothermia, the small oxygen reserves available can be depleted rapidly with the development of hypoxemia. Patients with compromised cardiorespiratory reserve or neuromuscular disease are likely to have difficulty compensating for increased demands imposed by shivering.

The best treatment for shivering, as with most other complications, begins with prevention. Most anesthetic techniques used in association with hypothermia use combinations of inhalation anesthetics, narcotics, and, especially, neuromuscular blocking agents to minimize, if not avoid shivering. Postanesthetic shivering can be treated with radiant or conductive heat,[103] microwave warming,[104] ventilation with warm, humidified oxygen,[105] narcotics such as meperidine,[106] and vasodilators such as nitroprusside.[107]

CARDIAC DYSRHYTHMIAS

Cardiac dysrhythmias are commonplace when the body temperature falls below 30°C and invariably occur below 28°C. The fact that the dysrhythmia is occurring during hypothermia should not prevent the clinician from considering and, if necessary, treating the many other potential etiologies: inadequate depth of anesthesia with endogenous catecholamine release; exogenous administration of a catecholamine; electrolyte imbalance (e.g., hypokalemia); hypotension with inadequate coronary perfusion; hypercarbia; and hypoxemia.

Once the more common etiologies have been excluded, the clinician should attempt conventional treatment for the specific dysrhythmia, if the disturbance is having a deleterious effect on blood pressure (see Chap. 14). Propranolol (in doses of 0.5 mg, to a total dosage of 1 mg–2 mg) has been advocated in anecdotal case reports,[108,109] but whether it is more effective than other therapies remains to be demonstrated. Clinical experience suggests that during hypothermia most rhythm disturbances are generally recalcitrant to therapy; this usually does not pose a problem because blood pressure and tissue perfusion are well maintained during short periods of well-monitored induced hypothermia. Ventricular fibrillation, the most serious complication of hypothermia, however, deserves treatment. Unfortunately, below about 27°C, defibrillation is invariably ineffective. Therapy for fibrillation occurring in the absence of cardiopulmonary bypass (which would maintain tissue perfusion) should be directed to raising the body temperature to 28°C to 30°C, where defibrillation is usually effective.

Anesthetic Overdosage

The narcosis accompanying hypothermia results, not unexpectedly, in a diminished anesthetic requirement. Minimal alveolar concentration (MAC) is reduced linearly as temperature falls, although the magnitude of this effect varies with the different anesthetics.[110–113] For example, a 10°C decrease in body temperature is associated with a 53 per cent decrease in the MAC for halothane.[112] Similarly, depression of liver function results in slower metabolism of drugs such as morphine.[114] In addition, because anesthetic gases are more soluble as temperature falls and both blood flow and ventilation are reduced by hypothermia, emergence from anesthesia is likely to be prolonged. The metabolism and elimination of nondepolarizing neuromuscular blocking agents are also depressed during hypothermia, but there is also an associated antagonism of their relaxant effect, the net result being a prolongation of neuromuscular blockade at moderate levels of hypothermia (28°C).[115] Although no prolongation is noted at lesser degrees of hypothermia, upon rewarming there is the possibility that residual relaxant can have a clinically important effect. Unless the reduced requirement for anesthetics is considered and depth of anesthesia is monitored more carefully, overdosage is likely.

REFERENCES

1. Armstrong Division, M. H.: Evolution of anaesthesia. Br. J. Anaesth., *31*:134, 1959.
2. Smith, L. W., and Fay, T.: Observations on human beings with cancer maintained at reduced temperature of 75–90 Fahrenheit. Am. J. Clin. Path., *10*:1, 1940.
3. Ciocatto, E., and Cattaneo, A. D.: Experimental and clinical results with clinical hypothermia. Anesthesiology, *17*:16, 1956.
4. Sedzimir, C. B., and Dundee, J. W.: Hypothermia in the treatment of cerebral tumors. J. Neurosurg., *15*:199, 1958.
5. Bigelow, W. G., Callaghan, J. C., and Hopps, J. A.: General hypothermia for experimental intracardiac surgery; use of electrophrenic respirations, artificial pacemaker for cardiac standstill, and radio-frequency rewarming in general hypothermia. Ann. Surg., *132*:531, 1950.
6. Bigelow, W. G., Lindsay, W. K., and Greenwood, W. F.: Hypothermia: Possible role in cardiac surgery: investigation of factors governing survival in dogs at low body temperature. Ann. Surg., *132*:948, 1950.
7. Hervey, G. R.: Hypothermia. Proc. Roy. Soc. Med., *66*:1053, 1973.
8. Reuler, J. B.: Hypothermia: Pathophysiology, clinical settings, and management. Ann. Intern. Med., *89*:519, 1978.
9. Coniam, S. W.: Accidental hypothermia. Anaesthesia, *34*:250, 1979.
10. Maclean, D., and Emslie-Smith, D.: Accidental Hypothermia. Oxford, Blackwell Scientific Publications, 1977.
11. Welton, D. E., Mattox, K. L., Miller, R. R., et al.: Treatment of profound hypothermia. J.A.M.A., *240*:2291, 1978.
12. Cannard, T. H., and Zaimis, E.: Effect of lowered muscle temperature on the action of neuromuscular blocking drugs in man. J. Physiol. (Lond.), *149*:112, 1959.
13. Little, D. M., Jr.: Hypothermia. Anesthesiology, *20*:842, 1959.
14. Collins, V. J.: Hypothermia—total body (refrigeration anesthesia). Anesthesiology. ed. 2. pp. 748–770. Philadelphia, Lea & Febiger, 1976.
15. Dills, D. B., and Forbes, W. H.: Respiratory and metabolic effects of hypothermia. Am. J. Physiol., *132*:685, 1941.
16. Spurr, G. B., Hutt, B. K., and Horwath, S. M.: Reponses of dogs to hypothermia. Am. J. Physiol., *179*:139, 1954.
17. Lougheed, W. H., Sweet, W. H., White, J. C., et al.: Use of hypothermia in surgical treatment of cerebral vascular lesions; Preliminary report. J. Neurosurg., *12*:240, 1955.
18. Severinghaus, J. W., Stupfel, M., and Bradley, A. F.: Alveolar dead space and arterial to end-tidal carbon dioxide differences during hypothermia in dog and man. J. Appl. Physiol., *10*:349, 1957.
19. Rosomoff, H. L.: Pathophysiology of the central nervous system during hypothermia. Acta Neurochirurgica, Suppl., *XIII*:11, 1964.
20. Blair, E.: Physiologic and metabolic effects of hypothermia in man. *In* Muschia, X. J., and Saunders, J. F. (eds.): Depressed Metabolism. Proceedings of the First International Conference on Depressed Metabolism, Washington, D. C., August 22–23, 1968. New York, American Elsevier, 1969.
21. Wolff, R. C., and Penrod, K. E.: Factors affecting the rate of cooling in immersion hypothermia in dogs. Am. J. Physiol., *163*:580, 1950.
22. Hegnauer, A. H., and D'Amoto, H. E.: Oxygen consumption and cardiac output in the hypothermic dog. Am. J. Physiol., *178*:138, 1954.
23. Bay, J., Nunn, J. F., and Prys-Roberts, C.: Factors influ-

encing arterial P_aO_2 during recovery from anaesthesia. Br. J. Anaesth., *40*:398, 1968.

24. Rosomoff, H. L.: Effects of hypothermia on physiology of the nervous system. Surgery, *40*:328, 1958.
25. Albert, S. N., and Fazekas, J. F.: Cerebral hemodynamics and metabolism during induced hypothermia. Anesth. Analg., *35*:381, 1956.
26. Michenfelder, J. D., and Theye, R. A.: Hypothermia: Effect on canine brain and whole-body metabolism. Anesthesiology, *29*:1107, 1968.
27. Lafferty, J. J., Keykhah, M. M., Shapiro, H. M., et al.: Cerebral hypometabolism obtained with deep pentobarbital anesthesia and hypotermia (30–°C). Anesthesiology, *49*:159, 1978.
28. Stone, H. H., Donnelly, C., and Frobese, A. S.: Effect of lowered body temperature on cerebral hemodynamics and metabolism of man. Surg. Gynecol. Obstet., *103*:313, 1956.
29. Rosomoff, H. L., and Holaday, D. A.: Cerebral blood flow and cerebral oxygen consumption during hypothermia. Am. J. Physiol., *179*:85, 1954.
30. Rosomoff, H. L., and Gilbert, R.: Brain volume and cerebrospinal fluid pressure during hypothermia. Am. J. Physiol., *183*:19, 1955.
31. Scott, J. W.: The EEG during hypothermia. EEG Clin. Neuro-Physiol., *7*:466, 1955.
32. Gasser, H. S.: Nerve activity as modified by temperature changes. Am. J. Physiol., *97*:254, 1931.
33. Chatfield, P. O., Battista, A. F., Lyman, C., et al.: Effects of cooling on nerve conduction in hibernator and nonhibernator. Am. J. Physiol., *155*:179, 1948.
34. Choh, L. L.: Effect of cooling on neuromuscular transmission in rat. Am. J. Physiol., *194*:200, 1958.
35. Hegnauer, A. H., Shriber, W. J., and Haterius, H. O.: Cardiovascular response of the dog to immersion hypothermia. Am. J. Physiol., *161*:455, 1950.
36. Hook, W. E., and Stormont, R. T.: Effect of lowered body temperature on heart rate, blood pressure and electrocardiogram. Am. J. Physiol., *133*:334, 1941.
37. Badeer, H.: Influence of temperature on S-A rate of dog's heart in denervated heart-lung preparation. Am. J. Physiol., *167*:76, 1951.
38. Cookson, B. A., and DiPalma, J. R.: Severe bradycardia of profound hypothermia in dog. Am. J. Physiol., *182*:447, 1955.
39. Bullard, R. W.: Cardiac output of the hypothermic rat. Am. J. Physiol., *196*:415, 1959.
40. Popovic, V., and Kent, K. M.: Cardiovascular responses in prolonged hypothermia. Am. J. Physiol., *209*:1069, 1965.
41. Jude, J. R., Haroutunian, L. M., and Folse, R.: Hypothermic myocardial oxygenation. Am. J. Physiol., *190*:57, 1957.
42. Berne, R. M.: Effect of immersion hypothermia on coronary blood flow. Circ. Res., *2*:236, 1954.
43. Edwards, W. S., Tuluy, S., Reber, W. E., et al.: Coronary blood flow and myocardial metabolism in hypothermia. Ann. Surg., *139*:275, 1954.
44. Sabiston, D. C., Theilen, E. O., and Gregg, D. E.: Relationship of coronary blood flow and cardiac output and other parameters in hypothermia. Surgery, *38*:498, 1955.
45. Mangiardi, J. L., Aiken, J. E., Behrer, A., et al.: Coronary blood flow during moderate and profound hypothermia. J. Cardiovasc. Surg., *6*:349, 1965.

46. Eiseman, B., and Spencer, F. C.: Effect of hypothermia on the flow characteristics of blood. Surgery, *52*:532, 1962.
47. Wells, R.: Microcirculation and the coronary blood flow. Am. J. Cardiol., *29*:847, 1972.
48. Prec, C. R., Roseman, K., Baun, S., et al.: The cardiovascular effects of acutely induced hypothermia. J. Clin. Invest., *28*:293, 1949.
49. Gunton, R. W., Scott, J. W., Lougheed, W. M., et al.: Changes in cardiac rhythm and in the form of the electrocardiogram resulting from induced hypothermia in man. Am. Heart J., *52*:419, 1956.
50. Johansson, B., Biorck, G., Heager, K., et al.: Electrocardiographic observations on patients operated upon in hypothermia. Acta Med. Scand., *155*:257, 1956.
51. Schwab, R. H., Lewis, D. W., Killough, J. H., et al.: Electrocardiographic changes occurring in rapidly induced deep hypothermia. Am. J. Med. Sci., *248*:290, 1964.
52. Osborn, J. J.: Experimental hypothermia. Respiratory and blood pH changes in relation to cardiac function. Am. J. Physiol., *175*:389, 1953.
53. Boba, A.: Abnormal electrocardiographic pattern and its relation to ventricular fibrillation; observations during clinical and experimental hypothermia. Am. Heart J., *57*:255, 1959.
54. Fleming, P. R., and Muir, F. H.: Electrocardiographic changes in induced hypothermia in man. Br. Heart J., *19*:59, 1957.
55. Emslie-Smith, D., Sladden, G. E., and Stirling, G. R.: The significance of changes in the electrocardiogram in hypothermia. Br. Heart J., *21*:343, 1959.
56. Abbott, J. A., and Chietlin, M.D.: The nonspecific camel-hump sign. J.A.M.A., *235*:413, 1976.
57. Lange, K., Weiner, D., and Gold, M. M. A.: Mechanism of Cardiac injury in experimental hypothermia. Ann. Intern. Med., *31*:989, 1949.
58. Falk, R. B., Jr., Denlinger, J. K., and O'Neill, M. J.: Changes in the electrocardiogram associated with intra-operative epicardial hypothermia. Anesthesiology, *46*:302, 1977.
59. Collins, V. J., and Granatelli, A. F.: Controlled hypothermia during anesthesia in human adults. Angiology, *6*:118, 1955.
60. Blair, M., Austin, R., Blount, S. G., et al.: A study of the cardiovascular changes during cooling and rewarming in human subjects undergoing total circulatory occlusion. J. Thorac. Surg., *33*:707, 1957.
61. Lynch, J. F., and Adolph, E. F.: Blood flow in small vessels during deep hypothermia. J. Appl. Physiol., *11*:192, 1957.
62. Keatinge, W. R.: Mechanism of adrenergic stimulation of mammalian arteries and its failure at low temperatures. J. Physiol., *174*:184, 1964.
63. D'Amato, H. E.: Thiocyanate space and distribution of water in musculature of hypothermic dog. Am. J. Physiol., *178*:143, 1954.
64. D'Amato, H. E., and Hegnauer, A. H.: Blood volume in hypothermic dog. Am. J. Physiol., *173*:100, 1953.
65. Rose, J. C., McDermott, T. F., Lilienfield, L. S., et al.: Cardiovascular function in hypothermic anesthetized man. Circulation, *15*:512, 1957.
66. Steen, P. A., and Michenfelder, J. D.: Deterimental effects of prolonged hypothermia in cats and monkeys

with and without regional cerebral ischemia. Stroke, 10:522, 1979.

67. Steen, P. A., and Michenfelder, J. D.: The deterimental effects of prolonged hypothermia and rewarming in the dog. Anesthesiology, 52:224, 1980.

68. Bigelow, W. G., Lindsay, W. K., Harrison, R. C., et al.: Oxygen transport and utilization in dogs at low temperatures. Am. J. Physiol., 160:125, 1950.

69. Rosenfeld, J. B.: Acid–base and electrolyte disturbances in hypothermia. Am. J. Cardiol., 12:678, 1963.

70. Salzano, J., and Hall, F. G.: Effect of hypothermia on ventilatory responses to carbon dioxide inhalation and carbon infusion in dogs. J. Appl. Physiol., 15:397, 1960.

71. Regan, M. J., and Eger, E. I., II: Ventilatory responses to hypercapnia and hypoxia at normothermia and moderate hypothermia during constant-depth halothane anesthesia. Anesthesiology, 27:624, 1966.

72. Sodipo, J. O., and Lee, D. C.: Comparison of ventilation responses to hypercapnia at normothermia and hypothermia during halothane anaesthesia. Can. Anaesth. Soc. J., 18:426, 1971.

73. Severinghaus, J. W., and Stupfel, M.: Respiratory dead space increases following atropine in man, and atropine, vagal or ganglionic blockade and hypothermia in dogs. J. Appl. Physiol., 8:81, 1955.

74. Nisbet, H. I. A.: Acid–base disturbance in hypothermia. Int. Anesthesiol. Clin., 2:829, 1964.

75. Miles, B. E., and Churchill-Davidson, H. C.: Effect of hypothermia on renal circulation of dog. Anesthesiology, 16:230, 1955.

76. Page, L. B.: Effects of hypothermia on renal function. Am. J. Physiol., 181:171, 1955.

77. Morales, P., Carberry, W., Morello, A., et al.: Alterations in renal function during hypothermia in man. Ann. Surg., 145:488, 1957.

78. Moyer, J. H., Greenfield, L., Heider, C., et al.: Hypothermia: Effect of agents which depress sympathetic nervous system on hypothermic induction time and on renal functional alterations due to hypothermia. Ann. Surg., 146:12, 1957.

79. Moyer, J. H., Morris, G. C., Jr., and DeBakey, M. E.: Hypothermia: I. Effect on renal hemodynamics and on excretion of water and electrolytes in dog and man. Ann. Surg., 145:26, 1957.

80. Carloss, H. W., and Tavassoli, M.: Acute renal failure from precipitation of cryoglobulins in a cool operating room. J.A.M.A., 244:1472, 1980.

81. Hallet, E. B.: Effect of decreased body temperature on liver function and splanchnic blood flow in dogs. Surg. Forum, 5:362, 1955.

82. Brauer, R. W., Holloway, R. J., Krebs, J. S., et al.: The liver in hypothermia. Ann. N.Y. Acad. Sci., 80:395, 1959.

83. Curry, D. L., and Curry, K. P.: Hypothermia and insulin secretion. Endocrinology, 87:750, 1970.

84. Blair, E.: Clinical Hypothermia. p. 49. New York, McGraw-Hill Book Company, 1964.

85. Bunker, J. P., and Goldstein, R.: Coagulation during hypothermia in man. Proc. Soc. Exp. Biol. Med., 97:199 1958.

86. Anstall, H. B., and Huntsman, R. G.: Influence of temperature upon blood coagulation in a cold- and a warm-blooded animal. Nature, 186:726, 1960.

87. Halinen, M. O., Suhonen, R. E., and Sarajas, H. S.: Characteristics ob blood clotting in hypothermia. Scand. J. Clin. Lab. Invest., 21 [suppl 101]:65, 1968.

88. Kopriva, C. J., Sreenivasan, N., Stefansson, S., et al.: Hypothermia can cause errors in activated coagulation time. Anesthesiology, 53:585, 1980.

89. Helmsworth, J. A., Stiles, W. J., and Elstun, W.: Changes in blood cellular elements in dogs during hypothermia. Surgery, 38:843, 1955.

90. Wensel, R. H., and Bigelow, W. G.: Use of haparin to minimize thrombocytopenia and bleeding tendency during hypothermia. Surgery, 45:223, 1959.

91. Von Kaulla, K. N., and Swan, H.: Clotting deviations in man associated with open-heart surgery during hypothermia. J. Thorac. Surg., 36:857, 1958.

92. Cooper, K. E., and Kenyon, J. R.: A comparison of temperatures measured in the rectum, oesophagus and on the surface of the aorta during hypothermia in man. Br. J. Surg., 44:616, 1957.

93. Whitby, J. D., and Dunkin, L. J.: Temperature differences in the oesophagus. The effects of intubation and ventilation. Br. J. Anaesth., 41:615, 1969.

94. Benzinger, T. H.: Clinical temperature: New physiological basis. J.A.M.A., 209:1200, 1969.

95. Benzinger, M.: Tympanic thermometry in surgery and anesthesia. J.A.M.A., 209:1207, 1969.

96. Webb, G. E.: Comparison of esophageal and tympanic temperature monitoring during cardiopulmonary bypass. Anesth. Analg., 52:729, 1973.

97. Whitby, J. D., and Dunkin, L. J.: Cerebral, oesophageal and nasopharyngeal temperatures. Br. J. Anaesth., 43:673, 1971.

98. Boere, L. A.: Ventricular fibrillation in hypothrmia. Anaesthesia, 12:299, 1957.

99. Severinghaus, J. W.: Blood gas calculator. J. Appl. Physiol., 21:1108, 1966.

100. Kelman, G. R., and Nunn, J. F.: Nomograms for correction of blood PO_2, PCO_2, pH, and base excess for time and temperature. J. Appl. Physiol., 21:1484, 1966.

101. Rahn, H., Reeves, R. B., and Howell, B. J.: Hydrogen ion regulation, temperature, and evolution. The 1975 J. Burns Amberson Lecture. Am. Rev. Resp. Dis., 112:165, 1975.

102. Hansen, J. E., and Sue, D. Y.: Should blood gas measurements be corrected for the patient's temperature? N. Engl. J. Med., 303:341, 1980.

103. Vaughan, M. S., Vaughan, R. W., and Cork, R. C.: Radiation vs. conduction for postop rewarming of adults. Anesthesiology, 53:S195, 1980.

104. Westenskow, D. R., Wong, K. C., Johnson, C. C., et al.: Physiologic effects of deep hypothermia and microwave rewarming: Possible application for neonatal cardiac surgery. Anesth. Analg., 58:297, 1979.

105. Pflug, A. E., Aasheim, G. M., Foster, C., et al.: Prevention of post-anaesthesia shivering. Can. Anaesth. Soc. J., 25:43, 1978.

106. Claybon, L. E., and Hirsh, R. A.: Meperidine arrests postanesthesia shivering. Anesthesiology, 53:S180, 1980.

107. Noback, C. R., and Tinker, J. H.: Hypothermia after cardiopulmonary bypass in man: Amelioration by nitroprusside-induced vasodilation during rewarming. Anesthesiology, 53:277, 1980.

108. Cole, A. F. D., and Jacobs, J. A.: Propranolol in the management of cardiac arrhythmias during hypothermia. Can. Anaesth. Soc. J., 14:44, 1967.

109. Finley, W. E. I., and Dykes, W. S.: Cardiac arrhythmias during hypothermia controlled by propranolol. Anaesthesia, *23*:631, 1968.
110. Cherkin, A., and Catchpoll, J. F.: Temperature dependence of anesthesia in goldfish. Science, *144*:1460, 1964.
111. Eger, E. I., II, Saidman, L. J., and Brandstater, B.: Temperature dependence of halothane and cyclopropane anesthesia in dogs: Correlation with some theories of anesthetic action. Anesthesiology, *26*:764, 1965.
112. Regan, M. J., and Eger, E. I., II: The effect of hypothermia in dogs on anesthetizing and apneic doses of inhalation agents. Anesthesiology, *28*:689, 1967.
113. Munson, E. S.: Effect of hypothermia on anesthetic requirement in rats. Lab. Anim. Sci., *20*:1109, 1970.
114. Rink, R. A., Gray, I., Rueckert, R. R., et al.: Effect of hypothermia on morphine metabolism in isolated perfused liver. Anesthesiology, *17*:377, 1956.
115. Ham, J., Miller, R. D., Benet, L. Z., et al.: Pharmacokinetics and pharmacodynamics of *d*-tubocurarine during hypothermia in the cat. Anesthesiology, *49*:324, 1978.

FURTHER READING

Benazon, D.: Hypothermia. *In* Scurr, C. and Feldman, S. (eds.): Scientific Foundations of Anaesthesia. ed 2. pp. 344–357. London, William Heinemann Medical Books, 1974.
Little, D. M., Jr.: Hypothermia. Anesthesiology, *20*:842, 1959.
Maclean, D., and Emslie-Smith, D.: The abnormal physiology of hypothermia. Accidental Hypothermia. pp. 76–132. Oxford, Blackwell Scientific Publications, 1977.
Popovic, V., and Popovic, P.: Hypothermia in Biology and in Medicine. New York, Grune & Stratton, 1974.

Part Twelve

Iatrogenesis

50 Equipment Malfunction

Robert E. Johnstone, M.D.

Anesthesia equipment includes high-pressure gas sources, pressure regulators, flow regulators, liquid vaporizers, breathing circuits, suction devices, and patient monitoring devices. The multiple parts, interconnections, and complexities of these anesthetic systems predispose them to malfunction and misuse. Eger and Epstein reviewed the hazards of anesthetic equipment in 1964[1]; more than a decade later, many of the problems they described still exist. Dorsch and Dorsch have written extensively on construction, care, and complications of anesthesia equipment.[2]

This chapter reviews some recent anesthetic complications related to equipment malfunction. Mechanical ventilator malfunctions, hazards of endotracheal tubes, electrical problems, and precautions for the use of explosive agents are discussed in Chapters 8, 9, 11, 52, and 53.

INCIDENCE OF EQUIPMENT MALFUNCTION

Anesthetic morbidity and mortality related to equipment malfunction are difficult to quantitate. Survey results depend on how malfunction is defined and how aggressively anesthetic deaths are investigated. Some reported series of anesthetic deaths fail to mention equipment malfunction.[3–5] Other series relate up to 7.6 per cent of anesthetic deaths to breathing system problems[6,7] or oxygen failure. Table 50-1 lists the causes of 29 anesthetic equipment-related deaths or permanent complications reported to the Medical Defence Union of England for the years 1964 to 1973.[8] Frequent publication of pertinent case reports of deaths and "near misses" shows that equipment hazards still exist.

Recently, using the technique of "critical incident reporting," Cooper examined preventable mishaps.[9] Though human error accounted for most of the mishaps, equipment malfunction was involved in 14 per cent. Monitors (24%), breathing circuits (20%), airway components (18%), and the anesthesia machine (12%) were the principal sources of malfunction. Frequent specific inci-

Table 50-1. Causes of Injuries or Death Related to Anesthesia Equipment

MALFUNCTION	NO. OF CASES
No oxygen owing to various causes	17
Apparatus disconnected	5
Equipment incorrectly used	3
Carbon dioxide excess	2
Contaminated nitrous oxide	2
Total no. of cases	29

(Wylie, W. D.: "There, but for the grace of God . . ." Ann R. Coll. Surg. Engl., 56:171, 1975)

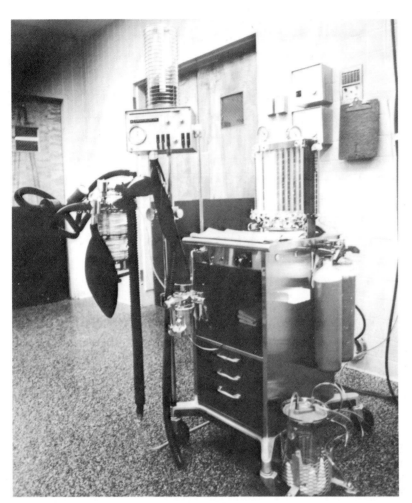

Fig. 50-1. A typical anesthesia machine with mechanical ventilator, inspired-oxygen meter, and waste-gas eliminator. If distracted, an anesthesiologist could confuse the 7 flowmeter columns, and 2 anesthetic filling columns, and several breathing tubes. Monitoring equipment and numerous operative team members may add to the confusion.

dents included breathing circuit disconnection, inadvertent gas flow changes, gas supply problems, laryngoscope malfunction, and disconnection of the intravenous administration set.

ANESTHESIA MACHINE

A modern anesthesia machine usually consists of sources of oxygen and nitrous oxide, pressure-reducing valves, meters to indicate gas flow rate and pressure, a liquid vaporizer, oxygen flush valve, carbon dioxide absorber, pressure relief (pop-off) valve, one-way flow valves, rebreathing bag, and tubing (Fig. 50-1). In addition, many anesthesia machines have additional gas tanks, flowmeters and vaporizers, a mechanical ventilator, waste-gas scavenger, suction apparatus, humidifier, monitoring devices, and shelves and drawers for drugs and equipment. The complexity of anesthesia systems has now increased to the extent that the equipment itself may confuse the anesthetist or distract attention from the patient and thereby contribute to error. This trend toward increasing complexity and distractions seems likely to continue as more safety and monitoring devices are incorporated. Current awareness of infection and pollution hazards of anesthetic machines requires frequent disassembly and cleaning of parts, so there is a possibility that the equipment may be reassembled in a faulty or incomplete manner.[10]

EXCESSIVE GAS PRESSURE

Oxygen is stored in cylinders at pressures of up to 100,000 torr* and liquid oxygen tanks at 3300 torr. Piping systems in hospitals usually operate at approximately 2600 torr. Pressure-reducing valves, a pop-off valve, and a compliant rebreathing bag lower gas pressures between source and patient. If pressure exceeding 60 torr is transmitted to a patient's lungs, pneumothorax and circulatory collapse may occur in seconds. Common causes of excessive airway pressure include sticking expiratory valves, opposed valves, foreign bodies in the breathing circuit, faulty pressure-reducing valves, oxygen flushing valves that are "stuck open," and excessive gas inflow rates in a noncompliant system.[11,12] Excessive gas pressure is hazardous primarily in intubated patients, in whom this pressure is transmitted directly to the lungs, in infants who have small total lung capacities, and in all patients breathing through closed circuits.[13] When gas flows into a closed breathing circuit with a shut pop-off valve, gas pressure depends on the relative compliances of lungs and rebreathing bag. Individual bags vary greatly, reaching maximum pressures of 22 to 120 torr before bursting. New disposable rebreathing bags are usually less compliant and thus exert higher pressures than reusable bags.[14] Prestretching a new rebreathing bag assures that with inadvertent overinflation, gas pressure will not exceed 30 to 35 torr. Misconnection of the manual handbag connector of an anesthesia ventilator to the universal gas delivery pipe of the anesthesia machine has resulted in several pneumothoraces[15] (see Chap. 12).

---

*Under most clinical circumstances, 1 atm. of pressure is the same as 760 mm. Hg, 760 torr, 1030 cm. H_2O, 101 kPa, or 14.7 p.s.i.

High-pressure gas systems also pose hazards to anesthetists and hospital employees. Tubing may become loose and whip through the operating room.[16] Faulty check valves in the cylinder yoke will allow transfilling of an empty cylinder on a multiple cylinder yoke; rapid gas compression in the empty cylinder creates high temperatures and may result in an explosion (see Chap. 52). Malfunctions of bulk oxygen delivery systems have led to pressures high enough to threaten hospital staff and rupture nitrous oxide reducing valves on anesthesia machines.[17] In one hospital, the oxygen system was not equipped with a high-pressure relief valve, and a serious situation was detected only by observation of rising pressure on the manometer located behind the anesthesia machine.[18]

INSUFFICIENT GAS FLOW

The problem posed by insufficient gas flow ranges in severity from annoying to dangerous. The worst complications are usually caused by unrecognized administration of hypoxic gas mixtures. Causes of insufficient gas flow include failure of bulk gas supply systems, empty gas cylinders, non-connection of the gas source to the anesthesia machine, leak, or misconnection within the anesthetic system and incompetent breathing tubes.

Feeley and Hedley-Whyte have reviewed the designs and dangers of bulk oxygen and nitrous oxide delivery systems.[19] Nearly one-third of 193 hospitals that they surveyed reported serious or potentially serious accidents, resulting in three deaths, related to their bulk gas delivery systems. More than half of these accidents involved decreases in oxygen pipeline pressure, often resulting in insufficient delivery of oxygen for clinical use. Causes of a reduction in or lack of oxygen pressure included pipeline damage during construction, pipeline obstruction, depletion of oxygen, freezing of the regulator during use, unannounced system shutdown, lightning damage to regulators, installation of the wrong wall connectors, and regulator malfunction.

Piped-in oxygen and nitrous oxide usually

connect to anesthesia machines by a spring-loaded, male-to-female, push-and-lock connection. These connections can be tight enough to hold the hose ends together but not permit gas flow, and they are often hidden from view behind the anesthesia machine. Oxygen cylinders may be empty, even though the pressure gauge on the anesthesia machine initially shows adequate pressure, or cylinder valves may not be opened enough to permit free flow of gas after the cylinder pressure falls.[20] Most modern anesthesia machines are equipped with oxygen-failure safety valves that cause the flow of anesthetic gases to cease when oxygen supply pressure falls.[20]

Leaks large enough to cause hypoxia can occur within anesthesia machines (e.g., when flowmeters are loose or vaporizer controls are broken).[21] The hose connecting the common outflow from the anesthesia machine to the breathing circuit may be unattached or misconnected, such as to a ventilator support post. Large leaks may occur at the pop-off valve, waste gas scavenger, and carbon dioxide absorber. Lastly, anesthesia bags may suddenly burst. Obstruction in the breathing circuit occurs when two one-way valves are placed in opposite directions, when a valve sticks, when tubing kinks or fills with condensed ‘water, or when a foreign body obstructs flow.[22]

DEFICIENT OXYGEN CONCENTRATION

The very serious complication of administration of deficient oxygen concentration is the subject of numerous case reports. Unfortunately, delivery of hypoxic gas mixtures is not usually obvious, and the first indication of trouble may be tachycardia, bradycardia, cyanosis, or cardiovascular collapse.

Cylinders of nitrous oxide or other gases can be placed on oxygen yokes despite pin-indexing systems. Multiple washers and bent pins defeat this safety system.[23,24] Inverted nitrous oxide yoke blocks are easily fitted on oxygen yokes.[25] Nitrous oxide and oxygen lines can be reversed during construction or repair before entering the operating suite; this mix-up recently resulted in a number of deaths.[26–29] Lastly, oxygen cylinders may not contain oxygen.

When high- and low-flow oxygen meters are both present, a low oxygen flow may be set and misread on the adjacent flowmeter scale as a higher flow, and, thus, an unknown, insufficient oxygen concentration is delivered to the patient.[30] Lack of standardization has led to placement of the oxygen flowmeter on the left of, on the right of, or between other flowmeters on the anesthesia machine; this contributes to human error. Flowmeters may indicate the wrong flow rate because they are incorrectly placed, calibrated for a different gas, or contain the wrong bobbin or a foreign body.[31–35] Alternatively, a correct amount of oxygen may be dialed and accurately delivered through an unused flowmeter to the cylinder yoke instead of the patient.[36]

EXCESSIVE ANESTHETIC CONCENTRATION

Vaporizers may deliver more or less than the intended anesthetic concentration.[37] Administration of too much anesthetic is a serious, potentially fatal hazard, and administration of too little may result in awareness during anesthesia or at least unsatisfactory operating conditions.

Increasing fresh gas inflow increases the anesthetic concentration delivered by some vaporizers. Oxygen-flushing systems usually bypass vaporizers, but in some anesthetic machines the build-up in circuit pressure with flushing can deliver boli of anesthetic vapor from vaporizers.[38] An overfilled vaporizer can deliver liquid anesthetic into the inspiratory line.[39] Vaporizers of new designs prevent overfilling but, even when filled to the "maximum safe level," can deliver liquid agent with high total gas flows.[40] Tipping free-standing vaporizers usually delivers liquid agent into the outflow line,[41] and connecting the vaporizer backwards approximately doubles the anesthetic concentration.[42] Imperfect temperature-compensating mechanisms in some vaporizers allow anesthetic output to fall as temperature decreases; refilling of the vaporizer with warm liquid suddenly increases the output.[43]

Many vaporizers deliver a lower concentration as they age, but the internal bypass can become occluded and cause administration of excessive concentrations.

ADMINISTRATION OF THE WRONG ANESTHETIC AGENT

Many people other than the anesthesiologist who administers an anesthetic may handle and fill his vaporizer. Once the vaporizer is filled, most anesthesiologists cannot reliably identify the contained anesthetic agent by smell. Substitution of a more volatile agent for a less volatile one, such as pouring trichloroethylene into a halothane vaporizer, leads to administration of excessive anesthetic concentrations. Halothane, when used in a methoxyflurane vaporizer, is delivered at dangerously high concentrations of over 15 per cent.[44] When vaporizers are connected in series, the upstream vaporizer may contaminate the downstream one, so that when the second vaporizer is used, two agents are delivered.[45,46] Finally, anesthetic cleaning fluids may be introduced into hospital piped-gas systems.[47]

HYPERCAPNIA

Failure to switch the carbon dioxide absorber into the breathing circuit, exhausted or no soda lime, and faulty connections allow carbon dioxide accumulation.[48] Defects in design of some absorbers allow internal bypass of soda lime.[49] Many non-rebreathing valves allow rebreathing; 10 to 76 per cent of inflation volumes with a bag-valve-mask arrangement may leak back into the rebreathing bag during exhalation.[50]

MISCELLANEOUS EQUIPMENT MALFUNCTIONS

Essentially every piece of equipment and interconnection that the anesthesiologist uses may fail. Many malfunctions are so common that they are considered normal annoyances, but better equipment design would prevent or reduce them. Laryngoscopes frequently fail to light because debris has covered the bulb contact plate, or the batteries are old. Operating tables may stick in an up, down, or tilted position because the gears are filled with debris. Anesthesia drawers make convenient foot rests but then may not open or shut because the drawer slide is off its railing. Suction tubing kinks easily or collapses under a foot. Small wheels on most anesthesia machines and portable equipment make movement difficult, especially in operating rooms with tubes and cords on the floor.

TREATMENT AND PREVENTION OF COMPLICATIONS OWING TO EQUIPMENT MALFUNCTION

As new anesthetic equipment is developed and marketed, new problems occur; as more equipment is attached to our anesthesia machines, more interfacing problems develop. More equipment and more sophistication sometimes prove counterproductive. Anesthesiologists of advanced age know that equipment failure was minimal during open-drop ether anesthesia with finger-on-the-pulse monitoring. Thus, when an equipment-related problem suddenly develops and the solution is not obvious, switching to the simplest techniques can save a life. If the patient is in trouble, mouth-to-mouth ventilation is nearly infallible.

It is better to concentrate on preventing equipment failure rather than on treating the ensuing complications. Regular maintenance by trained personnel and manufacturer's representatives prevents the development of some problems caused by wear. Information on maintenance is available from manufacturers and the anesthesia literature.[50] However, anesthesia equipment frequently functions in an all-or-none fashion, and even regular maintenance will not identify or prevent all problems.

Before each anesthetic, the anesthesiologist must check his suction, oxygen and gas supplies, breathing equipment, and essential drugs. Continuous monitoring of oxygen concentration in inspired gas should prevent the most common cause of equipment-related fatalities. Standardization committees, such as Committee Z-79 of the American National Standards Institute, National Fire Protection Association, and Compressed Gas Association, discuss and recommend design changes of gas systems and anesthesia machines and equipment. These changes might include non-interchangeable flowmeters, color-coded bobbins, pin-indexed vaporizer filling systems, a standardized location for oxygen-flow knobs, and touch identification of control knobs. Some changes will increase the cost of anesthetic equipment, and the change to new techniques might even be confusing initially. Ultimately, prevention and correction of equipment malfunction depends on the anesthesiologist, who must understand the function of each piece of equipment and remain (eternally) vigilant.

REFERENCES

1. Eger, E. I., and Epstein, R. M.: Hazards of anesthetic equipment. Anesthesiology, 25:490, 1964.
2. Dorsch, J. A., and Dorsch, S. E.: Understanding Anesthesia Equipment: Construction, Care and Complications. Baltimore, Williams and Wilkins, 1975.
3. Ament, R.: Classification of operating room mortality: review of cases in a pediatric medical center during the 10-year period, 1949 to 1958. Anesth. Analg., 39:158, 1960.
4. Dripps, R. D., Lamont, A., and Eckenhoff, J. E.: The role of anesthesia in surgical mortality. J.A.M.A., 178:261, 1961.
5. Phillips, O. C., Frazier, T. M., Graff, T. D., et al.: The Baltimore anesthesia study committee. Review of 1,024 postoperative deaths. J.A.M.A., 174:2015, 1960.
6. Dinnick, O. P.: Hazards in the operating theatre. Ann. R. Coll. Surg. Engl., 52:349, 1973.
7. Edwards, G., Morton, H. J. V., Park, E. A., et al.: Deaths associated with anaesthesia: a report of 1000 cases. Anaesthesia, 11:194, 1956.
8. Wylie, W. D.: "There, but for the grace of God . . ." Ann. R. Coll. Surg. Engl., 56:171, 1975.
9. Cooper, J. B., Newbower, R. S., Long, C. S., et al.: Preventable anesthetic mishaps—a human factors study. Anesthesiology, 49:399, 1978.
10. Duncalf, D.: Care of anesthetic equipment and other devices. Arch. Surg., 107:600, 1973.
11. Dogu, T. S., and Davis H. S.: Hazards of inadvertently opposed valves. Anesthesiology, 33:122, 1970.
12. Dean, H. N., Parsons, D. E., and Raphaely, R. C.: Bilateral tension pneumothorax from mechanical failure of anesthesia machine due to misplaced expiratory valve. Anesth. Analg., 50:195, 1971.
13. Arens, J. F.: A hazard in the use of the Ayre T-piece. Anesth. Analg., 50:943, 1971.
14. Johnstone, R. E., and Smith, T. C.: Rebreathing bags as pressure-limiting devices. Anesthesiology, 38:192, 1973.
15. Turndorf, H., Capan, L., and Kessel, J. W.: Prevention of misconnection of the Air-Shields ventimeter-ventilator. Anesth. Analg., 53:342, 1974.
16. Jones, R. J.: External vigilance. Anesthesiology, 32:566, 1970.
17. Eichhorn, J. H., Bancroft, M. L., Laasberg, H., et al.: Contamination of medical gas and water pipelines in a new hospital building. Anesthesiology, 46:286, 1977.
18. Feeley, T. W., McClelland, K. J., and Malhotra, I. V.: The hazards of bulk oxygen delivery systems. Lancet, 1:1416, 1975.
19. Feeley, T. W., and Hedley-Whyte, J.: Bulk oxygen and nitrous oxide delivery systems. Anesthesiology, 44:301, 1976.
20. Epstein, R. M., Rackow, H., Lee, A. S. J., et al.: Prevention of accidental breathing of anoxic gas mixtures during anesthesia. Anesthesiology, 23:1, 1962.
21. Mulroy, M., Ham, J., and Eger, E. I. II: Inflowing gas lead, a potential source of hypoxia. Anesthesiology, 45:102, 1976.
22. Rendell-Baker, L.: Another close call with "crossed valves." Anesthesiology, 31:194, 1969.
23. Hogg, C. E.: Pin-indexing failures. Anesthesiology, 38:85, 1973.
24. Steward, D. J., and Sloan, I. A.: Additional pin-indexing failures. Anesthesiology, 39:355, 1973.
25. Rawstron, R. E., and McNeill, T. D.: Pin-index failure. Br. J. Anaesth., 34:591, 1962.
26. Porter, K.: Gas fitter followed plan, Sudbury inquest is told. The Toronto Star, Feb. 7, 1974, page A7.
27. Deaths at Pennsylvania hospital laid to mixup in labelling gases. N. Y. Times, August 3, 1977, p. 1.
28. The Westminister inquiry. Lancet, 2:175, 1977.
29. Eichhorn, J. H., Bancroft, M. L., Laasberg, L. H., et al.: Contamination of medical gases and water pipelines in a new hospital building. Anesthesiology, 46:286, 1977.
30. Mazze, R. I.: Therapeutic misadventures with oxygen delivery systems: the need for continuous in-line oxygen monitors. Anesth. Analg., 51:787, 1972.
31. Walts, L. F., and Inglove, H.: Malfunction of a new anesthetic machine. Anesthesiology, 25:867, 1964.
32. Kelley, J. M., and Gabel, R. A.: The improperly calibrated flowmeter—another hazard. Anesthesiology, 33:467, 1970.
33. Chadwick, D. A.: Transposition of rotameter tubes. Anesthesiology, 40:102, 1974.
34. Slater, E. M.: Transposition of rotameter bobbins. Anesthesiology, 41:101, 1974.
35. Battig, C. G.: Unusual failure of an oxygen flowmeter. Anesthesiology, 37:561, 1972.
36. Liew, P. C., and Ganendran, A.: Oxygen failure: a potential danger with air flowmeters in anaesthetic machine with remote controlled needle valves. Br. J. Anaesth., 45:1165, 1973.
37. Latto, I. P.: Administration of halothane in the 0-0.5% concentration range with the Fluotec Mark 2 and Mark 3 vaporizers. Br. J. Anaesth., 45:563, 1973.
38. Greenhow, D. E., and Barth, R. L.: Oxygen flushing delivers anesthetic-vapor: a hazard with a new machine. Anesthesiology, 38:409, 1973.
39. Safar, P., and Galla, S. J.: Overdose with Ohio halothane vaporizer. Anesthesiology, 23:715, 1962.
40. Kopriva, C. J., and Lowenstein, E.: An anesthetic accident: cardiovascular collapse from liquid halothane delivery. Anesthesiology, 30:246, 1969.

41. Munson, W. M.: Cardiac arrest: hazard of tipping a vaporizer. Anesthesiology, *26*:235, 1965.
42. Marks, W. E., and Bullard, J. R.: Another hazard of free-standing vaporizers, increased anesthetic concentration with reversed flow of vaporizing gas. Anesthesiology, *45*:445, 1976.
43. Gartner, J., and Stoelting, R. K.: Laboratory comparison of Copper Kettle, Fluotec Mark 2 and Pentec vaporizers. Anesth. Analg., *53*:187, 1974.
44. Paull, J. D., and Sleeman, K. W.: An anaesthetic hazard. Br. J. Anaesth., *43*:1202, 1971.
45. Dorsch, S. E., and Dorsch, J. A.: Chemical cross-contamination between vaporizers in series. Anesth. Analg., *52*:176, 1973.
46. Murray, W. J., Zsigmond, E. K., and Fleming, P.: Contamination of in-series vaporizers with halothane-methoxyflurane. Anesthesiology, *38*:487, 1973.
47. Lackore, L. K., and Perkins, H. M.: Accidental narcosis. J.A.M.A., *211*:1846, 1970.
48. Eger, E. I. II, and Ethans, C. T.: The effects of inflow, outflow and valve placement on economy of the circle system. Anesthesiology, *29*:93, 1968.
49. Whitten, M. P., and Wise, C. C.: Design faults in commonly used carbon dioxide absorbers. Br. J. Anaesth., *44*:535, 1972.
50. Loehning, R. W., Davis, G., and Safar, P.: Rebreathing with "nonbreathing" valves. Anesthesiology, *25*:854, 1964.
51. Mayer, A.: Malfunctions of anesthesia machines: a guide for maintenance. Anesth. Analg., *52*:376, 1973.

FURTHER READING

Cooper, J. B., Newbower, R. S., Long, C. S., et al.: Preventable anesthetic mishaps—a human factors study. Anesthesiology, *49*:399, 1978.
Dorsch, J. A., and Dorsch, S. E.: Understanding Anesthesia Equipment: Construction, Care and Complications. Baltimore, Williams and Wilkins, 1975.
Rendell-Baker, L.: Some gas machine hazards and their elimination. Anesth. Analg., *55*:26, 1976.

51 Positioning Trauma

Beverley A. Britt, M.D., Nancy Joy, A.O.C.A., and Margot B. Mackay, B.Sc.A.A.M.

Incorrect positioning of a patient during anesthesia may cause trauma to nerves, spinal cord, eyes, skin, muscles, tendons, ligaments, and appendages and malfunctioning of the respiratory and cardiovascular systems. These untoward events are all preventable.[1-6] Nevertheless, they still constitute a major proportion of postanesthetic complications, even though they have been observed since shortly after the introduction of ether[7-9] and their true etiology has been known since the end of the last century.[8,10,11]

TRAUMA TO THE NERVES

Main Etiologic Factors

The principal cause of the majority of peripheral nerve injuries in anesthetized patients is ischemia of the intraneural vasa nervorum.[12-14] This results primarily from stretching of the nerve and secondarily from compression of a nerve already rendered vulnerable by stretching. Both stretching and compression of nerves are likely to occur in the anesthetized patient for two reasons. Firstly, muscle tonus is reduced, especially when muscle relaxants are employed, and thus susceptibility to unphysiological positions is increased.[15] Secondly, with perceptive powers no longer intact, the patient is unable to complain of postural insults that he normally would not tolerate.[9] Even in the conscious patient, abduction of the arm to more than 90 degrees in a steep Trendelenburg position becomes painful and intolerable after a few minutes, and the radial pulse disappears in 83 per cent of such volunteers.[6,16] Only 30 to 40 min. of anesthesia in an unfavorable position may be sufficient to result in nerve palsy.[6]

Factors Contributing to Trauma to the Nerves

In addition to ischemia of the vasa nervorum, there are several factors that contribute to peripheral nerve injuries.[17]

Congenital Anomalies. Certain congenital anomalies increase vulnerability of nerves to injury during anesthesia. For example, the brachial plexus is particularly susceptible to injury when there is preexisting hypertrophy of the scalenus anterior,[15,18,19]; hypertrophy of the scalenus medius*; cervical rib[15]; anomalous derivation of the plexus (higher or lower than normal)[15]; or an abnormal slope of the shoulder.[2]

Preexisting Diseases. Patients with diabetes mellitus are especially vulnerable to irreversible nerve injury during anesthesia. Jones, for instance, described a diabetic patient who, following anesthesia, developed an ulnar nerve palsy that progressively became worse rather than better.[20]

Malposition during anesthesia stresses not only nerves but also blood vessels, thus permitting

---

*Personal communication, R. MacKenzie.

hematoma formation in patients suffering from blood dyscrasias (e.g., factor VIII deficiency[21]) and in patients on anticoagulant therapy.[22-24] These hematomas, in turn, exacerbate nerve injuries induced directly by malposition.

Other preexisting conditions that may predispose patients to nerve palsies during anesthesia are anemia (e.g., pernicious anemia), hypovolemia, electrolyte imbalances,[25] and arteriosclerosis.[8]

Hypothermia of 30 minutes or more may be followed by a peripheral neuropathy,[26] because with surface cooling far lower temperatures (3–5°C) are recorded peripherally than in the core (27–31°C).[27,28] Even minimal concomitant stretching or compression (e.g., by the rubber straps of diathermy pads) greatly exaggerates the likelihood of hypoxia within nerve cells.[29]

Hypotension. Accidental or controlled hypotension may aggravate a nerve palsy primarily owing to malposition, by reducing blood flow into the nerves.[8]

Tourniquet. A tourniquet has been reported occasionally to cause damage to the nerves over which it was applied, if the pressure was excessive or continued for a prolonged period,[8,12,30,31] or if the patient had diabetes mellitus. In the properly positioned healthy patient, however, neuropathy following tourniquet application is extremely unlikely, because there is no stretching. The compression is dissipated around the entire circumference of the limb, being exerted generally through an abundance of soft tissues and not directly against a hard, bony point.

Differential Diagnosis

Before it is concluded that a peripheral nerve injury is the result of positioning trauma during anesthesia, several other diagnoses must be excluded.[17]

Trauma Sustained Prior to Hospitalization. Patients may arrive in the operating theatre already suffering from nerve injuries that remained undiagnosed prior to anesthesia. This is most likely in patients with injuries that are extremely painful or life-threatening: The comparatively painless nerve lesion goes unnoticed by both patient and surgeon until the postoperative period.

Blood Dyscrasias. Neuropathies that are entirely caused by compression from hematomas secondary to preexisting blood dyscrasias or excessive therapeutic anticoagulation may become evident in the immediate postoperative period. The sciatic,[21,24] median,[22,23] and femoral[24,32] nerves are frequently injured. For example, injury may be caused by hematoma formation in the retroperitoneal area that compresses the femoral nerve as it descends between the iliac and psoas muscles.[33]

Misplaced Needles. For medicolegal purposes, injuries caused by malposition of the patient during anesthesia should be differentiated from those caused by needles inserted by personnel other than anesthesiologists. Palsy may result from direct probing of a needle, from chemical irritation of injected drugs (e.g., thiopental, diazepam, chlorpromazine, and norepinephrine, bacterial contamination, or from local hematoma formation secondary to perforation of an adjacent vein.[34,35] For example, damage has followed percutaneous angiograms performed by the Seldinger technique[36] through the axillary artery.[37-39] Particularly uncooperative or pediatric patients are sometimes anesthetized for this procedure, or they are anesthetized for a major surgical procedure shortly after angiography. Therefore, determination of the exact mechanism of the injury is of extreme importance.

Premedication distal to rather than into the deltoid muscle may easily damage the radial nerve in the spiral groove.[40] Infusion of thiopental into the vein passing up the lateral side of the wrist has injured the underlying superficial radial nerve,[41] producing numbness of the dorsum of the thenar web.

The sciatic nerve can be traumatized if a nurse administers an intramuscular injection too medially and too deeply into the buttock.[41]

Spinal Anesthesia. The low cerebrospinal fluid pressure that follows a dural leak is probably the cause of the cranial nerve palsies that have been observed after spinal anesthesia.[42,43] The low pressure is presumed to result in descent of the medulla and pons, with secondary stretching of the cranial nerves.[44-48] Paralysis of every cranial

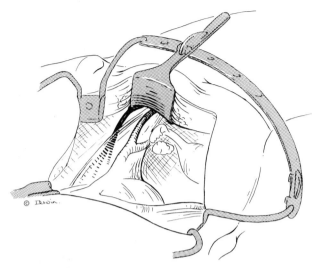

Fig 51-1. The femoral nerve is compressed and laterally deflected by the leg of a self-retaining retractor. (Britt, B. A., and Gordon, R. A.: Peripheral nerve injuries associated with anaesthesia. Can. Anaesth. Soc. J., *11*: 514, 1964)

nerve except the tenth has been reported, but in 90 per cent of cases, the sixth nerve is affected. The incidence is probably greater than reports indicate because a slight paresis is overlooked when the patient complains only of slight blurring of vision that clears up in a few days. In full-blown cases there is diplopia, preceded by severe headache, stiff neck, nausea, dizziness, and photphobia. The onset of the palsy varies up to 21 days postoperatively,[41] and recovery may not be complete for up to 2 years (see Chap. 5).[49]

Surgical Mal-manipulation. The femoral nerve has been damaged by pressure and lateral deflection by the leg of a self-retaining retractor used during a gynecological laparotomy (Fig. 51-1).[50] On examination, there is loss of flexion of the hip and extension of the knee owing to quadriceps femoris palsy. Sensation and autonomic function are lost over the anterior aspect of the thigh, as well as medial and anteromedial side of the calf.

Obturator nerve palsy with paralysis of the abductors and numbness over the medial side of the thigh was observed in a patient following an epidural anesthetic.* This patient had undergone

---

*Personal communication, R. A. Gordon.

a difficult forceps delivery, and the obstetrician recalled that he had to "pull harder" on the forceps than he had ever done before.

Toxic Effect of General Anesthetics. Damage to the nervous system may be produced by direct toxic action of the degradation products of anesthetics or by other impurities contained in them. As an example, phosgene is produced from chloroform on exposure to heat. In the presence of heat and alkali, trichloroethylene decomposes to form dichloroacetylene, which, in turn, is converted by heat to phosgene and carbon monoxide.[41,51,52] Soda lime is capable of triggering each of these reactions, since carbon dioxide absorption by soda lime is an exothermic reaction. Both dichloroacetylene and phosgene are extremely toxic to the CNS and to the cranial nerves, especially the fifth. Numbness and coldness around the lips begin 1 to 2 days after the anesthetic. During the next few days, the area of sensory loss spreads to involve the whole field supplied by the trigeminal nerve. Difficulty with chewing and jaw drop may be present. The mortality is high owing to a toxic encephalopathy. If the patient survives, complete recovery usually occurs in about 8 weeks (see Chap. 22).

SPECIFIC NEUROPATHIES

Trauma to the Brachial Plexus

Mechanism of Injury. For two reasons, the brachial plexus is the most susceptible of all nerve groups to damage from malpositioning during anesthesia.[1,2,4,5,6,7,9,10,11,15,16,27,35,38,53–60] First, the plexus has a relatively long, mobile, and superficial course in the axilla between two firm points of fixation: the vertebrae and prevertebral fascia above, and the axillary fascia below. Second, the plexus lies in close proximity to a number of freely moveable bony structures.

Stretching is usually the chief cause of injury to the brachial plexus.[10,61–63] Compression plays only a secondary role and acts as a fulcrum or stabilizing point; the nerves must then traverse a greater than normal distance around this fulcrum. Damage to the plexus is produced by any factor that increases the distance between the points of fixation above and below:

DORSAL EXTENSION AND LATERAL FLEXION OF THE HEAD to the opposite side in the supine (Fig. 51-2) or lateral (Fig. 51-3A,B) position widens the angle between the head and shoulder tip and thus stretches the plexus.[1,10,15,64]

PERMITTING THE ARM TO SAG off the side of the table so that it is abducted, externally rotated, and dorsally extended, especially if the extremity is at an angle of more than 60 degrees to the table, considerably elongates the plexus.[1,15]

THE PLEXUS MAY ALSO BE PINCHED between the clavicle and first rib when shoulder braces, used to prevent the patient from slipping downward in the Trendelenburg position, are not placed properly over the acromioclavicular joint, but instead are placed rather too far medially, where they depress the clavicle caudally and posteriorly into the retroclavicular space.[1,7,15] The plexus must now travel a devious "S-shaped" course, increasing the distance between the proximal and distal points of fixation. If, in addition, the patient's arm is abducted on an arm board, stretching becomes extreme (Fig. 51-4).

THE PLEXUS MAY BE DEPRESSED CAUDALLY by being stretched over the head of the humerus. This occurs in the Trendelenburg position with the arm abducted on an arm board. The shoulder-rests in this case are placed too far laterally and actually ride over the humeral head; thus drives it downward into the axilla, carrying the plexus with it (Fig. 51-5).[54,64] Thus, in the Trendelenburg position, shoulder braces should be padded well and placed over the acromia and not over the clavicles or the head of the humeri; the arms should always be kept close to the patient's sides,[58] with a metal arm guard or a draw sheet (Fig. 51-6). If a metal arm guard is used, its inner side must be well padded. If a draw sheet is employed, obese surgeons should be deterred from using the patient's arm as a resting place for their abdomens. The use of a steep Trendelenburg position must be discouraged.[65]

THE PLEXUS MAY BE DEVIATED POSTERIORLY by the tendon of pectoralis minor or even by the tip of the coracoid process in rather obese patients undergoing a cholecystectomy. This occurs when a gall bladder rest has been inserted, and the head of the humerus on the same side is allowed to sag down off the operating table mattress, onto an

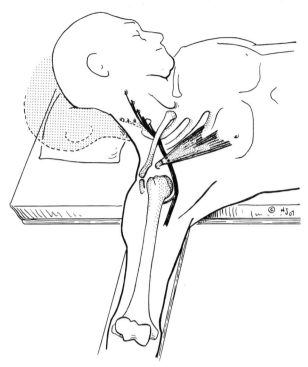

Fig. 51-2. Dorsal extension and lateral flexion of the head to the opposite side stretch the brachial plexus. (Britt, B. A., and Gordon, R. A.: Peripheral nerve injuries associated with anaesthesia. Can. Anaesth. Soc. J., *11:* 514, 1964)

arm board that is not padded up to the level of the mattress. The entire shoulder girdle is depressed posteriorly and laterally in relation to the rib cage. The attachment of the tendon of pectoralis minor to the coracoid process and, with it, the brachial plexus are, therefore, deviated in the same direction (Fig. 51-7).[2]

INTRANEURAL ISCHEMIA is likely when the patient is in the lateral position with an arm suspended from an "ether screen," so that the extremity is abducted to more than 90 degrees with the forearm pronated. The pronation twists the ulnar, radial, and medial nerves into a more circuitous course, and gravity accentuates the intraneural ischemia (Fig. 51-8). In the lateral position a suspended arm should be abducted to less than 90 degrees, and the forearm must be supinated slightly to ensure against brachial plexus injury.[61]

EXTREME ABDUCTION without anterior flexion

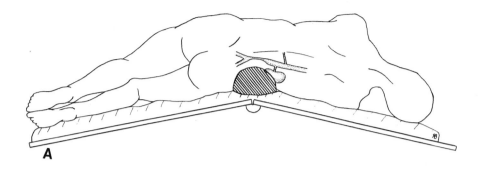

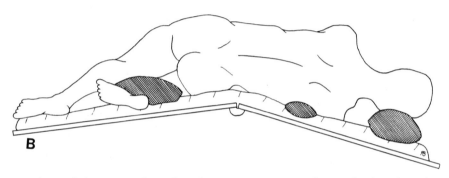

Fig. 51-3. (A) Incorrect lateral nephrectomy position. The top leg lies directly over the bottom leg, so that bony prominences are directly opposing each other, with inadequate padding between. Inadequate support under the head permits excessive lateral flexion of the head. A lack of padding behind the rib cage leaves the head of the humerus directly under the thorax. Exaggerated kidney rest constricts the inferior vena cava. The brachial plexus is consequently compressed. (B) Correct lateral nephrectomy position. The bottom leg is flexed more than the top leg, so that bony prominences are opposed by soft muscles. Padding between the legs is ample. A pillow prevents excessive lateral flexion of the head. Padding behind the lower rib cage permits slight posterior tilting of the upper part of the rib cage, so that the humeral head is anterior to the thorax, thus preventing compression of the brachial plexus. A small or no kidney rest ensures free flow of blood through the inferior vena cava.

of the arms, so that the hands rest beside, above, or behind the head, along with supination of the forearms, induces extreme stretching of the plexus. The patient may be either supine for a cardiac operation[56] (Fig. 51-9) or flexed prone (prone-jacknife) on an orthopaedic frame for spinal surgery (Fig. 51-10). In either of these positions, anterior flexion and abduction of the arms must be minimized (Figs. 51-11 and 51-12).

SUSPENSION OF A PATIENT BY THE WRISTS, to prevent slipping in an extreme Trendelenburg position, has been reported to some investigators to heighten tension of the plexus. Clausen believed that the first rib became a fulcrum, over which the plexus rubbed when anticephalad traction was placed on the abducted arm.[15] Ewing has disputed this,[54] and in the author's experience with the dissection of cadavers, there is not

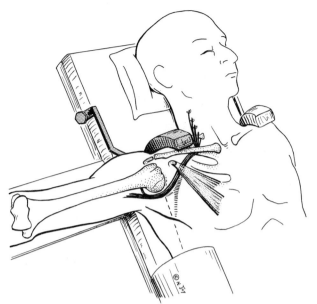

Fig. 51-4. Shoulder-rests placed too medially and abduction of the arm in the Trendelenburg position cause deviation and compression of the plexus between the depressed clavicle and first rib. (Britt, B. A., and Gordon, R. A.: Peripheral nerve injuries associated with anaesthesia. Can. Anaesth. Soc. J., *11:* 514, 1964)

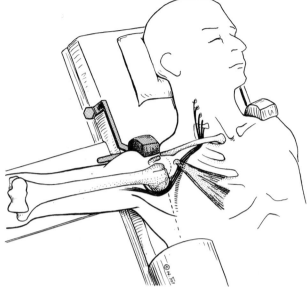

Fig. 51-5. Shoulder-rests placed too far laterally and abduction of the arm in Trendelenburg position cause deviation of the brachial plexus below the head of the humerus, which has been forced down into the axilla. (Britt, B. A., and Gordon, R. A.: Peripheral nerve injuries associated with anaesthesia. Can. Anaesth. Soc. J., *11:* 514, 1964)

significant increase in the tension of the plexus in such a position, nor does the first rib in any way compress the plexus.

COMPRESSION appears to play a predominant role in traumatizing the brachial plexus when the patient is in the lateral position with the lower shoulder and arm directly under the rib cage.[66,67] This injury can be prevented by ensuring that in the lateral position, the entire lower humerus, including the humeral head, is positioned anterior to the rib cage (Fig. 51-3A,B).

NEEDLES MISPLACED by anesthesiologists may

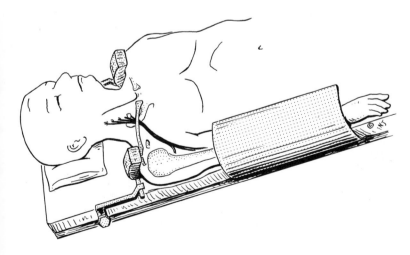

Fig. 51-6. Correct placement of the patient and supports in the Trendelenburg position. The arms are at the sides and protected by a well-padded metal arm guard or draw sheet. Shoulder-rests are placed over the acromioclavicular joint. (Britt, B. A., and Gordon, R. A.: Peripheral nerve injuries associated with anaesthesia. Can. Anaesth. Soc. J., *11:* 514, 1964)

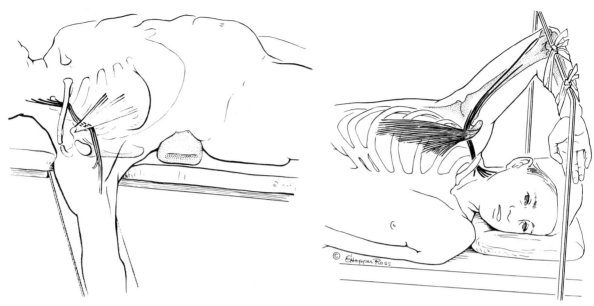

Fig. 51-7. In the obese patient, abduction of the arm and insertion of a gall bladder rest stretches and shifts the tendon of pectoralis minor backward, thus causing posterior deviation of the brachial plexus. (Britt, B. A., and Gordon, R. A.: Peripheral nerve injuries associated with anaesthesia. Can. Anaesth. Soc. J., *11*: 514, 1964)

Fig. 51-8. Suspension of the arm from an "ether screen" with extreme abduction of the arm and pronation of the forearm deviates the brachial plexus posteriorly, behind the tendon of pectoralis minor. (Britt, B. A., and Gordon, R. A.: Peripheral nerve injuries associated with anaesthesia. Can. Anaesth. Soc. J., *11*: 514, 1964)

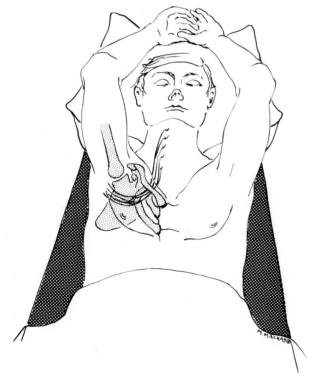

Fig. 51-9. Incorrect "arms-up" position for open heart surgery. Extreme abduction and anterior flexion of the arms radically stretches the brachial plexus behind the clavicle and tendon of pectoralis minor and below the head of the humerus.

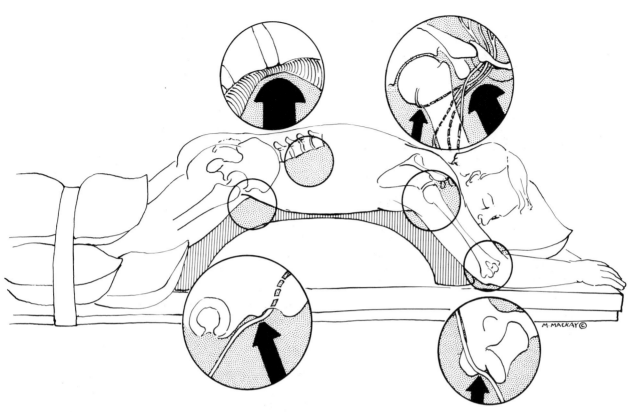

Fig. 51-10. Incorrect flexed prone position. Abduction and anterior flexion of the arms stretches the brachial plexus. Inadequate padding of the elbows compresses the ulnar nerve. A bolster under the anterosuperior and inferior iliac spine compresses the anterolateral femoral nerve of the thigh. Improper padding under the cheek and forehead permits compression of the lower eyelid. Exaggerated upward convexity of the orthopedic frame constricts the inferior vena cava, especially in obese patients.

be responsible for injury to the brachial plexus. For example, palsy resulting from irritation during attempted regional anesthesia of the plexus by the supraclavicular route has occurred in several patients[35] (see Chap. 6).

Clinical Features. Characteristically there is shoulder pain and tenderness in the supraclavicular area 1 to several days postoperatively.

The entire plexus may be involved, so that the arm hangs flaccid and the skin of the whole limb is numb. The upper roots (C5–7) only may be injured, with consequent internal rotation of the arm, extension of the forearm, and pronation of the hand (Erbs palsy). More rarely, the lower roots (C8 and T1) also may be affected, with loss of flexion of the fingers, paralysis of the hand muscles, and perhaps Horner's syndrome (Klumpke's paralysis).

Involvement may be confined chiefly to one of the cords. With posterior cord damage, there is loss of abduction of the arm and paralysis of the extensors of the elbow, wrist, and fingers. With lateral cord involvement, paralysis of the flexors of the elbow and wrist occur. With medial cord injury, the lesion is similar to that affecting the lower roots.

Determining exactly which area of the skin is numb may be very difficult, because there is extensive overlapping in the distribution of the cutaneous nerves. A simple method is to test the

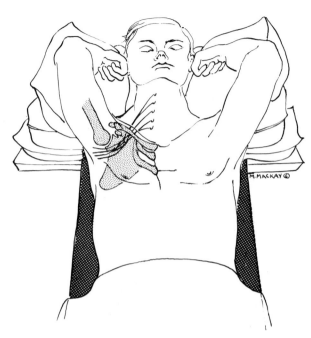

Fig. 51-11. Correct "arms-up" position for open heart surgery. Arms are abducted and anteriorly flexed to less than 90°.

dorsum of the first web space for posterior cord damage, the palmar pad of the distal phalanx of the index finger for lateral cord palsy, and the

palmar pad of the distal phalanx of the little finger for medial cord anesthesia.

Trauma to the Circumflex Nerve

The circumflex nerve was injured in a patient who was placed in the Trendelenburg position: The patient's arm, at right angles to the body, was allowed to press against the vertical portion of a metal "ether screen."[55,68] In such cases, the nerve is compressed between bone and metal as it circles lateral to the neck of the humerus. Gravity in the head-down position undoubtedly accentuates the pressure (Fig. 51-13). This injury causes inability to abduct the arm and loss of sensation over the upper half of the lateral aspect of the arm.

Trauma to the Radial Nerve

The radial nerve may be injured as it traverses the brachium if the arm is permitted to slip off the side of the operating table. If the patient is horizontal, the plexus rubs against the table edge. If the patient is in the Trendelenburg position, the arm tends to be pushed up against the "ether screen" (Fig. 51-14), thus squeezing the nerve between the screen and the spiral groove. Clinically, there is wrist drop, inability to extend the

Fig. 51-12. Correct flexed prone position. Arms are abducted and anteriorly flexed to less than 90°. Elbows, groin, and lower face and forehead are well padded. Upward convexity of orthopedic frame is minimal.

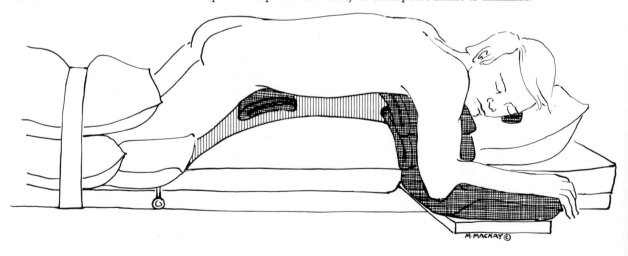

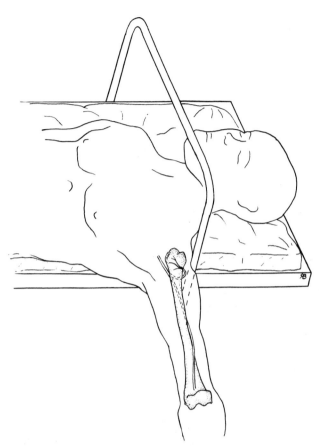

Fig. 51-13. Abduction of the arm against an "ether screen" in the Trendelenburg position pinches the circumflex nerve.

metacarpophalangeal joints, and weakness of abduction of the thumb. The dorsal surface of the lateral three and one-half fingers and adjacent hand show varying degrees of numbness, dryness, increased warmth, and redness.

Trauma to the Median Nerve

The median nerve, lying adjacent to the medial cubital and basilic veins in the antecubital fossa, may be traumatized during intravenous injection of thiopental,[69] either by the needle itself or by extravasation of thiopental (Fig. 51-15). On examination, there is inability to appose thumb and little finger, weakness of abduction of the thumb, and loss of flexion of the distal phalanx of the

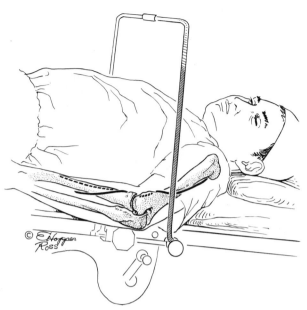

Fig. 51-14. When the arm slips off of the table against the "ether screen" in the Trendelenburg position, the radial nerve is pinched. (Britt, B. A., and Gordon, R. A.: Peripheral nerve injuries associated with anaesthesia. Can. Anaesth. Soc. J., *11*: 514, 1964)

index finger. Eventually, the thenar eminence becomes flattened. Sensation and sweating are diminished on the palmar surface of the lateral three and one-half digits and adjacent palm.

Trauma to the Ulnar Nerve

The ulnar nerve may be compressed against the posterior aspect of the medial epicondyle of the humerus.[70] The compression may be caused by the sharp edge of the table if the elbow is allowed to slip just slightly over its side. This may occur if the draw sheet used to keep the arm tucked to the patient's side is folded under, between mattress and table, rather than between patient and mattress. Injuries to the ulnar nerve have also been reported following operations in which the patient's arm was folded across the abdomen or chest; the stretching of the nerve around the medial epicondyle of the humerus by acute flexion of the elbow and the pressure exerted by the weight of the arm itself apparently are sufficient

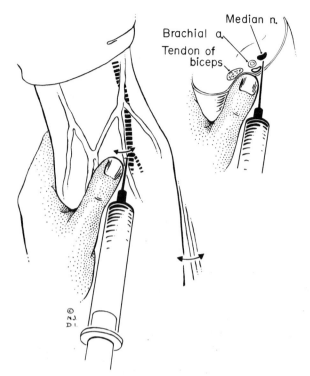

Fig. 51-15. The median nerve is traumatized by a misplaced needle during attempted puncture of a vein in the anticubital fossa. (Britt, B.A., and Gordon, R.A.: Peripheral nerve injuries associated with anaesthesia. Can. Anaesth. Soc. J., *11*: 514, 1964)

to produce ischemia. This occurs, perhaps, because in over 20 per cent of people, the ulnar nerve pursues a more medial course than that described in anatomy texts, passing behind the posteriorly projecting tip of the epicondyle, rather than in the more protected groove (Fig. 51-16).

As a result of ulnar nerve injury, the grip on the ulnar side of the fist is weak, as is flexion of the interphalangeal joints of the medial two digits. Flexion of the metacarpophalangeal and proximal interphalangeal joints, extension of the distal interphalangeal joints, and abduction and adduction of the medial four digits, when extended, are impaired. There is also inability to abduct or appose the little finger. Sensory and autonomic loss occurs over both surfaces of the medial one and one-half fingers and adjacent hand. Eventually the intrinsic hand muscles, except for the thenar eminence, become wasted, and contractures develop, resulting in a characteristic "claw-like" hand.

Trauma to the Sciatic Nerve

In a thin, emaciated patient who is lying on a poorly padded table, the sciatic nerve may be squeezed as it escapes from under cover of the piriformis when the opposite buttock is elevated, as in a hip-pinning procedure.

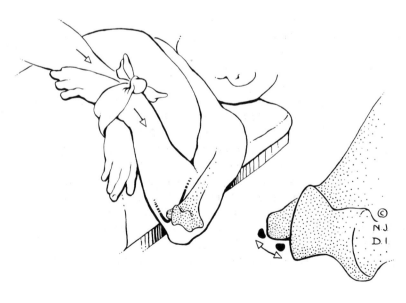

Fig. 51-16. When the elbow slips off of the side of the table, the ulnar nerve is squeezed between the sharp edge of the table and the medial epicondyle of the humerus. The anomalous course of the ulnar nerve behind the tip of the medial epicondyle predisposes it to injury. (Britt, B. A., and Gordon, R. A.: Peripheral nerve injuries associated with anaesthesia. Can. Anaesth. Soc. J., *11*: 514, 1964).

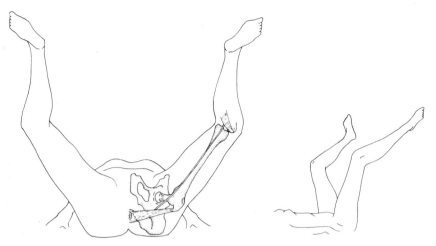

Fig. 51-17. Incorrect lithotomy position. Extreme external rotation of hips stretches the sciatic nerve.

A patient in the lithotomy position can suffer sciatic nerve damage if the thighs and legs are externally rotated (Fig. 51-17) or if the knees are extended (Fig. 51-18).[57] Both of these positions increase the distance between the points of fixation of the sciatic nerve in the sciatic notch proximally and in the neck of the fibula distally. To reduce stretch of the sciatic nerve, external rotation of the thighs and knees must be minimal, and the knees should be flexed (Fig. 51-19). Care should be exercised by assistants to avoid leaning on the inner aspect of the leg or thigh.[71]

Failure to flex the knees in the sitting position may also stretch the sciatic nerve, with unfortunate consequences.[72]

Clinically, all muscles below the knee and,

Fig. 51-18. Incorrect lithotomy position. Extension of the knees stretches the sciatic nerve.

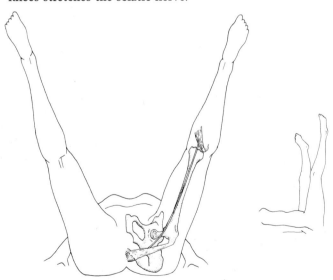

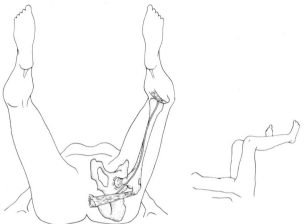

Fig. 51-19. Correct lithotomy position. External rotation of the hips is minimal. Knees are flexed.

perhaps, also the hamstrings are paralyzed, and there is numbness of the lateral half of the calf and almost all of the foot, with the exception of the inner border of the arch.

Trauma to the Common Peroneal Nerve

The common peroneal nerve is the most frequently damaged nerve in the lower limb,[73] although injuries to it are not nearly as common as those to the brachial plexus. It may be compressed against the head of the fibula in the lithotomy position.[74] In such a position, flexion of the hips and knees stretches the nerve.[75] The neck of the fibula rubs against the vertical metal brace, from which the supporting foot strap is slung, or against a curved metal support under the knee, so that the already overstretched nerve is pinched (Fig. 51-20). The common peroneal nerve, like the sciatic nerve, can also be stretched in the lithotomy position when the knees are extended or the thighs and legs externally rotated.[73] Damage to the common peroneal nerve may also follow undue, prolonged pressure against the nerve by a poorly padded table, with the patient in the lateral position.[68] In the supine position, similar injury may be produced by hard knee rolls. Finally, an improperly applied tourniquet may lead to common peroneal nerve neuropathy.[9] The physical findings are foot drop, loss of dorsal extension of the toes, inability to evert the foot,[75]

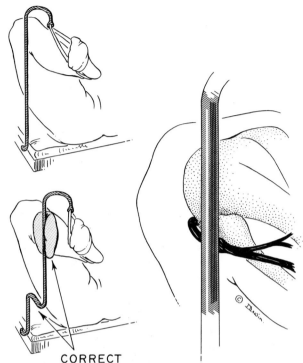

CORRECT

Fig. 51-20. The common peroneal nerve is compressed between the fibula and vertical metal brace in the lithotomy position when padding is inadequate. (Britt, B. A., and Gordon, R. A.: Peripheral nerve injuries associated with anaesthesia. Can. Anaesth. Soc. J., *11:* 514, 1964)

and numbness of the lateral and anterolateral aspects of the calf and medial half of the dorsum of the foot.

Trauma to the Anterior Tibial (Deep Peroneal) Nerve

Foot drop and anesthesia of the dorsum of the foot proximal to the first and second toes may occur if the feet are left plantar flexed for extended periods during anesthesia.[76] This position increases the distance that the anterior tibial nerve must travel over the anterior surface of the ankle joint and thereby stretches that portion of the nerve lying between its origin lateral to the head of the fibula above and the superior and inferior extensor retinacula below (Fig. 51-21). Patients in the sitting position should have a foot support under their feet, while patients in the prone

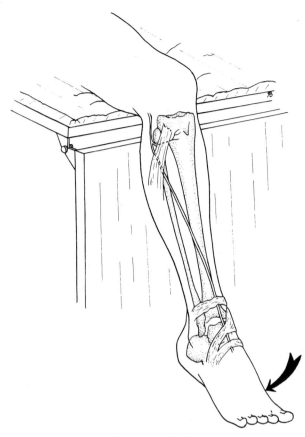

Fig. 51-21. Plantar flexion of the foot in sitting or prone positions stretches the anterior tibial nerves.

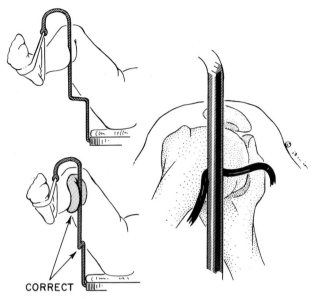

CORRECT

Fig. 51-22. The saphenous nerve is pinched between the medial condyle of the tibia and the vertical metal brace in the lithotomy position when padding is inadequate. (Britt, B. A., and Gordon, R. A.: Peripheral nerve injuries associated with anaesthesia. Can. Anaesth. Soc. J., *11*: 514, 1964)

position should have a roll placed under the anterior aspect of their ankles to maintain the feet in the dorsiflexed (extended) position.

Trauma to the Posterior Tibial Nerve

The posterior tibial nerve may be injured when the legs of a patient in the lithotomy position are placed on Bierhoff stirrups that support the posterior aspect of the knee. If undue weight is borne by the popliteal fossa, through which this nerve passes,[66,76] weakness of plantar flexion of the foot and anesthesia of the toes, sole, and lateral aspect of the foot result.

Trauma to the Saphenous Nerve

Similarly, the saphenous nerve can be compressed against the medial tibial condyle if the foot is suspended lateral to the vertical brace (Fig. 51-22).[9] Paresthesias develop along the medial and anteromedial side of the calf. Thus, in the lithotomy position, there should always be ample padding between the legs and vertical metal braces.

Trauma to the Lateral Femoral Cutaneous Nerve of the Thigh

In the flexed prone position the lateral femoral cutaneous nerve of the thigh has been damaged by hard bolsters. The nerve is pinched between the bolster and the ilium as it passes behind the inguinal ligament medial to the anterosuperior spine (Fig. 51-10).* The injury is characterized by anesthesia of the lower lateral portion of the anterior aspect of the thigh.

Trauma to the Pudendal Nerve

The pudendal nerve may be pressed against the ischial tuberosity owing to traction of both legs

---

*Personal communication, B. M. Marshall.

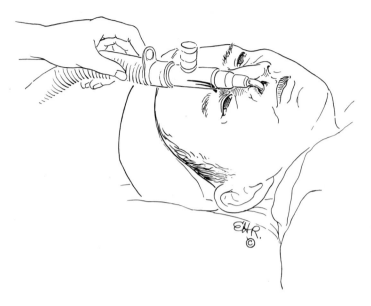

Fig. 51-23. The supraorbital nerve is squeezed between the metal connectors and bony forehead when padding is insufficient. (Britt, B. A., and Gordon R. A.: Peripheral nerve injuries associated with anaesthesia. Can. Anaesth. Soc. J., *11*: 514, 1964)

against a poorly padded orthopaedic post, resulting in loss of perineal sensation and incontinence of feces.[77]

Trauma to the Supraorbital Nerve

The supraorbital nerve can be compressed by the metal connector of a tracheal tube if insufficient padding is used (Fig. 51-23). The injury results in photophobia, numbness of the forehead, and pain in the eye.[78]

Trauma to the Facial Nerve

The facial nerve may be pinched between the anesthesiologist's fingers and the ascending ramus of the mandible if unusual forward pressure is required to maintain a clear airway (Fig. 51-24). The corner of the mouth sags, saliva drools, chewing is difficult, and the affected side of the face is smoother than normal, owing to loss of muscle tone.[79]

Trauma to the Buccal Branch of the Facial Nerve

There have been reports of injury to the buccal branch of the facial nerve caused by pressure from a head strap applied too tightly. This is especially likely to occur if the course of the nerve is superficial to the parotid gland. There is loss of function of the orbicularis oris muscle (Fig. 51-25).[41]

Prognosis

Recovery from a peripheral nerve injury may be complete within a few days, weeks, or months, or permanent weakness, wasting, and sensory and autonomic loss may remain.

TRAUMA TO THE SPINAL CORD

Compression and actual disruption of the cervical spinal cord, with subsequent quadriplegia, has been observed following anesthesia. The etiology appears to be excessive dorsal extension of the head, often in association with spondolytic spurs. Such gross distortion can occur during a tonsillectomy employing a Boyle-Davis mouth gag suspended from a Mayo stand adjusted too high, so that the patient's occiput is lifted (Figs. 51-26 and 51-27). These patients may also have retropharyngeal abscesses or hematomas that probably exacerbate the severity of the neurological deficit.

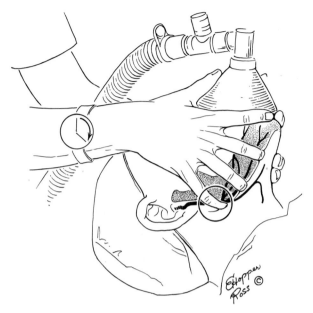

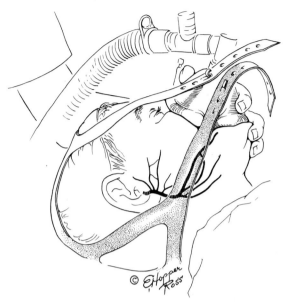

Fig. 51-24. The facial nerve is pinched between the finger and ascending ramus of the jaw when unusual foreward pressure is applied. (Britt, B. A., and Gordon, R. A.: Peripheral nerve injuries associated with anaesthesia. Can. Anaesth. Soc. J., *11*: 514, 1964)

Fig. 51-25. The buccal branch of the facial nerve is injured by a mask strap that is fitted too tightly. (Britt, B. A., and Gordon, R. A.: Peripheral nerve injuries associated with anaesthesia. Can. Anaesth. Soc. J., *11*: 514, 1964)

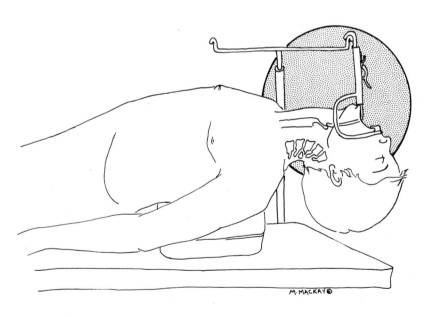

Fig. 51-26. Incorrect tonsillectomy position. Suspension of a Boyle-Davis mouth gag from a Mayo stand placed too high induces extreme dorsal extension of the head. Such distortion, when associated with spondylitic spurs, retropharyngeal abscesses, or hematomas, can disrupt the spinal cord.

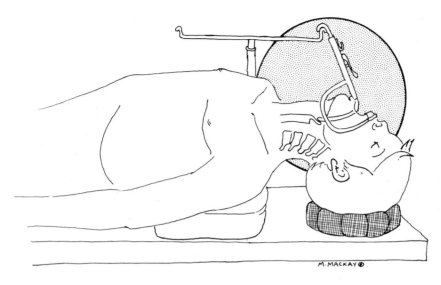

Fig. 51-27. Correct tonsillectomy position. The posterior aspect of the head is supported by a doughnut. The Mayo stand is sufficiently low that excessive dorsal extension of the head does not occur.

TRAUMA TO THE EYE

Damage to the eye has most serious consequences for the patient and unfortunately is not too uncommon. Pressure against the eyeball, especially during controlled or accidental hypotension, causes thrombosis of the central retinal artery, with permanent blindness upon awakening from the anesthetic. There may also be disorganization of the entire globe (see Chap.23).

Such pressure is very likely to occur in the prone position, and it is in this very position that controlled hypotension is often used, for instance, for a spinal fusion or a Harrington rod insertion. Walkup reports two cases of unilateral blindness following pressure on the eye; a horseshoe headrest had been used for pulmonary resection in the prone position.[80] We also know of a similar reaction produced by this type of headrest during a neurosurgical procedure. Eyeball compression has resulted from the pressure produced by a frontal bone flap that was turned down over the face and inadvertently into one or both eyes. Severe damage to the eye may occur if a Bailey head rest slips over the eye during surgery involving a posterior fossa bone flap, with the patient in the sitting position (Fig. 51-28). Blood flow in the central artery is likely to be already reduced,

because of the head-up position. Finally, a face mask that is too large for the patient may squeeze the eye (see Chap.48).

On examination within the first 24 hours, the pupil is dilated and reacts consensually but not directly to light. The cornea is slightly hazy and the lids are often edematous. The retinal arterioles are dilated and the venules engorged. The macula and the retina surrounding the optic disc are edematous. If the damage is severe, there may be a cherry red spot in the fovea. After several days, the optic disc becomes pearly white. The arterioles narrow to white threads. The macula and the peripapillary retina become diffusely pigmented, and faint radical scarring appears in the fovea.[81]

TRAUMA TO THE APPENDAGES

In the lithotomy position with the arms resting at the patient's side, fingers have been severed. As the foot of the table is rolled back up at the end of surgery, the digits become crushed if care is not taken to keep the fingers out of the progressively narrowing gap between the main portion and the foot of the table (Fig. 51-29).[82]

The ear may be necrosed by a head strap or by being folded forcibly between the patient's head

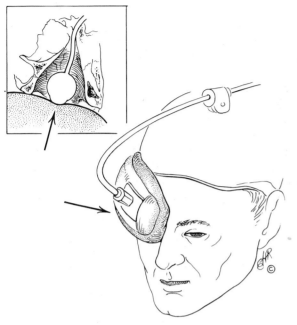

Fig. 51-28. The eyeball is compressed by a misplaced headrest in the sitting or prone positions. (Britt, B. A., and Gordon, R. A.: Peripheral nerve injuries associated with anaesthesia. Can. Anaesth. Soc. J, *11*: 514, 1964)

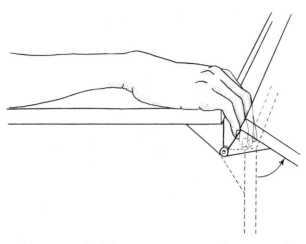

Fig. 51-29 In the lithotomy position with arms to the patient's side, fingers may be pinched as the foot of the table is being rolled up.

and a hard pillow during a long operation (Fig. 51-30).[82] Even in this era of long hair, cabbage ears are not acceptable in either sex.

The nose may be crushed by the elbow of a tired surgeon. This may occur when the head is completely covered by surgical drapes.

The tongue can be grossly lacerated so as to require sutures if the mouth gag is incorrectly positioned during electroshock therapy. The gag should be placed so that its flanges lie between the lips and the teeth (Fig. 51-31).

TRAUMA TO THE TEETH

Since patients value their teeth, metal objects must be positioned within the mouth with much gentleness. During a laryngoscopy or an endotracheal intubation, if a tooth crown, or bridge is chipped, lossened, or knocked out, (even if it is discolored, misshapen, decayed, or loose), the anesthesiologist will promptly discover the high value attached to that tooth. The value is corre-

spondingly greater if the tooth happens to be healthy or belongs to a child whose jaw development is incomplete.[83] When a tooth is knocked out or chipped, the tooth fragments *must* be located and recovered, by x-ray and bronchoscopy, if necessary [84] (see Chap. 34).

TRAUMA TO THE SKIN

Excessive pressure over a localized area of skin with resulting ischemia and even localized gangrene is a much too frequent complication that arises from improper positioning of the patient during anesthesia. Skin damage is worsened if the ischemic area is wet and macerated with water, sterilizing solutions, or electrode jelly.

Insufficiently padded headrests, placed posterior to the ears to maintain the patient in a sitting or semisitting position during a neurosurgical procedure, are liable to cause ischemia of the underlying skin. The hypotension that accompanies this position is a contributory factor. The end result may be permanent baldness of the ischemic areas. Scalp biopsy of such bald spots reveals an "obliterative vasculitis."[82] These unsightly cosmetic defects tend to cause marked dissatisfaction among female patients.

Facial skin may be damaged by an inadequately padded support when the patient is in the prone

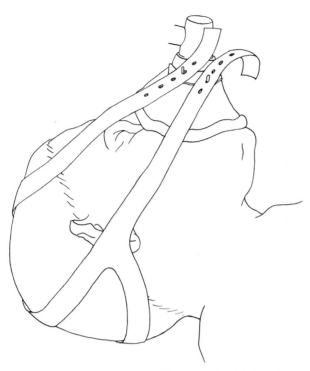

Fig. 51-30. An ear is necrosed by being buckled under a tightly fitted mask strap.

Fig. 51-31. Incorrect positioning of a mouth gag during electroconvulsive therapy permits the tongue to be lacerated by the teeth.

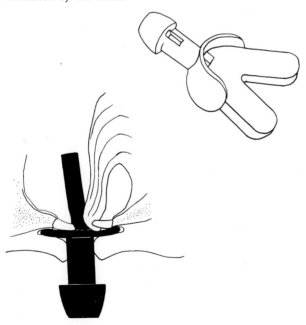

position. The "catcher face mask" type of support is particularly at fault. These supports are used to maintain the eyes free of pressure, but skin ischemia may ensue in the area of the chin if great care is not taken to provide enough extra padding. Unfortunately, the blackened spot is immediately visible to the patient during his first postoperative glance in the mirror.

Care must be taken when positioning a tracheal tube to ensure that it does not exert undue pressure on the angle of the mouth. This problem is seldom brought to the anesthesiologist's attention by the patient, because the only complaint is that of marked tenderness at the corner of the mouth.[66]

The posts of bolster-type orthopaedic frames used to support patients during spinal surgery must be padded well to prevent pressure necrosis of skin in the groin. The knees must also be padded amply in this position.[72]

Patients whose buttocks have been allowed to rest in a pool of alcoholic sterilizing solution throughout a long operation may subsequently develop a pressure sore in this area. Pressure sores may develop on the apposing surfaces of the legs, particularly over the medial tibial condyles and medial malleoli when the patient is lying in the lateral nephrectomy position, without pillows between the legs (Fig. 51-3A,B). The heels of very tall people require padding, as they are likely to sag over the end of the mattress onto the hard edge of the lower end of the table.[82]

TRAUMA TO THE TENDONS AND LIGAMENTS

Stresses, strains, and stretches of the back are most likely to occur when the position is extreme, when muscle relaxation is profound, and when the duration of the operation is long.[9,47,64] This combination of factors is common. In fact, postoperative low backache occurs in 12 to 37 per cent of all patients anesthetized in the supine, lithotomy, prone, and lateral nephrectomy positions.[82,85] Anesthesia relaxes paraspinal muscles. In the supine position, therefore, there is flattening of the convexity of the lumbar spine, and thus tension is applied to the interlumbar and lumbosacral ligaments. Moreover, the legs lie perfectly flat upon the table (which does not occur in the conscious patient), thus stretching the ligaments and muscles of the lower spine.[47] In the lithotomy position, rotation of the pelvis flattens the convexity of the lumbar spine to an even greater degree and again puts great tension on these ligaments.[82] Postoperatively, minor stretch is interpreted as pain, soreness, or stiffness localized to the lumbosacral area or radiating down the sciatic nerve.[66] Such discomfort may last from a few days to several months. To avoid such injury, the knees should be flexed slightly in the supine position; while in the lithotomy position, small pillows should be placed at the side of and slightly under the hips, and legs should be placed in the stirrups or removed from them at the *same* time.[82]

Whiplash injury in the cervical area is another common anesthetic complication. It can often be avoided by taking care during turning of the patient, to ensure that the head is turned at the same speed and in the same direction as the torso, so that undue tensions on the cervical ligaments are avoided. Prevention of markedly abnormal head position (torsion, lateral flexion, and extension) also lowers the incidence of whiplash injury.

TRAUMA TO THE MUSCLES

Edema, distortion, and disintegration of the myofibrils of the deltoid developed in a patient after a 7-hour heart operation in the lateral position. In this case, there were no rolls behind the dependent axilla to relieve pressure on the lower shoulder (Fig. 51-3A,B).[82]

EFFECTS ON THE RESPIRATORY SYSTEM

Ventilation

The single most important effect of posture upon respiration is mechanical interference with chest movements. The result is limitation of lung expansion, leading to progressive closure of the alveoli and abnormal distribution of inspired air.[47,86] Pulmonary compliance may also be low-ered because of increased stasis of blood in the lungs.[87] The longer the time an adverse surgical posture is maintained, the greater will be the deleterious effects of respiratory muscle fatigue and hypoventilation. Frank atelectasis may follow in the postoperative period.[82] It must not be forgotten that obesity, which constitutes one of the gravest hazards in anesthesia today, grossly exaggerates respiratory insufficiency induced by abnormal postures.[82,86,88] The lateral nephrectomy, flexed prone (jackknife), and Trendelenburg[65] positions cause the most marked falls in ventilation in the spontaneously breathing, anesthetized patient, while the reverse Trendelenburg and gall bladder positions lead to more modest impairments of ventilation.[47,82,89] Any position that compresses the abdomen, preventing descent of the diaphragm, is to be condemned. Thus during positioning of the patient in the prone position with rolls, bolsters, or padded frames, the anesthesiologist should palpate the abdomen to ensure its freedom from pressure.

Airway Obstruction

Extreme torsion, dorsal extension, or lateral or anterior flexion of the neck may obstruct a tracheal tube: for example, during an air encephalogram in a child in whom a small, highly flexible tube has been inserted. The use of armored (anode) tubes and careful taping of the tube into a secure position resistant to surgical manipulation greatly reduces the incidence of this sort of obstruction.

Change of position of a tracheal tube after the beginning of operation should be carried out with great care and not in the dark under a drape, as illustrated by a recent case:[90]

Case 51-1. A surgeon requested that the anesthesiologist change the position of a tube during repair of a deviated nasal septum. Almost immediately, difficulty was encountered in ventilating the patient, and the tube was found to be kinked. It was manipulated blindly from beneath the drapes. The difficulty lessened but did not disappear. At the end of the operation a cardiac arrest occurred. The patient survived, but with a major neurological disability.

EFFECTS ON THE CIRCULATORY SYSTEM

Untoward effects of surgical posture on the circulatory system can occur suddenly and, unlike neuropathies, are obvious during rather than after anesthesia. Anesthesia causes pooling of blood in the dependent portion of the peripheral vasculature, owing to dilatation of blood vessels,[91] to a lesser extent to direct depression of the myocardium, and to inhibition of the reflex compensatory mechanisms. Gravity and external obstruction of blood vessels further exacerbate pooling and sludging of blood. The degree to which a patient tolerates these effects depends upon his cardiovascular reserve. When the latter is reduced by heart disease, decreased blood volume, or peripheral vascular decompensation, the patient will be at a disadvantage in certain surgical postures, especially if he is moved into these positions rapidly rather than slowly.[47,82]

Supine and Lithotomy Positions

The supine position usually has fewer deleterious effects on the circulation than does any other position. It can be hazardous, however, when a large abdominal mass, such as a tumor, gravid uterus, or the contents of a large hernia sac recently returned to the abdomen, squeezes the inferior vena cava sufficiently to impede blood flow. Venous return to the heart and arterial blood pressure are reduced.[47,92–95] An abdominal mass may also obstruct the inferior vena cava when the patient is in the lithotomy position,[82] especially after hypotension has been induced by an epidural anesthetic (Fig. 51-32). During labor, such hypotension can be reversed by placing a roll under the right hip, which tilts the uterus to the left and away from the inferior vena cava. (The supine hypotensive syndrome is discussed further in Chap. 41.)

Trendelenburg Position

By decreasing arterial flow to the legs and increasing venous return from them, the Trendelenburg position engorges the blood vessels of the thorax and mediastinum, raises cerebrospinal fluid pressure in the cranial vault, and thereby compresses brain tissue.[65] Pressure of the viscera on the diaphragm lowers stroke volume and cardiac output and increases the work of breathing.[47,82] Some of these harmful results of the Trendelenburg position can be attenuated by intermittent positive pressure ventilation, with a negative pressure phase during expiration.

Flexed Prone Position

The flexed prone (jacknife) position causes pooling of blood in the dependent cephalad half of the body and in the legs. The abdominal contents are compressed dorsally, thus obstructing the inferior vena cava (Fig. 51-10).[82] In obese patients, a large panniculus of abdominal fat further obstructs the inferior vena cava.[47] There is therefore not only hypotension but also increased venous bleeding at the wound site in the lumbar area of the back. This occurs because blood is forced to return from the legs to the heart by way of collateral veins that course cephalad through the paravertebral area. This complication can be mitigated by refraining from too marked dorsal flexion of the torso (Fig. 51-12).[96] Quadriceps bolsters and long rolls placed vertically under the lateral part of each side of the body cause less flexion than does the MacKay frame. If bolsters are used, however, it must not be forgotten that they can exert excessive pressure in the groin and obstruct the femoral artery. It is of interest that the prone position with roll-supports is the only one in which the cardiac index rises rather than falls during anesthesia.[91]

Lateral Nephrectomy Positions

The right and, less often, the left lateral nephrectomy position causes similar pooling of the blood, but this time in the lower half of the body.[82,91,97] Again, there is marked compression of the inferior vena cava. Unwisely exaggerating this position with a high kidney rest can precipitate cardiovascular collapse (Fig. 51-3A,B). The left lateral nephrectomy position puts pressure on the lower chest, which may shift the position of the heart sufficiently to interfere with cardiac action.[47,82]

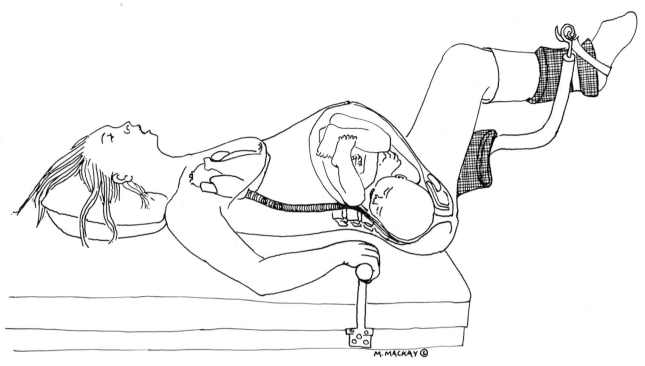

Fig. 51-32. An abdominal mass compresses the inferior vena cava in the supine or lithotomy positions. Compression is relieved by inserting a roll under the right hip.

Sitting and Reverse Trendelenburg Positions

The sitting position and the reverse Trendelenburg position lower blood pressure and cerebral blood flow through the effect of gravity. Consequently, oxygenation of the brain tissues may be endangered if a hyperventilation technique is employed or if the intracranial vasculature is already compromised by preexisting vascular disease.[98] Because of gravity, these positions are also associated with marked stasis of blood in the lower part of the body,[47,82,98,99] possibly with the formation of thrombi. The latter, of course, are highly likely to embolize to the lungs postoperatively. Wrapping the legs with elastic bandages during the operation may help to prevent body hypotension, as well as pulmonary emboli. Diathermy pads should be placed behind the buttock rather than bandaging them to the leg, where they will further exacerbate venous stasis of the leg.[100]

In the sitting position, sagging of the cerebellar hemispheres stretches and tears superior and inferior cerebellar veins that communicate with adjacent venous sinuses. Following such a tear, there is continuous bleeding from the superior surface of the cerebellum after excision of a posterior fossa mass. In this position, venous pressure may fall below atmospheric pressure. Thus, a tear in the vein can allow a fatal amount of air to be sucked in through the vessel to the heart. This complication is most likely to occur during expiration if the patient is being ventilated with a negative expiratory phase or during inspiration if the patient is breathing spontaneously. Sequelae are minimized through prompt diagnosis and treatment. Diagnosis is aided by the use of an esophageal stethoscope or an ultrasonic (Doppler) device placed on the chest over the precordial area. Treatment consists of compression of the open veins to prevent further air entry, movement of the patient into the recumbent lateral position, thereby washing the air out of the heart and through the lungs, ventilation with 100-per-cent oxygen, and support of the blood pressure.[98,101-104] (Air embolism is discussed in greater depth in Chap. 18.)

Abnormal Head Positions

Extreme extension or lateral flexion of the head sufficient to induce tension of the neck muscles—as in the supine position during thyroidectomy or in the lateral position with insufficient support under the head—may permit obstruction of venous return from the head, with resultant elevation of the intracerebral blood pressure and plethora and edema of the superficial blood vessels.[66] Sufficient extension of the head may occur in an aged patient with a prominent dorsal kyphosis lying on a gall bladder rest, so that compression of the vertebral artery develops with resultant cerebral ischemia.

OVERVIEW

The hazards and pitfalls of positioning an anesthetized patient are many for the unwary anesthesiologist. An understanding of the anatomy of the peripheral nervous system and of the physiology of the respiratory and cardiovascular systems is essential for the avoidance of potentially injury-producing positions. In addition, meticulous care must be taken during movement of a patient into the desired surgical position, to ensure that the change is carried out in a slow and gentle manner; to ascertain that all points of pressure caused by surgical and anesthetic apparatus are padded thoroughly, especially when situated over bony prominences; and, finally, to ensure that the patient is not contorted into any positions that induce strain on nerves, tendons, or ligaments that the patient would not tolerate if awake. Finally, it is the anesthesiologist's duty always to protect the patient from all of these hazards before permitting the surgeon to proceed.

REFERENCES

1. Dhuner, K. G.: Nerve injuries following operations: a survey of cases occurring during a six-year period. Anesthesiology, *11*:289, 1950.
2. Kiloh, L. G.: Brachial plexus lesions after cholecystectomy. Lancet, *258*:103, 1950.
3. Lincoln, J. R., and Sawyer, H. P., Jr.: Complications related to body positions in surgical procedures. Anesthesiology, *22*:800, 1961.
4. Magendie, J., Bergouignan, M., Royyere, R., et al.: Troubles sensitive-moteurs due plexus brachial dus a certains positions sur la table d'operation. Bordeaux Chir. p. 133. October, 1949.
5. Shaw, W. M.: Prevention of brachial plexus paralysis. Anesthesiology, *14*:206, 1953.
6. Westin, B.: Prevention of upper limb nerve injuries in Trendelenburg position. Acta Chir. Scand., *108*:61, 1954.
7. Budinger, K.: Ueber lahmungen nach chloroformnarkosen. Arch. Klin. Chir., *47*:121, 1894.
8. Garriques, H.: Anesthesia paralysis. Am. J. Med. Sci., *113*:81, 1897.
9. Slocum, H. C., O'Neal, K. C., and Allen, C. R.: Neurovascular complications from malposition on the operating table. Surg. Gynecol. Obstet., *86*:729, 1948.
10. Horsley, V.: On injuries to peripheral nerves. Practitioner, *113*:131, 1898.
11. Krumm, F.: Editorial on narcosis paralysis. Ann. Surg., *25*:203, 1897.
12. Denny-Brown, D., and Brenner, C.: Lesion in peripheral nerve resulting from compression by spring clip. Arch. Neurol. Psychiat., *52*:1, 1944.
13. Denny-Brown, D., and Doherty, M.: Effects of transient stretching of peripheral nerves. Arch. Neurol. Psychiat., *54*:116, 1945.
14. Sunderland, S.: Blood supply of the nerves of the upper limb in man. Arch. Neurol. Psychiat., *53*:91, 1945.
15. Clausen, E. G.: Postoperative ("anesthetic") paralysis of the brachial plexus. A review of the literature and report of nine cases. Surgery, *12*:933, 1942.
16. Wright, S.: The neurovascular syndrome produced by hyperabduction of the arms. Am. Heart J., *29*:1, 1945.
17. Staal, A.: The entrapment neuropathies. *In* Vinken, P. J., and Bruyn, G. W.(eds): Handbook of Clinical Neurology: Diseases of the Nerves. part 1, pp. 285–325. vol. 7. New York, Elsevier Publishing Co., 1971.
18. Pommerenke, W. T., and Risteen, W. A. scalenus anticus syndrome as a complication after gynecologic operations. Am. J. Obstet. Gynecol., *47*:395, 1944.
19. Turney, H. G.: Post anaesthetic paralysis. Clin. J., *14*:185, 1899.
20. Jones, H. D.: Ulnar nerve damage following general anaesthetic. A case possibly related to diabetes mellitus. Anaesthesia, *22*:471, 1967.
21. Patten, B. M.: Neuropathy induced by hemorrhage. Arch. Neurol., *21*:381, 1969.
22. Hartwell, S. W., and Kurtay, M.: Carpal tunnel compression caused by hematoma associated with anticoagulant therapy. Report of a case. Clev. Clin. Q., *33*:127, 1966.
23. Macon, W. L., and Futrell, J. W.: Median-nerve neuropathy after percutaneous puncture of the brachial artery in patients receiving anticoagulants. N. Engl. J. Med., *288*:1396, 1973.
24. Parkes, J. D., and Kidner, P. H.: Peripheral nerve and root lesions developing as a result of haematoma formation during anticoagulant treatment. Postgrad. Med. J., *46*:146, 1970.
25. Bartholomew, L. G., and Scholz, D. A.: Reversible post operative neurological symptoms: a report of five cases secondary to water intoxication and water depletion. J.A.M.A., *162*:22, 1956.

26. Delorme, E. J.: Hypothermia. Anaesthesia, *11*:221, 1956.
27. Stephens, J. W.: Neurological sequelae of congenital heart surgery. Arch. Neurol., 7:459, 1962.
28. Stephens, J., and Appleby, S.: Polyneuropathy following induced hypothermia. Trans. Am. Neurol. Assoc., *80*:102, 1955.
29. Swan, H., Virtue, R. W., Blout, S. G., et al.: Hypothermia in surgery. Ann. Surg., *142*:382, 1955.
30. Eckhoff, N. L.: Tourniquet paralysis. Lancet, *3*:343, 1931.
31. Roth, P. B.: Tourniquet paralysis. Lancet, *3*:554, 1931.
32. Kounis, N. G., Macauley, M. B., and Ghorbal, M. S.: Iliacus hematoma syndrome. Can. Med. Assoc. J., *112*:872, 1975.
33. Butterfield, W. C., Neviaser, R. J., and Roberts, M. P.: Femoral neuropathy and anticoagulants. Ann. Surg., *176*:58, 1972.
34. Johnson, P. S., and Greifenstein, F. E.: Brachial plexus block anesthesia. J. Mich. State Med. Soc., 53:1329, 1955.
35. Wooley, E. J., and Vandam, L. D.: Neurological sequellae of brachial plexus nerve block. Ann. Surg., *194*:53, 1959.
36. Seldinger, S. I.: Catheter replacement of the needle in percutaneous arteriography. Acta Radiologica, *39*:368, 1953.
37. Carroll, S. E., and Wilkins, W. W.: Two cases of brachial plexus injury following percutaneous arteriograms. Can. Med. Assoc. J., *102*:861, 1970.
38. Dudrick, S., Masland, W., and Mishkin, M.: Brachial plexus injury following axillary artery puncture. Radiology, *88*:271, 1967.
39. Staal, A., Van Voorthuisen, A. E., and Van Dijk, L. M.: Neurological complications following arterial catheterization by the axillary approach. Br. J. Radiol., *39*:115, 1966.
40. Mazzia, V. D. B.: Radial nerve palsy from intramuscular injection. N.Y. State J. Med., *62*:1674, 1962.
41. Conway, C.: Neurological and ophthalmic complications of anaesthesia. *In* Churchill-Davidson, H. C. (ed.): A Practice of Anaesthesia. ed. 3, p. 1021. London, Lloyd-Luke, 1978.
42. Cappe, B. E.: Prevention of postspinal headache with a 22-gauge pencil-point needle and adequate hydration. Anesth. Analg., *39*:462, 1960.
43. Enhorning, G., and Westin, B.: Aspects on the technique in giving spinal analgesia. Acta Chir. Scand., *108*:69, 1954.
44. Gilbert, R. G. B., and Brindle, G. F.: Spinal surgery and anesthesia. Int. Anesthesiol. Clin., *4*:863, 1966.
45. Atkinson, R. S., Rushman, G. B., and Lee, J. A.: A Synopsis of Anaesthesia. ed. 8. p. 453. Bristol, John Wright & Sons, 1977.
46. Letter to the Editor. Sixth nerve palsy after spinal analgesia. Br. Med. J., *4*:842, 1952.
47. Little, D. M., Jr.: Posture and anaesthesia. Can. Anaesth. Soc. J., 7:2, 1960.
48. Sadove, M. S., Levin, M. J., and Rant-Sejdinaj, I.: Neurological complications of spinal anaesthesia. Can. Anaesth. Soc. J., 8:405, 1961.
49. Hayman, I. R., and Wood, P. M.: Abducens nerve paralysis following spinal anesthesia. Ann. Surg., *115*:864, 1942.
50. Ruston, F. G., and Politi, V. L.: Femoral nerve injury from abdominal retractors. Can. Anaesth. Soc. J., 5:428, 1958.
51. Carden, S.: Hazards in the use of the closed circuit technique for trilene anaesthesia. Br. Med. J., *1*:319, 1944.
52. Humphrey, J. H., and McClelland, M.: Cranial nerve palsies with Herpes following general anaesthesia. Br. Med. J., *1*:315, 1944.
53. DeForest, H. P.: Krumm on narcosis paralysis. Ann. Surg., *25*:203, 1897.
54. Ewing, M. R.: Postoperative paralysis in the upper extremity. Report of five cases. Lancet, *1*:99, 1950.
55. Halstead, A. E.: Anesthesia paralysis. Surg. Gynecol. Obstet., 6:201, 1908.
56. Jackson, L., and Keats, A. S.: Mechanism of brachial plexus palsy following anesthesia. Anesthesiology, *26*:190, 1965.
57. Nicholson, M. J., and Eversole, U. H.: Nerve injuries incident to anesthesia and operation. Anesth. Analg., *36*:19, 1957.
58. Petrick, E. C.: Paralysis of the brachial plexus following elective surgical procedures. Anesth. Analg., *34*:119, 1955.
59. Raffan, A. W.: Post-operative paralysis of the brachial plexus. Br. Med. J., *3*:149, 1950.
60. Wood-Smith, F. F.: Post-operative brachial plexus paralysis. Br. Med. J., *2*:1115, 1952.
61. Britt, B. A., and Gordon, R. A.: Peripheral nerve injuries associated with anaesthesia. Can. Anaesth. Soc. J., *11*:514, 1964.
62. Gerdy, P.: *Quoted In* Clausen, E. G.: Postoperative ("anesthetic") paralysis of the brachial plexus. A review of the literature and report of nine cases. Surgery, *12*:933, 1942.
63. Stevens, J.: Brachial plexus paralysis. *In* Codman, E. A. (ed.): The Shoulder. Boston, 1934.
64. Brown, C.: *Quoted In* Garriques, H.: Anesthesia paralysis. Am. J. Med. Soc, *113*:81, 1897.
65. Inglis, J. M., and Brook, B. N.: Trendelenburg tilt: obsolete position. Br. Med. J., *2*:343, 1956.
66. Costley, D. O.: Peripheral nerve injury. Int. Anesthesiol. Clin., *10*:189, 1972.
67. Wisconsin Anesthesia Study Commission of the Wisconsin Society of Anesthesiologists. Crush syndrome. Wis. Med. J., *57*:185, 1958.
68. Ellul, J. M., and Notermans, S. L. H.: Paralysis of the circumflex nerve following general anesthesia for laparoscopy. Anesthesiology, *41*:520, 1974.
69. Pask, E. A., and Robson, J. G.: Injury to the median nerve. Anaesthesia, 9:94, 1954.
70. Wood, D. A.: Injuries to nerves during anesthesia. Calif. Western Med., *53*:267, 1940.
71. Burkhart, F. L., and Daly, J. W.: Sciatic and peroneal nerve injury: a complication of vaginal operations. Obstet. Gynecol., *28*:99, 1966.
72. Gilbert, R. G. B., and Brindle, G. F.: Posture. Int. Anesthesiol. Clin., *4*:815, 1966.
73. Sunderland, S.: Relative susceptibility to injury of medial and lateral popliteal divisions of sciatic nerve. Br. J. Surg., *41*:300, 1953.
74. Solnitzky, O.: Common peroneal nerve paralysis. Bull. Georgetown Univ. Med. Ctr., *1*:222, 1948.
75. Garland, H., and Moorhouse, D.: Compressive lesions of the external popliteal (common peroneal) nerve. Br. Med. J., *4*:1373, 1952.
76. Schwartz, A. I., and Rosenblum, E.: Management of the anaesthetized patient. Anesthesiology, 8:395, 1945.

77. Lembcke, W.: Rare nerve paralysis due to pressure while lying on an extension table: two cases. Chirurgie, *17*:264, 1947.
78. Barron, D. W.: Supraorbital neuropraxia. Anaesthesia, *10*:374, 1955.
79. Fuller, J. E., and Thomas, D. V.: Facial nerve paralysis after general anesthesia. J.A.M.A., *162*:645, 1956.
80. Walkup, H. E., Murphy, J. D., and Oteen, N. C.: Retinal ischemia with unilateral blindness, a complication occurring during pulmonary resection in the prone position. J. Thorac. Surg., *23*:174, 1952.
81. Hollenhorst, R. W., Svien, H. J., and Benoit, C. F.: Unilateral blindness occurring during anesthesia for neurosurgical operations. Arch. Ophthalmol., *52*:819, 1954.
82. Courington, F. W., and Little, D. M.: The role of posture in anesthesia. Clin. Anesth., *3*:24, 1968.
83. Canadian Medical Protective Association, 66th Annual Report, 1967.
84. Wasmuth, C. E.: Anesthesia and the Law. p. 22. Springfield, Charles C Thomas, 1961.
85. Brown, E. M., and Elman, D. S.: Postoperative backache. Anesth. Analg, *40*:683, 1961.
86. Gold, M. I., and Helrich, M.: Pulmonary compliance during anesthesia. Anesthesiology, *27*:281, 1965.
87. Kaneko, K., Milic-Emili, J., Dolovich, M. B., et al.: Regional distribution of ventilation and perfusion as a function of body position. J. Appl. Physiol., *21*:767, 1966.
88. Catenacci, A. J., Anderson, J. D., and Boersma, D.: Anesthetic hazards of obesity. J.A.M.A., *175*:657, 1961.
89. Wood-Smith, F. F., Horne, G. M., and Nunn, J. F.: Effect of position on ventilation of patients anaesthetized with halothane. Anaesthesia, *16*:340, 1961.
90. Canadian Medical Protective Association, 73rd Annual Report, 1974.
91. Eggers, G. W. N., Jr., DeGroot, W. J., Tanner, C. R., et al.: Hemodynamic changes associated with various surgical positions. J.A.M.A., *185*:1, 1963.
92. Eckstein, K. L., and Marx, G. F.: Aortocaval compression and uterine displacement. Anesthesiology, *40*:92, 1974.
93. Grennell, H. J., and Vanderwater, S. L.: The supine hypotensive syndrome during conduction anaesthesia for the near term gravid patient: case reports. Can. Anaesth. Soc. J., *8*:417, 1961.
94. Scott, D. B.: Inferior vena caval pressure. Changes occurring during anaesthesia. Anaesthesia, *18*:135, 1963.
95. ———: Inferior vena caval occlusion in late pregnancy and its importance in anaesthesia. Br. J. Anaesth., *40*:120, 1968.
96. Relton, J.E.S., and Conn, A.W.: Anaesthesia for the surgical correction of scoliosis by the Harrington method in children. Can. Anaesth. Soc. J., *10*:603, 1963.
97. Malatinsky, J., and Kadlic, T.: Inferior vena caval occlusion in the left lateral position. A case report. Br. J. Anaesth., *46*:165, 1974.
98. Tindall, G. T., Craddock, A., and Greenfield, J. C.: Effects of the sitting position on blood flow in the internal carotid artery of man during general anesthesia. J. Neurosurg., *26*:383, 1967.
99. Ward, R. J., Danziger, F. A., Bonica, J. J., et. al.: Cardiovascular effects of change of posture. Aerosp. Med., *37*:257, 1966.
100. Hodgson, D. C.: Venous stasis during surgery. Anaesthesia, *19*:96, 1964.
101. Hunter, A. R.: Air embolism in the sitting position. Anaesthesia, *4*:467, 1962.
102. Marshall, B. M.: Air embolus in neurosurgical anaesthesia, its diagnosis and treatment. Can. Anaesth. Soc. J., *12*:255, 1965.
103. Michenfelder, J. D., Miller, R. H., and Gronert, G. A.: Evaluation of an ultrasonic device (Doppler) for the diagnosis of venous air embolism. Anesthesiology, *36*:164, 1972.
104. Gildenberg, P. L., O'Brien, R. P., Britt, W. J., et al.: The efficacy of Doppler monitoring for detection of venous air embolism. J. Neurosurg., *54*:75, 1981.

FURTHER READING

Martin, J. T.: Positioning in Anesthesia and Surgery. Philadelphia, W. B. Saunders Co., 1978.
Omer, G. E., Jr., and Spinner, M.: Management of Peripheral Nerve Problems. Philadelphia, W. B. Saunders Co., 1980.
Sunderland, S.: Nerves and Nerve Injuries. ed 2. London, Longman Group Ltd, 1978.

52 Fires and Explosions

Gordon R. Neufeld, M.D.

Of the complications encountered in the practice of anesthesia, certainly a fire or an explosion is the most devastating. The development of nonflammable anesthetic gases and vapors has reduced the occurrence of this complication. However, a review of the literature reveals some interesting facts.[1-3]

A survey published in 1941 reported the causes of 230 operating room fires and explosions.[1] In 210 of these, the fuel was a flammable anesthetic, and in 70 per cent, the source of ignition was something other than a static spark. The incidence reported by the Ministry of Health in Britain was approximately 4.2 per 100,000 administrations in the 7-year period ending in 1956.[3]

Over the past 3 decades, considerable effort and expense have been directed toward the development of systems for the control of fires and explosions in operating rooms. Most of this effort, including the development of nonflammable anesthetics, has focused on the concept that flammable anesthetics served as fuel in the majority (80%) of cases. This, indeed, was true in the period before 1955. A current review of the English medical literature reveals, however, that this is no longer true. In the 15-year period from 1959 to 1974, a total of 36 fires or explosions in operating room settings were reported. Less than one-third (31%) of these were related to the use of a flammable anesthetic, although flammable agents were still the single most common source of fuel. The second most common type of fuel

(28%) included plastic, rubber, paper, fabric components of apparatus, and disposable products. The third most common (22%) was enteric gas, and this was most commonly ignited by electrosurgical apparatus. Volatile "prep" solutions were the fourth most common type of fuel (8%). The remaining materials included cleaning compounds, electrical apparatus and components, and oxygen line contaminants like oil and dust.

During this same period there were 11 fires or explosions from the use of flammable anesthetics. Current estimates show the usage of flammable anesthetics to be 5 per cent or less of total anesthetic administrations,[4] down from approximately 31 per cent in 1956.[3] It is difficult to evaluate from published data whether operating room fires and explosions have been reduced by the decline in use of the formerly common fuel sources or by other preventive measures.

An examination of the sources of ignition is also revealing. Electrocautery devices were the source of ignition in 53 per cent of operating room fires and explosions. Rapid compression of high-pressure gases accounted for 17 per cent, and electrical devices, another 17 per cent. The remaining 13 per cent were caused by static sparks (6%), open flames (6%), and unknown sources (1%).

Thus, in comparison to the 1950s, the number of fires and explosions is much reduced, based on the number of total anesthetics. Currently, the most common fuels are materials other than anesthetics, and they are most commonly ignited by electrosurgical sparks. This chapter reviews the fundamental physical processes involved in fires and explosions and presents methods for their control.

OXIDATION, COMBUSTION, AND FLAMES

In the strict chemical sense, oxidation is the loss of electrons from one molecular species to another. The species that gains electrons is "reduced." Oxidation processes are generally associated with the release of energy owing to the difference in the bond energies between the compounds that are oxidized and the new compounds that are formed. For example, there are two hydroxyl (O-H) bonds in water, each with a bond energy of 109 kilocalories. The bond energies of the water molecule, thus, are 218 kcal. per mol. of water. The bond energies between the two hydrogen atoms of the hydrogen molecule are 103 kcal. per mol. of hydrogen. Similarly, the O-O bond represents 117 kcal. per mol. From these bond energies, one can calculate the energy released from the oxidation of hydrogen to form water:

$$2\ H_2 + O_2\ \rightarrow 2\ H_2O$$
$$(2 \times 103) + 117 \rightarrow (2 \times 218)$$
$$\downarrow$$
$$\frac{\text{energy}}{\text{excess}} = 113\ \text{kcal.}$$
$$= 57\ \text{kcal./mol. } H_2O \text{ formed}$$

Oxidation processes may occur at ambient room temperatures, but generally the reaction rates are extremely slow, since they depend upon the random occurrence of collisions between the reactants. Not all collisions of reactants will cause the oxidation to occur. Only collisions that involve sufficient energy of impact to disrupt the existing molecular bonds and allow the formation of the product molecule will result in oxidation and the release of energy. The probability of these collisions occurring between a flammable material and oxygen can be enhanced by the following:

Occurrence of the Reactants (Fuel and Oxygen) in a Gas Phase. The gas phase allows complete mixing of the fuel, and molecular oxygen enhances the probability of collisions.

The Lack of Nonreactive Components in the Mixture, such as Nitrogen. Nonreactive components serve to dilute the mixture and reduce the probability of collisions between reactants.

Increasing the velocity of the molecules within the mixture raises the probability of collisions with sufficient energy to react. The velocities developed are directly proportional to the temperature.

As an oxidation process proceeds, the heat of reaction must be dissipated, or the temperature of the mixture rises. If the heat is rapidly conducted or convected away, the reaction temperature may drop to a point at which the oxidation stops (e.g., blowing out a match). If the heat is dissipated at a rate equal to the rate of combustion, then combustion proceeds at a steady level (e.g., a gas burner). If, on the other hand, conditions are such that heat is not dissipated as quickly as it is given off, then the temperature of the reaction rises. This increases the probability of collision among the reactants, generating more heat and higher temperatures. The result is an accelerating flame or an explosion.

FUEL-OXYGEN MIXTURES

When the proportions of a fuel-oxygen mixture are such that all fuel is oxidized by all of the oxygen present, leaving only oxidized products, the mixture is said to be stoichiometric. For example, a mixture of 2 mol. of hydrogen and 1 mol. of oxygen is stoichiometric, because oxidation yields 1 mol. of water vapor and no excess of either hydrogen or oxygen. Mixtures containing an excess of oxygen (e.g., oxygen remains in the mixture following oxidation of the fuel) are "lean." Mixtures with an excess of fuel (e.g., fuel plus combustion products remain after oxidation is complete) are "rich."

As a fuel-oxygen mixture becomes increasingly lean, a proportion is reached at which the heat of combustion of the mixture is dissipated faster than it can be generated by the available fuel, and the mixture becomes nonflammable. This proportion is the lower limit of flammability. Similarly, as a mixture is made richer, the reaction products formed dilute the available oxygen, and the heat

**Table 52-1. Ranges of Flammability and Stoichiometric Proportions
of Anesthetic Gases and Vapors**

| | FLAMMABILITY LIMITS | | | STOICHIOMETRIC CONCENTRATION | | |
| | (% V/V) | | | (% V/V) | | |
ANESTHETIC	IN AIR	IN O_2	IN N_2O	IN AIR	IN O_2	IN N_2O
Diethyl ether	1.9–48	2.0–82	1.5–24	3.4	13	8
Cyclopropane	2.4–10.4	2.5–60		4.5	18	10
Trichloroethylene	None	10–65	2.0–?			
Divinyl ether	1.7–2.7	0.8–45	1.4–25	4.0	17	9
Ethyl chloride	3.8–15.4	4.0–67	2.0–33	6.5	25	14
Ethylene	3.1–32	3.0–80	1.9–40	6.5	25	14
Methoxyflurane	9.0–28	5.2–28	4.0–?			
Fluoroxene	4.2–?	4.0–?				

is dissipated to a point at which combustion ceases and the mixture becomes nonflammable, defining the upper limit of flammability. Table 52-1 lists the ranges of flammability and the stoichiometric proportions of anesthetic gases and vapors.

FLAMES AND EXPLOSIONS

A combustion that proceeds with the generation of light is a flame. Depending upon the conditions, a flame may remain static and continue to burn at the source of fuel and oxygen (gas burner), or it may spread along the fuel-oxygen supply and cause a deflagration. Smith described an accident involving a Copper Kettle vaporizer that was being cleaned with liquid ether.[5] The ether vapor passed from the cleaning area to an adjacent room, where it was ignited by a cigarette, and deflagration was initiated; the flame traveled back to the cleaning room and ultimately caused an explosion in the copper kettle. Fortunately, the technician sustained only slight injuries, though the kettle was damaged extensively.

The accident illustrates a deflagration in which the explosion was limited to the vaporizer. The conditions necessary to cause an explosion must include those that favor the retention of heat. Explosions occur when the heat energy of combustion is retained by the mixture, causing a temperature rise sufficient to accelerate the combustion process. The rising temperature and accelerating combustion cause a rapid expansion of gas, resulting in a shock wave, a wave of compression traveling at supersonic speeds. The shock wave contains the mechanical energy necessary to cause damage (as illustrated by the vaporizer).

Just as fuel-oxygen mixtures have a range of flammability, they also have a range of explosivity or detonability. Table 52-2 gives the ranges of detonability of some inhalation anesthetics in oxygen, air, and nitrous oxide. As shown Table 52-2, the range of detonability is narrower than the range of flammability. It is also shown that the detonability of anesthetics is enhanced by the presence of nitrous oxide.

ROLE OF NITROUS OXIDE IN FIRES AND EXPLOSIONS

The ranges of flammability and detonability of fuel-air mixtures are much narrower than fuel-oxygen mixtures. The nitrogen in air acts as a diluent, absorbing energy without entering the

**Table 52-2. Ranges of Detonability
of Anesthetic Gases and Vapors**

| | LIMITS OF DETONABILITY (% V/V) | | |
ANESTHETIC	IN AIR	IN O_2	IN N_2O
Diethyl ether	1.7–27	1.8–85	1.5–24
Cyclopropane		2.5–60	1.6–30
Divinyl ether			1.4–25
Ethyl chloride	3.8–15	4.0–67	2–33
Ethylene		9–50	2–40

reaction, and as a medium for conducting heat. Nitrous oxide, on the other hand, not only supports the combustion process, but enhances it.

The chemical formation of nitrous oxide requires the input of energy (19 kcal./mol.); it is an endothermic chemical reaction. This energy of formation is released when nitrous oxide is broken down or enters a combustion process. On page 672, it was shown that the combustion of hydrogen and oxygen yields 57 kcal. per mol. of water formed. The same reaction using nitrous oxide in place of oxygen yields 76 kcal. per mol. of water; the extra 19 kcal. results from the breakdown of nitrous oxide.

Consequently, the ranges of flammability and detonability of fuel-nitrous oxide mixtures are wider than those of fuel-oxygen mixtures. These ranges can be extended still further by oxygen enrichment of nitrous oxide-fuel mixtures, as in clinical practice. Tables 52-1 and 52-2 show that flammable and detonable concentrations frequently lie in the clinically useful range.

TYPES AND SOURCES OF IGNITION

Chemical Ignition

The presence of ether, oxygen, and light in storage containers is conducive to the formation of ether peroxides, which are very labile oxidizers and resemble chemical detonators. Although peroxide formation was at one time a source of ignition, it has been eliminated by the presence of antioxidants (e.g., a copper lining) in light-tight ether containers.

Spontaneous Ignition

Mixtures of fuel and air or oxygen will ignite spontaneously if their temperature is raised to a certain minimum, at which it is high enough to start an oxidation reaction. The locally produced heat raises the temperature and accelerates the oxidation process until ignition occurs. (This is the mechanism of spontaneous ignition operative in haystacks and oil-saturated rags.) The temperature required to start the spontaneous ignition process is considerably lower than the temperature required for local ignition by an open flame or spark. For example, mixtures of some volatile anesthetics and oxygen have temperatures of spontaneous ignition that range from 350 to 400°C. Rich mixtures of diethyl ether and air can ignite spontaneously at temperatures as low as 200°C.

Local Ignition

Local ignition requires that a small zone of the flammable mixture be heated to the ignition temperature. This is, by far, the most common type of ignition and requires that only small amounts of heat be concentrated in a localized area.

Open flames are a source of local ignition. Examples include burners, matches, and cigarettes. Although these items are not found in the operating room, they may be found in peripheral areas (e.g., offices, waiting rooms, lounges, laboratories).

Light and heat sources also cause local ignition. Examples include projection lamps used in fiberoptic light sources, endoscopic bulbs, and hot wire cautery units.

Sparks are the most common source of ignition in operating room fires and explosions. A spark occurs when there is sufficient electrical potential or voltage between two points separated by insulation to cause a breakdown of that insulation. Electrical energy flows between the points through the gap. High temperatures are generated because the electrical energy flows through a material of high resistance (the air gap), which is the basis of all electrical heating devices. MacIntosh cites an example in which a spark develops 0.001 cal. of heat.[6] He states that if the spark passes through a volume of air equal to 1 mm.[3] in 1 msec., the temperature within the air volume could reach 1000°C. This temperature is sufficient, in the presence of a flammable mixture, to cause ignition. The major sources of sparks in operating rooms are electrosurgical devices, other electrical apparatus, and static electricity.

Static electricity is generated when two dissimilar nonconducting materials are in motion and in contact with each other. One material tends to give up electrons in the frictional process to the other material. As a result, a negative charge builds up on the material that gains electrons, and a positive charge, on the other material. The two materials then behave like the plates of a capacitor separated by an air gap. If the process continues, accumulation of charge and voltage continues until a spark jumps across the air gap. This is the mechanism by which the Van der Graaf generator operates. In the operating room, the equivalent of this is a patient roller with a nonconductive cover.

Electrical devices are the most common source of electrical sparks in the modern operating room. Sparks from electrical devices may be generated from "making" or "breaking" switch or relay contacts, electric motor brushes, commutators, loose or faulty electrical plugs and receptacles, and, most commonly, electrosurgical devices.

Mechanical sources of ignition energy include rapid gas compression, hammers, drills, and saws. A small explosion was reported by Garfield when an oxygen tank was opened into a pressure regulator contaminated with oil.[7] The rapid compression of gas within the regulator owing to oxygen release created sufficient heat to ignite the oil and explode the regulator.

CONTROL OF FIRE AND EXPLOSION HAZARDS

For fires and explosions to occur, the following must be present simultaneously: a source of fuel, a source of oxygen, and a source of ignition. Prevention is directed toward their control.

Elimination or Control of Flammable Materials

Investigations and discussions of operating room fires and explosions usually focus upon the use of flammable anesthetic drugs. The clinical issues that involve the use of flammable agents have been discussed by Ngai.[4] However, other flammable materials are commonly used in the operating room. These include alcohol, other organic volatile "prep" solutions (acetone, ether, tincture of iodine), aerosol adhesive sprays, tincture of benzoin, plastic coating sprays, and collodion. Many of these materials are not labelled as flammable. In addition, in the past decade use of disposable products has increased and brought large amounts of paper and plastic waste into the operating room. Although not explosive, these materials are readily flammable and will liberate dense smoke and/or toxic fumes. Volatile prep solutions and aerosols require adequate ventilation, as do the flammable anesthetics. These materials should be handled in such a way that pooling or saturation of patient drapes is avoided. Alcohol-saturated drapes on patients undergoing electrocautery are a significant fire hazard. Although complete elimination of flammable materials is not practical, some thought should be given to their control.

Flammable Anesthetics

If the use of a flammable anesthetic is required, then techniques should be geared toward low-flow or closed rebreathing systems. The hazard of fire and explosion is greatest during induction of anesthesia and during emergence. Induction is associated with the use of high-gas-flow rates and with periods during which the anesthetic circuit is completely opened (e.g., during tracheal intubation). During emergence, the anesthetic circuit is opened, and the patient exhales anesthetic gas into the room again; however, concentrations of the gas are lower than during induction.

The National Fire Protection Association (NFPA) code for locations where mixed or explosive anesthetizing agents are administered defines the hazardous zone as a portion of the operating room below the 5-foot level measured from the floor.[8] This zone is defined on the basis that most anesthetic gases are denser than air and tend to gravitate to floor level. For this reason, the NFPA also recommends that the return air grill be at the floor level.

Although NFPA codes are intellectually satisfying, they have not been backed up by any recent data. The modern operating room is a very dynamic place; doors are opened and closed, personnel move around, and there is little chance for gas to settle to the floor level in a room with turbulent air currents. Recent studies on trace levels have shown that anesthetic gases are widely dispersed, and "hot spots" (localized zones of concentration) can form above the floor level.[9] Unfortunately, the NFPA code does not specify a minimum ventilation requirement that will determine the rate of removal of anesthetics from an operating room, which is far more important than the location of the air grills alone. Clearly this is an example of a committee specifying a design rather than a performance standard.

Elimination or Control of Ignition Sources

Sources of chemical and spontaneous ignition are not common in operating room facilities, though local ignition sources are. Common sense dictates that sources of open flame (e.g., cigarettes) should be kept well away from operating rooms, recovery rooms, equipment, and storage areas.

Most of the effort to reduce ignition sources in anesthetic-related fires is directed to the control of sparks.

Conductive floors, anesthetic rubber goods, shoes, upholstery fabrics, and castors are meant to dissipate static charge and prevent the development of large potential differences between objects. These measures are defeated by waxes, coatings, and dirt. Regular checks of these materials must be made to ensure that they remain conductive. Shoe testers should be readily available and used.

An adequate relative humidity promotes the formation of a water film over surfaces and dissipation of static charges. The relative humidity should be at least 50 per cent. Operating room humidities may vary greatly with the prevailing weather, so that spot checks are an inadequate safeguard. Operating rooms used for flammable agents should have accurate hygrometers to ensure that they meet this standard.

Sparks from electrical apparatus can be avoided by the use of equipment specifically labelled "for use in hazardous atmospheres." Electrical equipment not so labelled should be mounted above the mythical 5-foot level in a well ventilated room.

Electrocautery should be banned during administration of agents that are highly flammable or explosive in clinical concentrations. Surgical personnel should be made aware that electrosurgical devices are currently the most common source of ignition in operating room fires and explosions, and that most fires and explosions now involve fuel other than anesthetics. Enteric gas is one of the most commonly reported. For this reason, the use of nitrous oxide as an insufflating gas for laparoscopy may be hazardous when electrocoagulation is used. The explosive properties of colonic gas have been discussed by Ragans and colleagues.[10] They found explosive concentrations of methane and/or hydrogen in 42 per cent of patients with unprepared intestines. Laparoscopic patients rarely have bowel preps. Enteric gas contains both methane and hydrogen, which can diffuse into the abdominal cavity. Nitrous oxide can diffuse into the bowel cavity, and this has been well documented in cases of intestinal obstruction. While carbon dioxide insufflation for laparoscopy causes mild peritoneal irritation and slightly increased propensity to cardiac arrhythmias, these disadvantages can be minimized by drugs and ventilatory support. In contrast, the consequences of an intra-abdominal fire or explosion are less easily treated. Although no cases of this type have been reported during laparoscopy, the possibility has been discussed, and some preliminary measurements have been made.[11,12]

REFERENCES

1. Greene, B. A.: The hazard of fire and explosion in anesthesia: report of a clinical investigation of 230 cases. Anesthesiology, 2:144, 1941.
2. Woodbridge, P. D.: Incidence of anesthetic explosions. J.A.M.A., 113:2308, 1939.
3. Ministry of Health: Anesthetic Explosions: Report of a working party. H. M. Stationary Office, London, 1956.
4. Ngai, S. H.: Explosive agents—are they needed? Surg. Clin. North Am., 55:975, 1975.
5. Smith, T. C.: Serious explosion during cleaning of a copper kettle. Anesthesiology, 29:386, 1968.
6. MacIntosh, R., Mushin, W. W., and Epstein, H. G.: Sources of ignition and explosion hazards. In Physics for the Anaesthetist. (ed. 3). Oxford, Blackwell Scientific Publications, 1963.
7. Garfield, J. M., Allen, G. W., Silverstein, P., et al.: Flash fire in a reducing valve. Anesthesiology, 34:578, 1971.
8. National Fire Protection Association: Bulletin 56A Standard for the use of inhalation anesthetics. NFPA, Boston, 1973.
9. Piziali, R. L., Whitcher, C., Sher, R., et al.: Distribution of waste anesthetic gases in the operating room air. Anesthesiology, 45:487, 1976.
10. Ragans, H., Shinya, H., and Wolff, W.: The explosive potential of colonic gas during colonoscopic electrosurgical polypectomy. Surg. Gynecol. Obstet., 138:554, 1974.
11. Robinson, J. C., Thompson, J. M., and Wood, A. W.: Laparoscopy explosion hazards with nitrous oxide. Br. Med. J., 3:764, 1975.
12. Drummond, G. B., and Scott, D. B.: Laparoscopy hazards with nitrous oxide. Br. Med. J., 1:586, 1976.

53 Burns and Electrocution

Gordon R. Neufeld, M.D.

The operating room is a unique, highly technical environment that poses complicating hazards to patients and to personnel. Interrelated control of these hazards constitutes the topic of "operating room safety." They can be divided into two broad categories: physical hazards and "toxic" hazards (environmental pollution). The physical hazards are further subdivided into electrical hazards, fires, and explosions.

All damage or injury results from the misapplication of energy. In the operating room, many sources of electrical energy are focused on the patient. The control of this energy forms the basis of electrical safety. The complications arising from electrical sources are cardiac arrest, burns, and the consequences of misinformation. This chapter reviews the physical principles underlying the flow of electrical current, the causes of damage, and the factors that should be considered in the use and control of electrical devices.

Over the past 3 decades, advances in technology have led to the use of a mass of electrical apparatus in the operating room. These devices can be grouped into three basic categories: labor-savers—electric tables, dermatomes, drills, saws, and pumps; energy conversion devices—hypothermia units, blood warmers, heat exchangers, transducers, and electrosurgical units; information display devices—cathode ray oscilloscopes, meters, and x-ray machines.

In the last decade, improvements in monitoring equipment have mushroomed. Technology has provided the means to continuous, instant display of information through the development of solid state electronics, integrated circuits, and computer techniques. However, as a result of technological innovations, the increased role of electronics in patient care has brought more electrical devices (and their related hazards) into an already dangerous environment. Although the risks of electrocution and burns have been recognized and discussed in the literature for many years, there is another less obvious electrical hazard, the "information hazard." Failure of monitoring equipment can manifest itself in the display of artifactual information that can mimic pathophysiologic change.

BASIC PRINCIPLES OF POWER AND CURRENT DENSITY

We are all familiar with the fact that a patient's blood pressure is a reflection of his cardiac output and peripheral resistance:

$$BP = CO \times PR$$

This is Ohm's law as applied to the circulation. Ohm's law for electrical energy relates voltage (electrical pressure) to current (electrical flow) and resistance (electrical resistance). Returning to the physiologic analog, for a patient to maintain a constant blood pressure in the face of dropping peripheral resistance (e.g., from loss of sympathetic tone), cardiac output must increase proportionately. The energy expenditure of the heart

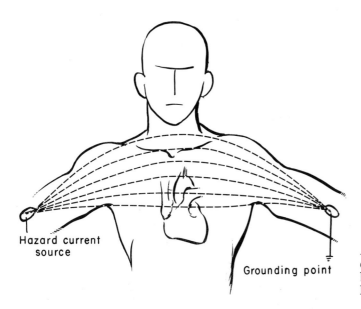

Hazard current source

Grounding point

Fig. 53-1. A very simplified view of electrical current flow in the human body, in which the body is considered to be a leather bag filled with a homogeneously conducting electrolyte solution.

increases to increase the flow. Power is a measure of energy consumption and is the product of flow and pressure. Similarly, the product of electrical flow and pressure is electrical power. It is the misapplication of electrical power that causes damage, and the type of damage is related to the power density.

If a patient has a cardiac output of 6 L. per min. and the aorta has a cross-sectional area of 10 cm.^{2}, then the flow density through the aorta is 0.6 L. per min. per cm.^{2} In electrical flow, if 1 milliampere (mamp.) of current flows through a conducting medium with a cross-sectional area of 10 cm.^{2}, the current density will be 0.1 mamp. per cm.^{2} However, if 1 mamp. flows through a fine wire or catheter of 0.1 cm.^{2} cross-sectional area, then the current density is increased one-hundred-fold, to 10 mamp. per cm.^{2}

The human body is a generator and conductor of electricity. It is sometimes considered, for purposes of understanding electrical current flow, to be an irregularly shaped leather bag, filled with an electrolyte solution (Fig. 53-1). This analogy, however, is grossly oversimplified and must be modified to serve as an effective model. The body is not a homogeneous electrical conducting medium. The skin is a better conductor than the underlying fat but not as good a conductor as

muscle. Thus, within the body there are preferential pathways for the flow of electrical energy (Fig. 53-2). Subsequently, when current is applied to this heterogeneous volume conductor, the current densities vary, depending upon the relative conductivity or resistivity of the components of the conductor.

In the typically diagrammed, saline-filled leather bag, the current density is depicted as being uniformly dispersed through the chest and arms. Here, the fraction of the current received by the myocardium is small compared to the total flow and relates to the ratio of cross-sectional areas of the heart to the area presented by the chest.

The real chest is not homogeneous. Within the arm, the highly conducting medium is the muscle mass. At the shoulder girdle, the available conductive pathways consist of the axillary vessels and the muscle mass of the shoulder girdle and chest walls. Thus, the current density through the chest is not uniformly distributed but is split between the chest wall and the great vessels, with direct access to the myocardium. It is this heterogeneity of conduction that results in the massive bulk tissue damage that occurs in the muscle below the skin in severe electrical burns, even when the points of entry and exit of the injury current may be small.

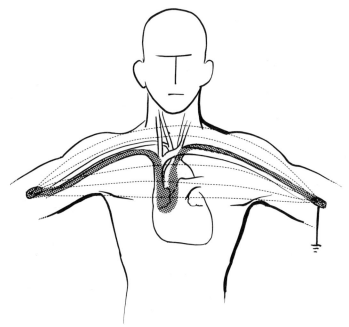

Fig. 53-2. Electrical current flows through the human body in preferential pathways which reflect the relative conductivity of the tissues. The highly conductive components are the great vessels and the muscle masses of the shoulder girdle and chest wall.

The previous diagrams and text exemplify what is called a *macroshock condition.* The total current flow is large (milliamperes or greater) and may cause tissue damage by burning. Ventricular fibrillation may be induced if the current density is sufficiently great through the myocardium to exceed the fibrillatory threshold. Macroshocks result from the application of large potentials from gross faults in equipment or wiring. Fortunately, they are rare. It is the microshock condition that is most insidious and most difficult to detect, and it represents a threat to the "electrically susceptible" patient.

The National Fire Protection Association has written a new tentative standard for the safe use of electricity in patient care facilities.[1] Within this bulletin, an attempt has been made to place patients into classes of electrical susceptibility. Three risk levels are defined:*

---

*Reproduced by permission from NFPA 76B-T, Tentative Standard for the Safe Use of Electricity in Patient Care Areas of Health Care Facilities. Copyright © 1973, National Fire Protection Association, Boston.

Risk I comprises patients without debilitating disease who are reasonably alert and mobile, and who are minimally exposed to electric monitoring or therapeutic appliances. Their hazard level is similar to that of the general public but somewhat increased, since they are likely to be in electric beds, have electric appliances such as lamps, radios, and call buttons close at hand and may be wet. Sick patients are less alert than usual and therefore prone to ill-advised actions. The contact of Risk I patients with electric conductors is likely to be external, accidental, temporary and easily interrupted. The occupational hazard of hospital personnel is comparable to Risk I.

The minimum hazardous current levels for external contacts range from the order of 4.5 milliamperes for "let go" level to 80 milliamperes which could induce ventricular fibrillation. These values are for 60 Hz current. With a typical patient resistance of 1,000 ohms, 4.5 to 80 volts are needed to produce these currents. In the range of 1 to 4.5 milliamperes or less, there may be a disturbing sensation.

The basic method of protection for Risk I is to reduce the possible contact with electric power by enclosing or insulating energized conductors, and by grounding exposed metal of electric appliances. The insulation of exposed conductive surfaces in the patient vicinity provides additional protection.

The design goal maximum leakage current in the grounding wire for each appliance used on such patients is 500 microamperes. Under normal operating conditions this leakage current is diverted from the patient by grounding conductors.

Risk II includes patients who are critically ill, less alert, perhaps obtunded, more likely to be monitored or connected to several therapeutic appliances, and subject to more manipulation by attendants. They are likely to have intentional conductive contacts, external or subcutaneous, that are firmly attached for long periods of time, and they are more likely to be wet. Because of their disease or medication, they may be subject to ventricular fibrillation at lower current levels. The inability of the patient to separate himself from his contacts and the low contact resistance make painful and paralyzing currents more likely to occur. Voltages from one to 10 V may cause such currents.

For Risk II patients, the basic protection is voltage reduction by means of an equipotential environment possibly augmented by insulation of the ungrounded exposed metal in the environment. Grounding circuit continuity testing can ensure the maintenance of grounding integrity. Appliances must be designed to stricter criteria; more frequent and intensive inspection and testing is required than with Risk I patients. Ground fault circuit interrupters or isolated power systems enhance protection against ground fault currents.

The design goal maximum leakage current in the grounding conductor for each appliance for Risk II patients is 100 microamperes. This applies particularly to appliances which are intimately associated with the patient, with intentional conductive contacts, such as electrodes, endoscopes, etc. Leakage currents in such patient contact (leads) shall be less than 50 μA. Under normal conditions even this current is diverted from the patient by the appliance grounding conductor. Additional protective mechanisms such as an equipotential environment, insulation of exposed metal, and use of current limiters further reduce the possible hazard.

Risk III patients have a direct low impedance electrical connection to the conduction system of the heart. This may be a transvenous or intrathoracic wire such as a pacing catheter, or a nonconductive catheter filled with conductive liquid or other device deliberately introduced for diagnostic, therapeutic, or investigative purpose. The increased electric hazard for Risk III patients results from the high current density at the tip of the externalized conductor when electricity is inadvertently applied to its exposed end. Current applied to the endocardium has been shown to cause fibrillation with as little as 20 microamperes at 60 Hz in the dog. It is estimated that an equal current may cause fibrillation in the human. Data obtained during open heart surgery indicate that minimum currents of about 200 microamperes applied to the epicardium are required to cause fibrillation. The design goal of 10 microamperes maximum current to the heart muscle probably provides a safety factor of at least two and perhaps ten.

It is difficult to provide an equipotential environment to protect against a 10 microampere hazard level under fault condition. The basic protection for cardiac catheterized patients is insulation of the exposed catheter terminal. Risk III patients require the same protection as Risk II patients, plus an equipotential or insulated environment or fault current limitation for ground fault protection to complement insulation of the catheter terminal.

For skin contact, current levels similar to Risk II patients are critical.

All anesthetized patients in operating rooms fall into Risk Category III. They are unconscious in an environment rich in electrical energy, often under wet conditions, and have, with increasing frequency, centrally placed intravenous catheters, monitoring electrodes, and thermistor probes. Patients of Risk Category III are prone to microshock.

MICROSHOCK

During microshock, all of the "hazard current" flows through the catheter system or endocardial electrode (Fig. 53-3). The current density at the catheter tip can thus be very high. The current is preferentially dissipated through the myocardium, blood, and great vessels. If the fibrillatory threshold is reached, cardiac arrest occurs, without other evidence of injury. These microshock hazard currents are in the microampere region. Starmer, Whalen, and McIntosh reported fibrillatory currents ranging from 20 to 800 μamp. in anesthetized dogs with intracardiac electrodes (mean = 258 μamp.).[2] Several investigators have found that catheter position was an important factor in the current level required for fibrillation, and that the most sensitive area is the inner aspect of the right ventricular wall near the apex. Other investigators have also observed that at current levels well below the fibrillatory threshold, ventricular activity ceased while the current flowed, but normal activity resumed when the current was turned off. This type of current flow probably mimics more closely the clinical situation in which the combined leakage of current of several devices or a single faulty device can cause

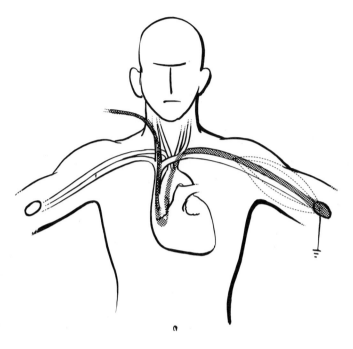

Fig. 53-3. Microshock results when electric current, inadvertently applied to the exposed end of an externalized conductor (saline-filled central venous catheter), is dissipated as a high current density from the tip of the conductor through the great vessels, blood, and myocardium.

ventricular arrest through an intracardiac or central venous catheter.

There is little data on fibrillatory thresholds of the human myocardium, but the data that do exist indicate a higher threshold than for dogs. Starmer found that the current necessary to fibrillate the heart during open heart procedures was 180 to 1500 μamp., with a mean of 583 μamp.[2] Other investigators have observed a similar range. No data exist on levels of sustained current flow necessary for ventricular standstill in humans, but from the data from dogs one can assume that the levels are much lower than for fibrillation.

Some recent work by Roy helps to clarify the discrepancies in fibrillatory thresholds observed by different investigators and in different species.[3] He has examined, in detail, the current density required to produce three phenomena. The first to be observed is rhythm disruption while current is applied. This occurs at the lowest current densities. The second phenomenon Roy calls *pump failure* (cardiac standstill), which is reversible (i.e., sinus rhythm resumes when the current is turned off). The third end-point is pump failure with fibrillation, which is not spontaneously reversible. Both pump failure and pump failure with fibrillation are related directly to the current density. Roy did not observe either effect at currents below 10 μamp., regardless of the contact area.

CONTROL OF SHOCK HAZARDS

Conductivity and Electrical Isolation

Operating room design includes specific measures to promote the dissipation of static electricity. The provision of conductive floors, the wearing of conductive shoes, and the use of conductive materials on surfaces are geared to this end. To reduce the electrical hazard of this conductive "bathtub" environment, several measures are incorporated into the power distribution system, materials, and design of operating room suites.

First, the conductive materials used in flooring, surface coverings, and shoes are designed to be sufficiently conductive to dissipate static charge, but to offer significant resistance to the flow of large or macroshock currents. The National Fire Protection Association standard for conductive flooring specifies that the resistance between two points on the floor spaced 3 ft. apart should not exceed 1 million ohms and should not be less than 25,000 ohms.[4] Using this minimum value and Ohm's law, one can calculate that, if 110 V are applied, the maximum current flow between the two points is as follows:

$$I = \frac{E}{R} = \frac{110}{25\ K} \simeq 4 \text{ mamp.}$$

A 4-mamp. current flow through the torso is easily perceived, though probably not dangerous; through a centrally placed catheter, it can easily be fatal. Thus, minimum resistivity protects against only macroshock.

Second, the electrical power distribution to operating rooms is "isolated." This means that the power distribution or power receptacles of the operating rooms are separated from the main hospital power by a transformer. The "isolation transformer" provides a warning system when a major electrical fault exists in the operating room and requires that there be two simultaneous electrical faults before a macroshock condition can exist. The purpose of the isolated power distribution is to provide a mechanism for detecting faulty equipment before a short circuit develops. The short circuit is a potential source of ignition for a fire or explosion, if a spark occurs, and is a macroshock hazard.

Normally the power supplied to a wall receptacle in the home or at the hospital bedside involves three wires. One of the wires is "hot" and color-coded with black insulation; it supplies the 110 V necessary to operate equipment. The second wire is "neutral"; it is not associated with a voltage but functions only to return the current used by an electrical device back to the distribution panel and, ultimately, to the utility company. The neutral wire is color-coded white. The third wire is the ground wire, which acts as a redundant neutral or return path for electrical current when a hazardous fault develops. The neutral and ground wires are bonded together at the distribution panel and firmly grounded through a cold water pipe. Thus, no electrical potential can, in theory, develop on the ground or neutral conductors in the receptacle; only the

"hot" wire supplies potentially injurious electrical power.

Hospital electrical equipment is supplied with a corresponding three-wire power cord and plug. The wires within the power cord are also color-coded. The black wire is the power supply line to the device, the white wire is the neutral or return path, and the green wire is the ground connection. The plug is designed so that these wires correspond properly at the receptacle. The correspondence can be overridden through the use of "cheater" plugs or improperly wired extension cords, neither of which should be used in hospitals. The green ground wire in the power cord is connected within the electrical device to the main frame and to any exposed metal parts. If a fault develops in the equipment so that the "hot" lead comes in contact with the frame or metal case of the device, a short circuit develops and a fuse or circuit breaker interrupts the supply of power, preventing a macroshock to the individual in contact with the device. This system, however, is not sufficient in a conductive operating room environment and is augmented by the isolation transformer (Fig. 53-4).

In the operating room, the isolation transformer supplies power between two leads from the secondary winding of the transformer. The ground wire is also provided, but there is no connection between the ground wire and the secondary winding of the transformer. Because of this, current can flow only from one lead of the secondary winding to the other lead. In other words, a 110-V potential exists only between the two secondary leads of the transformer, but not between any one secondary lead and ground. Consequently, touching a single, secondary lead and simultaneously touching ground will not complete a circuit that allows current to flow (Fig. 53-4A). This provides a level of protection to operating room personnel and patients from a macroshock. If a faulty piece of equipment is energized in the operating room and the fault is "a short" between one of the supply leads and the case or ground, the other supply lead then becomes "hot" with respect to ground. This constitutes a "first fault" condition. The first fault

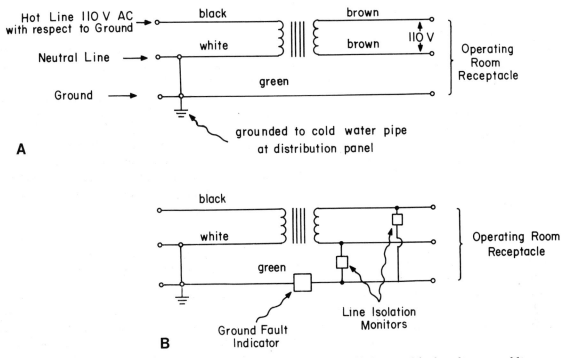

Fig. 53-4. Schematic diagrams of (*A*) isolation transformer and (*B*) ground fault indicator and line isolation monitors built into the isolation transformer.

condition is detected by warning systems, known as the line isolation monitor (LIM) and the ground fault indicator (GFI), built into the isolation transformer. These devices are depicted in Figure 53-4B. The offending equipment can be removed and repaired before a second fault, which represents a macroshock hazard, develops. Essentially, the first fault converts the isolated power system of the operating room into a conventional grounded power system. Subsequently, a second fault is necessary to create a macroshock hazard.

In planning new operating room facilities, there is often pressure applied to ban the use of flammable anesthetics, to reduce the building cost by eliminating the need for conductive flooring. Isolated power to each room is still required, however, for good reason. There are many opportunities for both patients and personnel to come in contact simultaneously with electrical apparatus and a low resistance path to ground in the operating room. A typical major operation may include the use of the following:

Apparatus Used in a Typical Major Operation

Electric operating table
Surgical lights
Electrosurgical units
Hypothermia units
X-ray equipment
Monitors
Blood warmers

Each of these devices has a metal case that is electrically "grounded" and commonly in contact with the patient and/or personnel under wet conditions. These grounded pieces of equipment do not have a minimum resistivity of 25 kilohms, as does a conductive floor. In fact, the ground pathway of an electrical device should be maintained at less than one-tenth of 1 ohm.

Thus, the added protection against macroshock provided by isolated power in the operating suite is probably worth the cost. It is possible that less expensive warning devices for electrical faults can be provided, but studies of comparative safety between isolated power distribution and ground fault detectors have not been done. Until these studies are undertaken, isolated power distribution provides reasonable protection from macroshock, as well as sparks, and acts as a warning device for defective electrical equipment.

Equipment Control Programs

The purpose of an equipment control program is to reduce electrical hazards from electrical equipment malfunctions. This purpose is best served by taking the following precautions:

Careful Selection of New Equipment. The considerations involve meeting minimum safety standards, ease of maintenance, simplicity and ruggedness of design, record of performance in the field, and compatibility with current equipment in the facility. It is desirable to reduce to a minimum the number of models or manufacturers for a specific device, because it simplifies maintenance and the training of operators.

Initial checkout of equipment ensures that it meets the specifications of the hospital and manufacturer.

Preventive Maintenance and Calibration (PMC). Good PMC requires the use of a tagging and inventory system. Such a system has been described by Nobel.[5] Outside contractors are available to provide such services, but the quality control and overall supervision of the contractor remains the primary responsibility of the hospital administration. Many hospitals are consolidating the control and service functions into departments of clinical engineering.

Safety Education in Hospitals

Although well recognized as an important aspect of safety in industrial settings, safety education in hospitals is generally haphazard and neglected. The best equipment and maintenance available may be completely offset if personnel do not realize that cracked or frayed insulation, broken strain reliefs, cracked plugs, and repairs with adhesive tape constitute an electrical hazard. The focus of educational programs must encompass the following: What constitutes an electrical hazard? What should be done when the proper functioning of a piece of electrical equipment is in doubt? What is the correct procedure for operating the device?

Safety education requires creativity and innovation in the hospital facility. Ultimately, education can be more effective in reducing electrical accidents than the most sophisticated preventive maintenance program.

ELECTRICAL BURNS AND ELECTROSURGERY

Electrical burns constitute the most common electrical hazard in the operating room. Virtually all electrical burns are associated with the use of electrosurgery or cautery units. In addition to electrical burns, electrosurgical devices are currently the most common source of ignition for operating room fires and explosions.

Principles of Electrocautery

The common electrosurgical device is a radio-frequency generator. It supplies alternating current to the active electrode tip at frequencies between 500,000 and 2 million Hz. The myocardium is not sensitive to frequencies in this range, and therefore, electrocautery does not constitute a fibrillatory hazard (in a properly functioning unit). The total power output of available units ranges from 40 to 400 watts. The current density at the electrode tip is very high, causing local heating and coagulation. The current density falls rapidly as the current is dissipated through the body. The current is returned to the instrument by way of the dispersive electrode, which provides a large surface of contact and, therefore, a low-current density.

Extraneous burns are always associated with the existence of alternate return pathways for the electrosurgical current through body contacts with small surface areas or inadequate contact of patient to the dispersive plate. Burns have been described at points of contact for EEG and ECG leads, and circumorbital burns have been experienced by operators of laparoscopic units. The burn hazards of electrosurgical devices have recently been reviewed by Becker and colleagues.[6] Their study was initiated after the occurrence of nine burns to patients over a period of 10 months. The most common site of these burns was at the attachment of ECG electrodes. In investigating these burns, they found a variety of causative faults in the devices used:

A defective alarm circuit in the electrosurgical unit was responsible in one case. Becker and colleagues observed that the resistance necessary to trip the alarm, in units that were not defective, ranged from 2,300 to 13,800 ohms, an overly broad tolerance in the design of these alarms. Furthermore, alarms may provide a false sense of security, since they can be "fooled" by the existence of other return paths to the machine.

Defective dispersive plate cables accounted for two burns. Out of 20 cables examined, three were completely broken and one partially broken, although all were visibly intact. An electrical continuity test was the only effective method for checking these cables.

The positioning of the ECG indifferent electrode with respect to the dispersive plate was found to affect the ratio of the electrocautery current carried by these two pathways. For example, during a median sternotomy procedure, if the dispersive plate was placed under the buttock of the patient and the ECG indifferent electrode was placed on the upper arm, Becker and colleagues measured 175 mamp. of radio-frequency current through the ECG electrode. This was reduced to 25 mamp. when the indifferent electrode of the ECG was shifted close to the patient plate by placing it on the calf.

Becker deduces from these studies that the amount of current dissipated through the ECG indifferent electrode is directly proportional to the proximity of the electrocautery knife to that electrode. The radio-frequency current is dissipated by way of the "paths of least impedance" through the body. Just as in microshock, the availability of an alternate pathway for current flow creates the hazard. *Unfortunately, in the case of electrosurgery, the alternate current path also satisfies the criterion for many patient alarm and fail-safe circuits.*

The interconnection of devices that are claimed to be compatible by different manufacturers, but that have been inadequately designed or tested for compatibility, is likely to cause extraneous burns.

Becker and colleagues conclude their study with the following recommendations:

A radio-frequency choke (inductor) should be incorporated into all ECG electrode leads used for operating room monitoring. This provides a high impedance for the flow of radio-frequency current in the electrode leads, thereby limiting the current flow in the electrode system, without affecting the quality of the ECG signal. (There is some controversy regarding this claim.)

All alarm systems should be inspected to ensure that they meet the manufacturer's specifications.

Alarm circuits should be routinely checked prior to each use of electrosurgery devices.

The indifferent electrode of the ECG should be kept as far as possible from the site of surgery, to minimize current division between it and the dispersive plate.

Clipping or coiling of ECG or electrosurgery cables should be avoided.

Regular preventive maintenance and calibration, along with personnel education in the safe use of electrocautery, should be undertaken.

Needle electrodes should be avoided in patients undergoing electrocautery.

Laparoscopy

Laparoscopic sterilization is a fairly new application of electrosurgery. Many devices are available, and techniques are recommended by manufacturers and surgeons. Some of these have not been adequately considered or tested under controlled laboratory conditions. The majority of surgeons are, unfortunately, at the mercy of these "expert" recommendations.

The principle behind laparoscopic sterilization is to locally heat the fallopian tube by grasping it with a forceps and applying radiofrequency current. The procedure is accomplished by direct visualization through the laparoscope, with the abdomen inflated with a gas, typically carbon dioxide. Some operators recommend the use of nitrous oxide as an insufflating gas, particularly when local anesthesia is used. Nitrous oxide is less irritating to the peritoneum, and patients tolerate it better. Precaution should be taken, however, because nitrous oxide supports combustion as well as pure oxygen. The presence of nitrous oxide in the abdomen, in combination with electrocoagulation, may constitute an intra-abdominal fire hazard. Nitrous oxide can readily diffuse into loops of bowel containing methane or hydrogen gas. Thus, the use of nitrous oxide as an insufflating gas should be confined to diagnostic laparoscopy or the application of clips, in which electrosurgical generators are not required. Gases have very low thermal capacities. Thus, temperatures generated locally during electrocautery may become high. The procedure differs from a transurethral prostatectomy in this respect. In the latter procedure, the area is surrounded by an irrigation solution that has a very high thermal capacity. Although bowel burns are a recognized complication, I am aware of only one study on the temperatures developed intra-abdominally during laparoscopy.[7] High temperatures on the electrode or laparoscope tip can cause a bowel burn during the withdrawal of the instrument from the abdomen.

Until the mid-1970s, almost all laparoscopic sterilizations were performed with unipolar electrocoagulating devices.[8] These instruments apply an electric current that proceeds through the instrument's grasping forceps (active electrode), coagulates the fallopian tube, courses through the patient's body, and exits the body via a ground plate (return electrode) affixed to the patient's skin. Thus, the patient is an integral part of the current circuit. More than 100 cases of thermal bowel injury have been reported,[9] occurring about once in every 2,000 cases of unipolar electrocoagulation.[10] In addition, there have been three deaths related to bowel injury.[9,11] Burns of the abdominal wall[12] and to the face and hands of the operator have also been reported.[13]

Extraneous burns can be reduced during laparoscopy by the use of low-power electrosurgical units (except for spark gap devices), bipolar grasping forceps, and isolated output stages on the electrocoagulator and by appropriately insulating the grasping forceps,[14] the trocar sheath, and the body of the laparoscope.

Since electrosurgical units are radio-frequency devices, insulation does not completely eliminate the transmission of current. For this reason, some investigators and manufacturers recommend multiple grounding points during laparoscopy. Such practices should be discouraged. If the body of the laparoscope is grounded or shares a pathway with the dispersive plate, a parallel pathway system is established through which current division will occur. If the dispersive plate path is poor or remote from the active electrode, then conditions are favorable for the bulk of the current to return by way of the body of the laparoscope. This, in turn, sets up a condition favorable for development of a burn to the bowel, to the puncture site, or to the operator. In addition, the abdominal contents provide many possible pathways for current flow. During the coagulation of the fallopian tube, the tube is heated, desiccated, and eventually charred. As heating and desiccation occur, the electrical resistance of the tube itself must increase. This sets the stage for current to seek alternate pathways of lower resistance within the abdomen. Direct contact of the electrode tip to adjacent tissue is not necessary for a bowel burn to occur, because radio-frequency current can be radiated through gas or along surfaces.

To reduce the incidence of burns, secondary pathways should be limited. The use of radio-frequency chokes in ECG electrodes serves this purpose; keeping the indifferent ECG electrode close to the dispersive plate and away from the active electrode also serves this purpose. Insulating the trocar sheath will reduce but not eliminate extraneous current flow through the body of a laparoscope. Grounding the body of the laparoscope, however, serves only to increase the potential for current flow through this inappropriate pathway and increases the likelihood of burns. Apart from using mechanical devices (e.g., spring clip[15] or silastic band[16]) to ligate the fallopian tube, greatest safety can be achieved through the use of the newer bipolar instruments during laparoscopic sterilization. Only one bowel burn has been reported with bipolar devices.[17]

There is an urgent need for adequate animal studies on these highly technical but poorly understood aspects of electrosurgery, particularly intra-abdominal use. The optics of laparoscopes allow for a very limited viewpoint by the operator (pun intended).

THE DANGER OF MISINFORMATION

Even the most sophisticated aircraft has a magnetic compass. When caring for the "highly monitored" patient, it is dangerous to rely solely or continuously on electronic information. Electronic components fail, and monitors are subject to artifact or miscalibration.

Gradual failure of a power supply in a large, multichannel, electronic monitor can mimic hypovolemia with a gradually falling arterial pressure, pulse pressure, and venous pressure. If vigorously treated, pulmonary edema may ensue from fluid overload.

Peripheral arterial pressure waveforms are notoriously "artifact-prone." The amplitude and shape of the radial artery pulse waveform is determined by mechanical characteristics of the myocardium, the peripheral vascular "tone," and the compliance and length of the catheter system between artery and transducer. When conditions are suitable (and the anesthesiologist cannot predict them in advance), the pulse pressure display may be grossly in error. The only clinically practical way to check this is to inflate a blood pressure cuff on the arm with the arterial line and then deflate the cuff and observe on the monitor the point when the arterial pressure trace first becomes apparent. The pressure in the cuff (using a manometer) at that point should agree approximately with the systolic pressure observed on the monitor after the cuff is totally deflated. If these do not agree, then a pressure artifact is being generated owing to pressure wave "reflections" within the vascular space and catheter system. Because of these effects, peripheral arterial pulse waveforms should never be used to diagnose or treat disorders of "myocardial contractility" in the absence of other supporting information.

CONCLUSION

The control and testing of medical devices, and the definition of standards for them, have, until recently, been virtually undefined. In the past, equipment manufacturers have not been required to provide data from laboratory tests or clinical trials prior to marketing devices. However, recent legislation on medical devices has changed this. The impact of this legislation, which is to be implemented by the Food and Drug Administration, has been reviewed by Geller.[18] Much of the current effort of the Food and Drug Administration is directed toward establishing standards for devices. Setting standards is easy when the problems and malfunctions are clearly understood. It becomes difficult when the relationship between several types of devices creates the hazard. The difficulties arise not so much from a lack of standards, but from a lack of data and the mechanisms needed to generate data. In this sense, it seems more appropriate to define standards for the testing of clinical devices and the analysis of their performance or failures in clinical use, rather than for the devices themselves. The problems that arise are not unlike the interaction of drugs; however, the mechanisms available for informing users and manufacturers are much less clearly defined. A great deal of this communication problem can be solved by the manufacturers.

The development of standards is not a panacea, and there is a real danger that standards developed by "armchair" experts with no basis in *controlled studies* may yield only an illusion of safety. Too often, standards become design specifications. The result is a rigid conformity that stifles solutions to problems. Creative design and well thought-out laboratory studies can yield more protection than the sometimes "tunnel vision" of standards committees. Committee activity should be directed toward criteria of performance, encompassing technical requirements (such as tolerances) and "human factors."

REFERENCES

1. National Fire Protection Association: Electricity in Patient Care Facilities. NFPA Bulletin 76B-T, Boston, 1973.
2. Starmer, C. F., Whalen, R. E., and McIntosh, H. D.: Hazards of electric shock in cardiology. Am. J. Cardiol., *14*:537, 1964.
3. Roy, O. Z., Scott, J. R., and Park, G. C.: 60 Hz ventricular fibrillation and pump failure thresholds versus electrode area. IEEE Trans. Biomed. Engin., *23*:45, 1976.
4. National Fire Protection Association: Standard for the use of inhalation anesthetics. NFPA Bulletin 56A, Boston, 1973.
5. Nobel, J. J.: Hospital equipment control programs. Health Devices, *1*:75, 1971.
6. Becker, C. M., Malhotra, I. V., and Hedley-Whyte, J.: The distribution of radio-frequency current and burns. Anesthesiology, *38*:106, 1973.
7. Stewart, K. S., Pearson, J. F., Docker, M. F., et al.: A possible hazard of laparoscopic sterilization. Am. J. Obstet. Gynecol., *115*:1154, 1973.
8. Phillips, J. M., Hulka, J., Hulka, B., et al.: American Association of Gynecologic Laparoscopists' 1976 membership survey. J. Reprod. Med., *21*:3, 1978.
9. Peterson, H. B., Ory, H. W., Greenspan, J. R., et al.: Deaths associated with laparoscopic sterilization by unipolar electrocoagulating devices. Am. J. Obstet. Gynecol., *139*:141, 1981.
10. Phillips, J. M., Keith, D., Hulka, J., et al.: Gynecologic laparoscopy in 1975. J. Reprod. Med., *16*:105, 1976.
11. Deaths following female sterilization with unipolar electrocoagulating devices. Morbid. Mortal., *30*(13):149, 1981.
12. Loffer, F. D., and Pent, D.: Indications, contraindications, and complications of laparoscopy. Obstet. Gynecol. Surv., *30*:407, 1975.
13. Neufeld, G. R., Johnstone, R. E., Garcia, C. R., et al.: Electrical burns during laparoscopy. J. A. M. A., *226*:1465, 1973.
14. Rioux, J. E., and Cloutier, D.: A new bipolar instrument for laparoscopic tubal sterilization. Am. J. Obstet. Gynecol., *119*:737, 1974.
15. Hulka, J. F., Fishburne, J. I., Mercer, J. P., et al.: Laparoscopic sterilization with a spring clip: a report of the first fifty cases. Am. J. Obstet. Gynecol., *116*:715, 1973.
16. Yoon, I. B., and King, T. M.: A preliminary and intermediate report on a new laparoscopic tubal ring procedure. J. Reprod. Med., *15*, 1975.
17. Hulka, J. F.: Relative risks and benefits of electric and nonelectric sterilization techniques. J. Reprod. Med., *21*:111, 1978.
18. Geller, J. H.: The regulation of medical devices: new tools for the FDA. J. Clin. Engin., *2*:231, 1977.

FURTHER READING

Bruner, J. M. R.: Hazards of electrical apparatus. Anesthesiology, *28*:396, 1967.
Leeming, M. N.: Protection of the "electrically susceptible patient." Anesthesiology, *38*:370, 1973.
Neufeld, G. R.: Principles and hazards of electrosurgery including laparoscopy. Surg. Gynecol. Obstet., *147*:705, 1978.

54 Unusual Iatrogenic Problems

Robert E. Johnstone, M.D.

Iatrogenic problems are those caused by the physician in treating a patient and include most of the complications discussed in this book. Although all possible complications of anesthesiology cannot be discussed or even listed here, several important problems are presented in this chapter.

IMPURITIES IN ANESTHETICS

Purity standards for oxygen and liquid and gaseous anesthetic agents are listed in the *U.S. Pharmacopoeia*[1] or *National Formulary*.[2] Cylinders of oxygen, for example, must contain more than 99.0 per cent oxygen and less than 300 p.p.m. carbon dioxide, 10 p.p.m. carbon monoxide, and 5 p.p.m. nitric oxide and nitrogen dioxide. Table 54-1 shows the typical analysis of medical-grade oxygen. Most anesthetic gases and agents well surpass their required purity standards, as does oxygen.

Some anesthetic impurities are clinically important. Thymol, the stabilizer added to halothane, is less volatile than halothane and accumulates in vaporizers. Thymol lowers vaporizer efficiency and reduces delivered halothane concentration. N-Phenylnapthylamine, the stabilizer added to fluroxene, may induce microsomal enzymes and accelerate the metabolism of some drugs. Dichlorohexafluorobutene, the most toxic impurity in halothane, was alleged to cause halothane-associated hepatitis.[3] Subsequently,

evidence to support this association with hepatitis has not been found.[4] Excessive amounts of nitric oxide and nitrogen dioxide contaminating cylinders of nitrous oxide have caused pulmonary edema, hypoxemia, and death.[5] At inspired concentrations of 0.5 per cent, both of these higher oxides of nitrogen kill dogs within 35 minutes.[6] At low concentrations, these oxides dissolve the plastic seals of pressure regulators in anesthesia machines.[7] Diethyl ether stored in a vaporizer for more than 2 days in a container not lined with copper allows formation of ether peroxide, an explosive compound.[8]

FOAMING OF ANESTHETICS

Bubble-through vaporizers, such as the Copper Kettle, occasionally produce anesthetic foam. This indicates contamination of the anesthetic,

Table 54-1. Analysis of Medical-Grade Oxygen

Oxygen	99.6%
Argon	0.2%
Hydrocarbons (90% methane)	10–25 p.p.m.
Nitrogen	5–15 p.p.m.
Krypton	10–20 p.p.m.
Water	5–10 p.p.m.
Nitrous oxide	0–1 p.p.m.
Carbon dioxide	0–1 p.p.m.
Carbon monoxide	0–1 p.p.m.

(Courtesy of Air Products and Chemicals, Inc., Allentown, Pa.)

because pure liquids do not foam. Foaming has occurred most commonly with methoxyflurane contaminated by polydimethyl siloxane-based silicone grease used for lubrication.[9] The problem is prevented by avoiding lubrication of the anesthesia machine and vaporizer or by using a wick vaporizer for all halogenated agents.[10]

INHALATION OF FOREIGN BODIES

During general anesthesia, laryngeal reflexes are depressed and frequently a tracheal tube is present, serving as a ready portal of entry for foreign bodies to the lungs. Teeth, tracheal tubes, syringes, needles, soda lime dust,[11] and metal flakes[12] from the anesthesia machine may be inhaled. When endotracheal tubes are reused, an array of foreign bodies may be found in the lumen after washing and storage.

CONTAMINATION OF SOLUTIONS AND EQUIPMENT

Sterile manufacturing conditions and quality control generally assure sterile intravenous solutions and catheters, although fungal and bacterial contaimination of solutions have occurred recently.[13,14] Small cracks in glass bottles, even those that are too small to see, allow entrance of bacteria. Bottles of intravenous fluids opened in unsterile air may be contaminated,[15] and insects may crawl into an air vent if present.[16] Single-dose drug ampules contain glass particles (Fig. 54-1), which may then be injected intravenously, intramuscularly, or intrathecally.[17] Every bottle of intravenous fluids must be swirled before use and discarded if particulate matter or cloudiness is present.

Hyperalimentation fluids are good culture media and should be mixed under a laminar flow hood. Use of in-line bacterial filters and frequent changing of sites of central venous cannulation prevent many infections.[18] The hazards of vascular cannulation are reviewed in Chapter 47. Breathing circuits, ventilators, and anesthesia machines are a source of corss-infections (see Chap. 50) and are difficult to sterilize.[19,20] Repeated refilling of disposable plastic syringes leads to bacterial contamination of the syringe contents.[21] If the plunger of a syringe is contaminated by soiled hands, these organisms can be transferred to the syringe contents.

HAZARDS OF STERILIZATION

To prevent cross-infection, anesthetic equipment is either used once and discarded or sterilized after use. Disposable equipment requires considerable storage space and may have an appreciable number of manufacturing flaws. Single use of items such as anesthetic breathing circuits and laryngoscopes also increases the expense of anesthesia.

Commonly used agents of sterilization include glutaraldehyde, isopropyl alcohol, ethylene oxide, and heat, and each of these has some disadvantages.[22] Liquid germicides are often ineffective against tubercle bacillae, bacterial spores, and viruses. Heat may damage rubber and plastic equipment and may cause rusting of valves and recording instruments. The local anesthetic bupivacaine and catecholamines decompose when regional anesthesia trays are steam-autoclaved.[23] Use of ethylene oxide is an effective, nondestructive method of sterilizing anesthetic equipment, but residual ethylene oxide and its by-products are highly toxic. Inadequately aired, gas-sterilized tracheal tubes and masks have caused burns of the face, as well as laryngotracheal inflammation and stenosis.[24] At least 7 days of storage must lapse between ethylene oxide sterilization and use of plastic or rubber material.[25] Items sterilized by gamma irradiation should not be sterilized by ethylene oxide, because ethylene chlorhydrin, a tissue irritant, may be formed.[26] Roberts has reviewed infections and sterilization problems in anesthesia.[27]

DERMATITIS

Some patients develop an allergic contact dermatitis after exposure to rubber, adhesive tape, and surgical sheets. Bromide ion released by the biometabolism of halothane may cause acneiform eruptions in patients and anesthetists.[28,29] Skin reactions may precede jaundice in patients devel-

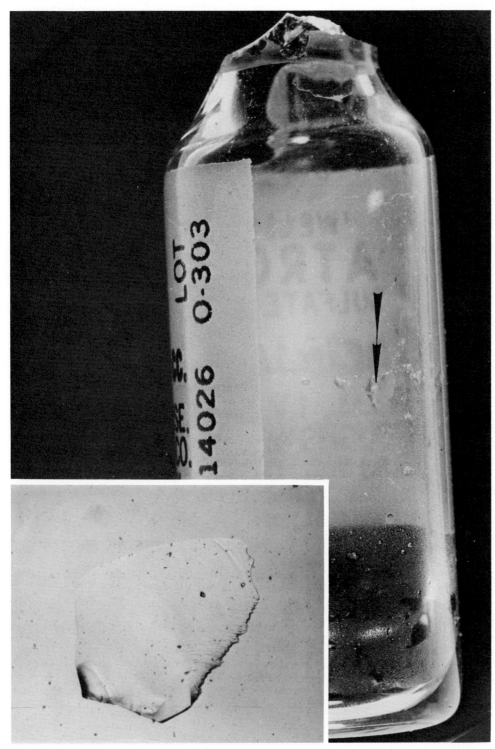

Fig. 54-1. Opening a single-dose ampule can result in glass particles that may then be injected along with the intended drug.

oping hepatitis associated with halogenated anesthetics. For patients with suspected hypersensitivity to a particular agent, the entire breathing circuit and carbon dioxide absorbent should be replaced with fresh equipment. The halogenated anesthetic agents are very soluble in rubber; as much as 300 ml. of anesthetic vapor may be transferred from the breathing circuit used during one anesthetic to a subsequent patient, for whom that agent was not intended.[30]

INTRA-ARTERIAL INJECTIONS

There are numerous case reports of accidental intra-arterial injection of drugs. These usually involve direct injection of thiopental by syringe and needle into an aberrantly located radial artery for induction of anesthesia. Intra-arterial thiopental causes red blood cell hemolysis, platelet aggregation, blockage of small arterioles by acid crystals, and vasospasm resulting in distal ischemia and necrosis.[31] This complication is prevented by starting an intravenous infusion prior to induction of anesthesia and injecting thiopental only into the free-flowing infusion. Complications are minimized if thiopental concentrations of 2.5 per cent or less are used; more concentrated solutions cause more tissue necrosis.[32] Drug addicts who have sclerosed their superficial veins occasionally inject drugs intra-arterially.[33] The most damage is caused by membrane-soluble drugs.[34] Once intra-arterial injection has occurred, continuous infusion of heparin into the artery and sympathetic blockade limit the area of ischemic injury.[35] Management of these patients should include antibiotics if gangrene develops, morphine to control pain, elevation of the arm, and prohibition of smoking.

A hazard of increasing importance to anesthesiologists is accidental injection of drugs into arterial cannulae placed for monitoring of blood pressure or gases.[36] This hazard is minimized by color-coding of arterial catheter tubing with red tape, by using tubing without injection sites, and by hanging bottles of fluids for intra-arterial infusion separately from intravenous bottles. Flushing radial artery catheters with large volumes causes the injected fluid to enter the cerebral circulation as a bolus.[37] Air bubbles or clots may embolize to the brain in this situation and cause neurologic damage (see Chap. 18).

EXTRAVASATION

Cutaneous sloughs may follow extravasation of vasopressors such as levarterenol, ephedrine, metaraminol, and phenylephrine.[38] Extravasation of tissue irritants such as thiopental, calcium chloride, and bromosulfophthalein may also cause tissue necrosis. Treatment consists of tissue infiltration with an anti-inflammatory corticosteroid and an alpha-adrenergic blocking agent, such as phentolamine, and sympathetic blockade.

ADMINISTRATION OF THE WRONG DRUG

Increasing sophistication of anesthetic practice, involving the administration of many drugs, has led to the problem of injection of the wrong drug.[39] The anesthesiologist's work table may contain ten different drugs in syringes and ampules for administration during the case. The similarity in size and design of ampules of different drugs and names that sound alike (such as methyldopa, dopamine, and levodopa) cause more confusion. Prevention involves orderliness, double-checking before injection, labeling of syringes, and color or size coding of syringes.

NOISE IN THE OPERATING ROOM

Operating room noises are intense enough to cause irritation and physiologic changes in exposed personnel and to interfere with speech communication. The opening of rubber glove packages, sliding of platforms along the floor, and open suction lines generate the most noise.[40]

REFERENCES

1. The U.S. Pharmacopoeia. ed. 18. Easton, Mack Printing, 1970.
2. National Formulary. ed. 13. Easton, Pa., Mack Printing, 1970.
3. Cohen, E. N., Bellville, J. W., Budzikiewicz, H., et al.: Impurity in halothane anesthetic. Science, *141*:899, 1963.
4. Raventos, J., and Lemon, P. G.: The impurities in Fluo-

thane: their biological properties. Br. J. Anaesth., *37*:716, 1965.

5. Clutton-Brock, J.: Two cases of poisoning by contamination of nitrous oxide with higher oxides of nitrogen during anaesthesia. Br. J. Anaesth., *39*:388, 1967.

6. Greenbaum, R., Bay, J., Hargreaves, M. D., et al.: Effects of higher oxides of nitrogen on the anaesthetized dog. Br. J. Anaesth., *39*:393, 1967.

7. Hamelberg, W., Mahaffey, J. S., and Bond, W. E.: Nitrous oxide impurities. Anesth. Analg., *40*:408, 1961.

8. Shukys, J. G., and Neeley, A. H.: Studies on the formation and decomposition of ether peroxides. Anesthesiology, *19*:671, 1958.

9. Larson, E. R.: The chemistry of modern inhalation anesthetics. *In* Handbook of Experimental Pharmacology. vol. 30., New York, Springer-Verlag, 1972.

10. Sweatman, F.: Foaming of methoxyflurane contaminated with silicone. Anesthesiology, *38*:407, 1973.

11. Debban, D. G., and Bedford, R. F.: Overdistention of the rebreathing bag, a hazardous test for circle-system integrity. Anesthesiology, *42*:365, 1975.

12. Austin, R. R.: Metallic flaking: a further hazard of anaesthetic apparatus. Anaesthesia, *27*:92, 1972.

13. Felts, S. K., Schaffner, W., Melley, A., et al.: Sepsis caused by contaminated intravenous fluids. Ann. Intern. Med., *77*:881, 1972.

14. Maki, E. G., Rhame, F. S., Mackel, D. C., et al.: Nationwide epidemic of septicemia caused by contaminated intravenous products. Am. J. Med., *60*:471, 1976.

15. Arnold, T. R., and Hepler, C. D.: Bacterial contamination of intravenous fluids opened in unsterile air. Am. J. Hosp. Pharm., *28*:614, 1971.

16. Rupp, C. A., and Formi, P.: Formic I.V. therapy. N. Engl. J. Med., *286*:894, 1972.

17. Particles in veins. Br. Med. J., *1*:307, 1973.

18. Maki, D. G., Goldmann, D. A., and Rhame, F. S.: Infection control in intravenous therapy. Ann. Intern. Med., *79*:867, 1973.

19. Joseph, J. M.: Disease transmission by inefficiently sanitized anesthesiology apparatus. J.A.M.A., *149*:1196, 1952.

20. Dryden, G. E.: Risk of contamination from the anesthesia circle absorber: an evaluation. Anesth. Analg., *48*:939, 1969.

21. Blogg, C. E., Ramsay, M. A. E., and Jarvis, J. D.: Infection hazard from syringes. Br. J. Anaesth., *46*:260, 1974.

22. Duncalf, D.: Care of anesthetic equipment and other devices. Arch. Surg., *107*:600, 1973.

23. DeLeo, B. C., Hamelberg, W., Stauffer, G. L., et al.: Instability of steam autoclaved bupivacaine with epinephrine. Anesthesiology, *40*:297, 1974.

24. LaDoge, L. H.: Facial "irritation" from ethylene oxide sterilization of anesthesia mask? Plast. Reconstr. Surg., *45*:179, 1970.

25. Lipton, B., Gutierrez, R., Blaugrund, S., et al.: Irradiated PVC plastic and gas sterilization in the production of tracheal stenosis following tracheostomy. Anesth. Analg., *50*:578, 1971.

26. Stetson, J. B., and Guess, W. L.: Causes of damage to tissues by polymers and elastomers used in the fabrication of tracheal devices. Anesthesiology, *33*:635, 1970.

27. Roberts, R. B. (ed.): Infections and sterilization problems. Int. Anesthesiol. Clin., *10*:1, 1972.

28. Johnstone, R. E., Kennell, E. M., Behar, M. G., et al.: Increased serum bromide concentration after halothane anesthesia in man. Anesthesiology, *42*:598, 1975.

29. Soper, L. E., Vitez, T. S., and Weinberg, D.: Metabolism of halogenated anesthetic agents as a possible cause of acneiform eruptions. Anesth. Analg., *52*:125, 1973.

30. Lowe, H. J., Titel, J. H., and Hagler, K. J.: Absorption of anesthetics by conductive rubber in breathing circuits. Anesthesiology, *34*:284, 1971.

31. Brown, S. S., Lyons, S. M., and Dundee, J. W.: Intra-arterial barbiturates. Br. J. Anaesth., *40*:13, 1968.

32. Kinmonth, J. B., and Shephard, R. C.: Accidental injection of thiopentone into arteries. Br. Med. J., *2*:914, 1959.

33. Birkhahm, H. J., and Heifetz, M.: Accidental intra-arterial injection of amphetamine: an unusual hazard of drug addiction. Br. J. Anaesth., *45*:761, 1973.

34. Knill, R. L., and Evans, D.: Pathogenesis of gangrene following intra-arterial injection of drugs: a new hypothesis. Can. Anaesth. Soc. J., *22*:637, 1975.

35. Albo, D., Cheung, L., Ruth, L., et al.: Effect of intra-arterial injections of barbiturates. Am. J. Surg., *120*:676, 1970.

36. Evans, J. M., Latto, I. P., and Ng, W. S.: Accidental intra-arterial injection of drugs: a hazard of arterial cannulation. Br. J. Anaesth., *46*:463, 1974.

37. Lowenstein, E., Little, J. W., and Lo, H. H.: Prevention of cerebral embolization from flushing radial artery cannulas. N. Engl. J. Med., *285*:1414, 1971.

38. Roberts, A. P., and Vandam, L. D.: Cutaneous slough after extravasation of phenylephrine. Anesthesiology, *23*:587, 1962.

39. Cooper, J. B., Newbower, R. S., Long, C. D., et al.: Preventable anesthesia mishaps: a study of human factors. Anesthesiology *49*:399, 1978.

40. Shapiro, R. A., and Berland, T.: Noise in the operating room. N. Engl. J. Med., *287*:1263, 1972.

Part Thirteen

Hazards to the Anesthesiologist

The Hazard of Viral Hepatitis to Anesthesiologists and Other Operating Room Personnel

55

Alix Mathieu, M.D., and Jules L. Dienstag, M.D.

Despite failure to cultivate human hepatitis viruses in vitro, there has been rapid progress in understanding these viruses during the last 10 to 15 years. Serologic and virologic tools have helped define the nature of these viruses, their modes of transmission, the prevalence of exposure to them, and the host immune response. Although hepatitis has been recognized as an occupational hazard of health professionals for many years,[1] many of the recent discoveries about hepatitis viruses have increased our awareness of and sensitivity to the problem of hepatitis transmission from patient to health care personnel. Risk of hepatitis exposure among hospital workers increases as a function of contact with patient's blood[2-5]; thus, clinical laboratory technologists and staffs of hemodialysis units are continuously at risk. Just as constant, often more difficult to control, and much less publicized is the exposure of operating room staff to hepatitis viruses in blood, feces, saliva, and other secretions. Moreover, while the risk to surgeons is well recognized,[6,7] there is also a substantial risk to anesthesiologists and other operating room personnel removed from the surgical field. These risks can be understood more clearly in the context of newer concepts of hepatitis virology and modes of transmission.

CLASSIFICATION OF HEPATITIS VIRUSES

The terms *infectious hepatitis* and *serum hepatitis* have been used to define what we call today *viral hepatitis type A* and *type B*, respectively. We know now, however, that epidemiologic and clinical patterns of infection with these viruses often overlap and that the older, descriptive terms are both inadequate and misleading. Viral hepatitis is now classified by etiologic agent, when serologic testing can implicate one of the following.

Hepatitis A Virus

Hepatitis A virus (HAV) is a 27-nm. virus of unusual stability to heat, acid, and ether inactivation. Although insufficient information is available to classify it, hepatitis A virus shares features in common with enteroviruses. Infection with HAV results in a relatively mild acute hepatitis after an incubation period of 15 to 50 days. In addition to its short incubation period and mild acute stage, HAV illness rarely lasts more than 2 to 4 weeks, and the subclinical attack rate far exceeds the frequency of overt clinical illness. Until recently, much of our information about this virus was generated in epidemiologic studies and transmission experiments in volunteers, such as those in which the MS-1 strain was studied.[8] Accelerated progress followed the identification of the virus by immune electron microscopy[9] and the development of animal models, using marmoset monkeys and chimpanzees.

Hepatitis B Virus

Much has been learned about hepatitis B virus (HBV) in the years since the discovery of Australia antigen.[10] What was originally called *Australia antigen* is actually the coat protein of HBV, the antigenic specificity on the surface of the 42-nm. virion (Dane particle) and on the 20-nm. spheres and tubules. The latter appear in great abundance in serum of infected persons. Hepatitis virus is an unclassified DNA virus containing a circular double-stranded DNA genome and an endogenous HBV-specific, DNA-dependent DNA polymerase. Viral hepatitis type B accounts for a large proportion of cases initially labeled "serum hepatitis" but can also be implicated by current serologic techniques in approximately half of cases unrelated to percutaneous exposure to contaminated blood products. Asymptomatic chronic carriers serve as the major reservoir of infection and constitute approximately 0.1 per cent of the population in the United States and Western Europe. (Higher frequencies are found in tropical and underdeveloped areas.) Illness occurs after a long incubation period of 30 to 180 days and not uncommonly is heralded by a serum-sickness-like prodrome of arthritis and/or rash, and fever. Duration of illness is quite variable, but most individuals recover within approximately 3 to 4 months. On the other hand, fulminant hepatitis, persistent hepatitis, and chronic active hepatitis, as well as a protracted carrier state, follow acute type B hepatitis in a small percentage of cases. Several subtypes of HBV have been identified, but the subtype does not determine severity or chronicity of the illness.

Epstein-Barr Virus and Cytomegalovirus

Both Epstein-Barr virus (EBV) and cytomegalovirus (CMV) can produce hepatitis in humans as part of a generalized systemic illness,[11] and occasionally these agents are implicated serologically in an isolated case or in small outbreaks of hepatitis. CMV may be an important pathogen in liver disease following renal transplantation[12] but is rarely implicated in post-transfusion hepatitis, despite its frequent transmission in blood.[13] Indeed, virologic and serologic evidence of CMV transmission is as common in transfused patients without hepatitis as in those developing hepatitis. CMV can be found also in patients with post-transfusion hepatitis B infection.[14] Still, it is worth keeping these viral agents in mind when considering etiologic agents for hepatitis. Other viruses occasionally implicated in hepatitis, such as *Herpes simplex*, contribute even less than CMV and EBV and can be discounted, except in very unusual circumstances (see p. 707).

Non-A, Non-B Hepatitis

Until recently, only two human hepatitis viruses, HAV and HBV, were recognized; however, in many patients with hepatitis, failure of sensitive serologic tests to detect these two viruses or CMV and EBV, as well, suggests that another pathogen, or pathogens, exist. The diagnosis of non-A, non-B viral hepatitis requires not only negative HAV and HBV serology; also, hepatotoxic drug exposure must be ruled out, and there must be an incubation period and mode of transmission epidemiologically associated with viral hepatitis. To date, non-A, non-B hepatitis has been found to contribute to transfusion-associated hepatitis, multiple bouts of hepatitis in illicit drug users, and hepatitis following renal transplantation. In addition, cases of non-A, non-B hepatitis have appeared in hemodialysis units, within families and institutions, and in occupationally exposed medical personnel. Both short (2–4 weeks) and long (1–3 months) incubation periods have been recorded for cases occurring after percutaneous exposure; this, plus the occasional occurrence of two separate bouts of non-A, non-B hepatitis in the same patient, suggest that there may be more than one such viral agent. Clinically and epidemiologically, non-A, non-B hepatitis resembles HBV infection: It occurs after parenteral exposure, is highly endemic in some groups, but is not readily spread from person to person; it probably perpetuates itself through a human carrier state and contributes to chronic hepatitis. All of these observations have been derived from epidemiologic investigation, for no viral agents or serologic marker for any of these agents have been identified.[15,16]

IMMUNOLOGIC FEATURES OF AND DIAGNOSTIC TESTS FOR HEPATITIS VIRUSES

Hepatitis A Virus: Immunology and Diagnosis

Only one antigen, hepatitis A virus antigen (HAAg or HAV), has been identified and is associated with the surface of the 27-nm. virion. No serologic subtypes have been described. The virus and its antibody (anti-HAV) can be identified by several in vitro techniques (Table 55-1). Because reagents containing HAV—feces and liver from infected humans or nonhuman primates—are so difficult to obtain and susceptible animals so limited, these tests had been restricted to a few research laboratories but now are unavailable for routine use. Information about hepatitis A generated in these research laboratories has been useful in defining its epidemiology and modes of spread (see p. 702). For practical purposes, it is important to realize that HAV is excreted in the feces during the late incubation period but not significantly after the development of jaundice; HAV is not readily detected in blood, even though blood may be infectious; there is probably no asymptomatic chronic carrier state; anti-HAV is detected shortly after acute illness and persists for many years; and, the prevalence of exposure to HAV increases as a function of age, rendering immune more than 70 per cent of urban adults older than 50 years of age.[17–19]

Hepatitis B Virus: Immunology and Diagnosis

The presence of immunologic markers for hepatitis B virus constitutes the basis of diagnostic tests used to identify acute or chronic infection with this virus. HBsAg is associated with three morphological forms: 20-nm. spheres, tubules of the same diameter but of variable length, and the surface of the 42-nm. virion (Dane particle). Within the Dane particle is a 27-nm. core, hepatitis B core antigen (HBcAg), immunologically distinct from HBsAg and to which the host mounts a specific immune response.

For the detection of these viral antigens and the corresponding antibodies, there is a wide variety of serological techniques of varying sensitivity.[20] Among the more commonly used tests for HBsAg, radioimmunoassay is the most sensitive and the method used most commonly to screen donated blood before transfusion. Despite its sensitivity, however, radioimmunoassay does not detect HBsAg in blood at a particle concentration less than 10^6 per ml. and, therefore, fails to identify all HBsAg-positive serum. Unfortunately, more sensitive techniques are not routinely available. Other tests for HBsAg that are occasionally used are, in order of decreasing sensitivity, immune adherence hemagglutination, passive hemagglutination inhibition, complement fixation, counterelectrophoresis, and agar gel diffusion (Table 55-1). Antibody to HBsAg can be detected by a number of techniques that include, in order of increasing sensitivity, agar gel diffusion, counterelectrophoresis, complement fixation, immune adherence hemagglutination, passive hemagglutination, solid-phase radioimmunoassay, and radioimmunoprecipitation. Of these, a commercially available radioimmunoassay and a passive hemagglutination test are most commonly used.

Free HBcAg is not found circulating in the blood of either acutely or chronically infected individuals, but antibody to HBcAg (anti-HBc) can be detected by a variety of immunologic techniques (Table 55-1). Routine anti-HBc testing, however, is hindered by difficulties in obtaining adequate supplies of purified HBcAg; such testing by radioimmunoassay is now commercially available (Abbott Laboratories, North Chicago, Ill.).

Using the diagnostic techniques available, we can detect the following sequence of serologic events during a typical case of acute viral hepatitis type B (Fig. 55-1): Approximately 1 month after exposure, HBsAg is detectable in the blood, predating clinical and biochemical evidence of illness by several weeks. During HBs antigenemia around the time of clinically apparent illness, anti-HBc becomes detectable, but not until HBsAg disappears (2–4 months after it is first detectable) can anti-HBs be detected. Although anti-HBs is produced earlier during illness and can circulate complexed to HBsAg, it cannot be detected by standard serologic techniques until antibody excess is achieved. For practical purposes, then, detectable anti-HBs is a serologic marker of previous experience with HBV and has been shown to correlate with immunity to reinfection. Antibody to HBcAg can be detected during acute illness, as mentioned above, but also persists as an indicator of past infection. Titers of anti-HBc discriminate between acute and previous infection. Serum anti-HBc titers sufficiently high for detection by complement fixation are achieved during the ongoing viral replication of acute

Table 55-1. Viruses Associated With Hepatitis in Man

TYPE	NOMEN-CLATURE	ANTIGENS AND CORRESPONDING ANTIBODIES		INCUBATION PERIOD	TRANSMISSION	SEROLOGIC TESTS
A	Infectious hepatitis, short incubation. MS-1	Hepatitis A virus antigen (HAAg or HAV)	anti-HAV	15–50 days	Predominantly fecal-oral	1. Immune electron microscopy 2. Complement fixation 3. Immune adherence 4. Radioimmunoassay
B	Serum hepatitis, long incubation. MS-2	Hepatitis B surface antigen (HBsAg)	anti-HBs	30–180 days	Percutaneous inoculation. Intimate contact	HBsAg 1, 2, 3, 4, 5. counter electro-phoresis 6. agar gel diffusion
		Hepatitis B core antigen (HBcAg)	anti-HBc		Blood and blood products	Anti-HBs 2, 3,4, 5, 6 7. radio-immuno precipitation
		Hepatitis B e antigen (HBeAg)			Vertical (maternal-fetal)	Anti-HBc 2, 3, 4, 5, 7 HBeAg & anti-HBe 5, 6
			anti-HBe			
Non-A, Non-B		None identified		2–22 weeks	Similar to hepatitis B	None
CMV		CMV	anti-CMV	variable, 2–13 weeks (hepatitis occurs 3–4 mo. after transplantation)	Neonatal Intimate contact Transfusion Transplantation	Complement fixation Fluorescent antibody Neutralization
EBV		Viral capsid antigen (VCA)	anti-VCA	2–8 weeks	Intimate contact Transfusion	Heterophile antibody Immunofluorescence Anti-VCA
		Cell membrane antigen (MA)	anti-MA			Anti- MA
		Early antigen (EA)	anti-EA			Anti-EA
		Nuclear antigen (EBNA)	anti-EBNA			Complement fixation Anti-EBNA

infection; however, in patients without acute illness, such as those who have recovered from hepatitis B, the titer of anti-HBc is lower, often beneath the sensitivity threshold for complement fixation but detectable by more sensitive tests (e.g., immune adherence hemagglutination and radioimmunoassay).

There are several notable variations on this theme of typical serologic events. First, the time course outlined may be protracted or contracted.

Second, occasionally a patient does not develop detectable HBs antigenemia; his HBV illness can be identified by the detection of a primary anti-HBc or anti-HBs response during convalescence. The third and most important variation involves the patient who does not clear HBsAg but becomes a chronic HBsAg carrier. In approximately 5 to 10 per cent of acutely infected persons, HBsAg persists in the circulation for several months to 1 year. A small percentage of these

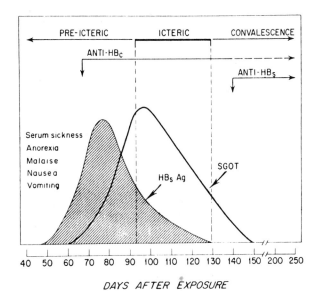

Fig. 55-1. Typical time relationships of clinical features, changes in SGOT levels, and appearance of hepatitis B antigen and antibodies. Anti-HB$_c$ is usually measurable during active infection and correlated with presence of HB$_s$Ag in serum. Anti-HB$_s$ has a variable appearance following recovery from acute hepatitis B. (Isselbacher, K. J., B. Adams, R. D., Braunwald, E., et al. (eds.): Harrison's Principles of Internal Medicine. ed. 9. p. 1462. New York, McGraw Hill, 1980)

become chronic HBsAg carriers indefinitely. In these persons, HBsAg remains detectable, and anti-HBc titers persist at a high level, consistent with a state of ongoing viral replication. Anti-HBs, however, the antibody that correlates with immunity, is not detectable.

A fourth serologic pattern worth mentioning is a secondary anti-HBs response: for example, an anamnestic antibody response that occurs when an anti-HBs-positive person is reexposed to HBV. Acute illness, HBs antigenemia, and anti-HBc titer rise do not occur, but there is a boost in serum anti-HBs titer.

In addition to HBsAg and HBcAg, a third antigen system has been identified with HBV infection. Hepatitis B associated e antigen (HBeAg) represents a group of antigens that have no known morphologic counterpart and that are immunologically distinct from HBsAg and HBcAg. Study of this system is hampered by the crudeness and insensitivity of tests for its identi-

fication (agar gel diffusion) and the paucity of potent reagents. If early acute phase serum is tested during HBV infection, HBeAg is present transiently in most cases; however, persistence of HBeAg correlates with other indicators of ongoing viral replication, infectivity, and ongoing liver disease. Preliminary reports indicate that the prognosis in HBeAg-positive cases of chronic HBV infection is less favorable than in HBeAg-negative or anti-HBe-positive cases. There is much to be learned about this new immunologic marker. Indeed, correlations with chronicity and severity of liver disease are not absolute, and tests of HBeAg cannot replace morphologic studies in estimating activity of chronic liver disease associated with HBV.

To reiterate the significance of detectable HBsAg, we should recall that HBs antigenemia can be seen in several different clinical settings: In patients with acute or chronic liver disease, the presence of HBsAg indicates HBV infection; asymptomatic HBsAg-positive persons may be carrying the virus during the prodromal period of an evolving acute illness, during the period of early convalescence after a symptomatic illness before antigen clearing, during an acute asymptomatic illness, or as chronic HBsAg carriers; among carriers, there is a clinical spectrum ranging from normal liver function, to minimal hepatocellular abnormalities, to chronic active liver disease, and to cirrhosis. Although there are reports linking infectivity with severity of liver disease in chronic carriers, these correlations have not been confirmed by other investigators. Indeed, asymptomatic HBsAg-positive hemodialysis patients with normal liver function and morphology are often highly infectious. For practical purposes, all HBsAg-positive patients and their secretions should be considered potentially infectious, for excess viral coat material and the complete infectious virion are almost always present together.

Epstein-Barr Virus and Cytomegalovirus: Immunology and Diagnosis

Unlike the hepatitis viruses, both of these herpes viruses can be cultivated in vitro, and a diagnosis can be made by virus isolation in cell culture. Like hepatitis viruses, EBV and CMV can be identified serologically. Several strains of CMV have been isolated that do not show complete antigenic homology, but a number of serologic tests are used for detection of anti-CMV (Table 55-1). For EBV, a complex array of antigens has been identified in various EBV lymphoblastoid lines (Table 55-1). Four major categories exist: viral capsid antigens; cell membrane antigens, both early and late; early antigens, both diffuse and restricted; and nuclear antigen, the reactive component in soluble complement fixing antigens. During acute EBV infection, the titers of antibody to the first three antigens appear, whereas antibody to nuclear antigen does not appear for weeks to months after acute illness. Immunofluorescence techniques are used to study the first three, and complement fixation, to study the latter antibody response.[21] Beyond the scope of this chapter, there are many complexities of the immune response to CMV and, especially, EBV.

In patients with hepatitis after transfusion or renal transplantation, EBV and CMV antibody responses are assessed by immunofluorescence and complement fixation, respectively; however, such studies have not implicated these viruses definitively in these settings (Table 55-1).

Non-A, Non-B Hepatitis: Immunology and Diagnosis

Because no viral agent or immunologic marker has been detected in these cases of hepatitis, no data are available to define the humoral immune response (Table 55-1).

TRANSMISSION OF VIRAL HEPATITIS AND ITS NOSOCOMIAL IMPLICATIONS

Traditional distinctions between fecal-oral transmission of "infectious" hepatitis A and parenterally spread "serum" hepatitis B were shattered by the application of new serologic techniques to epidemiologic investigation. Most striking is the finding that in approximately 50 per cent of cases without antecedent overt percutaneous inoculation, HBV can be implicated serologically.[22] Because of the high HBsAg serum titers achieved in HBV infection, because of the

development of sensitive serologic tests for detection of HBV infection, and because of wide availability of these tests, there is an enormous amount of new information about the ecology of this virus. Many inferences can be drawn from these new discoveries about the transmission of HBV. Hepatitis B surface antigen has been detected in virtually every body secretion, including saliva, urine, semen, cerebrospinal fluid, pleural fluid, sweat, and tears, and several non-percutaneous modes of spread have been suggested. These include oral, venereal, vertical (from mother to fetus), contact, aerosol, and arthropod-borne transmission. Although these potential modes of spread are unproven, and although covert percutaneous inoculation may be occurring in many of these situations, the epidemiologic evidence supporting the potential risk from these body fluids and modes of spread is growing progressively more convincing. Moreover, HBV is so stable that it can be recovered from contaminated environmental surfaces long after HBsAg-positive blood or body fluid has dried.[23]

Thus, aside from overt percutaneous inoculation with an HBsAg-contaminated needle or scalpel, there are many other avenues for infection of operating room staff exposed frequently to blood and body fluids. In support of this increased risk are anecdotal and published reports of hepatitis B among surgical teams[6] and a high prevalence of anti-HBs (indicative of prior HBV infection) in operating room personnel. In many serologic surveys of hospital personnel, surgeons and operating room staff ranked highest in serologic evidence of exposure. Pattison found the highest anti-HBs prevalence (29%) in operating room personnel[3]; surgical specialists compared to medical specialists had a much higher prevalence of HBV exposure (22.4 vs. 13.6%) in another study.[24] In a survey of 70 anesthesiologists on our staff, we found that 20 per cent gave a history of clinical hepatitis, 12 per cent had detectable anti-HBs by radioimmunoprecipitation, but none were HBsAg-positive.[25] This is not unexpected if possible modes of exposure are considered. Anesthesiologists often insert intravenous catheters, administer injections, obtain arterial blood gases, insert Foley catheters, administer spinal anesthesia, insert their hands into patients' mouths during intubation, and are present in the operating room where blood is aerosolized. Furthermore, as our survey showed, 96 per cent of 70 anesthesiologists reported that they sustained needle punctures during their work and noted frequent cuts on their hands, both of which are potential routes of virus inoculation.

Transmission of HBV is a risk not only when the surgical patient is a known HBsAg carrier, but also (and even more so) when that patient is an *unidentified* HBsAg carrier. In the latter situation, no special precautions are instituted. In studies of HBsAg among routine hospital admissions, investigators have reported prevalences of 0.8 to 1.5 per cent, far in excess of the 0.1 to 0.2 per cent found in the general population.[5,26,27] Furthermore, 90 per cent of these HBsAg-positive patients were admitted for reasons unrelated to hepatitis, and the risk to hospital personnel would have remained undetected if these HBsAg screening surveys had not been done. Certainly some of these unidentified carriers come to surgery and contribute to the insidious hazard. From these data, it seems wise to treat every patient's blood and secretions as potentially infectious for HBV. In addition, the possible presence of non-A, non-B hepatitis agents that we cannot identify makes scrupulous avoidance of unprotected contact with body fluids even more important.

As mentioned, non-A, non-B hepatitis appears to share many common modes of transmission and epidemiologic features with HBV. Most important, these agents are transmitted readily by blood transfusion (90% of transfusion-associated hepatitis today is non-A, non-B),[15] and epidemiologic evidence suggests that there is an asymptomatic chronic carrier state for non-A, non-B hepatitis. Given the correlation between blood contact and HBV exposure among health care personnel, and given the similarities between type B hepatitis and non-A, non-B hepatitis, it is reasonable to assume that hospital employees are exposed to the non-A, non-B hepatitis agent, or agents. Lacking a serologic tool to identify viral antigens and antibodies, however, we cannot speculate further about spread of these agents in the operating suite. Both EBV and CMV are transmitted by intimate contact and by blood transfusion and, therefore, theoretically can be a threat to hospital personnel; however, in practice, such occurrences are not common. For HAV, transmission by the fecal-oral route predominates. Because there appears to be no asymptomatic chronic carrier state and because natural transmission (except in experimental inoculation studies) has never been demonstrated by way of blood or percutaneous routes, the risk of HAV infection to operating room personnel is inconsequential. For hospital personnel, then, the major identified risk is from HBV, and susceptibility correlates directly with extent of exposure to patients' body fluids, most notably, blood.

PREVENTIVE MEASURES IN THE OPERATING ROOM

Although all body fluids should be handled with caution, surgeons and anesthesiologists should attempt to identify HBsAg carriers (see the list below).

Patients at High Risk for HBsAg Carriage

Drug abusers
Hemodialysis and renal transplant patients
Patients with diseases such as Down's syndrome, hepatic cancer, polyarteritis
Male homosexuals
Immunosuppressed patients (e.g., patients with immunodeficiency diseases, malignancies)
Patients with liver disease
Multiply transfused patients
Chronically institutionalized persons (e.g., prisoners, mentally retarded)
Immigrants or visitors from tropical areas

When known HBsAg-positive patients are treated in surgical suites, the following measures are thought to minimize infection of staff and other patients (see the list below):

All reusable contaminated instruments, including laryngoscopes, airways, and endotracheal tubes, and linens should be either autoclaved or gas-sterilized (with ethylene oxide), and disposable items should be autoclaved before discarding.

Contaminated surfaces that cannot be sterilized should be washed with 0.5- to 1.0-per-cent sodium hypochlorite, formalin, or gluteraldehyde.

Ungloved hand contact with the patient's skin, mucous membranes, and body fluids should be avoided.

Surgical specimens should be placed carefully in containers and labelled as biohazardous. Double-bagging in plastic is advisable.

Ideally, HBsAg and anti-HBs screening among operating room staff at regular intervals should be done to identify increases in exposure that require investigation and intervention.[28,29]

Measures to Minimize Risks of Handling Infected or High-Risk Patients in the Operating Room

Gowns, gloves, caps, plastic overshoes should be worn by anyone in contact with patients.

Disposable materials, such as syringes, sheets, pillows, and tracheal tubes, should be used whenever possible.

Unnecessary circulation in the room should be prevented.

Buckets containing hypochlorite should be used for all disposable and contaminated material; hypochlorite should be added to trap bottle on suction line.

Use of induction or recovery room should be avoided.

HBsAg-positive patients should be scheduled last to avoid exposure of other patients.

All disposable surgical and anesthetic items should be incinerated.

Special caution should be exercised when handling or disposing of contaminated sharp objects.

Surgical specimens should be carefully wrapped and labelled as biohazardous.

Reusable contaminated instruments (e.g., laryngoscopes, airways,) and linens should be autoclaved or gas-sterilized (with ethylene oxide) before washing.

Contaminated surfaces and equipment that cannot be sterilized (e.g., walls, floors, anesthesia machine, ventilator) should be washed with hypochlorite, formalin, or gluteraldehyde.

IMMUNOPROPHYLAXIS OF VIRAL HEPATITIS

Currently, trials are underway in experimental animals and humans to evaluate the safety and efficacy of a HBV vaccine prepared from HBsAg purified from the blood of chronic carriers. Although preliminary results are encouraging, several more years of testing must take place before HBV vaccination is approved for routine use in humans. In the interim, the alternatives of passive immunization with standard immune serum globulin or a hepatitis B hyperimmune globulin (containing very high titers of anti-HBs) are available.

Standard immune serum globulin is recommended for situations in which exposure at a relatively constant rate occurs, such as in hemodialysis units. Because such a high exposure rate has not been demonstrated in operating rooms, current recommendations do not include routine globulin administration to staffs of surgical theaters. On the other hand, should an operating room employee suffer a percutaneous exposure during surgery or ingest blood or secretions from a HBsAg-positive patient, he should be treated with high-titer anti-HBs hepatitis B immune globulin (HBIG), recently licensed for such use by the Food and Drug Administration. Recommended dosage is 0.06 ml. per kg., intramuscularly, immediately, repeated 1 month later.[30]

Although it is unlikely that exposure to HAV will occur in the operating room, should such exposure become apparent, immunoprophylaxis consists of standard immune serum globulin with an intramuscular dose of 0.02 ml. per kg.[30] Data concerning immunoprophylaxis of non-A, non-B hepatitis are insufficient, and recognition of the disease is too difficult at present for recommendation of passive immunization. There are no practical immunoprophylactic measures for EBV and CMV infection.

REFERENCES

1. Trumbull, M. L., and Greiner, D. J.: Homologous serum jaundice: an occupational hazard to medical personnel. J.A.M.A., *145*:965, 1951.
2. Williams, S. V., Huff, J. C., Feinglass, E. J., et al.: Epidemic viral hepatitis type B in hospital personnel. Am. J. Med., *57*:904, 1974.
3. Pattison, C. P., Maynard, J. E., Berquist, K. R., et al.: Epidemiology of hepatitis B in hospital personnel. Am. J. Epidemiol., *101*:59, 1975.
4. Leers, W. D., and Kouroupis, G. M.: Prevalence of hepatitis B antibodies in hospital personnel. Can. Med. Assoc. J., *113*:844, 1975.

5. Center for Disease Control. Hepatitis Surveillance Report #40. pp. 18–24. U.S. Department of Health, Education and Welfare Public Health Service, Atlanta, Georgia, 1977.
6. Rosenberg, J. L., Jones, D. P., Lipitz, L. R., et al.: Viral hepatitis: an occupational hazard to surgeons. J.A.M.A., *223*:395, 1973.
7. Jordan, G. L.: Hepatitis—the surgeons' disease. Am. J. Surg., *127*:629, 1974.
8. Krugman, S., Ward, R., and Giles, J. P.: The natural history of infectious hepatitis. Am. J. Med., *32*:717, 1962.
9. Feinstone, S. M., Kapikian, A. Z., and Purcell, R. H.: Hepatitis A: detection by immune electron microscopy of a virus-like antigen associated with acute illness. Science, *182*:1026, 1973.
10. Blumberg, B. S., Alter, H. J., and Visnich, S.: A "new" antigen in leukemia sera. J.A.M.A., *191*:541, 1965.
11. Stern, H.: Cytomegalovirus and EB virus infections of the liver. Br. Med. Bull., *28*:180, 1972.
12. Fiala, M., Payne, J. E., Berne, T. V., et al.: Epidemiology of cytomegalovirus infection after transplantation and immunosupression. J. Infect. Dis., *132*:421, 1975.
13. Prince, A. M., Szmuness, W., Millian, S. J., et al.: A serologic study of cytomegalovirus infections associated with blood transfusions. N. Engl. J. Med., *284*:1125, 1971.
14. Purcell, R. H., Walsh, J. H., Holland, P. V., et al.: Seroepidemiological studies of transfusion-associated hepatitis. J. Infect. Dis., *123*:406, 1971.
15. Feinstone, S. M., and Purcell, R. H.: Non-A, non-B hepatitis. Annu. Rev. Med., *29*:359, 1978.
16. Blumberg, B. S.: Non-A, non-B hepatitis. Ann. Intern. Med., *87*:111, 1977.
17. Dienstag, J. L., Feinstone, S. M., Kapikian, A. Z., et al.: Fecal shedding of hepatitis A antigen. Lancet, *1*:765, 1975.
18. Purcell, R. H., Dienstag, J. L., Feinstone, S. M., et al.: Relationship of hepatitis A antigen to viral hepatitis. Am. J. Med. Sci., *270*:61, 1975.
19. Dienstag, J. L., Szmuness, W., Stevens, C. E., et al.: Hepatitis A virus infection: new insights from seroepidemiologic studies. J. Infect. Dis., *137*:328, 1978.
20. Barker, L. F., Gerety, R. J., Hoofnagle, J. H., et al.: Viral hepatitis, type B: detection and prophylaxis. In Greenwalt, T. J., and Jamieson, G. A. (eds.): Transmissible Disease and Blood Transfusion. pp. 81–111. New York, Grune & Stratton, 1975.
21. Henle, W., Henle, G., and Horwitz, C. A.: Epstein-Barr virus diagnostic tests in infectious mononucleosis. Human Pathol., *5*:551, 1974.
22. Prince, A. M., Hargrove, R. L., Szmuness, W., et al.: Immunologic distinction between infectious and serum hepatitis. N. Engl. J. Med., *282*:987, 1970.
23. Favero, M. S., Bond, W. W., Petersen, N. J., et al.: Detection methods for study of the stability of hepatitis B antigen on surfaces. J. Infect. Dis., *129*:210, 1974.
24. Smith, J. L., Maynard, J. E., Berquist, K. R., et al.: Comparative risk of hepatitis B among physicians and dentists. J. Infect. Dis., *133*:705, 1976.
25. Mathieu, A., Battit, G. E., Huggins, C., et al.: Viral hepatitis—hazard to anesthesiologists—a prospective study. pp. 85–86. Abstracts of Scientific Papers, American Society of Anesthesiologists Annual Meeting, Washington, D.C., 1974.
26. Linneman, C. C., Hegg, M. E., Ramundo, N., et al.: Screening hospital patients for hepatitis B surface antigen. Am. J. Clin. Pathol., *67*:257, 1977.
27. Feinman, S. V., Krassnitzky, O., Sinclair, J. C., et al.: Prevalence and significance of hepatitis B surface antigen in a general hospital. Can. Med. Assoc. J., *112*:43, 1973.
28. Snydman, D. R., Bryan, J. A., and Dixon, R. E.: Prevention of nosocomial viral hepatitis, type B (hepatitis B). Ann. Intern. Med., *83*:838, 1975.
29. Committee on Viral Hepatitis, Division of Medical Sciences, National Academy Science—National Research Council, Public Health Service Advisory Committee on Immunization Practices: perspectives on the control of viral hepatitis, type B. Morbid. Mortal. Weekly Rep., *25* [Suppl.]:3, 1976.
30. ———:Immune globulins for protection against viral hepatitis. Morbid. Mortal. Weekly Rep., *30*:423, 1981.

FURTHER READING

Aach, R. D.: Viral Hepatitis—Update 1976. Viewpoints Dig. Dis., *8*:1, 1976.
Byas, G. N., Cohen, S. N., and Schmid, R. (eds.): Viral Hepatitis. Philadelphia, Franklin Institute Press, 1978.
Gerety, R. J. (ed.): Non-A, Non-B Hepatitis. New York, Academic Press, 1981.
Krugman, S., and Gocke, D. J.: Viral Hepatitis. Philadelphia, W. B. Saunders, Company, 1978.
Melneck, J. L., Dreesman, G. R., and Hollinger, F. B.: Viral Hepatitis. Sci. Am., *237*:44, 1977.
Proceedings of a Symposium on Viral Hepatitis. Am. J. Med. Sci., *270*:1, 1975.
WHO Expert Committee on Viral Hepatitis: Advances in viral hepatitis. WHO Technical Report Series 602 (WHO, Geneva, Switzerland), 1977.

56 Herpetic Whitlow

Fredrick K. Orkin, M.D.

Herpetic whitlow is an uncommon but painful and temporarily disabling finger infection caused by herpes simplex virus (HSV). Among the many curious facets of this infection is its occurrence almost exclusively among anesthesia personnel and other health-care personnel whose work exposes them to upper respiratory tract secretions. The lesion resembles a pyogenic infection so closely that it is usually subjected to unwarranted surgical intervention that only compounds the morbidity of what is a benign, self-limiting disease. This chapter reviews the epidemiology, clinical features, management, and prevention of this occupational hazard to anesthesia personnel.

THE PATHOGEN

A virus has been characterized as "the ultimate form of intracellular parasite, stripped to the barest essentials necessary for its own propagation."[1] Lacking metabolic systems, it is wholly dependent upon the host cell that it infects for the means to carry on activities characterizing living organisms, such as replication. The virus is essentially a small package of genes, which in the case of the HSV consists of double-stranded DNA of a specific composition, to program the host cell's metabolic systems for viral replication. Hence, the virus is an obligatory intracellular parasite.

The genetic material comprises the dense *core* of the virus. The core is surrounded by a protective coat composed of protein arranged in hexago-

nal clusters that collectively resemble a modern geodesic sphere; this coat is termed the *capsid*. It is surrounded, in turn, by a lipid-containing protein *envelope*. Small differences in DNA composition differentiate HSV type 1 from type 2.

Upon contact with a susceptible cell, the virus undergoes phagocytosis (viropexis) and once inside the cell, digestion of the capsid and envelope. The free viral DNA enters the cell's nucleus where the viral DNA is replicated by means of the host enzyme systems. The newly synthesized DNA is covered with viral protein synthesized in the cytoplasm from scavenged host protein. Within 10 hours, an infected cell lyses, releasing as many as 100 infectious virus particles which repeat the process.

PATHOGENESIS OF HERPETIC INFECTIONS

HSV has a predilection for cells of ectodermal origin (e.g., skin, mucous membrane, eye). The portal of entry and host factors determine the particular manifestation of the *primary illness*—for example, herpes labialis ("cold sore"), gingivostomatitis, keratoconjunctivitis, meningoencephalitis, vulvovaginitis, and generalized visceral disease. True to its ancient Greek name which means "to creep," herpes spreads locally and usually superficially from cell to cell. Multinucleated giant cells appear with balloon degeneration of the nucleus and Cowdry type A intranuclear inclusion bodies. Upon lysis of the infected cells, host white cells arrive to remove debris, and an inflammatory response results. In the midst of the debris, the lesion characteristic of superficial HSV infection appears, a thin-walled vesicle on an inflammatory base.

As infection proceeds, lymphatics drain infectious material and debris to regional lymph nodes. Protective antibodies, interferon, and sensitized "killer" lymphocytes are produced to stem the spread of infection. In the absence of competent immune mechanisms, viremia soon disseminates the infection throughout the body. Among the many disease states[2] characterized by impaired immune mechanisms and susceptibility to disseminated HSV infection are malignancy (especially hematologic[3–5]), other causes of malnutrition (e.g., kwashiorkor[6,7]), associated infectious disease (e.g., measles,[7,8] *H. influenzae*[9]), thermal burns,[10] defective cell-mediated immunity (e.g., Wiskott-Aldrich syndrome,[11] thymic dysplasia[12]), drug-induced immunosuppression (e.g., transplantation,[13–14] asthma[15]), prematurity,[16] and pregnancy.[17] Without vigorous supportive measures and specific antiviral chemotherapy, disseminated HSV infection is usually fatal. Mild immune deficiency can result in chronic herpetic infection.[18,19]

Under normal circumstances, this primary infection subsides any HSV cannot be detected. However, HSV persists in a *latent* state within the sensory nerve ganglion associated with the sensory nerves innervating the site of infection.[20–22] Within the ganglion the only identifiable portion of the virus is its DNA which, given an appropriate stimulus, migrates peripherally along the sensory nerve. Although various mechanisms have been advanced to explain HSV latency and reactivation,[23–27] none have been proven. Among the diverse factors associated with reactivation of latent HSV are fever,[28] menstruation,[29] corticosteriod[30] or foreign protein[29] administration, emotional stress,[31] and sunlight. Another factor worthy of particular note is surgery of the trigeminal nerve,[32–34] which Cushing first described.[35] Reactivation of HSV results in a *recurrent* infection in the vicinity of the primary infection. Generally, the symptomatology accompanying a recurrence is milder than that associated with the primary infection.

Figure 56-1 summarizes the possible courses that infection with HSV can take.

EPIDEMIOLOGY OF HERPETIC INFECTIONS

HSV is unbiquitous and worldwide in its distribution. Although experimental animals can be infected, man is the only known reservoir. The principal mode of spread is by direct contact with infected secretions. HSV type 1 is spread primarily by contact with oral secretions, whereas type 2 is spread by contact with genital secretions. Until recently it had been taught that HSV type 1 causes infections "above the belt" and type 2, "below the belt"; however, it is now recognized that there are no strict boundaries.[36–38] Hand infections are associated with either type.[36, 40, 41] The incubation period for both types ranges from 2 to 12 days, with illness usually appearing 3 to 9 days following infection.

The fetus and infant through about 6 months of age are protected by transplacental maternal antibodies. Between 6 months and 5 years of age, infections with and antibody response to HSV type 1 are frequent. By the age of 15, as much as 96 per cent of the population possesses type-specific antibody, depending upon the socioeconomic conditions.[42] Whereas 80 per cent to 100 per cent of adults in lower socioeconomic groups possesses antibodies to type 1, only 30 per cent to 50 per cent of those in higher classes exhibits seroconversion.[36] Infection with HSV type 2 is also related to age and socioeconomic status. Infection and seroconversion increase rapidly only after age 14; among adults of upper socioeconomic groups, type-specific antibody is found in 10 per cent, whereas it is present in 20 per cent to 60 per cent of those in lower classes.[36] Yet, perhaps only 10 per cent to 15 per cent of infected individuals have experienced clinical illness as a result of the primary infection.[28] Since most primary infections lead to *subclinical* disease, it is impossible to assess the susceptibility of a given person to HSV infection without antibody testing. Similarly, because virus continues to be shed

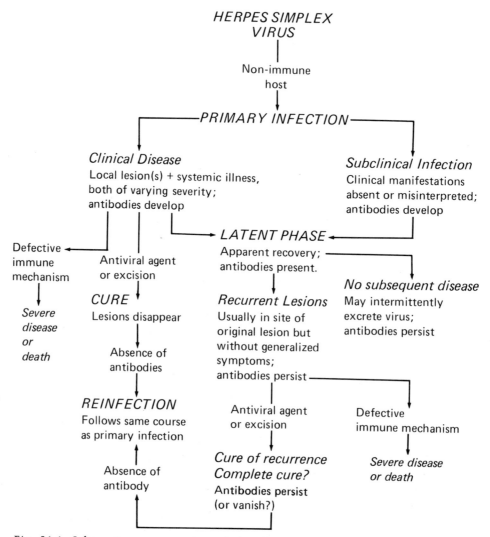

Fig. 56-1. Schematic representation of the diverse clinical courses HSV infection can take. (Modified from Juel-Jensen, B. E., and MacCallum, F. O.: Herpes Simplex, Varicella and Zoster: Clinical Manifestations and Treatment. p. 32. Philadelphia, J. B. Lippincott Company, 1972.)

for several months following recovery from infection, it is impossible to be certain that a given individual is definitely not a reservoir of HSV.

HERPETIC WHITLOW

Herpetic infection of the finger is probably not rare, although likely to be misdiagnosed. Recognized only during the past 20 years as an occupa-

tional hazard among certain health-care personnel, it was described decades earlier. Typically, the patient suffered an injury, inapparent or overt, to the finger which was then contaminated by oral secretions. One of the earliest reports described four children who had developed pinhead-sized vesicles resembling those usually seen with herpes febrilis ("cold sores") near the tips of a finger. Two of the children also had similar lesions of the lower lip, suggesting self-contamination, and another had had repeated eruptions at the same site.[43] Subsequent case reports highlighted other clinical aspects. The coalescence of several similar vesicles on the finger of a hairdresser, who probably traumatized it on a curling iron, resulted in a painful bullous lesion resembling bacterial infection; upon incision, however, no pus was found. The lesion recurred several times, sometimes with a prodromal neuralgia of the arm, and virus was isolated.[44] A similar lesion occurred in a child who had sucked her finger when she has gingivostomatitis.[45] Similarly, another report suggested that an eruption on an infant's hand following trauma resulted from contamination with either the child's own saliva or that of one of her parents (who had "kissed the hurt"). [46]

In contrast, the finger infection occurring in adults has been reported almost exclusively among health-care personnel who suffer trivial or inapparent injury and whose occupation exposes them to oral secretions. Stern was the first to identify the lesion as an occupational hazard after reviewing 54 such infections occurring in nurses between the ages of 18 and 29 years.[47] Reflecting their origin among the upper socioeconomic classes, half of the nurses had no antibody to HSV prior to beginning work, and one-third of this group developed lesions (primary illness) within a year. Other nurses with moderate antibody titers developed lesions (recurrence) as well. Most of the lesions developed during the care of patients lacking clinical evidence of HSV infection. Stern isolated HSV from 1.2 per cent of asymptomatic adults and 6.5 per cent of postoperative neurosurgical patients, many of whom were comatose and required frequent oropharyngeal suctioning. Seven nurses experienced recurrences.

Stern termed the lesion a *whitlow* (synonym—felon) to emphasize its resemblance to pyogenic infection such as the familiar paronychia. With or without surgical intervention, secondary bacterial infection was common but resistant to antibiotics even when isolates demonstrated *in vitro* sensitivity. Although most of his patients presented with vesicles that permitted a clinical diagnosis, others had large bullous lesions when

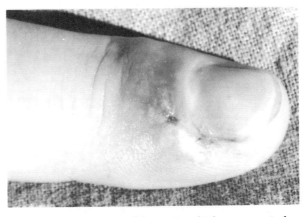

Fig. 56-2. Appearance of herpetic whitlow on an index finger of an intensive care nurse at day five when a periungual blister surrounded by erythema had formed from the coalescence of vesicles. Note the proximity of the lesion to the minor trauma in the cuticle.

first seen. Constitutional symptoms such as fever and lymphadenopathy were uncommon, though pain and the natural course of the illness resulted in a loss of an average of 3 weeks' work per nurse.

More recently, others have reported this lesion occurring in surgeons,[48–51] nurses,[41,48–50,52–55] dentists,[41,55–57] and anesthesiologists[58,59]—all personnel whose work exposed them to oral secretions. Usually the constitutional symptoms were more prominent than those in Stern's report, including fever, lymphangitis, lymphadenopathy, and malaise. This difference in symptomatology is probably more apparent than real since these reports described persons who sought care, whereas Stern's included all cases. The finger lesion can serve as the reservoir for self-inoculation of the eye[60] and oropharynx.[59,61, 62]

Although the development of the lesion can be insidious, a progression of symptomatology and signs is often evident. Intense itching and pain are followed within a day by the appearance of a vesicle with surrounding erythema at the site of minor injury at the finger tip (Fig. 56-2). Satellite vesicles appear during the next 7 to 10 days and often coalesce to form a yellow, honeycombed structure. Although the contained fluid is clear and yellowish at first, within a week if becomes cloudy, and the lesion becomes a grayish blister

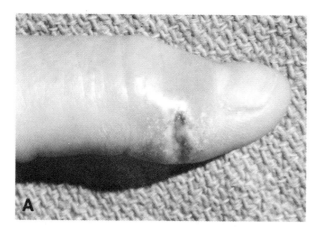

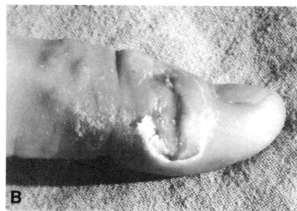

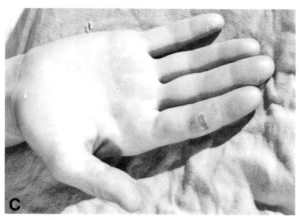

Fig. 56-3. Another early lesion on the thumb of an anesthesiology resident, which has been subjected to incision and drainage *(A)*, with subsequent bacterial infection and ulceration of the lesion one week later *(B)*, at which time satellite vesicles appeared proximal to the superinfected lesion. After two weeks, satellite lesions appeared over both the thumb and adjacent finger *(C)*. Note also the numerous sites of trauma on other fingers.

(Fig. 56-3). Throbbing pain becomes prominent as the distal portion of the involved finger, now erythematous, if not violaceous, swells. During the third week, the pain abates and the lesions become encrusted. Desquamation of superficial layers of the skin occurs, with complete healing after 3 weeks. Many reports emphasize that needless surgical intervention only ensures bacterial superinfection and prolongs the clinical course.

DIAGNOSIS OF HERPETIC WHITLOW

Generally the lesion can be identified upon clinical grounds alone such as the appearance of the lesion. Although often absent, a history of trauma at the site of infection and an exposure to a source of HSV are helpful. Definitive diagnosis is established by HSV isolation and identification with virus-specific antiserum, demonstration of multinucleated giant epithelial cells or nuclear inclusion bodies in smears taken from the base of a vesicle (Tzank technic), and a four-fold rise in HSV antibody titers in convalescent serum. If the presumed diagnosis of herpetic whitlow is not supported, then one must consider paronychia due to bacteria (e.g., *staphylococcus, streptococcus*) or fungus (e.g., *C albicans*), as well as deep fungal infections such as histoplasmosis, blastomycosis, or coccidiomycosis.

TREATMENT OF HERPETIC WHITLOW

GENERAL CONSIDERATIONS

Therapy should be conservative, consisting of immobilization, elevation, and analgesia. Although particularly tense, painful vesicles may be incised, deep incision is contraindicated. Should lymphangitis appear, penicillin administration is indicated.

SPECIFIC MEASURES

Much of what is known about specific therapy for herpetic whitlow has been gleaned from clinical experience and investigation with the more common and serious HSV infections, such as keratitis, meningoencephalitis, and visceral herpetic infection. Although controlled clinical trials have been conducted with specific therapy in these diseases, there have been no rigorous studies of the clinical efficacy of the potential specific therapies in herpetic whitlow. In addition, patients often do not present themselves for treatment at the onset of the illness when it is possible to alter and possibly abort the progression of signs and symptoms.[63]

ANTIVIRAL CHEMOTHERAPY

This category includes nucleoside derivatives that interfere with HSV DNA replication. The topical application of idoxuridine (IDU, 5-iodo-2'-deoxyuridine) has proved effective in the treatment of HSV keratitis[64]; but without a carrier substance, it does not appear to be efficacious in the treatment of herpetic whitlow. However, it has been effective when applied as a solution of 5% IDU in dimethyl sulfoxide (DMSO)[65]; unfortunately, DMSO is not available for clinical use in the United States. A nucleoside derivative that is effective in HSV keratitis[66,67] and meningoencephalitis,[68] and even against IDU-resistant infections, is adenine arabinoside (vidrabine Ara-A, 9-B-D-arabinofuranosyladenine). In currently available topical preparations, adenine arabinoside is not effective in the treatment of herpetic whitlow,[69,70] perhaps because of the low solubility of this substance in the solvent used. A glucose analog, 2-deoxy-D-glucose, has been found effective in genital skin infections when applied as a cream.[71] Other agents recently found to be effective in HSV keratitis—such as acyclovir (9-2[2-hydroxyethoxymethyl]guanine)[72] and trifluridine—have not been studied in HSV skin infections.

These nucleoside analogs are activated by a virus-specific enzyme (thymidine kinase); poor substrates for healthy cells, these substances are more selective for virus-infected cells and less toxic to normal cells. Acyclovir has recently been released in an ointment that deserves a trial in herpetic skin infections.

INTERFERON

This protein, produced by stimulated white cells, induces an antiviral state. It has been found effective in the topical therapy of herpetic keratitis[73] and, when administered intramuscularly, in the prevention of recurrence of skin lesions following surgery on the trigeminal root.[74] Limited supply of interferon has precluded its use in herpetic whitlow.

SURGERY

Superficial epidermal excision of recurrent herpetic whitlow within 36 hours of its appearance appears to prevent recurrence at the given site in almost all cases.[75]

A variety of potential therapies have been found to be ineffective in recent years: topical application of diethyl ether[76,77] and chloroform,[78] presumably to dissolve the lipid-containing viral envelope, parenteral administration of nonspecific immunoenhancers such as Bacillus Calmette-Guerin (BCG)[79] and levamisole,[80] and the application of heterotricyclic dyes with exposure to ultraviolet light (photodynamic inactivation).[81]

PREVENTION OF HERPETIC WHITLOW

Given the ubiquity of HSV and the frequency of minor or inapparent finger trauma, it is impossible to prevent the occurrence of herpetic whitlow in young, nonimmune health-care personnel without having them wear surgical gloves when working in contact with oropharyngeal secretions. However, such a practice is indefensible on economic grounds. Instead, one should be able to prevent the majority of potential exposures to infectious HSV by protecting one's hands when caring for patients particularly likely to be harboring HSV, as shown in the following.

Clinical Reservoir States for HSV

Malignant disease (especially hematologic)
Malnutrition (e.g., kwashiorkor)
Infectious disease (e.g., measles, *H. influenzae*)
Defective cell-mediated immunity
Thermal burns
Drug-induced immunosuppression (e.g., transplantation, asthma)
Overt HSV infection
Convalescence from recent HSV infection
Young children

Now that a potentially effective antiviral agent, acyclovir, is available, it is particularly important to treat the lesion at the earliest time in order to prevent its natural course, including the possibility of recurrence.[63] In addition, since unwarranted surgical intervention prolongs the course of this lesion, considerable morbidity can be avoided by resisting the urge to incise and drain the lesion.

REFERENCES

1. Fenwick, M. L.: Viruses and viral infection. 1. The nature of viruses and their growth. *In* Florey, L. (ed.): General Pathology, ed. 4. pp. 898–913. Philadelphia, W. B. Saunders Company, 1970.
2. Buss, D. H., and Scharyj, M.: Herpes virus infection of the esophagus and other visceral organs in adults: Incidence and clinical significance. Am. J. Med., 66:457, 1979.
3. Muller, S. A., Herrmann, E. C., Jr., and Winkelmann, R. K.: Herpes simplex infections in hematologic malignancies. Am. J. Med., 52:102, 1972.
4. Castleman, B., Scully, R. E., and McNeely, B. U.: Case 37-1975. N. Engl. J. Med., 293:598, 1975.
5. Castleman, B., Scully, R. E., and McNeely, B. U.: Case 12-1976. N. Engl. J. Med., 294:658, 1976.
6. McKenzie, D., Hansen, J. D. L., and Becker, W.: Herpes simplex virus infection: Dissemination in association with malnutrition. Arch. Dis. Child., 34:250, 1959.
7. Becker, W. B., Kipps, A., and McKenzie, D.: Disseminated herpes simplex virus infection: Its pathogenesis based upon virological and pathological studies in 33 cases. Am. J. Dis. Child., 115:1, 1968.
8. Kipps, A., Becker, W., Wainwright, J., et al.: Fatal disseminated primary herpes infection in children: Epidemiology based upon 93 non-neonatal cases. S. Afr. Med. J., 41:647, 1967.
9. Jaworski, M. A., Moffatt, M. E. K., and Ahronheim, G. A.: Disseminated herpes simplex associated with *H. influenzae* infection in a previously healthy child. J. Pediatr., 96:426, 1980.
10. Foley, F. D., Greenwald, K. A., Nash, G., et al.: Herpesvirus infection in burned patients. N. Engl. J. Med., 282:652, 1970.
11. St. Geme, J. W., Jr., Prince, J. T., and Burke, B. A.: Impaired cellular resistance to herpes-simplex virus in Wiskott-Aldrich syndrome. N. Engl. J. Med., 273:229, 1965.
12. Sutton, A. L., Smithwick, E. M., Seligman, S. J., et al.: Fatal disseminated herpesvirus hominis type 2 infection in an adult with associated thymic dysplasia. Am. J. Med., 56:545, 1974.
13. Montgomerie, J. Z., Becroft, D. M. O., Croxson, M. C., et al.: Herpes-simplex-virus infection after renal transplantation. Lancet, 2:867, 1967.
14. Rand, K. H., Rasmussen, L. E., Pollard, R. B., et al.: Cellular immunity and herpesvirus infections in cardiac-transplant patients. N. Engl. J. Med., 296:1372, 1976.
15. Diderholm, H., Stenram, U., Tegner, K. B., et al.: Herpes simplex hepatitis in an adult. Acta Med. Scand., 186:151, 1969.
16. Nahmias, A. J., Alford, C. A., and Korones, S. B.: Infection of the newborn with herpesvirus hominus. Adv. Pediatr., 17:185, 1970.
17. Goyette, R. E., Donowho, E. M., Jr., Hieger, L. R., et al.: Fulminant herpesvirus hominis hepatitis during pregnancy. Obstet. Gynecol., 43:191, 1974.
18. Arora, K. K., Karalakulasingam, R., Raff, M. J., et al.: Cutaneous herpesvirus hominis (Type 2) infection after renal transplantation. J. A. M. A., 230:1174, 1974.
19. Shneidman, D. W., Barr, R. J., and Graham, J. H.: Chronic cutaneous herpes simplex. J. A. M. A., 241:592, 1979.
20. Baringer, J. R., and Swoveland, P.: Recovery of herpes-simplex virus from human trigeminal ganglions. N. Engl. J. Med., 288:648, 1973.
21. Cook, M. L., Bastone, V. B., and Stevens, J. G.: Evidence that neurons harbor latent herpes simplex virus. Infect. Immunity, 9:946, 1974.
22. Warren, K. G., Brown, S. M., Wroblewska, Z., et al.: Isolation of latent herpes simplex virus from the superior cervical and vagus ganglions of human beings. N. Engl. J. Med., 298:1068, 1978.
23. Chang, T-W.: Recurrent viral infection (reinfection). N. Engl. J. Med., 284:765, 1971.
24. Roizman, B.: Herpesvirus, latency and cancer: A biochemical approach. J. Reticuloendo. Soc., 15:312, 1974.
25. Lehner, T., Walton, J. M. A., and Shillitoe, E. J.: Immunological bases for latency, recurrences and putative oncogenicity of herpes simplex virus. Lancet, 2:60, 1975.
26. Bierman, S. M.: The mechanism of recurrent infection by *Herpesvirus hominis*. Arch. Dermatol., 112:1459, 1976.
27. Openshaw, H., Puga, A., and Notkins, A. L.: Herpes simplex virus infection in sensory ganglia: Immune control, latency, and reactivation. Fed. Proc., 38(10):2660, 1979.
28. Warren, S. L., Carpenter, C. M., and Boak, R. A.: Symptomatic herpes, a sequela of artificially induced fever: Incidence and clinical aspects; recovery of virus from herpetic vesicles, and comparison with a known strain of herpes virus. J. Exp. Med., 71:155, 1940.
29. Scott, T. F.: Epidemiology of herpetic infections. Am. J. Ophthalmol., 43:134, 1957.
30. Thygeson, P., Hogan, M. J., and Kumura, S. J.: Cortisone and hydrocortisone in ocular infections. Trans. Am. Acad. Ophthalmol. Otolaryngol., 57:64, 1953.
31. Blank, H., and Brody, M. W.: Recurrent herpes simplex: A

psychiatric and laboratory study. Psychosom. Med., *12*:254, 1950.

32. Carton, C. A., and Kilbourne, E. D.: Activation of latent herpes simplex by trigeminal sensory-root section. N. Engl. J. Med., *246*:172, 1952.

33. Carton, C. A.: Effect of previous sensory loss on the appearance of herpes simplex: Following trigeminal sensory root section. J. Neurosurg., *10*:463, 1953.

34. Ellison, S. A., Carton, C. A., and Rose, H. M.: Studies of recurrent herpes simplex infections following section of the trigeminal nerve. J. Infect. Dis., *105*:161, 1959.

35. Cushing, H.: The surgical aspects of major neuralgia of the trigeminal nerve: A report of twenty cases of operations on the Gasserian ganglion, with anatomic and physiologic notes on the consequence of its removal. J. A. M. A., *44*:773, 860, 920, and 1002, 1905.

36. Nahmias, A. J., and Roizman, B.: Infection with herpes simplex virus types 1 and 2. N. Engl. J. Med., *289*:667, 719, and 781, 1973.

37. Morrison, R. R., Miller, M. H., Lyon, L. W., et al.: Adult meningoencephalitis caused by herpesvirus hominis type 2. Am. J. Med., *56*:540, 1974.

39. Young, E. J., Vainrub, B., Musher, D. M., et al.: Acute pharyngotonsilitis caused by herpesvirus type 2. J. A. M. A., *239*:1885, 1978.

40. Wolontis, S., and Jeanson, S. S.: Correlation of herpes simplex virus types 1 and 2 with clinical features of infection. J. Infect. Dis., *135*:28, 1977.

41. Giacobetti, R.: Herpetic whitlow. Dermatology, *18*:55, 1979.

42. Buddingh, G. J., Schrum, D. I., Lanier, J. C., et al.: Studies of the natural history of herpes simplex infections. Pediatrics, *11*:595, 1952.

43. Adamson, H. G.: Herpes febrilis attacking the fingers. Br. J. Dermatol., *21*:323, 1909.

44. Nicolau, S., and Poincloux, P.: Etude clinique et experimentale d'um cas d'herpes recidivant du doigt. Ann. Inst. Pasteur, *38*:977, 1924.

45. Burnet, F. M., and Williams, S. W.: Herpes simplex: A new point of view. Med. J. Austral., *1*:637, 1939.

46. Findlay, G. M., and MacCallum, F. O.: Recurrent traumatic herpes. Lancet, *1*:249, 1940.

47. Stern, H., Elek, S. D., Millar, D. M., et al.: Herpetic whitlow: A form of cross-infection in hospitals. Lancet, *2*:871. 1959.

48. Hambrick, G. W., Cox, R. P., and Senior, J. R.: Primary herpes simplex infection of fingers of medical personnel. Arch. Dermatol., *85*:583, 1962.

49. Rosato, F. E., Rosato, E. F., and Plotkin, S. A.: Herpetic paronychia—an occupational hazard of medical personnel. N. Engl. J. Med., *283*:804, 1970.

50. Berkowitz, R. L., and Hentz, V. R.: Herpetic whitlow—a non-surgical infection of the hand. Plast. Reconstr. Surg., *60*:125, 1977.

51. LaRossa, D., and Hamilton, R.: Herpes simplex infections of the digit. Arch. Surg., *102*:600, 1971.

52. Ward, J. R., and Clark, L.: Primary herpes simplex virus infection of the fingers. J.A.M.A., *176*:226, 1961.

53. Gavelin, G. E., and Knight, C. R.: Herpes simplex infection of the finger. Can. Med. Assoc. J., *93*:366, 1965.

54. Kanaar, P.: Primary herpes simplex infection of fingers in nurses. Dermatologica, *134*:346, 1967.

55. Chang, T-W., and Gorbach, S. L.: Primary and recurrent herpetic whitlow. Int. J. Dermatol., *16*:752, 1977.

56. Bart, B. J., and Fisher, I.: Primary herpes simplex infection of the hand: Report of case. J.A.D.A., *71*:74, 1965.

57. Brightman, V. J., and Guggenheimer, J. G.: Herpetic paronychia—primary herpes simplex infection of the finger. J. A. D. A., *80*:112, 1970.

58. DeYoung, G. G., Harrison, A. W., and Shapley, J. M.: Herpes simplex cross infection in the operating room. Can. Anaesth. Soc. J., *15*:394, 1968.

59. Orkin, F. K.: Herpetic whitlow—occupational hazard to the anesthesiologist. Anesthesiology, *33*:671, 1970.

60. Eiferman, R. A., Adams, G., Stover, B., et al.: Herpetic whitlow and keratitis. Arch. Ophthalmol., *97*:1079, 1979.

61. Muller, S. A., and Herrmann, E. C., Jr.: Association of stomatitis and paronychias due to herpes simplex. Arch. Dermatol., *101*:396, 1970.

62. Green, L. H., and Levin, M. P.: An unusual primary infection with herpes simplex virus: A case report. J. Peridontol., *42*:170, 1971.

63. Spotswood, S. L., Overall, J. C., Jr., Kern, E. R., et al.: The natural history of recurrent herpes simplex labialis. N. Engl. J. Med., *297*:69, 1977.

64. Kaufman, H. E.: Ocular antiviral therapy in perspective. J. Infect. Dis., *133(suppl)*:96, 1976.

65. MacCallum, F.O., and Juel-Jensen, B. E.: Herpes simplex virus skin infection in man treated with idoxuridine in dimethyl suphoxide. Results of double-blind controlled trial. Br. Med., J., *2*:805, 1966.

66. Pavan-Langston, D., and Dohlman, C. A.: A doublt-blind clinical study of adenine arabinoside therapy of viral keratoconjunctivitis. Am. J. Ophthalmol., *73*:932, 1972.

67. Pavan-Langston, D., and Buchanan, R. A.: Vidarabine therapy of simple and IDU-complicated herpetic keratitis. Trans. Am. Acad. Ophthalmol. Otolaryngol., *81*:813, 1976.

68. Whitley, R. J., Soong, S-J., Dolin, R., et al.: Adenine arabinoside therapy of biopsy-proved herpes simplex encephalitis. N. Engl. J. Med., *297*:189, 1977.

69. Goodman, E. L., Luby, J. P., and Johnson, M. T.: Prospective double-blind evaluation of topical adenine arabinoside in male herpes progenitalis. Antimicrob. Agents Chemother., *8*:693, 1975.

70. Adams, H. G., Benson, E. A., and Alexander, E. R.: Genital herpetic infection in men and women: Clinical course and effect of topical application of adenine arabinoside. J. Infect. Dis., *133(suppl)*:151, 1976.

71. Blough, H. A., and Guintoli, R. L.: Successful treatment of human genital herpes infections with 2-deoxy-D-glucose. J.A.M.A., *241*:2798, 1979.

72. Jones, B. R., Coster, D. J., Fison, P. N., et al.: Efficacy of acycloguanosine (Wellcome 248U) against herpes-simplex corneal ulcers. Lancet, *1*:243, 1979.

73. Jones, B. R., Coster, D. J., Falcon, M. G., et al.: Topical therapy of ulcerative herpetic keratitis with human interferon. Lancet, *2*:128, 1976.

74. Pazin, G. J., Armstrong, J. A., Lam, M. T., et al.: Prevention of reactivated herpes simplex infection by human leukocyte interferon after operation on the trigeminal root. N. Engl J. Med., *301*:225, 1979.

75. Shelley, W. B.: Surgical treatment for recurrent herpes simplex. Lancet, *2*:1021, 1978.

76. Corey, L., Reeves, W. C., Chiang, W. T., et al.: Ineffectiveness of topical ether for the treatment of genital herpes simplex virus infection. N. Engl. J. Med., *299*:237, 1978.

77. Guinan, M. E., MacCalman, J., Kern, E. R., et al.: Topical ether and herpes simplex labialis. J.A.M.A., *243*:1059, 1980.

78. Taylor, C. A., Hendley, J. O., Greer, K. E., et al.: Topical treatment of herpes labialis with chloroform. Arch. Dermatol., *113*:1550, 1977.

79. Bierman, S. M.: BCG immunoprophylaxis of recurrent herpes progenitalis. Arch. Dermatol., *112*:410, 1976.

80. Chang, T. W., and Fiumara, N.: Treatment with levamisole of recurrent herpes genitalis. Antimicrob. Agents Chemother., *13*:809, 1978.

81. Myers, M. G., Oxman, M. N., Clark, J. E., et al.: Failure of neutral-red photodynamic inactivation in recurrent herpes simplex virus infections. N. Engl. J. Med., *293*:945, 1975.

FURTHER READING

Hirsch, M. S.: Herpes simplex virus. *In* Mandell, G. L., Douglas, R. G., Jr., and Bennett, J. E. (eds.): Principles and Practice of Infectious Disease. pp. 1283–1294. New York, John Wiley & Sons, 1979.

Juel-Jensen, B. E., and MacCallum, F. O.: Herpes Simplex, Varicella and Zoster: Clinical Manifestations and Treatment. pp. 1–76 and 117–159. Philadelphia, JB Lippincott, 1972.

57 Problems of Trace Anesthetic Levels

John H. Lecky, M.D.

It has been known for sometime that occupational health hazards exist in many industries. These work-related diseases range from asbestosis secondary to the inhalation of particulate matter, to angiosarcoma of the liver following chronic inhalation of vinyl chloride monomer. Hepatitis is relatively common among physicians, nurses, and other allied health personnel and, as such, is also an occupational hazard. It has been only within the last decade, however, that data have appeared suggesting that chronic exposure to trace levels of anesthetic gases in the operating room can also constitute a medical health hazard.

This chapter addresses several aspects of this issue. The data that suggest that there is a health hazard for "exposed" operating room personnel are examined. The practical aspects of the problem include the following: How are trace anesthetic gas leakage sites identified? What methods are available to control and monitor equipment leakage? What hazards result from capturing (scavenging) excess anesthetic circuit gases? What long-term control measures are necessary to determine if—and to document that—low trace levels are being maintained in the operating room.

The potential impact of governmental regulation in managing trace anesthetic gas contamination in the operating room is significant. At present a National Institute of Occupational Safety and Health (NIOSH) Criteria Document is under review by the Occupation Safety and Health Administration (OSHA).[1] Its promulgation into law may have far-reaching consequences for the practice of anesthesia.

HEALTH HAZARDS OF EXPOSURE TO TRACE LEVELS OF ANESTHETICS

The possibility that chronic exposure to low levels of anesthetic agents constitutes a health hazard to medical personnel has attracted worldwide interest. The natural concern for self-protection, coupled with a growing awareness of a generalized environmental deterioration, makes this an intriguing topic for the health worker. It is also relatively easily understood and relevant when compared to more esoteric topics. Unfortunately, most of the health data on humans are derived from retrospective surveys. As such, the appealing simplicity of the problem is complicated by tenuous, confusing evidence. Laboratory studies in a variety of animal species have produced pathology similar to that suspected in man; yet, of necessity, these studies have been performed in many cases with much higher concentrations of anesthetic agent than those to which operating room workers are chronically exposed. Despite these limitations, the preponderance of data strongly suggest that there are health hazards associated with the chronic inhalation of trace amounts of anesthetic gases and vapors.

Toxicity of Chronic Anesthesia Exposure to Humans

In 1920 Hamilton reported "ether poisoning," characterized by a variety of gastrointestinal and CNS symptoms among workers exposed to ether vapor while making gunpowder during World War I.[2] In 1949, it was reported that a surgeon, nurse, and anesthetist recovered from a variety of symptoms, ranging from depression, headache, anorexia, and loss of memory, to peridontal disease and ECG abnormalities, by staying away from the operating room for an extended period of time.[3] They had been chronically exposed to high but unmeasured levels of ether vapor. Following the installation of better operating room ventilation equipment, they were able to resume practice without recurrence of symptoms. Until recently, with the exception of these anecdotal reports, the occupational health experiences of anesthesiologists and operating room workers had been virtually unstudied.

In the early 1960s, several studies investigated the toxicity of anesthetic agents on non-neural tissues in man. Chronic exposure to analgesic levels of nitrous oxide resulted in a dose-related depression of the bone marrow.[4,5] In 1968, a survey of causes of death among anesthesiologists between 1948 and 1967 identified an increased mortality rate from malignancies of the lymphoid and reticuloendothelial systems, as well as from suicide.[6]

In the same year, Vaisman surveyed the health of 303 Russian anesthesiologists (36% were women and 91% were younger than 40 years of age).[7] Administration of anesthesia for more than 2.5 hours per day was associated with headache in 96 per cent, increased irritability in 85 per cent, disturbance of sleep in 51 per cent, change of appetite in 48 per cent, and decreased resistance to alcohol in 33 per cent. The anesthetics most commonly used were ether, nitrous oxide, and halothane. Their operating rooms were characterized by poor or no ventilation and imperfect equipment. The latter undoubtedly produced gas

leakage and apparently also prompted these clinicians to inhale their vapor mixtures frequently to "verify" the administered concentration.

More disturbingly, Vaisman also noted a high incidence of spontaneous abortion among female anesthetists. Of 31 pregnancies, 18 ended in spontaneous abortion, and only seven had normal full-term deliveries. With only four exceptions, the women who aborted were working primarily with ether in poorly ventilated rooms. In those women who aborted, their average work week was 25 hours or more, compared with less than 15 hours per week in five of the seven women who had normal pregnancies. Subsequently, Askrog reported a 20-per-cent spontaneous abortion rate among actively practicing Danish female anesthetists.[8] Prior to operating room exposure, their abortion rate had been 10 per-cent. It was also suggested that there was an increased risk of abortion in the wives of working anesthesiologists.

A major weakness of these data lay in the choice of control group. The spontaneous abortion rate increases with maternal age. While the increased abortion rates seen in this study occurred following operating room exposure, they involved women who were older, so that the true cause was unknown. The increased abortion rate, however, appears to be greater than that expected on the basis of age alone.

Cohen compared the obstetric histories of anesthesiologists in California with those of physicians from other specialities, with female operating room nurses, and with general duty nurses.[9] The abortion rates were 38 per cent for the anesthesiologists, 30 per cent for operating room nurses, and 10 per cent for the corresponding control groups.

An increased abortion rate in British operating room personnel was also shown by Knill-Jones.[10] Five-hundred sixty-three married female anesthesiologists were compared with 828 married female physicians unexposed to anesthetics. The frequency of spontaneous abortion was 18.2 per cent when the anesthesiologists were working and 13.7 per cent when they did not work. The miscarriage rate of the control group was 14.7 per cent. An additional disturbing finding was an

Table 57-1. Spontaneous Abortion Rates Reported
by Women Belonging to Medical Societies*

"Exposed" Societies		"Unexposed" Societies		Statistical Significance
ASA	17.1 ± 2.0	AAP	8.9 ± 1.8	$p < .01$
AANA	17.0 ± 0.9	ANA	15.1 ± 0.9	$p = .07$
AORN/T	19.5 ± 0.9			$p < .01$

*Rate per 100 pregnancies, standardized for age and smoking

increased incidence of congenital anomalies in the live-born offspring of exposed women (6.5% in working anesthesiologists vs. 2.5% in those not working during pregnancy). Similarly, in another survey of British anesthesiologists, there was an increased incidence of congenital anomalies or developmental problems in their children (93% vs.4.3% in the children of anesthesiologists not exposed during pregnancy).[10a]

The American Society of Anesthesiologists (ASA), in a study cosponsored by NIOSH, surveyed 73,496 persons who were designated as "exposed" or "unexposed" according to whether they worked in an environment that contained anesthetic agents in the air.[11] "Exposed" personnel were drawn from membership lists of the ASA, American Association of Nurse Anesthetists (AANA), Association of Operating Room Nurses (AORN), and Association of Operating Room Technicians (AORT). Members of these societies were thought to represent persons with a spectrum of exposure to anesthetics, and the ASA and AANA members were thought to be exposed more consistently to higher levels of anesthetics than the AORN/T group. Specific questions relating to work practices identified those persons who, although they belonged to a society, were not working or were in administrative capacities and not exposed to the operating room environment during the period 1963 to 1972.

The choice of control groups was critical. "Unexposed" controls had to be of similar age and sex. Education and work schedule could differ only in absence from the operating room. A significant number of women had to belong to the "control society," as obstetric history was an important area of inquiry. Accordingly, pediatrics was selected as the physician control group, since

the American Academy of Pediatricians (AAP) had a membership similar to the ASA (7,024 men and 886 women in the AAP vs. 9,793 men and 1,399 women in the ASA). A randomly selected group of 15,681 women and 320 men belonging to the American Nursing Assocation (ANA) was chosen as the control for both the AANA and AORN/T groups.

Analysis revealed higher spontaneous abortion rates for personnel working in the operating room (Table 57-1). Although the rate of miscarriage among anesthesiologists was twice that of their control group, comparision of the groups of nurses was less striking, because the rate for the ANA control group was, itself, rather high. Were the ANA members reporting abortions that were actually misinterpretations of menstrual irregularities? This is but one of many questions that are difficult to resolve in such a survey. A separate comparison of abortions in nonworking (therefore, "unexposed") women in the AANA also revealed a fairly high rate, but which was still significantly lower than that of working female members (Table 57-2). A similar comparison of female members within ASA showed the same trend but was not statistically significant. This may be a result, in part, of the small size of the group of nonworking women in ASA. The ASA survey also examined abortion rates in the wives of "exposed" personnel. The only significant elevation was in the AORN/T groups; again, however, there were too few pregnancies among the control group for valid comparison. While the data in this study suggested an increased risk of spontaneous abortion among "exposed" women, there did not appear to be a significantly increased abortion rate in the wives of "exposed" men.

The data suggest a dose-dependent increase in the incidence of congenital anomalies in live-

Table 57-2. Spontaneous Abortion Rates Reported by Working and Nonworking Women Belonging to "Exposed" Medical Societies*

	AANA	AORN/T
Working mothers ("exposed")	17.0 ± 0.9	19.5 ± 0.9
Nonworking mothers ("unexposed")	14.4 ± 1.4	15.1 ± 1.2
Significance of differences	$p = .06$	$p < .01$

*Rate per 100 pregnancies, standardized for age and smoking

born children of "exposed" women in the three "exposed" groups (Table 57-3). Anesthesiologists and nurse anesthetists showed the greatest increase compared to controls, while the AORN/T members experienced almost the same incidence as general duty nurses. Congenital anomalies were reported to occur twice as often in offspring of women belonging to ASA as in offspring of pediatricians. This increase was not statistically significant. There was, however, a statistically significant increase in anomalies reported by wives of ASA members when compared to wives of AAP members (Table 57-4). Additionally, a comparison of working ("exposed") and nonworking ("unexposed") female nurse anesthetists showed that those exposed during pregnancy had a 60-per-cent greater incidence of anomalies among their live-born children than the "unexposed" group.

Combined data from the ASA study and two other retrospective studies in the United Kingdom demonstrated statistically significant increases in spontaneous abortions and congenital malformations in the children of female physicians working in the operating room.[12] In addition, offspring of male anesthesiologists had an increased incidence of hepatic disease and congenital malformations. Yet, the incidence of cancer in these men and the spontaneous abortion rate in their wives were similar to controls.

As an offshoot of the ASA survey, histories of "exposed" (those who administered anesthesia, primarily nitrous oxide, for more than 3 hours per week and "unexposed" dentists were compared.[13] In the "exposed" group, there were statistically significant increases in liver disease (5.9 vs. 2.3%) and spontaneous abortion (16 vs. 9%) in their wives.

The design and the limited size of many of these epidemilogic studies preclude statistical significance. Frequent obstetric mishaps, however, characterized by increased spontaneous abortion rates in "exposed" women and increased frequency of congenital anomalies in their offspring or in the offspring of "exposed" men are findings common to virtually all of the published epidemilogic surveys. These incidents strengthen our concern.

The ASA questionnaire also included questions about liver and kidney diseases, because of concerns for the potential toxicity of halogenated agents. Women of each "exposed" group who responded had a significantly higher rate of hepatic disease than the corresponding control group. For men, however, only the ASA–AAP comparison showed such a difference. Imprecision in the

Table 57-3. Rates of Congenital Anomalies* in Offspring of Women Belonging to Medical Societies†

"EXPOSED" SOCIETIES		"UNEXPOSED" SOCIETIES		STATISTICAL SIGNIFICANCE
ASA	5.9 ± 1.4	AAP	3.0 ± 1.1	$p = .07$
AANA	9.6 ± 0.8	ANA	7.6 ± 0.7	$p < .05$
AORN/T	7.7 ± 0.6			$p = .47$

*Skin abnormalities excluded
†Rate per 100 pregnancies, standardized for age and smoking

**Table 57-4. Rates of Congenital Anomalies* in Offspring of Men Belonging
to Medical Societies†**

"Exposed" Societies		"Unexposed" Societies		Statistical Significance
ASA	5.4 ± 0.4	AAP	4.2 ± 0.5	$p < .05$
AANA	8.2 ± 0.9	ANA	3.7 ± 2.5	$p = .13$
AORN/T	6.4 ± 2.5			$p = .22$

*Skin abnormalities excluded
†Rate per 100 pregnancies, standardized for age and smoking

diagnosis of hepatic disease (including the possibility that some respondents who indicated "hepatitis" actually had had serum hepatitis) makes this difficult to analyze. Whether hepatic disease is another health hazard associated with trace anesthetic inhalation has not been determined.

An increased incidence of renal disease was demonstrated only among nurse anesthetists and AORN/T members when compared to women in ANA. The higher incidence of renal disease among U.S. physicians, may be caused by diet or other cultural differences.[12] The ASA "cause of death" study[6] and a survey of Michigan nurses[14] suggested an increased cancer rate in anesthesia personnel. As shown in Table 57-5, while higher cancer rates were seen among "exposed" women, there was no significant difference among men who responded (Table 57-6). A 5-year update of the ASA mortality study,[15] however, has failed to reveal the increased death rate from lymphoid malignancies that had been previously noted. In addition, a survey of the American Cancer Society suggests that anesthesiologists live longer than other specialists and that the death rate from cancer is also lower. Cancer, then, may not be an occupational hazard. As a note of caution, however, it should be pointed out that the "lag time" for industrial carcinogens is 20 years. The carcino-

genic effects of halogenated agents, if any, may not yet be manifest. Additionally, new therapeutic modalities may result in higher cancer cure rates, and hence, there may be an increased incidence of cancer that is not reflected by mortality data.

Psychological Studies of Exposure to Trace Levels of Anesthetics

If the anesthetist inhales 0.001 MAC of anesthetic is he anesthetized to that degree? This question has led to several studies, in which volunteers inhaled trace concentrations of anesthetics and then took a series of psychological tests. The tests assessed behavioral modalities of particular importance in anesthesiology, such as recognition (perception), decision making (cognition), and action (motor activity).

Significant decrements in performance on such tests occur following exposure to nitrous oxide (500 p.p.m.*) plus halothane or enflurane (15 p.p.m.), as well as nitrous oxide (500 p.p.m.) alone. Nitrous oxide and halothane in concentrations as low as 50 p.p.m. and 1 p.p.m., respective-

---

*Trace gas levels are expressed in parts per million (p.p.m.), which is a volume per volume unit. A 100% concentration of gas = 1,000,000 p.p.m. and 1% = 10,000 p.p.m.

**Table 57-5. Cancer* Rates Reported
by Women Belonging to Medical Societies†**

"Exposed" Societies		"Unexposed" Societies		Statistical Significance
ASA	3.0 ± 0.6	AAP	1.6 ± 0.5	$p = .05$
AANA	2.6 ± 0.2	ANA	1.8 ± 0.2	$p < .01$
AORN/T	2.3 ± 0.2			$p = .07$

*Excluding skin cancer
†Rate per 100 members per 10 years, standardized for age and smoking

**Table 57-6. Cancer* Rates Reported
by Men Belonging to Medical Societies†**

"Exposed" Societies		"Unexposed" Societies		Statistical Significance
ASA	0.7 ± 0.1	AAP	0.7 ± 0.2	$p = .49$
AANA	1.5 ± 0.5	ANA	0.0	$p = .13$
AORN/T	0.3 ± 0.2			$p = .27$

*Excluding skin cancer
†Rate per 100 members per 10 years, standardized for age and smoking

ly, are also associated with significant decrements in visual perception, immediate memory, and performance on audiovisual ("divided attention") tests. These studies offer the only conclusive documentation of a causal relationship between trace anesthetic exposure and an undesirable effect in humans. These effects do not occur following exposure to nitrous oxide, 25 p.p.m., and halothane, 0.5 p.p.m., levels easily attainable in a standard operating room using current technology.[16–18] Other workers, however, have not been able to reproduce these results.[19–21] This failure may be caused by differences in experimental design. To date, these are the only laboratory studies in humans. The variable results are attributable to the minimal effects of trace levels of anesthetics on CNS function in humans and to the relatively poor resolving power of the tests available. The recurrent subjective complaints of mood alteration, fatigue, and irritability are even more difficult to assess objectively.

Studies of Chronic Exposure of Animals to Trace Levels of Anesthetics

A variety of laboratory studies in animals support the contention that a relationship exists between chronic exposure to trace levels of anesthetic agents and several disease entities. These studies have been performed using anesthetic concentrations ranging from clinical to trace levels. It is disturbing that relatively high levels of exposure are required to demonstrate detrimental effects in some studies. However, a short-term, relatively high level of exposure is an accepted technique in the investigation of industrial toxins when trying to determine if changes will be seen with lower-level, longer-term exposure. Exposure to many inhalation agents at a variety of concentrations has resulted in teratogenic effects in various species.[22] Similarly, following exposure, animals may show decreased survival,[20] CNS ultrastructural changes,[23] decrements in solving mazes following exposure in utero,[24] and testicular damage.[25,25a] and decreased ovulation and implantion efficiency.[25a] These effects closely parallel the obstetric mishaps suggested in the epidemiologic studies in humans. However, the chronic exposure of rats to trace concentrations of halothane and nitrous oxide is not associated with an increased incidence of malignancy.[25b]

While both epidemiologic and laboratory data support the contention that a cause-effect relationship exists between working in anesthetizing areas and the occurrence of a variety of disease entities, many investigators have urged that caution be taken in concluding that exposure to trace levels of anesthetic agents is the culprit.[26–28] They point out that other factors, such as work-related and emotional stress, smoking, and age can contribute variably to both obstetric mishap and the development and growth rate of cancer. They are skeptical, too, of epidemiologic studies in man. Data from such retrospective surveys often suffer from bias at several levels. Sophisticated statistical treatment and analysis usually required to achieve any degree of significance. A recent study that relied upon registry data, rather than mailed questionnaires or telephone interviews which can introduce bias, found no increase in the incidence of threatened abortion or congenital malformations in women working in the operating room.[28a]

Two studies that may resolve many of these issues are being planned. There will be a follow-up study by ASA in the early 1980s to determine if results are different after the installation of scavenging, with the attendant reduction of trace levels. A large scale study of dentists is also underway. This study will help resolve the question of whether nitrous oxide exposure is harmful. In addition, it will include a control group similar to the "exposed" group (e.g., male dentists with similar background and working conditions).

At present, the data, while equivocal, strongly suggest that there is a cause-effect relationship between anesthetic exposure and health hazards. The strength of these data results from the following: While individual studies may not be conclusive, the observed trends and disease entities, which closely parallel laboratory animal studies are noted repeatedly in different surveys. We must therefore address the issue of trace gas control until we obtain more reliable data that refute the existence of a health hazard.

ENVIRONMENT OF THE OPERATING ROOM

"Threshold limit values" (TLVs) have been established by industrial hygienists for many agents.[29] Such values are timeweighted upper limits of concentrations to which workers may be exposed daily, presumably without adverse effect. For example, the TLV for diethyl ether is 400 p.p.m. (0.04%) with a "permissible excursion factor" of 1.25, meaning that occasional 500-p.p.m. peaks are allowed. TLVs are usually based on data that suggests that these values are "safe" in animals. Until recently, nitrous oxide was rated as a "simple asphyxiant," and no TLV was given. Nitrous oxide levels were governed only by the limitation of available oxygen in the air, which must not fall below 18 per cent.

In 1929, ether was reported to be present at concentrations of 20 to 500 p.p.m. in operating rooms in which it was being given by open drop.[30] The next similar report was made 40 years later when, in 1969, average concentrations of 10-p.p.m. halothane and 130-p.p.m. nitrous oxide were found in operating rooms.[31] Subsequent studies have shown that nitrous oxide levels in unscavenged operating rooms, in which no attempt to control atmospheric levels of anesthetic gases are made, range from 300 to 500 p.p.m. for nitrous oxide and 5 to 15 p.p.m. for halogenated agents.[32,33] When high-flow techniques are employed in poorly ventilated areas, levels can be even higher.

A Danish report showed that 85-p.p.m. halothane and 7,000-p.p.m. nitrous oxide resulted when a non-rebreathing system was used to deliver anesthesia,[34] and nitrous oxide levels in dental operatories have also been reported to approach 10,000 p.p.m.[35–38]

Uptake of Anesthetics by Personnel

Of real concern is the exposure of personnel working in anesthetizing areas. Assays for end-expired levels of halogenated agents (gas chromatographic analyses for these compounds are easily performed) have served as "indices" of personnel exposure.[31,39–42]

Linde and Bruce found that end-expired halothane in anesthesiologists ranged from 0 to 12.2 p.p.m., with a mean value of 1.8 p.p.m.; similar values were reported by others. Corbett found end-expired methoxyflurane levels of 0.1 to 0.7 p.p.m. Serial measurements taken until the agent was no longer detectable allowed the determination of "breath decay curves." Wash out times were 10 to 29 hours for methoxyflurane, 7 to 64 hours for halothane, and 3 to 7 hours for nitrous oxide.[39] For the fat-soluble halogenated vapors, the corollary is obvious. After 8 hours of administering these agents, the anesthesiologist has only 16 hours to excrete them before reexposure. If clearance takes longer than 16 hours, then the anesthesiologist can progressively accumulate the agent.

It is clear, then, that measurable amounts of anesthetic gases and vapors are present in operating room air, that anesthesiologists inhale and retain these for some time, and that the slow rate of elimination of some vapors allows accumulation of retained trace anesthetic quantities from one day to the next. While the mechanism, or mechanisms, by which these health hazards occur are still unknown, it has been demonstrated that enzyme induction takes place in practicing anesthesiologists and that a given halothane load is metabolized to a greater extent by them than a control group of pharmacists.[43]

MEASURES TO CONTROL TRACE LEVELS OF ANESTHETICS IN THE OPERATING ROOM

Reduction and control of anesthetic trace levels in the operating room requires capturing (scavenging) of excess circuit gases, institution of an ongoing maintenance program to prevent leakage from equipment, and alteration of anesthetic technique to avoid gross spillage into the room.

The National Institute for Occupational Safety and Health (NIOSH) Criteria Document cites target levels of 25 p.p.m. for nitrous oxide and 0.5 p.p.m. for halogenated anesthetics (when used with N_2O) or 2.0 p.p.m. when used alone.* In an operating room in which excess circuit gases are not scavenged and no maintenance of equipment to prevent leaks has been performed, anesthetic levels in the breathing zone of the anesthesiologist are 300 to 500 p.p.m. for nitrous oxide and 5 to 15 p.p.m. for halogenated anesthetics; these concentrations are well above the target levels and within the range at which impairment on psychomotor testing has been demonstrated.

SCAVENGING OF EXCESS GASES

Installation of an effective excess gas disposal system is the most important factor in reducing trace gas levels. Elimination of excess circuit gas spillage into the operating room reduces levels approximately 90 per cent, depending on gas flows. Because anesthetic gases are heavier than air, it is a common misconception that they sink to the floor and flow out of the room by way of the ventilation system. In reality, ventilation system flow and personnel movement effectively mix the operating room air, producing a fairly uniform distribution of gases.[44] A scavenging system has three major components: a gas-capturing assem-

bly, or manifold, an interface, and a disposal system.[44a]

Gas-Capturing Assembly

Excess gases from the breathing circuit, ventilator, or extracorporeal pump oxygenator must be contained and conducted to the disposal system. Safety as well as performance is a major consideration, in the design and selection of a scavenging system. A "pop-off" valve equipped with a gas-capturing manifold and other devices used to capture waste anesthetic gases should not significantly alter ventilator or oxygenator function, anesthetic circuit dynamics, or delivered gas concentration.

Mechanical anesthesia ventilators should be equipped, when they are new or retrofitted, with the means to capture effluent gases. In some instances, the ventilator exhaust volume includes both excess circuit gases and the driving gas,[45] and this makes it necessary to determine if the disposal system has sufficient capacity to handle this additional volume of gas. Ventilator manufacturers, then, should clearly specify the scavenging system flow or capacity requirements necessary for effective scavenging when their ventilator is in use. Similarly, manufacturers of scavenging equipment should specify optimal operating conditions (e.g., liters per minute suction flow) and what the capacity limits are for their system.

In the event that anesthesia is administered during bypass, the gas flow from extracorporeal oxygenators should also be scavenged. At present, gas-capturing systems for oxygenators are still in the developmental stage, and a variety of "do-it-yourself" systems have been developed.[46–48]

Significant positive or negative pressure variation in the scavenger circuit can markedly alter function in the system to which it is attached. It is necessary, then, to regulate pressure in the scavenging system, so that swings are minimal. This pressure regulation is the major function of the interface and is discussed on page 723.

The use of closed-system anesthesia is often proposed as a money-saving alternative to scavenging. With the decreased use of cyclopropane,

---

*These should be time-weighted average (TWA) samples obtained in the breathing zone of the anesthesiologist during the administration of anesthesia.

such a system mandates the use of an oxygen analyzer for safety. While excess gas spill during a case would be minimal, the anesthetic must still be exhausted at the end of the procedure; thus, a scavenger is probably still necessary. Even if a closed system is used, other factors produce room contamination (see p. 726) and must be considered. It should be pointed out, too, that while low circuit gas inflows save money, a good scavenging system is effective in handling virtually any of the standard gas flows without spill.

Disposal System

There are several routes for the disposal of excess anesthetic gas. These include the non-recirculating portion of the air-conditioning system, the central vacuum system, a dedicated suction or blower system, a passive through-wall system, and an adsorber.

In operating rooms with non-recirculating ventilation systems (all air that enters the room is fresh), excess anesthetic gases can be piped to the exhaust grill fixture. Flow around the fixture flushes the waste anesthetic gas into the ventilation system and then outside the building. When possible, the disposal line to the exhaust grill should run overhead, so that the risk of occlusion is minimal. If such a routing is impractical, however, the tubing wall should be reinforced to avoid the possibility of occlusion by equipment wheels or by persons who stand on the tubing. For additional safety, a positive pressure relief device (interface; see below) should be included in the system, proximal to the breathing circuit.

Unless excess gas is exhausted downstream of the recirculation point, dumping of this gas into a recirculating air-conditioning system (in which only a small portion of the air entering a room is fresh) results in contamination of all rooms on the common manifold. In this case, then, the central vacuum is an alternate disposal route. It should be noted, however, that regulations of the National Fire Protection Association (NFPA) prohibit disposal of flammable agents into a central vacuum system.[49] A disposal route that can generate significant negative pressure necessitates that a device (interface) be included in the scavenging

system to prevent negative pressure from being applied to the anesthetic circuit.

If the central vacuum or a non-recirculating air-conditioning system is not available for gas disposal, then a dedicated disposal route must be employed. Such an independent gas evacuation system should also be an important consideration in the design of new operating rooms or the renovation of existing operating rooms. The system should be readily accessible to the anesthesia machine, and high volume (30–40 L./min.), low-pressure flow should be provided. The exhausted gases from this system (as well as other disposal systems) should be dumped at a point where there is no possibility of personnel exposure. Passive systems that dump excess gas through a wall fitting to the outside are also acceptable; however, the outlet of such a system should be protected from occlusion by dirt, ice, and insects.[50] If the central vacuum or independent blower system is to be used, the hospital engineering department should be consulted regarding the volume capacity of the pump and the resistance of the equipment to corrosive agents. Activated charcoal adsorbers can effectively remove halogenated agents from a stream of gas for a short (6–10 hours) period of time. They do not remove nitrous oxide, however, and as such are an expensive means of dealing with only part of the pollution problem.

Interface

Scavenging equipment adds complexity and, thus, hazards to the administration of anesthesia. In essence, the scavenging system extends the anesthetic circuit all the way to the disposal point. Pressure alteration in the scavenging system from unopposed vacuum or occlusion of the scavenging system can be transferred directly to the anesthesia circuit, ventilator, or oxygenator, thereby markedly altering their performance and potentially harming the patient. For safety purposes, then, the interface is the most important component of the scavenging system. This device can be effectively designed in a number of ways. It must relieve positive pressure ($+10$ cm. H_2O maximum), in the event of system occlusion, and negative pressure $(-0.5$ cm. H_2O maximum$(,$[51] when the central suction or other negative pressure route is used for excess gas disposal.

In addition, during anesthesia, the excess gas flow rate can transiently exceed the vacuum or blower flow capacity. For example, with an anesthetic system inflow of 5 L. per min. and 10 ventilatory cycles per min., 500 ml. of gas must leave the circuit during each respiratory cycle. If 500 ml. of excess gas enters the scavenging system in 1 second, the exhaust flow rate is 30 L. per min. If the vacuum flow rate is only 20 L. per min., then scavenger capacity will be transiently exceeded, and spillage can occur. Under these circumstances, the interface should have a reservoir to contain the transient overflow until the disposal system can catch up. There are a number of designs, ranging from a reservoir bag to a coaxial (tube within a tube) system. Considerations of interface design include means to protect the patient from extremes of positive or negative pressure and sufficient reservoir capacity to avoid spillage of anesthetic agents into the operating room when the disposal system flow capacity is transiently exceeded.

Equipment Maintenance for Leak Prevention

While effective excess gas scavenging reduces intraoperative trace levels markedly, an ongoing equipment maintenance program for leak prevention is also necessary if trace gas levels are to be well controlled.

The anesthesia machine should undergo routine servicing by a manufacturer's representative at 4- to 6-month intervals. In addition to the routine care offered by the manufacturers at these visits, both the high-pressure (upstream of the flow meters) and low-pressure (downstream of the flowmeters) systems should be examined carefully and leaks corrected.

Our experience has been, however, that routine manufacturer service has not adequately identified or corrected all of the high- or low-pressure leak points. In fact, after one such maintenance inspection at the University of Pennsylvania, significant leakage remained in 20 per cent of the low-pressure systems and 25 per cent of the high-pressure systems.[52] Ongoing in-house monitoring by departmental personnel has been necessary to ensure that equipment leakage is controlled. In terms of time and money, it is unrealistic to expect the manufacturer to maintain anesthetic equipment in a leak-free state in the field, particularly when leakage in some portions of the system develops frequently.

High-Pressure System Leakage

The high-pressure system includes the lines for piped-in nitrous oxide, the nitrous oxide tanks, and the anesthesia machine up to the flowmeters.

Baseline nitrous oxide measurements were made at the University of Pennsylvania prior to any attempt at equipment "clean-up."[52] Samples were obtained serially in each operating room at 5:00 AM Monday, when no anesthesia was being given in any operating room. Under these conditions, cross-contamination or residual anesthetic traces were not a factor. Surprisingly, it was found that the average nitrous oxide level in 20 rooms was 19 p.p.m., with a range of 0 to 66 p.p.m. (This was the average of eight weekly analyses per room.) This average level was virtually at the NIOSH suggested target level of 25-p.p.m. nitrous oxide, *without concurrent administration of anesthesia!* Some rooms, in fact, had baseline nitrous oxide levels *above* the target levels.

Background nitrous oxide levels are the net result of high-pressure system leakage and the ability (or inability) of the ventilation system to rid the operating room of the contaminant.

Testing Procedures. By submerging them in water, it was found that one-half of the nitrous oxide "quick connects" on the central inflow lines leaked significantly. The major leak sites (crimped joints, pipe threads, and spring seals) were easily identified and corrected.

The ability of the anesthesia machine to hold pressure was also examined by disconnecting the machine from the central nitrous oxide source, opening a nitrous oxide tank to pressurize the system, and then closing the tank. Gauge pressure was then recorded and observed for 1 hour to determine the pressure drop. Initially, pressure in 53 per cent of the machines fell to zero in 1 hour. The most common leak site was the nitrous oxide tank yoke connector. With the exception of one

HOSPITAL *of the* UNIVERSITY *of* PENNSYLVANIA

HIGH PRESSURE TEST

(1) PERFORM TEST DURING FIRST WEEK OF EACH MONTH
(2) RECORD N$_2$O CONNECTOR LEAKS ON A 0 TO 3 BASIS
(3) RECORD MACHINE PRESSURES IN PSI

TECHNICIAN ....

Date	Room No.	Machine No.	N$_2$O Connectors Mid	End	Machine Pressure Initial	After 1 Hr.	Comments

Fig. 57-1. High-pressure-leak reporting form. (Lecky, J. H.: The mechanical aspects of anesthetic pollution control. Anesth. Analg., 56:769, 1977.)

machine that had a leaky pressure regulator, all of these leaks were eliminated by replacing washers or merely tightening the yokes.

High-pressure leaks develop slowly and persist until corrected. At present, the high-pressure system is examined monthly by anesthesia technicians who report their findings to the responsible physician on the form shown in Figure 57-1. This equipment testing and maintenance program has reduced and maintained baseline nitrous oxide levels at an average of 0.2 p.p.m., with a range of 0 to 2 p.p.m. during 38 months of observation.

If leakage of the nitrous oxide line connector is eliminated and the high-pressure portion of the anesthesia machine is leak-free, then baseline nitrous oxide levels will be negligible. If nitrous oxide connectors leak visibly when immersed in water and the high-pressure side of the anesthesia machine fails to maintain its pressure over 1 hour, then sigificant baseline nitrous oxide levels can be anticipated.

Low-Pressure System Leakage

The low-pressure portion of the anesthesia machine (in which pressures rarely exceed 30 cm.H$_2$0) extends from the flowmeters to the patient. Leakage from this portion of the anesthesia apparatus can be of sufficient magnitude to negate scavenging. Nitrous oxide levels can reach the 200- to 300-p.p.m. range owing to low-pressure leakage alone! This can be significant during closed-system anesthesia. Even without spill into the room from the "pop-off" valve, room levels can still exceed the target levels owing to low-pressure leakage.

Testing Procedures. Low-pressure leakage is quantitated by closing the "pop-off" valve, removing the anesthesia bag, and occluding its port and the "Y" piece with rubber stoppers or one's hand. An oxygen flow is administered that will achieve and maintain a steady circuit pressure of 40 cm. H$_2$0. The oxygen inflow then equals the leak rate of 40 cm.H$_2$0. The leakage rate should be less than 200 ml. of oxygen per min.* The most common sources of leaks are presented below. Anesthesia department technicians test this portion of the anesthetic system weekly and every

---

*A leak of this size will produce < 4 p.p.m. N$_2$O in a room with normal circuit pressures and anesthetic concentrations.

HOSPITAL of the UNIVERSITY of PENNSYLVANIA

LOW PRESSURE TEST

REPORT LEAK RATE IN CC O_2/MIN AT A CIRCUIT PRESSURE OF 40 CM H_2O

TECHNICIAN ....

Date	Room No.	Machine No.	Initial Leak Rate	Corrected Rate	Leak Sites

Fig. 57-2. Low-pressure-leak reporting form. (Lecky, J. H.: The mechanical aspects of anesthetic pollution control. Anesth. Analg., 56: 769, 1977.)

time the soda lime is changed. This program departmental testing has kept rates of leakage in the low-pressure system at acceptable levels. The test recording form used at the University of Pennsylvania is shown in Figure 57-2. This portion of the anesthesia system develops leaks so frequently that anesthesiologists are urged to incorporate low-pressure leak testing as a routine part of their preinduction machine checkout.

Common Low-Pressure Leak Sites

Improperly connected or leaking circuit tubing
Improperly sealed valve domes
Deformed gas delivery line or machine connection joint
Leaking delivery line
Leaking "Y" connector joints
Improperly closed absorber
Torn, kinked, or soda lime-covered canister gaskets
Leaking bypass tubing
Improperly closed petcock

VENTILATION SYSTEM

Anesthetic contamination resulting from equipment leakage, technique error, or scavenger malfunction must be removed by the air-conditioning system. The efficiency of the ventilation system is described in room air turnovers per hour. This number can be obtained by using the following equation:[33]

$$\frac{\text{Turnover}}{\text{Hour}} = \frac{\text{Inflow air velocity (ft./min.)} \times \text{Ventilation grill effective area (sq. ft.)}}{\text{Room volume (cu. ft.)}}$$

Inflow air velocity can be measured with a sensitive flowmeter (velometer). Ten turnovers per hour is probably the minimal acceptable level. Room size is also a consideration. A standard contaminant load in a small room with 10 turnovers per hour will result in higher levels than in a large room with the same number of turnovers per hour. Interestingly, it was found that little correlation existed between room air turnover (as measured at the inflow grille) and anesthetic trace levels produced in a standard stress test.[53] In this test, 3 L. per min. of nitrous oxide were spilled from the anesthesia machine. After a period of equilibration, nitrous oxide levels in front of the machine were measured. The poor correlation resulted from ventilation flow channeling, which produces both high flow as well as stagnant areas.

As a corollary, because of the volume of excess circuit gases produced by common anesthesia practice and because gases that sink to the floor are swept up and distributed throughout the room, the ventilation system alone is unable to keep pollutant levels low. Thus, a scavenging system and a maintenance program for leak prevention are mandatory for pollution control. Recirculating operating room air saves considerable cost by eliminating the necessity to cool or warm all of the incoming air. Thus, for economic reasons, a recirculating system is favored in very hot or very cold climates, and the filters now available eliminate the problems of bacterial contamination. Such a system, however, can cause trace concentration buildup in all rooms on the common manifold, even if they are not being used for anesthetic administration. Usubiaga showed that by noon the concentration in the surgeon's lounge was nearly as great as that found in the operating rooms that morning.[41]

The ventilation system is an adjunct to an effective scavenging and maintenance program Hospital engineers should be contacted and urged to ensure that the system functions optimally and that filters are clean and dampers are properly adjusted. Where possible, the anesthesia machine should be placed near an exhaust grill to facilitate purging of spilled gases. Where ventilatory patterns produce significant flow channeling, the anesthesia machine should be placed in a high-flow area, not in a stagnant portion of the room.

ALTERATION OF ANESTHETIC TECHNIQUE

Errors in technique also contribute significantly to pollution levels within the operating room.

Contamination resulting from careless technique tends to be transient but can reach quite high levels. In the case of a poor mask fit, these levels can persist throughout an operation. Unopposed spill of anesthetic gas into the room rapidly leads to high contamination levels.

It is quite possible, however, to alter technique to avoid gross spill and, yet, not compromise the administration of anesthesia. There are several ways to alter technique, thereby avoiding unopposed spill of gases into the operating room:

Avoid turning on the nitrous oxide or the vaporizer until the mask is fitted to the patient's face or the patient is intubated and connected to the circuit. By doing this, all excess circuit gas enters the scavenging system, and spill into the room is avoided.

Discontinue anesthetic gas flows and empty the reservoir bag prior to suctioning or intubation, when possible.

Administer oxygen as long as possible at the end of an anesthetic, before extubation or removal of the mask. The scavenger system can then eliminate the majority of the washed out anesthetic gases. This practice keeps contamination to a minimum and is beneficial to the patient.

Avoid spilling volatile agents during vaporizer filling. Such spill results in markedly elevated trace gas levels in the operating room. (1 ml. of liquid halothane vaporizes to about 200 ml. of gas, which has a concentration of 1,000,000 p.p.m.!) The threshold of smell for halothane is greather than 50 p.p.m.; when the odor is apparent, the anesthesiologist is being exposed to at least 100 times the target levels.[54]

Mask fit is critical. A gas-tight fit is possible using a mask and assisted or controlled ventilation. Poor mask fit, however, results in significant ongoing spillage, with resultant high contaminant levels. Often, a very small change in mask angle can mean the difference between a good and a bad fit. It is interesting for the anesthesiologist to fit a mask to himself and determine how small of a change in pressure or angle is required to achieve a good fit.

Adherence to these suggestions for modification of anesthetic technique will significantly reduce the operating room contaminant load.

They are intended as suggestions only. These, as well as all other scavenging considerations, become of secondary importance when patient safety is in question. Our experience has been, however, that these principles can be followed most of the time without compromising the safe administration of anesthesia.

The mechanical aspects of reducing and controlling anesthetic pollution in the operating room are not expensive or difficult to understand and achieve. At our institution, the procedures outlined above were implemented and have been followed with a minimum of expense and effort. They have not interfered with the safe administration of anesthesia. The resultant reduction of baseline and intraoperative trace gas levels has been most dramatic and gratifying. Similar results should be possible in virtually any hospital. Using the techniques above, intraoperative levels well below NIOSH target levels are routinely achieved.

TRACE GAS MONITORING

Measurement of intraoperative trace gas levels is the final and most important assessment of the effectiveness of a pollution control program.

These trace levels are the net result of several factors: high- and low-pressure system leakage, technique error, scavenger system malfunction, and the effectiveness of the ventilation system. Intraoperative measurements have two objectives: They reflect how well the factors above are controlled, and they can document that low trace levels are being maintained.

This section discusses the considerations in selecting a trace gas monitoring system. Trace gas levels can be assayed by several methods, and each has its own advantages and disadvantages. Whether analysis is performed on site or the services of a central testing facility are used is a question of economic importance.

There are three different techniques for the sampling of gaseous atmospheric contaminants. In the "instantaneous" or "grab" sampling technique, a syringe or other leak-proof container is used to capture the sample. The sample is subse-quently analyzed by either chromatographic or infrared techniques. Glass syringes, which leak slightly, are suitable, if the analysis is to be performed soon after sampling; however, if samples are to be sent to a central testing facility, then an absolutely leak-proof, inert container that does not absorb or adsorb the contaminant is essential. The "grab" sample is best used for analysis of an equilibrium state (e.g., baseline N_2O sampling prior to starting anesthesia to detect high-pressure leakage). In this situation, there is a rough equilibrium between equipment leakage and ventilation system purging. Intraoperative levels, however, tend to rise in a fluctuating pattern during the early part of a case, then to roughly equilibrate at a level that represents the net effect of system leaks, air-conditioning flow, inflow gas rate, scavenging efficiency, and personnel movement. Under these conditions, a "grab" sample can serve as a spot check on intraoperative levels. However, in an operating room where poor technique is employed and where no attempt has been made to eliminate equipment leakage, pollution levels vary markedly. Under these conditions, the instantaneous sample can be quite misleading.

The time-weighted average (TWA) sampling technique is the industrial and governmental standard. The presumed toxicity of chronic exposure to trace anesthetic gases is probably a function of both *dose* and *length of exposure time;* hence, a sample that reflects an average exposure level is of great interest (and is analogous to the radiation safety badge). A TWA sample is obtained by pumping ambient air continuously into a Mylar or other inert bag, at low flow rates throughout the working period. The air concentration in the bag then reflects the average exposure in parts per million. If one is interested in sampling only halogenated agents, air can be pumped or drawn continuously through a tube containing activated charcoal, which adsorbs halogenated hydrocarbons. The halogenated agent is then eluted from the charcoal with heat, carbon disulfide, or some other solvent and analyzed chromatographically, to give the TWA level for the halogenated agent. Nitrous oxide cannot be assayed by this technique, because it is not adsorbed by activated charcoal. TWA sampling, then, eliminates the potential for errors to which instantaneous samples are subject, particularly when sampling is performed during a case in which trace levels fluctuate markedly.

Monitors capable of continuous sampling, while expensive in terms of initial cost and maintenance, are useful for the rapid detection of leaks and for demonstrating the effects of technique error on contamination levels. For the hospital with a large number of operating rooms or a teaching program that attempts to demonstrate the contaminating effects of poor technique, the convenience and the immediate feedback provided by a continuous monitor far outweigh its expense. In the small hospital with fewer than six or seven operating rooms or in the dental operatory, the time, expense, and staff required to maintain in-house analysis equipment (either infrared analyzers or gas chromatographs) probably dictate that a central testing facility be used for trace gas analysis. Gas chromatography is a reliable means of determining halogenated agent levels. However, nitrous oxide determination by gas chromatography is fraught with difficulty and is not a feasible technique for most institutions. Infrared analyzers readily detect nitrous oxide, and some have the capbility of measuring levels of halogenated agents.

SPECIFIC APPLICATIONS OF MONITORING TRACE CONCENTRATIONS

High- and Low-Pressure System Testing

The presence of baseline nitrous oxide levels (when no anesthesia is being given) indicates high-pressure system leakage (see p. 000). Analysis of baseline nitrous oxide levels can be used, then, to indicate that a problem exists. However, the simple tests (e.g., connector immersion in water and machine pressure testing) outlined above also accomplish this task effectively and far less expensively. Thus, frequent baseline measurements are not necessary if expense is a factor. Infrared analyzers can also be used to identify specific leakage sites, but again, water immersion

or application of soap solution is virtually as effective.

Intraoperative Monitoring

The NIOSH Criteria Document recommends that target levels of 25 p.p.m. for nitrous oxide and 0.5 p.p.m. for halogenated agents (2 p.p.m. if used alone) should be sought. To determine compliance, TWA or the equivalent should be obtained in the breathing zone of the anesthesiologist during the administration of anesthesia. Such measurements should be made every 3 months in each anesthetizing area or whenever there is a major renovation or alteration in equipment.

If values above target levels are obtained, then corrections should be made, and the area resampled. Some practical questions remain: Once a TWA sample has been obtained, how should it be analyzed? If two gases are being administered, do we need to test for both? Should all personnel in the operating room be monitored, or is a sample obtained in the breathing zone of the anesthesiologist representative of the highest level to which one is exposed in the operating room? Many of these questions with significant impact on public health and economics remain to be answered.

At this point, the NIOSH recommendations seem sound. Data from a large series of samples show that if one gas in a sample containing two gases is in compliance with target levels, then the paired gas in the sample will also be in compliance 85 to 90 per cent of the time.[55] Additional studies are necessary to confirm these findings. If one gas can indeed be used as a "marker," then analysis costs will be markedly reduced. Operating rooms at the University of Pennsylvania are monitored quarterly, and the results are recorded on the form shown in Figure 57-3.

ADDITIONAL IMPLICATIONS OF THE NIOSH CRITERIA DOCUMENT

The Criteria Document has been prepared by NIOSH and is still in review by the Occupational Safety and Health Administration (OSHA). If this document passes intact, the maintenance and

HOSPITAL of the UNIVERSITY of PENNSYLVANIA

INTRAOPERATIVE TRACE GAS MONITORING REPORT

DATE .... O.R. NO. .... MACHINE NO. .... TECHNICIAN ....

VENTILATOR .... LOW PRESSURE LEAK RATE .... SCAVENGER CHECKED ....

SINGLE SHOT SAMPLE

Time	PPM N$_2$O	PPM	PPM ......

TWA SAMPLE

Site	Time Span	PPM N$_2$O	PPM	PPM ......

(1) XEROX AND ATTACH ANESTHESIA RECORDS FOR THE DAY
(2) IF VALUES ABOVE 30 PPM N$_2$O OR 0.5 PPM HALOGENATED
    AGENT, CORRECT DEFECT AND REPORT STEPS ON BACK OF CARD

Fig. 57-3. Intraoperative trace gas monitoring form.

monitoring procedures outlined above will be requirements. In addition, workers potentially exposed to anesthetic agents will have to receive periodic written notice that a potential hazard exists. There will have to be preemployment and yearly physical examination and testing. Medical records will have to be kept for 20 years after employment. These requirements are an example of how such issues are handled in industry. At present, it is the policy of our department to inform women of childbearing age that there may be a hazard secondary to exposure to anesthetic agents. We point out that we do not know what safe levels are, but that we are making every effort to reduce and monitor levels. Should they become pregnant, we offer then the option of working somewhere other than the operating room during that period, if they so desire.

The fate of the Criteria Document is unknown. It may be passed as is, which will impose a good deal of burden on hospitals in terms of personnel management, record keeping, and follow-up.

However, it may well be modified. The American Society of Anesthesiologists has provided outstanding leadership in openly investigating the issues and in alerting its membership that health hazards may exist. In light of this, moderation of the fairly stringent requirements in the Criteria Document may occur.

In short, the data strongly suggest that a health hazard exists in medicine secondary to chronic exposure to trace levels of anesthetics. Much work must be done to prove conclusively that this is the case, and there is still room for some skepticism. The steps required to reduce ambient levels of anesthetic gas in the operating room, however, are straightforward and require only a modest investment for scavenging equipment and minimal labor to implement an ongoing maintenance program. Some education is required to demonstrate that alteration of anesthetic technique can avoid gross spill into the room. Time-weighted average monitoring of intraoperative trace gas levels will be an important factor in determining the effectiveness of an antipollution program following personnel exposure.

It is important to keep the entire issue of pollution control in perspective. Patient safety should not be compromised by any of the procedures mentioned herein.

REFERENCES

1. National Institute for Occupational Safety and Health (NIOSH): Criteria for a recommended Occupational Exposure to Waste Anesthetic Gases and Vapors. DHEW Pub. No. (NIOSH) 77-140.
2. Hamilton, A., and Minot, G. R.: Ether poisoning in the manufacture of smokeless powder. J. Indust. Hyg., 2:41, 1920.
3. Wertham, H.: Beitrag zur chronischen ather intoxikation der chirurgen. Beitr. Klin. Chir., 178:149, 1949.
4. Eastwood, D. W., Green, C. D., Lambdin, M. A., et al.: Effect of nitrous oxide on the white-cell count in leukemia. N. Engl. J. Med., 268:297, 1963.
5. Green, C. D., and Eastwood, D. W.: Effects of nitrous oxide-halothane on hemopoiesis in rats. Anesthesiology, 24:341, 1963.
6. Bruce, D. L., Eide, K. A., Linde, H. W., et al.: Causes of death among anesthesiologists: a 20-year survey. Anesthesiology, 29:565, 1968.
7. Vaisman, A. I.: Work in surgical theatres and its influence on the health of anesthesiologists. Eksp. Khir. Anesteziol., 3:44, 1967.
8. Askrog, V., and Harvald, B.: Teratogen effekt af inhalations anestetika. Nord. Med., 83:498, 1970.
9. Cohen, E. N., Bellville, J. W., and Brown, B. W.: Anesthesia, pregnancy and miscarriage: a study of operating room nurses and anesthetists. Anesthesiology, 35:343, 1971.
10. Knill-Jones, R. P., Moir, D. B., Rodrigues, I. V., et al.: Anaesthetic practice and pregnancy: a controlled survey of women anaesthetists in the United Kingdom. Lancet, 2:1326, 1972.
10a. Tomlin, P. J.: Health problems of anaesthetists and their families in the West Midlands. Br. Med. J., 1:779, 1979.
11. American Society of Anesthesiologists *Ad Hoc* Committee on the Effect of Trace Anesthetics on the Health of Operating Room Personnel: Occupational disease among operating room personnel: a national study. Anesthesiology, 41:321, 1974.
12. Spence, A. H., Cohen, E. N., Brown, B. W., et al.: Occupational hazard for operating room-based physician. Analysis of data from the United States and the United Kingdom. J.A.M.A., 238:955, 1977.
13. A survey of anesthetic health hazards among dentists. Report of ad hoc committee on the effects of trace anesthetics on the health of operating room personnel. J. Am. Dent. Assoc., 90:1291, 1975.
14. Corbett, T. H., Cornell, R. G., Lieding, K., et al.: Incidence of cancer among Michigan nurse-anesthetists. Anesthesiology, 38:260, 1973.
15. Bruce, D. L., Eide, K. A., Smith, N. J., et al.: A prospective survey of anesthesiologist mortality, 1967–1971. Anesthesiology, 41:71, 1974.
16. Bruce, D. L., Bach, M. J., and Arbit, J.: Trace anesthetic effects on perceptual, cognitive and motor skills. Anesthesiology, 40:453, 1974.
17. Bruce, D. L., and Bach, M. J.: Psychological studies of human performance as affected by traces of enflurane and nitrous oxide. Anesthesiology, 42:194, 1975.
18. Bruce, D. L., and Bach, M. J.: Effects of trace anaesthetic gases on behavioural performance of volunteers. Br. J. Anaesth., 48:871, 1976.
19. Smith, G., and Shirley, A. W.: Failure to demonstrate effect of trace concentrations of nitrous oxide and halothane on psychomotor performance. Br. J. Anaesth., 49:65, 1977.
20. Stevens, W. C., Eger, E. I., II, White, A., et al.: Comparative toxicities of halothane, isoflurane and diethyl ether at sub-anesthetic concentrations in laboratory animals. Anesthesiology, 42:408, 1975.
21. Frankhuizen, J. L., Vlek, C. A. J., Burm, A. G. L., et al.: Failure to replicate negative effects of trace anaesthetics on mental performance. Br. J. Anaesth., 50:229, 1978.
22. Fink, B. R.: Toxicity of anesthetics. Part IV teratogenic effects. p. 259. Baltimore, Williams & Wilkins, 1968.
23. Chang, W. C., Dudley, A. W., Jr., Lee, Y. K., et al.: Ultrastructural changes in the nervous system after chronic exposure to halothane. Exp. Neurol., 45:209, 1974.
24. Quimby, K. L., Katz, J., and Bowman, R. E.: Behavioral consequences in rats from chronic exposure to 10 ppm halothane during early development. Anesth. Analg., 54:628, 1975.
25. Kripke, B. J., Kelman, A. D., Shah, N. K., et al.: Testicular reaction to prolonged exposure to nitrous oxide. Anesthesiology, 44:104, 1976.
25a. Coate, W. B., Kapp, R. W., Jr., and Lewis, T. R.: Chronic exposure to low concentrations of halothane-nitrous oxide. Anesthesiology, 50:310, 1979.
25b. ——, Ulland, B. M., and Lewis, T. R.: Chronic exposure to low concentrations of halothane-nitrous oxide: lack of carcinogenic effect in the rat. Anesthesiology, 50:306, 1979.
26. Fink, B. R., and Cullen, B. F.: Anesthetic pollution: What is happening to us? Anesthesiology, 45:79, 1976.
27. Ferstandig, L. L.: Trace concentrations of anesthetic gases: a critical review of their disease potential. Anesth. Analg., 57:328, 1978.
28. Vessey, M. P.: Epidemiological studies of the occupational hazards of anaesthesia—a review. Anaesthesia, 33:430, 1978.
28a. Ericson, A., and Källén, B.: Survey of infants born to Swedish women working in operating rooms during their pregnancies. Anesth. Analg., 58:302, 1979.
29. International Labour Office. Encyclopaedia of Occupational Health and Safety. vol. 2. p. 1539. New York, McGraw Hill, 1974.
30. Hirsch, J., and Kappus, A. L.: Uber die mengen des narkoseathers in der luft von operationssalen. Z. Hyg., 110:391, 1929.
31. Linde, H. W., and Bruce, D. L.: Occupational exposure of anesthetists to halothane, nitrous oxide and radiation. Anesthesiology, 30:363, 1969.
32. Whitcher, C. E., Cohen, E. N., and Trudell, J. R.: Chronic exposue to anesthetic gases in the operating room. Anesthesiology, 35:348, 1971.
33. Whitcher, C., Piziali, R., Sher, R., et al.: Development and evaluation of methods for the elimination of waste

anesthetic gases and vapors in hospitals. DHEW Pub. (NIOSH) No. 75–137.

34. Nikki, P., Pfaffli, P., Ahlman, K., et al.: Chronic exposure to anaesthetic gases in the operating theatre and recovery room. Ann. Clin. Res., 4:266, 1972.

35. Swenson, R. D.: Scavenging of dental anesthetic gases. J. Oral Surg., 34:207, 1976.

36. Millard, R. I., and Corbett, T. H.: Nitrous oxide concentrations in the dental operatory. J. Oral Surg., 32:593, 1974.

37. Strunin, L., Strunin, J. M., and Mallios, C. C.: Atmospheric pollution with halothane during outpatient dental anaesthesia. Br. Med. J., 4:459, 1973.

38. Whitcher, C. E., Zimmerman, D. C., and Piziali, R. L.: Control of occupational exposure to N_2O in the dental operatory. Final report. Contract No. CDC 210-75-0007. Cincinnati, National Institute for Occupational Safety and Health, Division of Field Studies and Clinical Investigation, 1977.

39. Corbett, T. H.: Retention of anesthetic agents following occupational exposure. Anesth. Analg., 52:614, 1973.

40. Pfaffli, P., Nikki, P., and Ahlman, K.: Halothane and nitrous oxide in end-tidal air and venous blood of surgical personnel. Ann. Clin. Res., 4:273, 1972.

41. Usubiaga, L., Aldrete, J. A., and Fiserova-Bergerova, V.: Influence of gas flows and operating room ventilation on the daily exposure of anesthetists to halothane. Anesth. Analg., 51:968, 1972.

42. Corbett, T. H., and Ball, G. L.: Chronic exposure to methoxyflurane: a possible occupational hazard to anesthesiologists. Anesthesiology, 34:532, 1971.

43. Cascorbi, H. F., Blake, D. A., and Helrich, M.: Differences in the biotransformation of halothane in man. Anesthesiology, 32:119, 1970.

44. Piziali, R. L., Whitcher, C., Sher, R., et al.: Distribution of waste anesthetic gases in the operating room air. Anesthesiology, 45:487, 1976.

44a. Lecky, J. H.: The mechanical aspects of anesthetic pollution control. Anesth. Analg., 56:769, 1977.

45. Bruce, D. L.: Venting overflow gases from the Air Shields (Ventimeter) ventilator. Anesthesiology, 41:292, 1974.

46. Muravchick, S.: Scavenging enflurane from extracorporal pump oxygenators. Anesthesiology, 47:468, 1977.

47. Annis, J. P., Carlson, D. A., and Simmons, D. H.: Scavenging system for the Harvey blood oxygenator. Anesthesiology, 45:359, 1976.

48. Miller, J. D.: A device for the removal of waste anesthetic gases from the extracorporeal oxygenator. Anesthesiology, 44:181, 1976.

49. Publication No. 56A (Standard for use of inhalational anesthetics), National Fire Protection Association, Boston, Mass. 02210.

50. Hägerdal, M., and Lecky, J. H.: Anesthesia death in an experimental animal related to a scavenging system malfunction. Anesthesiology, 47:522, 1977.

51. Lecky, J. H. (Chairman): American National Standards Institute (ANSI) Draft Standard For Anesthetic Gas Scavenging Equipment. Z79, SC-4.

52. Lecky, J. H., Springstead, J. M., and Andrews, R. A.: Reduction of operating room anesthetic contamination: the time requirements and effectiveness of a two year program. p. 551. Abstracts of Scientific Papers, American Society of Anesthesiologists Annual Meeting, 1977.

53. Neufeld, G. R., Flemming, D. C., and Lecky, J. H.: Evaluation of operating room clearance of trace anesthetic gases. p. 371. Abstracts of Scientific Papers, American Society of Anesthesiologists Annual Meeting, 1975.

54. Flemming, D. C., and Johnstone, R. E.: Recognition thresholds for diethyl ether and halothane. Anesthesiology, 46:68, 1977.

55. Lecky, J. H., and Andrews, R.: Anesthetic trace levels in 161 hospitals: a presentation of data obtained over a four year period. p. 481. Abstracts of Scientific Papers, American Society of Anesthesiologists Annual Meeting, 1976.

FURTHER READING

American Society of Anesthesiologists *Ad Hoc* Committee on the Effect of Trace Anesthetics on the Health of Operating Room Personnel: Occupational disease among operating room personnel: a national study. Anesthesiology, 41:321, 1974.

Ferstandig, L. L.: Trace concentrations of anesthetic gases: a critical review of their disease potential. Anesth. Analg., 57:328, 1978.

Vessey, M. P.: Epidemiological studies of the occupational hazards of anaesthesia—a review. Anaesthesia, 33:430, 1978.

Index

Numbers followed by an *f* indicate a figure; *t* following a page number indicates tabular material.